JARVIS

Physical Examination & Health Assessment

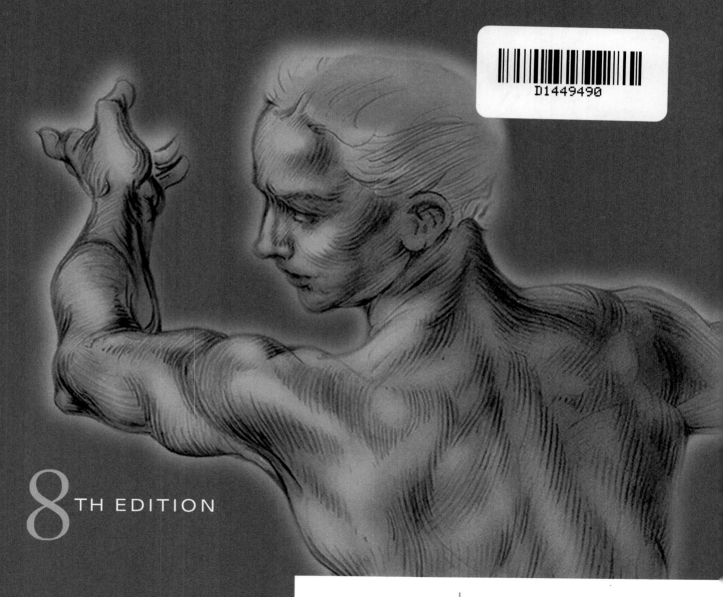

8TH EDITION

Evolve® | Student Resources on Evolve
Access Code Inside

ELSEVIER

Evolve®

YOU'VE JUST PURCHASED
MORE THAN A TEXTBOOK!

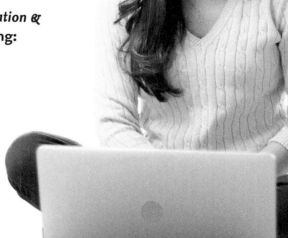

Evolve Student Resources for *Jarvis: Physical Examination & Health Assessment, Eighth Edition,* include the following:

- Animations
- Audio Clips
- Audio Glossary
- Case Studies
- Clinical Reference
  - Complete Inpatient Reassessment
  - Complete Older Person Evaluation
  - Complete Physical Examination
  - Physical Examination Summary Checklists
- Content Updates
- Key Points
- Review Questions
- Video Clips

Activate the complete learning experience that comes with each NEW textbook purchase by registering with your scratch-off access code at

http://evolve.elsevier.com/Jarvis/

If you rented or purchased a used book and the scratch-off code at right has already been revealed, the code may have been used and cannot be re-used for registration. To purchase a new code to access these valuable study resources, simply follow the link above.

REGISTER TODAY!

ELSEVIER

2018v1.0

CHAPTER ORGANIZATION

The following color bars are used consistently for each section within a chapter to help locate specific information.

STRUCTURE AND FUNCTION

Anatomy and physiology by body system

SUBJECTIVE DATA

Health history through questions (examiner asks) and explanation (rationale)

OBJECTIVE DATA

Core of the examination part of each body system chapter with skills, expected findings, and common variations for healthy people, as well as selected abnormal findings

HEALTH PROMOTION AND PATIENT TEACHING

Health promotion related to each body system.

DOCUMENTATION AND CRITICAL THINKING

Clinical case studies with sample documentation for subjective, objective, and assessment data

ABNORMAL FINDINGS

Tables of art and photographs of pathologic disorders and conditions; abnormal findings for clinical practice and advanced practice where appropriate

CONTENTS

Physical Examination & Health Assessment

Physical Examination & Health Assessment

CAROLYN JARVIS, PhD, APRN, CNP
Professor of Nursing
Illinois Wesleyan University
Bloomington, Illinois
and
Family Nurse Practitioner
Bloomington, Illinois

With Ann Eckhardt, PhD, RN
Associate Professor of Nursing
Illinois Wesleyan University
Bloomington, Illinois

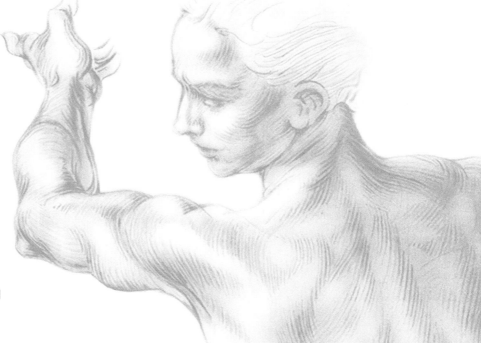

8TH EDITION

ELSEVIER

Original Illustrations by
Pat Thomas, CMI, FAMI
East Troy, Wisconsin

PHYSICAL EXAMINATION AND HEALTH ASSESSMENT, EIGHTH EDITION   ISBN: 978-0-323-51080-6

Notice

Practitioners and researchers must always rely on their own experience and knowledge in evaluating and using any information, methods, compounds or experiments described herein. Because of rapid advances in the medical sciences, in particular, independent verification of diagnoses and drug dosages should be made. To the fullest extent of the law, no responsibility is assumed by Elsevier, authors, editors or contributors for any injury and/or damage to persons or property as a matter of products liability, negligence or otherwise, or from any use or operation of any methods, products, instructions, or ideas contained in the material herein.

Previous editions copyrighted 2016, 2012, 2008, 2004, 2000, 1996, 1993.

International Standard Book Number: 978-0-323-51080-6

Executive Content Strategist: Lee Henderson
Senior Content Development Specialist: Heather Bays
Publishing Services Manager: Julie Eddy
Senior Project Manager: Jodi M. Willard
Design Direction: Brian Salisbury

Printed in Canada

Last digit is the print number: 9   8   7   6   5   4   3   2   1

ELSEVIER

3251 Riverport Lane
St. Louis, Missouri 63043

Working together to grow libraries in developing countries

www.elsevier.com • www.bookaid.org

To Paul, with love and thanks. You have read every word.

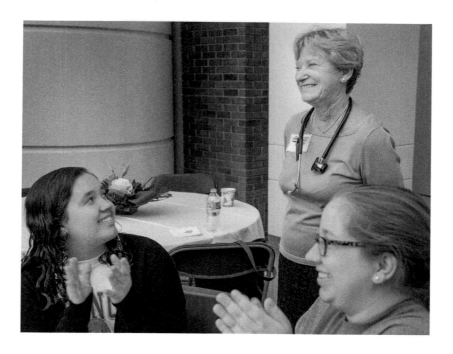

Carolyn Jarvis received her PhD from the University of Illinois at Chicago, with a research interest in the physiologic effect of alcohol on the cardiovascular system; her MSN from Loyola University (Chicago); and her BSN cum laude from the University of Iowa. She is Professor, School of Nursing at Illinois Wesleyan University, where she teaches Health Assessment, Pathophysiology, and Pharmacology. Dr. Jarvis has taught physical assessment and critical care nursing at Rush University (Chicago), the University of Missouri (Columbia), and the University of Illinois (Urbana). Her current research interest concerns alcohol-interactive medications, and she includes Honors students in this research.

In 2016, Illinois Wesleyan University honored Dr. Jarvis for her contributions to the ever-changing field of nursing with the dedication of the Jarvis Center for Nursing Excellence. The Jarvis Center for Nursing Excellence equips students with laboratory and simulation learning so that they may pursue their nursing career with the same commitment as Dr. Jarvis.

Dr. Jarvis is the Student Senate Professor of the Year (2017) and was honored to give remarks at commencement. She is a recipient of the University of Missouri's Superior Teaching Award; has taught physical assessment to thousands of baccalaureate students, graduate students, and nursing professionals; has held 150 continuing education seminars; and is the author of numerous articles and textbook contributions.

Dr. Jarvis has maintained a clinical practice in advanced practice roles—first as a cardiovascular clinical specialist in various critical care settings and as a certified family nurse practitioner in primary care. During the last 12 years, her enthusiasm has focused on Spanish language skills to provide health care in rural Guatemala and at the Community Health Care Clinic in Bloomington. Dr. Jarvis has been instrumental in developing a synchronous teaching program for Illinois Wesleyan students both in Barcelona, Spain, and at the home campus.

CHAPTER CONTRIBUTOR

Lydia Bertschi, DNP, APRN, ACNP-BC
The co-contributor for Chapter 22 (Abdomen), Dr. Bertschi is an Assistant Professor at Illinois Wesleyan University School of Nursing and a nurse practitioner in the intensive care unit at UnityPoint Health—Methodist.

ASSESSMENT PHOTOGRAPHERS

Chandi Kessler, BSN, RN
Chandi is a former Intensive Care Unit nurse and is an award-winning professional photographer. Chandi specializes in newborn and family photography in and around Central Illinois.

Kevin Strandberg
Kevin is a Professor of Art Emeritus at Illinois Wesleyan University in Bloomington, Illinois. He has contributed to all editions of *Physical Examination & Health Assessment*.

INSTRUCTOR AND STUDENT ANCILLARIES

Case Studies

Melissa M. Vander Stucken, MSN, RN
Clinical Assistant Professor
School of Nursing
Sam Houston State University
Huntsville, Texas

Key Points

Joanna Cain, BSN, BA, RN
Auctorial Pursuits, Inc.
President and Founder
Boulder, Colorado

PowerPoint Presentations

Daryle Wane, PhD, ARNP, FNP-BC
BSN Program Director—Professor of Nursing
Department of Nursing and Health Programs
Pasco-Hernando State College
New Port Richey, Florida

Review Questions

Kelly K. Zinn, PhD, RN
Associate Professor
School of Nursing
Sam Houston State University
Huntsville, Texas

TEACH for Nurses

Jennifer Duke
Freelancer
St. Louis, Missouri

Test Bank

Heidi Monroe, MSN, RN-BC, CAPA
Assistant Professor of Nursing
NCLEX-RN Coordinator
Bellin College
Green Bay, Wisconsin

Test Bank Review

Kelly K. Zinn, PhD, RN
Associate Professor
School of Nursing
Sam Houston State University
Huntsville, Texas

Valerie J. Fuller, PhD, DNP, AGACNP-BC, FNP-BC, FAANP, FNAP
Assistant Professor
School of Nursing
University of Southern Maine
Portland, Maine

Peggy J. Jacobs, DNP, RNC-OB, CNM, APRN
Instructional Support and Outcomes Coordinator
School of Nursing
Illinois Wesleyan University
Bloomington, Illinois

Marie Kelly Lindley, PhD, RN
Clinical Assistant Professor
Louise Herrington School of Nursing
Baylor University
Dallas, Texas

Jeanne Wood Mann, PhD, MSN, RN, CNE
Assistant Dean;
Associate Professor
School of Nursing
Baker University
Topeka, Kansas

Judy Nelson, RN, MSN
Nurse Educator
Nursing
Fort Scott Community College
Fort Scott, Kansas

Cheryl A. Tucker, DNP, RN, CNE
Clinical Associate Professor;
Undergraduate Level II BSN Coordinator
Louise Herrington School of Nursing
Baylor University
Dallas, Texas

Melissa M. Vander Stucken, MSN, RN
Clinical Assistant Professor
School of Nursing
Sam Houston State University
Huntsville, Texas

Kelly K. Zinn, PhD, RN
Associate Professor
School of Nursing
Sam Houston State University
Huntsville, Texas

This book is for those who still carefully examine their patients and for those of you who wish to learn how to do so. You develop and practice, and then learn to trust, your health history and physical examination skills. In this book, we give you the tools to do that. Learn to listen to the patient—most often he or she will tell you what is wrong (and right) and what you can do to meet his or her health care needs. Then learn to inspect, examine, and listen to the person's body. The data are all there and are accessible to you by using just a few extra tools. High-tech machinery is a smart and sophisticated adjunct, but it cannot replace your own bedside assessment of your patient. Whether you are a beginning examiner or an advanced-practice student, this book holds the content you need to develop and refine your clinical skills.

This is a readable college text. All 8 editions have had these strengths: a clear, approachable writing style; an attractive and user-friendly format; integrated developmental variations across the life span with age-specific content on the infant, child, adolescent, pregnant woman, and older adult; cultural competencies in both a separate chapter and throughout the book; hundreds of meticulously prepared full-color illustrations; sample documentation of normal and abnormal findings and 60 clinical case studies; integration of the complete health assessment in 2 photo essays at the end of the book, where all key steps of a complete head-to-toe examination of the adult, infant, and child are summarized; and a photo essay highlighting a condensed head-to-toe assessment for each daily segment of patient care.

NEW TO THE EIGHTH EDITION

The 8th edition has a new chapter section and several new content features. Cultural Assessment in Chapter 2 is rewritten to increase emphasis on cultural assessment, self-assessment, and a new section on spiritual assessment. The Interview in Chapter 3 has a new section on interprofessional communication; Mental Status Assessment in Chapter 5 now includes the Montreal Cognitive Assessment; Substance Use Assessment in Chapter 6 includes additional content on opioid/heroin epidemic and alcohol-interactive medications; Domestic and Family Violence Assessment in Chapter 7 includes all new photos, updates on the health effects of violence, added information on the health effects of violence, and additional content on child abuse and elder abuse. The former Vital Signs and Measurement chapter is now split into 2 chapters to increase readability; the Vital Signs chapter (Chapter 10) stands alone with updated information on blood pressure guidelines.

The Physical Examination chapters all have a new feature—Health Promotion and Patient Teaching—to give the reader current teaching guidelines. Many chapters have all new exam photos for a fresh and accurate look. The

focus throughout is evidence-based practice. Examination techniques are explained and included (and in some cases, rejected) depending on current clinical **evidence.**

Pat Thomas has designed 15 new art pieces in beautiful detail and 30 photo overlays. We have worked together to design new chapter openers and anatomy; note Fig. 11.4 on opioid targets, Figs. 14.1 and 14.2 on complex anatomy of skull and facial muscles, Fig. 15.5 on complex eye anatomy; Fig 23.8 on 3 images of complex shoulder anatomy showing muscle girdle, Fig. 27.2 on complex female internal anatomy, and many others. We have worked with Chandi Kesler and Kevin Strandberg in new photo shoots, replacing exam photos in Chapters 6 (Substance Use Assessment), 23 (Musculoskeletal System), 24 (Neurologic System), 28 (The Complete Health Assessment: Adult), and many others.

All physical examination chapters are **revised and updated,** with evidence-based data in anatomy and physiology, physical examination, and assessment tools. **Developmental Competence** sections provide updated common illnesses, growth and development information, and the Examination section of each body system chapter details **exam techniques and clinical findings for infants, children, adolescents, and older adults**.

Culture and Genetics data have been revised and updated in each chapter. Common illnesses affecting diverse groups are detailed. We know that some groups suffer an undue burden of some diseases, not because of racial diversity *per se*, but because these groups are overrepresented in the uninsured/poverty ranks and lack access to quality health care.

The **Abnormal Findings** tables located at the end of the chapters are revised and updated with many new clinical photos. These are still divided into two sections. The Abnormal Findings tables present frequently encountered conditions that every clinician should recognize, and the Abnormal Findings for Advanced Practice tables isolate the detailed illustrated atlas of conditions encountered in advanced practice roles.

Chapter references are up-to-date and are meant to be used. They include the best of clinical practice readings as well as basic science research and nursing research, with an emphasis on scholarship from the last 5 years.

DUAL FOCUS AS TEXT AND REFERENCE

Physical Examination & Health Assessment is a **text for beginning students** of physical examination as well as a **text and reference for advanced practitioners.** The chapter progression and format permit this scope without sacrificing one use for the other.

Chapters 1 through 7 focus on **health assessment of the whole person,** including health promotion for all age-groups, cultural environment and assessment, interviewing and complete health history gathering, the social environment of mental status, and the changes to the whole person on the occasions of substance use or domestic violence.

Chapters 8 through 12 begin the approach to the **clinical care setting,** describing physical data-gathering techniques, how to set up the examination site, body measurement and vital signs, pain assessment, and nutritional assessment.

Chapters 13 through 27 focus on the **physical examination and related health history** in a body systems approach. This is the most efficient method of performing the examination and is the most logical method for student learning and retrieval of data. Both the novice and the advanced practitioner can review anatomy and physiology; learn the skills, expected findings, and common variations for generally healthy people; and study a comprehensive atlas of abnormal findings.

Chapters 28 through 32 **integrate the complete health assessment.** Chapters 28, 29 and 30 present the choreography of the head-to-toe exam for a complete screening examination in various age-groups and for the focused exam in this **unique chapter on a hospitalized adult.** Chapters 31 and 32 present special populations—the assessment of the pregnant woman and the functional assessment of the older adult, including assessment tools and caregiver and environmental assessment.

This text is valuable to both advanced practice students and experienced clinicians because of its comprehensive approach. *Physical Examination & Health Assessment* can help clinicians learn the skills for advanced practice, refresh their memory, review a specific examination technique when confronted with an unfamiliar clinical situation, compare and label a diagnostic finding, and study the Abnormal Findings for Advanced Practice.

CONTINUING FEATURES

1. **Method of examination** (Objective Data section) is clear, orderly, and easy to follow. Hundreds of original examination illustrations are placed directly with the text to demonstrate the physical examination in a step-by-step format.

2. **Two-column format** begins in the Subjective Data section, where the running column highlights the rationales for asking history questions. In the Objective Data section, the running column highlights selected abnormal findings to show a clear relationship between normal and abnormal findings.

3. **Abnormal Findings tables** organize and expand on material in the examination section. The **atlas** format of these extensive collections of pathology and original illustrations helps students recognize, sort, and describe abnormal findings.

4. **Genetics and cultural variations** in disease incidence and response to treatment are cited throughout using current evidence. The Jarvis text has the richest amount of cultural-genetic content available in any assessment text.

5. **Developmental approach** in each chapter presents a prototype for the adult, then age-specific content for the infant, child, adolescent, pregnant female, and older adult so students can learn common variations for all age-groups.

6. **Stunning full-color art** shows detailed human anatomy, physiology, examination techniques, and abnormal findings.

7. **Health history** (Subjective Data) appears in two places: (1) in Chapter 4, The Complete Health History; and (2) in pertinent history questions that are repeated and expanded in each regional examination chapter, including history questions that highlight health promotion and self-care. This presentation helps students understand the relationship between subjective and objective data. Considering the history and examination data together, as you do in the clinical setting, means that each chapter can stand on its own if a person has a specific problem related to that body system.

8. Chapter 3, The Interview, has the most complete discussion available on the process of communication, interviewing skills, techniques and traps, and cultural considerations (for example, how nonverbal behavior varies cross-culturally and the use of an interpreter).

9. **Summary checklists** at the end of each chapter provide a quick review of examination steps to help develop a mental checklist.

10. **Sample recordings** of normal and abnormal findings show the written language you should use so that documentation, whether written or electronic, is complete yet succinct.

11. **60 Clinical Case Studies** of frequently encountered situations that show the application of assessment techniques to patients of varying ages and clinical situations. These case histories, in SOAP format ending in diagnosis, use the actual language of recording. We encourage professors and students to use these as critical thinking exercises to discuss and develop a Plan for each one.

11. **User-friendly design** makes the book easy to use. Frequent subheadings and instructional headings assist in easy retrieval of material.

12. **Spanish-language translations** highlight important phrases for communication during the physical examination and appear on the inside back cover.

SUPPLEMENTS

- The ***Pocket Companion for Physical Examination & Health Assessment*** continues to be a handy and current clinical reference that provides pertinent material in full color, with over 200 illustrations from the textbook.

- The ***Study Guide & Laboratory Manual*** with physical examination forms is a full-color workbook that includes for each chapter a student study guide, glossary of key terms, clinical objectives, regional write-up forms, and review questions. The pages are perforated so students can use the regional write-up forms in the skills laboratory or in the clinical setting and turn them in to the instructor.

- The revised *Health Assessment Online* is an innovative and dynamic teaching and learning tool with more than **8000 electronic assets**, including video clips, anatomic overlays, animations, audio clips, interactive exercises, laboratory/diagnostic tests, review questions, and **electronic charting activities**. Comprehensive **Self-Paced Learning Modules** offer increased flexibility to faculty who wish to provide students with tutorial learning modules and in-depth capstone case studies for each body system chapter in the text. The **Capstone Case Studies** include **Quality and Safety Challenge** activities. Additional **Advance Practice Case Studies** put the student in the exam room and test history-taking and documentation skills. The comprehensive **video clip library** shows exam procedures across the life span, including clips on the pregnant woman. Animations, sounds, images, interactive activities, and video clips are embedded in the learning modules and cases to provide a dynamic, multimodal learning environment for today's learners.
- The companion *EVOLVE Website* (http://evolve.elsevier.com/Jarvis/) for students and instructors contains learning objectives, more than 300 multiple-choice and alternate-format review questions, printable key points from the chapter, and a comprehensive physical exam form for the adult. **Case studies**—including a variety of developmental and cultural variables—help students apply health assessment skills and knowledge. These include 25 in-depth case studies with critical thinking questions and answer guidelines. Also included is a complete Head-to-Toe Video Examination of the Adult that can be viewed in its entirety or by systems.
- *Simulation Learning System.* The new *Simulation Learning System* (SLS) is an online toolkit that incorporates medium- to high-fidelity simulation with scenarios that enhance the clinical decision-making skills of students. The SLS offers a comprehensive package of resources, including leveled patient scenarios, detailed instructions for preparation and implementation of the simulation experience, debriefing questions that encourage critical thinking, and learning resources to reinforce student comprehension.
- For instructors, the Evolve website presents TEACH for Nursing, PowerPoint slides, a comprehensive Image Collection, and a Test Bank. **TEACH for Nurses** provides annotated learning objectives, key terms, teaching strategies for the classroom in a revised section with strategies for both clinical and simulation lab use and a focus on QSEN competencies, critical thinking exercises, websites, and performance checklists. The **PowerPoint** slides include 2000 slides with integrated images and Audience Response Questions. A separate 1200-illustration **Image Collection** is featured and, finally, the ExamView **Test Bank** has over 1000 multiple-choice and alternate-format questions with coded answers and rationales.

IN CONCLUSION

Throughout all stages of manuscript preparation and production, we make every effort to develop a book that is readable, informative, instructive, and vital. Thank you for your enthusiastic response to the earlier editions of *Physical Examination & Health Assessment*. I am grateful for your encouragement and for your suggestions, which are incorporated wherever possible. Your comments and suggestions continue to be welcome for this edition.

Carolyn Jarvis
c/o Education Content
Elsevier
3251 Riverport Lane
Maryland Heights, MO 63043

ACKNOWLEDGMENTS

These 8 editions have been a labor of love and scholarship. During the 38 years of writing these texts, I have been buoyed by the many talented and dedicated colleagues who helped make the revisions possible.

Thank you to the bright, hardworking professional team at Elsevier. I am fortunate to have the support of Lee Henderson, Executive Content Strategist. Lee coordinates communication with Marketing and Sales and helps integrate user comments into the overall plan. I am grateful to work daily with Heather Bays, Senior Content Development Specialist. Heather juggled all the deadlines, readied all the manuscript for production, searched out endless photos for abnormal examination findings, kept current with the permissions, and so many other daily details. Her work is pivotal to our success. Heather, you rock.

I had a wonderful production team and I am most grateful to them. Julie Eddy, Publishing Services Manager, supervised the schedule for book production. I am especially grateful to Jodi Willard, Senior Project Manager, who has been in daily contact to keep the production organized and moving. She works in so many extra ways to keep production on schedule. I am pleased with the striking colors of the interior design of the 8th edition and the beautiful cover; both are the work of Brian Salisbury, Book Designer. The individual page layout is the wonderful work of Leslie Foster, Illustrator/Designer. Leslie hand-crafted every page, always planning how the page can be made better. Because of her work, we added scores of new art and content, and we still came out with comparable page length for the 8th edition.

I am so happy and excited to welcome Dr. Ann Eckhardt to this 8th edition. Ann has revised numerous chapters in this edition and is gifted with new ideas. I hope her contributions continue and grow. It has been wonderful to have a budding partner down the hall to bounce ideas and share chapter ideas and photo shoots.

I have gifted artistic colleagues, who made this book such a vibrant teaching display. Pat Thomas, Medical Illustrator, is so talented and contributes format ideas as well as brilliant drawings. Pat and I have worked together from the inception of this text. While we cannot answer each other's sentences, we have every other quality of a superb professional partnership. Chandi Kesler and Kevin Strandberg patiently set up equipment for all our photo shoots and then captured vivid, lively exam photos of children and adults. Julia Jarvis and Sarah Jarvis also photographed our infant photos with patience and clarity.

I am fortunate to have dedicated research assistants. Ani Almeroth searched and retrieved countless articles and sources. She was always prompt and accurate and anticipated my every request. Nicole Bukowski joined as a second research assistant and has been helpful in many ways. I am most grateful to Paul Jarvis, who read and reread endless copies of galley and page proof, finding any errors and making helpful suggestions.

Thank you to the faculty and students who took the time to write letters of suggestions and encouragement—your comments are gratefully received and are very helpful. I am fortunate to have the skilled reviewers who spend time reading the chapter manuscript and making valuable suggestions.

Most important are the members of my wonderful family, growing in number and in support. You all are creative and full of boundless energy. Your constant encouragement has kept me going throughout this process.

Carolyn Jarvis, PhD, APRN

CONTENTS

CHAPTER 1

Evidence-Based Assessment

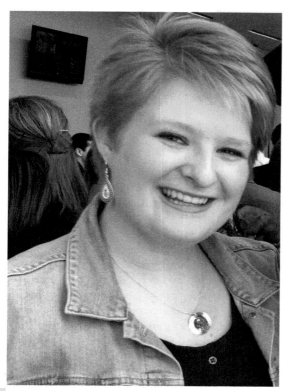

1.1

C.D. is a 23-year-old Caucasian woman who works as a pediatric nurse at a children's hospital. She comes to clinic today for a scheduled physical examination to establish with a new primary care provider (Fig. 1.1). On arrival the examiner collects a health history and performs a complete physical examination. The preliminary list of significant findings looks like this:

- Recent graduate of a BSN program. Strong academic record (A/B). Reports no difficulties in college.

Past medical history:

- Diagnosed with type 1 diabetes at age 12 years. Became stuporous during a family vacation. Rushed home; admitted to ICU with decreased level of consciousness (LOC) and heavy labored breathing; blood sugar 1200 mg/dL. Coma × 3 days; ICU stay for 5 days. Diabetic teaching during hospital stay; follow-up with diabetic educator as needed.
- Now uses insulin pump. Reports HbA1c <7%.
- Finger fracture and ankle sprains during childhood (unable to remember exact dates).
- Bronchitis "a lot" as a child.

- Tympanostomy tubes at age 5 due to frequent ear infections. No issues in adulthood.
- Diabetic seizures at ages 16 and 18 caused by hypoglycemia. Family gave glucagon injection. Did not go to emergency department (ED).
- Denies tobacco use. Reports having 1 glass of red wine approximately 5-6 days in the past month.
- Current medications: Insulin, simvastatin, birth control pills, fish oil, multivitamin, melatonin (for sleep).
- Birth control since age 16 because of elevated blood sugar during menstruation. Annual gynecologic examinations started at age 21 years. Last Pap test 6 months ago; told was "negative."
- Family history: Mother and paternal grandfather with hypertension; maternal grandfather transient ischemic attack, died at age 80 from a myocardial infarction; maternal grandmother died at age 49 of cervical and ovarian cancer; paternal grandmother with arthritis in the hands and knees; paternal grandfather with kidney disease at age 76; sister with migraine headaches.
- BP 108/72 mm Hg right arm, sitting. HR 76 beats/min, regular. Resp 14/min unlabored.
- Weight 180 lbs. Height 5 ft 6 in. BMI 29 (overweight).
- Health promotion: Reports consistently wearing sunscreen when outside and completing skin self-examination every few months. Consistently monitors blood glucose. Walks 2 miles at least 3 days per week and does strength training exercises 2 days per week. No hypoglycemic episodes during exercise. Reports weekly pedicure and foot check to monitor for skin breakdown. Biannual dental visits. Performs breast self-examination monthly.
- Relationships: Close relationship with family (mother, father, brother, and sister); no significant other. Feels safe in home environment and reports having close female friends.
- Health perception: "Could probably lose some weight," but otherwise reports "good" health. Primarily concerned with blood sugar, which becomes labile with life transitions.
- Expectations of provider: Establish an open and honest relationship. Listen to her needs and facilitate her health goals.

Physical examination:

- Normocephalic. Face symmetric. Denies pain on sinus palpation.
- Vision tested annually. Has worn corrective lenses since 4th grade. PERRLA.

- Scarring of bilateral tympanic membranes. Denies hearing problems. Whispered words heard bilaterally.
- Gums pink; no apparent dental caries except for 3 noticeable fillings. Reports no dental pain.
- Compound nevus on left inner elbow; patient reports no recent changes in appearance. No other skin concerns.
- Breath sounds clear and equal bilaterally. Heart S_1S_2, neither accentuated nor diminished. No murmur or extra heart sounds.
- Clinical breast exam done with annual gynecologic visit.
- Abdomen is rounded. Bowel sounds present. Reports BM daily.
- Extremities warm and = bilat. All pulses present, 2+ and = bilat. No lymphadenopathy.
- Sensory modalities intact in legs and feet. No lesions.

The examiner analyzed and interpreted all the data; clustered the information, sorting out which data to refer and which to treat; and identified the diagnoses. It is interesting to note how many significant findings are derived from data the examiner collected. Not only physical data but also cognitive, psychosocial, and behavioral data are significant for an analysis of C.D.'s health state. The findings are interesting when considered from a life-cycle perspective; she is a young adult who predictably is occupied with the developmental tasks of emancipation from parents, building an independent lifestyle, establishing a vocation, making friends, forming an intimate bond with another, and establishing a social group. C.D. appears to be meeting the appropriate developmental tasks successfully.

A body of clinical **evidence** has validated the use of the particular assessment techniques in C.D.'s case. For example, measuring the BP screens for hypertension, and early intervention decreases the risk of heart attack and stroke. Monitoring blood sugar levels and HbA1c facilitates management of her type 1 diabetes. Completing a skin assessment reveals a nevus on her elbow that needs to be watched for any changes. Collecting health promotion data allows the examiner to personalize risk reduction and health promotion information while reinforcing positive behaviors already in place. The physical examination is not just a rote formality. Its parts are determined by the best clinical evidence available and published in the professional literature.

ASSESSMENT—POINT OF ENTRY IN AN ONGOING PROCESS

Assessment is the collection of data about the individual's health state. Throughout this text you will be studying the techniques of collecting and analyzing **subjective data** (i.e., what the person *says* about himself or herself during history taking) and **objective data** (i.e., what you as the health professional *observe* by inspecting, percussing, palpating, and auscultating during the physical examination). Together with the patient's record and laboratory studies, these elements form the **database**.

From the database you make a clinical judgment or diagnosis about the individual's health state, response to actual or potential health problems, and life processes. Thus the purpose of assessment is to make a judgment or diagnosis.

An organized assessment is the starting point of diagnostic reasoning. Because all health care diagnoses, decisions, and treatments are based on the data you gather during assessment, it is paramount that your assessment be factual and complete.

Diagnostic Reasoning

The step from data collection to diagnosis can be a difficult one. Most novice examiners perform well in gathering the data (given adequate practice) but then treat all the data as being equally important. This leads to slow and labored decision making.

Diagnostic reasoning is the process of analyzing health data and drawing conclusions to identify diagnoses. Novice examiners most often use a diagnostic process involving hypothesis forming and deductive reasoning. This hypothetico-deductive process has four major components: (1) attending to initially available cues; (2) formulating diagnostic hypotheses; (3) gathering data relative to the tentative hypotheses; and (4) evaluating each hypothesis with the new data collected, thus arriving at a final diagnosis. A *cue* is a piece of information, a sign or symptom, or a piece of laboratory or imaging data. A *hypothesis* is a tentative explanation for a cue or a set of cues that can be used as a basis for further investigation.

Once you complete data collection, develop a preliminary list of significant signs and symptoms for all patient health needs. This is less formal in structure than your final list of diagnoses will be and is in no particular order.

Cluster or group together the assessment data that appear to be causal or associated. For example, with a person in acute pain, associated data are rapid heart rate, increased BP, and anxiety. Organizing the data into meaningful clusters is slow at first; experienced examiners cluster data more rapidly because they recall proven results of earlier patient situations and recognize the same patterns in the new clinical situation.[14] What is often referred to as nurses' intuition is likely skilled pattern recognition by expert nurses.[13]

Validate the data you collect to make sure they are accurate. As you validate your information, look for gaps in data collection. Be sure to find the missing pieces, because identifying missing information is an essential critical-thinking skill. How you validate your data depends on experience. If you are unsure of the BP, validate it by repeating it yourself, or ask another nurse to validate the finding. Eliminate any extraneous variables that could influence BP results such as recent activity or anxiety over admission. If you have less experience analyzing breath sounds or heart murmurs, ask an expert to listen. Even with years of clinical experience, some signs always require validation (e.g., a breast lump).

Critical Thinking and the Diagnostic Process

The standards of practice in nursing, traditionally termed the **nursing process**, include six phases: assessment, diagnosis, outcome identification, planning, implementation, and evaluation.[3] This is an iterative process, allowing practitioners to move back and forth while caring for the needs of complex patients (Fig. 1.2).

Although the nursing process is a problem-solving approach, the way in which we apply the process depends on our level and years of experience. The *novice* has no experience with a specified patient population and uses rules to guide performance. It takes time, perhaps 2 to 3 years in similar clinical situations, to achieve *competency*, in which you see actions in the context of patient goals or plans of care. With more time and experience the *proficient* nurse understands a patient situation as a whole rather than as a list of tasks. At this level you can see long-term goals for the patient. You understand how today's interventions will help the patient in the future. Finally it seems that *expert* nurses vault over the steps and arrive at a clinical judgment in one leap. The expert has an intuitive grasp of a clinical situation and zeroes in on the accurate solution.[5,6]

ASSESSMENT
- Collect data:
  - Review of the clinical record
  - Health history
  - Physical examination
  - Functional assessment
  - Risk assessment
  - Review of the literature
- Use evidence-based assessment techniques
- Document relevant data

DIAGNOSIS
- Compare clinical findings with normal and abnormal variation and developmental events
- Interpret data
  - Identify clusters of clues
  - Make hypotheses
  - Test hypotheses
  - Derive diagnoses
- Validate diagnoses
- Document diagnoses

OUTCOME IDENTIFICATION
- Identify expected outcomes
- Individualize to the person
- Identify expected culturally appropriate outcomes
- Establish realistic and measurable outcomes
- Develop a timeline

PLANNING
- Establish priorities
- Develop outcomes
- Set timelines for outcomes
- Identify interventions
- Integrate evidence-based trends and research
- Document plan of care

IMPLEMENTATION
- Implement in a safe and timely manner
- Use evidence-based interventions
- Collaborate with colleagues
- Use community resources
- Coordinate care delivery
- Provide health teaching and health promotion
- Document implementation and any modification

EVALUATION
- Progress toward outcomes
- Conduct systematic, ongoing, criterion-based evaluation
- Include patient and significant others
- Use ongoing assessment to revise diagnoses, outcomes, plan
- Disseminate results to patient and family

THE INDIVIDUAL

1.2

(Alfaro-LeFevre, 2009.)

Functioning at the level of expert in clinical judgment includes using intuition. Intuition is characterized by immediate recognition of patterns; expert practitioners learn to attend to a pattern of assessment data and act without consciously labeling it. Whereas the beginner operates from a set of defined, structured rules, the expert practitioner uses intuitive links, has the ability to see salient issues in a patient situation, and knows instant therapeutic responses.[5,6] The expert has a storehouse of experience concerning which interventions have been successful in the past.

For example, compare the actions of the nonexpert and the expert nurse in the following situation of a young man with *Pneumocystis jiroveci* pneumonia:

> He was banging the side rails, making sounds, and pointing to his endotracheal tube. He was diaphoretic, gasping, and frantic. The nurse put her hand on his arm and tried to ascertain whether he had a sore throat from the tube. While she was away from the bedside retrieving an analgesic, the expert nurse strolled by, hesitated, listened, went to the man's bedside, reinflated the endotracheal cuff, and accepted the patient's look of gratitude because he was able to breathe again. The nonexpert nurse was distressed that she had misread the situation. The expert reviewed the signs of a leaky cuff with the nonexpert and pointed out that banging the side rails and panic help differentiate acute respiratory distress from pain.[12]

The method of moving from novice to becoming an expert practitioner is through the use of critical thinking. We all start as novices, when we need the familiarity of clear-cut rules to guide actions. Critical thinking is the means by which we learn to assess and modify, if indicated, before acting. We may even be beginners more than once during our careers. As we transition to different specialties, we must rebuild our database of experiences to become experts in new areas of practice.[1]

Critical thinking is required for sound diagnostic reasoning and clinical judgment. During your career you will need to sort through vast amounts of data to make sound judgments to manage patient care. These data will be dynamic, unpredictable, and ever changing. There will not be any one protocol you can memorize that will apply to every situation.

Critical thinking is recognized as an important component of nursing education at all levels.[2,21] Case studies and simulations frequently are used to encourage critical thinking with students. As a student, be prepared to think outside the box and think critically through patient-care situations. Critical thinking goes beyond knowing the pathophysiology of a disease process and requires you to put important assessment cues together to determine the most likely cause of a clinical problem and develop a solution. Critical thinking is a multidimensional thinking process, not a linear approach to problem solving.

Remember to approach problems in a nonjudgmental way and to avoid making assumptions. Identify which information you are taking for granted or information you may overlook based on natural assumptions. Rates of incorrect diagnoses are estimated to be as high as 10% to 15%, and one

---

TABLE 1.1   Identifying Immediate Priorities

Principles of Setting Priorities

1. Complete a health history, including allergies, medications, current medical problems, and reason for visit.
2. Determine whether any problems are related, and set priorities. Priority setting evolves over time with changes in priority depending on the relationships between and severity of problems. For example, if the patient is having difficulty breathing because of acute rib pain, managing the pain may be a higher priority than dealing with a rapid pulse.

Steps to Setting Priorities

1. Assign high priority to **first-level** priority problems such as airway, breathing, and circulation.
2. Next attend to **second-level** priority problems, which include mental status changes, acute pain, infection risk, abnormal laboratory values, and elimination problems.
3. Address **third-level** priority problems such as lack of knowledge, mobility problems, and family coping.

Setting Priorities: Clinical Exemplar

You are working in the hospital and a patient is admitted to the emergency department with diabetic ketoacidosis as evidenced by a blood glucose of >1100 mg/dL. The patient is lethargic and cannot provide a history. Based on family report, he is 12 years old and has no significant medical, surgical, or medication history. Your first-level priorities include assuring a stable airway and adequate breathing. Your second-level priorities include addressing mental status changes and abnormal laboratory values by intervening to manage blood glucose levels. Once the patient has a stable blood sugar and is alert/oriented, you address third-level priorities, including diabetic education, nutritionist consults, and referral to community support groups as appropriate.

---

of the primary causes of misdiagnosis is the clinician's bias.[9] A 61-year-old man comes to your clinic with complaints of shortness of breath. His history reveals a 5-pound weight gain this week and a "fluttering in his chest." During the physical assessment you find 2+ pitting edema in bilateral lower extremities and an irregular apical pulse. Taken individually, ankle edema, weight gain, shortness of breath, and palpitations may appear unrelated, but together they are signs of an exacerbation of heart failure. Clustering of cues is extremely important in identifying a correct diagnosis. Another patient, an overweight 20-year-old female, comes to your office for a scheduled physical examination. Are you making assumptions about her lifestyle and eating habits? Make sure that you double-check the accuracy of your data (subjective and objective) and avoid assumptions that may bias your diagnosis.

Once you have clustered items that are related, you are ready to identify relevant information and anything that does not fit. In the case of your heart failure patient, his complaints of a headache may be viewed as unrelated to the primary diagnosis, whereas abdominal pain and difficulty buttoning his pants are related (presence of ascites). As you gather clinical cues and complete an assessment, also think about priority setting (Table 1.1).

- **First-level priority problems** are those that are emergent, life threatening, and immediate, such as establishing an airway or supporting breathing.
- **Second-level priority problems** are those that are next in urgency—those requiring your prompt intervention to forestall further deterioration (e.g., mental status change, acute pain, acute urinary elimination problems, untreated medical problems, abnormal laboratory values, risks of infection, or risk to safety or security).
- **Third-level priority problems** are those that are important to the patient's health but can be attended to after more urgent health problems are addressed. Interventions to treat these problems are long term, and the response to treatment is expected to take more time. These problems may require a collaborative effort between the patient and health care professionals (Fig. 1.3).

Patients often require the assistance of an interdisciplinary team of practitioners to treat complex medical problems. Throughout your career, look for opportunities to work in collaborative teams and consult other practitioners as appropriate to care for your patients. Remember, health is complex and requires input from a variety of specialties (e.g., physical therapy, speech therapy, occupational therapy). Once you have determined problems, you must identify expected outcomes and work with the patient to facilitate outcome achievement. Remember, your outcomes need to be measurable. Set small goals that can be accomplished in a given time frame. For your heart failure patient your goal may be to eliminate supplemental oxygen needs before discharge.

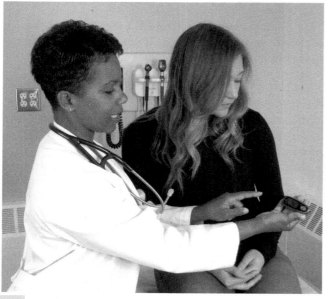

1.3

Include your patient and his or her input, as appropriate, in your outcome identification. Patients are more likely to participate actively in care and follow through with recommendations if they are part of developing the plan of care.

The final steps to the critical-thinking process include evaluation and planning. You must continuously evaluate whether you are on the right track and correct any missteps or misinterpretation of data. If you are not on the right path, reassess, reanalyze, and revise. The final step is the development of a comprehensive plan that is kept up to date. Communicate the plan to the multidisciplinary team. Be aware that this is a legal document and that accurate recording is important for evaluation, insurance reimbursement, and research.

EVIDENCE-BASED ASSESSMENT

Does honey help burn wounds heal more quickly? Do mobile health technologies improve patient compliance with medication administration? Does male circumcision reduce the risk of transmitting human immunodeficiency virus (HIV) in heterosexual men? Can magnesium sulfate reduce cerebral palsy risk in premature infants? Is aromatherapy an effective treatment for postoperative nausea and vomiting?

Health care is a rapidly changing field. The amount of medical and nursing information available has skyrocketed. Current efforts of cost containment result in a hospital population composed of people who have a higher acuity but are discharged earlier than ever before. Clinical research studies are continuously pushing health care forward. Keeping up with these advances and translating them into practice are very challenging. Budget cuts, staff shortages, and increasing patient acuity mean that the clinician has little time to grab a lunch break, let alone browse the most recent journal articles for advances in a clinical specialty.

The conviction that all patients deserve to be treated with the most current and best-practice techniques led to the development of **evidence-based practice (EBP)**. As early as the 1850s Florence Nightingale was using research evidence to improve patient outcomes during the Crimean War. It was not until the 1970s, however, that the term *evidence-based medicine* was coined.[16] In 1972 a British epidemiologist and early proponent of EBP, Archie Cochrane, identified a pressing need for systematic reviews of randomized clinical trials. In a landmark case, Dr. Cochrane noted multiple clinical trials published between 1972 and 1981 showing that the use of corticosteroids to treat women in premature labor reduced the incidence of infant mortality. A short course of corticosteroid stimulates fetal lung development, thus preventing respiratory distress syndrome, a serious and common complication of premature birth. Yet these findings had not been implemented into daily practice, and thousands of low-birth-weight premature infants were dying needlessly. Following a systematic review of the evidence in 1989, obstetricians finally accepted the use of corticosteroid treatment as standard practice for women in preterm labor. Corticosteroid treatment has since been shown to reduce the risk of infant mortality by 30% to 50%.[7]

EBP is more than the use of best-practice techniques to treat patients. The definition of EBP is multifaceted and reflects holistic practice. Once thought to be primarily clinical, EBP now encompasses the integration of research evidence, clinical expertise, clinical knowledge (physical assessment), and patient values and preferences.[16] Clinical decision making depends on all four factors: the best evidence from a critical review of research literature; the patient's own preferences; the clinician's own experience and expertise; and finally physical examination and assessment. Assessment skills must be practiced with hands-on experience and refined to a high level.

Although assessment skills are foundational to EBP, it is important to question tradition when no compelling research evidence exists to support it. Some time-honored assessment techniques have been removed from the examination repertoire because clinical evidence indicates that these techniques are not as accurate as once believed. For example, the traditional practice of auscultating bowel sounds was found to be a poor indicator of returning GI motility in patients having abdominal surgery.[17,18] Following the steps to EBP, the research team asked an evidence-based question (Fig. 1.4). Next, best research evidence was gathered through a literature search, which suggested that early postoperative bowel sounds probably do not represent return of normal GI motility. The evidence was appraised to identify whether a different treatment or assessment approach was better. Research showed the primary markers for returning GI motility after abdominal surgery to be the return of flatus and the first postoperative bowel movement. Based on the literature, a new practice protocol was instituted, and patient outcomes were monitored. Detrimental outcomes did not occur; the new practice guideline was shown to be safe for patients' recovery and a better allocation of staff time. The research led to a change of clinical practice that was safe, effective, and efficient.

Evidence shows that other assessment skills *are* effective for patient care. For example, clinicians should measure the ankle brachial index (ABI), as described in Chapter 21 of this text. Evidence is clear about the value of ABI as a screening measure for peripheral artery disease.

Despite the advantages to patients who receive care based on EBP, it often takes up to 17 years for research findings to be implemented into practice.[4] This troubling gap has led researchers to examine closely the barriers to EBP, both as individual practitioners and as organizations. As individuals, nurses lack research skills in evaluating quality of research studies, are isolated from other colleagues knowledgeable in research, and lack confidence to implement change. Other significant barriers are the organizational characteristics of health care settings. Nurses lack time to go to the library to read research; health care institutions have inadequate library research holdings; and organizational support for EBP is lacking when nurses wish to implement changes in patient care.[15]

Fostering a culture of EBP at the undergraduate and graduate levels is one way in which health care educators attempt to make evidence-based care the gold standard of practice. Students of medicine and nursing are taught how to filter through the wealth of scientific data and critique the findings. They are learning to discern which interventions would best serve their individual patients. Facilitating support for EBP at the organizational level includes time to go to the library; teaching staff to conduct electronic searches; journal club meetings; establishing nursing research committees; linking staff with university researchers; and ensuring that adequate research journals and preprocessed evidence resources are available in the library.[15] *"We have come to a time when the credibility of the health professions will be judged by which of its practices are based on the best and latest evidence from sound scientific studies in combination with clinical expertise, astute assessment, and respect for patient values and preferences."*[20]

COLLECTING FOUR TYPES OF PATIENT DATA

Every examiner needs to establish four different types of databases, depending on the clinical situation: complete, focused or problem-centered, follow-up, and emergency.

Complete (Total Health) Database

This includes a complete health history and a full physical examination. It describes the current and past health state and forms a baseline against which all future changes can be measured. It yields the first diagnoses.

The complete database often is collected in a primary care setting such as a pediatric or family practice clinic, independent or group private practice, college health service, women's health care agency, visiting nurse agency, or community health agency. When you work in these settings, you are the first health professional to see the patient and have primary responsibility for monitoring the person's health care. Collecting the complete database is an opportunity to build and strengthen your relationship with the patient. For the well person this database must describe the person's

Ask the clinical question

Acquire sources of evidence

Appraise and synthesize evidence

Apply relevant evidence in practice

Assess the outcomes

5 steps to evidence-based practice

1.4   (Eckhardt, 2018.)

health state; perception of health; strengths or assets such as health maintenance behaviors, individual coping patterns, support systems, and current developmental tasks; and any risk factors or lifestyle changes. For the ill person the database also includes a description of the person's health problems, perception of illness, and response to the problems.

For well and ill people, the complete database must screen for pathology and determine the ways people respond to that pathology or to any health problem. You must screen for pathology because you are the first, and often the only, health professional to see the patient. This screening is important to refer the patient to another professional, help the patient make decisions, and perform appropriate treatments. This database also notes the human responses to health problems. This factor is important because it provides additional information about the person that leads to nursing diagnoses.

In acute hospital care the complete database is gathered on admission to the hospital. In the hospital, data related specifically to pathology may be collected by the admitting physician. You collect additional information on the patient's perception of illness, functional ability or patterns of living, activities of daily living, health maintenance behaviors, response to health problems, coping patterns, interaction patterns, spiritual needs, and health goals.

Focused or Problem-Centered Database

This is for a limited or short-term problem. Here you collect a "mini" database, smaller in scope and more targeted than the complete database. It concerns mainly one problem, one cue complex, or one body system. It is used in all settings—hospital, primary care, or long-term care. For example, 2 days after surgery a hospitalized person suddenly has a congested cough, shortness of breath, and fatigue. The history and examination focus primarily on the respiratory and cardiovascular systems. Or in an outpatient clinic a person presents with a rash. The history follows the direction of this presenting concern such as whether the rash had an acute or chronic onset; was associated with a fever, new food, pet, or medicine; and was localized or generalized. Physical examination must include a clear description of the rash.

Follow-Up Database

The status of any identified problems should be evaluated at regular and appropriate intervals. What change has occurred? Is the problem getting better or worse? Which coping strategies are used? This type of database is used in all settings to follow up both short-term and chronic health problems. For example, a patient with heart failure may follow up with his or her primary care practitioner at regular intervals to reevaluate medications, identify changes in symptoms, and discuss coping strategies.

Emergency Database

This is an urgent, rapid collection of crucial information and often is compiled concurrently with lifesaving measures. Diagnosis must be swift and sure. For example, a person is brought into an ED with suspected substance overdose.

The first history questions are "What did you take?" "How much did you take?" and "When?" The person is questioned simultaneously while his or her airway, breathing, circulation, level of consciousness, and disability are being assessed. Clearly the emergency database requires more rapid collection of data than the episodic database. Once the person has been stabilized, a complete database can be compiled. An emergency database may be compiled by questioning the patient, or if the patient is unresponsive, health care providers may need to rely on family and friends.

EXPANDING THE CONCEPT OF HEALTH

Assessment is the collection of data about a person's health state. A clear definition of health is important because this determines which assessment data should be collected. In general the list of data that must be collected has lengthened as our concept of health has broadened.

Consideration of the whole person is the essence of **holistic health.** Holistic health views the mind, body, and spirit as interdependent and functioning as a whole within the environment. Health depends on all these factors working together. The basis of disease is multifaceted, originating from both within the person and from the external environment. Thus the treatment of disease requires the services of numerous providers. Nursing includes many aspects of the holistic model (i.e., the interaction of the mind and body, the oneness and unity of the individual). Both the individual human and the external environment are open systems, dynamic and continually changing and adapting to one another. Each person is responsible for his or her own personal health state and is an active participant in health care. Health promotion and disease prevention form the core of nursing practice.

In a holistic model, assessment factors are expanded to include such things as lifestyle behaviors, culture and values, family and social roles, self-care behaviors, job-related stress, developmental tasks, and failures and frustrations of life. All are significant to health.

Health promotion and disease prevention now round out our concept of health. Guidelines to prevention emphasize the link between health and personal behavior. The report of the U.S. Preventive Services Task Force[23] asserts that the great majority of deaths among Americans younger than 65 years are preventable. Prevention can be achieved through counseling from primary care providers designed to change people's unhealthy behaviors related to smoking, alcohol and other drug use, lack of exercise, poor nutrition, injuries, and sexually transmitted infections.[10] Health promotion is a set of positive acts that we can take. In this model the focus of the health professional is on teaching and helping the consumer choose a healthier lifestyle.

The frequency interval of assessment varies with the person's illness and wellness needs. Most ill people seek care because of pain or some abnormal signs and symptoms they have noticed, which prompts an assessment (i.e., gathering a complete, a focused, or an emergency database). In addition,

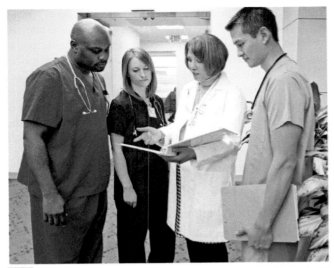

1.5 (Yoder-Wise, 2015.)

risk assessment and preventive services can be delivered once the presenting concerns are addressed. Interdisciplinary collaboration is an integral part of patient care (Fig. 1.5). Providers, nurses, dietitians, therapists and other health professionals must work together to care for increasingly complex patients.

For the well person opinions are inconsistent about assessment intervals. The term *annual checkup* is vague. What does it constitute? Is it necessary or cost-effective? How can primary-care clinicians deliver services to people with no signs and symptoms of illness? Periodic health checkups are an excellent opportunity to deliver preventive services and update the complete database. Although periodic health checkups could induce unnecessary costs and promote services that are not recommended, advocates justify well-person visits because of delivery of some recommended preventive services and reduction of patient worry.[11,19]

The *Guide to Clinical Preventive Services* is a positive approach to health assessment and risk reduction.[23] The *Guide* is updated annually and is accessible online or in print. It presents evidence-based recommendations on screening, counseling, and preventive topics and includes clinical considerations for each topic. These services include screening factors to gather during the history, age-specific items for physical examination and laboratory procedures, counseling topics, and immunizations. This approach moves away from an annual physical ritual and toward varying periodicity based on factors specific to the patient. Health education and counseling are highlighted as the means to deliver health promotion and disease prevention.

For example, the guide to examination for C.D. (23-year-old female, nonpregnant, not sexually active) would recommend the following services for preventive health care:

1. **Screening history** for dietary intake, physical activity, tobacco/alcohol/drug use, and sexual practices
2. **Physical examination** for height and weight, BP, and screening for cervical cancer and HIV
3. **Counseling** for physical activity and risk prevention (e.g., secondhand smoke, seatbelt use)
4. **Depression** screening
5. **Healthy diet** counseling, including lipid disorder screening and obesity screening
6. **Chemoprophylaxis** to include multivitamin with folic acid (females capable of or planning pregnancy)

C.D. is living successfully with a serious chronic condition. Because she has diabetes, including periodic checks of hemoglobin A1c and a fasting glucose level are important. In addition, you should ask how her pump is functioning and whether she is having any difficulties with blood sugar control.

CULTURE AND GENETICS

In a holistic model of health care, assessment factors must include culture. An introduction to cross-cultural concepts follows in Chapter 2. These concepts are developed throughout the text as they relate to specific chapters.

Metaphors such as *melting pot, mosaic,* and *salad bowl* have been used to describe the cultural diversity that characterizes the United States. The United States is becoming a majority-minority nation. Although non-Hispanic whites will remain the largest single group, they will no longer constitute a numeric majority. *Emerging minority* is a term that has been used to classify the populations, including African Americans, Latinos, and Asian Americans, that are rapidly becoming a combined numeric majority.[22] By 2060 the U.S. Census Bureau projects that minorities will constitute 56% of the population. The Latino and Asian populations are projected to nearly double by 2060, and all other racial groups are expected to increase as well. By 2060 nearly 29% of the population will be Latino, 14% African American, 9% Asian, and just over 1% American Indians or Alaska Natives. In 2040 the U.S. Census Bureau anticipates that there will be more people over the age of 65 years than under the age of 18 years for the first time in history.[8]

The United States is becoming increasingly diverse, making cultural competence more important and more challenging for health care providers. U.S. health care providers also travel abroad to work in a variety of health care settings in the international community. Medical and nursing teams volunteer to provide free medical and surgical care in developing countries (Fig. 1.6). International interchanges are increasing among health care providers, making attention to the cultural aspects of health and illness an even greater priority.

During your professional career you may be expected to assess short-term foreign visitors who travel for treatments, international university faculty, students from abroad studying in U.S. high schools and universities, family members of foreign diplomats, immigrants, refugees, members of more than 106 different ethnic groups, and American Indians from 510 federally recognized tribes. A serious conceptual problem exists in that nurses and physicians are expected to know, understand, and meet the health needs of people from

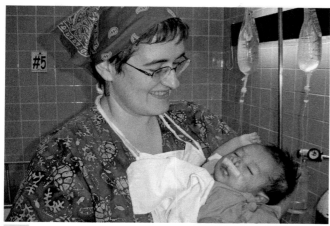

1.6

culturally diverse backgrounds with minimal preparation in cultural competence.

Culture has been included in each chapter of this book. Understanding the basics of a variety of cultures is important in health assessment. People from varying cultures may interpret symptoms differently; therefore, asking the right questions is imperative for you to gather data that are accurate and meaningful. It is important to provide culturally relevant health care that incorporates cultural beliefs and practices. An increasing expectation exists among members of certain cultural groups that health care providers will respect their "cultural health rights," an expectation that may conflict with the unicultural Western biomedical worldview taught in U.S. educational programs that prepare nurses, doctors, and other health care providers.

Given the multicultural composition of the United States and the projected increase in the number of individuals from diverse cultural backgrounds anticipated in the future, a concern for the cultural beliefs and practices of people is increasingly important.

REFERENCES

1. Alfaro-LeFevre, R. (2017). *Critical thinking, clinical reasoning and clinical judgment* (6th ed.). Philadelphia: Elsevier.
2. American Association of Colleges of Nursing. (2008). *Essentials of baccalaureate education for professional nursing practice.* Available at https://www.aacnnursing.org.
3. American Nurses Association. (2015). *Nursing: Scope and standards of practice* (3rd ed.). Washington, DC: American Nurses Publishing.
4. Balas, E. A., & Boren, S. A. (2000). Managing clinical knowledge for health care improvements. In J. Bemmel & A. T. McCray (Eds.), *Yearbook of medical informatics 2000.* Stuttgart, Germany: Schattauer.
5. Benner, P., Tanner, C. A., & Chesla, C. A. (1996). *Expertise in nursing practice.* New York: Springer.
6. Benner, P., Tanner, C. A., & Chesla, C. A. (1997). Becoming an expert nurse. *Am J Nurs, 97*(6), 16BBB–16DDD.
7. Cochrane Collaboration. (2018). Available at www.cochrane.org.
8. Colby, S. L., & Ortman, J. M. (2015). *Projections of the size and composition of the US population: 2014 to 2060.* Population Estimates and projections. US Census Bureau.
9. Croskerry, P. (2013). From mindless to mindful practice—cognitive bias and clinical decision making. *N Engl J Med, 368,* 2445–2450.
10. Ezzati, M., & Riboli, E. (2013). Behavioral and dietary risk factors for noncommunicable diseases. *N Engl J Med, 369*(10), 954–964.
11. Goroll, A. H. (2015). Toward trusting therapeutic relationships—in favor of the annual physical. *N Engl J Med, 373,* 1487–1489.
12. Hanneman, S. K. (1996). Advancing nursing practice with a unit-based clinical expert. *Image (IN), 28*(4), 331–337.
13. Harjai, P. K., & Tiwari, R. (2009). Model of critical diagnostic reasoning: Achieving expert clinician performance. *Nurs Educ Perspect, 30*(5), 305–311.
14. Koharchik, L., Caputi, L., Robb, M., et al. (2015). Fostering clinical reasoning in nursing students. *Am J Nurs, 115*(1), 58–61.
15. Lipscomb, M. (Ed.). (2016). *Exploring evidence-based practice: Debates and challenges in nursing.* New York: Routledge.
16. Mackey, A., & Bassendowski, S. (2017). The history of evidence-based practice in nursing education and practice. *J Prof Nurs, 33*(1), 51–55.
17. Madsen, D., Sebolt, T., Cullen, L., et al. (2005). Listening to bowel sounds: An evidence-based practice project. *Am J Nurs, 105*(12), 40–50.
18. Massey, R. L. (2012). Return of bowel sounds indicating an end of postoperative ileus: Is it time to cease this long-standing nursing tradition? *Medsurg Nurs, 21*(3), 146–150.
19. Mehrotra, A., & Prochazka, A. (2015). Improving value in health care—against the annual physical. *N Engl J Med, 373,* 1485–1487.
20. Melnyk, B. M., & Fineout-Overholt, E. (2011). *Evidence-based practice in nursing & healthcare* (2nd ed.). Philadelphia: Lippincott Williams & Wilkins.
21. National League for Nursing Accrediting Commission. (2006). *Accreditation manual and interpretive guidelines by program type for postsecondary and higher degree programs in nursing.* New York: Author.
22. Spector, R. E. (2016). *Cultural diversity in health and illness* (9th ed.). Indianapolis, IN: Pearson.
23. U.S. Preventive Services Task Force (USPSTF) (2017). Published recommendations. Available at https://uspreventiveservicestaskforce.org.

CHAPTER 2

Cultural Assessment

http://evolve.elsevier.com/Jarvis/

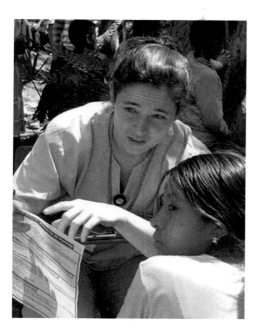

2.1

As a health professional, it is imperative that you learn to build trusting relationships with patients. Part of forming trust is listening to each patient's individual needs and establishing an awareness of his or her culture. You must be open to people who are different from you, have a curiosity about people, and work to become culturally competent (Fig. 2.1). A cultural assessment is an integral part of forming a full database of information about each patient. Serious errors can occur due to lack of cultural competence. If you fail to ask about traditional, herbal, or folk remedies, you may unknowingly give or prescribe a medication that has a significant interaction. For example, ginseng raises the serum digoxin level and can lead to adverse, even fatal, consequences.[18]

A key to understanding cultural diversity is self-awareness and knowledge of one's own culture. Your cultural identification might include the subculture of nursing or health care professionals. You might identify yourself as a Midwesterner, a college student, an athlete, a member of the Polish community, or a Buddhist. These multiple and often changing cultural and subcultural identifications help define you and influence your beliefs about health and illness, coping mechanisms, and wellness behaviors. Developing self-awareness will make you a better health care provider and ensure that you are prepared to care for diverse clients. Recognizing your own culture, values, and beliefs is an interactive and ongoing process of self-discovery.[18] A cultural assessment of each patient is important, but a cultural self-assessment is also an integral component of becoming culturally competent. To understand another person's culture, you must first understand your own culture.

Over the course of your professional education, you will study physical examination and health promotion across the life span and learn to conduct numerous assessments such as a health history, a physical examination, a mental health assessment, a domestic violence assessment, a nutritional assessment, and a pain assessment. However, depending on the cultural and racial background of the person, the data you gather in the assessments may vary. Therefore a cultural assessment must be an integral component of a complete physical and health assessment.

DEMOGRAPHIC PROFILE OF THE UNITED STATES

The estimates of the U.S. population illustrate the increasing diversity in the population and highlight the importance of cultural competence in health care.[40] The population of the United States exceeded 321 million people in 2015 with only 61.6% of the population identifying as white, non-Hispanic.[38] Over 13% of the U.S. population were born elsewhere, and over 21% of the U.S. population report speaking a language other than English in the home.[3,37] The national minority, actually *emerging majority*, population makes up 38% of the total. Among this emerging majority, the largest ethnic group is Hispanic, who make up 17.6% of the population and are the fastest-growing minority group. The largest racial minority group is African American or black (13.3%), followed by Asians (5.6%), two or more races (2.6%), American Indians and Alaska natives (1.2%), and native Hawaiians and other Pacific Islanders (0.2%).[38]

There are demographic differences between the emerging majority groups when compared with non-Hispanic whites. These demographic differences include age, poverty level, and household composition. The number of relatives living in the household is higher for all racial and ethnic minorities compared to non-Hispanic whites, as is the number of multigenerational families (Fig. 2.2). African Americans, American Indians, and Alaska natives are more likely to have grandparents who are responsible for the care of grandchildren compared with other groups.[37]

Asians and non-Hispanic whites have the highest median income, whereas African Americans have the lowest household income followed by Hispanics. All ethnic and racial minority

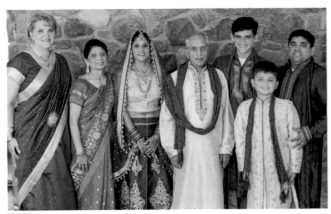

2.2   (Courtesy Holly Birch Photography.)

groups have poverty rates exceeding the national average of 14.8%. Non-Hispanic whites have the lowest reported poverty at 10%, whereas 25.2% of African Americans and 24.7% of Hispanics live at or below the poverty line.[11] Contributing to the high rates of poverty is low educational attainment. Approximately 33% of Hispanics and 13% of African Americans have less than a high school education compared with 6.7% of non-Hispanic whites.[33] Lower educational levels and lower income levels are also correlated with likelihood of disability. Approximately 20% of adults report having a disability. African Americans were the most likely to report a disability (29%), followed by Hispanics (25.9%).[6]

IMMIGRATION

Immigrants are people who are not U.S. citizens at birth. Some new immigrants have minimal understanding of health care resources and how to navigate the health care system. They may not speak or understand English, and they may not be literate in the language of their country of origin. Therefore it is imperative that health care providers address the needs of this growing population.

In 2014 the population of the United States included over 42.2 million foreign-born individuals, which accounted for 13.2% of the population. The number of foreign-born individuals residing in the United States has quadrupled since the 1960s and is expected to almost double by 2065.[3] During your career, you will care for foreign-born individuals who have unique health care needs. The United States health care system is complex and difficult to navigate for anyone. Keep in mind, the health care system may be even more difficult for foreign-born individuals with limited English proficiency. Make sure that you identify interpreter needs early and ask the appropriate cultural assessment questions when caring for each patient.

DETERMINANTS OF HEALTH AND HEALTH DISPARITIES

An individual's health status is influenced by a constellation of factors known as social determinants of health (SDOH).[15] The social determinants of health include economic stability,

education, social and community context, neighborhood and built environment, and health and health care (Fig. 2.3). The five social determinants of health are interconnected and affect a person's health from preconception to death. However, evidenced-based research has consistently shown that poverty has the greatest influence on health status.

For the past two decades the goals of *Healthy People* have been to eliminate health disparities. A health disparity is "a particular type of health difference that is closely linked with social, economic, and/or environmental disadvantage. Health disparities adversely affect groups of people who have systematically experienced greater obstacles to health based on their racial or ethnic group; religion; socioeconomic status; gender; age; mental health; cognitive, sensory, or physical disability; sexual orientation or gender identity; geographic location; or other characteristics historically linked to discrimination or exclusion."[12]

New health care delivery frameworks must strive for social and physical environments that promote quality of life free from preventable illness, disability, and premature death. Public health sectors must be encouraged to address the needs for safe and affordable housing; reliable transportation; nutritious food that is accessible to everyone; safe, well-integrated neighborhoods and schools; health care providers that are culturally and linguistically competent; and clean water and air.

Health Care Disparities Among Vulnerable Populations

Health disparities affect people who experience social, economic, and/or environmental disadvantage. These people are vulnerable populations and include ethnic and racial minorities, people with disabilities, and the LGBT community. Health care disparities are measured by comparing the percent of difference from one group to the best group rate for a disease. One study found a 33-year age difference

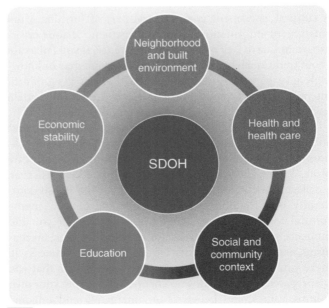

2.3   (USSDHS, 2018.)

between the longest- and shortest-living groups in the United States.[13] In another example, African American children are twice as likely to be hospitalized and four times as likely to die from asthma as non-Hispanic whites.[13] Overall infant mortality in the United States is 5.90 per 1,000 live births, but the mortality rate for African American infants is 10.93 per 1,000 live births.[27] Lack of health insurance may contribute to health disparities. An estimated 10.6% of non-Hispanic whites do not have health insurance, whereas more than 30% of Hispanics, nearly 19% of non-Hispanic blacks, and almost 14% of Asians lack basic insurance coverage.[7]

Few of the differences in health between ethnic and racial groups have a biologic basis but rather pertain to the social determinants of health. Disparities in exposure to environmental contaminants, violence, and substance abuse among some racial and ethnic minorities suggest the need for a major transformation of the neighborhoods and social contexts of people's lives. Although overall quality of health care is improving in the United States, access to care and health disparities are not showing any improvement.[14]

National Cultural and Linguistic Standards

Many forms of discrimination based on race or national origin limit the opportunities for people to gain equal access to health care services. Many health and social service programs provide information about their services in English only. Language barriers have a negative impact on the quality of care provided, and those patients with language barriers also have increased risk of noncompliance to treatment regimens.

Because immigration occurs at high levels and immigrants with limited English proficiency (LEP) have particular needs, the Office of Minority Health published the *National Standards for Culturally and Linguistically Appropriate Services in Health Care*. This set of 15 standards provides a blueprint to improve quality of care and eliminate health disparities for culturally diverse populations. Health disparities affect the health of individuals and communities, making this a major public health concern in the United States.[39]

Linguistic Competence

Under the provisions of Title VI of the Civil Rights Act of 1964, when people with LEP seek health care in settings such as hospitals, nursing homes, clinics, daycare centers, and mental health centers, services cannot be denied to them. English is the predominant language of the United States. However, among people at least 5 years old living in the United States, 21% spoke a language other than English at home.[38] Of those, 62% spoke Spanish, 18% reported speaking an Indo-European language, 16% spoke an Asian language, and 4% spoke a different language. Of people who spoke a language other than English at home, nearly 42% reported that they did not speak English "very well."[38]

When people with LEP seek health care, they are frequently faced with receptionists, nurses, and physicians who speak English only. Additional time and resources are necessary to adequately care for patients with LEP. The language barrier may lead to a decreased quality of care due to limited understanding of patient needs. To prevent serious adverse health outcomes for LEP persons, it is imperative that health care professionals communicate effectively and utilize resources such as interpreter services.

Chapter 3 describes in more detail how to communicate with people who do not understand English, how to interact with interpreters, and which services are available when no interpreter is available. It is vital that interpreters be present who not only serve to verbally translate the conversation but who can also describe to you the cultural aspects and meanings of the person's situation.

CULTURE-RELATED CONCEPTS

Culture is a complex phenomenon that includes attitudes, beliefs, self-definitions, norms, roles, and values. It is also a web of communication, and much of culture is transmitted nonverbally through socialization or enculturation (Fig. 2.4).[35] *Socialization* or *enculturation* is the process of being raised within a culture and acquiring the norms, values, and behaviors of that group. According to the Department of Health and Human Services Office of Minority Health, a person's culture defines health and illness, identifies when treatment is needed and which treatments are acceptable, and informs a person of how symptoms are expressed and which symptoms are important.[39]

Culture has four basic characteristics: (1) *learned* from birth through the processes of language acquisition and socialization; (2) *shared* by all members of the same cultural group; (3) *adapted* to specific conditions related to environmental and technical factors and to the availability of natural resources; and (4) *dynamic* and ever changing.

Culture is a universal phenomenon, yet the culture that develops in any given society is unique, encompassing all the knowledge, beliefs, customs, and skills acquired by members of that society. However, within cultures some groups of people share different beliefs, values, and attitudes. Differences occur because of ethnicity, religion, education, occupation, age, and gender. When such groups function within a large culture, they are referred to as *subcultural groups*.

Many people think about race and ethnicity as a part of the concept of culture. Race reflects self-identification and

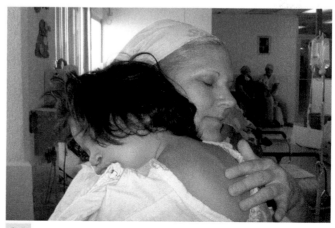

2.4

is typically a social construct referring to a group of people who share similar physical characteristics. The U.S. Census Bureau lists 15 racial categories for respondents to choose from: white, black (African American), American Indian or Alaskan native, Asian Indian, Chinese, Filipino, Japanese, Korean, Vietnamese, native Hawaiian, Guamanian or Chamorro, Samoan, other Pacific Islander, some other race, or more than one race. A growing number of respondents are identifying as more than one race, especially those in younger generations. An additional question asks respondents to identify whether they are of Hispanic origin. Hispanic origin includes the categories of Mexican, Puerto Rican, Cuban, and another Hispanic, Latino, or Spanish origin. People who self-identify as Hispanic can be of any racial category. For example, Dominicans typically identify as black Hispanics, whereas people from Argentina identify as white Hispanics. Because the terms *race* and *origin* cause confusion, the U.S. Census Bureau is considering changing the race and origin questions so that people can select all that apply, with racial categories and Hispanic origin combined in the same question.[8]

Race may be useful when determining disease prevalence, but does not typically refer to specific genetic or biologic characteristics that distinguish one group of people from another. Throughout the text, information on disease prevalence related to race is presented in the culture and genetics section of each chapter. As we learn more about the human genome, we may find that genetic variations become more important than overarching racial classifications.

Ethnicity refers to a social group that may possess shared traits, such as a common geographic origin, migratory status, religion, language, values, traditions or symbols, and food preferences. The ethnic group may have a loose group identity with few or no cultural traditions in common or a coherent subculture with a shared language and body of tradition. Similarly *ethnic identity* is one's self-identification with a particular ethnic group. This identity may be strongly adherent to one's country of origin or background or weakly identified.

Acculturation is the process of adopting the culture and behavior of the majority culture. During the late 1800s and early part of the 1900s when the United States experienced its greatest period of immigration, the expectation was that immigrants would take on the characteristics of the dominant culture, known as *assimilation*. Immigrants were discouraged

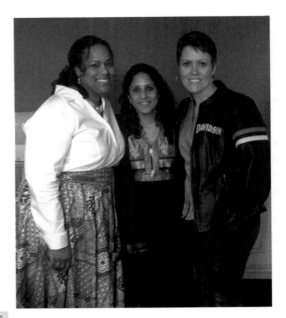

2.5

from having a unique ethnic identity in favor of the nationalist identity.

The recent wave of immigrants in the latter part of the 20th century has developed different strategies of acculturation. Rather than solely relying on assimilation, new immigrants developed new means of forging identities between the countries of origin and their host country, such as "biculturalism" and "integration."[34] Assimilation is unidirectional, proceeding in a linear fashion from unacculturated to acculturated. However, biculturalism and integration are bidirectional and bidimensional, inducing reciprocal changes in both cultures and maintaining aspects of the original culture in one's ethnic identity (Fig. 2.5).

Those who emigrate to the United States from non-Western countries may find the process of acculturation, whether in schools or society, to be an extremely difficult and painful process. The losses and changes that occur when adjusting to or integrating a new system of beliefs, routines, and social roles are known as **acculturative stress,** which has important implications for health and illness.[9,10,36] When caring for patients, please be aware of the factors that contribute to acculturative stress, as defined in Table 2.1.[5]

TABLE 2.1	**Dimensions of Acculturative Stress**		
INSTRUMENTAL/ENVIRONMENTAL		**SOCIAL/INTERPERSONAL**	**SOCIETAL**
Financial		Loss of social networks	Discrimination/stigma
Language barriers		Loss of social status	Level of acculturation
Lack of access to health care		Family conflict	Political/historical forces
Unemployment		Family separation	Legal status
Lack of education		Intergenerational conflict	
		Changing gender roles	

Modified from Caplan, S. (2007). Latinos, acculturation, and acculturative stress: a dimensional concept analysis. *Policy Politics Nurs Pract, 8*(2), 93-106.

RELIGION AND SPIRITUALITY

Other major aspects of culture are **religion and spirituality.** **Spirituality** is a broader term focused on a connection to something larger than oneself and a belief in transcendence. On the other hand, **religion** refers to an organized system of beliefs concerning the cause, nature, and purpose of the universe, as well as the attendance of regular services.[19] Religion is a shared experience of spirituality or the values, beliefs, and practices into which people either are born or that they may adopt to meet their personal spiritual needs through communal actions, such as religious affiliation; attendance and participation in a religious institution, prayer, or meditation; and religious practices (Fig. 2.6). Some people define their spirituality in terms of religion, whereas others identify spirituality outside a formal religion.[2]

The Landscape Survey detailed statistics on religion in America.[29] The study found that religious affiliation in the United States is both diverse and extremely fluid. The number of people who say they are not affiliated with any particular faith increased from 16.1% in 2007 to 22.8% in 2015. The number of people affiliated with Christian denominations fell from 78.4% to 70.6%, whereas those who belong to non-Christian faiths increased from 4.7% to 5.9%. The percentage of people who affiliate with a Christian faith has dropped, but American Christians are becoming increasingly diverse.[29]

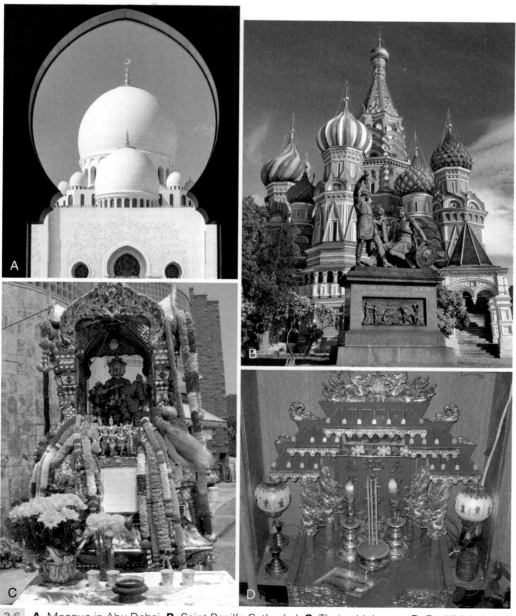

2.6 **A,** Mosque in Abu Dabai. **B,** Saint Basil's Cathedral. **C,** Thai spirit house. **D,** Buddhist shrine. (**C** and **D,** Spector, 2009.)

Although fewer individuals identify with a specific religion, spirituality assessment is important for all patients regardless of religious affiliation or nonaffiliation.

In times of crisis such as serious illness and impending death, spirituality may be a source of consolation for the person and his or her family. Religious dogma and spiritual leaders may exert considerable influence on the person's decision making concerning acceptable medical and surgical treatment such as vaccinations, choice of healer(s), and other aspects of the illness. Completion of a spiritual assessment is one component of a holistic patient assessment. Understanding a patient's spirituality can improve understanding of coping mechanisms, identify referral needs such as visits by a chaplain, identify social support after discharge, and open discussions about medical care (e.g., acceptance of certain treatments such as blood transfusion). Failure to assess spiritual needs has been shown to increase health care costs, especially at end of life, and unmet spiritual needs can lead to poor outcomes.[21] Religion and spirituality are associated with improved physical health, and attending to the religious and spiritual needs of patients is an important part of holistic patient care.[19]

HEALTH-RELATED BELIEFS AND PRACTICES

Healing and Culture

HEALTH is defined as the **balance** of the person, both within one's being (physical, mental, or spiritual) and in the outside world (natural, communal, or metaphysical). It is a complex, interrelated phenomenon. Before determining whether cultural practices are helpful, harmful, or neutral, you must first understand the logic of the traditional belief systems coming from a person's culture and then grasp the nature and meaning of the health practice from the person's cultural perspective. Wide cultural variation exists in the manner in which certain symptoms and disease conditions are perceived, diagnosed, labeled, and treated.

Beliefs About Causes of Illness

Throughout history people have tried to understand the cause of illness and disease. Theories of causation have been formulated on the basis of ethnic identity, religious beliefs, social class, philosophic perspectives, and level of knowledge.[23] Many people who maintain traditional beliefs would define HEALTH in terms of balance and a loss of this balance. This understanding includes the balance of mind, body, and spirit in the overall definitions of HEALTH and ILLNESS.

Disease causation may be viewed in three major ways: from a biomedical or scientific perspective, a naturalistic or holistic perspective, or a magicoreligious perspective.[22]

Biomedical

The **biomedical** or **scientific** theory of illness causation assumes that all events in life have a cause and effect. Among the biomedical explanations for disease is the germ theory, which holds that microorganisms such as bacteria and viruses cause specific disease conditions. Most educational programs for physicians, nurses, and other health care providers embrace the biomedical or scientific theories that explain the causes of both physical and psychological illnesses.[20]

Naturalistic

The second way in which people explain the cause of illness is from the **naturalistic** or **holistic** perspective, found most frequently among American Indians, Asians, and others who believe that human life is only one aspect of nature and a part of the general order of the cosmos. These people believe that the forces of nature must be kept in natural balance or harmony.

Some Asians believe in the **yin/yang theory,** in which health exists when all aspects of the person are in perfect balance.[25] Rooted in the ancient Chinese philosophy of *Tao,* the yin/yang theory states that all organisms and objects in the universe consist of yin and yang energy forces. The seat of the energy forces is within the autonomic nervous system, where balance between the opposing forces is maintained during health. Yin energy represents the female and negative forces such as emptiness, darkness, and cold, whereas yang forces are male and positive, emitting warmth and fullness. Foods are classified as hot and cold in this theory and are transformed into yin and yang energy when metabolized by the body. Yin foods are cold, and yang foods are hot. Cold foods are eaten with a hot illness, and hot foods are eaten with a cold illness. The yin/yang theory is the basis for *Eastern* or *Chinese* medicine.

Many Hispanic, Arab, and Asian groups embrace the **hot/cold theory** of health and illness, an explanatory model with origins in the ancient Greek humoral theory. The four humors of the body—blood, phlegm, black bile, and yellow bile—regulate basic bodily functions and are described in terms of temperature, dryness, and moisture. The treatment of disease consists of adding or subtracting cold, heat, dryness, or wetness to restore the balance of the humors. Beverages, foods, herbs, medicines, and diseases are classified as hot or cold according to their perceived effects on the body, not on their physical characteristics.

According to the hot/cold theory, the person is whole, not just a particular ailment. Those who embrace the hot/cold theory maintain that health consists of a positive state of total well-being, including physical, psychological, spiritual, and social aspects of the person.

Clinical case study: Y.L. is a 30-year-old female who delivered her first child via uncomplicated vaginal delivery yesterday. You notice that she has not been drinking, refused her shower, and that her family has been providing much of the baby's care. In an effort to promote healing, you encourage her to go for a walk, provide fresh ice water, and talk to her about the importance of bonding. Y.L. continues to rest, drinks only warm beverages, and allows her family to provide care. You are concerned for Y.L.'s well-being and decide to speak with a colleague.

You: I'm worried about Y.L. She isn't caring for her baby or herself, won't drink her water, and barely gets out of bed.

Colleague: Where is she from?

You: I'm not sure, but I think her family may have emigrated from China.

Colleague: It's common for the Chinese to believe in the hot/cold theory, wherein postpartum women need to avoid things that are cold and anything that might disrupt their yin. Have you asked her about her beliefs?

You: No. I didn't even think about it.

Colleague: We have pretty rigid standards of treatment in Western medicine, but we need to respect the beliefs of our patients. You should talk to her about her beliefs and any postpartum rituals we can support.

Magicoreligious

The third major way in which people explain the causation of Illness is from a **magicoreligious** perspective. The basic premise is that the world is an arena in which supernatural forces dominate.[16] The fate of the world and those in it depends on the action of supernatural forces for good or evil. Examples of magical causes of illness include beliefs in voodoo or witchcraft, whereas *faith healing* is based on religious beliefs.

Traditional Treatments and Folk Healers

All cultures have their own preferred lay or popular healers, recognized symptoms of ill health, acceptable sick role behavior, and treatments. In addition to seeking help from you as a biomedical/scientific health care provider, patients may also seek help from folk or religious healers (Fig. 2.7). Each culture has its own healers, most of whom speak the person's native tongue, make house calls, understand the person's cultural health beliefs, and cost significantly less than practitioners in the biomedical/scientific health care system. In some religions, spiritual healers may be found among the ranks of the ordained and official religious hierarchy. Spirituality is included in the perceptions of health and illness.

Hispanics may rely on *curandero(ra)*, *espiritualista* (spiritualist), *yerbo(ba)* (herbalist), or *partera* (lay midwife). Blacks may mention having received assistance from a *houngan* (a

voodoo priest or priestess), *spiritualist,* or *"old lady"* (an older woman who has successfully raised a family and who specializes in child care and folk remedies). American Indians may seek assistance from a *shaman* or a *medicine man* or *woman.* Asians may mention that they have visited *herbalists, acupuncturists,* or *bonesetters.* Among the Amish the term *braucher* refers to folk healers who use herbs and tonics in the home or community context. *Brauche,* a folk healing art, refers to sympathy curing, which is sometimes called *pow-wowing* in English.

Many cultures believe that the cure is incomplete unless healing of body, mind, and spirit is carried out. The division of the person into parts is itself a Western concept. If your patient refers to a lay healer that you are unfamiliar with or a practice you do not understand, ask for clarification. Be careful not to ask in a judgmental way that makes the person feel attacked for seeking help outside the medical community (e.g., "Why did you see a shaman instead of coming to the hospital?"). Instead ask in a way that communicates acceptance of their beliefs and allows for open communication (e.g., "Can you tell me more about your visit to the shaman? What did he/she recommend?").

The variety of healing beliefs and practices used by the many ethnocultural populations found in the United States far exceeds the limitations of this chapter. Fig. 2.8 presents samples of traditional amulets that may be seen in practice. In addition to folk practices, many other complementary healing practices exist. In the United States an estimated 38% of adults use some form of complementary therapy to treat an illness, including acupuncture, Ayurveda, biofeedback, chiropractic or osteopathic manipulation, deep-breathing exercises and guided imagery, diet-based therapies, homeopathy, hypnosis, meditation, tai chi, yoga, and traditional folk healers.[26] Furthermore, U.S. adults spend $30.2 billion out-of-pocket on visits to complementary and alternative medicine practitioners, to traditional healers, and for the purchase of related products each year.[26]

The availability of over-the-counter medications, the relatively high literacy level of Americans, the growing availability of herbal remedies, and the influence of the Internet and mass media in communicating health-related information to the general population have contributed to the high percentage of cases of self-treatment. Home treatments are attractive for their accessibility, especially compared with the inconvenience associated with traveling to a physician, nurse practitioner, or pharmacist, particularly for people from rural or sparsely populated areas. Furthermore, home treatment may mobilize the person's social support network and provide the sick person with a caring environment in which to convalesce.

A wide variety of alternative, complementary, or traditional interventions are gaining the recognition of health care professionals in the biomedical/scientific health care system. Acupuncture, acupressure, therapeutic touch, massage, therapeutic use of music, biofeedback, relaxation techniques, meditation, hypnosis, distraction, imagery, iridology, reflexology, and herbal remedies are examples of interventions that

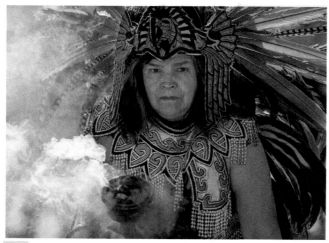

2.7 Aztec healer.   (US DoD, 2015.)

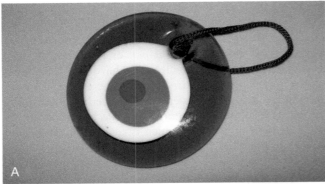

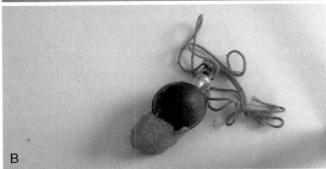

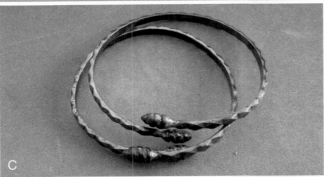

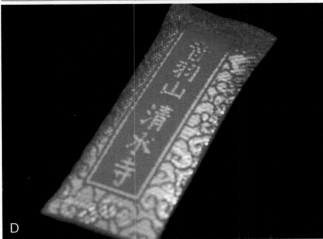

2.8 Amulets. **A,** The glass blue eye from Turkey seen here is an example of an amulet that may be hung in the home. **B,** A seed with a red string may be placed on the crib of a baby of Mexican heritage. **C,** These bangles may be worn for protection by a person of Caribbean heritage. **D,** This small packet is placed on a crib or in the room of a baby of Japanese heritage.[35]

people may use either alone or in combination with other treatments. Many pharmacies and grocery stores routinely carry herbal treatments for a wide variety of common illnesses. The effectiveness of complementary and alternative interventions for specific health problems has been studied (see National Center for Complementary and Integrative Health at www.nccih.nih.gov).

DEVELOPMENTAL COMPETENCE

Illness during childhood may pose a difficult clinical situation. Children and adults have spiritual needs that vary according to the child's developmental level and the religious climate that exists in the family. Parental perceptions about the illness of the child may be partially influenced by religious beliefs. For example, some parents may believe that a transgression against a religious law is responsible for a congenital anomaly in their offspring. Other parents may delay seeking medical care because they believe that prayer should be tried first. Certain types of treatment (e.g., administration of blood; medications containing caffeine, pork, or other prohibited substances) and selected procedures may be perceived as *cultural taboos* (i.e., practices to be avoided by both children and adults).

Values held by the dominant U.S. culture such as emphasis on independence, self-reliance, and productivity influence the aging members of society. North Americans define people as old at the chronologic age of 65 years and then limit their work, in contrast to other cultures in which people are first recognized as being unable to work and then identified as being "old."

Older adults may develop their own means of coping with illness through self-care, assistance from family members, and support from social groups. Some cultures have attitudes and specific behaviors for older adults that include humanistic care and identification of family members as care providers.

Older immigrants who have made major lifestyle adjustments in their move from their homelands to the United States or from a rural to an urban area (or vice versa) may not be aware of health care alternatives, preventive programs, health care benefits, and screening programs for which they are eligible. These people also may be in various stages of *culture shock* (i.e., the state of disorientation or inability to respond to the behavior of a different cultural group because of its sudden strangeness, unfamiliarity, and incompatibility with the newcomer's perceptions and expectations).

TRANSCULTURAL EXPRESSION OF PAIN

To illustrate how symptom expression may reflect the person's cultural background, let us use an extensively studied symptom—pain. Pain is a universally recognized phenomenon, and it is an important aspect of assessment. It is a private, subjective experience that is greatly influenced by cultural heritage. Expectations, manifestations, and management of pain are all embedded in a cultural context. The definition of pain, like that of health or illness, is culturally determined. The meaning of painful stimuli, the way people define their situations, and the impact of personal experience all help determine the experience of pain.

In addition to expecting variations in pain perception and tolerance, you also should expect variations in the expression of pain. While some patients will readily complain of pain, others will remain stoic and attempt to hide pain as much as possible. It is well known that people turn to their social environment for validation and comparison. A first important comparison group is the family, which transmits cultural norms to its children.

BECOMING A CULTURALLY COMPETENT PRACTITIONER

Cultural competency includes the attitudes, knowledge, and skills necessary for providing quality care to diverse populations.[4] The integration of cultural knowledge into day-to-day practice takes time because many practitioners in the health care system hesitate to adopt new ideas. Cultural competency does not come after reading a chapter or several books on this highly specialized area. It is complex and multifaceted, and many facets change over time. The areas of knowledge include sociology, psychology, theology, cultural anthropology, demography, folklore, and immigration history and policies. One must also have an understanding of poverty and environmental health. Cultural competency involves understanding your own culture and health. What cultural health practices do you use on a daily basis? What complementary or alternative therapies do you use?

One response to governmental mandates for cultural competency is the development of cultural care that describes professional health care as culturally sensitive, appropriate, and competent. There is a discrete body of knowledge, and much of the content is introduced in this chapter.

- *Culturally sensitive* implies that caregivers possess some basic knowledge of and constructive attitudes toward the diverse cultural populations found in the setting in which they are practicing.
- *Culturally appropriate* implies that the caregivers apply the underlying background knowledge that must be possessed to provide a given person with the best possible health care.
- *Culturally competent* implies that the caregivers understand and attend to the total context of the individual's situation, including awareness of immigration status, stress factors, other social factors, and cultural similarities and differences.[34]

Cultural care is the provision of health care across cultural boundaries; it considers the context both in which the patient lives and the situations in which the patient's health problems arise.[35] Each chapter in this text includes information necessary for the delivery of culturally appropriate care.

COMPLETING A CULTURAL ASSESSMENT

Lack of cultural knowledge has long been identified as a challenge to providing high-quality health care. Providing culturally congruent care is an integral part of providing holistic patient care. Many theories, frameworks, and models have been developed to facilitate understanding of culturally competent care. Instead of narrowly defining what to expect from a certain race or ethnic group, health care providers should complete a cultural assessment.

Categorical cultural knowledge related to language, food preferences, religion, and health care beliefs is limiting. Although health care providers have used this type of categorical information for years to inform practice, major limitations exist. The use of categorical knowledge can limit your perspective, putting you at risk for stereotyping.[15] As the United States continues to become increasingly diverse, health care providers are challenged to ignore previous assumptions and stereotypes in favor of asking the questions and completing a cultural assessment.

Cultural Self-Assessment

Although specific cultural self-assessment tools exist, a simple format is to think about and consider your culture: What influenced your life? Where is your family from? Do you or your family have cultural traditions? What led you to a career in health care? List your personal values, attitudes, and beliefs. Finally, answer the FICA questions presented in the upcoming section titled *Spiritual Assessment*. All too often, people state that they don't have a culture. Everyone has a culture, but individuals often don't think about the components of their culture in daily life. By purposefully exploring the areas of culture and understanding your personal history, you will develop cultural sensibility. **Cultural sensibility** is the "deliberate proactive behavior by health care providers who examine cultural situations through thoughtful reasoning, responsiveness, and discreet interactions."[15, p. 3]

Cultural Assessment

No one cultural assessment tool is identified as the gold standard of care. In addition to cultural assessment tools, there are a variety of theories, frameworks, and models of cultural competence. Each model identifies slightly different domains and perspectives on cultural competence, but all explicate the importance of completing a cultural assessment on every patient.

You should never assume an understanding of a person's culture; instead ask about cultural beliefs that may impact the care provided. Based on recommended domains from cultural experts,[17,24,32] the following is a list of domains you may consider assessing when caring for a patient. Please keep in mind that all domains may not be appropriate given your setting; however, each of the domains is an important component of understanding culture.

- Heritage. Country of ancestry; years in the United States, etc.

- Health practices. Use of a traditional healer; complementary/ alternative therapies; preventative medicine; any practices that are unacceptable (e.g., blood transfusion)
- Communication. Primary language; preferred name and method of communication; use of touch as a communication strategy
- Family roles and social orientation. Who makes health care decisions within the family; family priorities; role of extended family; relationship status
- Nutrition. Any forbidden foods; fasting rituals; foods avoided or consumed during illness and in the peripartum period
- Pregnancy, birth, child-rearing. Number of children in the family; beliefs surrounding pregnancy; beliefs surrounding childbirth and child-rearing; special rituals after delivery
- Spirituality/religion. Religious affiliation; religious beliefs; holidays; spirituality assessment
- Death. Rituals in preparation for death; meaning of death; grieving
- Health providers. What is the role of the nurse or doctor; preference for same sex provider; any healers besides physicians and nurses

Although all areas may not be appropriate in all settings, consider the aforementioned main areas as you complete a cultural assessment on each patient. Asking each patient about cultural beliefs will increase your cultural competence while decreasing the potential for stereotyping based on previous experiences with a client from a similar background.

Spiritual Assessment

All too often a singular question—"Do you have any religious or spiritual preferences that we can support?"—is the extent of the spiritual assessment. This one question can be answered with a dichotomous yes/no, does not allow for open discussion, and sometimes leads to confusion. Instead of a singular question, health care professionals can use a brief spiritual assessment tool. A number of tools exist that allow health care providers to open a discussion of spiritual care, and no one tool is recommended above others.

One easy-to-use spiritual assessment tool is the FICA Spiritual History Tool, which serves as a guide for conversations. Health care professionals are encouraged to use FICA as a guide for fostering open dialogue and not as a checklist of questions to ask a patient. Recommended questions for each area are provided, but should be adapted to the situation. Speaking with a person who is at the end of life requires very different questions than does speaking with a healthy person during a wellness visit. FICA stands for *faith, importance/influence, community,* and *address/action.*

F- "Do you consider yourself spiritual or religious? Do you have spiritual beliefs, values, or practices that help you cope with stress?"

I- "What importance does your faith or belief have in your life? Have your beliefs influenced you in how you

| TABLE 2.2 | Spirituality Assessment: The Brief RCOPE[a] |

The following items deal with how you coped with a significant trauma or negative event in your life. There are many ways to try to deal with problems. These items ask which part religion played in what you did to cope with this negative event. Obviously, different people deal with things in different ways, but we are interested in how you tried to deal with it. Each item says something about a particular way of coping. We want to know to what extent you did what the item says: *how much or how frequently.* Don't answer on the basis of what worked or not—just whether or not you did it. Use these response choices.

Try to rate each item separately in your mind. Make your answers as true *for you* as you can.

    1 = Not at all
    2 = Somewhat
    3 = Quite a bit
    4 = A great deal

1. Looked for a stronger connection with God. _____
2. Sought God's love and care. _____
3. Sought help from God in letting go of my anger. _____
4. Tried to put my plans into action together with God.

    _____

5. Tried to see how God might be trying to strengthen me in this situation. _____
6. Asked forgiveness for my sins. _____
7. Focused on religion to stop worrying about my problems. _____
8. Wondered whether God had abandoned me. _____
9. Felt punished by God for my lack of devotion. _____
10. Wondered what I did for God to punish me. _____
11. Questioned God's love for me. _____
12. Wondered whether my church had abandoned me.

    _____

13. Decided the devil made this happen. _____
14. Questioned the power of God. _____

From Pargament, K., Feuille, M., & Burdzy, D. (2011). The Brief RCOPE: current psychometric status of a short measure of religious coping. *Religions* 2, 51-76.
[a]The reproduction of any copyrighted material is prohibited without the express permission of the copyright holder.

handle stress? Do you have specific beliefs that influence your health care decisions? If so, are you willing to share those with your health care team?"

C- "Are you part of a spiritual or religious community?" If so, how does this group support you? "Is there a group of people you really love or who are important to you?"

A- "How should I address these issues in your health care?"[31]

In health care settings you frequently encounter people who are searching for a spiritual meaning to help explain their illnesses or disabilities. Some health care providers find spiritual assessment difficult because of the abstract and personal nature of the topic. The omission of questions about spiritual and religious practices can raise barriers to holistic care.

In addition to spiritual assessment tools, several well-validated questionnaires assess how a person is coping with loss, such as a serious illness. Perhaps the most well-known and widely used tool is the Brief RCOPE, a short 14-item assessment for use in clinical practice (Table 2.2).[28] The Brief RCOPE helps practitioners understand the patient's religious coping to enable them to integrate spirituality in treatment.[28] It examines whether a patient is using positive or negative religious coping. Positive religious coping mechanisms indicate that the person is strongly connected to a divine presence, is spiritually connected with others, and has a benevolent outlook on life, whereas negative religious coping methods reflect a spiritual struggle with one's self or with God. Illness may be attributed to God's punishment, to an act of the Devil, or totally within the hands of God. Just as positive religious coping has been linked to positive health, negative religious coping is associated with poor health outcomes.[28]

We need to understand a patient's cultural and religious beliefs because countless health-related behaviors are promoted by nearly all cultures and religions. Meditating, exercising and maintaining physical fitness, getting enough sleep, being willing to have the body examined, telling the truth about how one feels, maintaining family viability, hoping for recovery, coping with stress, being able to live with a disability, and caring for children are all related to one's core values and beliefs.

REFERENCES

1. Reference deleted in proofs.
2. Anandarajah, G., & Hight, E. (2001). Spirituality and medical practice: Using the HOPE questions as a practical tool for spiritual assessment. *Am Fam Physician, 63,* 81–89.
3. Brown, A., & Stepler, R. (2016). *Statistical portrait of the foreign-born population in the United States, 2014.* http://www.pewhispanic.org/2016/04/19/statistical-portrait-of-the-foreign-born-population-in-the-united-states-2014-key-charts/#2013-foreign-born-SP-int.
4. Campinha-Bacote, J. (2003). *The process of cultural competence in the delivery of healthcare services* (4th ed.). Cincinnati: Transcultural C.A.R.E. Associates.
5. Caplan, S. (2007). Latinos, acculturation, and acculturative stress: A dimensional concept analysis. *Policy Polit Nurs Pract, 8*(2), 93–106.
6. CDC. (2015). *53 million adults in the US live with a disability.* https://www.cdc.gov/media/releases/2015/p0730-us-disability.html.
7. CDC. *National Health Interview Survey.* https://www.cdc.gov/nchs/nhis/index.htm.
8. Cohn, D. (2015). *Census considers new approach to asking about race – by not using the term at all.* http://www.pewresearch.org/fact-tank/2015/06/18/census-considers-new-approach-to-asking-about-race-by-not-using-the-term-at-all/.
9. Cuellar, I., Bastida, E., & Braccio, S. M. (2004). Residency in the United States, subjective well-being, and depression in an older Mexican-origin sample. *J Aging Health, 16*(4), 447–466.
10. Dalla, R. I., & Christensen, A. (2005). Latino immigrants describe residence in rural Midwestern meatpacking communities. *Hispanic J Behav Sci, 27*(1), 23–41.
11. DeNavas-Walt, C., & Proctor, B. D. (2015). *U.S. Census Bureau, Current Population Reports, Income and poverty in the United States: 2014.* Washington, DC: U.S. Government Printing Office.
12. U.S. Department of Health and Human Services. (n.d.). https://www.healthypeople.gov/2020/topics-objectives/topic/social-determinants-of-health.
13. U.S. Department of Health and Human Services. (n.d.). *DHHS plan to reduce health disparities.* http://www.minorityhealth.hhs.gov/npa/files/Plans/HHS/HHS_Plan_complete.pdf.
14. *Disparities in healthcare quality among racial and ethnic minority groups.* (2010). http://archive.ahrq.gov/research/findings/nhqrdr/nhqrdr10/minority.html.
15. Ellis Fletcher, S. N. (2015). *Cultural sensibility in healthcare: A personal and professional guidebook.* Indianapolis, IN: Sigma Theta Tau International Honor Society for Nursing.
16. Fadiman, A. (1997). *The spirit catches you and you fall down: A Hmong child, her American doctors, and the collision of two cultures.* New York: Farrar, Straus and Giroux.
17. Giger, J. N., & Davidhizar, R. (2002). The Giger and Davidhizar Transcultural Assessment Model. *J Transcult Nurs, 13*(3), 185–188.
18. Jeffreys, M. R. (2010). *Teaching cultural competence in nursing and health care.* New York, NY: Springer Publishing Company.
19. Jim, S. L., Pustejovsky, J. E., Park, C. L., et al. (2015). Religion, spirituality, and physical health in cancer patients: A meta-analysis. *Cancer, 121,* 3760–3768.
20. Kleinman, A. (1978). Concepts and a model for the comparison of medical systems as cultural systems. *Social Sci Med, 12*(2–B), 85–95.
21. Koenig, H. G. (2012). Religion, spirituality, and health: The research and clinical implications. *ISRN Psychiatry.*
22. Kottak, C. P. (2008). *Cultural anthropology* (12th ed.). Boston: McGraw Hill.
23. Landrine, H., & Klonoff, E. A. (1994). Cultural diversity in causal attributions for illness: The role of the supernatural. *J Behav Med, 17,* 181–193.
24. Leininger, M. M., & McFarland, M. R. (2006). *Culture care diversity and universality: A worldwide nursing theory* (2nd ed.). Boston, MA: Jones and Bartlett Publishers.
25. Men, J., & Guo, L. (2010). *A general introduction to traditional Chinese medicine.* Boca Raton, FL: CRC Press.
26. Nahin, R. L., Barnes, P. M., & Stussman, B. J. (2016). *Expenditures on complementary health approaches: United States, 2012 National Health Statistics Reports.* Hyattsville, MD: National Center for Health Statistics.
27. National Center for Health Statistics. (2017). *Health, United States: 2016.* Hyattsville, MD.
28. Pargament, K., Feuille, M., & Burdzy, D. (2011). The Brief RCOPE. *Religions 2,* 51–76.
29. Pew Forum on Religion and Public Life. (2015). *America's changing religious landscape.* http://www.pewforum.org/2015/05/12/americas-changing-religious-landscape/.

30. Reference deleted in proofs.
31. Puchalski, C. M. (2014). The FICA spiritual history tool #274. *J Palliat Med*, *17*(1), 105–106.
32. Purnell, L. D. (2013). *Transcultural health care: A culturally competent approach* (4th ed.). Philadelphia, PA: FA Davis Company.
33. Ryan, C. L., & Bauman, K. (2016). *U.S. Census Bureau, Current Population Reports, Educational attainment in the United States: 2015*. Washington, DC: U.S. Government Printing Office.
34. Sam, D. L., & Berry, J. W. (2016). *The Cambridge handbook of acculturation psychology* (2nd ed.). Cambridge, UK: Cambridge University Press.
35. Spector, R. E. (2013). *Cultural diversity in health and illness* (8th ed.). Upper Saddle River, NJ: Pearson.
36. Torres, L., Driscoll, M. W., & Voell, M. (2012). Discrimination, acculturation, acculturative stress and Latino psychological distress: A moderated mediational model. *Cultur Divers Ethnic Minor Psychol*, *18*(1), 17–25.
37. U.S. Census Bureau. (n.d.). *American FactFinder*. factfinder. census.gov.
38. U.S. Census Bureau. (n.d.). *QuickFacts: United States*. www. census.gov/quickfacts.
39. US Department of Health and Human Services Office of Minority Health. *Think Cultural Health*. https://www. thinkculturalhealth.hhs.gov/Content/clas.asp.
40. Vespa, J., Lewis, J. M., & Kreider, R. M. (2013). *America's families and living arrangements: 2012: population characteristics P20-570. Source: U.S. Census Bureau, American Community Survey, 2011*. http://www.census.gov/prod/ 2013pubs/p20-570.pdf.

The Interview

http://evolve.elsevier.com/Jarvis/

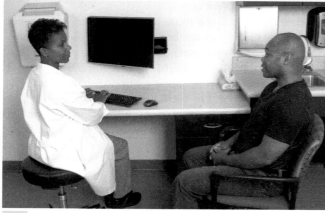

3.1

The interview is the first point of contact with a client[a] and the most important part of data collection. During the interview you collect **subjective data** (i.e., what the person says about himself or herself) (Fig. 3.1). Although the purpose of the interview isn't to collect **objective data** (i.e., what you obtain through physical examination), you will collect some objective data as you note the person's posture, physical appearance, ability to carry on a conversation, and overall demeanor. The interview is the best chance for a person to tell you what he or she perceives the health state to be. Once people enter the health care system, they relinquish some control, but during the interview the client remains in charge. The individual knows everything about his or her own health state, and you know nothing. Skilled interviewers are able to glean all necessary information while establishing a rapport with the client. Successful interviews allow you to:

1. Gather complete and accurate data about the person's health state, including the description and chronology of any symptoms.
2. Establish trust so that the person feels accepted and thus free to share all relevant data.
3. Teach the person about his or her health state.
4. Build rapport for a continuing therapeutic relationship.
5. Discuss health promotion and disease prevention.

---

[a]The term "client" is being used throughout this chapter to encompass the variety of settings in which you may encounter individuals where they are not considered patients, including the home setting.

Consider the interview a **contract** between you and your client. The contract concerns what the client needs and expects from health care and what you as a clinician have to offer. Your mutual goal is optimal health for the client. The terms of the contract include:

- Time and place of the interview and succeeding physical examination.
- Introduction of yourself and a brief explanation of your role.
- The purpose of the interview.
- How long it will take.
- Expectation of participation for each person.
- Presence of any other people (e.g., family, other health professionals, students).
- Confidentiality and to what extent it may be limited.
- Any costs to the client.

Although the person already may know some of this information through telephone contact with receptionists or the admitting office, the remaining points need to be stated clearly at the outset. Any confusion or unclear expectations can cause mistrust and resentment rather than the openness and trust required to facilitate the interview.

THE PROCESS OF COMMUNICATION

The vehicle that carries you and your client through the interview is communication. Communication is exchanging information so that each person clearly understands the other. If you do not understand one another, no communication has occurred.

It is challenging to teach the skill of interviewing because initially most people think it is common sense. They assume that if they can talk and hear, they can communicate. But much more than talking and hearing is necessary. Communication is based on behavior, conscious and unconscious, and all behavior has meaning.

Sending

Likely you are most aware of *verbal* communication—the words you speak, vocalizations, the tone of voice. *Nonverbal* communication is as important as verbal communication. This is your body language—posture, gestures, facial expression, eye contact, foot tapping, touch, even where you place your chair. Because nonverbal communication is under less conscious control than verbal communication, it may be more reflective of true feelings. A skilled interviewer will notice nonverbal behaviors and recognize the importance of potentially unconscious messages.

Receiving

Being aware of the messages you send is only part of the process. Your words and gestures must be interpreted by the receiver. Although you have a specific meaning in mind, the receiver may not understand the message as it was meant. The receiver uses his or her own interpretations of your words. These interpretations are based on past experiences, culture, and self-concept. Physical and emotional states also play a role in a person's interpretation. Your context and that of the receiver may not coincide, which can cause frustration and conflict. Your message can be sabotaged by the listener's bias or any preconceived notions. It takes mutual understanding by the sender and receiver to have successful communication.

Even greater risk for misunderstanding exists in the health care setting than in a social setting. The client's frame of reference is narrowed and focused on illness. The client usually has a health problem, and this factor emotionally charges your professional relationship. It intensifies the communication because the person feels dependent on you to get better.

Communication is one of the most important basic skills that can be learned and refined when you are a beginning practitioner. It is a tool, as basic to quality health care as the tools used in physical assessment. To maximize your communication skills, first you need to be aware of internal and external factors and their influence.

Internal Factors

Internal factors are those specific to you, the examiner. As you cultivate communication skills, you need to focus on the four inner factors of liking others, empathy, the ability to listen, and self-awareness.

Liking Others

One essential factor for a successful entry into a helping profession is a genuine liking of other people. This means a generally optimistic view of people—an assumption of strengths and a tolerance for weaknesses. An atmosphere of warmth and caring is necessary, and the client must believe that he or she is accepted unconditionally.

The respect for other people extends to respect for personal control over health and health care decision making. Your goal is to help clients be increasingly responsible for themselves. You wish to promote personal growth, and you have the health care resources to offer. Clients must choose how to apply resources and make health-related changes; you need to respect their choice to follow or disregard recommendations.

Empathy

Empathy means viewing the world from the other person's inner frame of reference while remaining you. It is a recognition and acceptance of the other person's feelings without criticism. Empathy is described as the ability to understand and be sensitive to the feelings of someone else. Empathy does not mean that you lose yourself in the other person at your own expense. By losing yourself, you cease to be useful. Empathy is the ability to recognize how someone perceives his or her world.

The Ability to Listen

Listening is not a passive role in the communication process; it is active and demanding. Listening requires complete and focused attention. You are not only hearing the person's words but also interpreting their meaning, asking follow-up questions, and ensuring a thorough understanding of what the person is telling you. If you are preoccupied with your own needs or those of other clients, you may miss important information. The needs of the person you are interviewing should be your sole concern.

Active listening is the route to understanding. Listen not only to what the person says but also to the way he or she says it. You also need to pay attention to what the person is not saying. Be aware of nonverbal communication and ask follow-up questions as appropriate, but do not interrupt. The story may not come out in the order you ask it, but it is important to allow the person to speak from his or her outline. As the person speaks, be aware of the way the story is told. Did he or she have any difficulty with language? What was the tone of voice? What is the person leaving out?

Self-Awareness

To effectively communicate with others, you must know yourself. Understanding your personal biases, prejudices, and stereotypes is an important part of developing your skills as an interviewer. By knowing your behaviors and responses, you become aware of how some unintentional actions can have a negative impact on your communication. You may have strong feelings about teen pregnancy, sexual orientation, or illicit drug use. By recognizing your biases and values, you can put them aside when dealing with people who may have a very different set of values. Part of your job as an interviewer is to recognize and set aside personal prejudices so that you can effectively care for all types of clients. If you recognize that you cannot put aside certain values, you may have to ask a colleague to step in and care for a client. For example, you are a devout Catholic who feels strongly that abortion is wrong. You are preparing to interview a 15-year-old who is 8 weeks pregnant. You know that she has made the appointment to discuss her options. If you are unable to put aside your belief that abortion is wrong and cannot counsel the young woman effectively, you may need to ask a colleague to complete the interview so that the young woman is presented with all options in an unbiased manner.

External Factors

Prepare the physical setting. The setting may be in a hospital room, an examination room in an office or clinic, or the person's home (where you have less control). In any location, optimal conditions are important to have a smooth interview.

Ensure Privacy

Aim for geographic privacy—a private room in the hospital, clinic, office, or home. If geographic privacy is unavailable, create "psychological privacy," using curtained partitions, but make sure that the person feels comfortable with the privacy provided. Privacy extends to ensuring that the client is comfortable with the people in the room. Consider a teenager being interviewed before an annual physical. You will need to ask questions about risky behaviors, including alcohol, illicit drugs, and sexual behaviors. Do you think the teenager is going to be forthright and honest with a parent or guardian in the room? He or she may not be comfortable asking the parent or guardian to leave; however, it is your job to advocate for the teenager, which may include asking a parent or guardian to step out during the interview.

Refuse Interruptions

Most people resent interruptions except in cases of an emergency. You need to concentrate and establish rapport. An interruption can destroy in seconds what you have spent many minutes building up. If you anticipate an interruption, let the person know ahead of time. Inform colleagues of the interview and the need to minimize interruptions.

Physical Environment

- Set the room temperature at a comfortable level.
- Provide sufficient lighting so that you can see each other clearly, but avoid strong, direct lighting that may cause squinting.
- Secure a quiet environment. Turn off televisions, radios, and any unnecessary equipment.
- Remove distracting objects or equipment. It is appropriate to leave some professional equipment (otoscope/ophthalmoscope, blood pressure manometer) in view, but avoid clutter such as stacks of mail, other files, or your lunch. The room should advertise a trained professional.
- Place the distance between you and the client at 4 to 5 feet. Personal space is any space within 4 feet of a person.

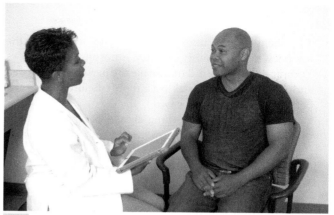

3.2 Equal-status seating.

Encroaching on personal space can cause anxiety, but if you position yourself farther away, you may seem aloof and distant. The personal reaction bubble depends on a variety of factors, including culture, gender, and age. (See Table 3.1 for information on personal space.)

- Arrange **equal-status seating** (Fig. 3.2). Both you and the client should be comfortably seated, at eye level. Placing the chairs at 90 degrees is good because it allows the person either to face you or to look straight ahead from time to time. Make sure that you avoid facing a client across a desk because this creates a barrier. Most important, avoid standing. Standing does two things: (1) it communicates your haste, and (2) it assumes superiority. Standing makes you loom over the client as an authority figure. When you are sitting, the person feels some control in the setting.
- When interviewing a hospitalized bedridden person, arrange a face-to-face position, and avoid standing over him or her (Fig. 3.3). The person should not be staring at the ceiling but should have access to eye contact. Without eye contact the person loses the visual message of your communication.

TABLE 3.1	Functional Use of Space
ZONE	**REMARKS**
Intimate zone (0 to 1½ ft)	Visual distortion occurs Best for assessing breath and body odors
Personal distance (1½ to 4 ft)	Perceived as an extension of the self, similar to a bubble Voice moderate Body odors inapparent No visual distortion Much of physical assessment occurs at this distance
Social distance (4 to 12 ft)	Used for impersonal business transactions Perceptual information much less detailed Much of interview occurs at this distance
Public distance (12+ ft)	Interaction with others impersonal Speaker's voice must be projected Subtle facial expressions imperceptible

From Hall, E. (1963). Proxemics: the study of man's spatial relations. In Galdston, I. (Ed.). *Man's image in medicine and anthropology.* New York: International University Press, pp. 109-120.

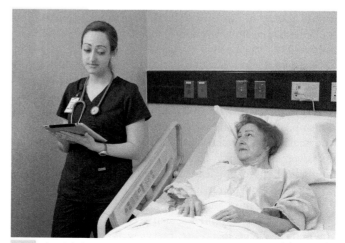

3.3 Avoid this position. (Potter et al., 2015.)

Dress

- The client should remain in street clothes during the interview except in an emergency. A hospital gown causes a power differential and may make the person feel exposed and uncomfortable. Establish rapport before asking the person to change into a gown.
- Your appearance and clothing should be appropriate to the setting and should meet conventional professional standards: a uniform or lab coat over conservative clothing, a name tag, and neat hair. Avoid extremes.

Note-Taking

Some use of history forms and note-taking may be unavoidable (see Fig. 3.2). When you sit down later to record the interview, you cannot rely completely on memory to furnish details of previous hospitalizations or the review of body systems. But be aware that excessive note-taking during the interview has disadvantages:

- It breaks eye contact too often.
- It shifts your attention away from the person, diminishing his or her sense of importance.
- Recording everything a person says may cause you to ask him or her to slow down, or the person may slow his or her tempo to allow for you to take notes. Either way, the client's natural mode of expression is lost.
- It impedes your observation of the client's nonverbal behavior.
- It is threatening to the client during the discussion of sensitive issues (e.g., alcohol and illicit drug use, number of sexual partners, or incidence of abuse).

Keep note-taking to a minimum and try to focus your attention on the person. Any recording you do should be secondary to the dialogue and should not interfere with the person's spontaneity. With experience you will rely less on note-taking. The use of standardized forms can decrease note-taking by providing check boxes for some of the information.

Electronic Health Record (EHR)

Direct computer recording of the health record has moved into nearly all health care settings. Mandates established by the federal government require health care organizations to utilize EHRs to improve quality and safety. The use of an EHR eliminates handwritten clinical data and provides access to online health education materials. Although computer entry facilitates data retrieval from numerous locations, this new technology poses problems for the provider-client relationship. EHR use improves documentation of biomedical information, but psychosocial and emotional information are not always captured.[13] Health care providers must capture biomedical, psychological, and emotional information in order to develop therapeutic relationships with clients. See Chapter 30 for more information about EHR.

Do not let the computer screen become a barrier between you and the client. Begin the interview as you usually would by greeting the person, establishing rapport, and collecting his or her narrative story in a direct face-to-face manner. Explain the computerized charting, and position the monitor so that the client can see it. Typing directly into the computer may ease entry of some sections of history such as past health occurrences, family history, and review of systems (see Chapter 4). Be aware that the client narrative, emotional issues, and complex health problems can only be addressed by the reciprocal communication techniques and client-centered interviewing presented in this chapter.

TECHNIQUES OF COMMUNICATION

Introducing the Interview

You may be nervous at the beginning of the interview. Keep in mind that the client probably is nervous as well. Keep the introduction short and formal. Address the person using his or her surname, and shake hands if appropriate. Unless the client directs you otherwise, avoid using the first name during the interview. Automatic use of the first name is too familiar for most adults and lessens dignity, but first names can be used with children and adolescents. You can also ask the person about his or her preference. If you are unsure how to correctly pronounce the name, ask. Interest in pronunciation shows respect.

Introduce yourself and state your role in the agency (if you are a student, say so). Give the reason for the interview:

> *"Mrs. Sanchez, I would like to talk about what caused you to come to the hospital today and get an update on your overall health status."*
> *"Mr. Craig, I want to ask you some questions about your previous medical history, family history, and any current complaints before we complete your physical examination."*

If the person is in the hospital, more than one health team member may be collecting a history. This repetition can be disconcerting because some people think that multiple clinicians asking the same questions indicates incompetence or a refusal to take the time to review the chart. Make sure that you indicate the reason for the interview to lessen the client's exasperation, and review notes from other health care team members before beginning the interview. Know which other team members the client has spoken to, and be able to tell him or her why your additional interview is necessary. Perhaps you are obtaining a full health history (including family history and review of systems) while your colleague obtained a focused history about the reason for seeking care.

After a brief introduction, ask an open-ended question (see the following section), and then let the person proceed. You do not need much friendly small talk to build rapport. This is not a social visit; the person wants to talk about some concern and wants to get on with it. You build rapport best by letting him or her discuss the concern early and by actively listening throughout the interview.

The Working Phase

The working phase is the data-gathering phase. Verbal skills for this phase include your ability to form questions appropriately and your responses to the answers given by the client. You will likely use a combination of open-ended and closed questions during the interview.

Open-Ended Questions

The **open-ended** question asks for narrative information. It states the topic to be discussed but only in general terms. Use it to begin the interview, to introduce a new section of questions, and whenever the person introduces a new topic.

> *"Tell me how I can help you."*
> *"What brings you to the hospital?"*
> *"You mentioned shortness of breath. Tell me more about that."*

The open-ended question is unbiased; it leaves the person free to answer in any way. This type of question encourages the person to respond in paragraphs and give a spontaneous account in any order chosen. It lets the person express himself or herself fully.

As the person answers, make eye contact and actively listen. Typically he or she will provide a short answer, pause, and then look at you for direction on whether to continue. How you respond to this nonverbal question is key. If you pose new questions on other topics, you may lose much of the initial story. Instead lean forward slightly toward the client and make eye contact, looking interested. With your posture indicating interest, the person will likely continue his or her story. If not, you can respond to his or her statement with "Tell me more about..." or "Anything else?"

Closed or Direct Questions

Closed or **direct** questions ask for specific information. They elicit a one- or two-word answer, a "yes" or "no," or a forced choice. Whereas the open-ended question allows the client to have free rein, the direct question limits his or her answer.

Direct questions help you elicit specific information and are useful to fill in any details that were initially left out after the person's opening narrative. For example, you may be interviewing a client who suffers from migraines. Your initial open-ended comment of "Tell me about your headaches" elicited narrative information about the headaches. You follow up with a direct question—"Where are your headaches located?"—to obtain specific information that was initially left out of the narrative.

Direct questions are also useful when you need specific facts such as past medical history or during the review of systems. You need direct questions to speed up the interview. Asking all open-ended questions would be unwieldy and extend the interview for hours, but be careful not to overuse closed questions. Follow these guidelines:

1. Ask only one direct question at a time. Avoid bombarding the client with long lists: "Have you ever had pain, double vision, watering, or redness in the eyes?" Avoid double-barreled questions, such as "Do you exercise and follow a diet for your weight?" The client will not know which question to answer. And if the client answers "yes," you will not know which question he or she has answered.
2. Choose language the client understands. You may need to use regional phrases or colloquial expressions. For example, "running off" means *running away* in standard English, but it means *diarrhea* to natives of the Appalachian region.

Verbal Responses—Assisting the Narrative

You have asked the first open-ended question, and the client begins to answer. Your role is to encourage free expression while keeping the person focused. Your responses help the teller amplify the story.

Some people seek health care for short-term or relatively simple needs. Their history is direct and uncomplicated; for these people you may require only a subset of your full communication arsenal. Other people have a complex story, a long history of a chronic condition, or accompanying emotions that will require you to pull out all the stops during your interaction. There are nine types of verbal responses. The first five responses (facilitation, silence, reflection, empathy, clarification) involve your reactions to the facts or feelings that the person has communicated (Fig. 3.4). In the last four responses (confrontation, interpretation, explanation, summary), you start to express your *own* thoughts and feelings. In the first five responses the client leads; in the last four responses you lead. Study the array of possible responses in Table 3.2.

Ten Traps of Interviewing

The verbal responses presented in Table 3.2 are productive and enhance the interview. Now we will consider *traps*, which

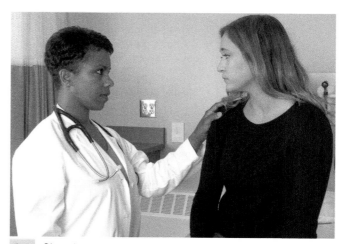

3.4 Showing empathy.

TABLE 3.2   Examiner's Verbal Responses

RESPONSE	REASON FOR USE	EXAMPLE(S)
Client's Perspective		
Facilitation, general leads, minimal cues	• Encourages client to say more • Shows person you are interested	• *Mm-hmmm, go on, uh-huh* • Maintaining eye contact, shifting forward • Nodding *yes*
Silence	• Communicates that client has time to think • Silence can be uncomfortable for novice examiner, but interruption can make client lose his or her train of thought • Provides you with chance to observe client and note nonverbal cues	• Waiting for response without interruption • Sitting quietly; **don't fidget** • Counting silently 1 to 10
Reflection	• Echoes client's words by repeating part of what person has just said • Can help express feelings behind words • Mirroring client's words can help person elaborate on problem	• Client: *It's so hard having to stay in bed during my pregnancy. I have kids at home I'm worried about.* • Response: *You feel worried and anxious about your children?*
Empathy	• Names a feeling and allows its expression • Allows person to feel accepted and strengthens rapport • Useful in instances when client hasn't identified the feeling or isn't ready to discuss it	• Client (sarcastically): *This is just great! I own a business, direct my employees; now I can't even go to the bathroom without help.* • Response: *It must be hard—one day having so much control and now feeling dependent on someone else.* • Other responses include: *This must be very hard for you* or just placing hand on person's arm (see Fig. 3.4)
Clarification	• Useful when person's word choice is ambiguous or confusing • Summarize person's words, simplify the statement, and ensure that you are on the right track	• Response: *The heaviness in your chest occurs with walking up 1 flight of stairs or more than 1 block, but it stops when you rest. Is that correct?* • Client: *Yes, that's it.*
Examiner's Perspective		
Confrontation	• Clarifying inconsistent information • Focusing client's attention on an observed behavior, action, or feeling	• *You look sad,* or *You sound angry.* • *Earlier you said that you didn't drink, but just now you said you go out every night after work for 1-2 beers.* • *When I press here, you grimace, but you said it doesn't hurt.*
Interpretation	• Links events, makes associations, and implies cause • Not based on direct observations but instead on inference or conclusion • Your interpretation may be incorrect but helps prompt further discussion	• *It seems that every time you feel the stomach pain, you have some type of stress in your life.* • Client: *I don't want any more treatment, but I can't seem to tell the doctor I'm ready to stop.* • Response: *Could it be that you're afraid of her reaction?*
Explanation	• Informing person • Sharing factual and objective information	• *You order your dinner from the menu provided, and it takes approximately 30 minutes to arrive.* • *You may not eat or drink for 12 hours before your blood test because the food may change the results.*
Summary	• Condenses facts and validates what was discussed during the interview • Signals that termination of interview is imminent • Both client and examiner should be active participants	• Review pertinent facts • Allow client time to make corrections

are nonproductive verbal and nonverbal messages. Because you want to help your client, it is easy to fall into the traps and send negative verbal messages that may do the opposite of what you intended by cutting off communication. Be aware of the following traps, and work to avoid them as you establish your communication style.

1. Providing False Assurance or Reassurance

A pregnant woman says, "I've been spotting on and off all day, and I haven't felt the baby kick. I just know I'm going to miscarry." Your automatic response may be to provide reassurance, "Don't worry. I'm sure you and the baby will be fine." Although this helps relieve your anxiety and gives you the sense that you have provided comfort, it actually trivializes the woman's anxiety and closes off communication. You have also just promised something that may not be true, which can diminish rapport. Consider these responses:

> *"You're really worried about your baby, aren't you?"*
> *"It must be hard to wait for the doctor. Is there anything I can get you or anything that you'd like to talk about?"*

These responses acknowledge the feeling and open the door for more communication.

A genuine, valid form of reassurance does exist. You *can* reassure clients that you are listening to them, that you understand them, that you have hope for them, and that you will take good care of them.

> Client: *"I feel so lost here since they transferred me to the medical center. My family lives too far away to visit, and no one here knows me or cares."*
> Response: *"I care what happens to you. I will be here all day today and for the next 3 days. Please call if you need anything."*

This type of reassurance makes a commitment to the client, and it can have a powerful impact.

2. Giving Unwanted Advice

It is important as a health care provider to recognize when giving advice is warranted and when it should be avoided. People often seek health care because they want professional advice. A parent may ask how to care for a child with chickenpox, or an older man may ask if it is appropriate to receive a pneumonia vaccine. These are straightforward requests for information, and you respond by providing the appropriate information.

But if advice is based on a hunch or feeling or is your personal opinion, then it is most likely inappropriate. Consider a young woman who has just met with her physician about her infertility issues: "Dr. Compton just told me I have to have surgery and that, if I don't, I won't be able to get pregnant. What would you do?" If you provide an answer, especially if the answer begins with "If I were you …" you would be falling into a trap. You are not your client and therefore cannot make decisions for her. Providing an

answer shifts accountability to you instead of the client. The woman must work out her own decision. So what do you do?

> *Response: What are your concerns about the recommendation?*
> *Woman: I'm terrified of being put to sleep. What if I don't wake up?*

Now you know her real concern and can help her deal with it. She will have grown in the process and may be better equipped to make her decision.

When asked for advice, other preferred responses are:

> *"What are the pros and cons of _____ [this choice] for you?"*
> *"What is holding you back?"*

Although it is quicker just to give advice, take the time to involve the patient in a problem-solving process.

3. Using Authority

"Your doctor/nurse knows best" is a response that promotes dependency and inferiority. You effectively diminish the client's concerns with one short sentence, and you cut off communication. Using authority should be avoided. Although you may have more professional knowledge than the client, you both have equally important roles since the client must make the final decision about his or her health.

4. Using Avoidance Language

People use euphemisms instead of discussing unpleasant topics. For example, people use "passed on" or "has gone to a better place" to avoid the reality of dying. Using euphemisms promotes the avoidance of reality and allows people to hide their feelings. Not talking about uncomfortable topics doesn't make them go away but instead makes them even more frightening. The best way to deal with frightening or uncomfortable topics is by using direct language.

5. Distancing

Distancing is the use of impersonal speech to put space between a threat and the self: "There is a lump in *the* left breast." By using "the" instead of "your," you are allowing the woman to deny any association with her diseased breast and protect herself from it. Health professionals use distancing to soften reality, but in actuality it may communicate that you are afraid of the procedure or disease. Clients use distancing to avoid admitting that they have a problem: "My doctor told me that the prostate was enlarged." Using specific language and blunt terms indicates that you are not fearful of the disease or procedure and may decrease anxiety and help the client cope with the reality of the situation.

6. Using Professional Jargon

The medical profession is fraught with jargon that sounds exclusionary and paternalistic. It is important to adjust your vocabulary to ensure understanding without sounding condescending. Just because your client uses medical jargon, don't assume that he or she understands the correct meaning. Some people think "hypertensive" means *tense*. This misunderstanding may cause them to take their medication only when they are feeling tense and stressed instead of taking it all the time. Misinformation must be corrected immediately to ensure compliance.

7. Using Leading or Biased Questions

Asking a client, "You don't smoke, do you?" or "You don't ever have unprotected sex, correct?" implies that one answer is "better" than another. If the client wants to please you, he or she will either answer in a way corresponding to your values or feel guilty when he or she must admit the other answer. The client feels that he or she risks your disapproval by not answering the question "correctly." If the client feels dependent on you for care, he or she won't want to alienate you and may not answer truthfully. Make sure that your questions are unbiased, and do not lead clients to a certain "correct" answer. For example, you might instead ask, "Do you smoke?" or "When you have sexual intercourse, do you use protection?"

8. Talking Too Much

Some examiners positively associate helpfulness with verbal productivity. If the air has been thick with their oratory and advice, these examiners leave thinking that they have met the client's needs. Just the opposite is true. Eager to please the examiner, the client lets the professional talk at the expense of his or her need to express himself or herself. A good rule for every interviewer is to listen more than you talk.

9. Interrupting

When you think you know what the client is going to say next, it is easy to cut him or her off and finish the statement. Unfortunately you are not proving that you are clever, but you are signaling impatience or boredom. Related to interruption is preoccupation with yourself. As the client speaks, you may be thinking about what to say next. If you are focused on your next statement instead of his or her statements, you are unable to fully understand what the person is saying. The goal of the interview is to include two people listening and two people speaking. Leave at least a second of space between the end of the client speaking and your next statement. This ensures that the client has finished.

10. Using "Why" Questions

Children ask why questions constantly. Why is the sky blue? Why can't I have a cookie for dinner? Their motive is an innocent search for information. The adult's use of "why" questions usually implies blame and condemnation; it puts the person on the defensive. Consider your use of "why" questions in the health care setting. "Why did you take so much medication?" Or "Why did you wait so long before coming to the hospital if you were having chest pain?" The use of a "why" question makes the interviewer sound accusatory and judgmental. By using a "why" question, the client must produce an excuse to rationalize his or her behavior. To avoid this trap, say, "I see you started to have chest pain early in the day. What was happening between the time the pain started and the time you came to the emergency department?"

Nonverbal Skills

As a novice interviewer you may be focused on what the client says, but listening with your eyes is just as important as listening with your ears. Nonverbal modes of communication include physical appearance, posture, gestures, facial expression, eye contact, voice, and touch. They are important in establishing rapport and conveying information.[1] They provide clues to understanding feelings. When nonverbal and verbal messages are congruent, the verbal message is reinforced. When they are incongruent, the nonverbal message tends to be the true one because it is under less conscious control.

Physical Appearance

We have all noted people who simply look sick without specific signs that lead to a precise diagnosis. As a health care provider, it is important that you consider physical appearance when you first encounter a client. Inattention to dressing or grooming suggests that the person is too sick to maintain self-care or has an emotional dysfunction such as depression. Choice of clothing also sends a message, projecting such varied images as role (student, worker, or professional) or attitude (casual, suggestive, or rebellious).

You are concerned with the client's image, and he or she is just as concerned with yours. Your appearance sends a message to the client. Professional dress varies among agencies and settings. Professional uniforms can create a positive or a negative image. Whatever your personal choice in clothing or grooming is, the aim should be to convey a competent, professional image and should follow agency guidelines (Fig. 3.5).

Posture

On beginning the interview, note the client's position. An open position with extension of large muscle groups shows relaxation, physical comfort, and a willingness to share information. A closed position with arms and legs crossed looks defensive and anxious. Changes in posture during the interview can also suggest a different comfort level with new topics. For example, if your client began the interview in an open posture but immediately assumes a closed posture when asked about his or her sexuality, he or she may be uncomfortable with the new topic.

Make sure that you are aware of your own posture. Assuming a calm, relaxed posture conveys interest. On the other hand, standing and hastily filling out forms while peeking at your watch communicates that you are busy with many more important things than interviewing this client. Even when your time is limited, it is important to appear unhurried. Sit down, even if it is only for a few minutes, and look as if nothing else matters except this client. If you are aware of a potential emergency that will require interruption, let the client know when you enter the room.

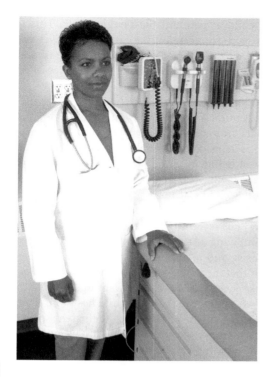

3.5

Gestures

Gestures send messages; therefore make sure that you are aware of your own gestures while also noting those of the client. Nodding the head or openly turning out the hand shows acceptance, attention, or agreement, whereas wringing the hands or picking the nails often indicates anxiety. Hand gestures can also reinforce descriptions of pain. When describing crushing substernal chest pain, the client often holds a fisted hand in front of the sternum. Sharply localized pain is often indicated by using one finger. Movements such as bouncing a leg, clicking a pen, playing with hair, or drumming fingers can distract the client and cause him or her to lose focus. Make sure that you know if you tend to fidget, and work on controlling that urge during interviews.

Facial Expression

Typically the face and facial expression are some of the first things we notice when we meet someone. The face reflects our emotions and conditions. As an interviewer it is important to note your client's facial expression. Does it match what he or she is saying, or is it incongruous?

As you pay attention to the client's expression, it is equally important that you are aware of your own facial expression. Your expression should reflect a person who is attentive, sincere, and interested. Avoid expressions that may be construed as boredom, disgust, distraction, criticism, or disbelief. A negative facial expression can severely damage your rapport with the client and may lead him or her to stop communicating.

Eye Contact

Lack of eye contact suggests that the person is shy, withdrawn, confused, bored, intimidated, apathetic, or depressed. This applies to examiners too. You should aim to maintain eye contact, but do not stare at the person. Do not have a fixed, penetrating look but rather an easy gaze toward the person's eyes, with occasional glances away. One exception to this is when you are interviewing someone from a culture that avoids direct eye contact.

Voice

Although spoken words have meaning, it is important that you are keenly aware of the tone of your voice and that of the client. Meaning comes not only from the words spoken, but also from the tone of voice, the intensity and rate of speech, the pitch, and any pauses. The tone of voice may show sarcasm, disbelief, sympathy, or hostility. People who are anxious often speak louder and faster than normal. A soft voice may indicate shyness or fear, whereas a loud voice may indicate that the person is hearing impaired.

Even the use of pauses conveys meaning. When your question is easy and straightforward, a client's long, unexpected pause indicates that the person is taking time to think of an answer. This raises some doubt as to the honesty of the answer or whether the client heard the question. When unusually frequent and long pauses are combined with speech that is slow and monotonous and a weak, breathy voice, it indicates depression.

Touch

The meaning of physical touch is influenced by the person's age, gender, cultural background, past experience, and current setting. The meaning of touch is easily misinterpreted. In most Western cultures physical touch is reserved for expressions of love and affection or for rigidly defined acts of greeting. Do not use touch during the interview unless you know the person well and are sure how it will be interpreted.

In summation, an examiner's nonverbal messages that show attentiveness and unconditional acceptance are productive and help build rapport. Defeating, nonproductive nonverbal behaviors are those of inattentiveness, authority, and superiority (Table 3.3).

Closing the Interview

The session should end gracefully. An abrupt or awkward closing can destroy rapport and leave the person with a negative impression of the interaction. To ease into the closing, ask the person:

"Is there anything else you would like to mention?"
"Are there any questions you would like to ask?"
"We've covered a number of concerns today. What would you most like to accomplish?"

This gives the person the final opportunity for self-expression. Once this opportunity has been offered, you will need to make a closing statement that indicates that the end of the

TABLE 3.3 Nonverbal Behaviors of the Interviewer	
Positive	**Negative**
Appropriate professional appearance	Appearance objectionable to client
Equal-status seating	Standing above the client
Close proximity to client	Sitting behind desk, far away, turned away
Relaxed, open posture	Tense posture
Leaning slightly toward person	Slouched in chair
Occasional facilitating gestures	Critical or distracting gestures: pointing finger, clenched fist, finger-tapping, foot-swinging, looking at watch
Facial animation, interest	Bland expression, yawning, tight mouth
Appropriate smiling	Frowning, lip biting
Appropriate eye contact	Shifty, avoiding eye contact, focusing on notes
Moderate tone of voice	Strident, high-pitched tone
Moderate rate of speech	Rate too slow or too fast
Appropriate touch	Too frequent or inappropriate touch

interview is imminent, such as, "Our interview is just about over." At this point no new topics should be introduced, and no unexpected questions should be asked. This is a good time to give your **summary** of what you have learned during the interview. The summary is a final statement of what you and the client agree the health state to be. It should include positive health aspects, any health problems that have been identified, any plans for action, and an explanation of the subsequent physical examination. As you part from clients, thank them for the time spent and for their cooperation.

❖ DEVELOPMENTAL COMPETENCE

Interviewing the Parent or Caregiver

When your client is a child, you must build rapport with two people—the child and the accompanying caregiver. Greet both by name, but with a younger child (1 to 6 years old) focus more on the caregiver. Ignoring the child temporarily allows him or her to size you up from a safe distance. The child can use this time to observe your interaction with the caregiver. If the child sees that the caregiver accepts and likes you, he or she will begin to relax (Fig. 3.6).

Begin by interviewing the caregiver and child together. If any sensitive topics arise (e.g., the parents' troubled relationship or the child's problems at school or with peers), explore them later when the caregiver is alone. Provide toys to occupy

a young child as you and the caregiver talk. This frees the caregiver to concentrate on the history and gives you information about the child's level of attention span and ability for independent play. Throughout the interview observe the caregiver-child interaction.

For younger children, the parent or caregiver will provide all or most of the history. Thus you are collecting the child's health data from the caregiver's frame of reference, which typically is considered reliable. Most caregivers have the child's well-being in mind and will cooperate with you to enhance it. Bias can occur when caregivers are asked to describe the child's achievements or when their ability to provide proper care seems called into question. For example, if you say "His fever was 103, and you didn't bring him in?" you are implying a lack of skills, which puts the caregiver on the defensive and increases anxiety. Instead use open-ended questions that increase description and defuse threat, such as "What happened when the fever went up?"

A parent with more than one child has more than one set of data to remember. Be patient as the parent sorts through his or her memory to pull out facts of developmental milestones or past history. A comprehensive history may be lacking if the child is accompanied by a family friend or daycare provider instead of the primary caregiver.

When asking about developmental milestones, avoid judgmental behavior or inferring that the behavior occurred late. Parents are understandably proud of their child's achievements and are sensitive to insinuations that these milestones occurred late. "So he didn't say any words until he was 15 months old? Did you take him to speech therapy?" Instead consider saying, "I see that Jon began speaking when he was 15 months old. How is his speech progressing now that he is 2 years old?"

Always refer to the child by name and ensure that he or she is included in the interview as appropriate. Refer to the parent by his or her proper surname instead of "Mom" or "Dad." Remember not to make any assumptions. The person

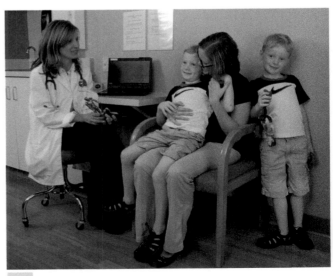

3.6

accompanying the child may not be the biological mother or father, so it is important to ask. Don't assume that a couple bringing in a child are mom and dad. Also don't assume that two women bringing a child in are mom and aunt; they may be the child's two mothers. If a same-sex couple brings the child, do not ask which one is the real parent. This downplays the importance of both parents. If you need a family history from the biological parent in order to develop a genogram (see Chapter 4), consider the following question: "We need to review family history, so I will be asking questions about medical conditions of family members biologically related to Jon."

Most of your communication is with the caregiver of a younger child, but make sure that you don't ignore the child completely. Allow him or her to size you up, but engage him or her in conversation as well. Contact made during the nonthreatening interview can ease the physical examination. Ask the child about the toy with which he or she is playing or about the special toy brought from home. Make sure that you stoop to meet the child at his or her eye level. Your size can seem overwhelming to young children, and standing at your full height may emphasize his or her smallness.

Nonverbal communication is even more important to children than it is to adults. Children are quick to pick up feelings, anxiety, or comfort from nonverbal cues. Keep your physical appearance neat and clean, and avoid formal uniforms that distance you. Keep your gestures slow, deliberate, and close to your body. Children are frightened by quick or grandiose gestures. Do not try to maintain constant eye contact; this feels threatening to a small child. Use a quiet, measured voice, and choose simple words in your speech. Considering the child's level of language development is valuable in planning your communication.

Stages of Cognitive Development

A child's thought process, perception of the world, and emotional responses to situations are very different from those of an adult. As an interviewer it is important that you consider the stage of development as you approach the child and converse with him or her. Piaget's cognitive-developmental theory can help you understand the child's current level and construct your approach to the interview (Table 3.4). Although this provides a guide, keep in mind that the ages are approximated and will differ slightly based on the maturity level of the child. Also keep in mind that you may be approaching children who are in crisis as a result of illness. Regression is a common response during times of acute stress; therefore a child may regress in his or her ability to communicate at this time.[1]

COMMUNICATING WITH DIFFERENT AGES

The Infant (Birth to 12 months)

Infants use coos, gurgles, facial expressions, and cries to identify their needs. Although you will not "interview" an infant, it is important to establish a rapport. Nonverbal communication is the primary method of communicating with infants. When their needs are met, most infants will be calm and relaxed. When they are frightened, hungry, tired, or uncomfortable, they will cry or be difficult to console. Respond quickly to changes in infant communication. If a baby begins to cry, respond to the communication. Use gentle handling and a quiet, calm voice. Face infants directly. They are fascinated by adult faces and enjoy looking at them, but remember that eyesight does not develop right away; thus you will need to hold them close. As infants get older, they may begin to exhibit stranger anxiety and will be more cooperative

TABLE 3.4	Stages of Cognitive Development		
AGE	**PIAGET'S STAGE**	**CHARACTERISTICS**	**LANGUAGE DEVELOPMENT**
Birth to 2 years	**Sensorimotor**	Infant learns by manipulating objects At birth reflexive communication, then moves through 6 stages to reach actual thinking	**Presymbolic** Communication largely nonverbal Vocabulary of more than 4 words by 12 months, increase to >200 words and use of short sentences before age 2 years
2-6 years	**Preoperational**	Beginning use of symbolic thinking Imaginative play Masters reversibility	**Symbolic** Actual use of structured grammar and language to communicate Uses pronouns Average vocabulary >10,000 words by age 6 years
7-11 years	**Concrete operations**	Logical thinking Masters use of numbers and other concrete ideas such as classification and conservation	Mastery of passive tense by age 7 years and complex grammatical skills by age 10 years
12+ years	**Formal operations**	Abstract thinking. Futuristic; takes broader, more theoretical perspective	Near adult-like skills

Adapted from Piaget J. (1972). *The child's conception of the world*, Savage, MD: Littlefield, Adams. In Arnold, E. C., & Boggs, K. U. (2016). *Interpersonal relationships: professional communication skills for nurses* (7th ed.). St. Louis: Saunders.

when the caregiver is kept in view or allowed to hold them during the examination.

The Toddler (12 to 36 months)

At this stage children are beginning to develop communication skills. At first they communicate with one- or two-word sentences and a limited vocabulary, which may include grunts and pointing intertwined with words. Language progresses from a vocabulary of about two words at 1 year to a spurt of about 200 words by 2 years. Then the 2-year-old begins to combine words into simple two-word phrases—"all gone," "me up," "baby crying." This is **telegraphic speech,** which is usually a combination of a noun and a verb and includes only words that have concrete meaning. Interest in language is high during the second year, and a 2-year-old seems to understand all that is said to him or her.

Older toddlers want to know why; therefore it is important that you provide a simple explanation of what you want. You can help them communicate by labeling their emotions and expanding on their one- or two-word sentences. Give toddlers one direction at a time, keeping it simple, and provide warnings before transitions when possible. Toddlers also struggle for control and autonomy; therefore provide simple choices when possible.[4]

The Preschooler (3 to 6 years)

A 3- to 6-year-old is egocentric. He or she sees the world mostly from his or her own point of view. Everything revolves around him or her. Only the child's own experience is relevant; thus telling what someone else is doing will not have any meaning.

A 3-year-old uses more complex sentences with more parts of speech. Between 3 and 4 years of age the child uses three- to four-word **telegraphic** sentences containing only essential words. By 5 to 6 years, the sentences are six to eight words long, and grammar is well developed.

Preschoolers' communication is direct, concrete, literal, and set in the present. Avoid expressions such as "climbing the walls," because they are easily misinterpreted by young children. Use short, simple sentences with a concrete explanation. Take time to give a short, simple explanation for any unfamiliar equipment that will be used on the child. Preschoolers can have *animistic* thinking about unfamiliar objects. They may imagine that unfamiliar inanimate objects can come alive and have human characteristics (e.g., that a blood-pressure cuff can wake up and bite or pinch). Preschoolers have active imaginations, so education and explanations can be provided through play (e.g., puppet shows, dress-up, drawings).

The School-Age Child (7 to 12 years)

A child 7 to 12 years old can tolerate and understand others' viewpoints. This child is more objective and realistic. He or she wants to know functional aspects—how things work and why things are done. At this age children are beginning to recognize that things they do can affect others. It is very important that you are nonjudgmental.

The school-age child can read. By using printed symbols for objects and events, the child can process a significant amount of information. At this age thinking is more stable and logical. School-age children can **decenter** and consider all sides of a situation to form a conclusion. They are able to reason, but this reasoning capacity still is limited because they cannot yet deal with abstract ideas.

Children of this age-group have the verbal ability to add important data to the history. Interview the caregiver and child together; but when a presenting symptom or sign exists, ask the child about it first and then gather data from the caregiver. For the well child seeking a checkup, pose questions about school, friends, or activities directly to the child.

The Adolescent

Adolescence begins with puberty. Puberty is a time of dramatic physiologic change. It includes a growth spurt—rapid growth in height, weight, and muscular development; development of primary and secondary sex characteristics; and maturation of the reproductive organs. A changing body affects a teen's self-concept.

Adolescents want to be adults, but they do not have the cognitive ability yet to achieve their goal. They are between two stages. Sometimes they are capable of mature actions, and other times they fall back on childhood response patterns, especially in times of stress. You cannot treat adolescents as children; yet you cannot overcompensate and assume that their communication style, learning ability, and motivation are consistently at an adult level.

Adolescents value their peers. They crave acceptance and sameness with their peers. Adolescents think that no adult can understand them. Because of this, some act with aloof contempt, answering only in monosyllables. Others make eye contact and tell you what they think you want to hear, but inside they are thinking, "You'll never know the full story about me." This knowledge about adolescents is apt to paralyze you in communicating with them. However, successful communication is possible and rewarding. The guidelines are simple.

The first consideration is your attitude, which must be one of respect. Respect is the most important thing you can communicate to the adolescent. The adolescent needs to feel validated as a person.

Second, your communication must be totally honest. The adolescent's intuition is highly tuned and can detect when information is withheld. Always give them the truth. Play it straight or you will lose them. Providing rationale for your questions will increase cooperation.

Stay in character. Avoid using language that is absurd for your age or professional role. It is helpful to understand the jargon used by adolescents, but you cannot use those words yourself to bond with the adolescent. You are not part of the adolescent's peer group, and he or she will not accept you as a peer.

Focus first on the adolescent, not on the problem. Although an adult wants to talk about the health concern immediately, the adolescent wants to talk about himself or herself as a

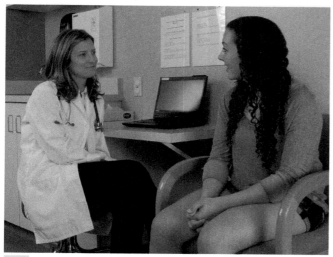

3.7

person. Show an interest in the adolescent (Fig. 3.7). Ask open, friendly questions about school, activities, hobbies, and friends. *"How are things at school?" "Are you in any sports or activities?" "Do you have any pets at home?"* Refrain from asking questions about parents and family for now—these topics can be emotionally charged during adolescence.

Do not assume that adolescents know anything about a health interview or a physical examination. Explain every step and give the rationale. They need direction. They will cooperate when they know the reason for the questions or actions. Encourage their questions. Adolescents are afraid that they will sound "dumb" if they ask a question to which they assume everybody else knows the answer.

Keep your questions short and simple. "Why are you here?" sounds brazen to you, but it is effective with the adolescent.[1] Be prepared for the adolescent who does *not* know why he or she is there. Some adolescents are pushed into coming to the examination by a caregiver.

The communication responses described for the adult need to be reconsidered when talking with the adolescent. Silent periods usually are best avoided. Giving adolescents a little time to collect their thoughts is acceptable, but silence for other reasons is threatening. Also avoid reflection. If you use reflection, the adolescent is likely to answer, "What?" They just do not have the cognitive skills to respond to that indirect mode of questioning. Adolescents are also more sensitive to nonverbal communication than are adults. Be aware of your expressions and gestures. Adolescents are struggling to develop their self-identity and may withdraw from you if you make a comment that they take as a criticism. It is important that you are cognizant of how the person may misinterpret your questions or comments.

Later in the interview, after you have developed rapport with the adolescent, you can address the topics that are emotionally charged, including smoking, alcohol and drug use, sexual behaviors, suicidal thoughts, and depression.

Adolescents undertake risky behaviors that may yield serious consequences.

Adolescents will assume that health professionals have similar values and standards of behavior as most of the other authority figures in their lives, and they may be reluctant to share this information. You can assure them that your questions are not intended to be curious or intrusive but cover topics that are important for most teens and on which you have relevant health information to share. You will want to ensure privacy during these questions. Adolescents may be more willing to share information without a caregiver in the room, but they may feel uncomfortable asking the caregiver for privacy. As the health professional, you can ask the caregiver to step out during the interview, explaining that privacy is important.

If confidential material is uncovered during the interview, consider what can remain confidential and what you believe you must share for the well-being of the adolescent. State laws vary about confidentiality with minors, and in some states caregivers are not notified about some health treatments such as birth control prescriptions or treatment for sexually transmitted infections (STIs). However, if the adolescent talks about an abusive home situation or risk of imminent physical harm, state that you must share this information with other health professionals for his or her own protection. Ask the adolescent, *"Do you have a problem with that?"* and then talk it through. Tell the adolescent, *"You will have to trust that I will handle this information professionally and in your best interest."*

Finally, take every opportunity for positive reinforcement. Praise every action regarding healthy lifestyle choices: *"That's great that you don't smoke. It will save you lots of money that you can use on other things, you won't smell like smoke, and your skin won't be so wrinkled when you get older."*

For lifestyle choices that are risky, this is a premium opportunity for discussion and early intervention. *"Have you ever tried to quit smoking?" "I'm concerned about your extra weight for someone so young. What kind of exercise do you like?" "What do you like to drink when you're at a party with your friends?" "Did you use a condom the last time you had sex?"* Providing information alone is not enough. Listen to their stories in an open, nonjudgmental way. Give them a small, achievable goal, and encourage another visit in a few weeks for follow-up on the behaviors of concern.

The Older Adult

The aging adult has the developmental task of finding the purpose of his or her own existence and adjusting to the inevitability of death. Some people have developed comfortable and satisfying answers and greet you with a calm demeanor and self-assurance, but be alert for the person who sounds hopeless and despairing about life and his or her future. Symptoms of illness and worries over finances are even more frightening when they mean physical limitation or threaten independence.

Always address the person by his or her proper surname, and avoid using the first name. Some older adults resent being called by their first name by younger people and think that it demonstrates a lack of respect. Above all, avoid "elderspeak,"[18] which consists of diminutives (honey, sweetie, dearie); inappropriate plural pronouns ("Are we ready for our interview?"); shortened sentences, slow speech rate, and simple vocabulary that sounds like baby talk; using a singsong voice or changing the pitch of your voice.

Older adults have a longer story to tell; therefore plan accordingly. The interview will likely take longer, and you don't want to appear rushed. Depending on the person's physical condition, you may need to break the interview into more than one session, making sure to cover the most important data during the first interview. You can also gather certain portions of the data such as past history or the review of systems on a form that is filled out at home, as long as the person's vision and handwriting are adequate. Take time to review any forms completed at home during the interview.

It is important to adjust the pace of the interview to the aging person (Fig. 3.8). The older person has a great amount of background material through which to sort, and this takes some time. Allow appropriate periods of silence during these times. Some aging people also need a greater amount of response time to interpret the question and process the answer, so schedule more time and avoid hurrying them. You will lose valuable data and not meet their needs if you urge them to go through information quickly or appear rushed.

Consider physical limitations when planning the interview. Make sure that you face the person with impaired hearing directly so that your mouth and face are fully visible. Do not shout; it does not help and actually distorts speech. For a person in a wheelchair, make sure you move the chairs so that an appropriate position is available for the client.

Touch is a nonverbal skill that is very important to older people. Their other senses may be diminished, and touch grounds you in reality. In addition, a hand on the arm or shoulder is an empathic message that communicates that you want to understand his or her problem.

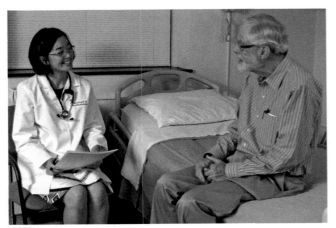

3.8

INTERVIEWING PEOPLE WITH SPECIAL NEEDS

Hearing-Impaired People

As the population ages, you will encounter more people who are deaf or hard of hearing. They see themselves as a linguistic minority, not as disabled.[14] People who are hearing impaired may feel marginalized and think that their intelligence is questioned because they cannot always understand what is being asked of them. Although some people will tell you in advance that they have a hearing impairment, others will not readily divulge the information. In the latter case you must use cues to recognize potential hearing loss, such as the client staring at your mouth, not answering unless looking at you, speaking in an unusually loud voice, or frequently requesting that you repeat a question. Full communication is important with every client. People with a hearing impairment may feel isolated and anxious because they cannot understand everything that is happening. Ask the person his or her preferred way to communicate—by signing, lipreading, or writing. If the person has hearing aids, make sure that he or she is using them properly. If you notice a hearing impairment but no hearing aids are in use, consider a referral for a hearing test and follow-up.

A complete health history of someone who is deaf requires a sign language interpreter. Because most health care professionals are not proficient in signing, try to find an interpreter through a social service agency or the person's own social network. You may use family members, but be aware that they sometimes edit for the person. Use the same guidelines as for the bilingual interpreter (see p. 40).

If the person prefers lipreading, be sure to face him or her squarely and have good lighting on your face. Examiners with a beard, mustache, or foreign accents are less effective. Do not exaggerate your lip movements because this distorts your words. Similarly, shouting distorts the reception of a hearing aid. Speak slowly and supplement your voice with appropriate hand gestures or pantomime. Nonverbal cues are important adjuncts because the lip reader understands at best only 50% of your speech when relying solely on vision. Be sure that the person understands your questions. Many hearing-impaired people nod "yes" just to be friendly and cooperative but really do not understand.

Written communication is efficient in sections such as past health history or review of systems when forms can easily be used. For the present history of illness, writing is very time-consuming and laborious. The syntax of the person's written words will read like English if the hearing impairment occurred after speech patterns developed. If the deafness occurred before speech patterns developed, the grammar and written syntax may follow that of sign language, which is different from that of English.

Acutely Ill People

Emergent situations require combining the interview with the physical examination. In this case focus the interview on pertinent information only, including history of present illness, medications, allergies, last meal, and basic health state. Subjective information is a crucial component of providing care; therefore, it is important that you try to interview as much as possible while performing lifesaving actions. Abbreviate your questioning. Identify the main area of distress and inquire about that. Family or friends often can provide important data.

A hospitalized person with a critical or severe illness is usually too weak, too short of breath, or in too much pain to talk. Focus on making him or her comfortable first and then ask priority questions about the history. Explore the first concern the person mentions. You will find that you ask closed, direct questions earlier in the interview to decrease response burden. Finally make sure that you are clear in your statements. When a person is very sick, even the simplest sentence can be misconstrued. The person will react according to preconceived ideas about what a serious illness means; thus anything you say should be direct and precise.

People Under the Influence of Street Drugs or Alcohol

It is common for people under the influence of alcohol or other mood-altering drugs to be admitted to a hospital; all of these drugs affect the central nervous system (CNS), increasing risk for overdose, accidents, and injuries. Also, chronic alcohol or drug use creates complex medical problems that require more care.

Many substance abusers are poly-drug abusers. The client's behavior depends on which drugs were consumed. Alcohol, benzodiazepines, and the opioids (heroin, methadone, morphine, oxycodone) are CNS depressants that slow brain activity and impair judgment, memory, intellectual performance, and motor coordination. Stimulants of the central nervous system (cocaine, amphetamine) can cause an intense high, agitation, and paranoid behavior. Hallucinogens (LSD, ketamine, PCP) cause bizarre, inappropriate, sometimes violent behavior accompanied by superhuman strength and insensitivity to pain.

When interviewing a person currently under the influence of alcohol or illicit drugs, ask simple and direct questions. Take care to make your manner and questions nonthreatening. Avoid confrontation while the person is under the influence, and avoid displaying any scolding or disgust because this may make the person belligerent.

The top priority is to find out the time of the person's last drink or drug, how much he or she took, and the name of each drug that was taken. This information will help assess any withdrawal patterns. (A full discussion of substance use assessment is presented in Chapter 6.) For your own protection, be aware of hospital security or other personnel who could be called on for assistance. Avoid turning your back, and make sure that you are aware of your surroundings.

Once a hospitalized substance abuser has been detoxified and is sober, he or she should be assessed for the extent of the problem and its meaning for the person and family. Initially you will encounter denial and increased defensiveness; special interview techniques are needed (see Chapter 6).

Personal Questions

Occasionally people will ask you questions about *your* personal life or opinions, such as "Are you married?" "Do you have children?" or "Do you smoke?" You do not need to answer every question, but you may supply information that you think is appropriate. Beware that there may be an ulterior motive to the questions, such as anxiety or loneliness. Try directing your response back to the person's frame of reference. You might say something like, *"No, I don't have children; I wonder if your question is related to how I can help you care for Jamie?"*

Sexually Aggressive People

On some occasions personal questions extend to flirtatious compliments, seductive innuendo, or sexual advances. Some people see illness as a threat to their self-esteem and sexual adequacy; this feeling creates anxiety that makes them act out in sexually aggressive ways.

Your response must make it clear that you are a health professional who can best care for the person by maintaining a professional relationship. It is important to communicate that you cannot tolerate sexual advances, but you should also communicate that you accept the person and understand his or her need to be self-assertive. This may be difficult, considering that the person's words or gestures may have left you shocked, embarrassed, or angry. Your feelings are normal. You need to set appropriate verbal boundaries by saying, *"I am uncomfortable when you talk to me that way; please don't."* A further response that would open communication is, *"I wonder if the way you're feeling now relates to your illness or to being in the hospital?"* If the behavior continues, you may need to remove yourself from the situation.

Crying

A beginning examiner may feel uncomfortable when the client starts to cry, but crying is a big relief to a person. Health problems come with powerful emotions, and it takes a good deal of energy to keep worries about illness, death, or loss bottled up. When you say something that "makes the person cry," do not think you have hurt the person. You have just broached a topic that is important. Do not go on to a new topic. It is important that you allow the person to cry and express his or her feelings fully before you move on. Have tissues available, and wait until the crying subsides to talk. Reassure the crying client that he or she does not need to be embarrassed and that you are there to listen.

Sometimes your client may look as if he or she is on the verge of tears but is trying hard to suppress them. Again, instead of moving on to something new, acknowledge the expression by saying, "You look sad." Don't worry that you will open an uncontrollable floodgate. The person may cry but will be relieved, and you will have gained insight to a serious concern. Use of appropriate therapeutic touch can help show empathy while a person is crying.

CLINICAL ILLUSTRATION

M.P., a 49-year-old male, is at the clinic today for a physical examination. He hasn't been seen in over 5 years and readily admits a dislike of doctors' offices.

M.P.: I haven't been seen in quite a while, but I thought I should come in soon.

Response: What made you decide to come see the doctor?

M.P.: (appears uncomfortable) My father died of a heart attack when he was 47 years old, so I figure I'm living on borrowed time (lip folds in; tears in eyes).

Response: You look sad. (places hand on forearm)

M.P.: (crying now) It's just that I have kids and a wife, and I worry about what's going to happen if I die. When my father died, my mother struggled so much to raise us. I don't want to leave my wife with that burden.

Response: I understand how worried you are, and I'm glad you came in for a checkup today. We'll take this one step at a time and work together to minimize your risk of having a heart attack.

Anger

Occasionally you will try to interview a person who is already angry. Don't take the anger personally; it typically doesn't relate to you. The person is showing aggression as a response to his or her own feelings of anxiety or helplessness. Do ask about the anger and hear the person out. Deal with the angry feelings before you ask anything else. An angry person cannot be an effective participant in a health interview.

Threats of Violence

Over 70% of nurses report physical or verbal abuse in the workplace,[12,16] and this number is likely low due to underreporting of incidents of violence. Patients are the primary source of abuse against health care professionals. Make sure you know your employer's policy on violent behavior, and be aware of resources, such as security personnel. Identifying red-flag behaviors of a potentially disruptive person is important. These behaviors include fist clenching, pacing, a vacant stare, confusion, statements out of touch with reality or that do not make sense, a history of recent drug use, or a recent history of intense bereavement (loss of partner, loss of job).

If you sense any suspicious or threatening behavior, act immediately to defuse the situation, or obtain additional support from others. Make sure that you leave the door to the examination room open, and never turn your back to a potentially aggressive person. You also want to make sure to position yourself between the person and door so that you can easily leave the room. Do not raise your own voice or try to argue with the threatening person. Act calm and talk to the person in a soft voice. Act interested in what the person is saying, and behave in an unhurried way. Your most important goal is safety; avoid taking any risks.

Anxiety

Finally take it for granted that nearly all sick people have some anxiety. This is a normal response to being sick. It makes some people aggressive and others dependent. Appearing unhurried and taking the time to listen to all of the client's concerns can help defuse some anxiety. Avoiding the traps to interviews and using therapeutic responses are other ways to help defuse anxiety.

 ## CULTURE AND GENETICS

Cultural Considerations on Gender

Violating cultural norms related to appropriate male-female relationships may jeopardize a professional relationship. Among some Arab Americans an adult male is never alone with a female (except his wife) and is generally accompanied by at least one other male when interacting with females. This behavior is culturally very significant; a lone male could be accused of sexual impropriety. Ask the person about culturally relevant aspects of male-female relationships at the beginning of the interview. When gender differences are important to the patient, try strategies such as offering to have a third person present. If a family member or friend has accompanied the patient, inquire whether the patient would like that person to be in the examination room during the history and/or physical examination. It is not unusual for a female to refuse to be examined by a male and vice versa. Modesty is another issue. It is imperative to ensure that the patient is carefully draped at all times, curtains are closed, and, when possible, doors are closed. Do not enter a room without knocking first and announcing yourself.

Cultural Considerations on Sexual Orientation

Lesbian, gay, bisexual, and transgender (LGBTQ) individuals are aware of heterosexist biases and the communication of these biases during the interview and physical examination. *Heterosexism* refers to the belief that heterosexuality is the only natural choice and assumes that everyone is or should be heterosexual. Heterosexism is a form of homophobia and leads to discrimination. Most admitting and health history forms are heterosexist. The form asks for marital status and does not include an option for a long-term committed relationship or partner. Many same-sex couples are in monogamous, committed relationships, but there is seldom a category that acknowledges their relationship on the form. Although technically and legally the person may be single, this trivializes the relationship with his or her significant other. If this type of form is in use, the interviewer may not realize that the person is in a relationship and may make inappropriate comments based on incorrect assumptions.

Simple, basic changes in your communication and nursing practice can help avoid heterosexism.[17]

- Do not marginalize a homosexual relationship. Ask the same questions of a homosexual couple that you would of a heterosexual couple as long as the questions are applicable.

- Know your state laws. For example, some states allow both same-sex parents to be listed on the birth certificate, whereas others do not.
- Use appropriate health teaching materials, including those that depict same-sex couples.
- Do not make assumptions about a person's sex based on his or her appearance.
- Avoid heterosexist assumptions. Make sure that you ask all appropriate questions while avoiding assumptions that heterosexism is the norm. For example, ask a sexually active woman, "Have you ever used birth control?" instead of, "Which type of birth control measures have you used?" The latter question assumes that the woman has had the need for birth control, which assumes that she has engaged in relations with a man.
- Make sure that registration and admitting forms allow for identification of a same-sex partner by using terms such as "partner" or "significant other" while avoiding terms such as "marital status."
- Ask new patients what their preferred pronoun is (e.g., her/hers, him/his, they/their, etc.). Do not assume because someone is biologically female that the preferred pronoun is her.
- Show a caring demeanor and ask open-ended questions.
- Avoid asking unnecessarily intrusive questions. For example, if you are updating a history for a client presenting with an upper respiratory infection, you have no need to inquire about sexual reassignment surgery or the genitalia of your transgender client.
- Don't assume that anyone knows the client's sexual orientation or status as a transgender individual. Always respect the person's privacy.
- Be nonjudgmental, and make sure that your workplace has adopted policies to avoid discrimination.

Most important, be aware of your personal bias and baggage. Being familiar with considerations for treatment of the LGBTQ community is the first step in providing culturally competent care.

Working With (and Without) an Interpreter

Over 62 million people in the United States report speaking a language other than English at home and over 25 million of those report speaking English "less than very well."[19] One of the greatest challenges in cross-cultural communication occurs when you and the client speak different languages (Fig. 3.9). After identifying a language barrier, you may find yourself trying to communicate effectively through an interpreter or trying to communicate effectively when there is no interpreter. Either way, it is important that you consider not only the meaning of the spoken language, but also nonverbal communication. See Chapter 2 for culturally competent care.

Clients with language barriers experience many negative health outcomes, especially if an interpreter is not used. Non–English-speaking clients have longer hospital stays, receive fewer preventive services, and are less satisfied. Clients who need but do not receive an interpreter are more likely to suffer adverse drug reactions, have a poor understanding of

the diagnosis, and are at greater risk for complications.[9,15] The use of trained interpreters has been linked to lower admission rates and increased use of preventive services. Trained interpreters can improve overall health outcomes, improve use of primary care, and increase client satisfaction. Their use may also result in a cost savings and reduced rate of complications.[8]

Interviewing the non–English-speaking person requires a bilingual interpreter for full communication. Even clients who seem to have a basic command of English as a second language may need an interpreter when faced with the anxiety-provoking situation of entering a hospital, describing a strange symptom, or discussing sensitive topics such as those related to reproductive or urologic concerns.

It is tempting to ask an ad hoc interpreter (e.g., a relative or friend) to interpret because this person is readily available. Although convenient, it is disadvantageous for a number of reasons to ask an untrained interpreter to translate. The client's confidentiality is violated by asking for an ad hoc interpreter because the client may not want his or her information shared. Furthermore, the friend or relative, although fluent in ordinary language usage, is unlikely to be familiar with medical terminology, hospital or clinic procedures, and medical ethics. Having a relative interpret adds stress to an already stressful situation and may disrupt family relationships. In some cultures full disclosure of a diagnosis such as cancer is taboo, so an ad hoc interpreter may edit the diagnosis or not fully disclose information.

Whenever possible, work with a bilingual team member or a trained medical interpreter. This person knows interpreting techniques, has a health care background, and understands clients' rights. A trained interpreter is also knowledgeable about cultural beliefs and health practices. They can help you bridge the cultural gap and advise you concerning the cultural appropriateness of your recommendations.

Many clients with limited English proficiency do not have access to interpreters. It is your responsibility to ensure that the provisions of Title VI as discussed in Chapter 2 are met. Few clinicians receive necessary preparation to practice with

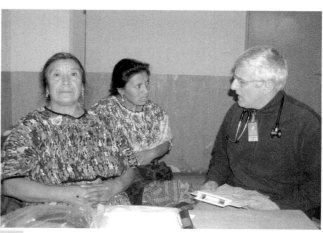

3.9

interpreters. As a first preference, language services should include the availability of a bilingual staff or on-site medical interpreters who can communicate directly with clients in their preferred language and dialect and have received adequate training.[5] When a trained interpreter is unavailable, telephone translation services such as AT&T LanguageLine Solutions (www.languageline.com) can be used 24 hours a day.

Although interpreters are trained to remain neutral, they can influence both the content of information exchanged and the nature of the interaction. Many trained medical interpreters are members of the linguistic community they serve. Although this is largely beneficial, it has limitations. For example, interpreters may know clients and details of their circumstances before the interview begins. Although acceptance of a code of ethics governing confidentiality and conflicts of interest is part of the training that interpreters receive, discord may arise if an interpreter relates information that the client has not volunteered to the examiner.

Note that being bilingual does not always mean that the interpreter is culturally aware. For example, the Latino culture is so diverse that a Spanish-speaking interpreter from one country, class, race, and gender does not necessarily understand the cultural background of a Spanish-speaking person from another country and different circumstances. Even trained interpreters, who are often from urban areas and represent a higher socioeconomic class than the clients whom they interpret, may be unaware of or embarrassed by rural attitudes and practices. Summarized in Table 3.5 are suggestions for the selection and use of an interpreter.

Although you will be in charge of the focus and flow of the interview, view yourself and the interpreter as a team. Ask the interpreter to meet the client beforehand to establish rapport and to determine the client's age, occupation, educational level, and attitude toward health care. This enables the interpreter to communicate on the client's level. Place the interpreter next to the client, but speak directly to the client. Although it can be difficult, focus on the client and address your questions to him or her. For example, do not say to the interpreter, "Ask him if he has pain," but rather ask the client directly, "Do you have pain?"

Although a trained interpreter is your best choice, you may find yourself in a situation in which the client insists on using a friend or family member or when you may have

---

TABLE 3.5 Use of an Interpreter

Choosing an Interpreter
- Before locating an interpreter, identify the language the person is most comfortable speaking.
- Use a *trained* interpreter, preferably one who knows medical terminology.
- Avoid interpreters from a rival tribe, state, region, or nation (e.g., a Palestinian who knows Hebrew may not be the best interpreter for a Jewish person).
- Be aware of gender differences between interpreter and client. In general the same gender is preferred.

Strategies for Effective Use of an Interpreter
- Plan what you want to say ahead of time. Meet privately with the interpreter before the interview to share your expectations and review the purpose of the appointment.
- Ask the interpreter to provide a verbatim account of the conversation.
- Be patient. When using an interpreter, interviews often take 2 to 3 times longer.
- Longer-than-expected explanatory exchanges are often required to convey the meaning of words such as *stress, depression, allergy, preventive medicine,* and *physical therapy* because there may not be comparable terms in the language the client understands.
- When discussing diagnostic tests, be sure to clarify the nature of the test to the interpreter. Indicate the purpose of the test, exactly what will happen to the client, approximately how long the test will take, whether the procedure is invasive or noninvasive, and which part(s) of the body will be tested.
- Avoid ambiguous statements and questions. Refrain from using conditional or indefinite phrasing such as "if," "would," and "could," especially for target languages such as Khmer (Cambodia) that lack nuances of conditionality or distinctions of time other than simple past and present. Conditional statements may be mistaken for actual agreement or approval of a course of action.
- Avoid abstract expressions, idioms, similes, metaphors, and medical jargon.
- Speak to the client, not the interpreter. Use positive nonverbal communication skills throughout the exchange to facilitate rapport.
- Use short, simple sentences, pausing frequently to allow for interpretation.
- Know what services are available at your workplace.

Recommendations for Institutions
- Maintain a current computerized list of interpreters who may be contacted as needed.
- Network with area hospitals, colleges, universities, and other organizations that may serve as resources.
- Use over-the-telephone interpretation services provided by telephone companies. For example, since 1989 AT&T has operated the LanguageLine Solutions, which provides interpretation in more than 140 languages. Services are available around the clock every day of the year. Call (800) 628-8486 or visit www.languageline.com for further information on services and charges.

no other choice. In either of these situations, make sure to document who was used as the interpreter and whether it was the client's choice. Unless there is an emergency, never use a minor as an interpreter. Make sure that you assess the ad hoc interpreter's ability to translate complex medical terminology. You may have to change your phrasing and terminology with an untrained interpreter. Keep your questioning in mind as well. If you are going to ask about sensitive topics such as domestic violence, sexually transmitted infections, illicit drugs, end-of-life care, or other controversial topics, the client may not be as forthcoming with a friend or family member as the interpreter.

You will need to allow more time for the interview. Having a third person repeat everything will take considerably longer than your interview with English-speaking clients. If you have limited time, focus on priority data.

There are two styles of interpreting: line-by-line and summarizing. Translating line-by-line takes more time, but it ensures accuracy. Use this style for most of the interview. Speak only 1 or 2 sentences at a time then allow for interpretation. Use simple language, not medical jargon that the interpreter must simplify before it can be translated. Summary translation progresses faster and is useful for teaching relatively simple health techniques with which the interpreter is already familiar. Be alert for nonverbal cues as the client talks. These cues can give valuable data. A good interpreter also notes nonverbal messages and passes them on to you.

Although use of an interpreter is the ideal, you may find yourself in a situation with a non–English-speaking client when no interpreter is available. Table 3.6 summarizes some suggestions for overcoming language barriers when no interpreter is present.

Health Literacy: Ensuring We Are Understood

You might have perfected the communication techniques described and feel fully prepared to interview the most challenging client, but are you sure that he or she understands everything you say? Literacy is the ability to read and write; however, **health literacy** refers to the ability to understand instructions, navigate the health care system, and communicate concerns with the health care provider.[7,11] A person can have adequate literacy yet lack adequate health literacy. In 2006 the U.S. Department of Education released the National Assessment of Adult Literacy, which estimated that only 12% of people have proficient health literacy. Said another way, nearly 9 out of 10 people that you encounter do not have adequate health literacy to navigate the health care system and understand health instructions.[10]

Health literacy encompasses a variety of factors beyond basic reading, including the ability to use quantitative (numeric) information and to understand and remember verbal instructions. People with low health literacy struggle to navigate the health care system and may be noncompliant because of a misunderstanding. Low health literacy has been associated with low medication compliance, more emergency department visits, increased readmission rates, inability to recall information after a clinic visit, and an inability to effectively manage chronic

TABLE 3.6 **What to Do When No Language Interpreter Is Available**
1. Be polite and formal.
2. Pronounce name correctly. Use proper titles of respect such as "Mr.," "Mrs.," "Ms.," "Dr." Greet the person using the last or complete name. Gesture to yourself and say your name. Offer a handshake or nod. Smile.
3. Proceed in an unhurried manner. Pay attention to any effort by the client or family to communicate.
4. Speak in a low, moderate voice. Avoid talking loudly. Remember that there is a tendency to raise the volume and pitch of your voice when the listener appears not to understand. The listener may perceive that you are shouting and/or angry. Speaking loudly will not help the person understand.
5. Use any words that you might know in the person's language. This indicates that you are aware of and respect his or her culture.
6. Use simple words such as "pain" instead of "discomfort." Avoid medical jargon, idioms, and slang. Avoid using contractions (e.g., *don't, can't, won't*). Use nouns repeatedly instead of pronouns. Do not say: "He has been taking his medicine, hasn't he?" Do say: "Does Juan take medicine?"
7. Pantomime words and simple actions while you verbalize them.
8. Give instructions in the proper sequence. Do not say: "Before you sterilize the bottle, rinse it." Do say: "First wash the bottle. Second, sterilize the bottle."
9. Discuss one topic at a time. Avoid using conjunctions. Do not say: "Are you cold and in pain?" Do say: "Are you cold (while pantomiming)? Are you in pain?"
10. Validate whether person understands by having him or her repeat instructions, demonstrate the procedure, or act out the meaning.
11. Write out several short sentences in English and determine the person's ability to read them.
12. Try a third language. Many Indochinese speak French. Europeans often know two or more languages. Try Latin words or phrases.
13. Ask who among the person's family and friends could serve as an interpreter.
14. Obtain phrase books from a library or bookstore, make or purchase flash cards, contact hospitals for a list of interpreters, and use both formal and informal networks to locate a suitable interpreter.

illness. Low health literacy leads to increased cost of care and poor outcomes for this population.

Tools for Determining Literacy

As a clinician you are on the front line in the battle for adequate health literacy for your clients. A wide variety of tools to measure health literacy exist—some more challenging than others. Although The Joint Commission requires that patient communication needs be identified, there is no requirement for actual assessment of health literacy. Multiple tools exist for the assessment of health literacy, each with varying strengths and weaknesses.

All health literacy tools can be used in the clinical setting, but incorporating them is challenging. The Test of Functional Health Literacy requires over 20 minutes to administer and measures numeracy and reading comprehension. The Rapid Estimate of Adult Literacy in Medicine takes only a few minutes but requires the person to read 68 medical terms while being scored on correct pronunciation. A Single-Item Literacy Screener has been suggested, but with only marginal effectiveness. The Newest Vital Sign assesses numeracy and comprehension by asking the person to answer questions based on an ice cream nutrition label. Some clinics simply ask standardized questions such as, "Do you have any limitations in learning?" or "What is the last grade level completed?" instead of requiring a specific assessment tool. No standard approach to measuring health literacy is currently recommended, but it is important that you know the policy at your place of work and take time to assess your client's health literacy to assure understanding of important information.

What Can You Do?
Oral Teaching

As a clinician there are steps you can take to ensure that your clients understand the information you are providing. Although completing a health literacy screener gives you objective data and can help you determine the appropriate level of information, most clients (regardless of literacy level) want to be provided with simple, easy-to-understand instructions; therefore the practice of giving all clients simple instructions at a lower reading level is acceptable. When discussing medical information with clients, keep it simple, use short sentences and words containing no more than two syllables (when possible), limit the number of messages you are giving the client, be sure to tell the person what they will gain by following your instructions, present only needed information, focus on the client, use the active voice, and avoid jargon. Although you may think using complex terms and sentences makes you sound more professional or smarter, it can confuse the client. You are better off speaking to them as you would to a friend, using a conversational structure that includes time for them to ask questions. A few examples follow:

Say: Feel for lumps about the size of a pea.
Don't say: Feel for lumps about 5 to 6 millimeters.
Say: Birth control
Don't say: Contraception
Say: Cook chicken until it is no longer pink.
Don't say: Cook chicken to an internal temperature of 165° F.

Written Materials

When preparing or using written materials, make sure to assess the appropriateness of the materials. Most client education materials are created at a reading level that is not suitable for the majority of clients. Written materials should be at the 5th-grade reading level or below. Reading level can be determined with a variety of formulas that use number of syllables per word and complexity of sentences to determine reading level. Materials should be at least 12-point font. Also avoid all capital letters, use headings and subheadings, use bullet points, and limit medical jargon.[3] Pictures are often used in written materials, but you must be careful to select appropriate graphics.

Teach-Back

Although ensuring appropriate verbal and written communication is important, one of the easiest things you can do when teaching a client is to use the teach-back approach. Teach-back is simple and free. It allows you to assess whether the person understands and to immediately correct misconceptions. Many health care professionals ask, "Do you understand?" or "Do you have any questions?" throughout the teaching sessions. Just because your client has no questions and indicates understanding with a nod doesn't mean that he or she actually understands the information. Using teach-back encourages the client to repeat in his or her own words what you have just said. This verbal discussion allows you to assess the understanding and may open the door for the client to ask questions.

COMMUNICATING WITH OTHER PROFESSIONALS

Throughout your career, you will work with professionals from a variety of health care disciplines. It is imperative that you learn to communicate effectively with other professionals. The use of therapeutic communication will not only help in your interactions with patients, but will also guide your interactions with other professionals. **Interprofessional communication** is communication that occurs between 2 or more individuals from different health professions (e.g., nursing, therapy services, physicians). Effective interprofessional communication requires an environment of mutual respect and collaboration among professionals of various disciplines.

Ineffective interprofessional communication has been linked to delays in treatment, medication errors, misdiagnosis, patient injury, and death.[6] Each health professional brings a different but necessary skill set to the treatment of a patient. Recognition and respect for each person's skills is necessary for effective teamwork, collaboration, and communication.[1]

Open lines of communication are necessary when caring for patients in any health care setting. Rarely will you work alone. Instead you will likely collaborate with other health care professionals as you care for patients throughout your career. When communicating with other health care professionals, make sure you provide timely updates, communicate in a clear, succinct manner, are polite and respectful, and use communication tools (e.g., SBAR).[2] Ineffective communication has negative consequences to patient care, but also impacts the job satisfaction of health care professionals.[20] It is important that health professionals work together to provide

TABLE 3.7   SBAR Communication

S	Situation	State your name, your unit, patient's name, room number, patient's problem, when it happened or when it started, and the severity.	This is Sue in the ortho unit. I am calling about pain control for Ms. Carpenter in room 15.
B	Background	Do not recite the patient's full history since admission. Do state the data pertinent to this moment's problem: admitting diagnosis, when admitted, and appropriate immediate assessment data (e.g., vital signs, pulse oximetry, change in mental status, allergies, current medications, IV fluids, laboratory results).	She has no significant medical history. Yesterday she had a right knee replacement. Her VS are: HR 126, respirations 20, BP 140/96. Her labs are within expected parameters. She has an order for Tylenol 650 mg every 4 hours for mild/moderate pain and morphine 1-4 mg every 2 hours for breakthrough pain. She has no medication allergies and has been consistently taking her pain medicine.
A	Assessment	State your assessment findings. This can include what you found and what you think may be wrong.	Ms. Carpenter is rating her pain at 10/10 with no relief from medication. She is reluctant to ambulate, refusing physical therapy. Pedal pulses are 2+, equal bilaterally, surgical site is within normal limits without signs of infection.
R	Recommendation or request	State what you want/need to continue caring for the patient.	I believe Ms. Carpenter would benefit from a different pain medication regimen such as scheduled tramadol with oral hydrocodone for more severe pain. What would you like to order for Ms. Carpenter?

the best possible patient experience and create the best work environment possible.

Standardized Communication

Standard communication formats are becoming more popular in the health care setting. A standardized communication report is similar to a checklist. Checklists are used to ensure safety and to prevent important steps from being missed due to fatigue or other factors. One of the most commonly used standardized communication tools in health care is the **Situation, Background, Assessment, Recommendation (SBAR).** SBAR was first developed in the U.S. military to standardize communication and prevent misunderstandings. In the hospital, communication errors contribute to most sentinel events. Thus SBAR is used at health care facilities all over the country to improve communication and reduce errors.

SBAR is a standardized framework to transmit important in-the-moment information. Using SBAR will keep your message concise and focused on the immediate problem yet give your colleague enough information to grasp the current situation and make a decision. Using a structured format allows for a common language among health professionals from a variety of disciplines. Nurses often communicate information in lengthy narratives, whereas physicians tend to use succinct bullet points. Using a standard tool which assures pertinent information is conveyed allows multiple disciplines to communicate more effectively (Table 3.7).

REFERENCES

1. Arnold, E., & Boggs, K. (2016). *Interpersonal relationships: Professional communication skills for nurses* (7th ed.). St. Louis: Elsevier.
2. Canadian Medical Practice Advisory Council. (2011). https://www.cmpa-acpm.ca/en/advice-publications/browse-articles/2011/strengthening-inter-professional-communication.
3. Centers for Disease Control and Prevention. (2009). *Simply put: a guide for creating easy-to-understand materials* http://www.cdc.gov/healthliteracy/learn/index.html.
4. Chalmers, D. (2017). *Communicating with children from birth to four years.* New York: Routledge.
5. Flores, G., Abreu, M., Barone, C. P., et al. (2012). Errors of medical interpretation and their potential clinical consequences: A comparison of professional versus ad hoc versus no interpreters. *Ann Emerg Med, 60*(5), 545–553.
6. Foronda, C., MacWilliams, B., & McArthur, E. (2016). Interprofessional communication in healthcare: An integrative review. *Nurse Educ Pract, 19*, 36–40.
7. Institute of Medicine. (2004). Health literacy: A prescription to end confusion. In L. Nielsen-Bohlman, A. Panzer, & D. Kindig (Eds.). Washington, DC: National Academies Press.
8. Interpreting Stakeholder Group. (2009). *How to work effectively with interpreters.* www.umtia.org.
9. Juckett, G., & Unger, K. (2014). Appropriate use of medical interpreters. *Am Fam Physician, 90*(7), 476–480.
10. Kutner, M., Greenberg, E., Jin, Y., et al. (2006). *The health literacy of America's adults.* Washington, DC: National Center for Education Statistics, U.S. Department of Education. http://nces.ed.gov/pubs2006/2006483.pdf. Sep. NCES 2006–483.
11. McCleary-Jones, V. (2016). A systematic review of the literature on health literacy in nursing education. *Nurse Educ, 41*(2), 93–97.
12. Occupational Safety and Health Administration. (2015). *Workplace violence in healthcare.* https://www.osha.gov/Publications/OSHA3826.pdf.
13. Rathert, C., Mittler, J. N., Banerjee, S., et al. (2017). Patient-centered communication in the era of electronic health records: What does the evidence say? *Patient Educ Couns, 100*, 50–64.

14. Richardson, K. J. (2014). DEAF CULTURE: Competencies and best practices. *Nurse Practitioner, 39*(5), 20–29.

15. Rorie, S. (2015). Using medical interpreters to provide culturally competent care. *AORN J, 101*(2), P7–P9.

16. Speroni, K. G., Fitch, T., Dawson, E., et al. (2014). Incidence and cost of nurse workplace violence perpetrated by hospital patients or visitors. *J Emerg Nurs, 40*(3), 218–228.

17. Sullivan, K., Guzman, A., & Lancellotti, D. (2017). Nursing communication and the gender identity spectrum. *Am Nurse Today, 12*(5), 6–11.

18. Touhy, T. A., & Jett, K. F. (2016). *Ebersole & Hess' toward healthy aging* (9th ed.). St. Louis: Elsevier.

19. U.S. Census Bureau. (n.d.). *American FactFinder.* factfinder. census.gov.

20. Vermeir, P., Vandijck, D., Degroote, S., et al. (2015). Communication in healthcare: A narrative review of the literature and practice recommendations. *Int J Clin Pract, 69*(11), 1257–1267.

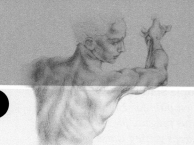

CHAPTER 4

The Complete Health History

ⓔhttp://evolve.elsevier.com/Jarvis/

The purpose of the health history is to collect **subjective data**—what the person says about himself or herself. This is different from **objective data**—what you observe through measurement, inspection, palpation, percussion, and auscultation. The history is combined with the objective data from the physical examination and laboratory studies to form the database. The database is used to make a judgment or a diagnosis about the health status of the individual (Fig. 4.1).

The health history provides a complete picture of the person's past and present health. It describes the individual as a whole and how the person interacts with the environment. It records health strengths and coping skills. The history should recognize and affirm what the person is *doing right:* what he or she is doing to help stay well. For the well person, the history is used to assess his or her lifestyle, including such factors as exercise, healthy diet, substance use, risk reduction, and health promotion behaviors.

For the ill person, the health history includes a detailed and chronologic record of the health problem. For everyone the health history is a screening tool for abnormal symptoms, health problems, and concerns; and it records ways of responding to the health problems.

In many settings the patient fills out a printed or electronic history form. This allows the person ample time to recall and consider such items as dates of health landmarks and relevant family history. You then review and validate the written data and collect more data on lifestyle management and current health problems.

Although history forms vary, most contain information in the sequence of categories listed to the right. This health history format presents a generic database for all practitioners. Those in primary care settings may use all of it, whereas those in a hospital may focus primarily on the history of present illness and the functional, or patterns of living, data.

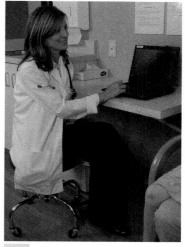

4.1

Health History Sequence
1. Biographic data
2. Reason for seeking care
3. Present health or history of present illness
4. Past history
5. Medication reconciliation
6. Family history
7. Review of systems
8. Functional assessment or activities of daily living (ADLs)

THE HEALTH HISTORY—THE ADULT

Record the date and time of day of the interview.

Biographic Data

Biographic data include name, address, and phone number; age and birth date; birthplace; gender; relationship status; race; ethnic origin; and occupation. If illness has caused a change in occupation, include both the usual occupation and the present occupation. Record the person's primary language. Try to find a language-concordant provider to collect the history or a medical interpreter fluent in the patient's language.

Source of History

1. Record who furnishes the information—usually the person himself or herself, although the source may be an interpreter or caseworker. Less reliable is a relative or friend.
2. Judge how reliable the informant seems and how willing he or she is to communicate. A reliable person always gives the same answers, even when questions are rephrased or repeated later in the interview.
3. Note whether the person appears well or ill; a sick patient may communicate poorly.

See sample recordings at right.

Sample Statements:
Patient herself, who seems reliable
Patient's son, John Ramirez, who seems reliable
Mrs. R. Fuentes, interpreter for Theresa Castillo, who does not speak English

Reason for Seeking Care[a]

This is a brief, spontaneous statement in the person's own words that describes the reason for the visit. Think of it as the "title" for the story to follow. It states one (possibly two) symptoms or signs and their duration. A **symptom** is a subjective sensation that the person feels from the disorder. A **sign** is an objective abnormality that you as the examiner could detect on physical examination or through diagnostic testing. Try to record whatever the person *says* is the reason for seeking care, enclose it in quotation marks to indicate the person's exact words, and record a time frame. See examples at right.

The reason for seeking care is not a diagnostic statement. Avoid translating it into the terms of a medical diagnosis. For example, Mr. J.S. enters with shortness of breath, and you ponder writing "emphysema." Even if he is known to have emphysema from previous visits, it is not the chronic emphysema that prompted *this visit* but, rather, the "increasing shortness of breath" for 4 hours.

Some people try to self-diagnose based on similar signs and symptoms in their relatives or friends or on conditions they know they have. Rather than record a woman's statement that she has "strep throat," ask her what symptoms she has that make her think this is present, and record those symptoms.

Occasionally a person may have *many* reasons for seeking care. After the first reason, ask, "Is there anything else we should take care of today?" The most important reason to the person may not necessarily be the one stated first. Try to focus on which is the most pressing concern by asking the person which one prompted him or her to seek help now.

Present Health or History of Present Illness

For the well person, this is a short statement about the general state of health: *"I feel healthy right now." "I am healthy and active."*

For the ill person, this section is a chronologic record of the reason for seeking care, from the time the symptom first started until now. Isolate each reason for care identified by the person and say, for example, "Please tell me all about your headache, from the time it started until the time you came to the hospital" (Fig. 4.2). If the concern started months or years ago, record what occurred during that time and find out why the person is seeking care now.

As the person talks, do not jump to conclusions and bias the story by adding your opinion. Collect all the data first. Although you want the person to respond in a narrative format without interruption from you, your final summary of any symptom the person has should include these eight critical characteristics:

1. **Location.** Be specific; ask the person to point to the location. If the problem is pain, note the precise site. "Head pain" is vague, whereas descriptions such as "pain behind the eyes," "jaw pain," and "occipital pain" are more precise and diagnostically significant. Is the pain localized to one site or radiating? Is the pain superficial or deep?

2. **Character or Quality.** This calls for specific descriptive terms such as burning, sharp, dull, aching, gnawing, throbbing, shooting, viselike when describing pain. You also need to ask about the character of other symptoms. Use similes: Blood in the stool looks like sticky tarm whereas blood in vomitus looks like coffee grounds.

3. **Quantity or Severity.** Attempt to quantify the sign or symptom, such as "profuse menstrual flow soaking five pads per hour." Quantify the symptom of pain using the scale shown on the right. With pain, avoid adjectives, and ask how it affects daily activities. Then record if the person says, "I was so sick I was doubled over and couldn't move" or "I was able to go to work, but then I came home and went to bed."

4. **Timing (Onset, Duration, Frequency).** When did the symptom first appear? Give the specific date and time or state specifically how long ago the symptom started prior to arrival (PTA). "The pain started yesterday" will not mean much when you return to read the record in the future. The report must include answers to questions such as the following: "How long did the symptom last (duration)?" "Was it steady (constant) or did it come and go (intermittent)?" "Did it resolve completely and reappear days or weeks later (cycle of remission and exacerbation)?"

Sample Statements:
"Chest pain for 2 hours"
"Sinus pressure for 3 days that keeps getting worse"
"Tugging at her ears and was fussy all night"
"Need annual physical for work"
"Want to start exercise program and need checkup"

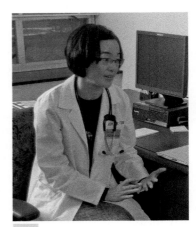

4.2

Pain Scale
Quantify the symptom of pain by asking: *"On a 10-point scale, with 10 being the most pain you can possibly imagine and 0 being no pain, tell me how your pain feels right now."* (See Chapter 11 for a full description.)

---

[a]In the past, this statement was called the chief complaint (CC). Avoid this title because it labels the person a "complainer" and, more important, does not include wellness needs.

5. **Setting.** Where was the person or what was the person doing when the symptom started? What brings it on? For example, "Did you notice the chest pain after shoveling snow, or did the pain start by itself?"

6. **Aggravating or Relieving Factors.** What makes the pain worse? Is it aggravated by weather, activity, food, medication, standing, fatigue, time of day, or season? What relieves it (e.g., rest, medication, or ice pack)? What is the effect of any treatment? Ask, "What have you tried?" or "What seems to help?"

7. **Associated Factors.** Is this primary symptom associated with any others (e.g., urinary frequency and burning associated with fever and chills)? Review the body system related to this symptom now rather than waiting for the Review of Systems section later. Many clinicians review the person's medication regimen now (including alcohol and tobacco use) because the presenting symptom may be a side effect or toxic effect of a chemical.

8. **Patient's Perception.** Find out the meaning of the symptom by asking how it affects daily activities (Fig. 4.3). "How has this affected you? Is there anything you can't do now that you could do before?" Also ask directly, "What do you think it means?" This is crucial because it alerts you to potential anxiety if the person thinks the symptom may be ominous.

You may find it helpful to organize this question sequence into the mnemonic **PQRSTU** to help remember all the points.

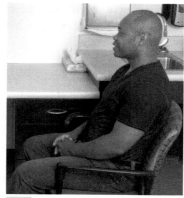

4.3

P: **Provocative or Palliative.** What brings it on? What were you doing when you first noticed it? What makes it better? Worse?

Q: **Quality or Quantity.** How does it look, feel, sound? How intense/severe is it?

R: **Region or Radiation.** Where is it? Does it spread anywhere?

S: **Severity Scale.** How bad is it (on a scale of 0 to 10)? Is it getting better, worse, staying the same?

T: **Timing.** Onset—Exactly when did it first occur? Duration—How long did it last? Frequency—How often does it occur?

U: **Understand Patient's Perception of the Problem.** What do you think it means?

Past Health

Past health events are important because they may have residual effects on the current health state. The previous experience with illness may also give clues about how the person responds to illness and the significance of illness for him or her.

Childhood Illnesses. Measles, mumps, rubella, chickenpox, pertussis, and strep throat. Avoid recording "usual childhood illnesses," because an illness common in the person's childhood (e.g., mumps) may be unusual today. Ask about serious illnesses that may have sequelae for the person in later years (e.g., rheumatic fever, scarlet fever, poliomyelitis).

Accidents or Injuries. Auto accidents, fractures, penetrating wounds, head injuries (especially if associated with unconsciousness), and burns.

Serious or Chronic Illnesses. Asthma, depression, diabetes, hypertension, heart disease, human immunodeficiency virus (HIV) infection, hepatitis, sickle cell anemia, cancer, and seizure disorder.

Hospitalizations. Cause, name of hospital, how the condition was treated, how long the person was hospitalized, and name of the physician.

Operations. Type of surgery, date, name of the surgeon, name of the hospital, and how the person recovered.

Obstetric History. Number of pregnancies (gravidity), number of deliveries in which the fetus reached full term (term), number of preterm pregnancies (preterm), number of incomplete pregnancies (miscarriages or abortions), and number of children living (living). For each complete pregnancy, note the course of pregnancy; labor and delivery; sex, weight, and condition of each infant; and postpartum course.

Recorded as:
Grav 3
Term 2
Preterm 1
Ab 0
Living 3

Immunizations. Routinely assess vaccination history and urge the recommended vaccines. Your strong recommendation increases compliance. Use the current Centers for Disease Control and Prevention (CDC) recommendations for adults, but be aware of primary contraindications and precautions, as well as the person's lifestyle, occupation, and travel. The recommendations for adults include the following[5]: influenza (annually), tetanus-diphtheria-pertussis (Tdap) once if not given previously then Td every 10 years, varicella (if no evidence of immunity), human papillomavirus (HPV), zoster (after 60 years), measles-mumps-rubella ([MMR], if not immunized as a child or no evidence of immunity), pneumococcal (after 65 years), meningococcal (based on exposure risk), and hepatitis A and B. Serologic proof of immunity may be required even if childhood vaccines were given. Consult current guidelines and counsel each patient appropriately. In addition to the recommendations above, repeat Tdap should be given with each pregnancy during 27 to 36 weeks' gestation.[5]

Advise gay and bisexual men to receive HPV, hepatitis A, and hepatitis B vaccinations. If they are not in a long-term monogamous relationship, they should have annual testing for HIV, syphilis, gonorrhea, and chlamydia.[3]

Last Examination Date. Physical, dental, vision, hearing, electrocardiogram (ECG), chest x-ray, mammogram, Pap test, stool occult blood, serum cholesterol.

Allergies. Note both the allergen (medication, food, or contact agent such as fabric or environmental agent) and the reaction (rash, itching, runny nose, watery eyes, difficulty breathing). For drug allergies, list only those that are true allergic reactions, not unpleasant side effects.

Current Medications. **Medication reconciliation** is a comparison of a list of current medications with a previous list, which is done at every hospitalization and every clinic visit. The purpose is to reduce errors and promote patient safety.[11] For all currently prescribed medications, note the name (generic or trade), dose, and schedule, and ask: "How often do you take it each day? What is it for? How long have you been taking it? Do you have any side effects?" and if not taking it, "What is the reason you stopped taking it?" This is an important opportunity for health teaching. Take a moment to teach the patient about medications as applicable.

Ask about nonprescription and over-the-counter (OTC) drugs. The average U.S. home medicine cabinet holds 24 OTC medications, and 40% of Americans take at least one OTC medicine every 2 days.[9] Specifically ask about aspirin (because many people do not consider it a medication even though they take it every day) and other medications: vitamins, birth control pills, antacids, cold remedies, acetaminophen. Be aware that acetaminophen is a component in many OTC pain and cold medications. It has close to 25 trade names, including Tylenol. Serious liver damage may ensue if a person unknowingly doubles or triples the maximum daily acetaminophen intake. For any pain reliever (e.g., acetaminophen, ibuprofen [Advil, Motrin]), ask how many milligrams the person takes. This is an opportunity to provide teaching about maximum safe doses of medications such as Tylenol. Always counsel patients to read medication labels and be mindful of maximum dosages.

Ask about herbal medications. Although not regulated by the Food and Drug Administration, they are popular because consumer advertising of these products often promises weight loss, improved memory, or relief from insomnia, depression, or other conditions. Many are considered safe, but some interact with prescribed medications. For example, St. John's wort is often taken for depression, but because it enters the CYP 450 enzyme metabolism, it has many herb-drug interactions.[9]

Inquire about substances (alcohol, tobacco, street drugs) here or later in Personal Habits (see p. 53).

Family History

In the age of genomics an accurate family history highlights diseases and conditions for which a particular patient may be at increased risk. A person who learns that he or she may be vulnerable for a certain condition may seek early screening and periodic surveillance. A person with significant coronary heart disease history (e.g., a cardiac event in a first-degree male relative <55 years or female relative <65 years) may be influenced to adopt a healthy lifestyle when possible to mitigate that risk.

The most fruitful way to compile a complete family history is to send home a detailed questionnaire before the health care/hospital encounter because the information takes time to compile and often comes from multiple family members. Then you can use the health visit to complete the pedigree. A **pedigree** or **genogram** is a graphic family tree that uses symbols to depict the gender, relationship, and age of immediate blood relatives in at least three generations such as parents, grandparents, and siblings (Fig. 4.4). Other relatives who are included in the genogram are aunts, uncles, nieces, nephews, and cousins. The health of

---

You can find a printable color-coded table of the adult immunization schedule at https://www.cdc.gov/vaccines/schedules/hcp/imz/adult.html.

A person could take furosemide from one prescriber and Lasix from another, not knowing that it is the same medication.

Family History Tools in Electronic and Print Format
U.S. Surgeon General (My Family Health Portrait): www.hhs.gov/familyhistory/
Utah Health Family Tree: www.health.utah.gov/genomics
American Medical Association: https://www.ama-assn.org/sites/default/files/media-browser/public/adult_history.pdf.

Drawing Your Family Tree:
- Make a list of all of your family members.
- Use this sample family tree as a guide to draw your own family tree.
- Write your name at the top of your paper and the date you drew your family tree.
- In place of the words *father, mother,* etc., write the names of your family members.

- When possible, draw your brothers and sisters and your parents' brothers and sisters starting from oldest to the youngest, going from left to right across the paper.
- If dates of birth or ages are not known, then estimate or guess ("50s," "late 60s").

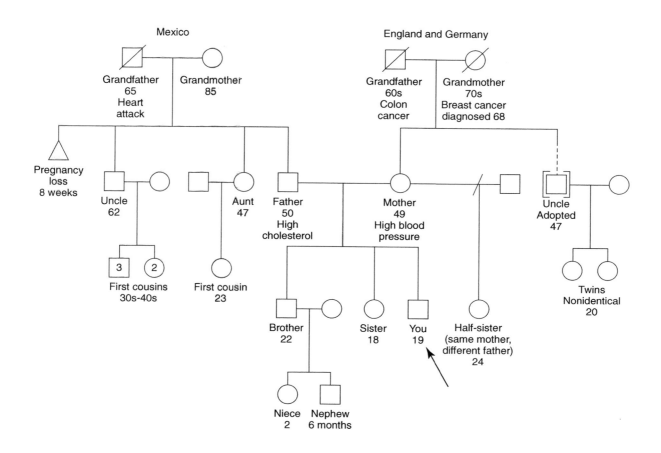

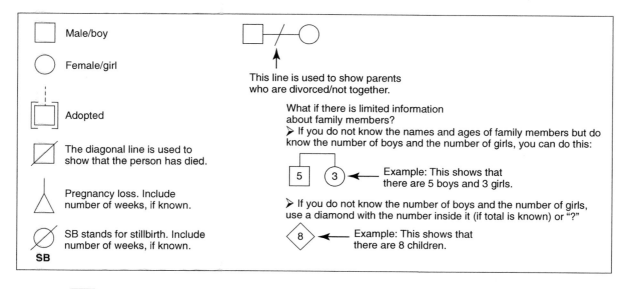

4.4   Genogram or family tree.   (American Society of Human Genetics, 2004.)

close family members, such as spouse or partner and children, is equally important to highlight the patient's prolonged contact with any communicable disease or environmental hazard such as tobacco smoke or to flag the effect of a family member's illness on this person.

Record the medical condition of each relative and other significant health data such as age and cause of death, twinning, tobacco use, and heavy alcohol use. When reviewing the family history data, ask specifically about coronary heart disease, high blood pressure, stroke, diabetes, obesity, blood disorders, breast/ovarian cancer, colon cancer, sickle cell anemia, arthritis, allergies, alcohol or drug addiction, mental illness, suicide, seizure disorder, kidney disease, and tuberculosis (TB).

🌐 CULTURE AND GENETICS

Add several questions to the complete health history when the person is a new immigrant:
- Biographic data—When did the person enter the United States and from what country? If a refugee, under which conditions did he or she come? Was there harassment or torture?
  - The older adult may have come to this country after World War II and may be a Holocaust survivor. Questions regarding family and history may evoke painful memories and must be asked carefully.
- Spiritual resources/religion—Assess whether certain procedures, such as administering blood to a Jehovah's Witness or drawing large amounts of blood from a Chinese patient, are prohibited.
- Past health—Which immunizations were given in the homeland (e.g., was the person given *bacillus Calmette-Guérin* [BCG])? This vaccine is used in many countries to prevent TB; it is not administered in the United States. If the person has had BCG, he or she will have a positive tuberculin skin test; further diagnostic procedures including a sputum test and chest x-ray must be done to rule out TB.
- Health perception—How does the person describe health and illness, and what does he or she see as the problem that he or she is now experiencing?
- Nutritional—Which foods and food combinations are taboo?

Many immigrants have significant health care needs (e.g., diabetes, accidents on the job, muscle pain) but are in the country without documentation. They may be reluctant to seek care and furnish biographic data for fear of deportation.

Review of Systems

The purposes of this section are (1) to evaluate the past and present health state of each body system, (2) to double-check in case any significant data were omitted in the Present Illness section, and (3) to evaluate health promotion practices. The order of the examination of body systems is roughly head to toe. The items within each system are not inclusive, and only the most common symptoms are listed. If the Present Illness section covered a body system, you do not need to repeat all the data here. For example, if the reason for seeking care is earache, the Present Illness section describes most of the symptoms listed for the auditory system. Just ask now what was not asked in the Present Illness section.

Medical terms are listed here, but they need to be translated for the patient. Do not ask the patient about polydipsia. Instead inquire about any unusual or severe thirst. (Note that symptoms and health promotion activities are merely listed here. These terms are repeated and expanded in each related physical examination chapter, along with suggested ways to pose questions and a rationale for each question.)

When recording information, avoid writing "negative" after the system heading. You need to record the *presence* or *absence* of all symptoms; otherwise the reader does not know about which factors you asked.

A common mistake made by beginning practitioners is to record some physical finding or objective data such as "skin warm and dry" in the review of systems. Remember that the history should be limited to patient statements or subjective data—factors that the person *says* were or were not present.

> ***General Overall Health State.*** Present weight (gain or loss, over what period of time, by diet or other factors), fatigue, weakness or malaise, fever, chills, sweats or night sweats.

> ***Skin, Hair, and Nails.*** History of skin disease (eczema, psoriasis, hives), pigment or color change, change in mole, excessive dryness or moisture, pruritus, excessive bruising, rash or lesion (Fig. 4.5).

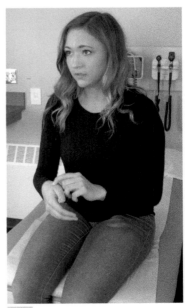

4.5

Recent hair loss or change in texture. Change in shape, color, or brittleness of nails.

Health Promotion. Amount of sun exposure; method of self-care for skin and hair.

Head. Any unusually frequent or severe headache; any head injury, dizziness (syncope), or vertigo.

Eyes. Difficulty with vision (decreased acuity, blurring, blind spots), eye pain, diplopia (double vision), redness or swelling, watering or discharge, glaucoma or cataracts.

Health Promotion. Wear glasses or contacts; last vision check or glaucoma test; how coping with loss of vision if any.

Ears. Earaches, infections, discharge and its characteristics, tinnitus or vertigo.

Health Promotion. Hearing loss, hearing aid use, how loss affects daily life, any exposure to environmental noise, and method of cleaning ears.

Nose and Sinuses. Discharge and its characteristics, any unusually frequent or severe colds, sinus pain, nasal obstruction, nosebleeds, allergies or hay fever, or change in sense of smell.

Mouth and Throat. Mouth pain, frequent sore throat, bleeding gums, toothache, lesion in mouth or tongue, dysphagia, hoarseness or voice change, tonsillectomy, altered taste.

Health Promotion. Pattern of daily dental care, use of dentures, bridge, and last dental checkup.

Neck. Pain, limitation of motion, lumps or swelling, enlarged or tender nodes, goiter. Recent injuries (Fig. 4.6).

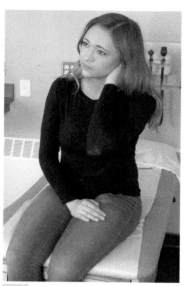

4.6

Breast. Pain, lump, nipple discharge, rash, history of breast disease, any surgery on breasts.

Health Promotion. Performs breast self-examination, including its frequency and method used; last mammogram.

Axilla. Tenderness, lump or swelling, rash.

Respiratory System. History of lung diseases (asthma, emphysema, bronchitis, pneumonia, TB), chest pain with breathing, wheezing or noisy breathing, shortness of breath, how much activity produces shortness of breath, cough, sputum (color, amount), hemoptysis, toxin or pollution exposure.

Health Promotion. Last chest x-ray, TB skin test.

Cardiovascular. Chest pain, pressure, tightness or fullness, palpitation, cyanosis, dyspnea on exertion (specify amount of exertion [e.g., walking one flight of stairs, walking from chair to bath, or just talking]), orthopnea, paroxysmal nocturnal dyspnea, nocturia, edema, history of heart murmur, hypertension, coronary heart disease, anemia.

Vigorously pursue all vague chest pain similarities. Consider a woman with fatigue or vague indigestion as a cardiac patient until proven otherwise.

Health Promotion. Date of last ECG or other cardiac tests, cholesterol screening.

Peripheral Vascular. Coldness, numbness and tingling, swelling of legs (time of day, activity), discoloration in hands or feet (bluish red, pallor, mottling, associated with position, especially around feet and ankles), varicose veins or complications, intermittent claudication, thrombophlebitis, ulcers.

Health Promotion. Does the work involve long-term sitting or standing? Does the patient frequently cross his or her legs at the knees? Wear support hose?

Gastrointestinal. Appetite, food intolerance, dysphagia, heartburn, indigestion, pain (associated with eating), other abdominal pain, pyrosis (esophageal and stomach burning sensation with sour eructation), nausea and vomiting (character), vomiting blood, history of abdominal disease (liver or gallbladder, ulcer, jaundice, appendicitis, colitis), flatulence, frequency of bowel movement, any recent change, stool characteristics, constipation or diarrhea, black stools, rectal bleeding, rectal conditions (hemorrhoids, fistula).

Health Promotion. Use of antacids or laxatives. (Alternatively, diet history and substance habits can be placed here.)

Urinary System. Frequency, urgency, nocturia (the number of times the person awakens at night to urinate, recent change); dysuria; polyuria or oliguria; hesitancy or straining, narrowed stream; urine color (cloudy or presence of hematuria); incontinence; history of urinary disease (kidney disease, kidney stones, urinary tract infections, prostate); pain in flank, groin, suprapubic region, or low back.

Health Promotion. Measures to avoid or treat urinary tract infections, use of Kegel exercises after childbirth.

Male Genital System. Penis or testicular pain, sores or lesions, penile discharge, lumps, hernia.

Health Promotion. Perform testicular self-examination? How frequently?

Female Genital System. Menstrual history (age at menarche, last menstrual period, cycle and duration, any amenorrhea or menorrhagia, premenstrual pain or dysmenorrhea, intermenstrual spotting), vaginal itching, discharge and its characteristics, age at menopause, menopausal signs or symptoms, postmenopausal bleeding.

Health Promotion. Last gynecologic checkup and last Pap test.

Sexual Health. Begin with: "I ask all patients about their sexual health." Then ask: "Are you presently in a relationship involving intercourse? Are the aspects of sex satisfactory to you and your partner? Are condoms used routinely (if applicable)? Is there any dyspareunia (for female) or are there any changes in erection or ejaculation (for male)? Are contraceptives used (if applicable)? Is the contraceptive method satisfactory? Are you aware of contact with a partner who has any sexually transmitted infection (chlamydia, gonorrhea, herpes, venereal warts, HIV/acquired immunodeficiency syndrome [AIDS], or syphilis)?"

Musculoskeletal System. History of arthritis or gout. In the joints: Pain, stiffness, swelling (location, migratory nature), deformity, limitation of motion, noise with joint motion? In the muscles: Any muscle pain, cramps, weakness, gait problems, or problems with coordinated activities? In the back: Any pain (location and radiation to extremities), stiffness, limitation of motion, or history of back pain or disc disease? Any recent injuries to the joints, muscles, or back? (Fig. 4.7)

Health Promotion. How much walking per day? What is the effect of limited range of motion on ADLs such as grooming, feeding, toileting, dressing? Are any mobility aids used?

Neurologic System. History of seizure disorder, stroke, fainting, blackouts. Motor function: Weakness, tic or tremor, paralysis, or coordination problems? Sensory function: Numbness, tingling (paresthesia)? Cognitive function: Memory disorder (recent or distant, disorientation)? Mental status: Any nervousness, mood change, depression, or history of mental health dysfunction or hallucinations? Conduct suicide screening on all patients. See p. 61 for adolescent screening and p. 70 in Chapter 5 for full description.

Health Promotion. Alternatively, data about interpersonal relationships and coping patterns are placed here.

Hematologic System. Bleeding tendency of skin or mucous membranes, excessive bruising, lymph node swelling, exposure to toxic agents or radiation, blood transfusion and reactions.

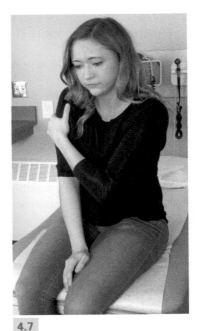

4.7

Endocrine System. History of diabetes or diabetic symptoms (polyuria, polydipsia, polyphagia), history of thyroid disease, intolerance to heat and cold, change in skin pigmentation or texture, excessive sweating, relationship between appetite and weight, abnormal hair distribution, nervousness, tremors, and need for hormone therapy.

Functional Assessment (Including Activities of Daily Living)

Functional assessment measures a person's self-care ability in the areas of general physical health; ADLs such as bathing, dressing, toileting, eating, walking; instrumental ADLs or those needed for independent living such as housekeeping, shopping, cooking, doing laundry, using the telephone, managing finances; nutrition; social relationships and resources; self-concept and coping; and home environment.

Functional assessment instruments may be used to objectively measure the person's present functional status and monitor changes over time (see Chapter 32 for more information).

Functional assessment questions listed here provide data on the lifestyle and type of living environment to which the person is accustomed. Because the person may consider these questions "private," they are best asked later in the interview after rapport is established.

Self-Esteem, Self-Concept. Education (last grade completed, other significant training), financial status (income adequate for lifestyle and/or health concerns), value-belief system (religious practices and perception of personal strengths).

Activity/Exercise. A daily profile reflecting usual daily activities. Ask, "Tell me how you spend a typical day." Note ability to perform ADLs: independent or needs assistance with feeding, bathing, hygiene, dressing, toileting, bed-to-chair transfer, walking, standing, or climbing stairs. Is there any use of a wheelchair, prostheses, or mobility aids?

Record leisure activities enjoyed and the exercise pattern (type, amount per day or week, method of warm-up session, method of monitoring the response of the body to exercise).

Sleep/Rest. Sleep patterns, daytime naps, any sleep aids used.

Nutrition/Elimination. Record the diet by a recall of all food and beverages taken over the past 24 hours. Ask, "Is that menu typical of most days?" Describe eating habits and current appetite. Ask, "Who buys food and prepares food? Are your finances adequate for food? Who is present at mealtimes?" Indicate any food allergy or intolerance. Record daily intake of caffeine (coffee, tea, cola drinks).

Ask about usual pattern of bowel elimination and urinating, including problems with mobility or transfer in toileting, continence, use of laxatives.

Interpersonal Relationships/Resources. Social roles: Ask, "How would you describe your role in the family? How would you say you get along with family, friends, and co-workers?" Ask about support systems composed of family and significant others: "To whom could you go for support with a problem at work, with your health, or a personal problem?" Include contact with spouse or partner, siblings, parents, children, friends, organizations, workplace. "Is time spent alone pleasurable and relaxing, or is it isolating?" (See Fig. 4.8.)

Spiritual Resources. Many people believe in a relationship between spirituality and health, and they may wish to have spiritual matters addressed in the traditional health care setting. Use the Faith, Influence, Community, and Address (FICA) questions to incorporate the person's spiritual values into the health history.[10] *Faith:* "Does religious faith or spirituality play an important part in your life? Do you consider yourself to be a religious or spiritual person?" *Influence:* "How does your religious faith or spirituality influence the way you think about your health or care for yourself?" *Community:* "Are you a part of any religious or spiritual community or congregation?" *Address:* "Would you like me to address any religious or spiritual issues or concerns with you?" See Chapter 2 for more information.

Coping and Stress Management. Types of stresses in life, especially in the past year; any change in lifestyle or any current stress; methods tried to relieve stress and whether these have been helpful.

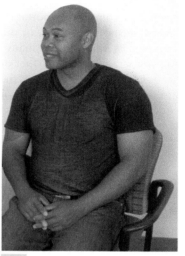

4.8

Personal Habits. Tobacco, alcohol, street drugs: Ask, "Do you smoke cigarettes (pipe, use chewing tobacco)? At what age did you start? How many packs do you smoke per day? How many years have you smoked?" Record the number of packs smoked per day (PPD) and duration (e.g., 1 PPD × 5 years). Then ask, "Have you ever tried to quit?" and "How did it go?" to introduce plans about smoking cessation.

Alcohol. Health care professionals often fail to question about alcohol unless problems are obvious. However, alcohol interacts adversely with all medications; is a factor in many social problems such as assaults, rapes, high-risk sexual behavior, and child abuse; contributes to half of all fatal traffic accidents; and accounts for 5% of all deaths in the United States. The latter figure is actually an underestimate because alcohol-related conditions are underreported on death certificates.

Therefore be alert to early signs of hazardous alcohol use. Ask whether the person drinks alcohol. If yes, ask specific questions about the amount and frequency of alcohol use: Ask, "When was your last drink of alcohol? How much did you drink that time? In the past 30 days, about how many days would you say that you drank alcohol? Has anyone ever said that you had a drinking problem?"

You may wish to use a screening questionnaire to identify excessive or uncontrolled drinking such as the **C**ut down, **A**nnoyed, **G**uilty, and **E**ye-opener (**CAGE**) test[6]:

- Have you ever thought you should **C**ut down your drinking?
- Have you ever been **A**nnoyed by criticism of your drinking?
- Have you ever felt **G**uilty about your drinking?
- Do you drink in the morning (i.e., an **E**ye opener)?

If the person answers "yes" to two or more CAGE questions, you should suspect alcohol abuse and continue with a more complete substance-abuse assessment (see Chapter 6, p. 90). If the person answers "no" to drinking alcohol, ask the reason for this decision (psychosocial, legal, health). Any history of alcohol treatment? Involved in recovery activities? History of a family member with problem drinking?

Illicit or Street Drugs. Ask specifically about prescription painkillers such as OxyContin or Norco, cocaine, crack cocaine, amphetamines, heroin, and marijuana. Indicate frequency of use and how use has affected work or family.

Environment/Hazards. Housing and neighborhood (living alone, knowledge of neighbors), safety of area, adequate heat and utilities, access to transportation, and involvement in community services (Fig. 4.9). Note environmental health, including hazards in workplace, hazards at home, use of seatbelts, geographic or occupational exposures, and travel or residence in other countries, including time spent abroad during military service.

Intimate Partner Violence. Begin with open-ended questions: "How are things at home?" and "Do you feel safe?" These are valuable initial screening questions because some people may not recognize that they are in abusive situations or may be reluctant to admit it because of guilt, fear, shame, or denial. If the person responds to feeling unsafe, follow up with closed-ended questions: "Have you ever been emotionally or physically abused by your partner or someone important to you? Within the past year, have you been hit, slapped, kicked, pushed, or shoved or otherwise physically hurt by your partner or ex-partner?" If yes, ask: "By whom? How many times? Does your partner ever force you into having sex? Are you afraid of your partner or ex-partner?" See Chapter 7 for more information.

Occupational Health. Ask the person to describe his or her job. Ever worked with any health hazard such as asbestos, inhalants, chemicals, repetitive motion? Wear any protective equipment? Any work programs in place that monitor exposure? Aware of any health problems now that may be related to work exposure?

Note the timing of the reason for seeking care and whether it may be related to change in work or home activities, job titles, or exposure history. Take a careful smoking history, which may contribute to occupational hazards. Finally ask the person what he or she likes or dislikes about the job.

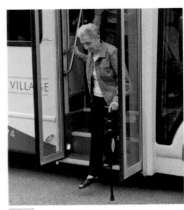

4.9

Perception of Health

Ask the person questions such as: "How do you define health? How do you view your situation now? What are your concerns? What do you think will happen in the future? What are your health goals? What do you expect from us as nurses or physicians (or other health care providers)?"

❖ DEVELOPMENTAL COMPETENCE

Children

The health history is adapted to include information specific for the age and developmental stage of the child (e.g., the mother's health during pregnancy, labor and delivery, the perinatal period, and the family unit) (Fig. 4.10). Note that the developmental history and nutritional data are listed as separate sections because of their importance for current health.

Biographic Data

Include the child's name, nickname, address and phone number, parents'/caregivers' names and work numbers, child's age and birth date, birthplace, sex, race, ethnic origin, and information about other children and family members at home.

Source of History

1. Person providing information and relation to child
2. Your impression of reliability of information
3. Any special circumstances (e.g., the use of an interpreter)

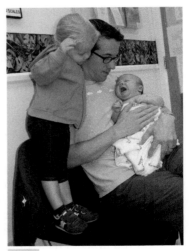

4.10

Reason for Seeking Care

Record the parent's/caregivers' spontaneous statement. Because of the frequency of well-child visits for routine health care, there will be more reasons such as "time for the child's checkup" or "she needs the next shot." Reasons for health problems may be initiated by the child, the parent/caregiver, or a third party such as a classroom teacher or social worker.

Sometimes the reason stated may not be the real reason for the visit. A parent/caregiver may have a "hidden agenda," such as the mother who brought her 4-year-old child in because "she looked pale." Further questioning revealed that the mother had heard recently from a former college friend whose 4-year-old child had just been diagnosed with leukemia.

Present Health or History of Present Illness

If the parent/caregiver or child seeks routine health care, include a statement about the usual health of the child and any common health problems or major health concerns.

Describe any presenting symptom or sign, using the same format as for the adult. Some additional considerations include:

- Severity of pain: "How does your child behave when he or she is in pain?" (e.g., pulling at ears alerts parent/caregiver to ear pain). Note the effect of pain on usual behavior (e.g., does it stop child from playing?).
- Associated factors such as relation to activity, eating, and body position.
- The parent's/caregiver's intuitive sense of a problem. As the constant caregiver, this intuitive sense is very accurate. Even if proved otherwise, this factor gives you an idea of the parent's/caregiver's area of concern.
- Parent's/caregiver's coping ability and reaction of other family members to child's symptoms or illness.

Past Health

Prenatal Status. Start with an open-ended question: "Tell me about this pregnancy." Then ask: "How was this pregnancy spaced? Was it planned? What was the mother's attitude toward the pregnancy? What was the partner's attitude? Was there prenatal care? At what month was prenatal care started? What was the mother's health during pregnancy? Were there any complications (bleeding, excessive nausea and vomiting, unusual weight gain, high blood pressure, swelling of hands and feet, falls, infections—rubella or sexually transmitted infections)? During which month were diet and medications prescribed and/or taken during pregnancy (dose and duration)?" Record the mother's use of alcohol, street drugs, or cigarettes and any radiographic studies taken during pregnancy.

Labor and Delivery. Parity of the mother, duration of the pregnancy, name of the hospital, course and duration of labor, use of anesthesia, type of delivery (vertex, breech, cesarean section), birth weight, Apgar scores, onset of breathing, any cyanosis, need for resuscitation, and use of special equipment or procedures.

Postnatal Status. Any problems in the nursery, length of hospital stay, neonatal jaundice, whether the baby was discharged with the mother, whether the baby was breastfed or bottle-fed, weight gain, any feeding problems, "blue spells," colic, diarrhea, patterns of crying and sleeping, the mother's health postpartum, the mother's reaction to the baby (Fig. 4.11), placement on back when sleeping.

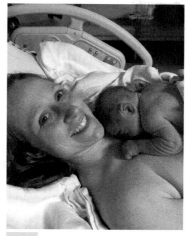
4.11

Childhood Illnesses. Age and any complications of measles, mumps, rubella, chickenpox, whooping cough, strep throat, and frequent ear infections; any recent exposure to illness.

Serious Accidents or Injuries. Age of occurrence, extent of injury, how the child was treated, and complications of auto accidents, falls, head injuries, fractures, burns, and poisonings.

Serious or Chronic Illnesses. Age of onset, how the child was treated, and complications of meningitis or encephalitis; seizure disorders; asthma, pneumonia, and other chronic lung conditions; rheumatic fever; scarlet fever; diabetes; kidney problems; sickle cell anemia; high blood pressure; and allergies.

Operations or Hospitalizations. Reason for care, age at admission, name of surgeon or primary care providers, name of hospital, duration of stay, how child reacted to hospitalization, any complications. (If child reacted poorly, he or she may be afraid now and will need special preparation for the examination that is to follow.)

Immunizations. Age when administered, date administered, and any reactions following immunizations (Fig. 4.12). Because of outbreaks of measles across the United States, the American Academy of Pediatrics recommends two doses of the measles-mumps-rubella vaccine, one at 12 to 15 months and one at age 4 to 6 years.[4]

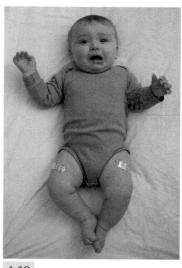
4.12

Pertussis (whooping cough) is on the rise, with periodic epidemics every 3 to 5 years.[12] The young infant is at high risk because of an immature immune system and because the schedule for the vaccination does not start until 6 to 8 weeks of age. The CDC recommends the *cocooning strategy*, which is the vaccination of parents/caregivers and others in close contact with the baby. Cocooning may prevent approximately 20% of infant pertussis cases; however, it does not prevent transmission from adults outside the home. In addition to cocooning, recommendations include immunization of the mother during the third trimester of pregnancy. Transplacental transfer of antibodies helps protect newborns until their first vaccine is given.[12]

The CDC recommends routine immunizations to protect against 15 childhood and adolescent diseases and cancers.[4] The impact of routine immunizations in the United States is enormous: more than 732,000 children's lives saved and over 322 million hospitalizations prevented in the past 20 years.[2] Yet many children are underimmunized: those living in poverty, children in certain ethnic subgroups, and even children of attentive parents/caregivers who gain misinformation from the Internet and have unwarranted concerns about vaccines. You should acknowledge these parents'/caregivers' concerns in a respectful way, yet teach the scientific basis of immunizations.[5]

Allergies. Any drugs, foods, contact agents, and environmental agents to which the child is allergic and the reaction to the allergens. A true *food allergy* is an immune response caused by exposure to a food substance. Common pediatric food allergies include cow's milk, eggs, peanuts, tree nuts, soybean, and fish. A true food allergy can be life threatening but should be differentiated from a *food intolerance*, which causes distress and illness yet is a nonimmunologic response and not life threatening.[13] Also note allergic reactions particularly common in childhood, such as allergic rhinitis, insect hypersensitivity, eczema, and urticaria.

Medications. Any prescription and OTC medications (or vitamins) that the child takes, including the dosage, daily schedule, why the medication is given, and any problems.

Developmental History

Growth. Height and weight at birth and at 1, 2, 5, and 10 years; any periods of rapid gain or loss (Fig. 4.13); process of dentition (age of tooth eruption and pattern of loss).

Milestones. Age when child first held head erect, rolled over, sat alone, walked alone, cut his or her first tooth, said his or her first words with meaning, spoke in sentences, was toilet trained, tied shoes, dressed without help. Does the parent/caregiver believe this development has been normal? How does this child's development compare with that of siblings or peers?

Current Development (Children 1 Month Through Preschool). Gross motor skills (rolls over, sits alone, walks alone, skips, climbs), fine motor skills (inspects hands, brings hands to mouth, has pincer grasp, stacks blocks, feeds self, uses crayon to draw, uses scissors), language skills (vocalizes, first words with meaning, sentences, persistence of baby talk, speech problems), and personal-social skills (smiles, tracks movement with eyes to midline, past midline, attends to sound by turning head, recognizes own name). If the child is undergoing toilet training, indicate the method used, age of bladder/bowel control, parents'/caregivers' attitude toward toilet training, and terms used for toileting.

School-Age Child. Gross motor skills (runs, jumps, climbs, rides bicycle, general coordination), fine motor skills (ties shoelace, uses scissors, writes letters and numbers, draws pictures), and language skills (vocabulary, verbal ability, able to tell time, reading level).

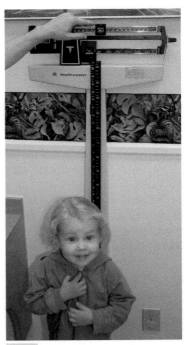

4.13

Nutritional History

The amount of nutritional information needed depends on the child's age; the younger the child, the more detailed and specific the data should be. For the infant, record whether breastfeeding or bottle-feeding. If the child is breastfed, record nursing frequency and duration, any supplements (vitamin, iron, fluoride, bottles), family support for nursing, and age and method of weaning. If the child is bottle-fed, record type of formula used, frequency and amount, any problems with feeding (spitting up, colic, diarrhea), and supplements used; discourage any bottle propping. Record introduction of solid foods (age when the child began eating solids, which foods, whether foods are home or commercially made, amount given, child's reaction to new food, parent's/caregiver's reaction to feeding).

For preschool and school-age children and adolescents, record the child's appetite, 24-hour diet recall (meals, snacks, amounts), vitamins taken, how much junk food is eaten, who eats with the child, food likes and dislikes, and parent's/caregiver's perception of child's nutrition.

A weeklong diary of food intake may be more accurate than a spot 24-hour recall. Also consider cultural practices in assessing child's diet.

Family History

As with the adult, diagram a family tree for the child, including siblings, parents, and grandparents (see p. 48). Ask specifically for the family history of heart disease, high blood pressure, diabetes, blood disorders, cancer, sickle cell anemia, arthritis, allergies, obesity, cystic fibrosis, mental illness, seizure disorder, kidney disease, developmental delay, learning disabilities, birth defects, and sudden infant death. Ask about biological relatives for the genogram. Never assume relationships. Always ask to assure you understand the family dynamic.

Review of Systems

General. Significant gain or loss of weight, failure to gain weight appropriate for age, frequent colds, ear infections, illnesses, energy level, fatigue, overactivity, and behavioral change (irritability, increased crying, nervousness).

Skin. Birthmarks, skin disease, pigment or color change, mottling, change in mole, pruritus, rash, lesion, acne, easy bruising or petechiae, easy bleeding, and changes in hair or nails (Fig. 4.14).

Head. Headache, head injury, dizziness.

Eyes. Strabismus, diplopia, pain, redness, discharge, cataracts, vision changes, reading problems. Is the child able to see the board at school? Does the child sit too close to the television?

Health Promotion. Use of eyeglasses, date of last vision screening.

Ears. Earaches, frequency of ear infections, myringotomy tubes in ears, discharge (characteristics), cerumen, ringing or crackling, and whether parent/caregiver perceives any hearing problems.

Health Promotion. How does the child clean his or her ears?

Nose and Sinuses. Discharge and its characteristics, frequency of colds, nasal stuffiness, nosebleeds, and allergies.

Mouth and Throat. History of cleft lip or palate, frequency of sore throats, toothache, caries, sores in mouth or tongue, tonsils present, mouth breathing, difficulty chewing, difficulty swallowing, and hoarseness or voice change.

Health Promotion. Child's pattern of brushing teeth and last dental checkup.

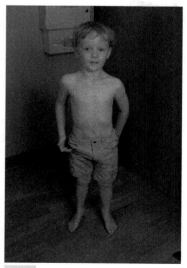

4.14

Neck. Swollen or tender glands, limitation of movement, or stiffness.

Breast. For preadolescent and adolescent girl, when did she notice that her breasts were changing? What is the girl's self-perception of development? Does the female older adolescent perform breast self-examination? (See Chapter 18 for suggested phrasing of questions.)

Respiratory System. Croup or asthma, wheezing or noisy breathing, shortness of breath, chronic cough.

Cardiovascular System. Congenital heart problems, history of murmur, and cyanosis (what prompts this condition). Is there any limitation of activity, or can the child keep up with peers? Is there any dyspnea on exertion, palpitations, high blood pressure, or coldness in the extremities?

Gastrointestinal System. Abdominal pain, nausea and vomiting, history of ulcer, frequency of bowel movements, stool color and characteristics, diarrhea, constipation or stool holding, rectal bleeding, anal itching, history of pinworms, and use of laxatives.

Urinary System. Painful urination, polyuria/oliguria, narrowed stream, urine color (cloudy, dark), history of urinary tract infection, whether toilet trained, when toilet training was planned, any problems, bed-wetting (when the child started, frequency, associated with stress, how child feels about it).

Male Genital System. Penile or testicular pain, whether told if testes are descended, any sores or lesions, discharge, hernia or hydrocele, or swelling in scrotum during crying. Has the preadolescent or adolescent boy noticed any change in the penis and scrotum? Is the boy familiar with normal growth patterns and nocturnal emissions? Screen for sexual abuse. (See Chapter 25 for suggested phrasing of questions.)

Female Genital System. Has the girl noted any genital itching, rash, vaginal discharge? For the preadolescent and adolescent girl, when did menstruation start? Was she prepared? Is the girl familiar with normal development patterns? Screen for sexual abuse. (See Chapter 27 for suggested phrasing of questions.)

Sexual Health. What is the child's attitude toward the opposite sex? Who provides sex education? How does the family deal with sex education, masturbation, dating patterns? Is the adolescent in a relationship involving intercourse? Does he or she have information on birth control and sexually transmitted infections? (See Chapters 25 and 27 for suggested phrasing of questions.)

Musculoskeletal System. In bones and joints: arthritis, joint pain, stiffness, swelling, limitation of movement, gait strength and coordination. In muscles: pain, cramps, and weakness. In the back: pain, posture, spinal curvature, and any treatment. Any recent injuries.

Neurologic System. Numbness and tingling. (Behavioral and cognitive issues are covered in the sections on development and interpersonal relationships.)

Hematologic Systems. Excessive bruising, lymph node swelling, and exposure to toxic agents or radiation.

Endocrine System. History of diabetes or thyroid disease; excessive hunger, thirst, or urinating; abnormal hair distribution; and precocious or delayed puberty.

Functional Assessment (Including Activities of Daily Living)

Interpersonal Relationships. Within the family constellation, record the child's position in family; whether the child is adopted; who lives with the child; who is the primary caregiver; who is the daycare provider if both parents/caregivers work outside the home; any support from relatives, neighbors, or friends; and the ethnic or cultural milieu.

Indicate family cohesion (Fig. 4.15). Does the family enjoy activities as a unit? Has there been a recent family change or crisis (death, divorce, move)? Record information on child's self-image and level of independence. Does the child use a security blanket or toy? Is there any repetitive behavior (bed-rocking, head-banging), pica, thumb-sucking, or nail-biting? Note method of discipline used. Indicate type used at home. How effective is it? Who disciplines the child? Is there any occurrence of negativism, temper tantrums, withdrawal, or aggressive behavior?

Provide information on the child's friends: whether the child makes friends easily. How does the child get along with friends? Does he or she play with same-age or older or younger children?

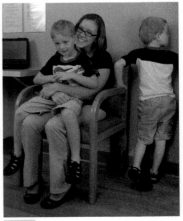

4.15

Activity and Rest. Record the child's play activities. Indicate amount of active and quiet play, outdoor play, time watching television, and special hobbies or activities. Record sleep and rest. Indicate pattern and number of hours at night and during the day and the child's routine at bedtime. Is the child a sound sleeper, or is he or she wakeful? Does the child have nightmares, night terrors, or somnambulation? How does the parent/caregiver respond? Does the child have naps during the day?

Record school attendance. Any experience with daycare or nursery school? In what grade is the child in school? Has the child ever skipped a grade or been held back? Does the child seem to like school? What is his or her school performance? Are the parent/caregiver and child satisfied with the performance? Were days missed in school? Provide a reason for the absence. (These questions give an important index to the child's functioning outside the home.)

Economic Status. Ask about the parents'/caregivers' occupations. Indicate the number of hours each person is away from home. Do parents/caregivers perceive their income to be adequate? What is the effect of illness on financial status?

Home Environment. Where does family live (house, apartment)? Is the size of the home adequate? Is there access to an outdoor play area? Does the child share a room, have his or her own bed, and have toys appropriate for his or her age?

Environmental Hazards. Inquire about home safety (precautions for poisons, medications, household products, presence of gates for stairways, and safe yard equipment). Inquire about the home structure (adequate heating, ventilation, bathroom facilities), neighborhood (residential or industrial, age of neighbors, safe play areas, playmates available, distance to school, amount of traffic, whether area is remote or congested and overcrowded, if crime is a problem, presence of air or water pollution), and automobile (child safety seat, seatbelts).

Coping/Stress Management. Is the child able to adapt to new situations? Record recent stressful experiences (death, divorce, move, loss of special friend). How does the child cope with stress? Any recent change in behavior or mood? Has counseling ever been sought?

Habits. Has the child ever tried cigarette smoking? How much did he or she smoke? Has the child ever tried alcohol? How much alcohol did he or she drink weekly or daily? Has the child ever tried other drugs (marijuana, cocaine, amphetamines, barbiturates)?

Health Promotion. Who is the primary health care provider? When was the child's last checkup? Who is the dental care provider and when was the last dental checkup? Provide date and result of screening for vision, hearing, urinalysis, phenylketonuria, hematocrit, TB skin test, sickle cell trait, blood lead, and other tests specific for high-risk populations.

The Adolescent

This section presents a psychosocial review of symptoms intended to maximize communication with youth. The **HEEADSSS** method of interviewing focuses on assessment of the Home environment, Education and employment, Eating, peer-related Activities, Drugs, Sexuality, Suicide/depression, and Safety from injury and violence (Fig. 4.16). The tool minimizes adolescent stress because it moves from expected and less-threatening questions to those that are more personal.[8] Interview the youth alone while the parent/caregiver waits outside and fills out past health questionnaires.

In addition ask, "How many hours of sleep do you get on most nights of the week? What time do you actually go to bed? What time do you wake up on school days? What time would you wake up if left alone? Which activities are you in at school or after school? Do your activities change the time that you go to bed or get up in the morning?"[7] Note that teens need about 9 hours of sleep per night, yet most U.S. teens get far less than that. Older teens report <6.5 to 7 hours per night; younger teens report 7.7 hours per night.[7]

Ask about driving; stress the importance of keeping hands on the wheel and paying attention to the road. Evidence shows the risk of crash increases significantly among novice drivers when they perform secondary tasks (e.g., dialing or reaching for a cell phone, texting, eating, reaching for another object, looking at a roadside object).[1]

The HEEADSSS psychosocial interview for adolescents

	Potential first-line questions	Questions if time permits or if situation warrants exploration
Home	Who lives with you? Where do you live? What are relationships like at home? Can you talk to anyone at home about stress? (Who?) Is there anyone new at home? Has someone left recently? Do you have a smart phone or computer at home? In your room? What do you use it for? (May ask this in the activities section.)	Have you moved recently? Have you ever had to live away from home? (Why?) Have you ever run away? (Why?) Is there any physical violence at home?
Education and employment	Tell me about school. Is your school a safe place? (Why?) Have you been bullied at school? Do you feel connected to your school? Do you feel as if you belong? Are there adults at school you feel you could talk to about something important? (Who?) Do you have any failing grades? Any recent changes? What are your future education/employment plans/goals? Are you working? Where? How much?	How many days have you missed from school this month/quarter/semester? Have you changed schools in the past few years? Tell me about your friends at school. Have you ever had to repeat a class/grade? Have you ever been suspended? Expelled? Have you ever considered dropping out? How well do you get along with the people at school? Work? Have your responsibilities at work increased? What are your favorite subjects at school? Your least favorite subjects?
Eating	Does your weight or body shape cause you any stress? If so, tell me about it. Have there been any recent changes in your weight? Have you dieted in the last year? How? How often?	What do you like and not like about your body? Have you done anything else to try to manage your weight? Tell me about your exercise routine. What do you think would be a healthy diet? How does that compare to your current eating patterns? What would it be like if you gained (lost) 10 lb? Does it ever seem as though your eating is out of control? Have you ever taken diet pills?
Activities	What do you do for fun? How do you spend time with friends? Family? (With whom, where, when?) Some teenagers tell me that they spend much of their free time online. What types of things do you use the Internet for? How many hours do you spend on any given day in front of a screen, such as a computer, TV, or phone? Do you wish you spent less time on these things?	Do you participate in any sports? Do you regularly attend religious or spiritual activities? Have you messaged photos or texts that you have later regretted? Can you think of a friend who was harmed by spending time online? How often do you view pornography (or nude images or videos) online? What types of books do you read for fun? How do you feel after playing video games? What music do you like to listen to?
Drugs	Do any of your friends or family members use tobacco? Alcohol? Other drugs? Do you use tobacco or electronic cigarettes? Alcohol? Other drugs, energy drinks, steroids, or medications not prescribed to you?	Is there any history of alcohol or drug problems in your family? Does anyone at home use tobacco? Do you ever drink or use drugs when you're alone? (Assess frequency, intensity, patterns of use or abuse, and how patient obtains or pays for drugs, alcohol, or tobacco.)

4.16

(Klein et al., 2014.)

	Potential first-line questions	Questions if time permits or if situation warrants exploration
Sexuality	Have you ever been in a romantic relationship? Tell me about the people that you've dated. Have any of your relationships ever been sexual relationships (such as involving kissing or touching)? Are you attracted to anyone now? OR: Tell me about your sexual life. Are you interested in boys? Girls? Both? Not yet sure?	Are your sexual activities enjoyable? Have any of your relationships been violent? What does the term "safer sex" mean to you? Have you ever sent unclothed pictures of yourself on e-mail or the Internet? Have you ever been forced or pressured into doing something sexual that you didn't want to do? Have you ever been touched sexually in a way that you didn't want? Have you ever been raped, on a date or any other time? How many sexual partners have you had altogether? (Girls) Have you ever been pregnant or worried that you may be pregnant? (Boys) Have you ever gotten someone pregnant or worried that might have happened? What are you using for birth control? Are you satisfied with your method? Do you use condoms every time you have intercourse? What gets in the way? Have you ever had a sexually transmitted infection or worried that you had an infection?
Suicide/ depression	Do you feel "stressed" or anxious more than usual (or more than you prefer to feel)? Do you feel sad or down more than usual? Are you "bored" much of the time? Are you having trouble getting to sleep? Have you thought a lot about hurting yourself or someone else? Tell me about a time when someone picked on you or made you feel uncomfortable online. (Consider the PHQ-2 screening tool to supplement.)	Tell me about a time when you felt sad while using social media sites like Facebook. Does it seem that you've lost interest in things that you used to really enjoy? Do you find yourself spending less time with friends? Would you rather just be by yourself most of the time? Have you ever tried to kill yourself? Have you ever had to hurt yourself (by cutting yourself, for example) to calm down or feel better? Have you started using alcohol or drugs to help you relax, calm down, or feel better?
Safety	Have you ever been seriously injured? (How?) How about anyone else you know? Do you always wear a seatbelt in the car? Have you ever met in person (or plan to meet) with anyone whom you first encountered online? When was the last time you sent a text message while driving? Tell me about a time when you have ridden with a driver who was drunk or high. When? How often? Is there a lot of violence at your home or school? In your neighborhood? Among your friends?	Do you use safety equipment for sports and/or other physical activities (for example, helmets for biking or skateboarding)? Have you ever been in a car or motorcycle accident? (What happened?) Have you ever been picked on or bullied? Is that still a problem? Have you gotten into physical fights in school or your neighborhood? Are you still getting into fights? Have you ever felt that you had to carry a knife, gun, or other weapon to protect yourself? Do you still feel that way? Have you ever been incarcerated?

Abbreviations: *HEEADSSS*, Home, Education and employment, Eating, Activities, Drugs, Sexuality, Suicide/depression, Safety; *PHQ-2*, Patient Health Questionnaire 2.

4.16, cont'd

REFERENCES

1. Adeola, R., Omorogbe, A., & Johnson, A. (2016). Get the message: A teen distracted driving program. *J Trauma Nurs, 23*(6), 312–320.
2. Centers for Disease Control and Prevention. (2014). *Report shows 20-year US immunization program spares millions of children from diseases.* https://www.cdc.gov/media/releases/2014/p0424-immunization-program.html.
3. Centers for Disease Control and Prevention. (2017). *Gay and bisexual men's health.* https://www.cdc.gov/msmhealth/for-your-health.htm.
4. Centers for Disease Control and Prevention (CDC). (2017). *Immunization schedules for health care professionals.* http://www.cdc.gov/vaccines/schedules/index.html.
5. Centers for Disease Control and Prevention. (2018). *Recommended immunization schedule for adults aged 19 years or older, United States 2018.* https://www.cdc.gov/vaccines/schedules/hcp/adult.html.
6. Ewing, J. A. (1984). Detecting alcoholism: The CAGE questionnaire. *JAMA, 252,* 1905–1907.
7. George, N. M., & Davis, J. E. (2013). Assessing sleep in adolescents through a better understanding of sleep physiology. *Am J Nurs, 113*(6), 26–32.
8. Klein, D. A., Goldenring, J. M., & Adelman, W. P. (2014). *HEEADSSS 3.0: The psychosocial interview for adolescents updated for a new century fueled by media.* Contemporary pediatrics. http://contemporarypediatrics.modernmedicine.com/contemporary-pediatrics/content/tags/adolescent-medicine/heeadsss-30-psychosocial-interview-adolesce?page=0,1.
9. Lehne, R. A. (2016). *Pharmacology for nursing care* (9th ed.). St. Louis: Elsevier.
10. Post, S. G., Puchalski, C. M., Larson, D. B., et al. (2000). Physician and patient spirituality: Professional boundaries, competency, and ethics. *Ann Intern Med, 132,* 578–583.
11. Rose, A. J., Fischer, S. H., & Paasche-Orlow, M. K. (2017). Beyond medication reconciliation: The correct medication list. *JAMA, 317*(20), 2057–2058.
12. Suryadevara, M., & Domachowske, J. B. (2015). Prevention of pertussis through adult vaccination. *Hum Vaccin Immunother, 11*(7), 1744–1747.
13. Turnbull, J. L., Adams, H. N., & Gorard, D. A. (2015). Review article: The diagnosis and management of food allergy and food intolerances. *Aliment Pharmacol Ther, 41*(1), 3–25.

CHAPTER 5

Mental Status Assessment

STRUCTURE AND FUNCTION

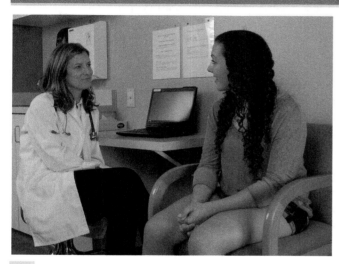

5.1

DEFINING MENTAL STATUS

Mental status is a person's emotional (feeling) and cognitive (knowing) function. Optimal functioning aims toward simultaneous life satisfaction in work, in caring relationships, and within the self (Fig. 5.1). Mental health is "a state of well-being in which every individual realizes his or her own potential, can cope with normal stresses of life, can work productively and fruitfully, and is able to make a contribution to her or his community."[27] Mental health is relative and ongoing. We all have days when we feel anxious or depressed or feel as if we cannot cope. Usually these feelings dissipate and we return to healthy function socially and occupationally.

The stress surrounding a traumatic life event (death of a loved one, serious illness) tips the balance, causing transient dysfunction. This is an expected response to a trauma. For example, bereavement may lead to someone feeling down or depressed, but is an expected emotional response to a major loss and does not usually induce a major depressive episode.[1] Most grieving people feel sadness, tearfulness, loss of appetite, and insomnia; these feelings last 2 to 6 months. The survivor needs social support but no medical treatment. Mental status assessment during a traumatic life event can identify remaining strengths and help the individual mobilize resources and use coping skills.

A **mental disorder** is apparent when a person's response is much greater than the expected reaction to a traumatic life event. It is a clinically significant behavioral, emotional, or cognitive *syndrome* that is associated with significant distress (a painful symptom) or disability (impaired functioning) involving social, occupational, or key activities.[1] For example, major depression is characterized by feelings that are unrelenting or include delusional or suicidal thinking, feelings of low self-esteem or worthlessness, or loss of ability to function.[1]

Mental disorders include **organic disorders** (caused by brain disease of *known* specific organic cause [e.g., delirium, dementia, alcohol and drug intoxication, and withdrawal]) and **psychiatric mental disorders** (in which an organic etiology has not yet been established [e.g., anxiety disorder or schizophrenia]). Mental status assessment documents a dysfunction and determines how that dysfunction affects self-care in everyday life.

Mental status cannot be scrutinized directly like the characteristics of skin or heart sounds. Its functioning is *inferred* through assessment of an individual's behaviors:

Consciousness: Being aware of one's own existence, feelings, and thoughts and of the environment. This is the most elementary of mental status functions.

Language: Using the voice to communicate one's thoughts and feelings. This is a basic tool of humans, and its loss has a heavy social impact on the individual.

Mood and affect: Both of these elements deal with the prevailing feelings. **Affect** is a temporary expression of feelings or state of mind, and **mood** is more durable, a prolonged display of feelings that color the whole emotional life.

Orientation: The awareness of the objective world in relation to the self, including person, place, and time.

Attention: The power of concentration, the ability to focus on one specific thing without being distracted by many environmental stimuli.

Memory: The ability to lay down and store experiences and perceptions for later recall. *Recent* memory evokes day-to-day events; *remote* memory brings up years' worth of experiences.

Abstract reasoning: Pondering a deeper meaning beyond the concrete and literal.

Thought process: The *way* a person thinks; the logical train of thought.

Thought content: *What* the person thinks—specific ideas, beliefs, the use of words.

Perceptions: An awareness of objects through the five senses.

❖ DEVELOPMENTAL COMPETENCE

Infants and Children

Emotional and cognitive functioning mature progressively from simple reflex behavior into complex logical and abstract thought. It is difficult to separate and trace the development of just one aspect of mental status. All aspects are interdependent. For example, consciousness is rudimentary at birth because the cerebral cortex is not yet developed; the infant cannot distinguish the self from the mother's body. Consciousness gradually develops along with language so that, by 18 to 24 months, the child learns that he or she is separate from objects in the environment and has words to express this. We also can trace language development: from the differentiated crying at 4 weeks, the cooing at 6 weeks, through one-word sentences at 1 year, to multiword sentences at 2 years. The concept of language as a social tool of communication occurs around 4 to 5 years of age, coincident with the child's readiness to play cooperatively with other children.

Attention gradually increases in span through preschool years so that by school age most children are able to sit and concentrate on their work for a period of time. Some children are late in developing concentration. School readiness coincides with the development of the thought process; around age 7 years thinking becomes more logical and systematic, and the child is able to reason and understand. Abstract thinking, the ability to consider a hypothetical situation, usually develops between ages 12 and 15 years, although a few adolescents never achieve it.

An estimated 1 in 7 children (14%) ages 2 to 8 years has a mental, behavioral, or developmental disorder, and that number increases to 1 in 5 (20%) for children and adolescents ages 9 to 17 years.[3] A childhood mental disorder is one that is diagnosed and begins in childhood (e.g., attention-deficit/hyperactivity disorder [ADHD], behavioral or conduct problems, anxiety, depression, autism spectrum disorders). Adolescents ages 12 to 17 years also experience illicit drug use or alcohol use disorder and cigarette dependence. Substance abuse disorders and cigarette dependence may present as changes in how children learn, behave, or handle emotions.[3]

Substance use disorders can interact with other factors, resulting in suicide, the second leading cause of death among adolescents ages 12 to 17 years.[3] Youth suicides are nearly twice as high in rural as compared to urban areas. Although the reason is unclear, potential causes include limited access to mental health services, increased access to firearms, increased social isolation, and increased economic hardships in rural areas. To address the urban-rural suicide disparity, increased access and acceptability of mental health services are imperative.[7] Although mental health is a prevalent problem among children and adolescents, only 15% to 25% of children receive the specialty care needed to treat their psychiatric illness.[24]

The Aging Adult

The aging process leaves the parameters of mental status mostly intact. There is no decrease in general knowledge and little or no loss in vocabulary. Response time is slower than in youth; it takes a bit longer for the brain to process information and to react to it. Thus performance on timed intelligence tests may be lower for the aging person—not because intelligence has declined, but because it takes longer to respond to the questions. The slower response time affects new learning; if a new presentation is rapidly paced, the older person does not have time to respond to it.[20]

Recent memory, which requires some processing (e.g., medication instructions, 24-hour diet recall, names of new acquaintances), is somewhat decreased with aging. Remote memory is not affected.

Age-related changes in sensory perception can affect mental status. For example, vision loss (as detailed in Chapter 15) may result in apathy, social isolation, and depression. Hearing changes are common in older adults (see the discussion of presbycusis in Chapter 16). Age-related hearing loss involves high-frequency sounds. Consonants are high-frequency sounds; therefore, older people who have difficulty hearing them have problems with normal conversation. This problem produces frustration, suspicion, and social isolation and may make the person look confused.

The era of older adulthood contains more potential for loss (e.g., loss of loved ones, job status and prestige, income, and an energetic and resilient body) than do earlier eras. In addition, living with chronic diseases (e.g., heart failure, cancer, diabetes, osteoporosis) may increase the fear of loss of independence or of death. The grief and despair surrounding these losses can affect mental status. The losses can result in disorientation, disability, or depression.

In a given year mental disorders affect an estimated 18.3% of U.S. adults ages 18 years and older. A smaller group, approximately 4.2%, suffers from a serious mental illness.[15] The global impact of mental illness is enormous, with an estimated 14.3% of deaths worldwide being attributed to mental illness.[25] The problem is lack of access to good-quality mental health services, both in the United States for poor, homeless, uninsured, or underinsured people and in the rest of the world for low- and middle-income countries. An estimated 76% to 85% of people with mental illness in low- and middle-income countries and 35% to 50% of people with mental illness in high-income countries receive no treatment.[26]

COMPONENTS OF THE MENTAL STATUS EXAMINATION

The full mental status examination is a systematic check of emotional and cognitive functioning. However, the steps described here rarely need to be taken in their entirety. Usually you can assess mental status through the context of the health history interview. During that time keep in mind the four main headings of mental status assessment:

**Appearance, Behavior, Cognition,
and Thought processes, or
A, B, C, T**

Integrating the mental status examination into the health history interview is sufficient for most people. You will collect ample data to be able to assess mental health strengths and coping skills and to screen for any dysfunction.

It is necessary to perform a full mental status examination when you discover any abnormality in affect or behavior and in the following situations:

- Patients whose initial brief screening suggests an anxiety disorder or depression.
- Family members concerned about a person's behavioral changes such as memory loss or inappropriate social interaction.
- Report of relevant organic behavioral symptoms, including bizarre behavior (e.g., nocturnal wandering), concentration problems, trouble with simple activities such as using the television remote, inappropriate judgment, or linguistic difficulty.
- Brain lesions (trauma, tumor, stroke). A mental status assessment documents any emotional or cognitive change associated with the lesion. Not recognizing these changes hinders care planning and creates problems with social readjustment.
- Aphasia (the impairment of language ability secondary to brain damage). A mental status examination assesses language dysfunction and any emotional problems associated with it, such as depression or agitation.

- Symptoms of psychiatric mental illness, especially with acute onset.

In every mental status examination, note these factors from the health history that could affect your interpretation of the findings:

- Any known illnesses or health problems such as alcohol use disorders or chronic renal disease.
- Current medications with side effects that may cause confusion or depression.
- The usual educational and behavioral level—note that factor as the normal baseline, and do not expect performance on the mental status examination to exceed it.
- Responses to personal history questions indicating current stress, social interaction patterns, sleep habits, drug and alcohol use.

In the following examination the sequence of steps forms a *hierarchy* in which the most basic functions (consciousness, language) are assessed first. The first steps must be assessed accurately to ensure validity for the steps to follow (i.e., if consciousness is clouded, the person cannot be expected to have full attention and to cooperate with new learning). Or if language is impaired, subsequent assessment of new learning or abstract reasoning (anything that requires language functioning) can give erroneous conclusions.

OBJECTIVE DATA

EQUIPMENT NEEDED
(Occasionally)
Pencil, paper, reading material

Normal Range of Findings	Abnormal Findings
Appearance	
Posture. *Posture* is erect, and *position* is relaxed.	Sitting on edge of chair or curled in bed, tense muscles, frowning, darting and watchful eyes, and restless pacing occur with anxiety and hyperthyroidism. Sitting slumped in chair, slow walk, dragging feet occur with depression and some organic brain diseases.
Body Movements. *Body movements* are voluntary, deliberate, coordinated, smooth, and even.	Restless, fidgety movement or hyperkinetic appearance occurs with anxiety. Apathy and psychomotor slowing occur with depression and dementia. Abnormal posturing and bizarre gestures occur with schizophrenia. Facial grimaces may occur with pain. Involuntary tics can occur with neurologic disorders (e.g., Tourette syndrome, tardive dyskinesia; see Table 24.4, Abnormalities in Muscle Movement, p. 672).

Normal Range of Findings	Abnormal Findings
Dress. *Dress* is appropriate for setting, season, age, gender, and social group. Clothing fits and is worn appropriately.	Inappropriate dress can occur with organic brain syndrome. Eccentric dress combination and bizarre makeup occur with schizophrenia or manic syndrome.
Grooming and Hygiene. The person is clean and well groomed; hair is neat and clean; women have moderate or no makeup; men are shaved, or beard or mustache is well groomed. Nails are clean (although some jobs leave nails chronically dirty). Note congruence between dress/grooming and age. NOTE: A disheveled appearance in a previously well-groomed person is significant. Use care in interpreting clothing that is disheveled, bizarre, or in poor repair; piercings; and tattoos because these sometimes reflect the person's economic status or a deliberate fashion trend (especially among adolescents).	Unilateral neglect (total inattention to one side of body) occurs following some strokes. Inappropriate dress, poor hygiene, and lack of concern with appearance occur with depression and severe Alzheimer disease. Meticulously dressed and groomed appearance and fastidious manner may occur with obsessive-compulsive disorders.
Pupils. Note pupil size and reaction to light.	Dilated or constricted pupils may be a sign of recent drug use. Recent anisocoria (unequal pupil size) can be the result of a brain tumor.

Behavior

Level of Consciousness. The person is awake, alert, and aware of stimuli from the environment and within the self and responds appropriately and reasonably soon to stimuli.	Loses track of conversation, falls asleep. Lethargic (drowsy), obtunded (confused) (see Table 5.1, Levels of Consciousness, p. 75).
Facial Expression. The look is appropriate to the situation and changes appropriately with the topic. There is comfortable eye contact unless precluded by cultural norm.	Flat, masklike expression occurs with parkinsonism and depression.
Speech. Judge the quality of speech by noting that the person makes laryngeal sounds effortlessly and shares conversation appropriately.	Dysphonia is abnormal volume, pitch (see Table 5.2, Speech Disorders, p. 76). Monopolizes interview or is silent, secretive, or uncommunicative.
The pace of the conversation is moderate, and stream of talking is fluent.	Slow, monotonous speech with parkinsonism or depression. Rapid-fire, pressured, and loud talking occurs with manic syndrome.
Articulation (ability to form words) is clear and understandable.	Dysarthria is distorted speech (see Table 5.2). Misuses words; omits letters, syllables, or words; transposes words; occurs with aphasia. Circumlocution or repetitive abnormal patterns: neologism, echolalia (see Table 5.6, p. 80).
Word choice is effortless and appropriate to educational level. The person completes sentences, occasionally pausing to think.	Unduly long word-finding or failure in word search occurs with aphasia.
Mood and Affect. Judge this by body language and facial expression and by asking directly, "How do you feel today?" or "How do you usually feel?" The mood should be appropriate to the person's place and condition and change appropriately with topics. The person is willing to cooperate with you.	See Table 5.3, Mood and Affect Abnormalities, p. 77, and Table 5.5, Delirium, Dementia, and Depression, p. 79.

Normal Range of Findings	Abnormal Findings

Cognitive Functions

Orientation. You can discern orientation through the course of the interview by asking about the person's address, phone number, and health history. Or ask for it directly, using tact, by saying, "Some people have trouble keeping up with the dates while in the hospital. Do you know today's date?" Assess:

Time: Day of week, date, year, season

Place: Where person lives, present location, type of building, name of city and state

Person: Own name, age, who examiner is

Many hospitalized people normally have trouble with the exact date but know the year and are fully oriented on the remaining items.

Disorientation occurs with delirium and dementia. Orientation is usually lost in this order: first to time, then to place, and rarely to person.

Attention Span. Check the person's ability to concentrate by noting whether he or she completes a thought without wandering. Note any distractibility or difficulty attending to you. Or give a series of directions to follow and note the correct sequence of behaviors, such as, "Please take this glass of water with your left hand, drink from it, shift it to your right hand, and set it on the table." Note that attention span commonly is impaired in people who are anxious, fatigued, or drug intoxicated.

Digression from initial thought. Irrelevant replies to questions. Easily distracted; "stimulus bound" (i.e., any new stimulus quickly draws attention). Confusion, negativism.

Recent Memory. Assess recent memory in the context of the interview by the 24-hour diet recall or by asking the time the person arrived at the agency. Ask questions you can corroborate. This screens for the occasional person who confabulates or makes up answers to fill in the gaps of memory loss.

Recent memory deficit occurs with delirium, dementia, amnestic syndrome, or Korsakoff syndrome in chronic alcoholism.

Remote Memory. In the context of the interview, ask the person verifiable past events (e.g., ask to describe past health, the first job, birthday and anniversary dates, and historical events that are relevant for that person).

Remote memory is lost when the cortical storage area for that memory is damaged (e.g., Alzheimer dementia or any disease that damages the cerebral cortex).

New Learning—The Four Unrelated Words Test. This tests the person's ability to lay down new memories. It is a highly sensitive and valid memory test. It requires more effort than does the recall of personal or historic events. It also avoids the danger of unverifiable material.

Say to the person: "I am going to say four words. I want you to remember them. In a few minutes I will ask you to recall them." To be sure the person has understood, have the person repeat the words. Pick four words with semantic and phonetic diversity:

1. brown	1. fun
2. honesty	2. carrot
3. tulip	3. ankle
4. eyedropper	4. loyalty

After 5 minutes, ask for the recall of the four words. To test the duration of memory, ask for a recall at 10 minutes and at 30 minutes. The normal response for people younger than 60 years is an accurate three- or four-word recall after a 5-, 10-, and 30-minute delay.[22]

People with Alzheimer dementia score a zero- or one-word recall. Impaired new learning ability also occurs with anxiety (because of inattention and distractibility) and depression (because of lack of effort mobilized to remember).

Additional Testing for Persons With Aphasia

Word Comprehension. Point to articles in the room, parts of the body, or articles from pockets and ask the person to name them.

Reading. Ask the person to read available print. Be aware that reading is related to educational level. Use caution that you are not testing literacy. Ensure that the person has reading glasses if needed, and use a large-print item if possible.

Aphasia is the loss of the ability to speak or write coherently or to understand peech or writing as a result of a stroke or brain damage (see Table 5.2, p. 76).

Objective Data

Normal Range of Findings

Writing. Ask the person to make up and write a sentence describing the weather or their job. Note coherence, spelling, and parts of speech (the sentence should have a subject and a verb).

Thought Processes and Perceptions

Thought Processes. Ask yourself, "Does this person make sense? Can I follow what the person is saying?" The *way* a person thinks should be logical, goal directed, coherent, and relevant. The person should complete a thought.

Thought Content. *What* the person says should be consistent and logical.

Perceptions. The person should be consistently aware of reality. The perceptions should be congruent with yours. Ask the following questions:
- How do people treat you?
- Do other people talk about you?
- Do you feel as if you are being watched, followed, or controlled?
- Is your imagination very active?
- Have you heard your name when alone?

Screen for Anxiety Disorders. Anxiety and depression are the two most common mental health problems seen in people seeking general medical care. Anxiety disorders are common, disabling, and often untreated. You can screen for core anxiety symptoms by administering the first 2 questions (GAD-2) from the 7-item generalized anxiety disorder scale (GAD-7) listed in Fig. 5.2.

Abnormal Findings

Reading and writing are important in planning health teaching and rehabilitation. Agraphia (inability to communicate through writing) often occurs in patients with aphasia.[22]

Illogical, unrealistic thought processes. Digression from initial thought. Ideas run together. Evidence of blocking (person stops in middle of thought) (see Table 5.6, Thought Process Abnormalities, p. 80).

Obsessions, compulsions (see Table 5.7, Thought Content Abnormalities, p. 81).

Illusions, hallucinations (see Table 5.8, Perception Abnormalities, p. 81). Auditory and visual hallucinations occur with psychiatric and organic brain disease and psychedelic drugs. Tactile hallucinations occur with alcohol withdrawal.

The four most common anxiety disorders are GAD, panic disorder, social anxiety disorder, posttraumatic stress disorder (PTSD) (see Table 5.4, Anxiety Disorders, p. 78).

GENERALIZED ANXIETY DISORDER SCALE (GAD-7)

Over the last 2 weeks, how often have you been bothered by the following problems?	Not at all	Several days	More than half the days	Nearly every day
1. Feeling nervous, anxious, or on edge	0	1	2	3
2. Not being able to stop or control worrying	0	1	2	3
3. Worrying too much about different things	0	1	2	3
4. Trouble relaxing	0	1	2	3
5. Being so restless that it is hard to sit still	0	1	2	3
6. Becoming easily annoyed or irritable	0	1	2	3
7. Feeling afraid as if something awful might happen	0	1	2	3

Total ____ = Add ____ + ____ + ____
score   columns

If you checked off any problems, how difficult have these problems made it for you to do your work, take care of things at home, or get along with other people?

Not difficult at all	Somewhat difficult	Very difficult	Extremely difficult
☐	☐	☐	☐

5.2   Screen for anxiety symptoms.   (Kroenke, 2007.)

A score of 10 on the GAD-7 identifies GAD; scores of 5, 10, and 15 represent mild, moderate, and severe levels of anxiety. More recently, research suggests that a score ≥8 on the GAD-7 may better identify patients with GAD.[17]

Normal Range of Findings

Scores on the GAD-2 range from 0 to 6; a score of 0 suggests that no anxiety disorder is present, whereas a score ≥3 is suggestive of GAD.[17] The full scale identifies probable GAD and is a severity measure in that increasing scores are associated with increasing impairment and disability.

Screen for Depression. Many formal screening tools are available. However, a shorter screening method is the Patient Health Questionnaire-2 (PHQ-2), which entails asking two questions about depressed mood and anhedonia (little interest or pleasure in doing things) that will detect a majority of depressed patients.[10] Thus you can ask: "Over the past 2 weeks have you felt down, depressed, or hopeless?" and "Over the past 2 weeks, have you felt little interest or pleasure in doing things?"

The PHQ-2 works as a screening tool for depression. If the person answers "several days" or higher, administer the full PHQ-9[19] (Fig. 5.3). Add the totals for each of the three columns together to obtain the severity score. If question 10 is answered "somewhat difficult" or greater, it indicates functional impairment.

Abnormal Findings

Finding positive answers to these questions then requires further diagnostic tools to assess specific depressive disorders (see Table 5.5).

A PHQ-9 score of 5 to 9 = minimal symptoms; 10 to 14 = minor depression; 15 to 19 = major depression, moderately severe; ≥20 = major depression, severe. Treatment recommendations and follow up for each score are available in the literature.

PATIENT HEALTH QUESTIONNAIRE-9 (PHQ-9)

Over the last 2 weeks, how often have you been bothered by any of the following problems? (Use "✓" to indicate your answer)	Not at all	Several days	More than half the days	Nearly every day
1. Little interest or pleasure in doing things	0	1	2	3
2. Feeling down, depressed, or hopeless	0	1	2	3
3. Trouble falling or staying asleep, or sleeping too much	0	1	2	3
4. Feeling tired or having little energy	0	1	2	3
5. Poor appetite or overeating	0	1	2	3
6. Feeling bad about yourself — or that you are a failure or have let yourself or your family down	0	1	2	3
7. Trouble concentrating on things, such as reading the newspaper or watching television	0	1	2	3
8. Moving or speaking so slowly that other people could have noticed? Or the opposite — being so fidgety or restless that you have been moving around a lot more than usual	0	1	2	3
9. Thoughts that you would be better off dead or of hurting yourself in some way	0	1	2	3

FOR OFFICE CODING   *0*   + ____ + ____ + ____

=Total Score: ____

If you checked off any problems, how difficult have these problems made it for you to do your work, take care of things at home, or get along with other people?

Not difficult at all	Somewhat difficult	Very difficult	Extremely difficult
☐	☐	☐	☐

5.3   (Developed by Spitzer, R. L., Williams, J. B. W, Kroenke, K., et al. 1999.)

Objective Data

Objective Data

Normal Range of Findings	Abnormal Findings

Normal Range of Findings

Screen for Suicidal Thoughts. When a person expresses feelings of sadness, hopelessness, despair, or grief, it is important to assess for any possible risk of physical harm to himself or herself. Begin with more general questions. If you hear affirmative answers, continue with more specific questions:

- Have you ever felt that life is not worth living?
- Have you ever thought of hurting yourself? If so, how often?
- Do you feel like hurting yourself now?
- Do you have a plan to hurt yourself?
- How would you do it?
- What would happen if you were dead?
- How would other people react if you were dead?
- Whom could you tell if you felt like killing yourself?

It is very difficult, especially for beginning examiners, to question people about possible suicidal wishes. Examiners fear an invasion of privacy and may have their own normal denial of death and suicide. However, the risk is *far greater* if you skip these questions when you have the slightest clue that they are appropriate. You may be the only health professional to pick up clues of suicide risk. You are responsible for encouraging the person to talk about suicidal thoughts.

Another recommendation is to have the person sign a contract that contains a plan not to act on suicidal thoughts if they happen again. The plan should contain the names and numbers of people the patient can call if suicidal ideations occur.[5]

Depression is painful and debilitating, and sometimes a depressed person really wishes to kill himself or herself. However, most suicidal people are ambivalent, and being able to discuss their feelings may give them the time needed to identify a coping mechanism for current stressors. Asking about suicidal thoughts does not increase suicidal behavior. Promptly share any concerns you have about a person's suicide ideation with a mental health professional.

Judgment

A person exercises judgment when he or she can compare and evaluate the alternatives in a situation and reach an appropriate course of action. You are interested in the person's judgment about daily or long-term life goals, the likelihood of acting in response to delusions or hallucinations, and the capacity for violent or suicidal behavior.

To assess judgment in the context of the interview, note what the person says about job plans, social or family obligations, and plans for the future. Job and future plans should be realistic, considering the person's health situation. In addition, ask the person to describe the rationale for personal health care and how he or she decided whether to comply with prescribed health regimens. The person's actions and decisions should be realistic.

Supplemental Mental Status Examination

The Mini-Mental State Examination (MMSE) is a test of the cognitive functions of the mental status examination (memory, orientation to time and place, naming, reading, copying or visuospatial orientation, writing, and the ability to follow a three-stage command). It requires paper and pencil; the person must be able to write and have no vision impairment. The MMSE is copyrighted and available for purchase from Psychological Assessment Resources, Inc.

The MMSE is quick and easy, includes a standard set of only 11 questions, and requires only 5 to 10 minutes to administer. It is useful for both initial and

Abnormal Findings

Suicide is preventable, but it is the 10th leading cause of death in the United States and the 2nd leading cause among those ages 15 to 34 years. Between 20% and 33% of suicide victims test positive for alcohol, antidepressants, or opiates. Although females are more likely to have suicidal thoughts, males are 4 times more likely to commit suicide (most often by firearms).[4]

A precise suicide plan to take place in the next 24 to 48 hours using a lethal method constitutes high risk. Important clues and warning signs of suicide:
   Prior suicide attempts
   Depression, hopelessness
   Firearms in the home
   Family history of suicide
   Incarceration
   Family violence, including physical or
      sexual abuse
   Self-mutilation
   Anorexia
   Verbal suicide messages (defeat,
      failure, worthlessness, loss, giving
      up, desire to kill self)
   Death themes in art, jokes, writing,
      behaviors
   Saying goodbye (giving away prized
      possessions)

Impaired judgment (unrealistic or impulsive decisions, wish fulfillment) occurs with developmental disability, emotional dysfunction, schizophrenia, and organic brain disease.

The MMSE is used with caution in people with low education, who may have problems copying intersecting pentagons, spelling "world" backward, or performing serial 7s. The MMSE also lacks sensitivity for mild cognitive impairment.[6]

Normal Range of Findings	Abnormal Findings

serial measurement; therefore you can demonstrate worsening or improvement of cognition over time and with treatment. It concentrates only on cognitive functioning, not on mood, thought processes, or executive function. It is a valid detector of organic disease but lacks sensitivity for mild cognitive impairment.

The maximum score on the test is 30; people with normal mental status average 27. Scores between 24 and 30 indicate no cognitive impairment.

An alternate assessment tool, the Montreal Cognitive Assessment (MoCA), is available to assess mental status. The MoCA examines more cognitive domains than the MMSE, is more sensitive to mild cognitive impairment, and can be obtained free of charge.[6] The MoCA includes items that measure visuo-constructive ability, language function, memory, auditory attention, conceptual thinking, working memory and calculations, as well as speech/language. The MoCA takes approximately 10 minutes to administer. The total score is 30 and a score of ≥26 is considered normal. One point is added to the score of any person with fewer than 12 years of formal education.

❖ DEVELOPMENTAL COMPETENCE

Infants and Children

The mental status assessment of infants and children covers behavioral, cognitive, and psychosocial development and examines how the child is coping with his or her environment. Essentially you follow the same A-B-C-T guidelines as for the adult, with special consideration for developmental milestones. Your best examination "technique" arises from thorough knowledge of developmental milestones. Abnormalities are often problems of *omission;* the child does not achieve a milestone you would expect.

The parent's health history, especially the sections on the developmental history and personal history, yields most of the mental status data.

In addition, the **Denver II screening** test gives you a chance to interact directly with the young child to assess mental status. The Denver II is designed to detect developmental delays in infants and preschoolers within four functions: gross motor, language, fine motor–adaptive, and personal-social skills. For mental status assessment, the Denver II helps identify young children who may be slow in development in behavioral, language, cognitive, and psychosocial areas. The test has 125 items arranged in chronologic order and displayed in groupings corresponding to recommended ages for health-maintenance visits.

In some settings, a caregiver-completed instrument may be used to assess developmental milestones. Caregiver-completed instruments include the Ages and Stages Questionnaire, the Modified Checklist for Autism in Toddlers Revised, or the Parents' Evaluation of Developmental Status. The tools ask about the child's development in a variety of areas and ask parents to identify any concerns. No one tool is recommended above others, but the American Academy of Pediatrics does recommend routine developmental screening for all infants and children.[12]

As you talk to the parent, listen for signs of irritability in the child (i.e., overreacting to a stimulus, leading to excitability or anger). This is expected in a child who is ill with a medical condition. Some irritability also is expected in some developmental stages (i.e., age 2 years and in adolescence as the teen struggles for independence).

Abnormal Findings column:

Scores that occur with dementia and delirium are classified as follows: 18-23 = mild cognitive impairment; 0-17 = severe cognitive impairment.

Any score <26 is indicative of mild cognitive impairment.

Denver II scoring avoids diagnostic labeling (e.g., developmental disability, language disorder). Instead the child's performance is scored either "normal," "abnormal," or "questionable."

See Table 5.10, Childhood Mental Disorders, p. 82.

In children and teens, note irritability that is more constant or obstructs performance in school or in social and family relationships. Note that irritability is a common sign in mental health disorders in childhood: anxiety, depression, ADHD, oppositional defiant disorder (ODD), and autism spectrum disorders.[8]

Objective Data

Normal Range of Findings	Abnormal Findings

For the adolescent, follow the same A-B-C-T guidelines as described for the adult. Keep your beginning questions open ended (i.e., "How are things at school? At home? How about friends—anyone close?"). Then you can ask more specific questions: "Do you feel any extra stress or anxiety at school? At home? With friends? How about your parents—do they think you act worried or anxious?" Review Fig. 4.16 for more information on interviewing adolescents.

Anxiety disorders are common in the teen years and are associated with GAD, social phobia, ADHD, PTSD (see Table 5.4, p. 78). In addition, anxiety and depression are seen together, two sides of a double-edged sword.

The Aging Adult

It is important to conduct even a brief examination of all older people admitted to the hospital. Confusion is common in aging people and is easily misdiagnosed. Delirium is present in 8% to 17% of elderly people who present to the emergency department (ED) and 40% of nursing home residents who present to the ED. Up to 50% of hospitalized elderly patients experience delirium.[9] Delirium can have deleterious effects after the acute episode, including increased risk of mortality, prolonged cognitive impairment (lasting up to a year), and physical impairment.[9]

Overall prevalence of dementia in those 65 years and older dropped significantly from 11.6% in 2000 to 8.8% in 2012.[11] Declining prevalence signals improved brain health in the elderly population. Although all factors related to the improvement are unknown, better control of cardiovascular risk factors and higher educational attainment are two contributing factors.[11,18] While the overall prevalence of dementia is declining, the burden of disease will increase as the baby boomer generation ages and life expectancy increases.[18]

Delirium is an acute confusional change or loss of consciousness and perceptual disturbance; it may accompany acute illness (e.g., pneumonia, alcohol/drug intoxication), and it is usually resolved when the underlying cause is treated.

In contrast, **dementia** is a gradual, progressive process, causing decreased cognitive function even though the person is fully conscious and awake; it is not reversible. Alzheimer disease accounts for about two-thirds of cases of dementia in older adults (see Table 5.5). Dementia is not part of normal aging. Risk factors for dementia include racial and ethnic groups other than Caucasians, advanced age, women, singles, living alone, lower educational attainment, and lower income.

Check sensory status before assessing any aspect of mental status. Vision and hearing changes caused by aging may alter alertness and leave the person looking confused. When older people cannot hear your questions, they cannot accurately complete cognitive screening examinations.

Follow the same A-B-C-T guidelines as described for the younger adult with the following *additional* considerations.

Behavior

Level of Consciousness. In a hospital or extended-care setting, the Glasgow Coma Scale (see Chapter 24) is a quantitative tool that is useful in testing consciousness. It gives a numeric value to the person's response in eye opening, best verbal response, and best motor response. This system avoids ambiguity when numerous examiners care for the same person.

Cognitive Functions

Orientation. Many aging persons experience social isolation, loss of structure without a job, a change in residence, or some short-term memory loss. These factors affect orientation, and this person may not provide the precise date or complete name of the agency. You may consider aging persons oriented if they know *generally* where they are and the present period (i.e., consider them oriented to time if the year and month are stated correctly). Orientation to place is accepted with the correct identification of the type of setting (e.g., the hospital) and the name of the town.

New Learning

In people of normal cognitive function, an age-related decline occurs in performance in the Four Unrelated Words Test described on p. 67. People in their 70s average two of four words recalled over 5 minutes. They will improve their performance at 10 and 30 minutes after being reminded by verbal cues (e.g., "one word was a color; a common flower in Holland is _____").

People with Alzheimer dementia do not improve their performance on subsequent trials.

Normal Range of Findings

Supplemental Mental Status Examination

The Mini-Cog. The Mini-Cog is a reliable, quick, and easily available instrument to screen for cognitive impairment in otherwise healthy older adults (Fig. 5.4).[23] It can be used with various cultural groups and literacy levels and takes only 3 to 5 minutes to administer. The Mini-Cog is not influenced by educational level or health literacy of the patient and can be used in a variety of settings, including the hospital.[14]

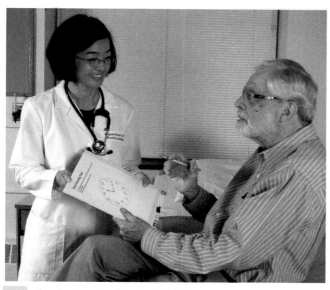

5.4 Clock drawing for the Mini-Cog.

The Mini-Cog consists of a 3-item recall test and a clock-drawing test. Begin by asking the older adult to listen carefully to, remember, and then repeat three words that you will say. Make sure that the person can hear you and that no distracting noises are present. Keep the words short and unrelated: "*Listen carefully. I am going to say three words. Say them back after I stop. Ready? Cup (pause), train (pause), blue. Now repeat those words to me. Good.*" Next give the adult a blank sheet of paper, saying, "*Now I want you to draw the face of a clock and write the numbers on the clock face. That's fine. Next I want you to draw the hands of the clock so it shows the time of 11:10.*" "*Remember the three words I told you earlier? Now I want you to repeat them.*"

The Mini-Cog tests the person's executive function, including the ability to plan, manage time, organize activities, and manage working memory.[13] A person with no cognitive impairment or dementia can recall all three words and draw a complete, round, closed clock circle, with all face numbers present and in correct position and sequence and with the hour and minute hands indicating the time you requested.

Abnormal Findings

A score of 0-5 is awarded based on the following criteria: 1 point is awarded for each word recalled (total of 3 points) and 2 points are awarded for a normal clock. A normal clock includes all numbers in the correct order with proper placement, and 2 hands pointing at 11 and 2. Hand length is not scored.

A score of <3 is indicative of dementia although some cognitive impairment cannot be ruled out with scores of 3, 4, or 5.[13]

DOCUMENTATION AND CRITICAL THINKING

Sample Charting

Appearance: Person's posture is erect, with no involuntary body movements. Dress and grooming are appropriate for season and setting.

Behavior: Person is alert, with appropriate facial expression and fluent, understandable speech. Affect and verbal responses are appropriate.

Cognitive functions: Oriented to time, person, place. Able to attend cooperatively with examiner. Recent and remote memory intact. Can recall four unrelated words at 5-, 10-, and 30-minute testing intervals. Future plans include returning home and to local university once individual therapy is established and medication is adjusted.

Thought process: Perceptions and thought processes are logical and coherent. No suicidal ideation.

Score on Mini-Mental State Examination is 28.

Clinical Case Study 1

L.P. is a 79-year-old married woman, with a recent hospitalization for evaluation of increasing memory loss, confusion, and socially inappropriate behavior. Her family reports that L.P.'s hygiene and grooming have decreased; she eats very little and has lost weight, does not sleep through the night, has angry emotional outbursts that are unlike her former demeanor, and does not recognize her younger grandchildren. Her husband reports that she has drifted away from the stove while cooking, allowing food to burn on the stovetop. He has found her wandering through the house in the middle of the night, unsure of where she was. She used to "talk on the phone for hours," but now he has to push her into conversations. During this hospitalization L.P. has undergone a series of medical tests, including a negative lumbar puncture test, normal electroencephalogram (EEG), and a negative head computed tomography (CT) scan. Her physician now suggests a diagnosis of Alzheimer dementia.

Appearance: Sitting quietly, somewhat slumped, picking on loose threads on her dress. Hooded, zippered sweatshirt top worn over dress. Hair is gathered in loose ponytail with stray wisps. No makeup.

Behavior: Awake and gazing at hands and lap. Expression is flat and vacant. Will make eye contact when called by name, although gaze quickly shifts back to lap. Speech is a bit slow but articulate; some trouble with word choice.

Cognitive function: Oriented to person and place. Can state the season but not the day of the week or the year. Is not able to repeat the correct sequence of complex directions involving lifting and shifting glass of water to the other hand. Scores a one-word recall on the Four Unrelated Words Test. Cannot tell examiner how she would plan a grocery shopping trip.

Thought process: Experiences blocking in train of thought. Thought content is logical. Acts cranky and suspicious with family members. No suicidal ideation.

Mini-Mental State Examination score is 17 and shows poor recall ability and marked difficulty with serial 7s.

ASSESSMENT

Chronic confusion
Impaired social interaction
Impaired memory
Wandering

Clinical Case Study 2

I.E. is a 64-year-old man with chronic hypertension who was admitted to the hospital 3 days ago with acute coronary syndrome. He underwent coronary artery bypass surgery 2 days ago and has been in the ICU. His preoperative score on the Mini-Mental State Examination was 26.

Appearance: Moves restlessly in hospital bed. Calms during family visits.

Behavior: Restlessness increases during evening and night hours. Speech is incoherent and rambling.

Cognitive function: Oriented to own name but not to time, place. No memory of surgery or recent events. Wants to leave and "get back to the plant." Verbalizes that nurses are keeping him here against his will. "They are in it together." Unable to recall words on Four Unrelated Words Test. Believes "little bugs" are crawling up wall by his bed.

Thought process: Thought content is illogical. Experiences hallucinations. Appears angry and suspicious with nurses.

ASSESSMENT

Postoperative delirium
Acute confusion
Impaired memory

ABNORMAL FINDINGS

TABLE 5.1	Levels of Consciousness

These terms are commonly used in clinical practice. They spread over a continuum from full alertness to deep coma. The terms are qualitative and therefore are not always reliable. (A *quantitative* tool that serves the same purpose and eliminates ambiguity is the Glasgow Coma Scale in Chapter 24.) However, these terms are widely accepted and are useful as long as all co-workers agree on definitions and are consistent in their application. To increase clarity when using these terms, record also:

1. The level of stimulus used, ranging progressively from:
   a. Name called in normal tone of voice
   b. Name called in loud voice
   c. Light touch on person's arm
   d. Vigorous shake of shoulder
   e. Painful stimuli
2. The person's response
   a. Amount and quality of movement
   b. Presence and coherence of speech
   c. Opening of eyes and making eye contact
3. What the person does on cessation of your stimulus

(1) Alert

Awake or readily aroused; oriented, fully aware of external and internal stimuli and responds appropriately; conducts meaningful interpersonal interactions.

(2) Lethargic (or Somnolent)

Not fully alert; drifts off to sleep when not stimulated; can be aroused to name when called in normal voice but looks drowsy; responds appropriately to questions or commands but thinking seems slow and fuzzy; inattentive; loses train of thought; spontaneous movements are decreased.

(3) Obtunded

(Transitional state between lethargy and stupor; some sources omit this level.)
Sleeps most of time; difficult to arouse—needs loud shout or vigorous shake; acts confused when is aroused; converses in monosyllables; speech may be mumbled and incoherent; requires constant stimulation for even marginal cooperation.

(4) Stupor or Semi-Coma

Spontaneously unconscious; responds only to persistent and vigorous shake or pain; has appropriate motor response (i.e., withdraws hand to avoid pain); otherwise can only groan, mumble, or move restlessly; reflex activity persists.

(5) Coma

Completely unconscious; no response to pain or any external or internal stimuli (e.g., when suctioned, does not try to push the catheter away); light coma has some reflex activity but no purposeful movement; deep coma has no motor response.

Delirium (Acute Confusional State)

Clouding of consciousness (dulled cognition, impaired alertness); inattentive; incoherent conversation; impaired recent memory and confabulatory for recent events; often agitated and having visual hallucinations; disoriented, with confusion worse at night when environmental stimuli are decreased.

Adapted from Strub, R. L., & Black, F. W. (2000). *Mental status examination in neurology.* (4th ed.). Philadelphia: Davis, with permission.

Abnormal Findings

TABLE 5.2	Speech Disorders	
Condition	**Disorder of**	**Description**
Dysphonia	Voice	Difficulty or discomfort in talking, with abnormal pitch or volume, caused by laryngeal disease. Voice sounds hoarse or whispered, but articulation and language are intact.
Dysarthria	Articulation	Distorted speech sounds; speech may sound unintelligible; basic language (word choice, grammar, comprehension) intact.
Aphasia	Language comprehension and production secondary to brain damage	True language disturbance; defect in word choice and grammar or defect in comprehension; defect is in *higher* integrative language processing.

Types of Aphasia

An earlier dichotomy classified aphasias as *expressive* (difficulty producing language) or *receptive* (difficulty understanding language). Because all people with aphasia have some difficulty with expression, beginning examiners tend to classify them all as expressive. The following system is more descriptive.

Condition	Description
Global aphasia	The most common and severe form. Spontaneous speech is absent or reduced to a few stereotyped words or sounds. Comprehension is absent or reduced to only the person's own name and a few select words. Repetition, reading, and writing are severely impaired. Prognosis for language recovery is poor. Caused by a large lesion that damages most of combined anterior and posterior language areas.
Broca aphasia	Expressive aphasia. The person can understand language but cannot express himself or herself using language. This is characterized by nonfluent, dysarthric, and effortful speech. The speech is mostly nouns and verbs (high-content words) with few grammatic fillers, termed *agrammatic* or *telegraphic* speech. Repetition and reading aloud are severely impaired. Auditory and reading comprehensions are surprisingly intact. Lesion is in anterior language area called the *motor speech cortex* or *Broca area*.
Wernicke aphasia	Receptive aphasia. The linguistic opposite of Broca aphasia. The person can hear sounds and words but cannot relate them to previous experiences. Speech is fluent, effortless, and well articulated but has many paraphasias (word substitutions that are malformed or wrong) and neologisms (made-up words) and often lacks substantive words. Speech can be totally incomprehensible. Often there is a great urge to speak. Repetition, reading, and writing also are impaired. Lesion is in posterior language area called the *association auditory cortex* or *Wernicke area*.

(For a discussion of other types of aphasia [e.g., conduction, anomic, transcortical] and speech disorders, please consult a neurology text.)

TABLE 5.3	Mood and Affect Abnormalities	
Type of Mood or Affect	Definition	Clinical Example
Flat affect (blunted affect)	Lack of emotional response; no expression of feelings; voice monotonous and face immobile	Topic varies, expression does not
Depression	Sad, gloomy, dejected; symptoms may occur with rainy weather, after a holiday, or with an illness; if the situation is temporary, symptoms fade quickly	"I don't enjoy anything anymore."
Depersonalization (lack of ego boundaries)	Loss of identity, feels estranged, perplexed about own identity and meaning of existence	"I don't feel real." "I feel like I'm not really here."
Elation	Joy and optimism, overconfidence, increased motor activity; not necessarily pathologic	"I'm feeling very happy." Can be a pathologic sign of mania.
Euphoria	Excessive well-being; unusually cheerful or elated, which is inappropriate considering physical and mental condition; implies a pathologic mood	"I'm high." "I feel like I'm flying." "I feel on top of the world."
Anxiety	Worried, uneasy, apprehensive from the anticipation of a danger whose source is unknown	"I feel nervous and high-strung." "I worry all the time." "I can't seem to make up my mind."
Fear	Worried, uneasy, apprehensive; external danger is known and identified	Fear of flying in airplanes
Irritability	Annoyed, easily provoked, impatient	Person internalizes a feeling of tension, and a seemingly mild stimulus "sets him (or her) off"
Rage	Furious, loss of control	Person has expressed violent behavior toward self or others
Ambivalence	The existence of opposing emotions toward an idea, object, person	A person feels love and hate toward another at the same time
Lability	Rapid shift of emotions	Person expresses euphoric, tearful, angry feelings in rapid succession
Inappropriate affect	Affect clearly discordant with content of person's speech	Laughs while discussing admission for liver biopsy

TABLE 5.4 | **Anxiety Disorders**

Panic Attack

A defined period of intense fear, anxiety, and dread accompanied by signs of dyspnea, choking, chest pain, increased heart rate, palpitations, nausea, and sweating. Also has fear of going crazy, dying, or impending doom. Sudden onset, lasts about 10 minutes, then subsides.

Specific Phobia

A pattern of debilitating fear when faced with a particular object or situation (e.g., dogs, spiders, thunder or storms, enclosed spaces, heights, blood). Person knows it is irrational yet studiously avoids the feared object, thus becoming restricted in social or occupational activities.

Generalized Anxiety Disorder (GAD)

A pattern of excessive worrying and morbid fear about anticipated "disasters" in the job, personal relationships, health, or finances. Characterized by restlessness, muscle tension, diarrhea, palpitations, tachypnea, hypervigilance, fatigue, or sleep disturbance. Person devotes much time to preparing for anticipated catastrophe, has difficulty making decisions, and practices avoidance.

Agoraphobia

An irrational fear of being out in the open or in a place from which escape is difficult (airport or airplane, car or bus, elevator, bridge). Fear is so intense that these places are avoided and person is reluctant to leave a safe place (home).

Social Anxiety Disorder (Social Phobia)

A persistent and irrational fear of being in social situations. Person anticipates being judged or criticized, feeling or looking foolish, feeling embarrassment, being unable to answer questions, or being unable to remember the lines or notes. Person studiously avoids social situations or endures them with intense anxiety.

Obsessive-Compulsive Disorder (OCD)

A pattern of recurrent obsessions (intrusive, uncontrollable thoughts) and compulsions (repetitive ritualistic actions) done to decrease anxiety and prevent a catastrophe (e.g., contamination [fear of germs], violence, perfectionism, and superstitions). Intrusive thoughts and actions are time consuming, interfere with daily activities, and make the person feel humiliated or ashamed for giving in to them.

Posttraumatic Stress Disorder (PTSD)

This follows a traumatic event outside the range of usual human experience involving actual or threatened death (e.g., military combat, natural disaster [flood, tornado, earthquake], plane or train accident, violence [mugging, rape, bombing]). The person relives the trauma many times, intrusively and unwillingly. The same feelings of helplessness, fear, or horror recur. Avoidance of any trigger associated with the trauma occurs, and the person has hypervigilance, sleep problems, and difficulty concentrating, leading to feelings of being permanently damaged.

Adapted from Halter, M. J. (2017). *Varcarolis' foundations of psychiatric mental health nursing.* (8th ed.). St. Louis: Elsevier; and *Stedman's medical dictionary.* (28th ed.). (2005). Philadelphia: Lippincott Williams & Wilkins.

Abnormal Findings

TABLE 5.5 | Delirium, Dementia, and Depression

Delirium is an acute confusional state, potentially preventable in hospitalized persons. (See Table 5.1.) Characterized by disorientation, disordered thinking and perceptions (illusions and hallucinations), defective memory, agitation, inattention.

Dementia is a chronic progressive loss of cognitive and intellectual functions, although perception and consciousness are intact. Characterized by disorientation, impaired judgment, memory loss. (See Table 24.1, 10 Warning Signs of Alzheimer Disease).

Depression is a long-term depressed mood (≥2 weeks) with lack of pleasure; disturbed sleep and appetite; feelings of hopelessness, guilt, worthlessness, sadness, loneliness, and despair; suicide ideation.

See the following comparisons.

	Delirium	Dementia	Depression
Onset	Sudden, over hours to days	Slowly, over months	May be gradual, with exacerbation during crisis or stress
Cause or contributing factors	Hypoglycemia, fever, dehydration, hypotension; infection, other conditions that disrupt body homeostasis; adverse drug reaction; head injury; change in environment (e.g., hospitalization); pain; emotional stress; substance abuse	Alzheimer disease, vascular disease, human immunodeficiency virus infection, neurologic disease, chronic alcoholism, head trauma	Lifelong history, losses, loneliness, crises, declining health, medical conditions
Cognition	Impaired memory, judgment, calculations, attention span; can fluctuate through the day	Impaired memory, judgment, calculations, attention span, abstract thinking; agnosia	Difficulty concentrating, forgetfulness, inattention
Level of consciousness	Altered	Not altered	Not altered
Activity level	Can be increased or reduced; restlessness; behaviors may worsen in evening (sundowning); sleep/wake cycle may be reversed	Not altered; behaviors may worsen in evening (sundowning)	Usually decreased; lethargy, fatigue, lack of motivation; may sleep poorly and awaken in early morning
Emotional state	Rapid swings; can be fearful, anxious, suspicious, aggressive, have hallucinations and/or delusions	Flat; agitation	Extreme sadness, apathy, irritability, anxiety, paranoid ideation
Speech and language	Rapid, inappropriate, incoherent, rambling	Incoherent, slow (sometimes due to effort to find the right word), inappropriate, rambling, repetitious	Slow, flat, low
Prognosis	Reversible with proper and timely treatment	Not reversible; progressive	Reversible with proper and timely treatment

From Halter, M. J. (2017). *Varcarolis' foundations of psychiatric mental health nursing* (8th ed.). St. Louis: Elsevier.

ABNORMAL FINDINGS
FOR ADVANCED PRACTICE

TABLE 5.6	Thought Process Abnormalities	
Type of Process	**Definition**	**Clinical Example**
Blocking	Sudden interruption in train of thought, unable to complete sentence, seems related to strong emotion.	"Forgot what I was going to say."
Confabulation	Fabricates events to fill in memory gaps.	Gives detailed description of his long walk around the hospital although you know Mr. J. remained in his room all afternoon.
Neologism	Coining a new word; invented word has no real meaning except for the person; may condense several words.	"I'll have to turn on my thinkilator."
Circumlocution	Round-about expression, substituting a phrase when unable to think of name of object.	Says "the thing you open the door with" instead of "key."
Circumstantiality	Talks with excessive and unnecessary detail, delays reaching point; sentences have a meaningful connection but are irrelevant (this occurs normally in some people).	"When was my surgery? Well I was 28, I was living with my aunt, she's the one with psoriasis, she had it bad that year because of the heat, the heat was worse than it was the summer of '92. ..."
Loosening associations	Shifting from one topic to an unrelated topic; person seems unaware that topics are unconnected.	"My boss is angry with me, and it wasn't even my fault. *(pause)* I saw that movie too, Lassie. I felt really bad about it. But she kept trying to land the airplane and she never knew what was going on."
Flight of ideas	Abrupt change, rapid skipping from topic to topic, practically continuous flow of accelerated speech; topics usually have recognizable associations or are plays on words.	"Take this pill? The pill is blue. I feel blue. *(sings)* She wore blue velvet."
Word salad	Incoherent mixture of words, phrases, and sentences; illogical, disconnected, includes neologisms.	"Beauty, red-based five, pigeon, the street corner, sort of."
Perseveration	Persistent repeating of verbal or motor response, even with varied stimuli.	"I'm going to lock the door, lock the door. I walk every day, and I lock the door. I usually take the dog, and I lock the door."
Echolalia	Imitation, repeats others' words or phrases, often with a mumbling, mocking, or mechanical tone	Nurse: "I want you to take your pill." Patient *(mocking):* "Take your pill. Take your pill."
Clanging	Word choice based on sound, not meaning; includes nonsense rhymes and puns.	"My feet are cold. Cold, bold, told. The bell tolled for me."

TABLE 5.7	Thought Content Abnormalities	
Type of Content	**Definition**	**Clinical Example**
Phobia	Strong, persistent, irrational fear of an object or situation; feels driven to avoid it	Cats, dogs, heights, enclosed spaces
Hypochondriasis	Morbid worrying about his or her own health; feels sick with no actual basis for that assumption	Preoccupied with the fear of having cancer; any symptom or physical sign means cancer
Obsession	Unwanted, persistent thoughts or impulses; logic will not purge them from consciousness; experienced as intrusive and senseless	Violence (parent having repeated impulse to kill a loved child); contamination (becoming infected by shaking hands)
Compulsion	Unwanted repetitive, purposeful act; driven to do it; behavior thought to neutralize or prevent discomfort or some dreaded event	Handwashing, counting, checking and rechecking, touching
Delusions	Firm, fixed, false beliefs; irrational; person clings to delusion despite objective evidence to contrary	Grandiose—Person believes that he or she is God; famous, historical, or sports figure; or other well-known person Persecution—"They're out to get me."

TABLE 5.8	Perception Abnormalities	
Type of Perception	**Definition**	**Clinical Example**
Hallucination	Sensory perceptions for which there are no external stimuli; may strike any sense: visual, auditory, tactile, olfactory, gustatory	Visual: seeing an image (ghost) of a person who is not there; auditory: hearing voices or music
Illusion	Misperception of an actual existing stimulus, by any sense	Folds of bedsheets appear to be animated

TABLE 5.9	Characteristics of Eating Problems	
Anorexia Nervosa	**Bulimia Nervosa**	**Binge Eating**

• Intense fear of weight gain
• Distorted body image
• Restricted calories with significantly low body mass index
• Subtypes:
  • Restricting (no consistent bulimic features)
  • Binge eating/purging type (primarily restriction, some bulimic behaviors)
	• Recurrent episodes of uncontrollable bingeing
	• Inappropriate compensatory behaviors: vomiting, laxatives, diuretics, or exercise
	• Self-image largely influenced by body image
		• Recurrent episodes of uncontrollable bingeing without compensatory behaviors
		• Bingeing episodes induce guilt, depression, embarrassment, or disgust

From Halter, M. J. (2017). *Varcarolis' foundations of psychiatric mental health nursing* (8th ed.). St. Louis: Elsevier.

TABLE 5.10 | Childhood Mental Disorders

Attention-Deficit/Hyperactivity Disorder (ADHD)

A common behavioral disorder with inappropriate inattention (short attention span, unable to complete tasks or follow directions, easily distracted), impulsiveness, and hyperactivity (restlessness and fidgeting, excess talking). Present in two settings, home and school. Nearly 12% of adolescents ages 12-17 and 9.5% of children ages 6-11 have ADHD. The highest prevalence is in non-Hispanic white males.[16]

Autism Spectrum Disorder

A complex neurologic and biological developmental disorder characterized by problems in social interactions and verbal and nonverbal communication. Dysfunctions range from mild to severe and include problems making and maintaining friends, strict adherence to rituals or routines, resistance to change, repetitive speech, poor eye contact, and motor mannerisms. Autism has a genetic component, appears in early childhood (by 2 or 3 years), is 4 times more common in boys than girls, and is not affected by race, family income, or educational level.

Oppositional Defiant Disorder (ODD)

A disruptive set of behaviors characterized by negative, aggressive, angry, and irritable mood. Children with ODD lose their temper, argue with adults, refuse to obey adults' requests or rules, deliberately annoy others, and blame their actions on others. They may be spiteful, vindictive, or malicious. Because they violate social norms, presence in school is difficult. It is also hard to make friends or to fit well in the family.

Eating Disorder

A group of serious and complex psychological disorders affecting primarily adolescents. (1) Anorexia nervosa presents as a severely low body weight for height (low body mass index) and an intense fear of gaining weight. The person may eat very little food or binge and then purge food by vomiting. (2) Bulimia nervosa is the hallmark of a young person who binge eats and then compensates with self-induced vomiting, misuse of laxatives or diuretics, fasting, or excessive exercise. Both disorders leave the person severely underweight and at risk for electrolyte disturbances and other medical comorbidities (see Table 5.9). (3) People with binge-eating disorder use excessive food for comfort or to relieve stress and then feel extreme remorse. This leads to obesity.

Adapted from Halter, M. J. (2017). *Varcarolis' foundations of psychiatric mental health nursing* (8th ed.). St. Louis: Elsevier; and *Stedman's medical dictionary*. (28th ed.). (2005). Philadelphia: Lippincott Williams & Wilkins.

Summary Checklist: Mental Status Assessment

1. **Appearance**
   Posture
   Body movements
   Dress
   Grooming and hygiene
   Pupils
2. **Behavior**
   Level of consciousness
   Facial expression
   Speech (quality, pace, articulation, word choice)
   Mood and affect

3. **Cognitive function**
   Orientation
   Attention span
   Recent and remote memory
   New learning—the Four Unrelated Words Test
   Judgment
4. **Thought process**
   Thought process
   Thought content
   Perceptions
   Screen for suicidal thoughts

5. **Perform the Mini-Mental State Examination, MoCA, or the Mini-Cog**

REFERENCES

1. American Psychiatric Association. (2013). *Diagnostic and statistical manual of mental disorders* (5th ed.). Washington, DC: The Association.

2. Reference deleted in proofs.

3. Centers for Disease Control and Prevention. (2017). *Children's mental health: Basics.* https://www.cdc.gov/childrensmentalhealth/basics.html.

4. Centers for Disease Control (CDC). (2015). *Suicide data sheet-facts at a glance.* https://www.cdc.gov/violenceprevention/pdf/suicide-datasheet-a.pdf.

5. Diggle-Fox, B. S. (2016). Assessing suicide risk in older adults. *Nurse Pract, 41*(10), 28–35.

6. Finney, G. R., Minager, A., & Heilman, K. M. (2016). Assessment of mental status. *Neurol Clin, 34,* 1–16.

7. Fontanella, C. A., et al. (2015). Widening rural-urban disparities in youth suicides, United States, 1996-2010. *JAMA Pediatr, 169,* 466–473.

8. Halter, M. J. (2017). *Varcarolis' foundations of psychiatric mental health nursing* (8th ed.). St. Louis: Elsevier.

9. Inouye, S. K., Westendorp, R. G. J., & Saczynski, J. S. (2014). Delirium in elderly people. *Lancet, 383,* 911–922.

10. Lakkis, N. A., & Mahmassani, D. M. (2015). Screening instruments for depression in primary care: A concise review for clinicians. *Postgrad Med, 127*(1), 99–106.

11. Langa, K. M., Larson, E. B., & Crimmins, E. M. (2017). A comparison of the prevalence of dementia in the United States in 2000 and 2012. *JAMA Intern Med, 177,* 51–58.

12. Lipkin, P. H., et al. (2017). Trends in standardized developmental screening: Results from national surveys of pediatricians, 2002-2016. *Pediatric Academic Societies Annual Meeting.*

13. *Mini-Cog screening for cognitive impairment in older adults.* mini-cog.com.

14. Mion, L. C., & Sandhu, S. K. (2014). Screening for dementia in hospitalized older adults: Try the Mini-Cog. *Geriatr Nurs (Minneap), 35*(4), 313–315.

15. National Institute of Mental Health. *Statistics.* https://www.nimh.nih.gov/health/statistics/index.shtml.

16. Pastor, P. N. (2015). QuickStats: Percentage of Children and Adolescents Aged 5–17 Years with Diagnosed Attention-Deficit/Hyperactivity Disorder (ADHD), by Race and Hispanic Ethnicity — National Health Interview Survey, United States, 1997–2014. *MMWR Morb Mortal Wkly Rep, 64,* 925.

17. Plummer, F., et al. (2016). Screening for anxiety disorders with the GAD-7 and GAD-2: A systematic review and diagnostic metaanalysis. *Gen Hosp Psychiatry, 39,* 24–31.

18. Satizabal, C. L., et al. (2016). Incidence of dementia over three decades in the Framingham Heart Study. *N Engl J Med, 374,* 523–532.

19. Savoy, M., & O'Gurek, D. (2016). Screening your adult patients for depression. *Fam Pract Manag, 23*(2), 16–20.

20. Schaie, K. W., & Willis, S. L. (2016). *Handbook of the psychology of aging* (8th ed.). London: Academic Press, Elsevier.

21. Reference deleted in proofs.

22. Strub, R. L., & Black, F. W. (2000). *Mental status examination in neurology* (4th ed.). Philadelphia: Davis.

23. Tsoi, K. F., et al. (2015). Cognitive tests to detect dementia: A systematic review and meta-analysis. *JAMA Intern Med, 175*(9), 1450–1458.

24. Tyler, E. T., Hulkower, R. L., & Kaminski, J. W. (2017). *Behavioral health integration in pediatric primary care: Considerations and opportunities for policymakers, planners, and providers.* https://www.milbank.org/wp-content/uploads/2017/03/MMF_BHI_Executive-Summary-FINAL.pdf.

25. Walker, E. R., McGee, R. E., & Druss, B. G. (2015). Mortality in mental disorders and global disease burden implications. *JAMA Psychiatry, 72*(4), 334.

26. World Health Organization. (2017). *Mental disorders.* http://www.who.int/mediacentre/factsheets/fs396/en/.

27. World Health Organization (WHO). (December 2013). *Mental health: a state of well-being.* http://www.who.int/features/mental_health/en/index.html.

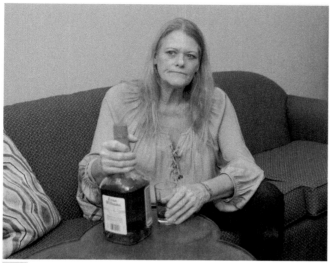

6.1

ALCOHOL USE AND ABUSE

Over half (56%) of Americans ages 18 and older report being current alcohol drinkers.[25] For adults ages 18 to 25 years, almost 40% report binge drinking ≥5 drinks/occasion, and almost 11% report heavy alcohol use (binge drinking on ≥5 days in past 30 days)[25] (Fig. 6.1). Thus alcohol is the most used and abused psychoactive drug. People like to drink!

In the 11 years between 2001-2002 and 2012-2013, the 12-month alcohol use by adults ages 18 years and older increased by 11.2%, high-risk drinking increased by almost 30%, and diagnosed alcohol use disorders (AUD) increased by almost 50%.[13] The highest increases are found among women, older adults, racial/ethnic minorities, and those with lower family income and educational level.[13] Most adults are able to drink low-to-moderate amounts of alcohol safely (≤2 drinks per day for men and ≤1 drink/day for women). But given the high rates of alcohol use, you will encounter many patients in the hospital and primary care setting with an alcohol use disorder.

Morbidity and mortality data reflect the adverse consequences of alcohol use. An estimated 88,000 people die annually from alcohol-related causes; thus alcohol use is the 4th leading preventable cause of death in the United States.[19] Alcohol-related driving deaths account for 31% of overall driving fatalities.[19] Emergency departments see over 500,000 visits each year for drugs with alcohol. For alcohol alone, it is over 800 ED visits for every 100,000 people under

age 21 years.[14] A surprisingly high number of prescription medications—591, or 45%—are classified as alcohol interactive (AI).[3] This means that their combination with alcohol changes the metabolism of the alcohol or the activity or metabolism of the medication, with a risk of adverse drug reactions (ADRs). This is especially significant with drugs that depress the central nervous system (CNS) (e.g., opioid pain relievers, heroin, benzodiazepines, antihistamines, antidepressants).[5]

Drinking a moderate amount of alcohol (i.e., ≤2 drinks per day for men and ≤1 drink per day for women) (Table 6.1) has a causal adverse effect on the risk for breast cancer and oral and esophageal cancers.[18] This is dose-dependent; the more a person drinks, the higher the risk. Drinking ≥30 grams/day (2.1 standard drinks) increases the rate of breast cancer by 32% compared with those with no alcohol intake.[17] The mechanism in causing breast cancer is likely an increase in estrogen steroids, increasing the risk for hormone-sensitive tumors.[18]

Heavy drinking (≥15 drinks per week for men and ≥8 drinks per week for women)[6] increases the risks for chronic diseases such as hypertension, heart disease, and stroke; the cancers listed earlier plus liver and colorectal cancer[8]; mental illness such as depression and anxiety; learning and memory dysfunction; social issues such as family problems and unemployment; and certainly alcohol dependence or alcoholism.[6] Alcoholism is a major cause of liver cirrhosis, which is the 8th leading cause of death in the United States.[12] The latest established causal relationship is between heavy drinking and infectious disease such as tuberculosis and the course of HIV/AIDS.[32] There is no safe limit of drinking for pregnant women as alcohol drinking causes fetal alcohol syndrome and preterm birth problems.[32]

Binge drinking (≥5 drinks per occasion for men and ≥4 drinks per occasion for women) increases the risk for injuries (motor vehicle accidents, falls, drownings, burns); violence (sexual assault, homicide, suicide); alcohol poisoning, which is a medical emergency; and risky sexual behaviors (unprotected sex or sex with multiple partners), which increases risk for sexually transmitted diseases and unintended pregnancy.[6]

Alcohol has many effects on the cardiovascular (CV) system. Evidence from multiple studies shows that in men and women, consuming more than 1 or 2 drinks of alcohol a day is associated with hypertension.[21] There are biological mechanisms postulated for this: arterial plaque buildup; baroreceptor reflex changes; body fluid changes through the renin-angiotensin-aldosterone system[21]; and activation of the

TABLE 6.1   What Is a Standard Drink?

A standard drink in the United States is any drink that contains about 14 grams of pure alcohol (about 0.6 fl oz or 1.2 tbsp). Below are U.S. standard drink equivalents. These are approximate because different brands and types of beverages vary in their actual alcohol content.

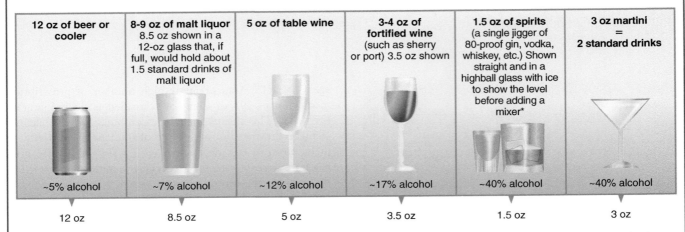

12 oz of beer or cooler	**8-9 oz of malt liquor** 8.5 oz shown in a 12-oz glass that, if full, would hold about 1.5 standard drinks of malt liquor	**5 oz of table wine**	**3-4 oz of fortified wine** (such as sherry or port) 3.5 oz shown	**1.5 oz of spirits** (a single jigger of 80-proof gin, vodka, whiskey, etc.) Shown straight and in a highball glass with ice to show the level before adding a mixer*	**3 oz martini = 2 standard drinks**
~5% alcohol	~7% alcohol	~12% alcohol	~17% alcohol	~40% alcohol	~40% alcohol
12 oz	8.5 oz	5 oz	3.5 oz	1.5 oz	3 oz

Many people do not know what counts as a standard drink; therefore they do not realize how many standard drinks are in the containers in which these drinks are often sold. Some examples:

For **beer,** the approximate number of standard drinks in:
- 12 oz = 1
- 16 oz = 1.3
- 22 oz = 2
- 40 oz = 3.3

For **malt liquor,** the approximate number of standard drinks in:
- 12 oz = 1.5
- 16 oz = 2
- 22 oz = 2.5
- 40 oz = 4.5

For **table wine,** the approximate number of standard drinks in:
- A standard 750-mL (25-oz) bottle = 5

For **80-proof spirits,** or "hard liquor," the approximate number of standard drinks in:
- A mixed drink = 1 to 3 or more*
- A pint (16 oz) = 11
- A fifth (25 oz) = 17
- 1.75 L (59 oz) = 39

Adapted from National Institute on Alcohol Abuse and Alcoholism (NIAAA). (Reprinted 2007). *Helping patients who drink too much: a clinician's guide.* Available at http://pubs.niaaa.nih.gov/publications/Practitioner/CliniciansGuide2005/clinicians_guide.htm.
***NOTE:** It can be difficult to estimate the number of standard drinks in a single mixed drink made with hard liquor. Depending on factors such as the type of spirits and the recipe, a mixed drink can contain from 1 to 3 or more standard drinks.

sympathetic nervous system, which constricts blood vessels and increases contractility. Also, ingestion of >2 drinks/day and especially >3 drinks/day increases the risk for all types of stroke. Heavy daily drinking (>5 drinks/day) increases the risk of heart failure and cardiomyopathy.[21] Finally, alcohol drinking is positively associated with risk for atrial fibrillation (AF), the most common cardiac arrhythmia. Consuming 15 to 21 drinks/week increases the risk of AF by 14% and >21 drinks/week increases risk by 39%.[16a] Binge drinking is especially to be avoided (increasing AF risk by 29%), but even habitual moderate intake poses a small and significant risk of developing AF.[16a,30]

Because of alcohol-related morbidity, many patients you encounter in primary care settings and in the hospital will have a significant drinking history. People visiting primary care providers have a significantly higher rate of past or present alcohol abuse than those in the general population. Alcohol abuse and alcohol withdrawal are involved in trauma, violence, suicides, motor vehicle accidents, and other conditions leading to intensive care unit (ICU) admissions. Among ICU patients an alcohol use disorder is present in 20% of patients and is higher with specific subpopulations: 40% of veterans and ED admissions, 60% to 70% of trauma patients, and up to 80% of patients with head and neck surgery.[11]

DEFINING ILLICIT DRUG USE

There are 7 categories of illicit drug use: marijuana,[a] cocaine, heroin, hallucinogens, inhalants, methamphetamine, and the nonmedical use of psychotherapeutics (prescription pain relievers, tranquilizers, stimulants, and sedatives). The prevalence of Americans ages 12 years or older reporting the use

---

[a]Recreational marijuana is legal in 10 states and the District of Columbia; medical marijuana is legal in 33 states.

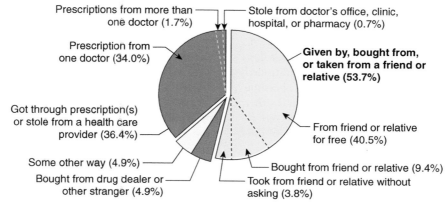

Source Where Pain Relievers Were Obtained for Most Recent Misuse Among People
12 Years of Age or Older Who Misused Prescription Pain Relievers in the Past Year:
Percentages, 2015

Prescriptions from more than one doctor (1.7%)

Stole from doctor's office, clinic, hospital, or pharmacy (0.7%)

Prescription from one doctor (34.0%)

Given by, bought from, or taken from a friend or relative (53.7%)

Got through prescription(s) or stole from a health care provider (36.4%)

From friend or relative for free (40.5%)

Some other way (4.9%)

Bought from friend or relative (9.4%)

Bought from drug dealer or other stranger (4.9%)

Took from friend or relative without asking (3.8%)

**12.5 Million People 12 Years of Age or
Older Who Misused Pain Relievers in the Past Year**

Note: The percentages do not add to 100% due to rounding.
Note: Respondents with unknown data for the Source for Most Recent Misuse or who reported Some Other Way but did not specify a valid way were excluded.

6.2

(SAMHSA, 2016.)

of any of the categories is 10.1%.[25] Marijuana use is the most common, used by almost 80% of drug users. Among youth ages 12 to 17 years, 17.5% used illicit drugs in the past year. This warrants our alarm and intervention. Any amount of illicit drug use has serious legal consequences and consequences for health, trauma, brain maturation, relationships, school, and career.

The United States now faces epidemics of prescription drug abuse and opioid-related deaths. Over 2.4 million Americans have a severe opioid-use disorder, including dependence on pain medications, heroin, or both.[31] Since 2013, rates of drug overdose death in the United States have exceeded mortality from motor vehicle accidents! Of those who obtained pain relievers nonmedically for misuse, more than half (53.7%) got them from a friend or relative. Among prescription abusers, 34% got their pain relievers from one doctor (Fig. 6.2).

Many people who abuse prescription opioids switch to heroin as prescription opioids become harder to obtain and to mix for ingestion, and for cost. Abuse of prescription opioids only was high but stable from 2008 to 2010, and then decreased annually by 6.1%.[7] At the same time, concurrent abuse of both prescription opioids and heroin increased by about 10.3% yearly from 2008 to 2014.[7] Still the abuse of pain relievers is alarmingly high, with 17.2% of people ages 12 years or older misusing in the past year.[25]

Contributing factors include an increase in prescriptions for pain relief in response to the past practice of undertreatment of pain in the mid- to late 20th century. The pendulum swung in the 2000s, with aggressive marketing by drug companies for an oxycodone product; the marketing strategies included paid speaker-training conferences; pain "education" programs; sales representatives who, encouraged by

bonuses, targeted high-volume opioid prescribers; and a misrepresentation of the addiction risk of the oxycodone product.[22] The dangers of prescription opioids (oxycodone, hydrocodone, methadone) are dose-dependent and include abuse and addiction, overdose, trauma and motor vehicle accidents, pneumonia, CV events, and death.[22]

Finally, the combination of drinking alcohol and taking alcohol-interactive (AI) drugs is alarmingly high (Fig. 6.3). In the United States 41% of current alcohol drinkers ages 20 years and over also take prescription AI medications. The most widely used medications are cardiovascular and CNS drugs.[3] Preventing alcohol-related ADRs and accidental overdose is a crucial concern.

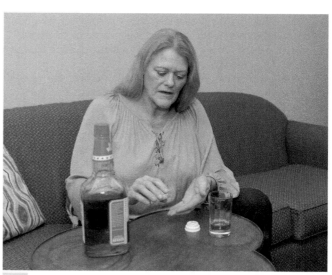

6.3

DIAGNOSING SUBSTANCE ABUSE

Substance abuse and ultimately addiction are diseases of the brain. The use of alcohol and other drugs activates reward circuits in the brain by releasing dopamine, and the users feel pleasure.[29] With continued use, the reward circuits are desensitized, pleasure is no longer felt, and the user feels less motivation to engage in everyday activities. The conditioned response (environmental cues that precede drug use) become more important, leading to cravings for alcohol and other drugs. Continued use leads to brain changes involved in executive function (decision making, control of inhibition, self-monitoring), and repeated relapse occurs.[29]

Not all drug use leads to addiction; although it is a brain disease, it is influenced by genetic, environmental, and developmental factors. The rate of Americans classified with substance abuse disorder is 8.8% of those ages 12 years and older; 5.9% had an alcohol use disorder, and 2.9% had an illicit drug use disorder.[25] It is important to note now that more and more people are poly-drug users.

The continuum of alcohol drinking ranges from special occasion use through low-to-moderate drinking to heavy drinking. Alcohol dependence, or alcoholism, is a chronic progressive disease that is not curable but is highly treatable. Accurate diagnosis is needed to provide advice, brief intervention, appropriate treatment, and follow-up. The gold standard of diagnosis is well defined by the American Psychiatric Association (APA) in its *Diagnostic and Statistical Manual of Mental Disorders*, 5th edition. Table 6.2 gives the criteria for Alcohol Use Disorder. Unfortunately alcohol problems are underdiagnosed in both primary care settings and hospitals. Excessive alcohol use often is unrecognized until patients develop serious complications.

 DEVELOPMENTAL COMPETENCE

Adolescents

Among youth 12 to 17 years of age who are diagnosed with substance use disorders, 3.4% have an illicit drug disorder and 2.5% have an alcohol disorder. For young adults ages 18

TABLE 6.2 **Alcohol Use Disorder**

Diagnostic Criteria

A. A problematic pattern of alcohol use leading to clinically significant impairment or distress, as manifested by at least two of the following occurring within a 12-month period:
1. Alcohol is often taken in larger amounts or over a longer period than was intended.
2. There is a persistent desire or unsuccessful efforts to cut down or control alcohol use.
3. A great deal of time is spent in activities necessary to obtain alcohol, use it, or recover from its effects.
4. Craving or a strong desire or urge to use alcohol.
5. Recurrent alcohol use results in a failure to fulfill major role obligations at work, school, or home.
6. Continued alcohol use despite having persistent or recurrent social or interpersonal problems caused or exacerbated by the effects of alcohol.
7. Important social, occupational, or recreational activities are given up or reduced because of alcohol use.
8. Recurrent alcohol use in situations in which it is physically hazardous.
9. Alcohol use is continued despite knowledge of having a persistent or recurrent physical or psychological problem that is likely to have been caused or exacerbated by alcohol.
10. Tolerance, as defined by either of the following:
    a. A need for markedly increased amounts of alcohol to achieve intoxication or desired effect
    b. A markedly diminished effect with continued use of the same amount of alcohol
11. Withdrawal, as manifested by either of the following:
    a. The characteristic withdrawal syndrome for alcohol
    b. Alcohol (or a closely related substance such as a benzodiazepine) taken to relieve or avoid withdrawal symptoms

Specify if:
  In early remission: After full criteria for alcohol use disorder were previously met, none of the criteria for alcohol use disorder have been met for at least 3 months but for less than 12 months (with the exception that criterion A4, "Craving, or a strong desire or urge to use alcohol," may be met).
  In sustained remission: After full criteria for alcohol use disorder were previously met, none of the criteria for alcohol use disorder have been met at any time during a period of 12 months or longer (with the exception that criterion A4, "Craving, or a strong desire or urge to use alcohol," may be met).

Specify if:
  In a controlled environment: This additional specifier is used if the individual is in an environment where access to alcohol is restricted.

Specify current severity:
  Mild: Presence of 2-3 symptoms.
  Moderate: Presence of 4-5 symptoms.
  Severe: Presence of 6 or more symptoms.

From American Psychiatric Association (2013). *Diagnostic and statistical manual of mental disorders.* (5th ed.). Washington, DC: The Association.

to 25 years, 7.2% have an illicit drug disorder and 10.9% have an alcohol disorder.[25] It is well known that alcohol retards brain development and maturity levels in adolescents. It is estimated that 4.7% of 16- or 17-year-olds and nearly 13% of 18- to 20-year-olds drive under the influence of alcohol. Youth who abuse alcohol also engage in high-risk sexual behavior and have academic problems in school, injuries from trauma, and alcohol problems that carry over to adulthood.

The Pregnant Woman

The dangers of alcohol use to the growing fetus during pregnancy are well known. Alcohol slips easily through the placenta; a defined dose that is easily metabolized by an adult woman is toxic to a fetus who weighs only grams or a few pounds. Alcohol toxicity results in physical, learning, and behavioral problems in a fetus that are defined in the Fetal Alcohol Spectrum Disorder (see Table 14.2, p. 268). Public awareness and health teaching have reduced the number of U.S. pregnant women who drink alcohol. During the 1st trimester, 19% of pregnant women ages 15 to 44 years drink alcohol, perhaps not knowing they are pregnant; this drops to 5% and 4.4% in the 2nd and 3rd trimesters, respectively.[28] The bottom line is that no amount of alcohol is safe during pregnancy.

No illicit drugs are safe during pregnancy either, yet 9% of pregnant women ages 15 to 44 years were current illicit drug users during the 1st trimester, 4.8% during the 2nd trimester, and 2.4% during the 3rd trimester.[28]

The Aging Adult

The number of older adults in the U.S. population is exploding; those over 60 years of age will number an estimated 77.6 million in 2020, and the total is projected to reach 112.5 million by 2060.[27] In 2015 the percentage of adults ages 60 to 64 years with alcohol use was 50.9%, with binge alcohol use 17%, and with heavy alcohol use 4.5%. Of those 65 years and older, the percentage with alcohol use was 42.7%, with binge alcohol use 10%, and with heavy alcohol use 2.5%.[25] Thus the projected population increase will yield a huge increase in the number of older drinkers by 2060.[2]

At the same time, older adults have numerous characteristics that can increase the risks associated with alcohol use. Liver metabolism, body water, and kidney function are decreased, which increases the bioavailability of alcohol in the blood for longer periods. Aging people lose muscle mass; less tissue to which the alcohol can be distributed means an increased alcohol concentration in the blood. Older adults may be on multiple medications, which can interact adversely with alcohol (e.g., benzodiazepines, antidepressants, antihypertensives, pain relievers, aspirin). Thus drinking alcohol increases the risk for falls, depression, gastrointestinal problems, toxic reactions, and fatal overdoses. Older adults may avoid detection of their alcohol problems; they may avoid alcohol-related consequences such as driving under the influence (DUI) because they no longer drive, or they may avoid job problems because they no longer work.

In addition, alcohol drinking increases the risk of cognitive decline in older adults.[1] All these factors are concerning because Americans over age 60 years are drinking more now than 20 years ago.[15] Both men and women have a higher prevalence of current drinking, and older women have significantly more binge drinking.[2] It may be more difficult for providers to isolate the symptoms of alcohol use disorders in the aging population, especially when considering the denial and fear of stigma that exist to a higher degree in this age group.[9]

SUBJECTIVE DATA

If the patient currently is intoxicated or going through substance withdrawal, collecting any history data is difficult and unreliable. However, when sober, most people are willing and able to give reliable data, provided the setting is private, confidential, and nonconfrontational.

Examiner Asks	Rationale
1. Ask about alcohol use: "Do you sometimes drink beer, wine, or other alcoholic beverages?" If the answer is "Yes," ask the screening question about heavy drinking days: "How many times in the past year have you had 5 or more drinks a day *(for men)* or 4 or more drinks a day?" *(for women)*	One or more heavy drinking days means that this person is an "at-risk" drinker.
To complete a picture of the person's drinking pattern, ask: "On average, how many days a week do you have an alcoholic drink?" and "On a typical drinking day, how many drinks do you have?" Recommend that the person stay at **low-to-moderate** drinking patterns: for men, ≤2 drinks/day; for women, ≤1 drink/day; for older than 65 years, ≤1 drink/day. Recommend even lower limits or abstinence for patients who take medications that interact with alcohol, have a health condition exacerbated by alcohol, or are pregnant (advise abstinence here).	For men, ≥15 drinks/week = **heavy or at-risk** drinking. For women, ≥8 drinks/week = **heavy or at-risk** drinking.[6]

Subjective Data

Examiner Asks	Rationale

2. Use brief screening instruments to help identify problem drinking and people who need a more thorough assessment. Ask the patient to respond to the AUDIT questionnaire (Table 6.3). A quantitative form has the advantage of letting you document a number for a response so it is not open to individual interpretation. The AUDIT helps detect both less severe alcohol problems (hazardous and harmful drinking) and alcohol abuse and dependence disorders. It is helpful with ED and trauma patients because it is sensitive to current as opposed to past alcohol problems. It is useful in primary care settings with adolescents and older adults. It is relatively free of gender and cultural bias.

Hazardous drinking—Pattern is high risk for future damage to physical or mental health. Harmful drinking—Alcohol use already results in problems.

TABLE 6.3 The Alcohol Use Disorders Identification Test—AUDIT*

Questions	0	1	2	3	4
1. How often do you have a drink containing alcohol?	Never	Monthly or less	2-4 times a month	2-3 times a week	4 or more times a week
2. How many drinks containing alcohol do you have on a typical day when you are drinking?	1 or 2	3 or 4	5 or 6	7 to 9	10 or more
3. How often do you have 5 or more drinks on one occasion?	Never	Less than monthly	Monthly	Weekly	Daily or almost daily
4. How often during the last year have you found that you were not able to stop drinking once you had started?	Never	Less than monthly	Monthly	Weekly	Daily or almost daily
5. How often during the last year have you failed to do what was normally expected of you because of drinking?	Never	Less than monthly	Monthly	Weekly	Daily or almost daily
6. How often during the last year have you needed a first drink in the morning to get yourself going after a heavy drinking session?	Never	Less than monthly	Monthly	Weekly	Daily or almost daily
7. How often during the last year have you had a feeling of guilt or remorse after drinking?	Never	Less than monthly	Monthly	Weekly	Daily or almost daily
8. How often during the last year have you been unable to remember what happened the night before because of your drinking?	Never	Less than monthly	Monthly	Weekly	Daily or almost daily
9. Have you or someone else been injured because of your drinking?	No		Yes, but not in the last year		Yes, during the last year
10. Has a relative, friend, doctor, or other health care worker been concerned about your drinking or suggested that you cut down?	No		Yes, but not in the last year		Yes, during the last year
					Total

*__NOTE:__ This questionnaire (the AUDIT) is reprinted with permission from the World Health Organization. To reflect standard drink sizes in the United States, the number of drinks in question 3 was changed from 6 to 5. A free AUDIT manual with guidelines for use in primary care settings is available online at www.who.org.

Examiner Asks	Rationale

Note that the AUDIT covers three domains: alcohol consumption (questions 1 to 3); drinking behavior or dependence (questions 4 to 6); and adverse consequences from alcohol (questions 7 to 10). Record the score at the end of each line and total; the maximum total is 40.

A cut point of ≥8 points for men or ≥4 points for women, adolescents, and those older than 60 years indicates hazardous alcohol consumption.

The AUDIT-C is a shorter form that is helpful for acute and critical care units. The AUDIT-C is a valid screening test for heavy drinking and/or active alcohol abuse.[5] It uses the three alcohol consumption questions (numbers 1 to 3), including question number 3, which is itself a brief screening test for heavy drinking. This helps examiners discriminate heavy, at-risk drinking from low-risk drinking in a very short time (less than 2 minutes). The possible score is 0 to 12; a low-risk response is ≤2 points.

A cut point of ≥3 is a measure of heavy or at-risk drinking. In addition, a "Yes" to drinking 6 or more drinks on one occasion *ever* in the past year warrants further assessment.

The CAGE questionnaire (**C**ut down, **A**nnoyed, **G**uilty, **E**ye-opener)[10] described in Chapter 4 (p. 53) works well in busy primary care settings because it takes less than 1 minute to complete and the 4 straightforward yes/no questions are easy for clinicians to remember. The CAGE tests for lifetime alcohol abuse and/or dependence but does not distinguish past problem drinking from active present drinking.[4] It may not detect low but risky levels of drinking and is less effective with women and minority groups.[24]

Answering "Yes" to ≥2 CAGE questions signals possible alcohol abuse and a need for further assessment.

3. Assess for alcohol use disorders using the standard clinical diagnostic criteria. Determine whether there is a maladaptive pattern of alcohol use causing clinically significant impairment or distress.[20] Ask, "In the past 12 months has your drinking repeatedly caused or contributed to:

- **Risk** for bodily harm (drinking and driving, operating machinery, swimming)?
- **Relationship** trouble (family or friends)?
- **Role failure** (interference with home, work, or school obligations)?
- **Run-ins** with the law (arrests or other legal problems)?"

If "Yes" to one or more points, it means that the person has been abusing alcohol. Warrants advice and brief intervention for assistance.

Ask, "In the past 12 months have you:
- **Not been able to stick to drinking limits** (repeatedly gone over them)?
- **Not been able to cut down or stop** (repeated failed attempts)?
- **Shown tolerance** (needed to drink a lot more to get the same effect)?
- **Shown signs of withdrawal** (tremors, sweating, nausea, or insomnia when trying to quit or cut down)?
- **Kept drinking despite problems** (recurrent physical or psychological problems)?
- **Spent a lot of time drinking** (or anticipating or recovering from drinking)?
- **Spent less time on other matters** (activities that had been important or pleasurable)?"

If "Yes" to 2 or more →, person may have alcohol use disorder. Warrants counseling and brief intervention for treatment or mutual help meetings (AA, NA).

If "No" →, patient is still at risk for developing alcohol-related problems. Warrants advice and brief intervention for assistance and close follow-up.

Ask about use of illicit substances: "Do you sometimes take illicit or street drugs such as marijuana, cocaine, hallucinogens, narcotics?" If "Yes," "When was the last time you used drugs? How much did you take that time?"

Screening Women for Alcohol Problems

The TWEAK questions[23] are a combination of items of two other questionnaires that help identify at-risk drinking in women, especially pregnant women. Instead of the guilt question from the CAGE questionnaire, the TWEAK includes a question that measures tolerance:
- **Tolerance:** How many drinks can you hold? Or how many drinks does it take to make you feel high?

Taking ≥3 drinks to feel high = Tolerance.

Examiner Asks	Rationale
• **Worry:** Have close friends or relatives worried or complained about your drinking in the past year? • **Eye-opener:** Do you sometimes take a drink in the morning when you first get up? • **Amnesia:** Has a friend or family member ever told you about things you said or did that you could not remember? • **Kut down:** Do you sometimes feel the need to cut down on your drinking?	
Score 2 points each for Tolerance and Worry, 1 point each for the rest. A low-risk response is ≤1 point.	Scoring ≥2 points = a drinking problem.
### Screening Aging Adults Use the SMAST-G questionnaire for older adults who report social or regular drinking of any amount of alcohol. Older adults have specific emotional responses and physical reactions to alcohol, and the 10 questions with yes/no responses address these factors. A low-risk response is zero or 1 point (Table 6.4).	Scoring ≥2 points indicates an alcohol problem and a need for more in-depth assessment.

4. Advise and Assist (brief intervention). Although it is beyond the scope of this text to present treatment plans, the consequences of substance abuse are so debilitating and destructive to patients and their families that a short statement of assistance and concern is given here. If your assessment has determined the patient to have at-risk drinking or illicit substance use, state your conclusion and recommendation clearly.[20]
    "You're drinking more than is medically safe." Relate to the person's concerns and medical findings, if present. *"I strongly recommend that you cut down (or quit), and I'm willing to help."*
Or, if you determine the person to have an alcohol use disorder, state your conclusion and recommendation clearly:
    "I believe that you have an alcohol use disorder. I strongly recommend that you quit drinking, and I'm willing to help." Relate to the person's concerns and medical findings if present.	

TABLE 6.4   Short Michigan Alcoholism Screening Test—Geriatric Version (SMAST-G)

	Yes (1)	No (0)
1. When talking with others, do you ever underestimate how much you drink?		
2. After a few drinks, have you sometimes not eaten or been able to skip a meal because you didn't feel hungry?		
3. Does having a few drinks help decrease your shakiness or tremors?		
4. Does alcohol sometimes make it hard for you to remember parts of the day or night?		
5. Do you usually take a drink to relax or calm your nerves?		
6. Do you drink to take your mind off your problems?		
7. Have you ever increased your drinking after experiencing a loss in your life?		
8. Has a doctor or nurse ever said they were worried or concerned about your drinking?		
9. Have you ever made rules to manage your drinking?		
10. When you feel lonely, does having a drink help?		
TOTAL SMAST-G-SCORE (0-10)	_____	

SCORING: 2 OR MORE **"YES"** RESPONSES IS INDICATIVE OF AN ALCOHOL PROBLEM.

Subjective Data

OBJECTIVE DATA

Normal Range of Findings	Abnormal Findings

Clinical laboratory findings (called **biomarkers**) give objective evidence of problem drinking. These are less sensitive than self-report questionnaires, but they are useful data to corroborate the subjective data and are unbiased. The serum protein **gamma glutamyl transferase (GGT)** is a commonly used biomarker of alcohol drinking. Occasional alcohol drinking does not raise this measure, but chronic heavy drinking does. Be aware that nonalcoholic liver disease also can increase GGT levels in the absence of alcohol.

The GGT is helpful in detecting relapses for alcohol-dependent people who are in recovery.

The **carbohydrate-deficient transferrin (CDT)** is used together with the GGT, which may increase detection of alcohol abuse. Healthy women have higher CDT levels than men; therefore combining it with GGT may improve accuracy.[26]

Serum **aspartate aminotransferase (AST)** is an enzyme found in high concentrations in the heart and liver.

From the complete blood count, the **mean corpuscular volume (MCV)** is an index of red blood cell (RBC) size. MCV is not sensitive enough to use as the only biomarker for problem drinking.

A direct serum biomarker, **phosphatidylethanol (PEth),** is a more sensitive and specific method to evaluate abstinence and sober living.[16] It the only biomarker that can detect moderate alcohol intake. PEth is a phospholipid produced only in the presence of alcohol.

Breath alcohol analysis detects any amount of alcohol in the end of exhaled air following a deep inhalation until all ingested alcohol is metabolized. This measure can be correlated with blood alcohol concentration (BAC) and is the basis for legal interpretation of drinking. Normal values indicating no alcohol are 0.00.

When caring for people experiencing alcohol withdrawal, the **Clinical Institute Withdrawal Assessment (CIWA)** is the most sensitive scale for objective measurement (Table 6.5). It is quantified to measure the progress of withdrawal. Intervention with appropriate pharmacotherapy avoids advanced withdrawal stages such as delirium tremens. Most withdrawing persons do not progress to advanced stages; thus using the CIWA scale also avoids overmedicating.

Take the vital signs: blood pressure (BP), pulse, respirations, oxygen saturation. Assess and rate each of the 10 criteria of the CIWA scale. Each criterion has a range from 0 to 7, except for "Orientation," which is rated 0 to 4. Add the scores for the total CIWA-Ar score. A score of 0 to 7 means that you can assess every 4 hours for 72 hours. If all the scores are <8 for 72 hours, you can safely discontinue use of the CIWA assessment.

Clinical appearance and behavioral signs of commonly abused substances are presented in Table 6.6. Note that clinical signs are described for both the intoxicated person and the person in withdrawal.

Abnormal Findings

Chronic alcohol drinking of ≥4 drinks/day for 4 to 8 weeks significantly raises GGT, but many chronic drinkers no longer have increased GGT.

A sudden elevated GGT after normal GGT levels may indicate relapse and prompts discussion with the person.

CDT is elevated after drinking 50 to 80 g alcohol/day for 1 week. CDT normalizes during abstinence with a half-life of 15 days.

Chronic drinking for months increases AST.

Heavy alcohol drinking for 4 to 8 weeks increases MCV.

PEth elevates after 3 weeks of drinking and remains elevated 14 days after abstinence.[26]

A BAC ≥0.08% = legal intoxication in most states (3 standard drinks), with loss of balance and motor coordination.

Withdrawal symptoms: craving for alcohol, irritability, anorexia, abdominal pain, fatigue. Signs are chills, muscle cramps, palpitations, tachycardia, hypertension, fever, disorientation, slurred speech, staggered gait, poor dexterity.

Scores of 0 to 9 = absent or minimal withdrawal; 10 to 19 = mild-to-moderate withdrawal; ≥20 = severe withdrawal.

If initial score is ≥8, take vital signs every hour for 8 hours. A score of 8 may trigger PRN medication. A score of ≥15 triggers scheduled medication.

Objective Data

ABNORMAL FINDINGS

TABLE 6.5	Clinical Institute Withdrawal Assessment of Alcohol Scale, Revised (CIWA-Ar)

Patient: _____ Date: _____ Time: _____:_____

Pulse (1 minute): _____ Blood pressure: _____/_____ Resp _____ O$_2$ Sat _____

Nausea and vomiting. Ask, "Do you feel sick to your stomach? Have you vomited?" Observation:
0 – No nausea and no vomiting
1 – Mild nausea with no vomiting
2 –
3 –
4 – Intermittent nausea with dry heaves
5 –
6 –
7 – Constant nausea, frequent dry heaves, and vomiting

Tremor. Ask patient to extend arms and spread fingers apart. Observation:
0 – No tremor
1 – Tremor not visible but can be felt, fingertip to fingertip
2 –
3 –
4 – Moderate tremor with arms extended
5 –
6 –
7 – Severe tremor, even with arms not extended

Paroxysmal sweats. Observation:
0 – No sweat visible
1 – Barely perceptible sweating; palms moist
2 –
3 –
4 – Beads of sweat obvious on forehead
5 –
6 –
7 – Drenching sweats

Anxiety. Ask, "Do you feel nervous?" Observation:
0 – No anxiety (at ease)
1 – Mildly anxious
2 –
3 –
4 – Moderately anxious or guarded; thus anxiety is inferred
5 –
6 –
7 – Equivalent to acute panic states as occur in severe delirium or acute schizophrenic reactions

Agitation. Observation:
0 – Normal activity
1 – Somewhat more than normal activity
2 –
3 –
4 – Moderately fidgety and restless
5 –
6 –
7 – Paces back and forth during most of the interview or constantly thrashes about

Tactile Disturbances. Ask, "Do you have any itching, pins-and-needles sensations, burning, or numbness, or do you feel like bugs are crawling on or under your skin?" Observation:
0 – None
1 – Very mild itching, pins-and-needles sensation, burning, or numbness
2 – Mild itching, pins-and-needles sensation, burning, or numbness
3 – Moderate itching, pins-and-needles sensation, burning, or numbness
4 – Moderately severe hallucinations
5 – Severe hallucinations
6 – Extremely severe hallucinations
7 – Continuous hallucinations

Auditory disturbances. Ask, "Are you more aware of sounds around you? Are they harsh? Do they frighten you? Do you hearing anything that is disturbing to you? Are you hearing things you know are not there?" Observation:
0 – Not present
1 – Very mild harshness or ability to frighten
2 – Mild harshness or ability to frighten
3 – Moderate harshness or ability to frighten
4 – Moderately severe hallucinations
5 – Severe hallucinations
6 – Extremely severe hallucinations
7 – Continuous hallucinations

Continued

TABLE 6.5	Clinical Institute Withdrawal Assessment of Alcohol Scale, Revised (CIWA-Ar)—cont'd

Visual disturbances. Ask, "Does the light appear to be too bright? Is its color different? Does it hurt your eyes? Are you seeing anything that is disturbing to you? Are you seeing things you know are not there? Observation:
0 – Not present
1 – Very mild sensitivity
2 – Mild sensitivity
3 – Moderate sensitivity
4 – Moderately severe hallucinations
5 – Severe hallucinations
6 – Extremely severe hallucinations
7 – Continuous hallucinations

Headache, fullness in head. Ask, "Does your head feel different? Does it feel like there is a band around your head?" Do not rate for dizziness or light-headedness; otherwise rate severity.
0 – Not present
1 – Very mild

2 – Mild
3 – Moderate
4 – Moderately severe
5 – Severe
6 – Very severe
7 – Extremely severe

Orientation and clouding of sensorium. Ask, "What day is this? Where are you? Who am I?" Observation:
0 – Oriented and can do serial additions
1 – Cannot do serial additions or is uncertain about date
2 – Date disorientation by no more than 2 calendar days
3 – Date disorientation by more than 2 calendar days
4 – Disorientated for place and/or person

Total score: _____ (Maximum = 67)

Rater's initials: _____

From Bayard, M., McIntyre, J., Hill, K.R., et al. (2004). Alcohol withdrawal syndrome. *Am Fam Physician, 69*(6), 1443-1550.

TABLE 6.6	Clinical Signs of Substance Use Disorders

"Substances" refer to agents taken nonmedically to alter mood or behavior.

Intoxication: Ingestion of substance produces maladaptive behavioral changes because of effects on the central nervous system

Abuse: Daily use needed to function, inability to stop, impaired social and occupational functioning, recurrent use when it is physically hazardous, substance-related legal problems

Dependence: Physiologic dependence on substance

Tolerance: Requires increased amount of substance to produce same effect

Withdrawal: Cessation of substance produces syndrome of physiologic symptoms

Substance	Intoxication	Withdrawal
Alcohol	**Appearance.** Unsteady gait, incoordination, nystagmus, flushed face **Behavior.** Sedation; relief of anxiety; dulled concentration; impaired judgment; expansive, uninhibited behavior; talkativeness; slurred speech; impaired memory; irritability; depression; emotional lability	**Uncomplicated.** (Shortly after cessation of drinking, peaks at 2nd day, improves by 4th to 5th day.) Coarse tremor of hands, tongue, eyelids; anorexia; nausea and vomiting; malaise; autonomic hyperactivity (tachycardia, sweating, elevated blood pressure); headache; insomnia; anxiety; depression or irritability; transient hallucinations or illusions **Withdrawal delirium, "delirium tremens."** (Much less common than uncomplicated, occurs within 1 week of cessation.) Coarse, irregular tremor; marked autonomic hyperactivity (tachycardia, sweating); vivid hallucinations; delusions; agitated behavior; fever

Continued

TABLE 6.6	Clinical Signs of Substance Use Disorders—cont'd	
Substance	Intoxication	Withdrawal
Sedatives, hypnotics (benzodiazepines)	Similar to alcohol **Appearance.** Unsteady gait, incoordination **Behavior.** Talkativeness, slurred speech, inattention, impaired memory, irritability, emotional lability, sexual aggressiveness, impaired judgment, impaired social or occupational functioning	Anxiety or irritability; nausea or vomiting; malaise; autonomic hyperactivity (tachycardia, sweating); orthostatic hypotension; coarse tremor of hands, tongue, and eyelids; marked insomnia; grand mal seizures
Nicotine	**Appearance.** Alert, increased systolic blood pressure, increased heart rate, vasoconstriction **Behavior.** Nausea, vomiting, indigestion (first use); loss of appetite; head rush; dizziness; jittery feeling; mild stimulant	Vasodilation, headaches, anger, irritability, frustration, anxiety, nervousness, awakening at night, difficulty concentrating, depression, hunger, impatience or restlessness, desire to smoke
Cannabis (marijuana)	**Appearance.** Reddened eyes; tachycardia; dry mouth; increased appetite, especially for "junk" food; loss of coordination and balance **Behavior.** Euphoria, pleasant state of relaxation and tranquility, slowed time perception, increased perceptions, impaired judgment, social withdrawal, anxiety, suspiciousness or paranoid ideation	No withdrawal with occasional use. Chronic heavy use may → mild withdrawal: irritability, sleep disturbances, weight loss, loss of appetite, sweating
Cocaine (including crack)	**Appearance.** Pupillary dilation, tachycardia or bradycardia, elevated or lowered blood pressure, sweating, chills, nausea, vomiting, weight loss **Behavior.** Euphoria, talkativeness, hypervigilance, pacing, psychomotor agitation, impaired social or occupational functioning, fighting, grandiosity, visual or tactile hallucinations	Dysphoric mood (anxiety, depression, irritability), fatigue, insomnia or hypersomnia, psychomotor agitation
Amphetamines	Similar to cocaine **Appearance.** Pupillary dilation, tachycardia or bradycardia, elevated or lowered blood pressure, sweating or chills, nausea and vomiting, weight loss **Behavior.** Elation, talkativeness, hypervigilance, psychomotor agitation, fighting, grandiosity, impaired judgment, impaired social and occupational functioning	Dysphoric mood (anxiety, depression, irritability), fatigue, insomnia or hypersomnia, psychomotor agitation
Opiates (morphine, heroin, meperidine)	**Appearance.** Pinpoint pupils; decreased blood pressure, pulse, respirations, and temperature **Behavior.** Lethargy; somnolence; slurred speech; initial euphoria followed by apathy, dysphoria, and psychomotor retardation; inattention; impaired memory; impaired judgment; impaired social or occupational functioning	Dilated pupils, lacrimation, runny nose, tachycardia, fever, elevated blood pressure, piloerection, sweating, diarrhea, yawning, insomnia, restlessness, irritability, depression, nausea, vomiting, malaise, tremor, muscle and joint pains; symptoms remarkably similar to clinical picture of influenza

BIBLIOGRAPHY

1. Bos, I., Vos, S. J., Frolich, L., et al. (2017). The frequency and influence of dementia risk factors in prodromal Alzheimer's disease. *Neurobiol Aging, 56*(8), 33–40.

2. Breslow, R. A., Castle, I., Chen, C. M., et al. (2017). Trends in alcohol consumption among older Americans: National health interview surveys, 1997 to 2014. *Alcohol Clin Exp Res, 41*(5), 976–986.

3. Breslow, R. A., Dong, C., & White, A. (2015). Prevalence of alcohol-interactive prescription medication use among current drinkers: United States, 1999 to 2010. *Alcohol Clin Exp Res, 39*(2), 371–379.

4. Bush, K., Kivlahan, D. R., McDonell, M. B., et al. (1998). The AUDIT alcohol consumption questions. *Arch Intern Med, 158*, 1789–1795.

5. Castle, I., Dong, C., Haughwout, S. P., et al. (2016). Emergency department visits for adverse drug reactions involving alcohol: United States, 2005 to 2011. *Alcohol Clin Exp Res, 40*(9), 1913–1925.

6. Centers for Disease Control and Prevention (CDC). (2016). *Alcohol use and your health.* https://www.cdc.gov/alcohol/fact-sheets/alcohol-use.htm.

7. Cicero, T. J., Ellis, M. S., & Harney, J. (2015). Shifting patterns of prescription opioid and heroin abuse in the United States. *N Engl J Med, 373*(18), 1789–1790.

8. Connor, J. (2017). Alcohol consumption as a cause of cancer. *Addiction, 112*(2), 222–228.

9. DiBartolo, M. C., & Jarosinski, J. M. (2017). Alcohol use disorder in older adults. *Issues Ment Health Nurs, 38*, 25–32.

10. Ewing, J. A. (1984). Detecting alcoholism: the CAGE questionnaire. *JAMA, 252*(14), 1905–1907.

11. Ferreira, J. A., Wieruszewski, P. M., Cunningham, D. W., et al. (2017). Approach to the complicated alcohol withdrawal patient. *J Inten Care Med, 32*(1), 3–14.

12. Ge, P. S., & Runyon, B. A. (2016). Treatment of patients with cirrhosis. *N Engl J Med, 375*(8), 767–777.

13. Grant, B. F., Chou, P., Saha, T. D., et al. (2017). Prevalence of 12-month alcohol use, high-risk drinking and DSM-IV alcohol use disorder in the United States, 2001-2002 to 2012-2013. *JAMA Psychiatry, 74*(9), 911–923.

14. Hack, J. B., Goldlust, E. J., Gibbs, F., et al. (2014). The H-Impairment index (HII): A standardized assessment of alcohol-induced impairment in the emergency department. *Am J Drug Alcohol Abuse, 40*(2), 111–117.

15. Han, B. H., Moore, A. A., Sherman, S., et al. (2017). Demographic trends of binge alcohol use and alcohol use disorders among older adults in the United States, 2005-2014. *Drug Alcohol Dep, 170*, 198–207.

16. Kechagias, S., Dernroth, D. N., Blomgren, A., et al. (2015). Phosphatidylethanol compared with other blood tests as a biomarker of moderate alcohol consumption in healthy volunteers. *Alcohol Alcohol, 50*(4), 399–406.

16a. Larsson, S. C., Drca, N., Wolk, A. (2014). Alcohol consumption and risk of atrial fibrillation. *J Am Coll Cardiol, 64*(3), 281–289.

17. Mostofsky, E., Mukamal, K. J., Giovannucci, E. L., et al. (2016). Key findings on alcohol consumption and a variety of health outcomes from the Nurses' Health Study. *Am J Public Health, 106*(9), 1586–1591.

18. Mukamal, K. J., Clowry, C. M., Murray, M. M., et al. (2016). Moderate alcohol consumption and chronic disease. *Alcohol Clin Exp Res, 40*(11), 2283–2291.

19. National Institute on Alcohol Abuse and Alcoholism (NIAAA). (2017). *Alcohol facts and statistics.* https://www.niaaa.nih.gov/alcohol-health/overview-alcohol-consumption/alcohol-facts-and-statistics.

20. National Institute on Alcohol Abuse and Alcoholism. (2007). *Helping patients who drink too much: a clinician's guide.* http://pubs.niaaa.nih.gov/publications/Practitioner/CliniciansGuide2005/Clinicians_guide.htm.

21. Piano, M. R. (2017). Alcohol's effects on the cardiovascular system. *Alcohol Res, 38*(2), e1–e24.

22. Psaty, B. M., & Merrill, J. O. (2017). Addressing the opioid epidemic. *N Engl J Med, 376*(16), 1502–1503.

23. Russell, M., Martier, S. S., & Sokol, R. J. (1994). Screening for pregnancy risk-drinking. *Alcohol Clin Exp Res, 18*(5), 1156–1161.

24. Steinbauer, J. R., Cantor, S. B., Holzer, C. E., et al. (1998). Ethnic and sex bias in primary care screening tests for alcohol use disorders. *Ann Int Med, 129*(5), 353–362.

25. Substance Abuse and Mental Health Services Administration (SAMHSA). (2016). *2015 National Survey on Drug Use and Health (NSDUH).* https://www.samhsa.gov/data/sites/default/files/NSDUH-DetTabs-2015/NSDUH-DetTabs-2015/NSDUH-DetTabs-2015.htm.

26. Tavakoli, H. R., Hull, M., & Okasinski, L. M. (2011). Review of current clinical biomarkers for the detection of alcohol dependence. *Innov Clin Neurosci, 8*(3), 26–33.

27. U.S. Census Bureau. (2014). *Projections of the population by sex and age for the United States; 2015 to 2060. Table 9. Projections of the Population by Sex and Age for the United States: 2015 to 2060.* https://www.census.gov/programs-surveys/popproj/data/tables.2014.html.

28. U.S. Department of Health and Human Services. (2014). *Results from the 2013 national survey on drug use and health.* https://www.samhsa.gov/data/sites/default/files/NSDUHresultsPDFWHTML2013/Web/NSDUHresults2013.pdf.

29. Volkow, N. D., Koob, G. F., & McLellan, T. (2016). Neurobiologic advances from the brain disease model of addiction. *N Engl J Med, 374*(4), 363–370.

30. Voskoboinik, A., Prabhu, S., Ling, L., et al. (2016). Alcohol and atrial fibrillation: A sobering review. *JACC, 68*(23), 2567–2576.

31. Williams, A. R., & Bisaga, A. (2016). From AIDS to opioids—How to combat an epidemic. *N Engl J Med, 375*(9), 813–815.

32. World Health Organization (WHO). (2015). *Alcohol fact sheet.* http://www.who.int/mediacentre/factsheets/fs349/en/.

Domestic and Family Violence Assessment

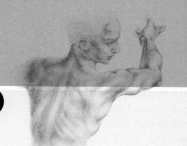

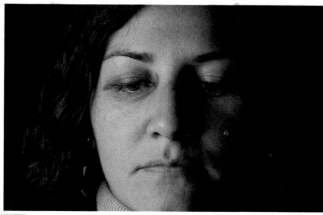

7.1 (© Nicolesy/iStock/Thinkstock.)

In the United States, approximately 20 people per minute are abused by an intimate partner, over 20,000 calls per day are placed to a domestic violence hotline,[20] and half of all female homicide victims are killed by a current or former intimate partner.[23] An average of 5 children die every day as a result of abuse and neglect,[8] and a report of child abuse is made every 10 seconds.[29] **Intimate partner violence, child abuse,** and **elder abuse** are important health problems that you must recognize the signs of and assess for in every patient (Fig. 7.1). The Joint Commission has set standards that all health care settings have policies and procedures to assess, document, and make referrals for family violence, including intimate partner abuse, child abuse, and elder abuse.

TYPES OF VIOLENCE

Intimate Partner Violence

In the United States, approximately 10 million people are physically abused by intimate partners annually, which equates to an average of 20 people every minute. Approximately 33% of women and 25% of men report being abused by an intimate partner.[20] An intimate partner is any partner (i.e., girlfriend/boyfriend, spouse, dating partner, sexual partner) with whom the person has a close relationship that may include emotional connectedness and physical/sexual contact. Intimate partner violence (IPV) includes both current and former partners, so the person need not currently be in a relationship to experience IPV. IPV can be divided into 4 main categories[2]:

- **Physical violence** is the use of force that could cause death, disability, or injury.

- **Sexual violence** includes any attempted or completed sex acts without the consent of the other person. Acts of sexual violence include, but are not limited to, rape, unwanted sexual contact, and exposure to sexual situations (e.g., pornography).
- **Stalking** is repeated, unwanted attention that leads to fear (e.g., repeated phone calls, spying, damaging personal property).
- **Psychological aggression** is a form of emotional abuse wherein the aggressor uses verbal or nonverbal communication to exert control or harm the person emotionally.

IPV also includes **teen dating violence,** which is physical, sexual, psychological, or emotional violence that occurs in a dating relationship during the adolescent years. Before the age of 18, 8.5 million female adolescents report being raped and 1.5 million male adolescents report being made to penetrate. Youth who experience dating violence are more likely to experience depression or anxiety, to engage in unhealthy behaviors (e.g., smoking and alcohol use), and to have thoughts about suicide.[5] It is important to note that, with advances of technology, new types of relationship violence are emerging, such as "sexting" or cyber abuse, which can be perpetrated 24/7 from a distance.

Child Abuse and Neglect

An average of 5 children die every day from child abuse and neglect.[8] Approximately 683,000 children are victims of child abuse and/or neglect each year, and that number is steadily increasing.[29] Child abuse and neglect are defined at both the federal and state levels. The Child Abuse and Prevention Treatment Act sets forth a federal definition of abuse and neglect, and it was recently amended to include sex trafficking and human trafficking in the definition and to enhance protections for infants affected by withdrawal symptoms and Fetal Alcohol Spectrum Disorder.[7] Some general definitions of child abuse and neglect include the following[6]:

- **Neglect** is the failure to provide for a child's basic needs (physical, medical, and supervision). Prenatal drug exposure, child abandonment, and the manufacturing of methamphetamines in the presence of a child are considered neglect in some states. Failure to educate the child is included as neglect in approximately 25 states.
- **Physical abuse** is nonaccidental physical injury caused by punching, beating, kicking, biting, burning, shaking, or otherwise harming a child. Even if the parent or caregiver did not intend to harm the child, such acts are considered abuse when done purposefully. Human

trafficking, including labor trafficking and involuntary servitude, is considered physical abuse in approximately 7 states.

- **Sexual abuse** includes fondling a child's genitals, incest, penetration, rape, sodomy, indecent exposure, and commercial exploitation through prostitution or the production of pornographic materials. Sexual abuse includes human trafficking (sex trafficking) in 21 states.
- **Emotional abuse** is any pattern of behavior that harms a child's emotional development or sense of self-worth. It includes frequent belittling, rejection, threats, and withholding of love and support.

Every state and U.S. territory has a definition of child abuse and neglect that may expand upon the federal definition. As a health care provider, it is important that you know the state definition and state laws related to child abuse and neglect since you are a mandatory reporter. As a mandatory reporter, you are required by law to report any known or suspected child abuse or neglect.

Elder Abuse and Neglect

Approximately 10% of Americans ages 60 years and older have experienced elder abuse, with estimates as high as 5 million people per year. Elder abuse is underreported, with some estimates that only 1 in 14 cases are actually reported to the authorities. In nearly 60% of the elder abuse and neglect incidents, the perpetrator is a family member, most commonly an adult child or spouse.[21] Elder abuse includes both intentional acts and failure to act by a caregiver or trusted person. Forms of elder abuse include the following[11]:

- **Physical abuse** is when an elder is intentionally injured, assaulted, threatened with a weapon, or inappropriately restrained.
- **Sexual abuse or abusive sexual contact** includes any sexual contact against the elder's will, including sexual contact with a person unable to understand the act or communicate consent.
- **Psychological or emotional abuse** includes verbal and nonverbal behavior meant to inflict fear and distress. It includes humiliation, embarrassment, controlling behavior, social isolation, and damaging/destroying property.
- **Neglect** is the failure of the caregiver to prevent harm. Neglect includes failure to meet basic needs such as hygiene, nutrition/hydration, clothing, shelter, and medical care.
- **Financial abuse or exploitation** is the unauthorized or improper use of the elder's resources for monetary or personal benefit, profit, or gain, such as forgery, theft, or improper use of guardianship or power of attorney.

Almost every state has some form of mandatory reporting of abused older adults and other vulnerable patients (the developmentally disabled and the mentally ill). You need to be familiar with the reporting requirements in the state in which you practice. Those who work in communities that border two states need to be informed about mandatory reporting statutes in both states. In some communities the reporting mechanism is established county by county, whereas other states have a statewide hotline. As mandatory reporters of abuse, you need only have suspicion that elder abuse and/or neglect may have occurred to generate a call to the authorities. You are not required to have proof before reporting suspected abuse.

HEALTH EFFECTS OF VIOLENCE

Violent experiences have significant immediate and long-term effects. The most obvious immediate health care problem is injury, but an increase in annual health care cost may persist for up to 15 years after the violence ends. Traumatic brain injury, headaches, and pain are directly associated with the injury received; however, victims of abuse also have significantly more chronic health problems, including significantly more cardiovascular, endocrine, immune, and gastrointestinal problems.[3,10] Women who are victims of abuse have more gynecologic problems and negative consequences during pregnancy (e.g., preterm birth, low-birth-weight babies, perinatal deaths). Abuse during pregnancy is also a significant health problem, with serious consequences for both the pregnant mother (e.g., depression, substance abuse) and infant (low birth weight, increased risk of child abuse).[3]

Abuse victims have significantly more depression, suicidality, posttraumatic stress disorder (PTSD), and problems with substance abuse (Fig. 7.2). Rape survivors are 3 times more likely to use marijuana and 6 times more likely to use cocaine than nonvictims.[30] Forced sex contributes to a host of reproductive health problems, including chronic pelvic pain, unintended pregnancy, sexually transmitted infections, and urinary tract infections.[3]

Child maltreatment can have deleterious effects on a child's quality of life and may lead to overall poor health, which

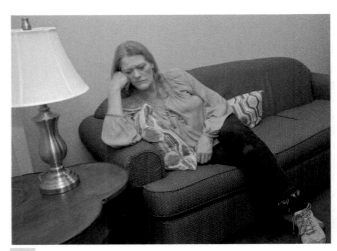

7.2

can last into adulthood. Children who are abused have an increased incidence of improper brain development, cerebral palsy due to head trauma, delayed language development, and mental health issues (e.g., depression, anxiety), and they are at higher risk for chronic diseases such as obesity, cardiovascular disease, cancer, and high blood pressure. Childhood abuse and neglect increase the likelihood of juvenile arrest, teen pregnancy, and adult criminal behavior.[4]

CULTURE AND GENETICS

IPV is a phenomenon that occurs universally in all populations.[1] However, lifetime prevalence of IPV (including rape, physical violence, and stalking) is significantly higher among ethnic and racial minorities than among non-Hispanic white women and men. Multiracial, American Indian/Alaskan native, and non-Hispanic black women and men are at higher risk for IPV than non-Hispanic white women and men. Unfortunately, little research exists about the effectiveness of screening and prevention efforts among racial and ethnic minorities and the effectiveness of therapeutic interventions to help survivors with resultant mental health problems.

Although there are wide differences among distinct cultural groups and within any given culture, some common themes create barriers to treatment for all. These barriers are societal stressors, legal issues, and lack of access to culturally appropriate care.

Societal stressors contribute to daily struggles and conflict in relationships. For example, poverty is a risk factor for IPV. All ethnic and racial minority groups have poverty rates exceeding the national average for non-Hispanic whites. In addition, help-seeking often is deferred because of fears of racism and discrimination. Because of past experiences of prejudice and discrimination by health care providers and lack of knowledge of the culture, many immigrants and members of racial and ethnic minorities are reluctant to seek help in the health care setting.

Legal status in the United States creates a barrier to care for many immigrant families. If a woman does not have legal status or citizenship within the United States, she may fear that she will be deported and lose her children.[26] Many immigrant women are unaware of their legal rights in situations of IPV. The Violence Against Women Act (VAWA) offers assistance to IPV survivors and includes protections for immigrant survivors. VAWA includes stipulations for coordinating services between law enforcement, victim services, and attorneys; training personnel to provide services; and funding programs to help victims.[17]

A **lack of access to culturally appropriate care** is a continual problem. In spite of the widespread growth of IPV services and the widely distributed availability of translation services, immigrants and ethnic minorities are less likely than non-Hispanic whites to use social service resources. Traditional gender roles reinforce dependency and may increase the risk for IPV against women. Women are often financially dependent on their husbands, and this dependency is reinforced by religious and cultural values, which identify men as the providers within the family. In some cultures, the traditional belief is that a man has the right to physically discipline his wife. In these cases, the women may not report violence because they expect it as a social norm. In other cases, women may feel stigmatized if they speak out against violence.[32]

To address barriers to care, recommendations for culturally sensitive approaches to screening and treatment are available.[14] These recommendations include access to bilingual bicultural providers, access to translators, education about legal rights, incorporation and acknowledgment of the importance of religion and training of religious leaders, and involvement of the family and outreach to the community to raise awareness of the prevalence of IPV. However, the most important aspects of treatment are to understand the meaning and experiences of IPV for each person and to account for her or his cultural beliefs and values.

DOCUMENTATION

Documentation of IPV, child abuse, and elder abuse must include detailed, nonbiased progress notes, injury maps, and photographic documentation as appropriate. Written documentation of histories needs to be verbatim but within reason. It may be unrealistic to transcribe everything the person tells you, but it is important to capture exceptionally poignant phrases. Phrases that identify the reported perpetrator and severe threats of harm made by the reported perpetrator are important. Other aspects of the abuse history, including reports of past abusive incidents, can be paraphrased with the use of partial direct quotations.

When quoting or paraphrasing the history, you should not sanitize the words reportedly heard by the victim. Verbatim documentation of the reported perpetrator's threats interlaced with curses and expletives can be useful in future court proceedings. Also be careful to use the exact terms that an abused patient uses to describe sexual organs or sexually assaultive behaviors. If you are unsure what the person means, ask for clarification.

Documentation of the physical examination needs to be thorough and unbiased. Do not speculate on what caused an injury; instead, document what you observed and what the victim said. Document any lesions using appropriate terminology. Table 7.1 lists common forensic terms with definitions.

Digital photographic documentation in the medical record can be invaluable. Prior written consent to take photographs should be obtained from all cognitively intact, competent adults. Most health facilities have standardized consent-to-photograph forms. If a patient is unconscious or cognitively impaired, taking photographs without consent is generally viewed as ethically sound because it is a noninvasive, painless intervention that has high potential to help a suspected abuse victim.

Subjective Data

TABLE 7.1 Forensic Terminology

Abrasion A wound caused by rubbing the skin or mucous membrane.

Avulsion The tearing away of a structure or part.

Bruise Superficial discoloration caused by hemorrhage into the tissues from ruptured blood vessels beneath the skin surface, without the skin itself being broken; also called a *contusion.*

Contusion A bruise; injury to tissues without breakage of skin; blood from broken blood vessels accumulates, producing pain, swelling, tenderness.

Cut See "Incision."

Ecchymosis A hemorrhagic spot or blotch, larger than petechia, in the skin or mucous membrane, forming a nonelevated, rounded or irregular blue or purplish patch.

Hematoma A localized collection of extravasated blood, usually clotted in an organ, space, or tissue.

Hemorrhage The escape of blood from a ruptured vessel, which can be external, internal, and/or into the skin or other organ.

Incision A cut or wound made by a sharp instrument; the act of cutting.

Laceration The act of tearing or splitting; a wound produced by the tearing and/or splitting of body tissue, usually from blunt impact over a bony surface.

Lesion A broad term referring to any pathologic or traumatic discontinuity of tissue or loss of function of a part.

Patterned injury An injury caused by an object that leaves a distinct pattern on the skin and/or organ (e.g., being whipped with an extension cord) or an injury caused by a unique mechanism of injury (e.g., immersion burns to the hands [glove burns] or feet [sock burns]).

Pattern of injuries Usually bruises and fractures in various stages of healing.

Petechiae Minute, pinpoint, nonraised, perfectly round purplish-red spots caused by intradermal or submucous hemorrhage, which later turn blue or yellow.

Puncture The act of piercing or penetrating with a pointed object or instrument.

Stab wound A penetrating, sharp, cutting injury that is deeper than it is wide.

Traumatic alopecia Loss of hair from pulling and yanking or by other traumatic means.

Wound A general term referring to a bodily injury caused by physical means.

Adapted from Merriam-Webster's *Medical Desk Dictionary Revised Edition.* (2005). Springfield, Ma: Merriam-Webster; and Sheridan, D. J., & Nash, K. R. (2007). Acute injury patterns of intimate partner violence victims. *Trauma Violence Abuse, 8*(3), 281-289.

When documenting the history and physical findings of child abuse and neglect, use the words the child has given to describe how his or her injury occurred. Remember that the possibility arises that the abuser may be accompanying the child. You will need to separate the child from the abuser for the interview. If the child is nonverbal, use statements from caregivers. It is important to know your employer/institutional protocol for obtaining a history in cases of suspected child maltreatment. Some protocols may delay a full interview until it can be done by a forensically trained interviewer.

SUBJECTIVE DATA

According to the latest guidelines published by the U.S. Preventive Services Task Force[18] (USPSTF), all women of childbearing age (14 to 46 years) should be screened for IPV. Screening should take place regardless of whether the person has any signs of abuse or neglect. Early detection is key in preventing long-term negative health outcomes associated with IPV. The USPSTF cites insufficient evidence to recommend routine screening of elderly or vulnerable adults (physically or mentally disabled). The USPSTF does not currently have recommendations on whether all children under the age of 18 years should be screened for abuse in the primary care setting; however, the scope of the problem is noted, and early community-based intervention, such as home visitation, is identified as a potential preventive measure.

While the USPSTF recommends screening for certain populations, we will discuss screening for every patient encountered in the health care setting. As a health care provider, you are a mandatory reporter, and it is important that you understand how to screen and assess for potential violence.

Examiner Asks	Rationale

IPV, elder abuse, and child abuse will be discussed separately, with recommendations for screening as well as screening tools identified in each section. It is important that you are familiar with the tools used in your facility so that you can screen for abuse based on your facility's policy. In any case of suspected

Examiner Asks	Rationale

abuse, an open-ended question such as "Tell me what happened" can be useful. In all cases, it is important to interview the victim separately from the potential perpetrator. Listen for cues of abuse, such as explanations that don't match the injury or inability to keep the story straight. Frequently seeking care for suspicious injuries is another potential indicator of abuse. Know your state laws, and do not hesitate to report suspected abuse per your state law and institutional policy. Remember, you don't need to prove the abuse in order to file a report.

Intimate Partner Violence

It is important that you normalize the questions by asking every patient about IPV. While women are at higher risk for IPV, men are also victims of abuse. Some clinicians express concern that screening everyone may cause unintended harm, but no research evidence supports that concern.[15]

Treat every patient the same in the screening process. Do not single out any gender or ethnic group.

History questions, including prior hospitalizations, treatment for injuries, and delayed treatment, may give some cues, especially if the person has been injured multiple times. If the person is seeing you for an injury, ask about the circumstances surrounding the injury and make sure the circumstances match the type of damage.

Cumulative trauma has been associated with more severe mental and physical health problems.

It is imperative that you know the IPV screening tool used in your setting. Some hospitals have a single question (e.g., "Do you feel safe at home?"), whereas others may use a standardized tool. The USPSTF reviewed IPV screening tools for sensitivity and specificity. Those with the highest levels of sensitivity and specificity were Hurt, Insult, Threaten, Scream (HITS); Ongoing Abuse Screen/ Ongoing Violence Assessment Tool (OAS/OVAT); Slapped, Threatened, and Throw (STaT); Humiliation, Afraid, Rape, Kick (HARK); Modified Childhood Trauma Questionnaire-Short Form (CTQ-SF); and Woman Abuse Screening Tool (WAST).[18]

Assessing risk for IPV and presence of IPV can aid in early intervention in the clinical setting. Early intervention may result in fewer long-term physical and mental health consequences. Using a tool with high levels of sensitivity and specificity will allow clinicians to better screen for and recognize clients who are victims of violence. Each of the recommended tools is a brief questionnaire that can be administered in minutes.

HITS is a 4-item tool that asks clients to answer the following questions from *never* to *frequently*.[27]

How often does your partner:
1- Physically hurt you
2- Insult or talk down to you
3- Threaten you with harm
4- Scream or curse at you

Each question is scored from 0 (never) to 5 (frequently) and the answers are totaled. A score greater than 10 on the HITS tool is indicative of IPV.[28]

STaT is a 3-item tool that includes the following questions[22]:
1- Have you ever been in a relationship where your partner has pushed or **slapped** you?
2- Have you ever been in a relationship where your partner **threatened** you with violence?
3- Have you ever been in a relationship where your partner has **thrown,** broken, or punched things?

Answering yes to any of the STaT questions constitutes a positive screen for IPV.

The HITS tool can also be used to screen adolescents for teen dating violence. When screening an adolescent, make sure to use age-appropriate language and provide examples. Instead of referring to IPV, ask about specifics (e.g., punched, hit, or slapped). Nurses play a critical role in identification of teen dating violence. All teens who come to the ED with an injury should be screened.[25]

Approximately 10% of teens report being victims of physical violence and 10% report sexual victimization.[31] Teens who experience dating violence are at higher risk for mental and physical health consequences. Early identification and intervention is needed.

Subjective Data

Examiner Asks	Rationale

Elder Abuse and Neglect

The USPSTF did not recommend a specific screening for elder abuse; however, The Joint Commission, National Center on Elder Abuse, National Academy of Sciences, and American Academy of Neurology all recommend routine screening. While validated screening tools are available, insufficient evidence is available to suggest whether one tool should be recommended. The Elder Abuse Suspicion Index (Fig. 7.3) has been validated in primary care and can be used with cognitively intact patients.[12]

By 2030, the elderly population in the United States is expected to top 30 million. With an increase in the number of elderly patients, an increase in the number of elder abuse cases is expected.

Elder Abuse Suspicion Index© (EASI)

EASI Questions Q.1-Q.5 asked of patient; Q.6 answered by doctor (*Within the last 12 months*)			
1) Have you relied on people for any of the following: bathing, dressing, shopping, banking, or meals?	YES	NO	Did not answer
2) Has anyone prevented you from getting food, clothes, medication, glasses, hearing aids, or medical care or from being with people you wanted to be with?	YES	NO	Did not answer
3) Have you been upset because someone talked to you in a way that made you feel shamed or threatened?	YES	NO	Did not answer
4) Has anyone tried to force you to sign papers or to use your money against your will?	YES	NO	Did not answer
5) Has anyone made you afraid, touched you in ways that you did not want, or hurt you physically?	YES	NO	Did not answer
6) **Doctor**: Elder abuse <u>may</u> be associated with findings such as poor eye contact, withdrawn nature, malnourishment, hygiene issues, cuts, bruises, inappropriate clothing, or medication compliance issues. Did you notice any of these today or in the last 12 months?	YES	NO	Not sure

7.3   (Copyright © 2006 M.J. Yaffe, M. Lithwick, & C. Wolfson.)

As with other populations, types of abuse may vary. In the elderly, it is important to consider financial or material abuse along with physical, emotional, and sexual abuse. Elders are at risk for financial abuse, including theft, forcible transfer of property, and coercion to steal assets.

Child Abuse and Neglect

Health care providers should monitor for signs of abuse and neglect during visits to the clinic or hospital. The primary health care provider is in an ideal position to screen for and prevent child abuse and neglect. By providing anticipatory guidance, health care providers can support caregivers of young children. During your contact with children, watch the interaction between the caregiver and child. Does the child appear to trust the caregiver? Does the child appear anxious? Overly quiet?

The use of developmental screening tools can identify risk for abuse and provide a platform for educating the caregiver. When a caregiver is aware of expected development and upcoming developmental changes (e.g., the normal periods of excessive crying in the newborn period), they may be less likely to become frustrated with the child.

For nonverbal children, subjective data will come from the caregiver. During the interview, be attentive to the interaction between the caregiver and child. If an injury is reported or abuse is suspected, be mindful of whether the information provided surrounding the injury/event matches what you observe clinically.

Health care providers have contact with infants and children multiple times a year and are able to monitor the child's development and interaction with caregivers.

Screening tools allow the provider to identify whether normal developmental milestones are being met. Children who are developmentally delayed are at higher risk for abuse.

Examiner Asks	Rationale
If the child is verbal, a history should be obtained away from the caregivers through open-ended questions or spontaneous statements. It is important to remember that children may have suffered significant trauma yet respond only minimally to open-ended questions. Keeping the questions short and using age-appropriate language and familiar words can help enrich the history taking. Children older than 11 years can generally be expected to provide a history at the level of most adults.	Separating the caregiver from the child is a necessary part of screening for child abuse and neglect. The child needs to feel safe answering the questions and may not be willing to answer truthfully if under the influence of a caregiver.
The medical history is an important part of screening for abuse and neglect in children. In addition to basic medical history questions, you will want to ask specific questions related to hospitalization, recent injuries, and delay in seeking care. Consider including the following questions: Has the child had previous hospitalizations or injuries? Does he or she suffer from any chronic medical conditions? Does the child take any medication or have a condition that may cause easy bruising? Is there a history of substance abuse in the family or any financial or social stressors in the home? What are the typical methods of discipline used in the home? Do you routinely use any specific cultural practices to promote healing (e.g., cupping, coining)?	Some medical conditions can mimic child abuse. Obtaining a thorough medical history is necessary to rule out a medical condition that mimics abuse.

Certain cultural practices may leave bruises on the skin, and some are not considered effective unless bruising is apparent[13] (Fig. 7.4). These are not acts of child abuse. |

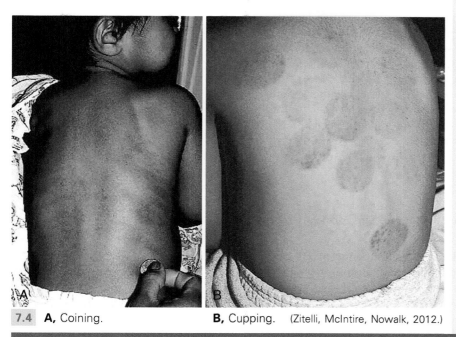

7.4 A, Coining.   **B,** Cupping.   (Zitelli, McIntire, Nowalk, 2012.)

OBJECTIVE DATA

Normal Range of Findings	Abnormal Findings

A thorough head-to-toe examination is imperative for any patient with suspected or known abuse. A visual examination of the entire body is necessary in order to document any lesions.

Keep in mind the following guidelines when documenting the physical examination:
- *Bruise* can be used interchangeably with *contusion.*
- *Laceration* is related to *avulsion.*
- *Ecchymosis* is related to *(senile) purpura.*

Normal Range of Findings	Abnormal Findings

- *Petechia* is related to *purpura*.
- *Rug burn* is more accurately described as a *friction abrasion*.
- *Incision* can be used interchangeably with *cut*.
- *Cut* can be used interchangeably with *sharp injury*.
- *Stab wounds* are penetrating, deep, sharp injuries.
- *Hematoma* is a collection of blood that is often but not always caused by blunt-force trauma.

Many practitioners try to date bruises based on the color; however, there is no scientific evidence to support the accurate dating of injuries based on color of the contusion.[19] Some guidelines can help to determine if the approximate age of the bruise is consistent with the history being provided by the patient and/or caregiver. A new bruise is usually red and often develops a purple or purple-blue appearance 12 to 36 hours after blunt-force trauma. The color of bruises (and ecchymoses) generally progress from purple-blue to bluish-green to greenish-brown to brownish-yellow before fading away. The color of bruises is the same on all people, but skin color may increase or decrease visibility of bruises.[19]

Document the size, color, and pattern of any bruises, but do not try to determine timing of the injury based solely on the color of the bruise.

Multiple factors can contribute to older adults bruising more readily or more severely than younger people. Medications (e.g., aspirin, anticoagulants, nonsteroidal anti-inflammatory drugs) and abnormal blood values can cause a person to bruise more easily. Nutritional supplements (e.g., garlic, ginkgo) also contribute to hematologic complications, especially if the person is already taking a blood-thinning or platelet-altering medication.

Any health evaluation for known or suspected elder abuse and neglect should include these baseline laboratory tests: a complete blood count (CBC) with platelet level, basic blood chemistries (including blood urea nitrogen [BUN], creatinine, protein, and albumin), serum liver function tests, a coagulation panel, and a urinalysis.

Infants and Children

A full visual inspection of children is necessary because clothing, diapers, socks, and long hair can hide significant injuries.

Accidental bruising in healthy, active children is common, but infants who are not yet walking with support (e.g., cruising around furniture) typically should not have bruises. Bruising in infants who are not yet cruising, usually infants younger than 9 months, should alert you to possible abusive mechanisms to the injury or an underlying medical condition.

Although any area of the body can be injured intentionally, certain locations are more concerning for inflicted injury. Bruising in atypical places, such as the buttocks, hands, feet, and abdomen, is exceedingly rare and should arouse concern. In children younger than 4 years, bruising on the torso, ears, and neck and any bruising on a precruising infant are significantly correlated with abuse in the absence of a compelling history.[24] Any bruise that takes the shape of an object is highly concerning for abuse. Bruising found in immobile children should raise your concern and should be the basis for a comprehensive evaluation for abuse or an underlying medical condition.

Bruising in a suspicious area of the body without a compelling history warrants further evaluation for abuse.

In a young child, a radiologic survey to look for occult injuries may be warranted. This includes a skeletal survey (series of x-ray images of all bones) or a bone scan (nuclear medicine).

Radiographic images that show multiple fractures in various stages of healing are suspicious for abuse.

ABNORMAL FINDINGS

TABLE 7.2 Abusive Burns

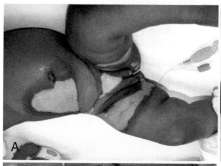

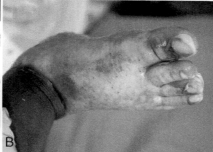

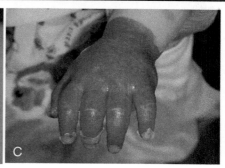

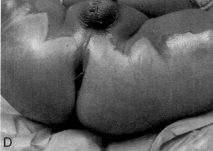

Immersion Injury Patterns

A, Immersion in hot water; note sparing of the flexor creases. **B,** Immersion stocking burn of an infant's foot. **C,** Immersion glove burn of an infant's hand. **D,** Immersion buttocks burn.

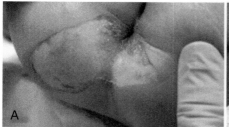

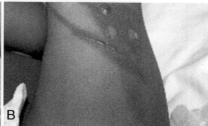

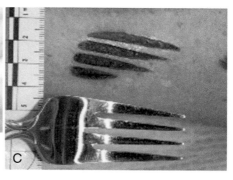

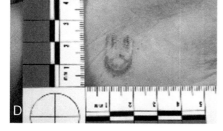

Pattern Burn Injury

A, Hair straightening iron burn on the buttocks. **B,** Burn caused by a steam iron. **C,** Burn caused by fork tines. **D,** Burn caused by a lighter.

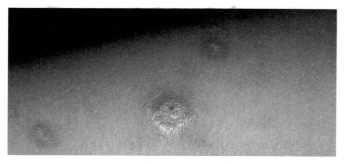

◄ Cigarette Burns

These burns demonstrate classic abuse with lesions in various stages of healing.

See Illustration Credits for source information.

TABLE 7.3	Suspicious Bruising

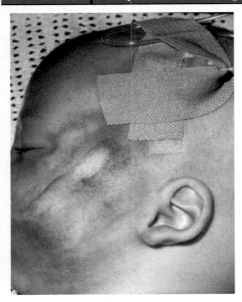

Fingers
Abusive bruise on the left cheek demonstrating the imprint of fingers.

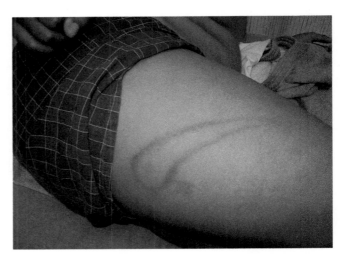

Belt Loop
Bruising in the pattern of a belt loop.

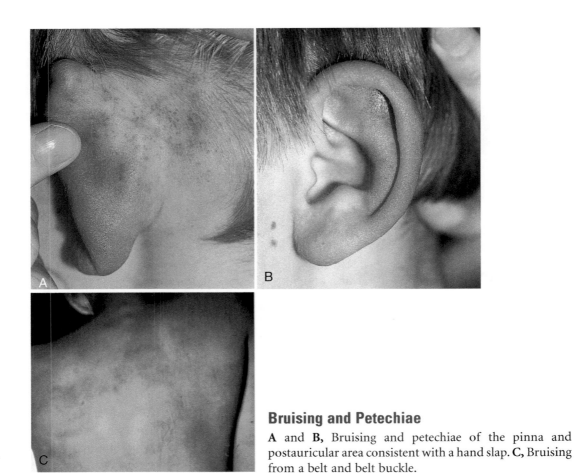

Bruising and Petechiae
A and **B,** Bruising and petechiae of the pinna and postauricular area consistent with a hand slap. **C,** Bruising from a belt and belt buckle.

Continued

TABLE 7.3	Suspicious Bruising—cont'd

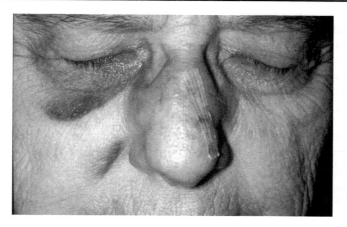

Nasal Fracture

Periorbital ecchymoses and fracture nasal bone.

Thigh Bruises

Inner thigh bruises on a woman with severe dementia. The placement of bruises is suspicious for sexual abuse.

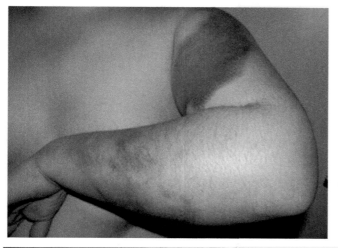

◄ **Defensive Wounds**

Defensive wounds are often found on the hands and forearms as the victim tries to protect his or her body from the assailant.

TABLE 7.4	Signs of Neglect

Pressure Ulcers

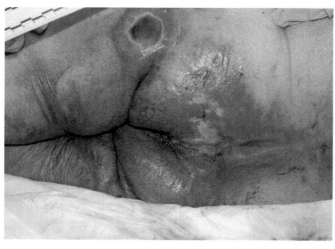

Case of elder abuse showing moisture-associated skin damage.

TABLE 7.5	Assessing Homicide Risk

Just over 55% of all female homicides are related to IPV, and over 11% of victims experienced violence in the month preceding the homicide. Non-Hispanic black women and American Indian/Alaskan native women experience the highest rate of homicide.[23] Failing to routinely assess for IPV in medical settings is a missed opportunity for health care professionals to identify IPV and intervene to decrease the danger. The Danger Assessment (DA) (Fig. 7.5) (http://www.dangerassessment.org/) begins with a calendar so that women can see for themselves how frequent and severe the violence has become over the past year. The calendar is followed by a series of 20 yes/no items. Although there are no predetermined cutoff scores on the DA, the more "yes" answers there are, the more serious the danger of the woman's situation.

DANGER ASSESSMENT Jacquelyn C. Campbell, Ph.D., R.N. Copyright 1985, 1988, 2001

Several risk factors have been associated with homicides (murders) of both batterers and battered women in research conducted after the murders have taken place. We cannot predict what will happen in your case, but we would like you to be aware of the danger of homicide in situations of severe battering and for you to see how many of the risk factors apply to your situation.

Using the calendar, please mark the approximate dates during the past year when you were beaten by your husband or partner. Write on that date how bad the incident was according to the following scale:

1. Slapping, pushing; no injuries and/or lasting pain
2. Punching, kicking; bruises, cuts, and/or continuing pain
3. "Beating up"; severe contusions, burns, broken bones
4. Threat to use weapon; head injury, internal injury, permanent injury
5. Use of weapon; wounds from weapon

(If **any** of the descriptions for the higher number apply, use the higher number.)

Mark **Yes** or **No** for each of the following. ("He" refers to your husband, partner, ex-husband, ex-partner, or whoever is currently physically hurting you.)

_____ 1. Has the physical violence increased in severity or frequency over the past year?
_____ 2. Has he ever used a weapon against you or threatened you with a weapon?
_____ 3. Does he ever try to choke you?
_____ 4. Does he own a gun?
_____ 5. Has he ever forced you to have sex when you did not wish to do so?
_____ 6. Does he use drugs? By drugs, I mean "uppers" or amphetamines, speed, angel dust, cocaine, "crack," street drugs or mixtures.
_____ 7. Does he threaten to kill you and/or do you believe he is capable of killing you?
_____ 8. Is he drunk every day or almost every day? (In terms of quantity of alcohol.)
_____ 9. Does he control most or all of your daily activities? (For instance, does he tell you who you can be friends with, when you can see your family, how much money you can use, or when you can take the car?)
     (If he tries, but you do not let him, check here: _____)
_____ 10. Have you ever been beaten by him while you were pregnant? (If you have never been pregnant by him, check here: _____)
_____ 11. Is he violently and constantly jealous of you? (For instance, does he say, "If I can't have you, no one can"?)
_____ 12. Have you ever threatened or tried to commit suicide?
_____ 13. Has he ever threatened or tried to commit suicide?
_____ 14. Does he threaten to harm your children?
_____ 15. Do you have a child that is not his?
_____ 16. Is he unemployed?
_____ 17. Have you left him during the past year? (If you have *never* lived with him, check here: _____)
_____ 18. Do you currently have another (different) intimate partner?
_____ 19. Does he follow or spy on you, leave threatening notes, destroy your property, or call you when you don't want him to?

_____ Total "Yes" Answers

Thank you. Please talk to your nurse, advocate, or counselor about what the Danger Assessment means in terms of your situation.

7.5	Danger assessment.	(Courtesy Jacquelyn C. Campbell.)

REFERENCES

1. Asay, S. M., DeFrain, J., Metzger, M., et al. (2016). Implementing a strengths-based approach to intimate partner violence worldwide. *J Fam Violence*, 31, 349–360.
2. Breiding, M. J., et al. (2015). *Intimate partner violence surveillance: Uniform definitions and recommended data elements, Version 2.0*. Atlanta, GA: National Center for Injury Prevention and Control, Centers for Disease Control.
3. Centers for Disease Control and Prevention. (2017). *Intimate partner violence: Consequences*. https://www.cdc.gov/violence prevention/intimatepartnerviolence/consequences.html.
4. Centers for Disease Control and Prevention. (2017). *Child abuse and neglect: Consequences*. https://www.cdc.gov/ violenceprevention/childmaltreatment/consequences.html.
5. Centers for Disease Control and Prevention. (2017). *Teen dating violence*. https://www.cdc.gov/violenceprevention/ intimatepartnerviolence/teen_dating_violence.html.

6. Child Welfare Information Gateway. (2016). *Definitions of child abuse and neglect*. Washington, DC: U.S. Department of Health and Human Services, Children's Bureau.

7. Child Welfare Information Gateway. (2017). *About CAPTA: A legislative history*. Washington, DC: U.S. Department of Health and Human Services, Children's Bureau.

8. Child Welfare Information Gateway. (2017). *Child abuse and neglect fatalities 2015: Statistics and interventions*. Washington, DC: U.S. Department of Health and Human Services, Children's Bureau.

9. Reference deleted in proofs.

10. Duffy, M. (2017). *Domestic violence and chronic health conditions: Are they linked?*. National Center for Health Research. http://www.center4research.org/domestic-violence -chronic-health-conditions-linked/.

11. Hall, J., Karch, D. L., & Crosby, A. (2016). *Uniform definitions and recommended core data elements for use in elder abuse surveillance, Version 1.0*. Atlanta, GA: National Center for Injury Prevention and Control, Centers for Disease Control.

12. Hoover, R. M., & Polson, M. (2014). Detecting elder abuse and neglect: Assessment and intervention. *Am Fam Physician, 89*, 453–460.

13. Killion, C. M. (2017). Cultural healing practices that mimic child abuse. *Ann Forensic Res Anal, 4*, 1042.

14. Marrs Fuchsel, C. L., & Hysjulien, B. (2013). Exploring a domestic violence intervention curriculum for immigrant Mexican women in a group setting. *Soc Work Groups, 36*(4), 304–320.

15. Miller, E., McCaw, B., Humphreys, B. L., et al. (2015). Integrating intimate partner violence assessment and intervention into healthcare in the United States: A systems approach. *J Womens Health, 24*, 92–99.

16. Reference deleted in proofs.

17. Modi, M. N., Palmer, S., & Armstrong, A. (2014). The role of Violence Against Women Act in addressing intimate partner violence: A public health issue. *J Womens Health, 23*, 253–259.

18. Moyer, V. A. (2013). Clinical guidelines: Screening for intimate partner violence and abuse of elderly and vulnerable adults: U.S. Preventive Services Task Force Recommendation Statement. *Ann Intern Med, 158*, 478–486.

19. Nash, K. R., & Sheridan, D. J. (2009). Can one accurately date a bruise: State of the science. *J Forensic Nurs, 5*, 31–37.

20. National Coalition Against Domestic Violence. (2015). *Domestic violence national statistics*. www.ncadv.org.

21. National Council on Aging. (2017). *Elder abuse facts*. https:// www.ncoa.org/public-policy-action/elder-justice/elder-abuse -facts/.

22. Paranjape, A., & Liebschutz, J. (2003). STaT: A three-question screen for intimate partner violence. *J Womens Health, 12*, 233–239.

23. Petrosky, E., Blair, J. M., Betz, C. J., et al. (2017). Racial and ethnic differences in homicides of adult women and the role of intimate partner violence—United States, 2003-2014. *MMWR Morb Mortal Wkly Rep, 66*, 741–746.

24. Pierce, M. C., Kaczor, K., Aldridge, S., et al. (2010). Bruising characteristics discriminating physical child abuse from accidental trauma. *Pediatrics, 125*(1), 67–74.

25. Potera, C. (2014). Screening teens for dating violence in EDs. *Am J Nurs, 114*(10), 14.

26. Rana, S. (2013). *Immigrant women and domestic violence*. https://vawnet.org/sc/immigrant-women-and-domestic -violence.

27. Sherin, K. M. (2017). *The HITS Tool*. http://thehitstool.com.

28. Sherin, K. M., Sinacore, J. M., Li, X. Q., et al. (1998). HITS: A short domestic violence screening tool for use in a family practice setting. *Fam Med, 30*, 508–512.

29. U.S. Department of Health & Human Services, Administration for Children and Families, Administration on Children, Youth and Families, Children's Bureau. (2017). *Child Maltreatment 2015*. http://www.acf.hhs.gov/programs/ cb/research-data-technology/statistics-research/child -maltreatment.

30. US Department of Veterans Affairs. (2016). *Sexual assault against females*. https://www.ptsd.va.gov/professional/trauma/ other/sexual_assault_against_females.asp.

31. Vagi, K. J., Olsen, E. O., Basile, K. C., et al. (2015). Teen dating violence (physical and sexual) among US high school students: Findings from the 2013 National Youth Risk Behavior Survey. *JAMA Pediatr, 169*, 474–482.

32. World Health Organization. (2009). *Changing cultural and social norms that support violence*. http://www.who.int/ violence_injury_prevention/violence/norms.pdf.

CHAPTER 8

Assessment Techniques and Safety in the Clinical Setting

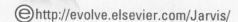

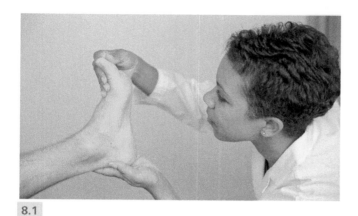

8.1

CULTIVATING YOUR SENSES

The physical examination requires you to develop technical skills and a knowledge base. The technical skills are the tools to gather data. You use your senses—sight, smell, touch, and hearing—to gather data during the physical examination (Fig. 8.1). The skills requisite for the physical examination are **inspection, palpation, percussion,** and **auscultation.** They are performed one at a time and typically in this order.

Inspection

Inspection is concentrated watching. It is close, careful scrutiny, first of the individual as a whole and then of each body system. Inspection begins the moment you first meet the person and develop a "general survey." Specific data to consider for the general survey are presented in Chapter 9. Your initial impression of the person can be helpful as you proceed through your assessment. Something as simple as a greeting and handshake can yield important assessment data.[2] As you proceed through the examination, start the assessment of each body system with inspection.

Inspection always comes first. Initially you may feel embarrassed "staring" at the person without also "doing something." A focused inspection takes time and yields a surprising amount of data. Train yourself not to rush through inspection by holding your hands behind your back.

Learn to use each person as his or her own control, and compare the right and left sides of the body. The two sides are nearly symmetric. Inspection requires good lighting, adequate exposure, and occasional use of certain instruments (otoscope, ophthalmoscope, penlight, nasal and vaginal specula) to enlarge your view.

Palpation

Palpation follows and often confirms what you noted during inspection. Palpation applies your sense of touch to assess the following factors: texture; temperature; moisture; organ location and size; and any swelling, vibration or pulsation, rigidity or spasticity, crepitation, presence of lumps or masses, and presence of tenderness or pain. Different parts of the hands are best suited for assessing different factors:

- Fingertips—Best for fine tactile discrimination, as of skin texture, swelling, pulsation, and determining presence of lumps
- A grasping action of the fingers and thumb—To detect the position, shape, and consistency of an organ or mass
- The dorsa (backs) of hands and fingers—Best for determining temperature because the skin is thinner than on the palms
- Base of fingers (metacarpophalangeal joints) or ulnar surface of the hand—Best for vibration

Your palpation technique should be slow and systematic, calm and gentle. Warm your hands by kneading them together or holding them under warm water. Identify any tender areas and palpate them last.

Start with light palpation to detect surface characteristics and to accustom the person to being touched. Then perform deeper palpation. Keep in mind that the person needs to be relaxed to allow adequate palpation. You might find it helpful to encourage the person to use relaxation techniques such as imagery or deep breathing. With deep palpation (as for abdominal contents), intermittent pressure is better than one long, continuous palpation. Avoid any situation in which deep palpation could cause internal injury or pain.

Bimanual palpation requires the use of both of your hands to envelop or capture certain body parts or organs such as the kidneys, uterus, or adnexa for more precise delimitation (see Chapters 22 and 27).

Percussion

Percussion is tapping the person's skin with short, sharp strokes to assess underlying structures. The strokes yield an audible vibration and a characteristic sound that depicts the location, size, and density of the underlying organ. While x-ray images are more accurate than percussion, they are not always available. Your hands are always available, are easily portable, and give instant feedback. Percussion has the following uses:

- Mapping out the *location* and *size* of an organ by exploring where the percussion note changes between the borders of an organ and its neighbors

- Signaling the *density* (air, fluid, or solid) of a structure by a characteristic note
- Detecting an abnormal mass if it is fairly superficial; the percussion vibrations penetrate about 5 cm (2 inches) deep—a deeper mass would give no change in percussion
- Eliciting a deep tendon reflex using the percussion hammer

The Stationary Hand

Hyperextend the middle finger (the *pleximeter)* and place its distal joint and tip *firmly* against the person's skin. Avoid placement over the ribs, scapulae, and other bony prominences. Percussing over a bone yields no data because it always sounds "dull." Lift the rest of the stationary hand up off the person's skin (Fig. 8.2). A hand resting on the skin will dampen the produced vibrations, making them difficult to interpret. Check your technique to assure that only the distal joint and tip of your middle finger are touching the person.

The Striking Hand

Use the middle finger of your dominant hand as the *striking finger* (the *plexor)* (Fig. 8.3). Hold your forearm close to the skin surface, with your upper arm and shoulder steady. Scan your muscles to make sure that they are steady but not rigid. The action is all in the wrist, and it *must* be relaxed. Spread your fingers, swish your wrist, and bounce your middle finger off the stationary one. Aim for just behind the nail bed or at the distal interphalangeal joint; the goal is to hit the portion of the finger that is pushing the hardest into the skin surface.

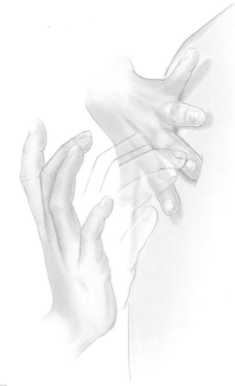

8.3

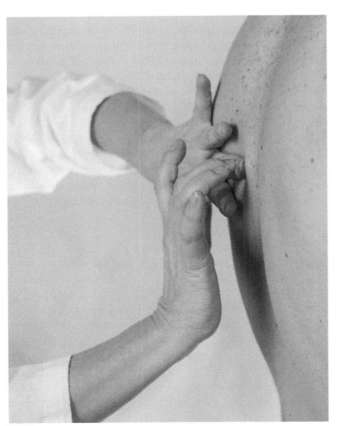

8.2

Flex the striking finger so that its tip, not the finger pad, makes contact. It hits directly at right angles to the stationary finger.

Percuss 2 times in each location using even, staccato blows. Lift the striking finger off quickly; a resting finger dampens vibrations. Then move to a new body location and repeat, keeping your technique even. The force of the blow determines the loudness of the note. You do not need a very loud sound; use just enough force to achieve a clear note. The thickness of the person's body wall will be a factor. You need a stronger percussion stroke for persons with obese or very muscular body walls.

Production of Sound

All sound results from vibration of some structure. Percussing over a body structure causes vibrations that produce characteristic waves and that are heard as "notes" (Table 8.1), which are differentiated by the following components: (1) **amplitude** (or intensity), a loud or soft sound; (2) **pitch** (or frequency), the number of vibrations per second; (3) **quality** (timbre), a subjective difference caused by the distinctive overtones of a sound; and (4) **duration**, the length of time the note lingers.

A basic principle is that a structure with relatively more air (e.g., the lungs) produces a louder, deeper, and longer sound because it vibrates freely, whereas a denser, more solid structure (e.g., the liver) gives a softer, higher, shorter sound because it does not vibrate as easily. Although Table 8.1 describes five "normal" percussion notes, variations occur in clinical practice. The "note" you hear depends on the nature

TABLE 8.1	**Characteristics of Percussion Notes**				
	AMPLITUDE	PITCH	QUALITY	DURATION	SAMPLE LOCATION
Resonant	Medium-loud	Low	Clear, hollow	Moderate	Over normal lung tissue
Hyperresonant	Louder	Lower	Booming	Longer	Normal over child's lung. Abnormal in the adult, over lungs with increased amount of air as in emphysema
Tympany	Loud	High	Musical and drumlike (like the kettledrum)	Sustained longest	Over air-filled viscus (e.g., the stomach, the intestine)
Dull	Soft	High	Muffled thud	Short	Relatively dense organ as liver or spleen
Flat	Very soft	High	A dead stop of sound, absolute dullness	Very short	When no air is present, over thigh muscles or bone or over tumor

of the underlying structure, the thickness of the body wall, and your technique.

Auscultation

Auscultation is listening to sounds produced by the body, such as the heart and blood vessels and the lungs and abdomen. You have probably already heard certain body sounds with your ear alone (e.g., the gurgling of a hungry stomach). However, most body sounds are very soft and must be channeled through a **stethoscope** for you to evaluate them. The stethoscope does not magnify sound but does block out extraneous room sounds. Of all the equipment you use, the stethoscope quickly becomes a very personal instrument. Take time to learn its features and to fit one individually to your needs.

The fit and quality of the stethoscope are important. You cannot assess what you cannot hear through a poor instrument. The slope of the earpiece should point forward toward your nose. This matches the natural slope of your ear canal and efficiently blocks out environmental sound. If necessary, twist the earpieces to parallel the slope of your ear canals. The earpieces should fit snugly, but if they hurt, they are inserted too far. Adjust the tension and experiment with different rubber or plastic earplugs to achieve the most comfort. The tubing should be of thick material, with an internal diameter of 4 mm ($\frac{1}{8}$ in), and about 36 to 46 cm (14 to 18 in) long. Longer tubing may distort the sound.

Choose a stethoscope with two endpieces—a diaphragm and a bell (Fig. 8.4). You will use the **diaphragm** most often because its flat edge is best for high-pitched sounds—breath, bowel, and normal heart sounds. Hold the diaphragm firmly against the person's skin, firm enough to leave a slight ring afterward. The **bell** endpiece has a deep, hollow, cuplike shape. It is best for soft, low-pitched sounds such as extra heart sounds or murmurs. Hold it lightly against the person's skin, just enough that it forms a perfect seal. Holding it any harder causes the person's skin to act as a diaphragm, obliterating the low-pitched sounds.

Some newer stethoscopes have one endpiece with a "tunable diaphragm." This enables you to listen to both low- and high-frequency sounds without rotating the endpiece. For low-frequency sounds (traditional bell mode), hold the endpiece very lightly on the skin; for high-frequency sounds (traditional diaphragm mode), press the endpiece firmly on the skin. Make sure that you familiarize yourself with your stethoscope to assure proper use.

Before you can evaluate body sounds, you must eliminate any confusing artifacts:
- Any extra room noise can produce a "roaring" in your stethoscope; therefore the room must be quiet.
- Keep the examination room warm, and warm your stethoscope. If the person starts to shiver, the involuntary

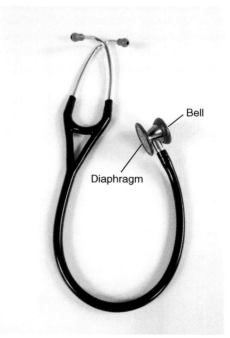

8.4 Stethoscope diaphragm (*left*) and bell (*right*).

muscle contractions could drown out other sounds. Clean your stethoscope endpiece with an alcohol wipe, and warm it by rubbing the endpiece in your palm.

- The friction on the endpiece from a man's hairy chest causes a crackling sound that mimics an abnormal breath sound called *crackles*. To minimize this problem, wet the hair before auscultating the area.
- **Never listen through a gown** (Fig. 8.5). Even though you see this on television, listening through clothing creates artifactual sound and muffles any diagnostically valuable sound from the heart or lungs. Therefore reach under a gown to listen, and take care that no clothing rubs on the stethoscope.
- Finally avoid your own "artifact," such as breathing on the tubing or the "thump" from bumping the tubing. Jewelry such as earrings and necklaces can also cause artifact.

Auscultation is a skill that beginning examiners are eager to learn but one that is difficult to master. First you must learn the wide range of normal sounds. Once you can recognize normal sounds, you can distinguish the abnormal and "extra" sounds. Be aware that in some body locations you may hear more than one sound, which can be confusing. You need to listen selectively to only one thing at a time. As you listen, ask yourself: What am I *actually hearing*? What *should* I be hearing at this spot?

These technical skills will help you gather data to add to your knowledge base and previous experience. A sturdy knowledge base enables you to look *for* rather than merely look *at*. The chapters that follow present the specific content for each body system and will help you determine what you are looking *for*.

SETTING

The examination room should be warm and comfortable, quiet, private, and well lit. When possible, stop any distracting noises such as humming machinery, radio or television, or talking that could make it difficult to hear body sounds. Your time with the individual should be secure from interruptions from other health care personnel.

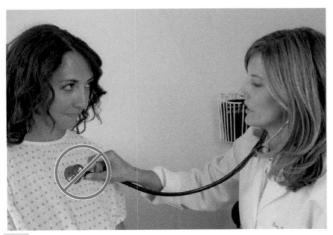

8.5

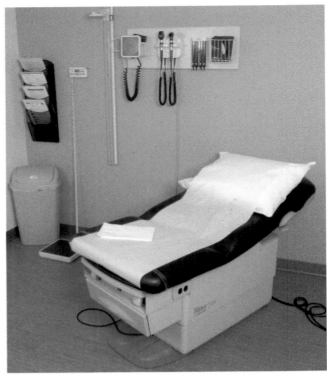

8.6

Lighting with natural daylight is best, although it is often not available; artificial light from two sources suffices and prevents shadows. A wall-mounted or gooseneck stand lamp is needed for high-intensity lighting. This provides *tangential* lighting (directed at an angle), which highlights pulsations and body contours better than perpendicular lighting.

Position the examination table so that both sides of the person are easily accessible (Fig. 8.6). The table should be at a height at which you can stand without stooping and should be equipped to raise the person's head up to 45 degrees. A roll-up stool is used for the sections of the examination for which you must be sitting. A bedside stand or table is needed to lay out all your equipment.

EQUIPMENT

During the examination you do not want to be searching for equipment or need to leave the room to find an item. Have all your equipment easily accessible and laid out in an organized fashion (Fig. 8.7). The following items are usually needed for a screening physical examination:

- Platform scale with height attachment
- Sphygmomanometer
- Stethoscope with bell and diaphragm endpieces
- Thermometer
- Pulse oximeter (in hospital setting)
- Flashlight or penlight
- Otoscope/ophthalmoscope
- Tuning fork

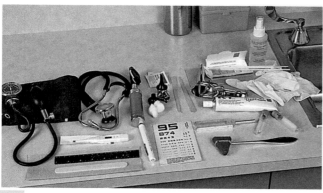

8.7

- Nasal speculum (if a short, broad speculum is not included with the otoscope)
- Tongue depressor
- Pocket vision screener
- Skin-marking pen
- Flexible tape measure and ruler marked in centimeters
- Reflex hammer
- Sharp object (split tongue blade)
- Cotton balls
- Bivalve vaginal speculum (for female persons)
- Clean gloves
- Alcohol wipes
- Hand sanitizer
- Materials for cytologic study (if applicable)
- Lubricant
- Fecal occult blood test materials

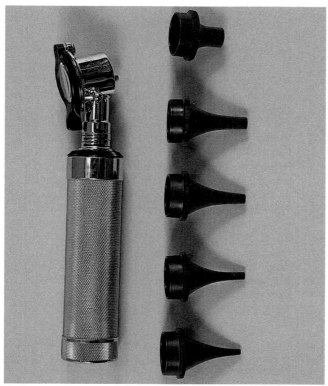

8.8 Otoscope.

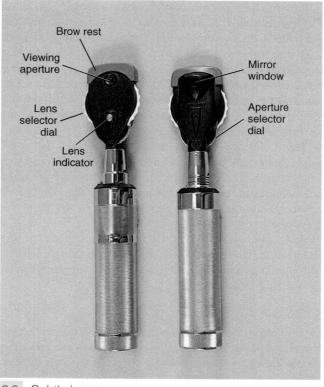

8.9 Ophthalmoscope.

Most of the equipment is described as it comes into use throughout the text. However, consider these introductory comments on the otoscope and ophthalmoscope.

The **otoscope** funnels light into the ear canal and onto the tympanic membrane. The base serves both as the power source by holding a battery and as the handle. To attach the head, press it down onto the male adaptor end of the base and turn clockwise until you feel a stop. To turn the light on, press the red button rheostat down and clockwise. (Always turn it off after use to increase the life of the bulb and battery.) Five specula, each a different size, are available to attach to the head (Fig. 8.8). The short, broad speculum is for viewing the nares. Choose the largest one that will fit comfortably into the person's ear canal. See Chapter 16 for technique on use of the otoscope.

The **ophthalmoscope** illuminates the internal eye structures. Its system of lenses and mirrors enables you to look through the pupil at the fundus (background) of the eye, much like looking through a keyhole at a room beyond. The ophthalmoscope head attaches to the base male adaptor just as the otoscope head does (Fig. 8.9). The head has five different parts:

1. Viewing aperture, with five different apertures
2. Aperture selector dial on the front
3. Mirror window on the front
4. Lens selector dial
5. Lens indicator

Select the aperture to be used, most often the small spot for undilated pupils or the large full spot for dilated pupils.

Rotating the lens selector dial brings the object into focus. The lens indicator shows a number, or *diopter,* that indicates the value of the lens in position. The black numbers indicate a positive lens, from 0 to +40. The red numbers indicate a negative lens, from 0 to −20. The ophthalmoscope can compensate for myopia (nearsightedness) or hyperopia (farsightedness) but does not correct for astigmatism. See Chapter 15 for details on how to hold the instrument, how to use the instrument, and what to inspect.

The following equipment occasionally will be used, depending on the individual's needs: goniometer to measure joint range of motion, Doppler sonometer to augment pulse or blood pressure measurement, pain rating scale (in numbers or faces), monofilament to test sensation in the foot, and bladder scanner to assess urine retention.

For a child you also will need appropriate pediatric-size endpieces for stethoscope and otoscope specula, materials for developmental assessment, age-appropriate toys, and a pacifier for an infant.

A Clean Field

Do not let your stethoscope become a *staph*-oscope! Stethoscopes and other equipment that are frequently used on many people are common vehicles for transmission of infection. Clean your stethoscope endpiece with an alcohol wipe before and after every person. The best routine is to combine stethoscope cleaning with every episode of hand hygiene.

Designate a "clean" versus a "used" area for handling your equipment. You can use two separate tables (e.g., an over-bed table and a side table) or use two separate areas of the same table. Distinguish the clean area by one or two disposable paper towels. On the towels place all the new or newly alcohol-swabbed equipment that you will use for this person (e.g., your stethoscope endpieces, the reflex hammer, ruler). As you proceed through the examination, pick up each piece of equipment from the clean area; after use on the person, relegate it to the used area or (as in the case of tongue blades, gloves) throw it directly in the trash.

A SAFER ENVIRONMENT

In addition to monitoring the cleanliness of your equipment, take all steps to avoid any possible transmission of infection between persons or between person and examiner (Table 8.2). A health care–associated (nosocomial) infection is a hazard because hospitals have sites that are reservoirs for virulent microorganisms. Some of these microorganisms (such as methicillin-resistant *Staphylococcus aureus* (MRSA), vancomycin-resistant *Enterococcus* (VRE), and multidrug-resistant tuberculosis) are resistant to antibiotics and difficult to treat.

The single most important step to decrease the risk of microorganism transmission is to wash your hands promptly and thoroughly: (1) **before and after** every physical patient encounter; (2) after contact with blood, body fluids, secretions, and excretions; (3) after contact with any equipment contaminated with body fluids; and (4) after removing gloves (see Table 8.2). Using alcohol-based hand sanitizer takes less time than soap-and-water handwashing; it also kills more organisms more quickly and is less damaging to the skin because of emollients added to the product. Alcohol is highly effective against both gram-positive and gram-negative bacteria; *Mycobacterium tuberculosis;* and most viruses, including

---

TABLE 8.2 Standard Precautions for Use With All Persons

STANDARD PRECAUTIONS are based on the principle that all blood, body fluids, secretions, excretions (except sweat), nonintact skin, and mucous membranes may contain transmissible infectious agents. Precautions apply to all patients, regardless of suspected or confirmed infection status, and in any setting in which health care is delivered. Components are:

- **Hand hygiene.** (1) Avoid unnecessary touching of surfaces in close proximity to the patient. (2) When hands are visibly dirty, contaminated with proteinaceous material, or visibly soiled with blood or body fluids, wash them with soap and water. (3) If not visibly soiled, decontaminate hands with an alcohol-based hand rub. Perform hand hygiene: (a) before having direct contact with patients; (b) after contact with blood, body fluids or excretions, mucous membranes, nonintact skin, or wound dressings; (c) after contact with a patient's intact skin (e.g., taking a pulse or blood pressure or lifting a patient); (d) after contact with medical equipment in the immediate vicinity of the patient; (e) after removing gloves.
- **Use of gloves, gown, mask, eye protection, or face shield.** (1) Wear gloves when you anticipate that contact with blood or other potentially infectious materials, mucous membranes, nonintact skin, or potentially contaminated intact skin (e.g., patient incontinent of stool or urine) could occur. (2) Wear a gown to protect skin and clothing when you anticipate contact with blood, body fluids, secretions, or excretions. (3) Use mouth, nose, and eye protection to protect the mucous membranes during procedures that are likely to generate splashes or sprays of blood, body fluids, secretions, and excretions (e.g., suctioning a patient).
- **Respiratory hygiene/cough etiquette** is targeted at patients and accompanying persons with undiagnosed transmissible respiratory infections. Elements include: (1) education of staff, patients, and visitors; (2) posted signs in language(s) appropriate to the population; (3) source control measures (e.g., covering the mouth/nose with a tissue when coughing and promptly disposing of used tissues, using surgical masks on the coughing person); (4) hand hygiene after contact with respiratory secretions; and (5) spatial separation of >3 feet from people with respiratory infections in common waiting areas.

Adapted from Centers for Disease Control and Prevention. (2007). Standard precautions—excerpt from the guidelines for isolation precautions: preventing transmissions of infectious agents in health-care settings. (2007). https://www.cdc.gov/infectioncontrol/basics/standard-precautions.html.

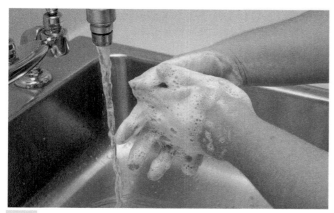

8.10   (Zakus, 2001.)

hepatitis B and C viruses, HIV, and enteroviruses.[1] Rub all hand surfaces with 3 to 5 mL of alcohol for 20 to 30 seconds. Use the mechanical action of soap-and-water handwashing (Fig. 8.10) when hands are visibly soiled and when the person is infected with spore-forming organisms (e.g., *Clostridium difficile* and noroviruses).[1]

Wear gloves when the potential exists for contact with any body fluids (e.g., blood, mucous membranes, body fluids, drainage, open skin lesions). However, wearing gloves is *not* a protective substitute for washing hands because gloves may have undetectable holes or become torn during use, or hands may become contaminated as gloves are removed. Wear a gown, mask, and protective eyewear when the potential exists for any blood or body fluid spattering (e.g., suctioning, arterial puncture).

THE CLINICAL SETTING

General Approach

Consider your emotional state and that of the person being examined. The person may be anxious about being examined by a stranger and about the unknown outcome of the examination. Try to reduce any anxiety so that the data will more closely describe the person's natural state. Anxiety can be reduced by an examiner who is confident and self-assured, considerate, and unhurried.

Usually a beginning examiner feels anything *but* self-assured! Most worry about technical skill, missing something significant, or forgetting a step. Many are embarrassed themselves about encountering a partially dressed individual. All these fears are natural and common. The best way to minimize anxiety is by practicing on a healthy willing subject, usually a fellow student. You have to feel comfortable with your motor skills before you can absorb what you are actually seeing or hearing in a "real" patient. This comes with practice under the guidance of an experienced practitioner and in an atmosphere in which it is acceptable to make mistakes and ask questions. Your subject should "act like a patient" so that you can deal with the "real" situation while still in a safe setting. After you feel comfortable in the laboratory setting, accompany

an experienced practitioner as he or she examines an actual patient so that you can observe an experienced examiner.

Hands On

With preparation it is possible to interact with your own patient in a confident manner. Begin by measuring the person's height, weight, blood pressure, temperature, pulse, and respirations (see Chapters 9 and 10). If needed, measure visual acuity at this time using the Snellen eye chart (see Chapter 15). All of these are familiar, relatively nonthreatening actions; they will gradually accustom the person to the examination. Sometimes an icebreaker about an irrelevant topic will help the person feel that he or she is seen as an individual. You might say, "Interesting cap. Does that mean you are a baseball fan?" or "I see you are from Michigan. How was the winter there?" These irrelevant openers signal that you have shared experiences and also that you are willing to have a conversation—a good warm-up for the examination data and shared decision making that come next.[4]

Then ask the person to change into an examining gown, leaving his or her underwear on. This will feel more comfortable, and the underwear can easily be removed just before the genital examination. Unless your assistance is needed, leave the room as the person undresses. Teens can remain in street clothes.

As you reenter the room, clean your hands in the person's presence. This indicates that you are protective of this person and are starting fresh for him or her. Explain each step in the examination and how the person can cooperate. Encourage the person to ask questions. Keep your own movements slow, methodical, and deliberate.

Begin by touching the person's hands, checking skin color, nail beds, and metacarpophalangeal joints (Fig. 8.11; see

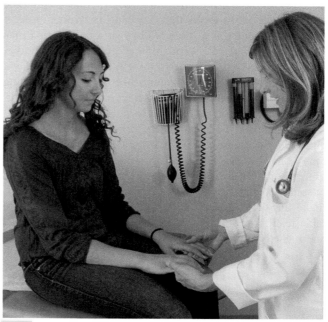

8.11

Chapters 13 and 23). Again this is a less threatening way to ease a person into being touched. Most people are used to having relative strangers touch their hands.

As you proceed through the examination, avoid distractions and concentrate on one step at a time. The sequence of the steps may differ, depending on the age of the person and your own preference. However, you should establish a system that works for you and stick to it to avoid omissions. Organize the steps so that the person does not change positions too often. Although proper exposure is necessary, use additional drapes to maintain the person's privacy and prevent chilling.

Do not hesitate to write out the examination sequence and refer to it as you proceed. The person will accept this as quite natural if you explain that you are making brief notations to ensure accuracy. Many agencies use a form that is printed or computerized, depending on the documentation system. You will find that you will glance at the form less and less as you gain experience. Even with a form, you sometimes may forget a step in the examination. When you realize this, perform the maneuver in the next logical place in the sequence. (See Chapter 28 for the sequence of steps in the complete physical examination.)

As you proceed through the examination, occasionally offer some brief teaching about the person's body. For example, you might say, "Everyone has two sounds for each heartbeat, something like this—lub-dup. Your own beats sound healthy and normal." Do not do this with every single step or you will be hard pressed to make a comment when you do come across an abnormality. But some sharing of information builds rapport and increases the person's confidence in you as an examiner. It also gives the person a little more control in a situation in which it is easy to feel completely helpless.

At some point you will want to linger in one location to concentrate on some complicated findings. To avoid anxiety, tell the person, "I always listen to heart sounds on a number of places on the chest. Just because I am listening a long time doesn't necessarily mean that anything is wrong." And it follows that sometimes you *will* discover a finding that may be abnormal and you want another examiner to double-check. You need to give the person some information, yet you should not alarm him or her unnecessarily. Say something like, "I don't have a complete assessment of your heart sounds. I want Stephanie to listen to you, too."

At the end of the examination, summarize your findings and share the necessary information with the person. Thank him or her for the time spent. In a hospital setting, apprise the person of what is scheduled next. Before you leave a hospitalized patient, lower the bed to reduce the risk for falls; make the person comfortable and safe; return the bedside table, television, or any equipment to the way it was originally; and make sure the call button is available.

❖ DEVELOPMENTAL COMPETENCE

Children are different from adults—not only in size, but also in their overall development. Children's bodies grow in a predictable pattern that is assessed during the physical examination. However, their behavior is also different. Behavior grows and develops through predictable stages, just as the body does.

With all children the goal is to increase their comfort in the setting. This approach reveals their natural state as much as possible and will give them a more positive memory of health care providers. Remember that a "routine" examination is anything but routine to the child. You can increase his or her comfort by attending to the following developmental principles and approaches. The *order* of the developmental stages is more meaningful than the exact chronologic age. Each child is an individual and will not fit exactly into one category. For example, if your efforts to "play games" with the preschooler are rebuffed, modify your approach to the security measures used with the toddler. For more detailed information on pediatric assessment and communication in the health care setting, please refer to *Wong's Essentials of Pediatric Nursing* (Hockenberry, Wilson, & Rodgers, 2017).[3]

The Infant

Erikson defines the major task of infancy as establishing trust. An infant is completely dependent on the caregiver for his or her basic needs. If these needs are met promptly and consistently, the infant feels secure and learns to trust others.

Position

- The caregiver should be present to understand normal growth and development and for the child's feeling of security.
- Place the neonate or young infant flat on a padded examination table (Fig. 8.12). The infant also may be held against the caregiver's chest for some steps.
- Once the baby can sit without support (around 6 months), as much of the examination as possible should be performed while the infant is in the caregiver's lap.

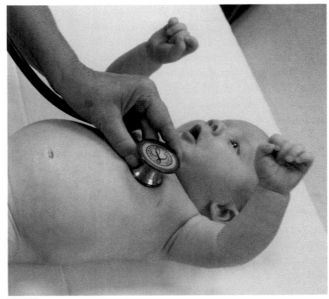

8.12

- By 9 to 12 months the infant is acutely aware of the surroundings. Anything outside the infant's range of vision is "lost"; thus the caregiver must be in full view.

Preparation

- Timing should be 1 to 2 hours after feeding, when the baby is not too drowsy or too hungry.
- Maintain a warm environment. A neonate may require an overhead radiant heater.
- An infant will not object to being nude. Have the caregiver remove outer clothing, but leave a diaper on.
- An infant does not mind being touched, but make sure that your hands and stethoscope endpiece are warm.
- Use a soft, crooning voice during the examination; the baby responds more to the feeling in the tone of the voice than to what is actually said.
- An infant likes eye contact; lock eyes from time to time.
- Smile; a baby prefers a smiling face to a frowning one. Often beginning examiners are so absorbed in their technique that they look serious or stern. Be mindful of facial expressions and take time to play.
- Keep movements smooth and deliberate, not jerky.
- Use a pacifier for crying or during invasive steps.
- Offer brightly colored toys for a distraction when the infant is fussy.
- Let an older baby touch the stethoscope or tongue blade.

Sequence

- Seize the opportunity with a sleeping baby to listen to heart, lung, and abdominal sounds first.
- Perform least distressing steps first. See the sequence in Chapter 29. Save the invasive steps of examination of the eye, ear, nose, and throat until last.
- If you elicit the Moro or "startle" reflex, do it at the end of the examination because it may cause the baby to cry.

The Toddler

This is Erikson's stage of developing autonomy. However, the need to explore the world and be independent is in conflict with the basic dependency on the caregiver. This often results in frustration and negativism. The toddler may be difficult to examine; do not take this personally. Because he or she is acutely aware of the new environment, the toddler may be frightened and cling to the caregiver (Fig. 8.13). The toddler also has fear of invasive procedures and dislikes being restrained.

Position

- The toddler should be sitting up on the caregiver's lap for all of the examination. When he or she must be supine (as in the abdominal examination), move chairs to sit knee-to-knee with the caregiver. Have the toddler lie in the caregiver's lap with his or her legs in your lap.
- Enlist the aid of a cooperative caregiver to help position the toddler during invasive procedures such as using the otoscope or taking a rectal temperature.

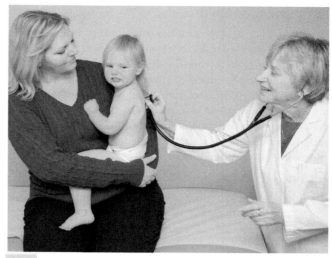

8.13

Preparation

- Children 1 or 2 years of age can understand symbols; thus a security object such as a special blanket or teddy bear is helpful.
- Begin by greeting the child and the accompanying caregiver by name, but with a child 1 to 6 years old focus more on the caregiver. By essentially "ignoring" the child at first, you allow him or her to adjust gradually and size you up from a safe distance. Then turn your attention gradually to the child, at first to a toy or object the child is holding or perhaps to compliment a dress, the hair, or what a big girl or boy the child is. If the child is ready, you will note these signals: eye contact with you, smiling, talking with you, or accepting a toy or a piece of equipment.
- A 2-year-old child does not like to take off his or her clothes; have the caregiver undress the child one part at a time.
- Children 1 or 2 years of age like to say "No." Do not offer a choice when there really is none. Avoid saying, "May I listen to your heart now?" When the 1- or 2-year-old child says "No" and you go ahead and do it anyway, you lose trust. Instead use clear, firm instructions in a tone that expects cooperation, "Now it is time for you to lie down so I can check your tummy."
- Also, 1- or 2-year-old children like to make choices. When possible, enhance autonomy by offering the *limited option:* "Shall I listen to your heart next or your tummy?"
- Demonstrate the procedures on the caregiver.
- Praise the child when he or she is cooperative.

Sequence

- Collect some objective data during the history, which is a less stressful time. While you are focusing on the caregiver, note the child's gross motor and fine motor skills and gait. A great deal of information can be gained through watching a child.
- Begin with "games" such as the Denver II test or cranial nerve testing.
- Start with nonthreatening areas. Save distressing procedures such as examination of the head, ear, nose, or throat for last.

The Preschool Child

The child at this stage displays developing initiative. The preschooler takes on tasks independently, plans the tasks, and sees them through. A child of this age is often cooperative, helpful, and easy to involve. However, he or she may have fantasies and see illness as punishment for being "bad." The concept of body image is limited. The child fears any body injury or mutilation; therefore he or she will recoil from invasive procedures (e.g., tongue blade, rectal temperature, injection, and venipuncture).

Position

- With a 3-year-old child the caregiver should be present and may hold the child on his or her lap.
- A 4- or 5-year-old child usually feels comfortable on the Big Girl or Big Boy (examining) table with the caregiver present.

Preparation

- A preschooler can talk. Verbal communication becomes helpful now, but remember that the child's understanding is still limited. Use short, simple explanations.
- The preschooler is usually willing to undress. Leave underpants on until the genital examination.
- Talk to the child and explain the steps in the examination exactly.
- Do not allow a choice when there is none.
- As with the toddler, enhance the autonomy of the preschooler by offering choice when possible.
- Allow the child to play with equipment to reduce fears (Fig. 8.14).
- A preschooler likes to help; have the child hold the stethoscope for you.

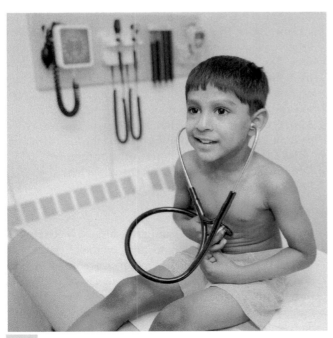

8.14

- Use games. Have the child "blow out" the light on the penlight as you listen to the breath sounds. Or pretend to listen to the heart sounds of the child's teddy bear first. One technique that is absorbing to a preschooler is to trace his or her shape on the examining table paper. You can comment on how big the child is, then fill in the outline with a heart or stomach and listen to the paper doll first. After the examination the child can take the paper doll home as a souvenir.
- Use a slow, patient, deliberate approach. Do not rush.
- During the examination give the preschooler needed feedback and reassurance: "Your tummy feels just fine."
- Compliment the child on his or her cooperation.

Sequence

- Examine the thorax, abdomen, extremities, and genitalia first. Although the preschooler is usually cooperative, continue to assess head, eye, ear, nose, and throat last.

The School-Age Child

During the school-age period the major task of the child is to develop industry. The child is developing basic competency in school and social networks and desires the approval of caregivers and teachers. When successful, the child has a feeling of accomplishment. During the examination the child is cooperative and interested in learning about the body. Language is more sophisticated now, but do not overestimate and treat the school-age child as a small adult. The child's level of understanding does not match that of his or her speech.

Position

- The school-age child should be sitting or lying on the examination table (Fig. 8.15).
- A 5-year-old child has a sense of modesty but will typically allow caregivers and siblings to be present during an examination. To maintain privacy, let the older child (an 11- or 12-year-old child) decide whether caregivers or siblings should be present.

Preparation

- Break the ice with small talk about family, school, friends, music, or sports.
- The child should undress himself or herself, leave underpants on, and use a gown and drape.
- Demonstrate equipment; a school-age child is curious to know how equipment works (Fig. 8.16).
- Comment on the body and how it works. An 8- or 9-year-old child has some understanding of the body and is interested to learn more. It is rewarding to see the child's eyes light up when he or she hears the heart sounds.

Sequence

- As with the adult, progress from head to toe.

The Adolescent

The major task of adolescence is to develop a self-identity. This takes shape from various sets of values and different

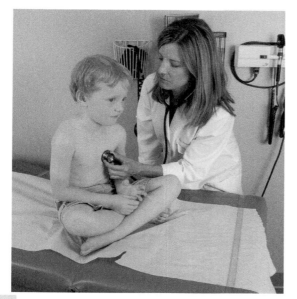

8.15

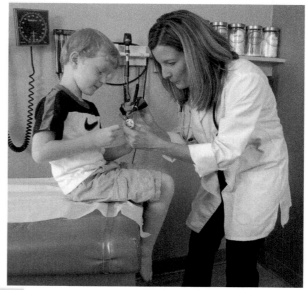

8.16

social roles (son or daughter, sibling, and student). In the end each person needs to feel satisfied and comfortable with who he or she is. In the process the adolescent is increasingly self-conscious and introspective. Peer group values and acceptance are important.

Position

- The adolescent should be sitting on the examination table. Try to keep street clothes on and work around them as much as possible (Fig. 8.17).
- Examine the adolescent alone, without parent or sibling present.

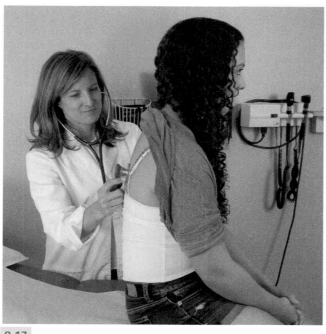

8.17

Preparation

- The body is changing rapidly. During the examination the adolescent needs feedback that his or her own body is healthy and developing normally.
- The adolescent has keen awareness of body image, often comparing himself or herself to peers. Apprise the adolescent of the wide variation among teenagers on the rate of growth and development (see Sexual Maturity Rating [SMR], Chapters 18, 25, and 27).
- Communicate with some care. Do not treat the teenager like a child, but do not overestimate and treat him or her like an adult either.
- Because the person is idealistic at this age, the adolescent is ripe for health teaching. Positive attitudes developed now may last through adult life. Focus your teaching on ways the adolescent can promote wellness.

Sequence

- As with the adult, a head-to-toe approach is appropriate. Examine genitalia last and do it quickly.

The Aging Adult

During later years the tasks are to develop the meaning of life and one's own existence and to adjust to changes in physical strength and health (Fig. 8.18).

Position

- The older adult should be sitting on the examination table; a frail older adult may need to be supine.
- Arrange the sequence to allow as few position changes as possible.
- Allow rest periods when needed.

Preparation

- Adjust the examination pace to meet the possible slowed pace of the aging person. It is better to break the complete examination into a few visits than to rush through the examination and turn off the person.
- Use physical touch (unless there is a cultural contra-indication). This is especially important with the aging person because other senses such as vision and hearing may be diminished.
- Do not mistake diminished vision or hearing for confusion. Confusion of sudden onset may signify a disease state. It is noted by short-term memory loss, diminished thought process, diminished attention span, and labile emotions (see Mental Status Assessment in Chapter 5).
- Be aware that aging years contain more life stress. Loss is inevitable, including changes in physical appearance of the face and body, declining energy level, loss of job through retirement, loss of financial security, loss of longtime home, and death of friends or spouse. How the person adapts to these losses significantly affects health assessment.

Sequence

- Use the head-to-toe approach, as in the younger adult.

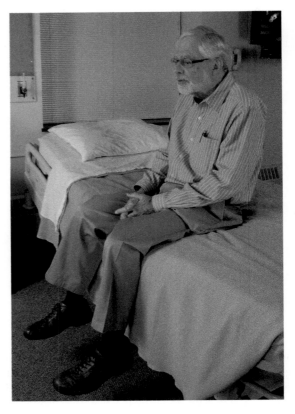

8.18

The Sick Person

For the person in some distress, alter the position during the examination. For example, a person with shortness of breath or ear pain may want to sit up, whereas a person with faint-ness or overwhelming fatigue may want to be supine. Adapt your assessment to the person's comfort level. Initially it may be necessary just to examine the body areas appropriate to the problem, collecting a **mini-database.** You may return to finish a complete assessment after the initial distress is resolved.

REFERENCES

1. Centers for Disease Control and Prevention (CDC). (2002). Guideline for hand hygiene in health-care settings. *MMWR Recomm Rep, 51*(RR–16). https://www.cdc.gov/mmwr/PDF/rr/rr5116.pdf.
2. Gupta, S., Saint, S., & Detsky, A. S. (2017). Hiding in plain sight—resurrecting the power of inspecting the patient. *JAMA Intern Med, 177,* 757–758.
3. Hockenberry, M., Wilson, D., & Rodgers, C. (2017). *Wong's essentials of pediatric nursing* (10th ed.). St. Louis, MO: Elsevier.
4. Wolpaw, D. R., & Shapiro, D. (2014). The virtues of irrelevance. *N Engl J Med, 370*(13), 1282–1285.

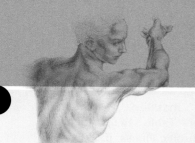

CHAPTER 9

General Survey and Measurement

http://evolve.elsevier.com/Jarvis/

OBJECTIVE DATA

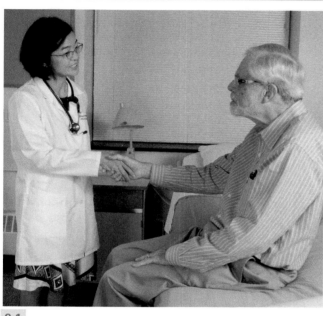

9.1

The general survey is a study of the whole person, covering the general health state and any obvious physical characteristics. It is an introduction for the physical examination that will follow; it gives an overall impression of the person. The general survey includes objective parameters that apply to the whole person, not just one body system.

Begin a general survey at the moment you first encounter the person. What leaves an immediate impression? Does the person stand promptly as his or her name is called and walk easily to meet you? Or does the person look sick, rising slowly or with effort, with shoulders slumped and eyes without luster or downcast? Is the hospitalized person conversing with visitors, involved in reading or television, or lying perfectly still? Even as you introduce yourself and shake hands, you collect data (Fig. 9.1). Does the person fully extend the arm, shake your hand firmly, make eye contact, or smile? Are the palms dry or wet and clammy? As you proceed through the health history, the measurements, and the vital signs, consider and make note of these four areas: **physical appearance, body structure, mobility,** and **behavior.**

Normal Range of Findings	Abnormal Findings

The General Survey

Physical Appearance

Age—The person appears his or her stated age.

Appears older than stated age, as with chronic illness or chronic alcoholism.

Sex—Sexual development is appropriate for sex and age. If the individual is transgender, note the stage of transformation.

Delayed or precocious puberty.

Level of consciousness—The person is alert and oriented to person, place, time, and situation. Attends to and responds appropriately to your questions.

Confused, drowsy, lethargic (see Table 5.1, Levels of Consciousness, p. 75).

Skin color—Color tone is even, pigmentation varying with genetic background; skin is intact with no obvious lesions. Make note of tattoos and piercings and stage of healing.

Pallor, cyanosis, jaundice, erythema, any lesions (see Chapter 13, p. 206).

Normal Range of Findings	Abnormal Findings
Facial features—Facial features are symmetric with movement.	Immobile, masklike, asymmetric, drooping (see Table 14.5, Abnormal Facies with Chronic Illness, p. 272).
Overall appearance—No signs of acute distress are present.	Cardiac or respiratory signs— Diaphoresis, clutching the chest, shortness of breath, wheezing. Pain, indicated by facial grimace, holding body part.

Body Structure

Stature—The height appears within normal range for age, genetic heritage (see Measurement, p. 127).	Excessively short or tall (see Table 9.2, Abnormalities in Body Height and Proportion, p. 136).
Nutrition—The weight appears within normal range for height and body build; body fat distribution is even.	Cachectic, emaciated. Simple obesity, with even fat distribution. Centripetal (truncal) obesity—Fat concentrated in face, neck, trunk, with thin extremities, as in Cushing syndrome (see Table 9.2).
Symmetry—Body parts look equal bilaterally and are in relative proportion to each other.	Unilateral atrophy or hypertrophy. Asymmetric location of a body part.
Posture—The person stands comfortably erect as appropriate for age. Note the normal "plumb line" through anterior ear, shoulder, hip, patella, ankle. Exceptions are the standing toddler, who has a normally protuberant abdomen ("toddler lordosis"), and the aging person, who may be stooped with kyphosis.	Rigid spine and neck; moves as one unit (e.g., arthritis). Stiff and tense, ready to spring from chair, fidgety movements. Shoulders slumped; looks deflated (e.g., depression).
Position—The person sits comfortably with arms relaxed at sides and head turned to examiner.	Tripod—Leaning forward with arms braced on chair arms; occurs with chronic pulmonary disease. Sits straight up and resists lying down (e.g., heart failure). Curled up in fetal position (e.g., acute abdominal pain).
Body build, contour—Proportions are: 1. Arm span (fingertip to fingertip) equals height. 2. Body length from crown to pubis roughly equal to length from pubis to sole.	Elongated arm span (e.g., Marfan syndrome, hypogonadism) (see Table 9.2).
Obvious physical deformities—Note any congenital or acquired defects.	Missing extremities or digits; webbed digits; shortened limb.

Mobility

Gait—Feet approximately shoulder width apart; foot placement is accurate; walk is smooth and even, and person can maintain balance without assistance. Associated movements such as symmetric arm swing are present.	Exceptionally wide base. Staggering, stumbling. Shuffling, dragging, nonfunctional leg. Limping with injury. Propulsion—Difficulty stopping (see Table 24.6, Abnormal Gaits, p. 675).

Objective Data

Normal Range of Findings	Abnormal Findings

Range of motion—Note full mobility for each joint and that movement is deliberate, accurate, smooth, and coordinated. (See Chapter 23 for information on more detailed testing of joint range of motion.)

No involuntary movement.

Limited joint range of motion.
Paralysis—Absent movement.
Jerky, uncoordinated movement.
Tics, tremors, seizures (see Table 24.4, Abnormalities in Muscle Movement, p. 672).

Behavior

Facial expression—The person maintains eye contact (if culturally appropriate); expressions are appropriate to the situation (e.g., thoughtful, serious, or smiling). (Note expressions both while the face is at rest and while the person is talking.)

Flat, depressed, angry, sad, anxious. However, note that anxiety is common in ill people. Also, some people smile when they are anxious.

Mood and affect—The person is comfortable and cooperative with the examiner and interacts pleasantly.

Hostile, distrustful, suspicious, crying.

Speech—Articulation (the ability to form words) is clear and understandable.

Dysarthria and dysphasia (see Table 5.2, Speech Disorders, p. 76). Speech defect, monotone, garbled speech.

Speech pattern—The stream of talking is fluent with an even pace. The person conveys ideas clearly. Word choice is appropriate for culture and education. Communicates in prevailing language easily by himself or herself or with an interpreter.

Extremes of few words or constant talking.

Dress—Clothing is appropriate to the climate, looks clean and fits the body, and is appropriate to the person's culture and age-group (e.g., normally Amish women wear clothing from the 19th century; Indian women may wear saris). Culturally determined dress should not be labeled as inappropriate by Western standards or adult expectations.

Clothing too large and held up by belt suggests weight loss, as does the addition of new holes in belt. Clothing too tight may indicate obesity or ascites.

Consistent wear of certain clothing may provide clues: long sleeves may conceal needle marks of drug abuse or thin arms of anorexia; Velcro fasteners instead of buttons may indicate chronic motor dysfunction.

Personal hygiene—The person appears clean and groomed appropriately for his or her age, occupation, and socioeconomic group. (Note that a wide variation of dress and hygiene is "normal." Many cultures do not include use of deodorant or women shaving legs.) Hair is groomed, brushed. Makeup is appropriate for age and culture.

Body odor, scent of alcohol.
Unkempt appearance in an individual who previously had good hygiene may indicate depression, malaise, or illness.

Measurement

Weight

Use a standardized *balance* or electronic standing scale (Fig. 9.2). Instruct the person to remove his or her shoes and heavy outer clothing before standing on the scale. When a sequence of repeated weights is necessary, aim for approximately the same time of day and the same type of clothing worn each time. Record the weight in kilograms and in pounds.

An unexplained weight loss may be a sign of a short-term illness (e.g., fever, infection, disease of the mouth or throat) or a chronic illness (e.g., endocrine disease, malignancy, depression, anorexia nervosa, bulimia). Unexplained weight gain may indicate fluid retention (e.g., heart failure).

Objective Data

Normal Range of Findings	Abnormal Findings

Objective Data

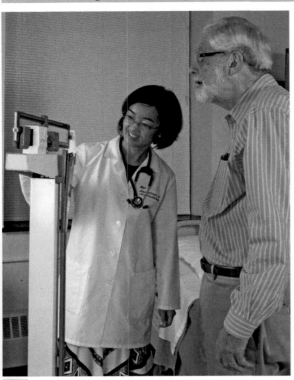

9.2

Height

Use a wall-mounted device or the measuring pole on the balance scale. Align the extended headpiece with the top of the head. The person should be shoeless, standing straight with gentle traction under the jaw, and looking straight ahead. Feet, shoulders, and buttocks should be in contact with the wall or measuring pole.

Body Mass Index

Body mass index (BMI) is a practical marker of optimal healthy weight for height and an indicator of obesity or malnutrition. Traditionally, BMI is used to guide patient progress toward a healthy weight and is used to identify people at high risk for developing health problems such as cardiovascular disease. BMI expresses the relationship between height and weight, but does not consider other variables such as muscle mass. BMI also may be less effective in children or in older adults.

Researchers recommend using BMI in conjunction with other measures such as waist circumference.[3] Using BMI alone, nearly 75 million adults in the United States are misclassified as cardiometabolically healthy or unhealthy.[4]

A healthy BMI is a level of 19 or greater to less than 25. Show the person how his or her own weight matches up to the national guidelines for optimal BMI (see Table 9.1). Compare the person's current weight with that from the previous health visit. Discuss the importance of other cardiometabolic risk factors such as healthy diet, exercise, and laboratory studies (e.g., lipids). Note that BMI overestimates body fat in people who are very muscular and underestimates body fat in older adults who have lost muscle mass. While BMI is a useful tool, it should not be used alone. You will need to consider other markers of overall health along with BMI.

The cause of weight gain is usually excess caloric intake; occasionally it is endocrine disorders, drug therapy (e.g., corticosteroids), or depression. BMI classifications for adults:
Underweight < 18.5 kg/m^2
Normal weight 18.5 to 24.9 kg/m^2
Overweight 25 to 29.9 kg/m^2
Obesity (class 1) 30 to 34.9 kg/m^2
Obesity (class 2) 35 to 39.9 kg/m^2
Extreme obesity (class 3) ≥40 kg/m^2

In the United States more than $\frac{2}{3}$ of adults and $\frac{1}{3}$ of children are overweight or obese. Overweight and obesity affect more Hispanics and non-Hispanic Blacks than non-Hispanic Whites, whereas Asian Americans have a much lower prevalence than other ethnic groups.[2]

TABLE 9.1   Body Mass Index Table

BMI	NORMAL						OVERWEIGHT					OBESE									
	19	20	21	22	23	24	25	26	27	28	29	30	31	32	33	34	35	36	37	38	39
HEIGHT (inches)	BODY WEIGHT (pounds)																				
58	91	96	100	105	110	115	119	124	129	134	138	143	148	153	158	162	167	172	177	181	186
59	94	99	104	109	114	119	124	128	133	138	143	148	153	158	163	168	173	178	183	188	193
60	97	102	107	112	118	123	128	133	138	143	148	153	158	163	168	174	179	184	189	194	199
61	100	106	111	116	122	127	132	137	143	148	153	158	164	169	174	180	185	190	195	201	206
62	104	109	115	120	126	131	136	142	147	153	158	164	169	175	180	186	191	196	202	207	213
63	107	113	118	124	130	135	141	146	152	158	163	169	175	180	186	191	197	203	208	214	220
64	110	116	122	128	134	140	145	151	157	163	169	174	180	186	192	197	204	209	215	221	227
65	114	120	126	132	138	144	150	156	162	168	174	180	186	192	198	204	210	216	222	228	234
66	118	124	130	136	142	148	155	161	167	173	179	186	192	198	204	210	216	223	229	235	241
67	121	127	134	140	146	153	159	166	172	178	185	191	198	204	211	217	223	230	236	242	249
68	125	131	138	144	151	158	164	171	177	184	190	197	203	210	216	223	230	236	243	249	256
69	128	135	142	149	155	162	169	176	182	189	196	203	209	216	223	230	236	243	250	257	263
70	132	139	146	153	160	167	174	181	188	195	202	209	216	222	229	236	243	250	257	264	271
71	136	143	150	157	165	172	179	186	193	200	208	215	222	229	236	243	250	257	265	272	279
72	140	147	154	162	169	177	184	191	199	206	213	221	228	235	242	250	258	265	272	279	287
73	144	151	159	166	174	182	189	197	204	212	219	227	235	242	250	257	265	272	280	288	295
74	148	155	163	171	179	186	194	202	210	218	225	233	241	249	256	264	272	280	287	295	303
75	152	160	168	176	184	192	200	208	216	224	232	240	248	256	264	272	279	287	295	303	311
76	156	164	172	180	189	197	205	213	221	230	238	246	254	263	271	279	287	295	304	312	320

BMI	EXTREME OBESITY														
	40	41	42	43	44	45	46	47	48	49	50	51	52	53	54
HEIGHT (inches)	BODY WEIGHT (pounds)														
58	191	196	201	205	210	215	220	224	229	234	239	244	248	253	258
59	198	203	208	212	217	222	227	232	237	242	247	252	257	262	267
60	204	209	215	220	225	230	235	240	245	250	255	261	266	271	276
61	211	217	222	227	232	238	243	248	254	259	264	269	275	280	285
62	218	224	229	235	240	246	251	256	262	267	273	278	284	289	295
63	225	231	237	242	248	254	259	265	270	278	282	287	293	299	304
64	232	238	244	250	256	262	267	273	279	285	291	296	302	308	314
65	240	246	252	258	264	270	276	282	288	294	300	306	312	318	324
66	247	253	260	266	272	278	284	291	297	303	309	315	322	328	334
67	255	261	268	274	280	287	293	299	306	312	319	325	331	338	344
68	262	269	276	282	289	295	302	308	315	322	328	335	341	348	354
69	270	277	284	291	297	304	311	318	324	331	338	345	351	358	365
70	278	285	292	299	306	313	320	327	334	341	348	355	362	369	376
71	286	293	301	308	315	322	329	338	343	351	358	365	372	379	386
72	294	302	309	316	324	331	338	346	353	361	368	375	383	390	397
73	302	310	318	325	333	340	348	355	363	371	378	386	393	401	408
74	311	319	326	334	342	350	358	365	373	381	389	396	404	412	420
75	319	327	335	343	351	359	367	375	383	391	399	407	415	423	431
76	328	336	344	353	361	369	377	385	394	402	410	418	426	435	443

Adapted from *Clinical guidelines on the identification, evaluation, and treatment of overweight and obesity in adults: the evidence report.* Available at https://www.nhlbi.nih.gov/health/educational/lose_wt/BMI/bmi_tbl.htm.

Objective Data

You may calculate BMI by using an online BMI calculator, or you can calculate it with the following formula:

$$\text{BMI} = \frac{\text{Weight (in pounds)}}{\text{Height (in inches)}^2} \times 703 \qquad Or \qquad \text{BMI} = \frac{\text{Weight (in kilograms)}}{\text{Height (in meters)}^2}$$

Normal Range of Findings	Abnormal Findings

Waist Circumference

Excess abdominal fat is an important independent risk factor for disease. If most of the weight is carried around the waist instead of around the hips, the person is at higher risk for heart disease and type 2 diabetes.

With the person standing, locate the hip bone—the very top is the iliac crest. Place a measuring tape around the waist, parallel to the floor, at the level of the iliac crest. The tape should be snug but not pinch in the skin. Note the measurement at the end of a normal expiration (Fig. 9.3).

A waist circumference (WC) ≥35 inches in women and ≥40 inches in men increases the risk for type 2 diabetes, dyslipidemia, hypertension, and cardiovascular disease (CVD) in people with a BMI between 25 and 35.

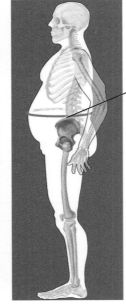

Iliac crest

Measuring tape position for abdominal circumference

 9.3

❖ DEVELOPMENTAL COMPETENCE

Infants and Children
General Survey

Physical appearance, body structure, mobility—Note the same basic elements as for the adult, with consideration to age and development. Remember that children just learning to walk have a wide gait and that normal toddler posture shows a protruding abdomen (lordosis).

Behavior—Note the response to stimuli and level of alertness appropriate for age. Infants usually look toward your voice and may mimic facial expressions.

Parental bonding—Note the child's interactions with caregivers (i.e., that caregiver and child show a mutual response and are warm and affectionate, appropriate to the child's condition). The parent provides appropriate physical care of child and promotes new learning.

Some signs of child abuse are that the child avoids eye contact; the child exhibits no separation anxiety when you would expect it for age; the parent is disgusted by child's odor, sounds, drooling, or stools.

For information on deprivation of physical or emotional care see Chapter 7.

Normal Range of Findings	Abnormal Findings

Measurement

Weight. Weigh an infant on a platform-type scale (Fig. 9.4). To check calibration of a balance scale, set the weight at zero and observe the beam balance. A digital scale should read zero before each use. You may need to press the zero/tare button before placing the infant on the scale. Follow agency guidelines for calibration of scales. Place the infant on the scale. Guard the infant so that he or she does not fall. Weigh to the nearest 10 g (½ oz) for infants and 100 g (¼ lb) for toddlers.

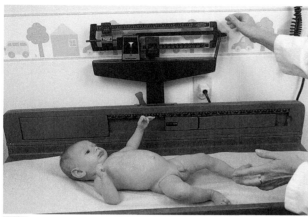

9.4

By age 2 or 3 years use the upright scale. Leave underpants on the child. Some young children are fearful of the rickety standing platform and may prefer sitting on the infant scale. Use the upright scale with preschoolers and school-age children, maintaining modesty with light clothing (Fig. 9.5).

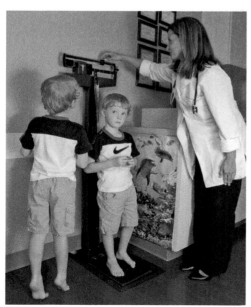

9.5

Objective Data

Normal Range of Findings	Abnormal Findings

Objective Data

Length. Until age 2 years measure the infant's body length supine by using a horizontal measuring board (Fig. 9.6). One person holds the top of the head against the head plate. Because the infant normally has flexed legs, extend them momentarily by gently stretching the spine and legs with the feet touching the perpendicular footplate. You may need to repeat the measure to ensure accuracy.

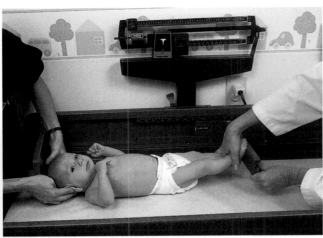

9.6

Height. Measure the child's height by standing against a ruler mounted on the scale or wall (Fig. 9.7). Encourage the child to stand straight and tall and to look straight ahead without tilting the head. The shoulders, buttocks, and heels ideally should touch the ruler. Hold a level on the child's head at a right angle and note the measure to the nearest 1 mm ($\frac{1}{8}$ in).

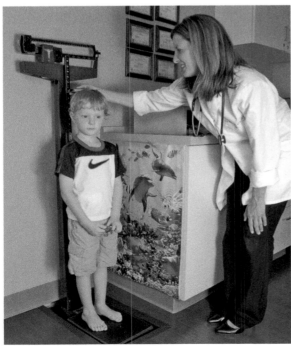

9.7

Normal Range of Findings

Physical growth is perhaps the best index of a child's general health. The child's height and weight are recorded at every health care visit to determine normal growth patterns. The results are plotted on growth charts based on data from the Centers for Disease Control and Prevention (CDC).[1] You can view these charts at www.cdc.gov. In addition to the weight, height, and head circumference charts, BMI-for-age charts are available for boys and girls ages 2 to 20 years.

Healthy childhood growth is continuous but uneven, with rapid growth spurts occurring during infancy and adolescence. Growth chart results are more reliable when comparing numerous growth measures over time. These charts also compare the individual child's measurements against the general population. Normal limits range from the 5th to the 95th percentile on the standardized charts.

Use your judgment and consider the genetic background of the small-for-age child. Explore the growth patterns of the parents and siblings. The differences in size and growth among the major racial/ethnic groups in the United States appear to be small and inconsistent.[1] You can use the revised 2000 CDC growth charts on all infants and children in the United States, regardless of race or ethnicity. The CDC notes that the most important evidence for growth potential appears to be economic, nutritional, and environmental.

Head Circumference. Measure the infant's head circumference at birth and at each well-child visit up to age 2 years and then annually up to 6 years (Fig. 9.8). A retractable plastic tape measure is more accurate than a paper tape measure. Circle the tape around the head aligned with the eyebrows at the prominent frontal and occipital bones; the widest span is correct. Plot the measurement on standardized growth charts. Compare the infant's head size with that expected for age. A series of measurements is more valuable than a single figure to show the *pattern* of head growth.

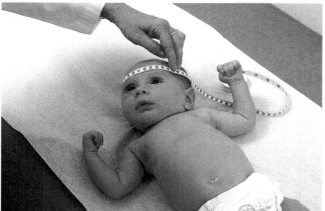

9.8

Abnormal Findings

Further explore any growth measure that:
- Falls below the 5th or above the 95th percentile with no genetic explanation
- Shows a wide percentile difference between height and weight (e.g., a 10th percentile height with a 95th percentile weight)
- Shows that growth has suddenly stopped when it had been steady
- Fails to show normal growth spurts during infancy and adolescence

Objective Data

Normal Range of Findings	Abnormal Findings

The newborn's head measures about 32 to 38 cm (average around 34 cm) and is about 2 cm larger than the chest circumference. The chest grows at a faster rate than the cranium; at some time between 6 months and 2 years both measurements are about the same; after age 2 years the chest circumference is greater than the head circumference.

Measurement of the chest circumference is valuable in a comparison with the head circumference but not necessarily by itself. Encircle the tape around the chest at the nipple line. It should be snug but not so tight that it leaves a mark (Fig. 9.9).

Enlarged head circumference occurs with increased intracranial pressure (see Chapter 14).

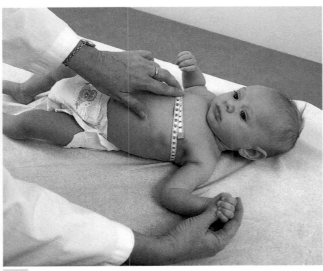

9.9

The Aging Adult

General Survey

Physical appearance—By the eighth and ninth decades, body contour is sharper with more angular facial features, and body proportions are redistributed. (See measuring weight and height, p. 127.)

Posture—A general flexion occurs by the eighth or ninth decade.

Kyphosis is the humpback appearance common in the very old and in those with osteoporosis.

Gait—Older adults often use a wider base to compensate for diminished balance, arms may be held out to help balance, and steps may be shorter or uneven.

Measurement

Weight. The older adult appears sharper in contour, with more prominent bony landmarks than the younger adult. Body weight decreases during the 80s and 90s. This factor is more evident in males, perhaps because of greater muscle shrinkage. The distribution of fat also changes during the 80s and 90s. Even with good nutrition, subcutaneous fat is lost from the face and periphery (especially the forearms), whereas additional fat is deposited on the abdomen and hips (Fig. 9.10).

Normal Range of Findings	Abnormal Findings

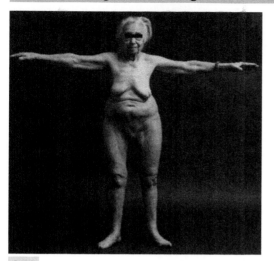

9.10 (Rossman, 1986.)

This change in fat distribution and loss in muscle mass can affect the BMI interpretation in older adults. For any given BMI, an older adult has more fat tissue than lean tissue when compared with a younger adult. As an aging person becomes shorter, the BMI reflecting the shorter height may overestimate the body fat content.

Height. By their 80s and 90s many people are shorter than they were in their 70s because of thinning of the vertebral disks, shortening of the individual vertebrae, postural changes of kyphosis, and slight flexion in the knees and hips. Because long bones do not shorten with age, the overall body proportion looks different—a shorter trunk with relatively long extremities (see Fig. 9.10).

DOCUMENTATION AND CRITICAL THINKING

Sample Charting

SUBJECTIVE

J.M. is a 95-year-old retired professor who appears healthy and of stated age. Alert, oriented, and cooperative during health history.

OBJECTIVE

Skin tone is even with senile lentigines on dorsa of hands and forearms bilaterally. Gait smooth; feet slightly wider than shoulders. No obvious physical deformities. Intention tremor noted when completing history form. Speech appropriate, clear, and understandable. Kempt appearance. Height 152 in (5 ft 10 in), weight 75 kg (165 lb). BMI 23 (healthy). Waist circumference 30 in.

Documentation and
Critical Thinking

ABNORMAL FINDINGS

TABLE 9.2	Abnormalities in Body Height and Proportion

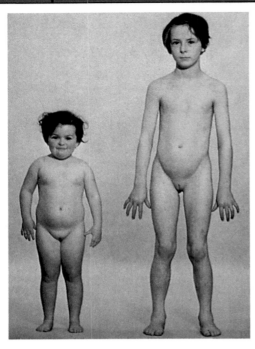

Hypopituitary Dwarfism

Deficiency in growth hormone in childhood results in retardation of growth below the 3rd percentile, delayed puberty, hypothyroidism, and adrenal insufficiency. The 9-year-old girl at left appears much younger than her chronologic age, with infantile facial features and chubbiness. The age-matched girl at right shows increased height, more mature facial features, and loss of infantile fat.

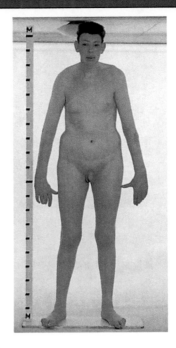

Gigantism

Excessive secretion of growth hormone by the anterior pituitary results in overgrowth of the entire body. When this occurs during childhood before closure of bone epiphyses, it causes increased height (here 2.09 m, or 6 ft 9 in), as well as increased weight and delayed sexual development.

◄ **Acromegaly (Hyperpituitarism)**

Excessive secretion of growth hormone in adulthood after normal completion of body growth causes overgrowth of bone in face, head, hands, and feet but no change in height. Internal organs also enlarge (e.g., cardiomegaly), and metabolic disorders (e.g., diabetes mellitus) may be present.

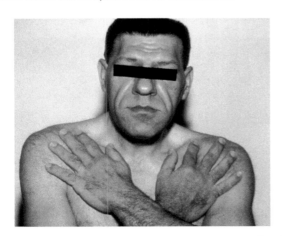

Continued

TABLE 9.2	Abnormalities in Body Height and Proportion—cont'd

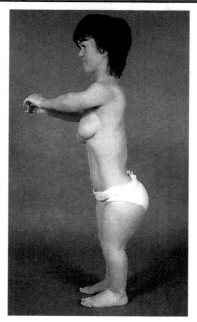

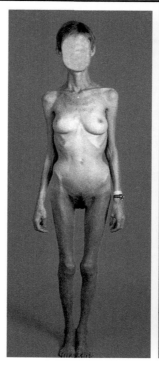 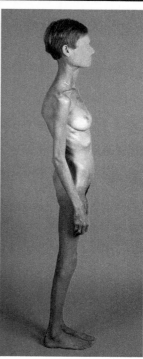

Achondroplastic Dwarfism

A genetic disorder in converting cartilage to bone results in normal trunk size, short arms and legs, and short stature. It is characterized by a relatively large head with frontal bossing; midface hypoplasia (small); and often thoracic kyphosis, prominent lumbar lordosis, and abdominal protrusion. The mean adult height in men is about 131.5 cm (4 ft 4 in) and in women about 125 cm (4 ft 1 in).

Anorexia Nervosa

This serious mental health disorder is characterized by severe and life-threatening weight loss in an otherwise healthy person. Behavior is characterized by fanatic concern about weight, aversion to food, distorted body image (perceives self as fat despite skeletal appearance), starvation diets, frenetic exercise patterns, and striving for perfection. Results in amenorrhea in females.

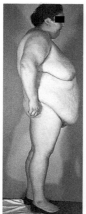 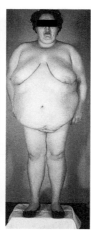 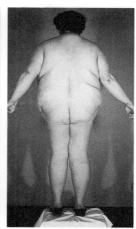

◄ Endogenous Obesity—Cushing Syndrome

Either administration of adrenocorticotropin (ACTH) or excessive production of ACTH by the pituitary stimulates the adrenal cortex to secrete excess cortisol. This causes Cushing syndrome, characterized by weight gain and edema with central trunk and cervical obesity (buffalo hump) and round, plethoric face (moon face). Excessive catabolism causes muscle wasting; weakness; thin arms and legs; reduced height; and thin, fragile skin with purple abdominal striae, bruising, and acne. Note that the obesity here is markedly different from *exogenous obesity* caused by excessive caloric intake, in which body fat is evenly distributed and muscle strength is intact. (See Chapter 12, Nutrition Assessment, p. 179.)

Continued

TABLE 9.2	Abnormalities in Body Height and Proportion—cont'd

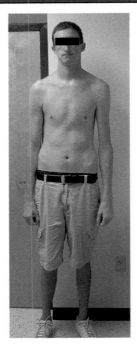

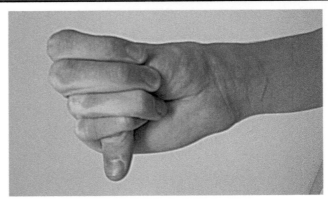

◀ Marfan Syndrome

This inherited connective tissue disorder is characterized by tall, thin stature (≥95th percentile), arachnodactyly (long, thin fingers), hyperextensible joints, arm span greater than height, pubis-to-sole measurement exceeding crown-to-pubis measurement, sternal deformity (note pectus excavatum), high-arched narrow palate, narrow face, and pes planus (flat feet). Early morbidity and mortality occur as a result of cardiovascular complications such as mitral regurgitation and aortic dissection.

See illustration credits for source information.

REFERENCES

1. Centers for Disease Control and Prevention (CDC). (2016). *CDC growth charts.* Available at: www.cdc.gov.
2. National Institute of Diabetes and Digestive and Kidney Diseases. (2017). *Overweight & obesity statistics.* https://www.niddk.nih.gov/health-information/health-statistics/overweight-obesity.
3. Nazare, J., Smith, J., Borel, A., et al. (2015). Usefulness of measuring both body mass index and waist circumference for the estimation of visceral adiposity and related cardiometabolic risk profile (from the INSPIRE ME IAA Study). *Am J Cardiol, 115,* 307–315.
4. Tomiyama, A. J., Hunger, J. M., Nguyen-Cuu, J., et al. (2016). Misclassification of cardiometabolic health when using body mass index categories in NHANES 2005-2012. *Int J Obes, 40,* 883–886.

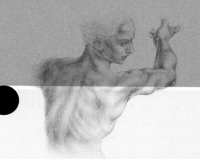

CHAPTER 10

Vital Signs

OBJECTIVE DATA

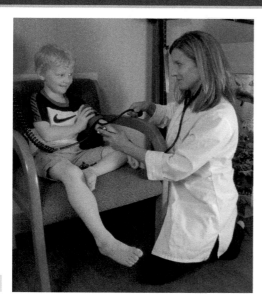

10.1

You will use vital signs as an objective measure of the body's basic functions. When measuring vital signs, you will include temperature, respiratory rate, pulse, and blood pressure (Fig. 10.1). Vital signs help you monitor your patient's health and indicate deterioration, especially in the acute care setting. Vital signs are monitored in the hospital setting, obtained at clinic visits, and monitored at home. You will need to follow the guidelines at your facility for vital sign frequency and normal range; however, you will use your [nursing] judgment to determine whether vital signs need to be taken more frequently or whether a provider should be notified. The normal vital sign values in this chapter are based on the current literature; however, patient condition may dictate a different vital sign range. Always follow provider orders for vital sign range and understand that each patient is different. If your patient is monitoring vital signs at home, you must provide teaching so that the patient knows how to use their home equipment and when to notify the provider.

Normal Range of Findings	Abnormal Findings

Vital Signs

Temperature

Cellular metabolism requires a stable core, or "deep body," temperature of a mean of 37.2°C (99°F). The body maintains a steady temperature through a thermostat, or feedback mechanism, regulated in the hypothalamus of the brain. The thermostat balances heat production (from metabolism, exercise, food digestion, external factors) with heat loss (through radiation, evaporation of sweat, convection, conduction).

The various routes of temperature measurement reflect the core temperature of the body. The normal oral temperature in a resting person is 37°C (98.6°F), with a range of 35.8° to 37.3°C (96.4° to 99.1°F). The rectal temperature measures 0.4° to 0.5°C (0.7° to 1°F) higher than an oral measurement.

The normal temperature is influenced by:
- A diurnal cycle of 1° to 1.5°F, with the trough occurring in the early morning hours and the peak occurring in late afternoon to early evening.
- The menstruation cycle in women. Progesterone secretion, occurring with ovulation at midcycle, causes a 0.5° to 1°F rise in temperature that continues until menses.
- Exercise. Moderate-to-hard exercise increases body temperature.

The thermostatic function of the hypothalamus may become scrambled during illness or central nervous system (CNS) disorders.

Hyperthermia, or fever, is caused by pyrogens secreted by toxic bacteria during infections or from tissue breakdown such as that following myocardial infarction, trauma, surgery, or malignancy. Neurologic disorders (e.g., a stroke, cerebral edema, brain trauma, tumor, or surgery) also can

Normal Range of Findings

- Age. Wider normal variations occur in the infant and young child because of less effective heat control mechanisms. In older adults temperature is usually lower than in other age-groups, with a mean of 36.2°C (97.2°F) via the oral route.

The **oral temperature** is the most convenient and accurate site. The sublingual pocket has a rich blood supply from the carotid arteries that quickly responds to changes in inner core temperature.

The Procedure: Oral Temperature

Shake a glass thermometer down to 35.5°C (96°F) and place it at the base of the tongue in either of the posterior sublingual pockets—*not* in front of the tongue. Instruct the person to keep his or her lips closed. Leave in place 3 to 4 minutes if the person is afebrile and up to 8 minutes if febrile. (Take other vital signs during this time.) Wait 15 minutes if the person has just taken hot or iced liquids and 2 minutes if he or she has just smoked.

The **electronic thermometer** has the advantages of swift and accurate measurement (usually less than 20 to 30 seconds). The instrument must be fully charged and correctly calibrated. Children may enjoy watching the numbers advance on the thermometer during measurement. Electronic thermometers can be used for both oral and rectal temperatures. Blue-tipped probes are for the oral route, whereas red-tipped probes are rectal.

The Procedure: Rectal Temperature

Rectal temperatures are the most accurate route, and the result is as close to core temperature as possible without using more invasive measures reserved for the operating room and critical care environments. Although the rectal temperature provides the closest approximation to core temperature, it is more invasive than other measures; therefore you must weigh the risks and benefits. Peripheral thermometers (e.g., tympanic, temporal artery) have poor sensitivity for detecting low-grade fever, a potentially important indicator of infection; therefore it may be advantageous to use a more sensitive method, such as a rectal temperature.[11] The rectal temperature is the preferred route when the other routes are impractical (e.g., for the comatose or confused patient; for patients in shock; or for those who cannot close their mouths or who have a wired mandible or other facial dysfunction). The primary disadvantages to the rectal route are patient discomfort and the invasive nature of the procedure.

Begin by positioning your patient appropriately, left lateral decubitus if possible. Wear gloves, place a cover on the thermometer and apply lubricant to the probe. Insert the lubricated rectal probe 2 to 3 cm (1 in) into the rectum, directed toward the umbilicus. For infants <6 months insert approximately ½ inch. Leave in place until the electronic thermometer beeps or for 2½ minutes if using a glass thermometer. Do not let go of the temperature probe while it is inserted into the rectum.

Abnormal Findings

reset the thermostat of the brain at a higher level, resulting in heat production and conservation. A body temperature >38.0°C is generally accepted as hyperthermia.

Hypothermia is usually caused by accidental, prolonged exposure to cold. It also may be purposefully induced to lower the body's oxygen requirements during heart or peripheral vascular surgery, neurosurgery, amputation, postcardiac arrest, or gastrointestinal (GI) hemorrhage. A body temperature below 36.0°C is typically accepted as hypothermia.

Glass thermometers are infrequently used due to inefficiency; however, they remain available for use, so it is important that you know the appropriate procedure.

Normal Range of Findings	Abnormal Findings

The Procedure: Tympanic Membrane Temperature

The **tympanic membrane thermometer (TMT)** senses infrared emissions of the tympanic membrane (eardrum). The tympanic membrane shares the same vascular supply that perfuses the hypothalamus (the internal carotid artery); thus it is an accurate measurement of core temperature.

The TMT is a noninvasive, nontraumatic device that is extremely quick and efficient. The probe tip has the shape of an otoscope, the instrument used to inspect the ear. Gently place the covered probe tip in the person's ear canal, and aim the infrared beam at the tympanic membrane. Do not occlude the canal. Activate the device and read the temperature in 2 to 3 seconds.

There is minimal chance of cross-contamination with the tympanic thermometer because the ear canal is lined with skin and not mucous membrane. Current evidence suggests that TMT measurement is not as accurate as other devices.[2] TMT has fallen out of favor in many acute care settings but is still used by some clinics.

The Procedure: Temporal Artery Thermometer

The newest noninvasive temperature measurement method uses infrared emissions from the temporal artery. The **temporal artery thermometer (TAT)** is used by sliding the probe across the forehead and behind the ear. The thermometer works by taking multiple readings and providing an average. The reading takes approximately 6 seconds. This approach is well tolerated and is more accurate than TMTs; however, there are conflicting reports about its accuracy.[2,11] Assuring that thermometers are calibrated and used per manufacturer instructions can help maintain accuracy.

Report the temperature in degrees Celsius unless your agency uses the Fahrenheit scale. Familiarize yourself with both scales. Note that it is far easier to learn to *think* in the centigrade scale than to take the time for conversions. Begin by memorizing these convenient equivalents:

$$104° \text{ F} = 40° \text{ C}; \quad 98.6° \text{ F} = 37° \text{ C}; \quad 95° \text{ F} = 35° \text{ C}$$

Along with your results, make sure to note the route used to obtain the temperature reading.

Pulse

With every beat the heart pumps an amount of blood—the **stroke volume**—into the aorta. This is about 70 mL in the adult. The force flares the arterial walls and generates a pressure wave, which is felt in the periphery as the **pulse.** Palpating the peripheral pulse gives the rate and rhythm of the heartbeat and local data on the condition of the artery.

Using the pads of your first three fingers, palpate the radial pulse at the flexor aspect of the wrist laterally along the radius bone (Fig. 10.2). If the rhythm is regular, count the number of beats in 30 seconds and multiply by 2. Although the 15-second interval is frequently practiced, any one-beat error in counting results in a recorded error of 4 beats/min. The 30-second interval is most accurate and efficient when heart rates are normal or rapid and when rhythms are regular.[6] However, if the rhythm is irregular, count for a full minute. As you begin the counting interval, start your count with "zero" for the first pulse felt. The second pulse felt is "one," and so on. Beginning the count at "one" overestimates the heart rate.[6] Assess the pulse, including (1) rate, (2) rhythm, and (3) force.

Objective Data

| Normal Range of Findings | Abnormal Findings |

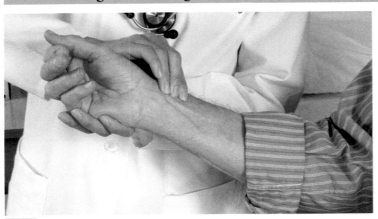

10.2 Palpate radial pulse.

Rate

In the adult at physical and mental rest, recent clinical evidence shows the normal resting heart range of 95% of healthy individuals at 50 to 95 beats/min.[10] Traditional resting heart rate limits established in the 1950s are 60 to 100 beats/min. This range is still used; however, no research evidence supports it.

The rate normally varies with age, being more rapid in infancy and childhood (Table 10.1) and more moderate during adult and older years. The rate also varies with gender; after puberty females have a slightly faster rate than males.

Many medications affect heart rate, with nearly all heart disease patients taking at least one medication that slows the heart rate.

TABLE 10.1 Normal Heart Rate (beats per minute) in Infants and Children			
AGE	**RESTING (AWAKE)**	**RESTING (ASLEEP)**	**EXERCISE/ FEVER**
Newborn	100-180	80-160	Up to 220
1 wk to 3 mo	100-220	80-200	Up to 220
3 mo to 2 yr	80-150	70-120	Up to 220
2 to 10 yr	70-100	60-90	195-215
10 to 20 yr	55-90	50-90	195-215

From Burns, C. Dunn, A., Brady, M., et al. (2017). *Pediatric primary care* (6th ed.). Philadelphia: Saunders.

In the adult a resting heart rate less than 50 beats/min is **bradycardia**. Heart rates in the 50s/min occur normally in the well-trained athlete, whose heart muscle develops along with the skeletal muscles. The stronger, more efficient heart muscle pushes out a larger stroke volume with each beat, thus requiring fewer beats per minute to maintain a stable cardiac output.

A more rapid heart rate, variably defined as over 95 beats/min or over 100 beats/min, is **tachycardia**. Rapid rates occur normally with anxiety or with increased exercise to match the body's demand for increased metabolism.

For descriptions of abnormal rates and rhythms, see Table 21.1, Variations in Pulse Contour, on p. 522.

Bradycardia may be normal in patients with heart disease who are taking one or more medications with negative chronotropic effects.

Tachycardia occurs with fever and also with sepsis, pneumonia, myocardial infarction, and pancreatitis. Tachycardia predicts complications and worse survival rates in the latter conditions.[10]

Normal Range of Findings	Abnormal Findings

Rhythm

The pulse normally has a regular, even tempo. One irregularity that is commonly found in children and young adults is **sinus arrhythmia.** In sinus arrhythmia the heart rate varies with the respiratory cycle, speeding up at the peak of inspiration and slowing to normal with expiration. Inspiration momentarily causes a decreased stroke volume from the left side of the heart; to compensate the heart rate increases. (See Chapter 20 for a full discussion on sinus arrhythmia.) If any other irregularities are felt, auscultate heart sounds for a more complete assessment (see Chapter 20).

Force

The force of the pulse shows the strength of the heart's stroke volume. A "full, bounding" pulse denotes an increased stroke volume (e.g., as with anxiety, exercise, and some abnormal conditions). The pulse force is recorded using a three-point scale:

> 3+—Full, bounding
> 2+—Normal
> 1+—Weak, thready
> 0—Absent

A "weak, thready" pulse reflects a decreased stroke volume (e.g., as occurs with hemorrhagic shock).

Some agencies use a four-point scale; make sure that your system is consistent with that used by your agency. Either scale is somewhat subjective. Experience will increase your clinical judgment. Most healthy adults have a force of 2+.

Record the rate, rhythm, and force of the pulse in the medical record.

Respirations

Normally a person's breathing is relaxed, regular, automatic, and silent. Because most people are unaware of their breathing, do not mention that you will be counting the respirations, because sudden awareness may alter the normal pattern. Maintain your position of counting the radial pulse and unobtrusively count the respirations. Count for 30 seconds, but count for a full minute if you suspect an abnormality. Avoid the 15-second interval. The result can vary by a factor of +4 or −4, which is significant with such a small number. If you are having difficulty seeing the chest rise, which can be especially difficult in obese individuals and children, you can place a hand on the upper chest or abdomen to help you "feel" the respiratory rate. Report the number of breaths per minute as well as the character of breathing (i.e., relaxed, even).

Report additional objective data (e.g., labored, shallow, or deep breathing; retractions in infants and children; and accessory muscle use in adults).

Note that respiratory rates (Table 10.2) normally are more rapid in infants and children. Also, a fairly constant ratio of pulse rate to respiratory rate exists, which is about 4:1. Normally both pulse and respiratory rates rise as a response to exercise or anxiety. More detailed assessment on respiratory status is presented in Chapter 19.

TABLE 10.2	Normal Respiratory Rates
AGE (YEARS)	**RESPIRATORY RATE (BREATHS/MINUTE)**
0-1	24-38
1-3	22-30
4-6	20-24
7-9	18-24
10-14	16-22
15-18	14-20
Adult	10-20

Table adapted from Burns, C. Dunn, A., Brady, M., et al. (2017). *Pediatric primary care* (6th ed.). Philadelphia: Saunders.

Objective Data

Normal Range of Findings	Abnormal Findings

Objective Data

Blood Pressure

Blood pressure (BP) is the force of the blood pushing against the side of its container, the vessel wall. The strength of the push changes with the event in the cardiac cycle. The **systolic** pressure is the maximum pressure felt on the artery during left ventricular contraction, or systole. The **diastolic** pressure is the elastic recoil, or resting, pressure that the blood exerts constantly between each contraction. The **pulse pressure** is the difference between the systolic and diastolic pressures and reflects the stroke volume (Fig. 10.3).

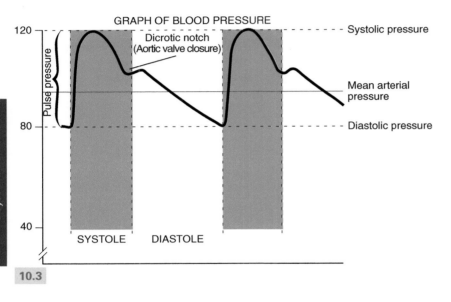

10.3

The **mean arterial pressure (MAP)** is the pressure forcing blood into the tissues averaged over the cardiac cycle. This is not an arithmetic average of systolic and diastolic pressures because diastole lasts longer. MAP can be calculated using a variety of formulas:

$$MAP = \frac{[(2 \times Diastolic) + Systolic]}{3}$$

Or

$$MAP = Diastolic + \tfrac{1}{3} Pulse\ pressure$$

The average BP varies with many factors such as:

- **Age.** Normally a gradual rise occurs through childhood and into the adult years.
- **Sex.** Before puberty no difference exists between males and females. After puberty females usually show a lower BP reading than do male counterparts. After menopause BP in females is higher than in male counterparts.
- **Race.** In the United States an African-American adult's BP is often higher than that of a non-Hispanic white person of the same age. The incidence of hypertension is twice as high in African Americans as in non-Hispanic whites.[3] The reasons for this difference are not understood fully, but we do know that genetic profile and environmental factors are involved. (See Chapter 20, p. 462.)

A MAP ≥60 mm Hg is needed to maintain adequate tissue and organ perfusion.

Normal Range of Findings	Abnormal Findings

- **Diurnal rhythm.** A daily cycle of a peak and a trough occurs: the BP climbs to a high in late afternoon or early evening and then declines to an early-morning low.
- **Weight.** BP is higher in obese people than in people of normal weight of the same age (including adolescents).
- **Exercise.** Increasing activity yields a proportionate increase in BP. Within 5 minutes of terminating the exercise, the BP normally returns to baseline.
- **Emotions.** The BP momentarily rises with fear, anger, and pain as a result of stimulation of the sympathetic nervous system.
- **Stress.** The BP is elevated in people feeling continual tension because of lifestyle, occupational stress, or life problems.

The level of **BP** is determined by five factors (Fig. 10.4):

FACTORS CONTROLLING BLOOD PRESSURE

FACTOR	CONDITION		RESULT
Cardiac output	↑ with heavy exercise to meet body demand for increased metabolism		↑ BP
	↓ with pump failure (weak pumping action after myocardial infarction, or in shock)		↓ BP
Vascular resistance	↑ resistance (vasoconstriction)		↑ BP
	↓ resistance (vasodilation)		↓ BP
Volume	↓ volume (hemorrhage)		↓ BP
	↑ volume (increased sodium and water retention, intravenous fluid overload)		↑ BP
Viscosity	↑ viscosity (increased hematocrit in polycythemia)		↑ BP
Elasticity of arterial walls	↑ rigidity, hardening as in arteriosclerosis (heart pumping against greater resistance)		↑ BP

10.4

1. **Cardiac output.** If the heart pumps more blood into the container (i.e., the blood vessels), the pressure on the container walls increases.
2. **Peripheral vascular resistance.** Peripheral vascular resistance is the opposition to blood flow through the arteries. When the container becomes smaller (e.g., with constricted vessels), the pressure needed to push the contents becomes greater. Conversely, if the container becomes larger (e.g., vasodilation), less pressure is needed.
3. **Volume of circulating blood.** Volume of circulating blood refers to how tightly the blood is packed into the arteries. Increasing the contents in the container (e.g., with a blood transfusion) increases the pressure.

Many medications used in the treatment of critically ill people affect peripheral vascular resistance.

Blood volume is increased via blood transfusions or volume expanders and decreased through hemorrhage.

Normal Range of Findings	Abnormal Findings

4. **Viscosity.** The "thickness" of blood is determined by its formed elements, the blood cells. When the contents are thicker, the pressure increases.
5. **Elasticity of vessel walls.** When the container walls are stiff and rigid, the pressure needed to push the contents increases.

BP is measured with a stethoscope and an aneroid *sphygmomanometer*. The aneroid gauge is subject to drift; it must be recalibrated at least once each year, and it must rest at zero.

> If the gauge doesn't rest at zero, the readings obtained will either be high or low, depending on the direction of the drift.

The cuff consists of an inflatable rubber bladder inside a cloth cover. The width of the rubber bladder should equal 40% of the circumference of the person's arm. The length of the bladder should equal 80% of the arm circumference.

Available cuffs include 6 sizes, a range that fits newborn infants to the extra-large adult, as well as tapered cuffs for the cone-shaped obese arm and thigh cuffs. Match the appropriate-size cuff to the person's arm size and shape and not to his or her age (Fig. 10.5).

> The cuff size is important; using a cuff that is too narrow yields a falsely high BP because it takes extra pressure to compress the artery.

Thigh cuff or large arm cuff

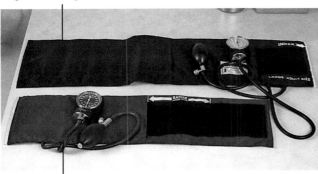

Standard adult arm cuff

10.5

The Procedure: Arm Pressure

A comfortable, relaxed person yields a valid BP. Many people are anxious at the beginning of an examination; allow at least a 5-minute rest before measuring the BP. Then take two or more BP measurements separated by 1 to 2 minutes.

For each person, verify BP in both arms once, either on admission or for the first complete physical examination. It is not necessary to continue to check both arms for screening or monitoring. Occasionally a 5- to 10-mm Hg difference may occur in BP in the two arms, which is caused by artifact or subtle differences in technique. If values are different, use the higher value. A normal BP reading is <120/<80 in adults.[13]

The person may be sitting or lying, with the **bare arm** supported at heart level. When sitting, the patient's feet should be flat on the floor because BP has a false-high measurement when legs are crossed versus uncrossed.[12]

Palpate the brachial artery, which is located just above the antecubital fossa, medial to the biceps tendon. With the cuff deflated, center it about 2.5 cm (1 in) above the brachial artery and wrap the cuff evenly.

> A reproducible difference in the two arms of more than 10 to 15 mm Hg may indicate arterial obstruction on the side with the lower reading. This warrants further evaluation.

Objective Data

Normal Range of Findings

Now palpate the brachial or radial artery (Fig. 10.6). Inflate the cuff until the artery pulsation is obliterated. Note that number. When you inflate the cuff to auscultate the blood pressure, you will add 20 to 30 mm Hg to the number you noted to identify the maximal inflation level. This maximal inflation pressure helps you to avoid missing an **auscultatory gap,** which is a period when Korotkoff sounds disappear during auscultation (Table 10.3).

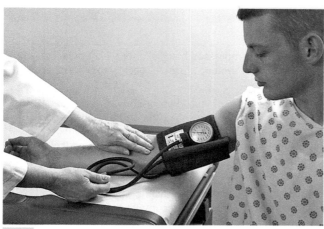

10.6

Deflate the cuff quickly and completely; then wait 15 to 30 seconds before reinflating so that the blood trapped in the veins can dissipate. Place the bell or diaphragm of the stethoscope over the site of the brachial artery, making a light but airtight seal (Fig. 10.7). The diaphragm endpiece is usually adequate, but the bell is designed to pick up low-pitched sounds such as the sounds of a BP reading. Most novice practitioners find it easier to use the diaphragm than the bell. You can use either side to obtain an accurate reading.[9]

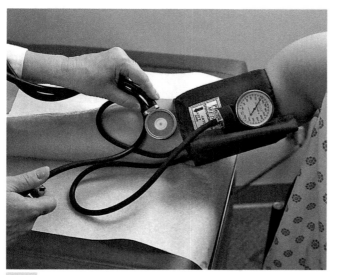

10.7

Abnormal Findings

An auscultatory gap occurs in about 5% of people, most often in hypertension caused by a noncompliant arterial system.

Objective Data

Normal Range of Findings	Abnormal Findings

Rapidly inflate the cuff to the maximal inflation level that you determined. Then deflate the cuff slowly and evenly, about 2 mm Hg per heartbeat. If the heartbeat is rapid, aim for approximately 2 mm Hg per second. Note the points at which you hear the first appearance of sound, the muffling of sound, and the final disappearance of sound. These are phases I, IV, and V of **Korotkoff sounds,** which are the components of a BP reading first described by a Russian surgeon in 1905 (see Table 10.3).

Objective Data

TABLE 10.3 Korotkoff Sounds

PHASE	QUALITY	DESCRIPTION	RATIONALE
Cuff correctly inflated	No sound		Cuff inflation compresses brachial artery. Cuff pressure exceeds heart systolic pressure, occluding brachial artery blood flow.
I	Tapping	Soft, clear tapping, increasing in intensity	**Systolic** pressure. As cuff pressure lowers to reach intraluminal systolic pressure, the artery opens and blood first spurts into brachial artery. Blood is at very high velocity because of small opening of artery and large pressure difference across opening. This creates turbulent flow, which is audible.
Auscultatory gap	No sound	Silence for 30 to 40 mm Hg during deflation; an abnormal finding	Sounds temporarily disappear during end of phase I and reappear in phase II. May occur with hypertension. If undetected, results in falsely low systolic or falsely high diastolic reading.
II	Swooshing	Softer murmur follows tapping	Turbulent blood flow through still partially occluded artery.
III	Knocking	Crisp, high-pitched sounds	Longer duration of blood flow through artery. Artery closes just briefly during late diastole.
IV	Abrupt muffling	Sound mutes to a low-pitched, cushioned murmur; blowing quality	Artery no longer closes in any part of cardiac cycle. Change in quality, not intensity.
V	Silence		Decreased velocity of blood flow. Streamlined blood flow is silent. The disappearance of sound is **diastolic** pressure. The fifth Korotkoff sound is used to define diastolic pressure in all age-groups.

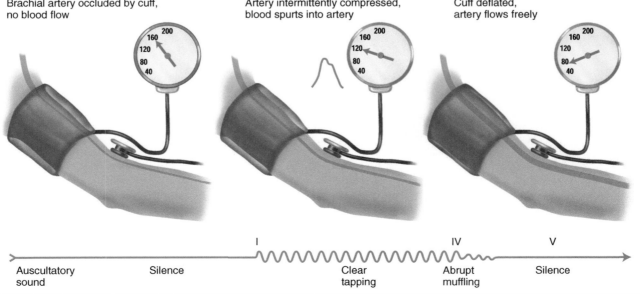

Brachial artery occluded by cuff, no blood flow

Artery intermittently compressed, blood spurts into artery

Cuff deflated, artery flows freely

| Auscultatory sound | Silence | | Clear tapping | Abrupt muffling | Silence |

Normal Range of Findings

For all age-groups the fifth Korotkoff phase is used to define diastolic pressure. However, when a variance greater than 10 to 12 mm Hg exists between phases IV and V, record *both* phases along with the systolic reading (e.g., 142/98/80). Clear communication is important because the results significantly affect diagnosis and planning of care. See Table 10.4 for a list of common errors in BP measurement.

Record the BP using even numbers since each line on the sphygmomanometer is 2 mm Hg. Also record the person's position, the arm used, and the cuff size if different from the standard adult cuff.

Abnormal Findings

Hypotension, abnormally low BP (Table 10.5 on p. 158); **hypertension,**[7,13] abnormally high BP (Table 10.6 on p. 159).

TABLE 10.4   Common Errors in Blood Pressure Measurement

COMMON ERROR	RESULT	RATIONALE
Taking blood pressure reading when person is anxious or angry or has just been active	Falsely high	Sympathetic nervous system stimulation
Faulty arm position:		
Above level of heart	Falsely low	Eliminates effect of hydrostatic pressure
Below level of heart	Falsely high	Additional force of gravity added to brachial artery pressure
Person supports own arm	Falsely high diastolic	Sustained isometric muscular contraction
Faulty leg position (e.g., person's legs are crossed)	Falsely high systolic and diastolic	Translocation of blood volume from dependent legs to thoracic area
Inaccurate cuff size (most common error):		
Cuff too narrow for extremity	Falsely high	Needs excessive pressure to occlude brachial artery
Cuff wrap is too loose or uneven, or bladder balloons out of wrap	Falsely high	Needs excessive pressure to occlude brachial artery
Failure to palpate radial artery while inflating:		
Inflating cuff not high enough	Falsely low systolic	Misses initial systolic tapping or may tune in during *auscultatory gap* (tapping sounds disappear for 30 to 40 mm Hg and then return; may occur with hypertension)
Inflating cuff too high	Pain	
Pushing stethoscope too hard on brachial artery	Falsely low diastolic	Excessive pressure distorts artery, and sounds continue
Deflating cuff:		
Too quickly	Falsely low systolic or falsely high diastolic	Insufficient time to hear tapping
Too slowly	Falsely high diastolic	Venous congestion in forearm makes sounds less audible
Halting during descent and reinflating cuff to recheck systolic	Falsely high diastolic	Venous congestion in forearm
Failure to wait 1-2 min before repeating entire reading	Falsely high diastolic	Venous congestion in forearm
Any observer error:		
Examiner's "subconscious bias"; a preconceived idea of what BP reading *should* be because of person's age, race, gender, weight, history, or condition	Error anywhere	Never assume that because a person appears healthy, his or her BP will be within normal limits
Examiner's haste	Error anywhere	
Faulty technique		
Examiner's digit preference; "hears" more results that end in zero than would occur by chance alone (e.g., 130/80)		
Diminished hearing acuity		
Defective or inaccurately calibrated equipment		

Objective Data

Normal Range of Findings	Abnormal Findings

Orthostatic (or Postural) Vital Signs

Take serial measurements of pulse and BP when (1) you suspect volume depletion, (2) when the person is known to have hypertension or is taking antihypertensive medications, or (3) when the person reports fainting or syncope. Have the person rest supine for at least 3 minutes, then take baseline BP and pulse readings. Have the patient sit up and assess BP and pulse; then have the patient stand and assess BP and pulse. Finally, after the patient has been standing for 3 minutes, assess BP and pulse.[1,4] For the person who is too weak or dizzy to stand, assess supine and then sitting with legs dangling. When the position is changed from supine to standing, normally a slight decrease (less than 10 mm Hg) in systolic pressure may occur.

Orthostatic hypotension refers to a drop in systolic pressure of ≥20 mm Hg or diastolic pressure ≥10 mm Hg after changing to a standing position. These changes are caused by abrupt peripheral vasodilation without a compensatory increase in cardiac output. Orthostatic changes occur with prolonged bed rest, older age, hypovolemia, and some medications. New recommendations suggest that the BP measurement within 1 minute of standing is most strongly related to identifying orthostatic hypotension.[8]

Thigh Pressure

When BP measured at the arm is excessively high, particularly in adolescents and young adults, compare it with the thigh pressure to check for **coarctation of the aorta** (a congenital form of narrowing). Normally the *thigh pressure is higher* than in the arm. If possible, help the person to a prone position. (If the person must remain in the supine position, bend the knee slightly.) Wrap a large cuff around the lower third of the thigh, centered over the popliteal artery on the back of the knee. Auscultate the popliteal artery for the reading (Fig. 10.8). Normally the systolic value is 10 to 40 mm Hg higher in the thigh than in the arm, and the diastolic pressure is the same.

With **coarctation of the aorta,** arm pressures are high. Thigh pressure is *lower* because the blood supply to the thigh is below the constriction.

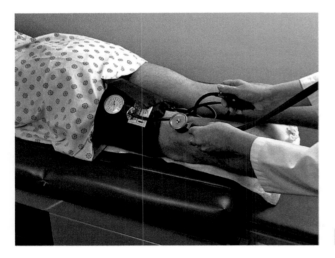

10.8

❖ DEVELOPMENTAL COMPETENCE

Infants and Children

Measure vital signs to monitor clinical condition in children, but follow agency guidelines for frequency. Note that blood pressure is not regularly assessed in children less than 3 years old. With an *infant,* reverse the order of vital sign measurement to respiration, pulse, and temperature. Taking a rectal temperature may cause the infant to cry, which will increase the respiratory and pulse rate, thus masking the normal resting values. A *preschooler's* normal fear of body mutilation is increased with any invasive procedure. Whenever possible avoid the rectal route and take a tympanic or temporal artery temperature. Remember

Objective Data

Normal Range of Findings	**Abnormal Findings**

that you may have to use the rectal route for an accurate core measure. It is important to weigh risks and benefits when deciding on the appropriate temperature route for a child. Promote the cooperation of the *school-age child* by explaining the procedure completely and encouraging the child to handle the equipment. Your approach to measuring vital signs with the *adolescent* is much the same as with the adult.

Temperature

Tympanic Membrane and Temporal Artery. TMT and TAT measurements are useful with toddlers who squirm at the restraint needed for the rectal route and with preschoolers who are not yet able to cooperate for an oral temperature yet fear the disrobing and invasion of a rectal temperature. TMT and TAT measure temperature so rapidly that the measurement is over before the child realizes it (Fig. 10.9).

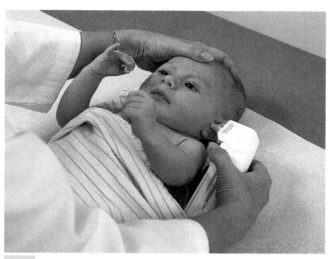

10.9

Axillary. The axillary route is safer and more accessible than the rectal route; however, its accuracy and reliability have been questioned. When cold receptors are stimulated, brown fat tissue in the area releases heat through chemical energy, which artificially raises skin temperature. When the axillary route is used, place the tip of the thermometer well into the axilla and hold the child's arm close to the body.

Oral. Use the oral route when the child is old enough to keep his or her mouth closed. This is usually at age 5 or 6 years, although some 4-year-old children can cooperate. When available, use an electronic thermometer because it is unbreakable and it registers quickly.

Rectal. Use this route with infants or other age-groups when other routes are not feasible, such as with the child who is unable to cooperate or is agitated, unconscious, or critically ill. An infant may be supine or side-lying, with the examiner's hand flexing the knees up onto the abdomen. (When supine, cover the boy's penis with a diaper.) An infant also may lie prone across the adult's lap. Separate the buttocks with one hand, and insert the lubricated electronic rectal probe *no farther than* 2.5 cm (1 in) for children >6 months and approximately ½ inch for children <6 months. Insertion >1 inch risks rectal perforation because the colon curves posteriorly at 3 cm (1¼ in). Do not let go of the thermometer probe.

Objective Data

Normal Range of Findings

Normally rectal temperatures measure higher in infants and young children than in adults, with an average of 37.8°C (100°F) at 18 months. In addition, the temperature normally may be elevated in the late afternoon, after vigorous playing, or after eating.

Pulse

Palpate or auscultate an apical rate with infants and toddlers. (See Chapter 20 for location of apex and technique.) In children older than 2 years, use the radial site. Count the pulse for a full minute to take into account normal irregularities such as sinus arrhythmia. The heart rate normally fluctuates more with infants and children than with adults in response to exercise, emotion, and illness. Note normal pulse rate in Table 10.1 on p. 142.

Respirations

Watch the infant's abdomen for movement because an infant's respirations are normally more diaphragmatic than thoracic (Fig. 10.10). The sleeping respiratory rate is the most accurate. Count a full minute because the pattern varies significantly from rapid breaths to short periods of apnea. Note the normal rate in Table 10.2 on p. 143.

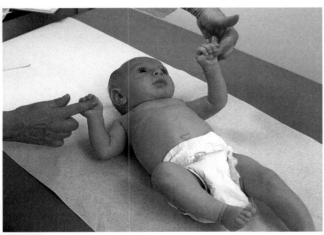

10.10

Blood Pressure

In children ages 3 years and older, measure a routine BP at least annually and more frequently in children with certain medical conditions. BP should be checked more frequently in children and adolescents if they have certain conditions such as obesity, renal disease, or diabetes.[5] For accurate measurement in children, make some adjustment in the choice of equipment and technique. The most common error is to use the incorrect size cuff. The cuff width must cover at least 40% of the upper arm, and the cuff bladder must be 80% to 100% the circumference of the arm.[5]

Use a pediatric-size endpiece on the stethoscope. Best practice dictates that the child should be seated 3 to 5 minutes before measurement. If possible, allow a crying infant to become quiet for 5 to 10 minutes before measuring the BP; crying may elevate the systolic pressure by 30 to 50 mm Hg. Children should be

Abnormal Findings

Up to ages 6 to 8 years, children have higher fevers with illness than adults do. Even with minor infections, fevers may elevate to 39.5° to 40.5°C (103° to 105°F).

Tachypnea, or rapid respiratory rate, is >60/min for newborns to 2 months, and >50/min for 2 to 12 months. This occurs with fever and may indicate infection. Tachypnea and labored respirations may indicate pneumonia.

Children who are obese, have an abnormal birth history (e.g., preterm birth and low birth weight), suffer from chronic kidney disease or sleep-disordered breathing are at higher risk for hypertension than children without the aforementioned conditions.[5]

Developing evidence shows that primary hypertension is detectable in children and occurs commonly. BP between the 90th and 94th percentiles

Normal Range of Findings

seated with their back supported and feet on the floor during measurement. For consistency and comparison to normative tables, BP in children should be taken in the right arm. The arm should be supported, at the level of the heart. Use the disappearance of sound (phase V Korotkoff) for the diastolic reading in both children and adults.

Note the guidelines for BP standards based on sex, age, and height.[5] These standards give a more precise classification of BP according to body size and avoid misclassifying children who are very tall or very short.

Children younger than 3 years have such small arm vessels that it is difficult to hear Korotkoff sounds with a stethoscope. Instead use an electronic BP device that uses *oscillometry*, such as Dinamap, and gives a digital readout for systolic, diastolic, MAP, and pulse. Or use a *Doppler* ultrasound device to amplify the sounds. This instrument is easy to use and can be used by one examiner. (Note the technique for using the Doppler device on p. 155.)

The Aging Adult

Vital Signs

Temperature. Changes in the body's temperature regulatory mechanism leave the older adult less likely to have fever but at a greater risk for hypothermia. Thus the temperature is a less reliable index of the older person's true health state. Sweat gland activity is also diminished.

Pulse. The normal range of heart rate is 50 to 95 beats/min, but the rhythm may be slightly irregular. The radial artery may feel stiff, rigid, and tortuous in an older person, although this condition does not necessarily imply vascular disease in the heart or brain. The increasingly rigid arterial wall needs a faster upstroke of blood, so the pulse is actually easier to palpate.

Respirations. Aging causes a decrease in vital capacity and a decreased inspiratory reserve volume. You may note a shallower inspiratory phase and an increased respiratory rate.

Blood Pressure. The aorta and major arteries tend to harden with age. As the heart pumps against a stiffer aorta, the systolic pressure increases, leading to a widened pulse pressure. With many older people, both the systolic and diastolic pressures increase, making it difficult to distinguish expected aging values from abnormal hypertension.

Additional Techniques

Measurement of Oxygen Saturation

The **pulse oximeter** is a noninvasive method to assess arterial oxygen saturation (SpO_2). A sensor attached to the person's finger, forehead, or earlobe has a diode that emits light and a detector that measures the relative amount of light absorbed by oxyhemoglobin (HbO_2) and unoxygenated (reduced) hemoglobin (Hb). The pulse oximeter compares the ratio of light emitted with light absorbed and converts this ratio into the percentage of oxygen saturation. Because it measures only light absorption of pulsatile flow, the result is SpO_2. A healthy person with no lung disease normally has a SpO_2 of 97% to 99% on room air, but a value of >95% is clinically acceptable in the presence of a normal hemoglobin.[14]

Abnormal Findings

is elevated blood pressure. In adolescents BP ≥120/80 mm Hg is considered elevated. BP ≥95th percentile may be hypertension. It should be measured on 3 separate occasions to confirm the diagnosis. Similar to adults, hypertension in children and adolescents is associated with obesity, hyperlipidemia, and diabetes.[5]

While oscillometric devices are commonly used in the health care setting, auscultation remains the gold standard. In studies, oscillometric devices consistently overestimate systolic blood pressure and diastolic blood pressure. If elevated BP is identified based on oscillometric readings, confirmation through auscultation is recommended.[5]

Objective Data

Normal Range of Findings	**Abnormal Findings**

Select the appropriate pulse oximeter probe. The finger probe is spring-loaded and feels like a clothespin attached to the finger, but it does not hurt (Fig. 10.11). An infant usually has a probe taped to the large toe. Some clinics use single-use probes that stick to the finger, forehead, or ear instead of the multipatient-use spring-loaded model. If you are using a finger, make sure that the hand is warm to prevent false low readings caused by vasoconstriction. At lower oxygen saturations, the earlobe probe is more accurate.

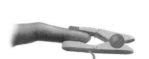 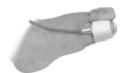

10.11

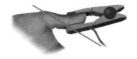

(© Pat Thomas, 2014.)

The probe will show both the oxygen saturation and the pulse. Make sure that the pulse reading you see on the pulse oximeter matches the palpated pulse. If it does not correlate with the palpated pulse, question the accuracy of the result.

Pulse oximetry readings are less accurate in patients with low perfusion (e.g., hypothermia, vasoconstriction), low hemoglobin, and dyshemoglobinemias. Dark nail polish is reported in some studies to negatively impact pulse oximetry readings. In low perfusion states, using the ear or forehead is preferred.[14]

Electronic Vital Signs Monitor

An automated vital signs monitor is in frequent use in hospital and clinic settings, especially when frequent BP measurement is needed. The artery pulsations create vibrations that are detected by an electronic sensor. The BP mode is noninvasive, fast, and has automatic measurement intervals and a bright numeric display. As with manual BP equipment, accuracy depends on correct cuff selection and placement. If the numeric display does not fit with the patient's clinical picture, always validate the measurement with a manual sphygmomanometer and your own stethoscope. Some electronic BP devices also have probes for thermometry and pulse oximetry (Fig. 10.12).

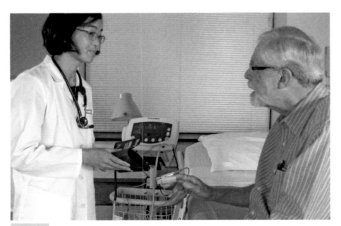

10.12

Normal Range of Findings	Abnormal Findings

The Doppler Technique

In many situations pulse and BP measurement are enhanced by using an electronic device, the *Doppler ultrasonic flowmeter*. The Doppler technique works by a principle discovered in the 19th century by an Austrian physicist, Johannes Doppler. Sound varies in pitch in relation to the distance between the sound source and the listener; the pitch is higher when the distance is small, and the pitch lowers as the distance increases. Think of a railroad train speeding toward you; its train whistle sounds higher the closer it gets, and the pitch of the whistle lowers as the train fades away.

In this case the sound source is the blood pumping through the artery in a rhythmic manner. A handheld transducer picks up changes in sound frequency as the blood flows and ebbs, and it amplifies them. The listener hears a whooshing pulsatile beat.

The Doppler technique is used to locate the peripheral pulse sites (see Chapter 21 for further discussion). For BP measurement the Doppler technique will augment Korotkoff sounds (Fig. 10.13). Through this technique you can evaluate sounds that are hard to hear with a stethoscope such as those in critically ill individuals with a low BP, infants with small arms, and obese persons in whom the sounds are muffled by layers of fat. In addition, proper cuff placement is difficult on the obese person's cone-shaped upper arm. In this situation you can place the cuff on the more even forearm and hold the Doppler probe over the radial artery. For either location, use the following procedure:

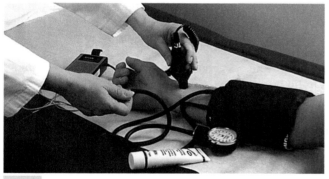

10.13

- Apply coupling gel to the transducer probe.
- Turn Doppler flowmeter on.
- Touch the probe to the skin, holding it perpendicular to the artery.
- A pulsatile whooshing sound indicates location of the artery. You may need to rotate the probe, but maintain contact with the skin. Do not push the probe too hard or you will occlude the pulse.
- Inflate the cuff until the sounds disappear; then proceed another 20 to 30 mm Hg beyond that point.
- Slowly deflate the cuff, noting the point at which the first whooshing sounds appear. This is the systolic pressure.
- It is difficult to hear the muffling of sounds or a reliable disappearance of sounds indicating the diastolic pressure (phases IV and V of Korotkoff sounds). However, the systolic pressure alone gives valuable data on the level of tissue perfusion and blood flow through patent vessels.

Objective Data

DOCUMENTATION AND CRITICAL THINKING

Sample Charting

K.A. is a 56-year-old male construction worker who appears healthy and of stated age. Alert, oriented, cooperative, with no signs of distress. Ht 170 cm (5 ft 7 in). Wt 83 kg (182 lb). BMI 28.5 (overweight). Temp 98.6° F (37° C). Pulse 84 bpm, regular rhythm, force 2+. Resp 14/min, easy, unlabored. BP 146/84 mm Hg right arm, sitting.

Clinical Case Study 1[a]

G.S. is a 76-year-old female retired secretary, previously in good health, who is brought to the ED by her 83-year-old husband. G.S. and her husband report nausea, vomiting, diarrhea, and abdominal cramping since last night. Symptoms began after eating "bad food" at a buffet-style restaurant. G.S.'s husband reports that his symptoms have improved. G.S. continues to have diarrhea and dry heaving.

[a]Please note that space does not allow a detailed plan for each clinical case study in this text. Please use these case studies as critical-thinking exercises and consult the appropriate text for current treatment plan.

SUBJECTIVE

G.S. reports extreme fatigue, weakness, and dizziness with position changes: "Feels like I'm going to black out." Severe nausea and vomiting; thirsty but cannot keep anything down; even sips of water result in "dry heaves." Cramping, intermittent abdominal pain. Watery brown diarrhea, profuse during the night, somewhat diminished now.

OBJECTIVE

Vital signs: Temp 100.1° F (37.8° C). BP (supine) 102/64 mm Hg. Pulse (supine) 70 bpm, regular rhythm. Resp 18/min, unlabored. Helped to seated, leg-dangling position. Vitals: BP 74/52 mm Hg. Pulse 138 bpm, regular rhythm. Resp 20/min, unlabored. Skin pale and moist (diaphoretic). Reports light-headed and dizzy in seated position. Returned to supine.
Respiratory: Breath sounds clear in all fields; no adventitious sounds.
Cardiovascular: Regular rate (70 bpm) and rhythm when supine, S_1 and S_2 are not accentuated or diminished, no extra sounds. All pulses present, 2+ and equal bilaterally. Carotids 2+ with no carotid bruit.
Abdomen: Bowel sounds hyperactive, skin pale and moist, abdomen soft and mildly tender to palpation. No enlargement of liver or spleen.
Neuro: Level of consciousness alert and oriented; pupils equal, round, react to light and accommodation. Sensory status normal. Mild weakness in arms and legs. Gait and standing leg strength not tested because of weakness. Deep tendon reflexes 2+ and equal bilaterally. Babinski reflex → down-going toes.

ASSESSMENT

Orthostatic hypotension, orthostatic pulse increase, and syncopal symptoms
Hypovolemia
Diarrhea
Fever
Deficient fluid volume

Clinical Case Study 2

G.H. is a 31-year-old male with no significant past medical history. Family history includes a mother with diabetes; father with hypertension diagnosed at age 40 years; and paternal grandfather with myocardial infarction at age 50, stroke at age 62, and heart failure diagnosed at age 51. G.H. presents to the ED with blurred vision and headache for the past 24 hours. He appears anxious but denies pain other than his headache.

SUBJECTIVE

Blurred vision for the past 24 hours that gets worse with activity. Frontal lobe headache that "comes and goes" for the past 24 hours. Denies nausea, vomiting. Reports occasional dizziness.

OBJECTIVE

Vital signs: Temp 98.6° F (37° C). BP 210/112 mm Hg right arm, sitting; 220/120 mm Hg left arm, sitting. Pulse 110 bpm, regular rhythm, force 3+. RR 20/min, unlabored.

Respiratory: Breath sounds clear throughout; no adventitious sounds.

Cardiovascular: Regular rate and rhythm. S_1 and S_2 not accentuated or diminished, no extra sounds. Pulses bounding 3+ bilateral. 2+ pitting edema bilateral lower extremities.

Abdomen: Rounded abdomen. Bowel sounds active. Abdomen soft, nontender.

Neuro: Level of consciousness alert and oriented. Pupils equal; sluggish reaction to light. Optic disc swollen. Deep tendon reflexes 2+ and equal bilaterally. Babinski reflex → down-going toes.

ASSESSMENT

Hypertensive urgency
Risk for stroke and myocardial ischemia
Pain
Decreased cardiac output

Clinical Case Study 3

J.T. is a 4-month-old girl brought to the pediatric clinic by her mother. Until 2 days PTA, she has been in good health. She has had diarrhea, vomiting, and decreased intake for 2 days. J.T.'s mother, father, and 3-year-old brother all had the same symptoms but are now improved.

SUBJECTIVE

J.T. has less diarrhea and no vomiting today, but she doesn't want to breastfeed and still appears to be "more sleepy than usual and just not herself." Her mother reports, "Now that I think about it, J.T. has only had 1 or 2 wet diapers since yesterday."

OBJECTIVE

Vital signs: Temp 99.5° F (37.5° C, rectally). BP 68/46 mm Hg (while lying being held). Pulse (apical) while sleeping 164 bpm, rhythm regular, force 2+. Resp 56/min. Weight 11 lb, 4 oz (5.2 kg).

General appearance: Listless, pale; appears to be sleeping in mother's arms and awakens to physical stimuli but does not cry.

HEENT: Anterior fontanel sunken; dry oral mucosa; no tear production.

Cardiovascular: Tachycardia; no abnormal heart sounds; femoral pulses 1+ = bilat.

Respiratory: Tachypnea. Pulse oximetry 94% on room air. Breath sounds clear in all fields and = bilat; no adventitious sounds.

Abdomen: Hyperactive bowel sounds; no palpable masses.

Extremities: Cool, decreased pulse, cap refill 4 sec.

ASSESSMENT

Dehydration
Diarrhea
Electrolyte imbalance
Fever

ABNORMAL FINDINGS

TABLE 10.5	Hypotension

In normotensive adults: <95/60 mm Hg
In hypertensive adults: < The person's average reading, but >95/60 mm Hg
In children: < Expected value for age

Occurs With	*Rationale*
Acute myocardial infarction	Decreased cardiac output
Shock	Decreased cardiac output
Hemorrhage	Decrease in total blood volume
Vasodilation	Decrease in peripheral vascular resistance
Addison disease (hypofunction of adrenal glands)	Decrease in circulating aldosterone

Associated Symptoms and Signs

In conditions of decreased cardiac output, a low BP is accompanied by an increased pulse, dizziness, diaphoresis, confusion, and blurred vision. The skin feels cool and clammy because the superficial blood vessels constrict to shunt blood to the vital organs. An individual having an acute MI may also complain of substernal chest pain, epigastric pain, shoulder or jaw pain, and any number of nonspecific symptoms (e.g., fatigue).

TABLE 10.6 | Essential or Primary Hypertension

Primary hypertension has no known cause but is responsible for about 95% of cases of hypertension in adults. Normal BP in adults is <120/<80. BP 120-129/<80 is considered elevated, and lifestyle modifications should be implemented.

Summary of Blood Pressure Guidelines

	Target BP	Initial Treatment	Special Considerations
ACC/AHA Task Force[a]	<130/80 mm Hg	In patients without cardiovascular disease (CVD) and 10-year atherosclerotic CVD risk of <10%, begin treatment ≥140/90 mm Hg. In patients with CVD or 10-year atherosclerotic CVD risk ≥10%, begin treatment ≥130/80 mm Hg	Consider lower BP targets for high-risk individuals, such as those with diabetes or chronic kidney disease (CKD).
JNC-8 Guidelines[b]	Adults ≥60 yr: <150/90 mm Hg; Adults <60 yr with diabetes or CKD: <140/90 mm Hg; Adults <60 yr: <140/90 mm Hg	Lifestyle modification and pharmacologic therapy, beginning with thiazide diuretics, CCB, ACEI, or ARB in non–African-American patients	Initial treatment for African-American patients is a CCB or a thiazide diuretic. CKD patients should begin with an ACEI or ARB.

Cardiovascular Risk Stratification in Patients With Hypertension

Major Risk Factors	Target Organ Damage/Clinical Cardiovascular Disease
Smoking	Heart diseases
Dyslipidemia	Left ventricular atrophy
Diabetes mellitus	Angina or prior myocardial infarction
Age >60 yr	Prior coronary revascularization
Gender (men and postmenopausal women)	Heart failure
Family history of cardiovascular disease: women <65 yr or men <55 yr	Stroke or transient ischemic attack
	Nephropathy
	Peripheral arterial disease
	Retinopathy

Lifestyle Modifications for Hypertension Prevention and Management

- Lose weight if overweight
- Limit alcohol intake to no more than 1 oz (30 mL) of ethanol (e.g., 24 oz [720 mL] of beer, 10 oz [300 mL] of wine, or 2 oz [60 mL] of 100-proof whiskey) per day or 0.5 oz (15 mL) of ethanol per day for women and lighter-weight people.
- Increase aerobic physical activity (30-45 min most days of the week).
- Reduce sodium intake to no more than 100 mmol/day (2.4 g of sodium or 6 g of sodium chloride).
- Maintain adequate intake of dietary potassium (approximately 90 mmol/day).
- Maintain adequate intake of dietary calcium and magnesium for general health.
- Stop smoking and reduce intake of dietary saturated fat and cholesterol for overall cardiovascular health.

ACEI, Angiotensin-converting enzyme inhibitor; *ARB,* angiotensin II receptor blocker; *CCB,* calcium channel blocker.
[a]Whelton, P. K., Carey, R. M., Aronow, W. S., et al. (2017). 2017 ACC/AHA/AAPA/ABC/ACPM/AGS/APhA/ ASH/ASPC/NMA/PCNA Guideline for the prevention, detection, evaluation, and management of high blood pressure in adults. *Journal of the American College of Cardiology.* doi: 10.1016/j.jacc.2017.11.006
[b]James, P. A., Oparil, S., & Carter, B. L. (2014). 2014 Evidence-based guidelines for the management of high blood pressure in adults: report from the panel members appointed to the Eighth Joint National Committee (JNC 8). *JAMA, 311,* 507-520.

REFERENCES

1. Agency for Healthcare Research and Quality. (2013). *Tool 3F: Orthostatic vital sign measurement.* https://www.ahrq.gov/professionals/systems/hospital/fallpxtoolkit/fallpxtk-tool3f.html.

2. Allegaert, K., Casteels, K., van Gorp, I., et al. (2014). Tympanic, infrared skin, and temporal artery scan thermometers compared with rectal measurement in children: A real-life assessment. *Curr Ther Res Clin Exp, 76,* 34–38.

3. Benjamin, E. J., Blaha, M. J., Chiuve, S. E., et al. (2017). Heart disease and stroke statistics—2017 update: A report from the American Heart Association. *Circulation, 135,* e146–e603.

4. CDC. (2017). *Assessment: Measuring orthostatic blood pressure.* https://www.cdc.gov/steadi/pdf/measuring_orthostatic_blood_pressure-a.pdf.

5. Flynn, J. T., Kaelber, D. C., Baker-Smith, C. M., et al. (2017). *Clinical practice guideline for screening and management of high blood pressure in children and adolescents.* http://pediatrics.aappublications.org/content/pediatrics/early/2017/08/21/peds.2017-1904.full.pdf.

6. Hollerbach, A. D., & Sneed, N. V. (1990). Accuracy of radial pulse assessment by length of counting interval. *Heart Lung, 19*(3), 258–264.

7. James, P. A., Oparil, S., & Carter, B. L. (2014). 2014 Evidence-based guidelines for the management of high blood pressure in adults: Report from the panel members appointed to the Eighth Joint National Committee (JNC 8). *JAMA, 311,* 507–520.

8. Juraschek, S. P., Daya, N., Rawlings, A. M., et al. (2017). Comparison of early versus late orthostatic hypotension assessment times in middle-age adults. *JAMA Intern Med, 177,* 1316–1323.

9. Liu, C., Griffiths, C., Murray, A., et al. (2016). Comparison of stethoscope bell and diaphragm, and of stethoscope tube length, for clinical blood pressure measurement. *Blood Press Monit, 21*(3), 178–183.

10. McGee, S. (2018). *Evidence-based physical diagnosis* (4th ed.). St. Louis: Elsevier.

11. Niven, D. J., Gaudet, J. E., Laupland, K. B., et al. (2015). Accuracy of peripheral thermometers for estimating temperature: A systematic review and meta-analysis. *Ann Intern Med, 163,* 768–777.

12. van Velthoven, M. H., Holewijn, S., van der Wilt, G. J., et al. (2014). Does wave reflection explain the increase in blood pressure during leg crossing? *Blood Press Monit, 19*(3), 129–133.

13. Whelton, P. K., Carey, R. M., Aronow, W. S., et al. (2017). 2017 ACC/AHA/AAPA/ABC/ACPM/AGS/APhA/ASH/ASPC/NMA/PCNA Guideline for the prevention, detection, evaluation, and management of high blood pressure in adults. *J Am Coll Cardiol,* doi:10.1016/j.jacc.2017.11.006.

14. Wiegand, D. L. (Ed.). (2016). *AACN procedure manual for high acuity, progressive, and critical care* (7th ed.). St. Louis: Elsevier.

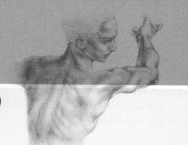

CHAPTER 11

Pain Assessment

http://evolve.elsevier.com/Jarvis/

STRUCTURE AND FUNCTION

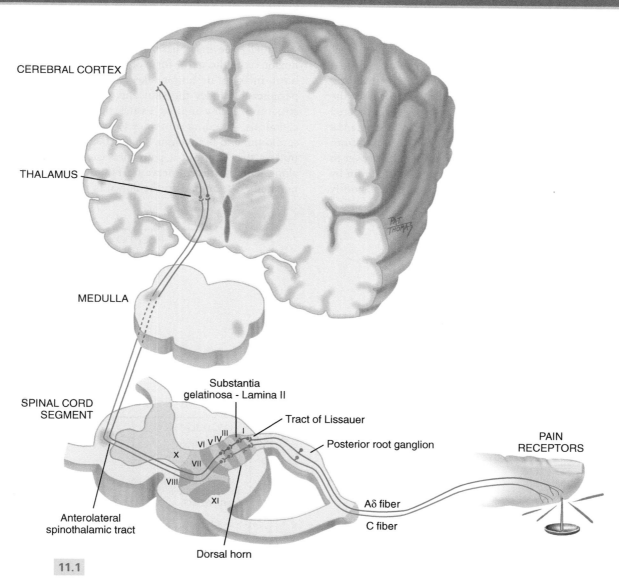

CEREBRAL CORTEX

THALAMUS

MEDULLA

SPINAL CORD SEGMENT

Substantia gelatinosa - Lamina II

Tract of Lissauer

Posterior root ganglion

PAIN RECEPTORS

VI V IV III I

X

VII

VIII

XI

Anterolateral spinothalamic tract

Aδ fiber

C fiber

Dorsal horn

11.1

Pathologic pain develops by two main processes: **nociceptive** (Fig. 11.1) and/or **neuropathic** processing. It is important to understand how these two types of pain develop because patients present with distinguishing sensations and respond differently to analgesics. An accurate pain assessment allows clinicians to more accurately select effective pharmacologic and nonpharmacologic strategies to interrupt the pain processing along multiple points within the pain messaging system and ultimately provide improved pain relief.

NEUROANATOMIC PATHWAY

Pain is a highly complex and subjective experience that originates from the central nervous system (CNS) and/or peripheral nervous system (PNS). Specialized nerve endings called **nociceptors** are designed to detect painful sensations from the periphery and transmit them to the CNS. Nociceptors are located primarily within the skin; joints; connective tissue; muscle; and thoracic, abdominal, and pelvic viscera. These nociceptors can be stimulated directly by mechanical or thermal trauma or secondarily by chemical mediators that are released from the site of tissue damage.

Nociceptors carry the pain signal to the CNS by two primary sensory (or afferent) fibers: **Aδ and C fibers** (see Fig. 11.1). **Aδ** fibers are myelinated and larger in diameter; thus they transmit the pain signal rapidly to the CNS. The sensation is localized, short term, and sharp in nature because of the **Aδ** fiber stimulation. In contrast, **C** fibers are unmyelinated and smaller, and they transmit the signal more slowly. The "secondary" sensations are diffuse and aching, and they last longer after the initial injury.

Peripheral sensory **Aδ** and **C** fibers enter the spinal cord by posterior nerve roots within the dorsal horn by the tract of Lissauer. The fibers synapse with **interneurons** located within a specified area of the cord called the **substantia gelatinosa.** A cross section shows that the gray matter of the spinal cord is divided into a series of consecutively numbered laminae (layers of nerve cells) (see Fig. 11.1). The substantia gelatinosa is lamina II, which receives sensory input from various areas of the body. The pain signals then cross over to the other side of the spinal cord and ascend to the brain by the **anterolateral spinothalamic tract.** When pain is poorly controlled over an extended period of time, structural plasticity and reorganization of pain pathways occur. Cells within the dorsal horn become altered in size and function, and this damage is associated with nociceptive hypersensitivity.[15]

NOCICEPTIVE PAIN

Nociceptive pain develops when *functioning and intact* nerve fibers in the periphery and the CNS are stimulated. It is triggered by events outside the nervous system from actual or potential tissue damage. Nociception can be divided into four phases: (1) transduction, (2) transmission, (3) perception, and (4) modulation (Fig. 11.2).

Initially the first phase of **transduction** occurs when a noxious stimulus in the form of traumatic or chemical injury, burn, incision, or tumor takes place in the periphery. The periphery includes the skin and the somatic and visceral structures. These injured tissues then release a variety of chemicals, including substance P, histamine, prostaglandins, serotonin, and bradykinin. These chemicals are neurotransmitters that transmit a pain message, or action potential, along sensory afferent nerve fibers to the spinal cord. These nerve fibers terminate in the dorsal horn of the spinal cord.

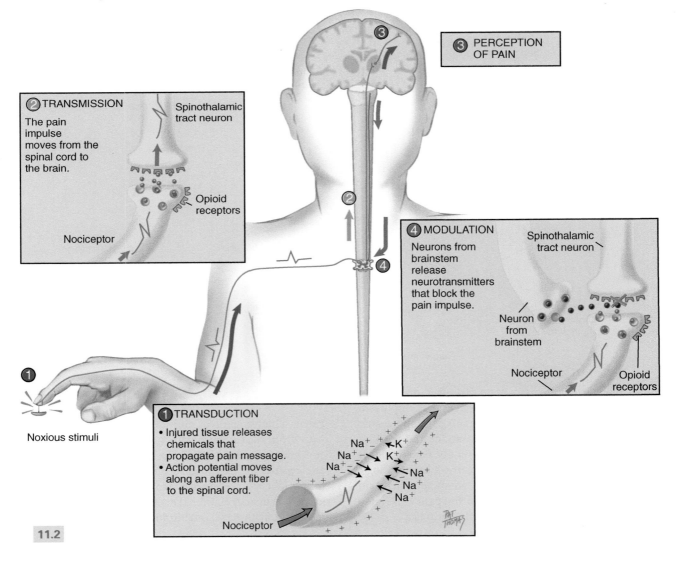

③ PERCEPTION OF PAIN

② TRANSMISSION
The pain impulse moves from the spinal cord to the brain.

Spinothalamic tract neuron

Opioid receptors

Nociceptor

④ MODULATION
Neurons from brainstem release neurotransmitters that block the pain impulse.

Spinothalamic tract neuron

Neuron from brainstem

Nociceptor

Opioid receptors

① TRANSDUCTION
• Injured tissue releases chemicals that propagate pain message.
• Action potential moves along an afferent fiber to the spinal cord.

Na^+ K^+
Na^+ K^+
Na^+ Na^+
Na^+
Na^+

Noxious stimuli

Nociceptor

Because the initial afferent fibers stop in the dorsal horn, a second set of neurotransmitters carries the pain impulse across the synaptic cleft to the dorsal horn neurons. These neurotransmitters include substance P, glutamate, and adenosine triphosphate (ATP).

In the second phase, known as **transmission,** the pain impulse moves from the level of the spinal cord to the brain. At the site of the synaptic cleft within the spinal cord are opioid receptors that can block pain signaling with endogenous opioids or with exogenous opioids if they are administered. However, if not stopped, the pain impulse moves to the brain via various ascending fibers within the spinothalamic tract to the thalamus. Once the pain impulse moves through the thalamus, the message is dispersed to higher cortical areas via mechanisms that are not clearly understood at this time.

The third phase, **perception,** signifies the conscious awareness of a painful sensation. Cortical structures such as the limbic system account for the emotional response to pain, and somatosensory areas can characterize the sensation. Only when the noxious stimuli are interpreted in these higher cortical structures can the sensation be identified as "pain."

Last, the pain message is inhibited through the phase of **modulation.** Fortunately our bodies have a built-in mechanism that will eventually slow down and stop the processing of a painful stimulus. If not for pain modulation, the experience of pain would continue from childhood injuries to adulthood. To inhibit and block the pain impulse, descending pathways from the brainstem to the spinal cord release a third set of neurotransmitters that produce an analgesic effect. These neurotransmitters include serotonin, norepinephrine, neurotensin, γ-aminobutyric acid (GABA), and our own endogenous opioids—β-endorphins, enkephalins, and dynorphins.

Normal nociceptive processing is protective and can be a warning signal that injury is about to or has taken place.[1] We quickly learn to move our hand away from a hot stove. Other examples of nociceptive pain include a skinned knee, kidney stones, menstrual cramps, muscle strain, venipuncture, or arthritic joint pain. Nociceptive pain is typically predictable and time limited based on the extent of the injury.

NEUROPATHIC PAIN

Neuropathic pain is pain that does not adhere to the typical and rather predictable phases in nociceptive pain. It is pain due to a lesion or disease in the somatosensory nervous system.[13] Neuropathic pain implies an abnormal processing of the pain message from an injury to the nerve fibers. This type of pain is the most difficult to assess and treat. Pain is often perceived long after the site of injury heals, and it evolves into a chronic condition.

Nociceptive pain can change into a neuropathic pain pattern over time when pain has been poorly controlled. This is because of the constant irritation and inflammation caused by a pain stimulus, which alters nerve cells, making them more sensitive to any future stimulus.

Conditions that may cause neuropathic pain include diabetes mellitus, herpes zoster (shingles), HIV/AIDS, sciatica, trigeminal neuralgia, phantom limb pain, and chemotherapy. Further examples include CNS lesions such as stroke, multiple sclerosis, and tumor. Pain sustained on a neurochemical level cannot be identified by x-ray image, computerized axial tomography (CAT) scan, or traditional magnetic resonance imaging (MRI). Recent advances in noninvasive neuroimaging techniques allow us to study the structural, functional, and neurochemical changes in the brain caused by nociception.[20] Pain researchers are using functional MRI (fMRI) to visualize changes in brain activity while patients experience pain. When these images are shown to patients in real time, patients can learn to use neurofeedback to help control pain. Researchers are able to better understand how pain is processed and how cognitive influences (e.g., fear, anxiety) impact the experience of pain.[20]

The abnormal processing of the neuropathic pain impulse can be continued by the PNS or CNS. An injury to peripheral neurons can result in spontaneous and repetitive firing of nerve fibers, almost seizurelike in activity (Fig. 11.3). Neuropathic

PERIPHERAL NERVES   DORSAL HORN NERVES

Tingling

Repetitive firing

Shooting
sensation

- Spontaneous firing of
  nerve fibers
- Hyperexcitability of dorsal
  horn neurons
- Hypersensitivity to typically
  innocuous stimuli

WIND-UP
Hyperexcitability

Pain report
"unequal" to
physical findings

Burning
sensation

11.3   NEUROPATHIC MECHANISMS

pain may be sustained centrally in a phenomenon known as neuronal "wind-up." Central neuron hyperexcitability leads to maintenance of neuropathic pain. In neuropathic pain, minor stimuli cause significant pain.[2]

SOURCES OF PAIN

Physical pain sources are based on their origin. **Visceral** pain originates from the larger internal organs (i.e., stomach, intestine, gallbladder, pancreas). It often is described as dull, deep, squeezing, or cramping. The pain can stem from direct injury to the organ or stretching of the organ from tumor, ischemia, distention, or severe contraction. Examples of visceral pain include ureteral colic, acute appendicitis, ulcer pain, and cholecystitis. The pain impulse is transmitted by ascending nerve fibers along with nerve fibers of the autonomic nervous system (ANS). That is why visceral pain often presents along with autonomic responses such as vomiting, nausea, pallor, and diaphoresis.

Somatic pain originates from musculoskeletal tissues or the body surface. **Deep somatic pain** comes from sources such as the blood vessels, joints, tendons, muscles, and bone. Pain may result from pressure, trauma, or ischemia. **Cutaneous pain** is derived from skin surface and subcutaneous tissues. Deep somatic pain often is described as aching or throbbing, whereas cutaneous pain is superficial, sharp, or burning. Whether somatic pain is sharp or dull, it is usually well localized and easy to pinpoint. Somatic pain, like visceral pain, can be accompanied by nausea, sweating, tachycardia, and hypertension caused by the ANS response.

Pain that is felt at a particular site but originates from another location is known as **referred pain.** Both sites are innervated by the same spinal nerve, and it is difficult for the brain to differentiate the point of origin. Referred pain may originate from visceral or somatic structures. Various structures maintain their same embryonic innervation. For example, an inflamed appendix in the right lower quadrant of the abdomen may have referred pain in the periumbilical area, or the pain from acute coronary syndrome may be felt in the left arm or neck. Please know the areas of referred pain for diagnostic purposes (see Table 22.3, Common Sites of Referred Abdominal Pain).

TYPES OF PAIN

Pain can be classified by its duration into acute or chronic categories (*chronic* is called *persistent* because it carries a less negative, malingering connotation). The duration provides information on possible underlying mechanisms and treatment decisions.

Acute pain is short term and self-limiting, often follows a predictable trajectory, and dissipates after an injury heals. Examples of acute pain include surgery, trauma, and kidney stones. Acute pain has a self-protective purpose; it warns the individual of actual or threatened tissue damage. *Incident pain* is an acute type that happens predictably when certain movements take place. Examples include pain in the lower back on standing or whenever turning a hospitalized patient from side to side.

In contrast, **chronic (persistent) pain** is diagnosed when the pain continues for 6 months or longer. Chronic pain can be divided into *malignant* (cancer-related) and *nonmalignant*. Malignant pain often parallels the pathology created by the tumor cells. The pain is induced by tissue necrosis or stretching of an organ by the growing tumor. It fluctuates within the course of the disease. Chronic nonmalignant pain is often associated with musculoskeletal conditions such as arthritis, low back pain, or fibromyalgia.

Chronic pain does not stop when the injury heals. It persists after the predicted trajectory. It outlasts its protective purpose, and the level of pain intensity does not correspond with the physical findings. Unfortunately many chronic pain sufferers are not believed by clinicians and are labeled as malingerers, attention seekers, or drug seekers. Chronic pain originates from abnormal processing of pain fibers from peripheral or central sites.[2]

Finally **breakthrough pain** is a transient spike in pain level, moderate to severe in intensity, in an otherwise controlled pain syndrome. It can result from end-of-dose medication failure. This occurs when a patient taking a long-acting opioid has a recurrence of pain before the next scheduled dose. Treatment of end-of-dose failure includes shortening the interval between doses or increasing the dose of medication. Breakthrough pain can also be the result of incident or episodic pain. This is a predictable breakthrough pain that may be triggered by a physical stimulus such as a return to activity after a surgery or from a psychosocial event.

The experience of pain is a complex biopsychosocial phenomenon. We are just now developing an understanding of pain at the cellular level, but more research is needed to fully understand the complexities of the pain experience. We still rely on patient report as the best indicator of pain, but researchers continue to explore whether pain and certain objective measures (e.g., biomarkers) are associated with one another.[9] When treating patients with acute or chronic pain, it is important to frequently reassess pain scores to evaluate the effectiveness of the therapy used. It is also important to talk to the patient about what pain score they consider tolerable.

❖ DEVELOPMENTAL COMPETENCE

Infants have the same capacity for pain as adults. In fetal development ascending sensory fibers, neurotransmitters, and connections to the thalamus are developed by 20 weeks' gestation. However, the immaturity of the cortex and lack of conscious awareness may prevent the fetus from experiencing emotional "pain" until 30 weeks' gestation. Conscious or not, pain-producing invasive fetal procedures elicit a stress response, and pain during gestation should be avoided until more is known about fetal pain. If invasive procedures must be performed on a developing fetus, adequate analgesia is necessary.[24]

Inhibitory neurotransmitters are insufficient until birth at full term. Therefore the preterm infant is rendered more sensitive to painful stimuli. Preverbal infants are at high risk for undertreatment of pain in part because of persistent myths and beliefs that infants do not remember pain. In fact, current evidence suggests that repetitive and poorly controlled pain in infants can result in changes in the CNS that lead to pain hypersensitivity later in life. Regardless of age, adequate analgesia use during painful procedures is necessary.[2]

The Aging Adult

No evidence exists to suggest that older individuals perceive pain to a lesser degree or that sensitivity is diminished. Although pain is a common experience among individuals 65 years of age and older, it is *not* a normal process of aging. Pain indicates pathology or injury. It should never be considered something to tolerate or accept in one's later years.

Unfortunately many clinicians and older adults wrongfully assume that pain should be expected in aging, which leads to underreporting of pain and less aggressive treatment. Older adults may have additional fears about becoming dependent, undergoing invasive procedures, taking pain medications, and having a financial burden. The most common pain-producing conditions for aging adults include pathologies such as osteoarthritis, osteoporosis, peripheral vascular disease, cancer, peripheral neuropathies, angina, and chronic constipation.

Dementia does not impact the ability to feel pain, but it does impact the person's ability to effectively use self-report instruments. Approximately 50% of patients with dementia experience pain.[10] In patients with dementia we can assess body language instead of verbal communication (e.g., a clenched fist may indicate pain; agitation may mean hunger or cold). See further discussion on pain assessment with dementia on p. 173.

Gender Differences

Gender differences are influenced by societal expectations, hormones, and genetic makeup. Traditionally men have been raised to be more stoic about pain, and more affective or emotional displays of pain are accepted for women. Hormonal changes have strong influences on pain sensitivity for women. Regarding migraine, the prevalence is equal in prepubertal girls and boys, but after puberty migraine headaches are 2 to 3 times more common in women.[4] Women have greater pain sensitivity than men with multiple biopsychosocial mechanisms contributing to differences in pain. Chronic pain is also more prevalent in women than in men.[16]

CULTURE AND GENETICS

When clinicians speak a language or belong to a culture different from their patient in pain, the risk increases for misunderstanding, underreporting, and undertreating. Please review the methods for working with an interpreter in Chapter 3 and the discussion on cultural variations in Chapter 2. Also adopt the habit of asking each patient how he or she typically behaves when in pain.

Most of the research conducted on racial differences and pain has focused on the disparity in the management of pain for various racial groups (i.e., comparing pain treatment for minority individuals [e.g., African Americans, Asians, Latinos] with the standard treatment for all individuals with similar injuries or diseases). Pain-related disparities continue to exist, with members of minority groups receiving less quality pain care than non-Hispanic whites.[22,25] Poorly treated pain has devastating results for the patient, with huge costs to society in losses of wages and productivity.

The experience of pain is more layered than just physical suffering. Pain and the expression of pain are influenced by social, cultural, emotional, and spiritual concerns. It is imperative that you do a thorough pain assessment on all patients, recognizing that a lack of outward signs of pain does not indicate an absence of pain. Ask open-ended questions and develop rapport before pain screening.[22]

The Opioid Epidemic

In 2017 the U.S. Department of Health and Human Services declared the opioid crisis a public health emergency and announced a strategy to combat the epidemic. The use of opioids began to increase in the late 1990s as drug companies assured the medical community that prescription opioids were safe and effective. While opioid medications are effective in the management of severe pain, they also cause a variety of side effects based on the mechanism of action and location of receptors.

Opioid medications must connect with mu-opioid receptors to achieve pain-relieving effects. Mu-opioid receptors are located throughout the body. There are high concentrations of mu-opioid receptors in the brain, including in the periaqueductal gray region, the thalamus, the cingulate cortex, and the insula; these receptors regulate pain perception.[28] Further, mu receptors in the amygdala mediate the emotional response to pain, and mu receptors in the ventral tegmental area and nucleus accumbens mediate the perception of well-being and pleasure. Thus, opioid medications produce pain relief and euphoria. As to the side effects of opioid medications, mu receptors in the brainstem lead to the concern of respiratory depression, and mu receptors in the small intestine produce troublesome constipation (Fig. 11.4). Mu receptors in the dorsal horn of the spinal cord and peripheral nerves modulate the perception of pain.

Mu receptors are also responsible for the physical dependence associated with continued use of opioid pain medications.[23,28] Physical dependence means only that repeated dosing will lead to a predictable physical reaction when the drug is withdrawn abruptly; this is **not** the same as addiction. Certainly the stimulation of mu receptors in the reward center of the brain can lead to addiction, especially when opioids are delivered rapidly, as happens when persons use opioids for pleasure and reward or can happen to persons in pain after months of opioid medication exposure.[28]

As prescription of opioid medications increased, misuse of the medications also increased. While research on pain indicates that the amount of pain experienced is stable, the

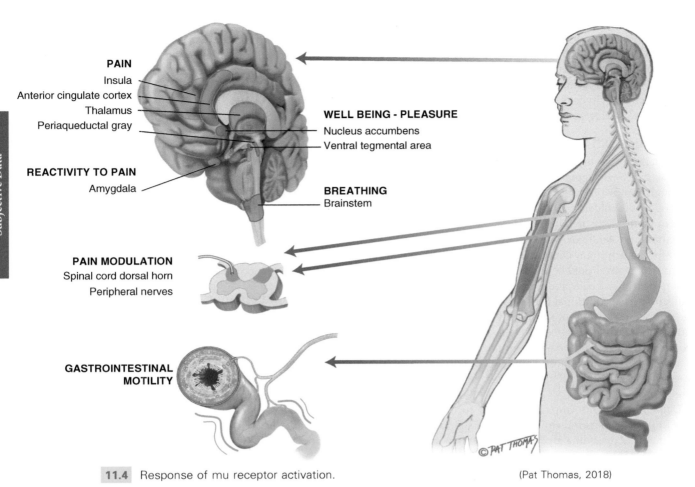

PAIN
Insula
Anterior cingulate cortex
Thalamus
Periaqueductal gray

WELL BEING - PLEASURE
Nucleus accumbens
Ventral tegmental area

REACTIVITY TO PAIN
Amygdala

BREATHING
Brainstem

PAIN MODULATION
Spinal cord dorsal horn
Peripheral nerves

GASTROINTESTINAL MOTILITY

11.4 Response of mu receptor activation. (Pat Thomas, 2018)

prescription of opioids has quadrupled. In 2016, 116 people died every day due to opioid-related overdose, and 11.5 million Americans misused prescription opioids.[5,21,26] In addition to overuse of opioid pain medications, the use of heroin has tripled since 2010,[8] and 75% of new heroin users report abusing prescription opioids first.[5]

Opioid pain medications are indispensable in treating certain types of pain (e.g., cancer pain, end-of-life pain). Providers are now advised not to use opioid pain medications as a first line for chronic pain, but instead to look to other treatment options.[8] While the opioid epidemic is a public health crisis, we must also recognize that patients in pain need adequate pain management. Refusing to prescribe appropriate medications to those in severe pain will not end the epidemic.[6,11] Ensuring adequate pain management competencies and appropriate education on opioid prescribing is necessary for all providers to stop the epidemic while assuring that patients receive appropriate treatment.[6]

SUBJECTIVE DATA

Pain is defined as an "unpleasant sensory and emotional experience associated with actual or potential tissue damage, or described in terms of such damage."[12]

Pain is a subjective experience and as such the person's report is the most reliable indicator of pain. Because pain occurs on a neurochemical level, the diagnosis of pain cannot be made exclusively on physical examination findings, although these findings can lend support. Self-report is the gold standard of pain assessment.

Examiner Asks	Rationale
Initial Pain Assessment	
1. **Do you have pain?** Discomfort or soreness? Ouch? Tell me in your own words.	Some people report pain only when it is severe. Try a variety of words.

2. **Where is your pain?** Tell me about *all* of the places that have pain.

Pain may be localized or occur in *multiple* sites.

3. **When did your pain start?** What were you doing when the pain started? Is it constant or does it come and go?

Identifies onset and duration. Chronic pain persists after injury heals; it is pain that occurs for 6 months or longer.

4. **What does your pain feel like?**
   - Burning, stabbing, aching
   - Throbbing, firelike, squeezing
   - Cramping, sharp, itching, tingling
   - Shooting, crushing, sharp, dull

Identifies quality of pain and helps differentiate between nociceptive and neuropathic pain mechanisms.

Neuropathic pain is described as burning, shooting, and tingling. Nociceptive pain originating from visceral sites is described as aching if localized and cramping if poorly localized; from somatic sites, it is described as throbbing/aching.

5. **How much pain do you have now?**

Identifies intensity (refer to various intensity scales).

6. **What makes your pain better or worse?** (Include behavioral, pharmacologic, and nonpharmacologic interventions.) What medications control your pain? Are doses adequate? How often do you take pain medication?

Identifies alleviating and aggravating factors. Evaluates effectiveness of current treatment.

7. **How does pain limit your function or activities?** What does pain prevent you from doing?

Identifies degree of impairment and quality of life.

8. **How do you usually react when you are in pain?** Any other symptoms along with the pain (nausea, vomiting, dizziness, heart racing)? How would others know that you are in pain?

Nonverbal behaviors are extremely variable, especially for chronic pain syndromes. Aids in detection and assessment.

9. **What does this pain mean to you?** Why do you think you are having pain?

Can identify myths, misconceptions, beliefs such as "I'm getting old"; "It's a punishment from God."

Alternatively you can collect a complete pain health history using the PQRST mnemonic described in Table 11.1.

TABLE 11.1 PQRST Method of Pain Assessment

P = Provocation/Palliation
What were you doing when the pain started? What caused it? What makes it better? Worse? What seems to trigger it? Stress? Position? Certain activities?
What relieves it? Medications, massage, heat/cold, changing position, being active, resting?
What aggravates it? Movement, bending, lying down, walking, standing?

Q = Quality/Quantity
What does it feel like? Use words to describe the pain, such as sharp, dull, stabbing, burning, crushing, throbbing, nauseating, shooting, twisting, or stretching.

R = Region/Radiation
Where is the pain located? Does it radiate? Where? Does it feel as if it travels/moves around? Did it start elsewhere and is now localized to one spot?

S = Severity Scale
How severe is the pain on a scale of 0 to 10, with zero being no pain and 10 being the worst pain ever? Does it interfere with activities? How bad is it at its worst? Does it force you to sit down, lie down, slow down? How long does an episode last?

T = Timing
When/at what time did the pain start? How long did it last? How often does it occur: hourly? daily? weekly? monthly? Is it sudden or gradual? What were you doing when you first experienced it? When do you usually experience it: daytime? night? early morning? Are you ever awakened by it? Does it lead to anything else? Is it accompanied by other signs and symptoms? Does it ever occur before, during, or after meals? Does it occur seasonally?

From Crozer Keystone Center for Nursing Excellence: Best practices: PQRST method facilitates accurate pain assessment. www.crozerkeystone.org/healthcare-professionals/nursing.

Subjective Data

PAIN ASSESSMENT TOOLS

Pain is multidimensional in scope, encompassing physical, affective, and functional domains. Various tools have been developed to capture unidimensional aspects (i.e., intensity) or multidimensional components. Select the pain assessment tool based on its purpose, time involved in administration, and the patient's ability to comprehend and complete the tool.

Ask the patient to rate and evaluate all of the pain sites. Some forms allow for only one number; therefore be sure to add additional sites to your documentation. Make sure you use the pain tool consistently before and after treatment to see whether the treatment was effective. Reassessment of pain following intervention, whether pharmacologic or nonpharmacologic, is essential to document pain trajectories alongside various treatments to achieve optimum pain control.

Standardized **overall pain assessment tools** are more useful for chronic pain conditions or particularly problematic acute pain problems. A few examples include the Initial Pain Assessment, the Brief Pain Inventory, and the McGill Pain Questionnaire.

The **Initial Pain Assessment**[17] asks the patient to answer 8 questions concerning location, duration, quality, intensity, and aggravating/relieving factors. Further, the clinician adds

---

Initial Pain Assessment Tool

Date _____

Patient's Name _____ Age _____ Room _____
Diagnosis _____ Physician _____
Nurse _____

1. LOCATION: Patient or nurse mark drawing.

2. INTENSITY: Patient rates the pain. Scale used _____
   Present: _____
   Worst pain gets: _____
   Best pain gets: _____
   Acceptable level of pain: _____

3. QUALITY: (Use patient's own words, e.g., prick, ache, burn, throb, pull, sharp.) _____

4. ONSET, DURATION, VARIATION, RHYTHMS: _____

5. MANNER OF EXPRESSING PAIN: _____

6. WHAT RELIEVES THE PAIN? _____

7. WHAT CAUSES OR INCREASES THE PAIN? _____

8. EFFECTS OF PAIN: (Note decreased function, decreased quality of life.)
   Accompanying symptoms (e.g., nausea) _____
   Sleep _____
   Appetite _____
   Physical activity _____
   Relationship with others (e.g., irritability) _____
   Emotions (e.g., anger, suicidal, crying) _____
   Concentration _____
   Other _____

9. OTHER COMMENTS: _____

10. PLAN: _____

11.5

(McCaffery, 1999.)

questions about the manner of expressing pain and the effects of pain that impair one's quality of life (Fig. 11.5).

The Brief Pain Inventory[5a,21a] asks the patient to rate the pain within the past 24 hours using graduated scales (0 to 10) with respect to its impact on areas such as mood, walking ability, and sleep. **The short-form McGill Pain Questionnaire**[18] asks the patient to rank a list of descriptors in terms of their intensity and to give an overall intensity rating to his or her pain.

Pain-rating scales are unidimensional and intended to reflect pain intensity. They come in various forms. They can indicate baseline intensity, track changes, and give some degree of evaluation to a treatment modality. **Numeric rating scales** ask the patient to choose a number that rates the level of pain for each painful site, with 0 being no pain and 10 indicating the worst pain ever experienced (Fig. 11.6). The use of a numeric rating scale makes the recording of results easy and consistent between numerous clinicians. The **Verbal Descriptor Scale** uses words to describe the patient's feelings and the meaning of the pain for the person. The **Visual Analogue Scale** lets the patient make a mark along a 10-cm horizontal line from "no pain" to "worst pain imaginable."

In general older adults find the numeric rating scale abstract and have difficulty responding, especially with a fluctuating chronic pain experience. An alternative is the simple **descriptor scale** that lists words that describe different levels of pain intensity such as *no pain, mild pain, moderate pain,* and *severe pain.* Older adults often respond to scales in which words are selected. Again it is essential to teach the person how to use the scale to enhance accuracy.

Tools for Infants and Children

Because infants are preverbal and incapable of self-report, pain assessment depends on behavioral and physiologic cues. Refer to the Objective Data section. It is important to underscore the point that infants *do* feel pain.

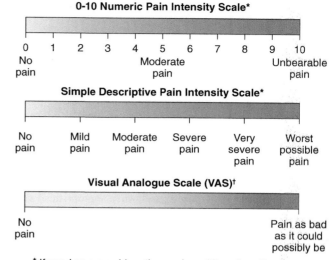

0-10 Numeric Pain Intensity Scale*

| 0 | 1 | 2 | 3 | 4 | 5 | 6 | 7 | 8 | 9 | 10 |

No pain   Moderate pain   Unbearable pain

Simple Descriptive Pain Intensity Scale*

No pain | Mild pain | Moderate pain | Severe pain | Very severe pain | Worst possible pain

Visual Analogue Scale (VAS)†

No pain   Pain as bad as it could possibly be

* If used as a graphic rating scale, a 10-cm baseline is recommended.
† A 10-cm baseline is recommended for VAS scales.

11.6   (Acute Pain Management Guideline Panel, 1992.)

Children 2 years of age can report pain and point to its location. They cannot rate pain intensity at this developmental level. It is helpful to ask the parent or caregiver what words the child uses to report pain (e.g., boo-boo, owie). Be aware that some children try to be "grown up and brave" and often deny having pain in the presence of a stranger or if they are fearful of receiving a "shot."

Rating scales can be introduced at 4 to 5 years of age. The Faces Pain Scale–Revised (FPS-R) has six drawings of faces that show pain intensity, from "no pain" on the left (score of 0) to "very much pain" on the right (score of 10) (Fig. 11.7). The FPS-R has realistic facial expressions, with a furrowed brow and horizontal mouth. It avoids smiles or tears so that children will not confuse pain intensity with happiness or sadness.[12]

Faces Pain Scale — Revised (FPS-R)
In the following instructions, say "hurt" or "pain," whichever seems right for a particular child.
"These faces show how much something can hurt. This face [point to left-most face] **shows no pain. The faces show more and more pain** [point to each from left to right] **up to this one** [point to right-most face] **— it shows very much pain. Point to the face that shows how much you hurt** [right now]."

  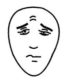

Score the chosen face 0, 2, 4, 6, 8, or 10, counting left to right, so '0' = 'no pain' and '10' = 'very much pain.' Do not use words like 'happy' and 'sad.' This scale is intended to measure how children feel inside, not how their face looks.

Sources. Hicks, C. L., von Baeyer, C. L., Spafford, P. van Korlaar, I., Goodenough, B. The Faces Pain Scale—Revised: toward a common metric in pediatric pain measurement. *Pain, 93,* 173-183. Bieri, D., Reeve, R., Champion, G. D. et al. The Faces Pain Scale for the self-assessment of the severity of pain experienced by children: development, initial validation and preliminary investigation for ratio scale properties. *Pain, 41,* 139-150.

11.7

OBJECTIVE DATA

PREPARATION

The physical examination process can help you understand the nature of the pain. Consider whether this is an acute or a chronic condition. Recall that physical findings may not always support the patient's pain reports, particularly for chronic pain syndromes. Based on the patient's pain report, make every effort to reduce or eliminate the pain with appropriate analgesic and nonpharmacologic intervention. According to the American Pain Society[1, p.5]:

> When the cause of acute pain is uncertain, establishing a diagnosis is a priority. However, consideration should be given to starting symptomatic pain treatment as the diagnostic workup progresses, when appropriate. A comfortable patient is better able to cooperate with diagnostic procedures.

EQUIPMENT NEEDED

Tape measure to measure circumference of swollen joints or extremities
Tongue blade
Penlight

Normal Range of Findings	Abnormal Findings
Joints	
Note the size and contour of the joint. Measure the circumference of the involved joint for comparison with baseline. Check active or passive range of motion (see discussion of complete technique beginning on p. 582 in Chapter 23). Joint motion normally causes no tenderness, pain, or crepitation.	Swelling, inflammation, injury, deformity, diminished range of motion, increased pain on palpation, crepitation (audible and palpable crunching that accompanies movement)
Observe posture; normally it is erect and relaxed.	Slumped posture or abdominal guarding with pain
Muscles and Skin	
Inspect the skin and tissues for color, swelling, and any masses or deformity.	Bruising, lesions, open wounds, tissue damage, atrophy, bulging, change in hair distribution
To assess for changes in sensation, ask the person to close his or her eyes. Test the person's ability to perceive sensation by breaking a tongue blade in two lengthwise. Lightly press the sharp and blunted ends on the skin in a random fashion and ask to identify it as sharp or dull (see Fig. 24.23). This test will help you identify location and extent of altered sensation.	Absent pain sensation (analgesia); increased pain sensation (hyperalgesia); severe pain sensation evoked with a stimulus that does not normally induce pain (e.g., the blunt end of the tongue blade, cotton ball, clothing) (allodynia)
Abdomen	
Observe for contour and symmetry. Palpate for muscle guarding and organ size (see discussion of complete technique beginning on p. 544 in Chapter 22). Note any areas of referred pain (see Table 22.3).	Swelling, bulging, herniation, inflammation, organ enlargement

Table 11.2 lists physiologic changes resulting from poorly controlled pain. Be aware that tachycardia and tachypnea also occur with anxiety and fear and are not specific to pain.[7]

NONVERBAL BEHAVIORS OF PAIN

When the individual cannot verbally communicate the pain, you can (to a limited extent) identify it using behavioral cues. Recall that individuals react to painful stimuli with a wide variety of behaviors. Behaviors are influenced by a wide variety of factors, including the nature of the pain (acute versus chronic), age, and cultural and gender expectations.

Acute Pain Behaviors

Because acute pain involves autonomic responses and has a protective purpose, individuals experiencing moderate-to-intense levels of pain *may* exhibit the following behaviors: guarding, grimacing, vocalizations such as moaning, agitation, restlessness, stillness, diaphoresis, or change in vital signs. This list of behaviors is not exhaustive because it should not be used exclusively to deny or confirm the presence of pain. For example, in a postoperative patient pulse and blood pressure can be altered by fluid volume, medications, and blood loss.

Chronic (Persistent) Pain Behaviors

People with chronic pain live with the experience for months or years. People adapt to chronic pain over time, and clinicians cannot look for or anticipate the same acute pain behaviors to exist to confirm a pain diagnosis.

Chronic pain behaviors have even more variability than acute pain behaviors. People with chronic pain typically try to give little indication that they are in pain and therefore are at higher risk for underdetection (Fig. 11.8). Behaviors associated with chronic pain include bracing, rubbing, diminished activity, sighing, and change in appetite. Whenever possible, it

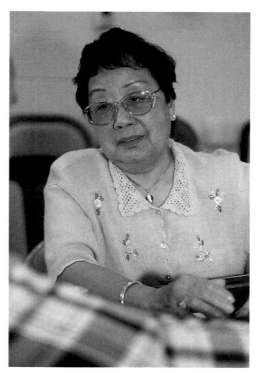

11.8   (Courtesy Rick Brady, Riva, MD.)

is best to ask the person how he or she acts or behaves when in pain. Chronic pain behaviors such as spending time with other people, movement, exercise, prayer, sleeping, or inactivity underscore the more subtle, less anticipated ways in which people behave when they are experiencing chronic pain (e.g., they use sleeping to self-distract). Unfortunately, clinical staff may inadvertently interpret this behavior as "comfort" and fail to follow up with an appropriate pharmacologic intervention.

❖ DEVELOPMENTAL COMPETENCE

Infants

Most pain research on infants has focused on acute procedural pain. We have a limited understanding of how to assess chronic pain in the infant. At this time no one assessment tool adequately identifies pain in the infant. Using a multidimensional approach for the whole infant is encouraged. Changes in facial activity and body movements may help. Much effort and time is spent on decoding facial expressions (e.g., taut tongue, bulging brow, closing of eye fissures), which may be difficult for the general practitioner to do in a busy clinical setting.

The CRIES score is one tool for postoperative pain in preterm and term neonates.[14] It measures physiologic and behavioral indicators on a three-point scale (Fig. 11.9).

A second tool often used is the FLACC scale.[19] This is a nonverbal assessment tool for infants and young children under 3 years. The FLACC scale is designed to be simple for practitioners to administer while providing a reliable and objective assessment of pain.[27] The tool assesses five behaviors

TABLE 11.2 Physiologic Changes from Poorly Controlled Pain	
Pain is not a benign symptom. Poorly controlled acute pain and chronic pain have a negative impact on physiologic systems.	
PHYSIOLOGIC SYSTEM	**ACUTE PAIN RESPONSES**
Cardiac	Tachycardia
	Elevated blood pressure
	Increased myocardial oxygen demand
	Increased cardiac output
Pulmonary	Hypoventilation
	Hypoxia
	Decreased cough
	Atelectasis
Gastrointestinal	Nausea
	Vomiting
	Ileus
Renal	Oliguria
	Urinary retention
Musculoskeletal	Spasm
	Joint stiffness
Endocrine	Increased adrenergic activity
Central nervous system	Fear
	Anxiety
	Fatigue
Immune	Impaired cellular immunity
	Impaired wound healing
Poorly controlled chronic pain	Depression
	Isolation
	Limited mobility and function
	Confusion
	Family distress
	Diminished quality of life

Objective Data

CRIES Neonatal Postoperative Pain Measurement Score

	0	1	2
Crying	No	High-pitched	Inconsolable
Requires O_2 for sat >95%	No	<30% from baseline	>30% from baseline
Increased vital signs	HR and BP = or < preop	HR or BP ↑ <20% of preop	HR or BP ↑ >20% of preop
Expression	None	Grimace	Grimace/grunt
Sleepless	No, continuously asleep	Wakes at frequent intervals	Constantly awake

11.9 (Krechel, 1995.)

of pain: facial expression, leg movement, activity level, cry, and consolability (Fig. 11.10).

Because the sympathetic nervous system is engaged particularly in acute episodes of pain, physiologic changes take place that may indicate the presence of pain. These include sweating, increases in blood pressure and heart rate, vomiting, nausea, and changes in oxygen saturation. However, as in the adult, these physiologic changes cannot be used exclusively to confirm or deny pain because of other factors, such as stress, medications, and fluid balance.

Note that these measures target acute pain. No biological markers have been identified for long-term chronic pain in infants or children. Therefore evaluate the whole individual. Look for changes in temperament, expression, and activity. If a procedure or disease process is known to induce pain in

adults (e.g., circumcision, surgery, sickle cell disease, cancer), it *will* induce pain in the infant or child.

The Aging Adult

Although pain should not be considered a "normal" part of aging, it is prevalent. When an older adult reports a history of conditions such as osteoarthritis, peripheral vascular disease, cancer, osteoporosis, angina, or chronic constipation, be alert and anticipate pain. Older adults often deny having pain for fear of dependency, further testing or invasive procedures, cost, and fear of taking pain killers or becoming a drug addict. During the interview you must establish an empathic and caring rapport to gain trust.

When you look for behavioral cues, look at changes in functional status. Observe for changes in dressing, walking,

FLACC Behavioral Pain Scale (Infants and Toddlers)

	DATE/TIME							
Face 0 - No particular expression or smile 1 - Occasional grimace or frown, withdrawn, disinterested 2 - Frequent to constant quivering chin, clenched jaw								
Legs 0 - Normal position or relaxed 1 - Uneasy, restless, tense 2 - Kicking, or legs drawn up								
Activity 0 - Lying quietly, normal position, moves easily 1 - Squirming, shifting back and forth, tense 2 - Arched, rigid, or jerking								
Cry 0 - No cry (awake or asleep) 1 - Moans or whimpers; occasional complaint 2 - Crying steadily, screams or sobs, frequent complaints								
Consolability 0 - Content, relaxed 1 - Reassured by occasional touching, hugging or being talked to, distractible 2 - Difficult to console or comfort								
TOTAL SCORE								

11.10 (Voepel-Lewis, 2010.)

Pain Assessment In Advanced Dementia (PAINAD) Scale

	0	1	2	Score
Breathing Independent of Vocalization	Normal	Occasional labored breathing, short period of hyperventilation	Noisy labored breathing, long period of hyperventilation, Cheyne-Stokes respirations	
Negative Vocalization	None	Occasional moan or groan, low level of speech with a negative or disapproving quality	Repeated troubled calling out, loud moaning or groaning, crying	
Facial Expression	Smiling or inexpressive	Sad, frightened, frown	Facial grimacing	
Body Language	Relaxed	Tense, distressed pacing, fidgeting	Rigid, fists clenched, knees pulled up, pulling or pushing away, striking out	
Consolability	No need to console	Distracted or reassured by voice or touch	Unable to console, distract, or reassure	
			TOTAL	

11.11   A score of 4 or greater should be reported to the RN for pain intervention. (Warden, 2003.)

toileting, or involvement in activities. A slowness and rigidity may develop, and fatigue may occur. Look for a sudden onset of acute confusion, which may indicate poorly controlled pain. However, you will need to rule out other competing explanations, such as infection or adverse reaction from medications.

People with dementia become less able to identify and describe pain over time, although pain is still present and destructive. They communicate pain through their behavior. Agitation, pacing, and repetitive yelling may indicate pain and not a worsening of the dementia. People who are comfortable do not yell, cry, moan, hit, or kick.

When these behaviors occur, consider pain as a primary explanation.

When asked whether they are having pain, people with dementia may say "no" when in fact they are very uncomfortable. Words have lost their meaning. Use the PAINAD scale (Fig. 11.11), which evaluates five common behaviors: breathing, vocalization, facial expression, body language, and consolability.[29] Specific behaviors in these categories are quantified from 0 to 2, with a total score ranging from 0 to 10. This is consistent with the commonly used 0-to-10 metric on other pain tool scores. For the PAINAD, a score of 4 or more indicates a need for pain management.

DOCUMENTATION AND CRITICAL THINKING

Sample Charting

SUBJECTIVE

Complains of severe epigastric pain within a half-hour of eating greasy, fatty foods, which began approximately 2 weeks prior to admission. Pain is stabbing and squeezing in nature with radiation to right shoulder blade. Rates pain as a 10 on a 0-to-10 scale. Nausea accompanies pain. Takes antacids with minimal relief. Pain diminishes after bringing knees to chest and "not moving" for a 1-hour period.

OBJECTIVE

Patient diaphoretic, grimacing, and having difficulty concentrating. Breathless during history. Arms guarding upper abdominal area. Abdomen distended. Severe tenderness noted on light LUQ and epigastric palpation. Bowel sounds hyperactive in all 4 quadrants.

ASSESSMENT

Acute episodic pain

Clinical Case Study 1

J.T. is an 18-year-old male living with sickle cell anemia. Admitted to the ED by his parents following 4 hours of increasing pain at home.

SUBJECTIVE

Within the past 48 hours J.T. reports increasing pain in upper- and lower-extremity joints and swelling of right knee. Reports having "stomach flu" 1 week before with periods of vomiting and diarrhea. Pain is aching and constant in nature. Rates pain as 10 on a 0-to-10 scale. Reports difficulty walking and climbing stairs. Taking acetaminophen, two tablets every 4 hours, and using ice packs with no relief. States, "I have had these before. I always need Dilaudid."

OBJECTIVE

Temp 98.6° F (37° C) oral. BP 118/68 mm Hg. Pulse 112 bpm. Resp 24/min.
Facial grimacing and moaning.
Requiring assistance to sit on exam table. Unable to bear weight on right leg. Affect flat; clenches jaw during position changes. Tenderness localized in elbow, wrist, finger, and knee joints. Diminished ROM in wrists and knees (right knee 36 cm, left knee 30 cm circumference). Right knee warm and boggy to touch.
Lungs: Clear to auscultation and percussion.
Heart: S_1 and S_2 not diminished or accentuated; no murmur.
Abdomen: Bowel sounds present, guarding with tenderness to palpation, RUQ pain with enlarged spleen at anterior axillary line.
Lab: Hb 9 g/dL. Hct 30%. Indices show sickling with RBCs of varying shapes.
Metabolic panel: Serum bilirubin 2 mg/dL, rest in normal limits.

ASSESSMENT

Acute pain
Risk for venous or arterial thromboembolism
Anemia

Clinical Case Study 2

H.S. is a 78-year-old female with a 10-year history of osteoarthritis. Comes for routine checkup today, stating, "Feeling pain in right knee now, and pain pills not working."

SUBJECTIVE

H.S. reports increased pain and stiffness in her neck, lower back, and right knee for the past month. Denies radiation of pain. Denies tingling or numbness in upper or lower extremities.

Having difficulty getting in and out of bathtub and dressing herself. Describes pain as aching, with good and bad days. Becomes frustrated when asked to rate her pain intensity. Replies, "I don't know what number to give; it hurts a lot, on and off." Takes acetaminophen, extra strength, two tablets, when the pain "really gets the best of me," with some degree of relief. Does not take part in "field trips" offered by assisted-living facility because she "hurts too much." Does not use cane or walker. No physical therapy.

OBJECTIVE

Localized tenderness noted on palpation to C3 and C4; unable to flex neck to chest. Crepitus noted in bilateral shoulder joints. No swelling noted. Muscle strength 1+ and equal for upper extremities. Lumbar area tender to moderate palpation. Rubs lower back frequently; limited flexion at the waist. Right knee swollen with circumference 2 cm > left knee but no redness or warmth. Left knee not enlarged, and normal ROM. Gait slow and unsteady. Facial expression stoic.

ASSESSMENT

Chronic pain that is now increased in intensity
Decreased ROM in neck, shoulders, back, R knee

Clinical Case Study 3

T.H. is a 7-year-old boy who has just experienced a laparoscopic appendectomy. On entering the room you see that he is awake, but his eyes are closed and he is lying flat on the bed without movement.

SUBJECTIVE

When asked if he is in pain, T.H. states "a little"; however, he rates pain as a +8 using a Faces Pain Scale.

OBJECTIVE

Requires assistance to move in the bed. Speaks only when spoken to.
Vital signs: Temp 98.6° F (37° C) (oral). BP: 122/72 mm Hg (supine). Pulse 126 bpm (while quiet but awake). Resp 22/min.
General appearance: Diaphoretic, flushed, grimaces with slight touch.
Cardiovascular: Tachycardic at rest; no abnormal heart sounds.
Respiratory: Tachypneic at rest; pulse ox 98% on room air; breath sounds clear in all fields, no adventitious sounds.
Abdomen: Hypoactive bowel sounds, tenderness localized to abdomen, dressing dry and intact at surgical site.

ASSESSMENT

Acute postoperative pain

Acute Pain Clinical Case Study 4

J.Y. is a 53-year-old male who fell approximately 10 feet from a ladder. Landed in a "funny" sitting position and is now experiencing severe back pain. Imaging studies in ED show herniated lumbar disk.

SUBJECTIVE

J.Y. reports pain rated at 10/10. Pain is sharp, constant, and shoots down left leg. Reports bilateral leg weakness.

OBJECTIVE

J.Y. required assistance to sit on exam table. Clenches jaw with position changes. Supports lower back with hands. Significant tenderness of lumbar spine. Unable to perform hip flexion/extension or spinal ROM because of pain.

ASSESSMENT

Herniated lumbar disk
Acute pain

Documentation and
Critical Thinking

ABNORMAL FINDINGS

TABLE 11.3	Summary of Pain Types			
Types of Pain	Etiology	Pain Descriptors	Associated Disorders	Treatment Options
Nociceptive (somatic or visceral)	Activity of nociceptors in cutaneous and deep musculoskeletal tissue in response to tissue-damaging stimuli Inflammation	Somatic: Dull Aching Well-localized Nocturnal Visceral: Deep, squeezing pressure Local tenderness and referred Poorly localized	Somatic: Postoperative pain Bone metastases Arthritis Sports injury Mechanical back pain Visceral: Liver metastases Pancreatic cancer	Treat the underlying cause Nonsteroidal anti-inflammatory drug (NSAID) Opioid Muscle relaxant Corticosteroid Bisphosphonate
Neuropathic	Primary lesion (neuroma) or dysfunction in nervous system causing ectopic charges within the nervous system	Constant dull ache Burning Stabbing Viselike Electric shock–like Numbness Tingling Allodynia Hyperalgesia Hyperpathia	Distal polyneuropathy (diabetes, HIV) Central poststroke pain Herpes zoster Trigeminal neuralgia Neuropathic back pain Complex regional pain syndrome	Tricyclic antidepressant (TCA) Anticonvulsant Antidepressant Antineuroleptic Local anesthetic Bisphosphonate Corticosteroid Opioid Interventional techniques
Cancer pain	Infiltration of lesion Nerve injury from periphery or central nervous system	Dependent on underlying pathology	Bone metastases neuropathy	Symptom control— any of the above

Data from Miller-Saultz, D. (2008). Identifying chronic pain: Awareness important. *Nurse Pract*, 33(9), 7.

TABLE 11.4	Peripheral Neuropathy

Peripheral neuropathy (PN) is symmetric damage to peripheral nerves (feet or hands), resulting in pain without stimulation of the nerves. This is a common neuropathic pain characterized by numbness and tingling, with interspersed shooting or lancinating pain that is not attributed to a specific nociceptive source. Diabetic neuropathy is a common complication of diabetes and may relate to demyelination of the larger peripheral nerves, with an increase in smaller myelinated nerves. Other etiologies may include ischemic damage to nerves or hyperglycemia, causing changes in nerve microenvironment.[2] Patients experience burning pain in feet bilaterally, which is often worse at night.

Chemotherapy-induced PN (CIPN) occurs during or after chemotherapy treatment for cancer. The risk increases with the number of agents used in the course of treatment, higher cumulative doses of neurotoxic agents, preexisting neuropathy from diabetes or other causes, and older age. A symptom is numbness or burning, shooting pain in a glove-and-stocking distribution.[3] NOTE: With any cancer survivor, you must address new onset of pain promptly to rule out pathologic recurrence of the cancer.

TABLE 11.5 | Reflexive Sympathetic Dystrophy

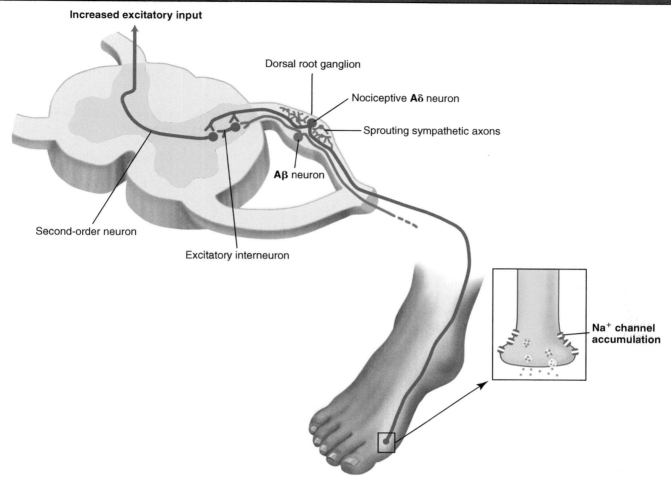

Increased excitatory input

Dorsal root ganglion

Nociceptive **Aδ** neuron

Sprouting sympathetic axons

Aβ neuron

Second-order neuron

Excitatory interneuron

Na⁺ channel accumulation

Complex Regional Pain Syndrome (CRPS) or Reflexive Sympathetic Dystrophy (RSD)

CRPS/RSD is a chronic progressive nerve condition characterized by burning pain, swelling, stiffness, and discoloration of the affected extremity. It affects both men and women, usually around 40 to 60 years old, and occurs weeks to months after a nerve injury (e.g., carpal tunnel syndrome, broken leg, cerebral lesions). Pathophysiology involves a complex interaction of sensory, motor, and autonomic nerves and the immune system. The nerve injury may modify the usual pain pathway, causing a neuropathic "wind-up" or "short-circuit" mechanism.

A key feature is that a typically innocuous stimulus (e.g., a light brush of a cotton ball or clothing) can create a severe, intense painful response. Other subjective data include burning pain often disproportionate to the degree of injury and joint pain during movement. Objective data include swelling, disappearance of skin wrinkles, cool skin temperature, discoloration, brittle nails, and finally atrophic changes (pale, dry, shiny skin and muscle atrophy). Treatment includes high doses of drugs (e.g., prednisone, amitriptyline, pregabalin, clonidine) to decrease symptoms and physical therapy to regain limb function.

Image © Pat Thomas, 2010.

REFERENCES

1. American Pain Society (APS). (2016). *Principles of analgesic use* (7th ed.). Chicago: American Pain Society.
2. Banasik, J. L., & Copstead, L. E. (2019). *Pathophysiology* (6th ed.). St. Louis: Elsevier.
3. Brewer, J. R., Morrison, G., Dolan, M. E., et al. (2015). Chemotherapy-induced peripheral neuropathy: Current status and progress. *Gynecol Oncol, 140*(1), 176–183.
4. Burch, R. C., Loder, S., Loder, E., et al. (2015). The prevalence and burden of migraine and severe headache in the United States: Updated statistics from government health surveillance studies. *Headache, 55*, 21–34.
5. Centers for Disease Control and Prevention. (2017). *Understanding the epidemic.* https://www.cdc.gov/drugoverdose/epidemic/index.html.
5a. Cleeland, C. S., & Ryan, K. M. (1994). Pain assessment: Global use of the Brief Pain Inventory. *Ann Acad Med Singapore, 23*(2), 129–138.
6. Curtiss, C. P. (2016). I'm worried about people in pain. *Am J Nurs, 116*(1), 11.
7. D'Arcy, Y. (2012). Treating acute pain in the hospitalized patient. *Nurse Pract, 37*(8), 23–30.
8. Davis, C., Green, T., & Beletsky, L. (2017). Action, not rhetoric, needed to reverse the opioid overdose epidemic. *J Law Med Ethics, 45*(S1), 20–23.
9. DeVon, H. A., Piano, M. R., & Hoppensteadt, D. A. (2014). The association of pain with protein inflammatory biomarkers: A review of the literature. *Nurs Res, 63*(1), 51–62.
10. Gagliese, L., Gauthier, L. R., Narain, H., et al. (2017). Pain, aging and dementia: Towards a biopsychosocial model. *Prog Neuropsychopharmacol Biol Psychiatry, 87*, 207–215.
11. Glod, S. A. (2017). The other victims of the opioid epidemic. *N Engl J Med, 376*, 2101–2102.
12. International Association for the Study of Pain (IASP). (2018). *Faces Pain Scale-Revised.* https://www.iasp-pain.org/Education/Content.aspx?ItemNumber=1519.
13. International Association for the Study of Pain. (2018). *Neuropathic pain.* https://www.iasp-pain.org/Advocacy/GYAP.aspx?ItemNumber=5054.
14. Krechel, S. W., & Bildner, J. (1995). CRIES: A new neonatal postoperative pain measurement score—initial testing of validity and reliability. *Paediatr Anaesth, 5*(1), 53–61.
15. Kuner, R., & Flor, H. (2017). Structural plasticity and reorganisation in chronic pain. *Nat Rev Neurosci, 18*, 20–30.
16. Legato, M. J. (2017). *Principles of gender-specific medicine: Gender in the genomic era* (3rd ed.). St. Louis: Elsevier.
17. McCaffery, M., & Pasero, C. (1999). *Pain: Clinical manual* (2nd ed.). St. Louis: Mosby.
18. Melzack, R. (1987). The short-form McGill Pain Questionnaire. *Pain, 30*, 191–197.
19. Merkel, S. I., Voepel-Lewis, T., Shayevitz, J. R., et al. (1997). The FLACC: A behavioral scale for scoring postoperative pain in young children. *Pediatr Nurs, 23*, 293–297.
20. Morton, D. L., Sandhu, J. S., & Jones, A. K. P. (2016). Brain imaging of pain: State of the art. *J Pain Res, 9*, 613–624.
21. NIH National Institute on Drug Abuse. (2018). *Opioid overdose crisis.* https://www.drugabuse.gov/drugs-abuse/opioids/opioid-overdose-crisis.
21a. Poquet, N., & Lin, C. (2010). The Brief Pain Inventory (BPI). *J Physiother, 62*, 52.
22. Robinson-Lane, S. G., & Booker, S. Q. (2017). Culturally responsive pain management for Black older Americans. *J Gerontol Nurs, 43*(8), 33–41.
23. Rosenjack Burchum, J., & Rosenthal, L. D. (2016). *Lehne's pharmacology for nursing care* (9th ed.). St. Louis: Elsevier.
24. Sekulic, S., Gebauer-Bukurov, K., Cvijanovic, M., et al. (2016). Appearance of fetal pain could be associated with maturation of the mesodiencephalic structures. *J Pain Res, 9*, 1031–1038.
25. Stein, K. D., Alcaraz, K. I., Kamson, C., et al. (2016). Sociodemographic inequalities in barriers to cancer pain management: A report from the American Cancer Society's Study of Cancer Survivors- II (SCS-II). *Psychooncology, 2016*, 1212–1221.
26. U.S. Department of Health and Human Services. (2018). *About the U.S. opioid epidemic.* https://www.hhs.gov/opioids/about-the-epidemic/index.html.
27. Voepel-Lewis, T., Zanotti, J., Dammeyer, J. A., et al. (2010). Reliability and validity of the face, legs, activity, cry, consolability behavioral tool in assessing acute pain in critically ill patients. *Am J Crit Care Nurses, 19*(1), 55–61.
28. Volkow, N. D., & McLellan, A. T. (2016). Opioid abuse in chronic pain—misconceptions and mitigation strategies. *N Engl J Med, 374*, 1253–1263.
29. Warden, V., Hurley, A. C., & Volicer, L. (2003). Development and psychometric evaluation of the Pain Assessment in Advanced Dementia (PAINAD) scale. *J Am Med Dir Assoc, 4*(1), 9–15.

STRUCTURE AND FUNCTION

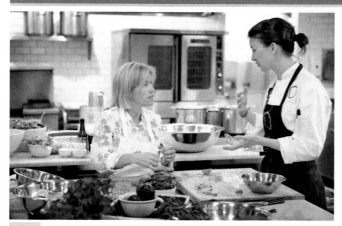

12.1 (© Cavan Images.)

DEFINING NUTRITIONAL STATUS

Nutritional status is the balance between nutrient intake and nutrient requirements. This balance is affected by physiologic, psychosocial, developmental, cultural, and economic factors.

Optimal nutritional status is achieved when sufficient nutrients are consumed to support day-to-day body needs and any increased metabolic demands caused by growth, pregnancy, or illness (Fig. 12.1). People having optimal nutritional status are more active, have fewer physical illnesses, and live longer than people who are malnourished.

Undernutrition occurs when nutritional reserves are depleted and/or when nutrient intake is inadequate to meet day-to-day needs or added metabolic demands. Vulnerable groups (i.e., infants, children, pregnant women, recent immigrants, people with low incomes, hospitalized people, and aging adults) are at risk for impaired growth and development, lowered resistance to infection and disease, delayed wound healing, longer hospital stays, and higher health care costs.

Overnutrition is caused by the consumption of nutrients, especially calories, sodium, and fat, in excess of body needs. A major nutritional problem today, overnutrition can lead to obesity and is a risk factor for many diseases, including heart disease, type 2 diabetes, osteoarthritis, sleep apnea, chronic kidney disease, gallstones, and gastroesophageal reflux.[9,14]

OBESITY

An estimated one-third of children and adolescents (ages 2 to 19 years) in the United States are overweight or obese, with nearly one-sixth (17%) being obese. Approximately two-thirds of adults in the United States are either overweight or obese, and more than one-third are obese.[14] For children the term "overweight" applies to a body mass index (BMI) at or above the 85th percentile based on age- and gender-specific BMI charts, and obesity is defined as a BMI equal to or greater than the 95th percentile.[4,14] Adults may be classified as overweight when they have a BMI of 25 or greater, and as obese when their BMI is 30 or greater.[14] Being overweight during childhood and adolescence is associated with an increased risk of chronic health problems (e.g., asthma, bone and joint problems, heart disease), an increased risk of being bullied, and an increased likelihood of depression and social isolation. Being overweight during childhood is also associated with an increased risk of being overweight or obese as an adult.[4]

Obesity is caused by multiple factors, including genetic predisposition, dietary intake, physical inactivity, and an *obesogenic* environment. An obesogenic environment is one that encourages large portions of high-fat, energy-dense food and fails to encourage healthy behaviors such as physical activity.[10] Consider the number of television ads geared toward fast, supersized food that is convenient or the amount of time children and adolescents spend watching television or playing video games. It is important that health care providers advocate for positive environmental changes that will support maintenance of a healthy weight, such as removing soda and candy machines from schools, advocating for the placement of grocery stores in food deserts, and assuring safe spaces where people can exercise and children can play outside.

✸ DEVELOPMENTAL COMPETENCE

Infants and Children

The time from birth to 4 months of age is the most rapid period of growth in the life cycle. Although infants lose weight during the first few days of life, they usually regain birth weight within 7 to 10 days after birth. Thereafter infants double their birth weight by 4 months and triple it by 1 year of age.

Breastfeeding is recommended for full-term infants for the first year of life because breast milk is ideally formulated to promote normal infant growth and development and natural immunity through IgA antibodies. Other advantages of breastfeeding are (1) fewer food allergies and intolerances, (2) reduced likelihood of overfeeding, (3) less cost than commercial infant formulas, and (4) increased mother-infant interaction time. Because cow's milk may cause gastrointestinal (GI) and kidney problems and is a poor source of iron and vitamins C and E, it is not recommended for infants until 1 year of age.

Infants increase their length by 50% during the first year of life and double it by 4 years of age. Brain size also increases very rapidly during infancy and childhood. By 2 years of age the brain has reached 50% of its adult size; by age 4, 75%; and by age 8, 100%. For this reason infants and children younger than 2 years should not drink skim or low-fat milk or be placed on low-fat diets; fat (calories and essential fatty acids) is required for proper growth and central nervous system development.

Adolescence

After a period of slow growth in late childhood, adolescence presents rapid physical growth and endocrine and hormonal changes. Caloric and protein requirements increase to meet this demand, and because of bone growth and increasing muscle mass (and in girls the onset of menarche), calcium and iron requirements also increase. Typically these increased requirements cannot be met by three meals per day; therefore nutritious snacks play an important role. Consider the following factors when working with adolescents to select healthier food choices: skipped meals, excessive fast food and sweetened beverage consumption, limited fruit and vegetable intake, peer pressure, alternative dietary patterns, eating disorders, hectic schedules, and possible experimentation with drugs and alcohol. Sugar-sweetened beverages interact with the genes that affect weight and increase a person's risk of obesity. The risk is especially high in people who are genetically predisposed to obesity.[2,16]

In general, boys grow taller and have less body fat than girls. The percentage of body fat increases in females to about 25% and decreases in males (replaced by muscle mass) to about 12%. Typically girls double their body weight between the ages of 8 and 14 years; boys double their body weight between the ages of 10 and 17 years.

Childhood is the most active period in the life span, with levels of physical activity decreasing in following decades; however, recent evidence from the Youth Risk Behavior Survey indicates that not all adolescents are physically active. In fact, 15% reported not engaging in 60 minutes of physical activity on any day during the past week, and 52% reported not attending physical education classes. Perhaps more alarming is that 33% reported watching 3 or more hours of television per day and nearly 42% reported playing computer or video games more than 3 hours per day.[3] Inactivity contributes to the development of overweight and obesity and the associated negative health outcomes.

Pregnancy and Lactation

To support the synthesis of maternal and fetal tissues, sufficient calories, protein, vitamins, and minerals must be consumed during pregnancy. In particular, iron, folate, and zinc are essential for fetal growth, and vitamin and mineral supplements are often required. The National Academy of Sciences (NAS) recommends a weight gain of 25 to 35 lb during pregnancy for women of normal weight, 28 to 40 lb for underweight women, 15 to 25 lb for overweight women, and 11 to 20 lb for obese women.[13]

Adulthood

During adulthood, growth and nutrient needs stabilize (Fig. 12.2). Most adults are in relatively good health. However, lifestyle factors such as cigarette smoking; stress; lack of exercise; excessive alcohol intake; and diets high in saturated fat, cholesterol, salt, and sugar and low in fiber can be factors in the development of hypertension, obesity, atherosclerosis, cancer, osteoporosis, and diabetes mellitus. Therefore the adult years are an important time for education to preserve health and prevent or delay the onset of chronic disease.

Lifestyle factors contribute to obesity, which is one risk factor in the development of **metabolic syndrome.** This syndrome carries increased cardiac risk and is diagnosed when a person has 3 of the following 5 biomarkers: elevated BP, increased fasting plasma glucose, elevated triglycerides, increased waist circumference, and low high-density lipoprotein (HDL) cholesterol (see exact parameters in Table 12.5 on p. 194).

The Aging Adult

Older adults have an increased risk for undernutrition or overnutrition. The nutritional status of older adults may be impacted by cognitive, social, economic, and psychological factors. Older adults are also at higher risk for medication-nutrient interactions. Physical changes also lead to nutritional issues in older adults.[11]

Normal physiologic changes in aging adults that directly affect nutritional status include poor dentition, decreased

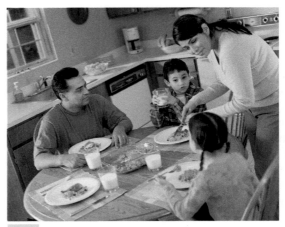

12.2   (Agricultural Research Service, 2012.)

visual acuity, decreased saliva production, slowed GI motility, decreased GI absorption, and diminished olfactory and taste sensitivity. Important nutritional features of the older years are a decrease in energy requirements caused by loss of lean body mass (the most metabolically active tissue) and an increase in fat mass. Because protein, vitamin, and mineral needs remain the same or increase (e.g., vitamin D and calcium), nutrient-dense food choices (e.g., milk, eggs, cheese, and peanut butter) are important to offset lower energy/calorie needs.

Socioeconomic conditions frequently affect the nutritional status of the aging adult. The decline of extended families and the increase in the mobility of families reduce available support systems. Facilities for meal preparation and eating, transportation to grocery stores, physical limitations, reduced income, and social isolation are frequent problems that interfere with acquiring a balanced diet. Medications must also be considered because aging adults frequently take multiple medications that have a potential for interaction with nutrients and with one another.

The age-related loss of muscle mass is termed **sarcopenia. Sarcopenic obesity** is characterized by low muscle mass with excess fat and can be attributed to a poor diet and low levels of physical activity.[19] Sarcopenic obesity results in a loss of muscle strength and function, decreased quality of life, physical frailty, and increased mortality rates. Aerobic exercise plays its part for cardiac fitness, but resistance training is needed to treat weakened muscles. A resistance training program with free weights, machines, or elastic bands two to three times per week is recommended. Obviously financial resources and access to safe exercise gyms are factors in meeting this need.

 ## CULTURE AND GENETICS

Because foods and eating customs are culturally distinct, each person has a unique cultural heritage that may affect nutritional status. Immigrants commonly maintain traditional eating customs (especially for holidays and religious observances) long after the language and manner of dress of an adopted country become routine (Fig. 12.3). Occupation, socioeconomic level, religion, gender, and health awareness also have an impact on eating customs.

Newly arriving immigrants may be at nutritional risk because they frequently come from countries with limited food supplies resulting from poverty, poor sanitation, war, or political strife. General undernutrition, hypertension, diarrhea, lactose intolerance, osteomalacia (soft bones), scurvy, and dental caries are among the more common nutrition-related problems of new immigrants from developing countries.

When immigrants arrive in the United States, other factors such as unfamiliar foods, food storage, food preparation, and food-buying habits contribute to their nutritional problems. Foods from the native country are difficult to obtain, and low income limits the access to familiar foods. When traditional

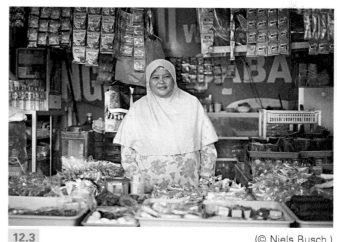

12.3 (© Niels Busch.)

food habits are disrupted by a new culture, borderline deficiencies or adverse nutritional consequences may result.

The cultural factors to consider are the cultural definition of food, frequency and number of meals eaten away from home, form and content of ceremonial meals, amount and types of foods eaten, and regularity of food consumption. The 24-hour dietary recalls or 3-day food records used traditionally for assessment may be inadequate when dealing with people from culturally diverse backgrounds. Standard dietary handbooks may not provide culture-specific diet information because nutritional content and exchange tables are generally based on Western diets. Another source of error may be cultural patterns of eating. For example, some ethnic groups eat sparingly or moderately during the week (i.e., simple rice or bean dishes), whereas weekend meals are markedly more elaborate (i.e., meats, fruits, vegetables, and sweets are added). Make sure that you adequately assess the nutritional status of all individuals. During the cultural assessment (see Chapter 3), ask about nutrition, including forbidden foods, fasting rituals, and foods typically avoided or consumed. Asking questions about dietary practices can help you identify any potential nutritional issues.

DIETARY PRACTICES OF SELECTED CULTURAL GROUPS

Cultural food preferences are often interrelated with religious dietary beliefs and practices. Many religions use foods as symbols in celebrations and rituals. Knowing the person's religious practices related to food enables you to suggest improvements or modifications that do not conflict with dietary laws. Table 12.1 summarizes dietary practices for selected religious groups, but make sure you ask the client about dietary practices. Do not make assumptions about diet based on the person's religious or ethnic background.

Other issues are fasting and other religious observations that may limit a person's food or liquid intake during specified times. For example, many Catholics fast and abstain from meat on Ash Wednesday and the Fridays of Lent. Muslims fast from dawn to sunset during the month of Ramadan in

TABLE 12.1	Religious Dietary Practices
RELIGIOUS GROUP	**FOOD RESTRICTIONS**
Buddhism	Will vary depending on the Buddhist sect All meat (some sects) Alcohol Pungent spices (garlic, onion, scallions, chives, leeks)
Catholicism	Meat by some denominations on Ash Wednesday, Good Friday, and other holy days Alcoholic beverages by some denominations
Hinduism	Lacto-vegetarianism often favored Alcohol and intoxicating substances Garlic, onion, and spicy foods by some Fasting on some holy days
Islam	All pork and pork products Meat not slaughtered according to ritual Alcoholic beverages and alcohol products (e.g., vanilla extract), coffee, and tea Food and beverages before sunset during Ramadan
The Church of Jesus Christ of Latter-Day Saints	Alcoholic beverages Hot beverages, specifically coffee and tea Food and beverages for 2 consecutive meals on fast Sunday
Orthodox Judaism	All pork and pork products Meat not slaughtered according to ritual All shellfish (e.g., crab, lobster, shrimp, oysters) Dairy products and meat at the same meal Leavened bread and cake during Passover Food and beverages on Yom Kippur
Seventh-Day Adventist	All pork and pork products Shellfish Meat, dairy products, and eggs by some Alcoholic beverages, coffee, and tea

the Islamic calendar and eat only twice a day—before dawn and after sunset. Members of some Jewish faiths observe a 24-hour fast on Yom Kippur.

TYPES OF NUTRITIONAL ASSESSMENT

Nutritional assessment techniques are noninvasive, inexpensive, and easy to perform. **Nutrition screening** is the first step in assessing nutritional status. Based on easily obtained data, nutrition screening is a quick and easy way to identify individuals at nutrition risk such as those with weight loss, inadequate food intake, or recent illness. Parameters used for nutrition screening typically include weight and weight history, conditions associated with increased nutritional risk, diet information, and routine laboratory data. A variety of

valid tools are available for screening different populations. For example, the Malnutrition Screening Tool[5] was validated for use in adult acute-care patients, and the Mini Nutritional Assessment (MNA®)[20] was designed and validated for use in older adults in long-term care and community settings.

Malnutrition in hospitalized patients is associated with negative patient outcomes, including increased length of stay, increased readmission rates, and increased mortality. Nurses are often the first health care provider to assess a newly hospitalized patient and, as such, are in an ideal position to identify patients who are malnourished or at risk for malnutrition.[18] Individuals identified to be at nutritional risk during screening should undergo a **comprehensive nutritional assessment,** which includes dietary history and clinical information, physical examination for clinical signs, anthropometric measures, and laboratory tests. The skills needed to collect the clinical and dietary history and to perform the physical examination are described in the Subjective and Objective Data sections that follow. Various methods for collecting current dietary intake information are available: 24-hour recall, food frequency questionnaire, and food diary. During hospitalization, documentation of nutritional intake is achieved through calorie counts of nutrients consumed and/or infused.

The easiest and most popular method for obtaining information about dietary intake is the **24-hour recall.** The individual or family member completes a questionnaire or is interviewed and asked to recall everything eaten within the last 24 hours. An advantage is that the 24-hour recall can elicit specific information about dietary intake over a specific period of time. However, there are several significant sources of error: (1) the individual or family member may not be able to recall the type or amount of food eaten; (2) intake within the last 24 hours may be atypical of usual intake; (3) the individual or family member may alter the truth for a variety of reasons; and (4) snack items and the use of gravies, sauces, and condiments may be underreported. It is important to also prompt the individual to report liquid intake as some individuals will omit drinks and simply report food consumed.

To counter some of the difficulties inherent in the 24-hour recall method, you can use a **food frequency questionnaire.** With this tool, information is collected on how many times per day, week, or month the individual eats particular foods, providing an estimate of usual intake. Drawbacks to the use of the food frequency questionnaire are: (1) it does not always quantify amount of intake, and (2) like the 24-hour recall, it relies on the individual's or family member's memory for how often a food is eaten.

Food diaries or records ask the individual or family member to write down everything consumed for a certain period. Three days (i.e., two weekdays and one weekend day) are customarily used. A food diary is most complete and accurate if you teach the individual to record information immediately after eating. Potential problems with the food diary include (1) noncompliance, (2) inaccurate recording,

(3) atypical intake on the recording days, and (4) conscious alteration of diet during the recording period.

Direct observation of the feeding and eating process can detect problems not readily identified through standard nutrition interviews. For example, observing the typical feeding techniques used by a parent or caregiver and the interaction between the individual and caregiver can help when assessing failure to thrive in children or unintentional weight loss in older adults. Increasingly, mobile devices and applications are being used to assess and monitor intake, including taking photos of meals and tracking weight changes and dietary adherence. Unfortunately, the applications lack evidence-based features and do not undergo rigorous scientific testing. Collaborative efforts among application developers, scientists, and end users are needed to enhance the usefulness of applications and assure quality.[17]

ChooseMyPlate, Dietary Guidelines, and the Dietary Reference Intakes (DRIs) are three guides commonly used to determine an adequate diet. Please access the websites ChooseMyPlate.gov and Dietaryguidelines.gov for additional information. The DRIs are recommended amounts of nutrients to prevent deficiencies and reduce the risk for chronic diseases. In addition to recommending adequate intakes, they also specify upper limits of nutrients to avoid toxicity. With an increase in the use of dietary supplements, the risk for nutrient toxicities is on the rise. Examples of specific DRIs and interactive tools can be found at fnic.nal.usda.gov/dietary-guidance/dietary-reference-intakes.

SUBJECTIVE DATA

1. Eating patterns
2. Usual weight
3. Changes in appetite, taste, smell, chewing, swallowing
4. Recent surgery, trauma, burns, infection
5. Chronic illnesses
6. Nausea, vomiting, diarrhea, constipation
7. Food allergies or intolerances
8. Medications and/or nutritional supplements
9. Patient-centered care
10. Alcohol or illegal drug use
11. Exercise and activity patterns
12. Family history

Examiner Asks	Rationale
1. Eating patterns • Number of meals/snacks per day? • Type and amount of food eaten? • Fad, special, or alternative diets? • Where is food eaten? • Food preferences and dislikes? • Religious or cultural restrictions? • Able to feed self?	Most individuals know about or are interested in the foods they consume. If misconceptions are present, begin gradual instruction to build self-care of healthy eating patterns. Many alternative diets are not supported by scientific safety or efficacy data.
2. Usual weight • What is your usual weight? • 20% below or above desirable weight? • Recent weight change? How much lost or gained? Over what time period? • Reason for loss or gain?	People with a recent weight loss or who are obese are at risk. Underweight individuals are vulnerable because their fuel reserves are depleted. Excess weight carries the risk of hypertension, diabetes, heart disease, and cancer.
3. Changes in appetite, taste, smell, chewing, swallowing • Type of change? • When did change occur?	These changes interfere with adequate nutrient intake.
4. Recent surgery, trauma, burns, infection • When? Type? How treated? • Conditions that increase nutrient loss (e.g., draining wounds, effusions, blood loss, dialysis)?	These conditions have caloric and nutrient needs that are 2 or 3 times greater than normal.

Examiner Asks	Rationale
5. Chronic illnesses • Type? When diagnosed? How treated? • Dietary modifications? • Recent chemotherapy or radiation therapy?	Cancer treatment or chronic illnesses that affect nutrient use (e.g., diabetes mellitus, pancreatitis, or malabsorption) carry twice the risk for nutritional deficits.
6. Nausea, vomiting, diarrhea, constipation • Any problems? Caused by? How long?	GI symptoms interfere with nutrient intake or absorption.
7. Food allergies or intolerances • Any problematic foods? Type of reaction? How long?	Food allergies, especially peanut allergies, are on the rise and are a major health concern. Intolerances such as gluten and lactose may cause nutrient deficiencies.
8. Medications and/or nutritional supplements • Prescription medications? • Nonprescription? • Use over a 24-hour period?	Analgesics, antacids, anticonvulsants, antibiotics, diuretics, laxatives, antineoplastic drugs, steroids, and oral contraceptives are drugs that interact with nutrients, impairing their digestion, absorption, metabolism, or use.
• Type of vitamin/mineral supplement? Amount? Duration of use?	Vitamin/mineral supplements have harmful side effects if taken in large amounts. An estimated 23,000 emergency room visits each year are the result of dietary supplements. The majority are due to cardiovascular effects of weight loss and energy supplements in younger adults and swallowing problems among older adults.[7]
• Herbal and botanical products? Functional foods or foods enhanced with nutrients? Specific type/brand and where obtained? How often used? Who recommended? How does it help you? Any problems?	Use of herbal/botanical supplements is often not reported; therefore ask and discuss proper use and potential adverse effects. Refer to www.nccam.nih.gov.
9. Patient-centered care • Meal-preparation facilities? • Transportation to grocery store? • Adequate income for food purchase? • Who prepares meals and does shopping? • Environment during mealtimes?	Poverty and lack of access to nutritious groceries interfere with ingestion of adequate amounts of food or usual diet.
10. Alcohol or illegal drug use • When was last drink of alcohol? • Amount taken that episode? • Amount of alcohol each day? Each week? • Duration of use? • Repeat questions for each drug used.	Alcoholic beverages contain "empty calories" devoid of nutrients. Alcohol and drugs block absorption of some nutrients. Pregnant women who smoke, drink alcohol, or use illegal drugs give birth to infants with low birth weights, failure to thrive, and other serious complications.
11. Exercise and activity patterns • Amount? • Type?	Caloric and nutrient needs increase with competitive sports and manual labor. Inactive or sedentary lifestyles lead to excess weight gain.

Examiner Asks	Rationale

12. Family history
- Heart disease, osteoporosis, cancer, gout, GI disorders, obesity, or diabetes?
- Effect of each on eating patterns?
- Effect on activity patterns?

Rationale: Long-term nutritional deficiencies or excesses may first appear as diseases such as these. Early identification permits dietary and activity modifications when the body can recover.

Additional History for Infants and Children

Dietary histories of infants and children are obtained from the parents, caregiver, or daycare center. Usually the person responsible for food preparation provides a fairly accurate dietary history. Having the caregivers keep a thorough daily food diary and occasionally requesting 24-hour recalls during clinic visits are the usual techniques.

1. Gestational nutrition
- Maternal history of alcohol or illegal drug use?
- Any diet-related complications during gestation?
- Infant's birth weight?
- Any evidence of delayed physical or mental growth?

Rationale: Low birth weight (<2500 g) is a major factor in infant morbidity and mortality.

Poor gestational nutrition, low maternal weight gain, and maternal alcohol and drug use—all factors in low birth weight—can lead to birth defects and delayed growth and development.

2. Infant breastfed or bottle-fed
- Type, frequency, amount, and duration of feeding?
- Any difficulties encountered?
- Timing and method of weaning?

Rationale: Well-nourished infants have appropriate physical and social growth and development. Inexperienced mothers may have problems with feeding or questions about whether the infant is receiving adequate food.

3. Child's willingness to eat what you prepare
- Any special likes or dislikes?
- How much will child eat?
- How do you control non-nutritious snack foods?
- How do you avoid food aspiration?

Rationale: Lifelong food habits form during childhood. The use of small portions, finger foods, simple meals, and nutritious snacks improve dietary intake. Avoid foods likely to be aspirated (e.g., hot dogs, nuts, grapes, round candies, popcorn).

4. Overweight and obesity risk factors
- Overweight or obese parent?
- Low-income family?
- Maternal smoking during pregnancy?
- Large-for-gestational-age birth weight?
- Rapid weight gain from birth to 5 months?

Rationale: Risk factors for overweight and obesity may be present during gestation, at birth, or during infancy. Overweight and obesity during childhood often lead to obesity during the adult years.[8]

Additional History for the Adolescent

1. Your present weight
- What would you like to weigh?
- How do you feel about your present weight?
- On any special diet to lose weight?
- On other diets to lose weight? If so, were they successful?
- Constantly think about "feeling fat?" Constantly exercising?
- Intentionally vomit or use laxatives or diuretics after eating?

Rationale: Obesity, particularly in girls, may precipitate fad dieting and malnutrition. Adolescents' increased body awareness and self-consciousness may cause eating disorders (anorexia nervosa or bulimia) when the real or perceived body image does not compare favorably to an ideal image in advertisements or among peers.

Examiner Asks	Rationale

2. Use of anabolic steroids or other agents to increase muscle size and physical performance
- When?
- How much?
- Any problems?

- Use of caffeinated, energy-boosting drinks? When? Type? Duration?

Once confined to male professional athletes, the use of performance-enhancing agents now extends to junior high, high school, and college. Adverse effects include personality disorders (aggressiveness) and liver and other organ damage.

Energy-boosting drinks such as Red Bull contain large amounts of caffeine, stimulants, and/or herbal products. Side effects include dehydration, elevated BP and heart rate, and sleep problems.

3. Overweight and obesity risk factors
- Are large amounts of food eaten in a short period of time or for hours on end?
- Which meals do you skip? How often? Which snacks, fast foods, and sweetened beverages do you like? How often do you eat/drink them?

Binge eating is now the most common eating disorder across all age-groups. Consuming fast foods and sweetened beverages is associated with increased weight gain.[6,12]

4. Age first started menstruating
- What is your menstrual flow like?

Malnutrition delays menarche. Likewise, amenorrhea or scant menstrual flow occurs with nutritional deficiency.

Additional History for the Pregnant Woman

1. Number of pregnancies
- How many times have you been pregnant?
- When?
- Any problems encountered during previous pregnancies?
- Problems this pregnancy?
- Do you take prenatal vitamins or supplements?

A multiparous mother with pregnancies less than 1 year apart has risk for depleted nutritional reserves. Note previous complications of pregnancy (excessive vomiting, anemia, or gestational diabetes). Slower GI motility and pressure from the fetus may cause constipation, hemorrhoids, and indigestion. A history of a low-birth-weight infant suggests past nutritional problems. Giving birth to an infant weighing 4.5 kg (10 lb) or more may signal *latent* diabetes in the mother.

2. Food preferences when pregnant
- What foods do you avoid?
- Crave any particular foods?

The expectant mother is vulnerable to familial, cultural, and traditional influences for food choices. Cravings for or aversions to particular foods are common; evaluate their contribution to, or interference with, dietary intake.

- How much fish do you eat each week?

Large amounts of fish consumption may be associated with maternal, fetal, and newborn mercury toxicity.

Additional History for the Aging Adult

1. Any diet differences from when you were in your 40s and 50s?
- Why?
- Which factors affect the way you eat?

Note any physiologic or psychological changes of aging or socioeconomic changes that affect nutritional status.

- Adequate vitamin D and calcium intake?

Vitamin D and calcium can help prevent osteoporosis.

OBJECTIVE DATA

CLINICAL SIGNS

The general appearance (i.e., obese, cachectic [fat and muscle wasting], or edematous) can provide clues to overall nutritional status. More specific clinical signs of nutritional deficiencies can be detected through a physical examination. Because clinical signs are late manifestations of malnutrition, only in areas of rapid turnover of epithelial tissue (i.e., skin, hair, mouth, lips, and eyes) are the deficiencies readily detectable. These signs may also be non-nutritional in origin. Therefore laboratory testing is required to make an accurate diagnosis. Clinical signs of various nutritional deficiencies are summarized in Table 12.2 and depicted in the section on abnormalities at the end of this chapter (see Tables 12.3 and 12.4).

EQUIPMENT NEEDED

Ross insertion tape or other measurement tape
Anthropometer
Pen or pencil
Nutritional assessment data form

TABLE 12.2   Clinical Signs of Malnutrition

AREA OF EXAMINATION	NORMAL APPEARANCE	SIGNS ASSOCIATED WITH MALNUTRITION	NUTRIENT DEFICIENCY
Skin	Smooth, no signs of rashes, bruises, flaking	Dry, flaking, scaly	Vitamin A, vitamin B–complex, linoleic acid
		Petechiae/ecchymoses	Vitamins C and K
		Follicular hyperkeratosis (dry, bumpy skin)	Vitamin A, linoleic acid
		Cracks in skin; lesions on hands, legs, face, or neck	Niacin, tryptophan
		Eczema	Linoleic acid
		Xanthomas (excessive deposits of cholesterol)	Excessive serum levels of LDLs or VLDLs
Hair	Shiny, firm, does not fall out easily; healthy scalp	Dull, dry, sparse	Protein, zinc, linoleic acid
		Color changes	Copper or protein
		Corkscrew hair	Copper
Eyes	Corneas are clear, shiny; membranes are pink and moist; no sores at corners of eyelids	Foamy plaques (Bitot spots)	Vitamin A
		Dryness (xerophthalmia)	Vitamin A
		Softening (keratomalacia)	Vitamin A
		Pale conjunctivae	Iron, vitamins B_6, B_{12}
		Red conjunctivae	Riboflavin
		Blepharitis	Vitamin B–complex, biotin
Lips	Smooth, not chapped or swollen	Cheilosis (vertical cracks in lips)	Riboflavin, niacin
		Angular stomatitis (red cracks at sides of mouth)	Riboflavin, niacin, iron, vitamin B_6
Tongue	Red in appearance, not swollen or smooth, no lesions	Glossitis (beefy red)	Vitamin B–complex
		Pale	Iron
		Papillary atrophy	Niacin
		Papillary hypertrophy	Multiple nutrients
		Magenta or purplish-colored	Riboflavin
Gums	Reddish-pink, firm, no swelling or bleeding	Bleeding	Vitamin C
Nails	Smooth, pink	Brittle, ridged, or spoon-shaped (koilonychia)	Iron
		Splinter hemorrhages	Vitamin C
Musculoskeletal	Erect posture, no malformations, good muscle tone, can walk or run without pain	Pain in calves, thighs	Thiamine
		Osteomalacia	Vitamin D, calcium
		Rickets	Vitamin D, calcium
		Joint pain	Vitamin C
		Muscle wasting	Protein, carbohydrate, fat
Neurologic	Normal reflexes, appropriate affect	Peripheral neuropathy	Thiamine, vitamin B_6
		Hyporeflexia	Thiamine
		Disorientation or irritability	Vitamin B_{12}

LDL, Low-density lipoprotein; *VLDL,* very low–density lipoprotein.

Objective Data

| Normal Range of Findings | Abnormal Findings |

Anthropometric Measures

Derived Weight Measures

The **percent usual body weight** is calculated as follows:

$$\text{Percent usual body weight} = \frac{\text{Current weight}}{\text{Usual weight}} \times 100$$

Recent weight change is calculated using the following formula:

$$\frac{\text{Usual weight} - \text{Current weight}}{\text{Usual weight}} \times 100$$

A current weight of 85% to 95% of usual body weight indicates mild malnutrition; 75% to 84%, moderate malnutrition; and <75%, severe malnutrition.

An unintentional loss of >5% of body weight over 1 month, >7.5% of body weight over 3 months, or >10% of body weight over 6 months is clinically significant.

Body Mass Index

BMI is a practical marker of optimal weight for height and an indicator of obesity or undernutrition (see p. 128 in Chapter 9). It is calculated by:

$$\text{Body mass index} = \frac{\text{Weight (kilograms)}}{\text{Height (meters)}^2}$$

$$\text{Or } \frac{\text{Weight (pounds)}}{\text{Height (inches)}^2} \times 703$$

BMI interpretation for adults:

<18.5	Underweight
18.5-24.9	Normal weight
25-29.9	Overweight
30-39.9	Obesity
≥40	Extreme obesity

BMI interpretation for children ages 2 to 20 years:

<5th percentile	Underweight
5th-85th percentile	Healthy weight
85th-95th percentile	Overweight
≥95th percentile	Obese

Waist-to-Hip Ratio

The waist-to-hip ratio assesses body fat distribution as an indicator of health risk. Obese people with a greater proportion of fat in the upper body, especially in the abdomen, have android obesity; obese people with most of their fat in the hips and thighs have gynoid obesity. The equation is:

$$\text{Waist-to-hip ratio} = \frac{\text{Waist circumference}}{\text{Hip circumference}}$$

where waist circumference is measured in inches just above the iliac crests of the hips, and hip circumference is measured in inches at the largest circumference of the buttocks. In addition, **waist circumference (WC)** alone can be used to predict greater health risk (Fig. 12.4).

A waist-to-hip ratio of 1.0 or greater in men or 0.8 or greater in women indicates android (upper body) obesity and increasing risk for obesity-related diseases and early mortality.

A WC >35 inches in women and >40 inches in men increases risk for heart disease, type 2 diabetes, and metabolic syndrome.

Although not routinely done, triceps skinfold (TSF) measurement estimates the body fat stores or the extent of undernutrition. A TSF value 10% below the standard suggests malnutrition. See www.massgeneral.org/crc/assets/Forms/skinfold/pdf for procedure.

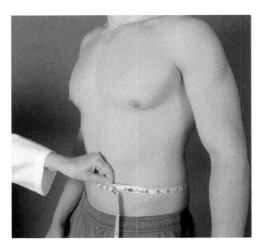

12.4

Normal Range of Findings	Abnormal Findings

Arm Span or Total Arm Length

Measurement of arm span is useful for situations in which height is difficult to measure, such as in children with cerebral palsy or scoliosis or in aging patients with spinal curvature. Arm span, which is nearly equivalent to height, is sometimes used clinically instead of height. Measure the distance from the sternal notch to the tip of the middle finger and multiply the number by 2.[15]

Height measures may not be accurate in individuals confined to a bed or wheelchair or in those older than 60 years (because of osteoporotic changes). Therefore arm span, which is correlated with height, may be a better measure.

Serial Assessment

To monitor nutritional status in malnourished individuals or individuals at risk for malnutrition, serial measurements are made at routine intervals. At a minimum, weight and dietary intake should be evaluated weekly. Because the other nutritional assessment parameters change more slowly, data on these indicators may be collected biweekly or monthly.

Based on the findings of the nutritional assessment, the type of malnutrition can be diagnosed. The four major types of malnutrition are obesity, marasmus, kwashiorkor, and marasmus-kwashiorkor mix (see Table 12.3). Each type of malnutrition has characteristic clinical and laboratory findings and a distinct cause.

Approaches to weight loss for overweight and obesity must be tailored to the individual, be culturally sensitive, and consider the patient's readiness to lose weight and his or her health care and self-care beliefs. Weight-loss programs that provide fewer than 1000 to 1200 calories per day may not provide adequate nutrients. Regardless of macronutrient composition, any diet that reduces caloric intake or contains 1400 to 1500 calories per day results in weight loss. In other words, it is not eating too much of any particular nutrient such as carbohydrate or fat that makes us gain weight, but rather the overall number of calories ingested. The **cardinal features** of a successful long-term weight loss plan are (1) getting regular physical exercise (i.e., 4 to 5 times/week for 30 minutes); (2) eating a low-calorie ($\approx$1400 to 1500 kcal/day), low-fat (20% to 25% of total calories) diet; and (3) monitoring daily food intake (e.g., food diary, portion size) and weight.

DOCUMENTATION AND CRITICAL THINKING

Sample Charting

SUBJECTIVE

A.J. is a 70- year-old retired teacher with no history of diseases or surgery that would alter intake/requirements; no recent weight changes; no appetite changes. Socioeconomic history is noncontributory. Does not smoke; drink alcohol; or use illegal, prescription, or over-the-counter drugs. No food allergies. Sedentary lifestyle; plays golf twice per week using riding cart. Reports losing 40 lb during past 6 months through monitored commercial weight-loss program.

OBJECTIVE

Dietary intake is adequate to meet protein and energy needs. No clinical signs of nutrient deficiencies. Height 70 in, weight 209 lb, BMI 30, and screening laboratory tests within normal ranges.

ASSESSMENT

Obesity, improving through monitored program
Sedentary lifestyle

Documentation and Critical Thinking

Case Study 1

K.L. is a 44-year-old female who has been overweight most of her life. Recently diagnosed with hypertension and type 2 diabetes. Comes to the clinic today for a nutritional assessment.

SUBJECTIVE

K.L. reports a lifelong struggle with obesity. Multiple failed diet attempts. Daily calorie intake approximately 3000 calories/day. Typical day: pastry or doughnut with coffee for breakfast, fast-food meal with soft drink for lunch, and "whatever I can find" for dinner. Lives in a low-income neighborhood. Nearest grocery store with fresh produce approximately 25 minutes by car. Few safe places in neighborhood for outdoor exercise.

OBJECTIVE

Inspection: General appearance is obese for age and height.
Anthropometric: Height 157.5 cm (62 in). Weight 120 kg (265 lb). BMI 48.5 (obese).
Laboratory: Hemoglobin, hematocrit, and albumin within normal limits. Hemoglobin A1c 12%. Fasting glucose 213 mg/dL.

ASSESSMENT

Morbid obesity; uncontrolled type 2 diabetes

Case Study 2

S.A. is a 14-year-old girl who has been overweight most of her life. She now has a weight gain of 12 pounds since starting high school 6 months PTA. She lives in a low-income neighborhood where the nearest grocery store with fresh fruits and vegetables is a bus ride away. There are no parks or well-lit areas with sidewalks near her home.

SUBJECTIVE

Based on S.A.'s diet recall, estimated daily calorie intake averages 2500 to 3000 calories/day. States, "I either skip breakfast or eat a doughnut on the way to school. At lunch, I eat what they give me that I don't have to pay for." Dinner is usually items from a fast-food restaurant such as a double cheeseburger, fries, and soft drink. Enjoys snacking on toaster pastries, instant ramen noodles, potato chips, and macaroni and cheese at home and consumes fruit punch and sweet tea throughout the day.

OBJECTIVE

Vital signs: Temp 98.6° F (37° C) (oral); BP 118/68 mm Hg (sitting); Pulse 82 bpm (resting); Resp 18/min.
Anthropometric: Height 162.6 cm (64 in). Weight 68.6 kg (151 lb). BMI 26.
General appearance: Appears overweight for age and height; moderate amount of open and closed comedones and acne lesions generalized to face, neck, and back.

ASSESSMENT

Overweight with BMI of 26

Documentation and Critical Thinking

TABLE 12.3 | **Classification of Malnutrition**

Type/Etiology	Clinical Features	Anthropometric Measures	Laboratory Findings
Obesity caused by caloric excess refers to weight more than 20% above ideal body weight or body mass index (BMI) of 30.0-39.9. The causes are complex and multifaceted—genetic, social, cultural, pathologic, psychological, and physiologic factors. In most cases a small caloric surplus over a long period results in the extra pounds. Although visceral protein levels are normal in the obese individual, anthropometric measures are above normal.	Obese appearance	Weight >120% standard for height BMI >30 Triceps skinfold (TSF) >10% above standard Waist-to-hip ratio >1 (men) or >0.8 (women) BMI ≥40 is morbid or extreme obesity (see Table 9.1, p. 129)	Serum cholesterol >200 mg/dL Serum triglycerides >250 mg/dL
Marasmus (protein-calorie malnutrition) is caused by inadequate intake of protein and calories or prolonged starvation. Anorexia, bowel obstruction, cancer cachexia, and chronic illness are among the clinical conditions leading to marasmus. It is characterized by decreased anthropometric measures (i.e., weight loss and subcutaneous fat and muscle wasting). Visceral protein levels may remain within normal ranges.	Starved appearance 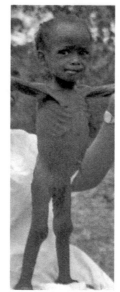	Weight ≤80% standard for height TSF <90% standard Mid–upper arm muscle circumference (MAMC) ≤90% standard	
Kwashiorkor (protein malnutrition) is caused by diets high in calories but little or no protein (e.g., low-protein liquid diets, fad diets, and long-term use of dextrose-containing intravenous fluids). In contrast to individuals with marasmus, those with kwashiorkor have decreased visceral protein levels but adequate anthropometric measures. Therefore they may appear well nourished or even obese.	Well-nourished appearance Edematous 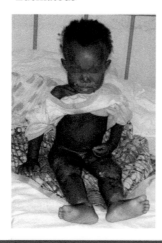	Weight ≥100% standard for height TSF ≥100% standard	Serum albumin <3.5 g/dL Serum transferrin <150 mg/dL

Continued

TABLE 12.3	Classification of Malnutrition—cont'd		
Type/Etiology	Clinical Features	Anthropometric Measures	Laboratory Findings
Marasmus/kwashiorkor mix is caused by prolonged inadequate intake of protein and calories such as severe starvation and severe catabolic states. Nutritional assessment findings include muscle, fat, and visceral protein wasting. Individuals have usually undergone acute catabolic stress such as major surgery, trauma, or burns in combination with prolonged starvation or have AIDS wasting. Without nutritional support, this type of malnutrition is associated with the highest risk for morbidity and mortality.	Emaciated appearance	Weight ≤70% standard TSF ≤80% standard MAMC ≤60% standard	Serum albumin <2.8 g/dL Serum transferrin <100 mg/dL

See Illustration Credits for source information.

TABLE 12.4	Abnormalities Caused by Nutritional Deficiencies

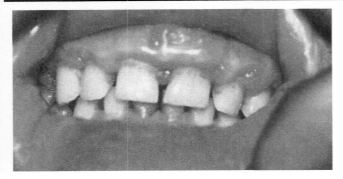

Scorbutic Gums

Deficiency of vitamin C. Gums are swollen, ulcerated, and bleeding because of vitamin C–induced defects in oral epithelial basement membrane and periodontal collagen fiber synthesis.

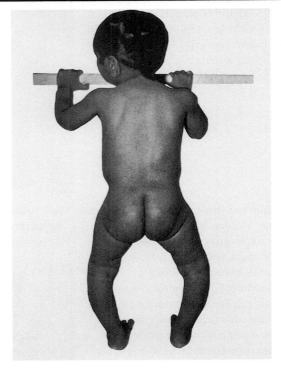

Rickets

Sign of vitamin D and calcium deficiencies in children (disorders of cartilage cell growth, enlargement of epiphyseal growth plates) and adults (osteomalacia).

Continued

TABLE 12.4	Abnormalities Caused by Nutritional Deficiencies—cont'd

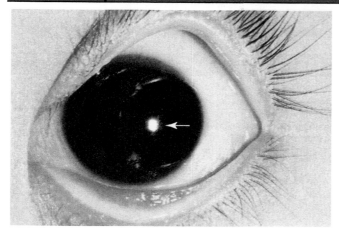

◀ **Bitot Spots**

Foamy plaques of the cornea are the accumulations of keratin that are a sign of vitamin A deficiency. Severe depletion may result in conjunctival xerosis (drying) and progress to corneal ulceration and finally destruction of the eye (keratomalacia).

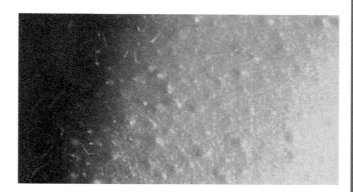

Follicular Hyperkeratosis

Dry, bumpy skin associated with vitamin A and/or linoleic acid (essential fatty acid) deficiency. Linoleic acid deficiency may also result in eczematous skin, especially in infants.

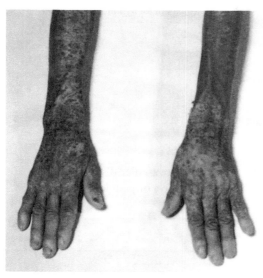

Pellagra

Pigmented keratotic scaling lesions resulting from a deficiency of niacin. These lesions are especially prominent in areas exposed to the sun such as hands, forearms, neck, and legs.

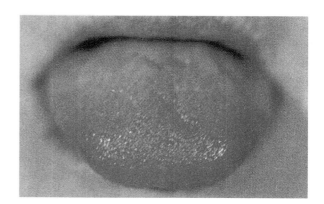

Magenta Tongue

A sign of riboflavin deficiency. In contrast, a pale tongue is probably attributable to iron deficiency; a beefy red–colored tongue is caused by vitamin B–complex deficiency.

Abnormal Findings

ABNORMAL FINDINGS
FOR ADVANCED PRACTICE

TABLE 12.5	Metabolic Syndrome (MetS)

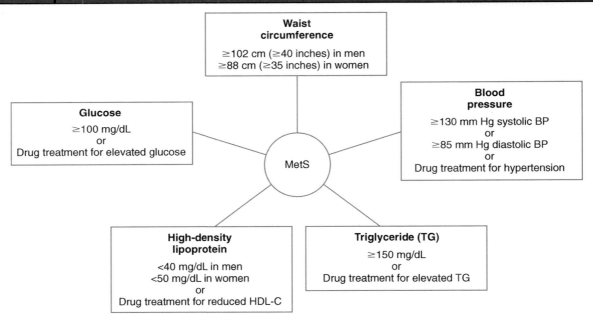

Having 3 of these 5 biomarkers signifies MetS. MetS is associated with increased risk for cardiovascular disease, type 2 diabetes mellitus, and mortality. Its prevalence is estimated to be nearly 35% of adults and 50% of people 60 years of age and older.[1]

TABLE 12.6	Nutritional Consequences of Bariatric Surgery[a,b]	
Potential Nutritional Consequences	**Related Dietary Changes**
Malabsorption of protein and calories caused by decreased absorptive surface and availability of digestive enzymes	Eating small, nutrient-dense meals
Malabsorption of vitamins and minerals caused by achlorhydria or loss of site of absorption	Taking vitamin and mineral supplements
Weight regain	Avoiding excessive intake of calorically dense liquids/foods
Obstruction of bypassed sections or pouch	Avoiding chunks of food that could cause blockage

[a]Vertical and adjustable gastric banding, Roux-en-Y gastric bypass.
[b]People who are 100% or more above ideal body weight or have a body mass index (BMI) ≥40 are categorized as morbidly or extremely obese and are possible candidates for bariatric or weight-loss surgery, as are people with BMIs ≥35 and comorbid conditions.

Summary Checklist: Nutritional Assessment

1. Obtain a **health history** relevant to nutritional status.
2. Elicit **dietary history** if indicated.
3. **Inspect** skin, hair, eyes, oral cavity, nails, and musculoskeletal and neurologic systems for clinical signs and symptoms suggestive of nutritional deficiencies.
4. **Measure** height, weight, BMI, WC, and other anthropometric parameters as indicated.
5. Review relevant **laboratory tests.**
6. Offer **health promotion** teaching.

REFERENCES

1. Aguilar, M., Bhuket, T., Torres, S., et al. (2015). Prevalence of metabolic syndrome in the United States, 2003-2012. *JAMA, 313,* 1973–1974.
2. Brunkwall, L., Chen, Y., Hindy, G., et al. (2016). Sugar-sweetened beverage consumption and genetic predisposition to obesity in 2 Swedish cohorts. *Am J Clin Nutr, 104,* 809–815.
3. Centers for Disease Control and Prevention. (2016). *Nutrition, physical activity, & obesity data & statistics.* https://www.cdc .gov/healthyyouth/data/topics/npao.htm.
4. Centers for Disease Control and Prevention. (2018). *Childhood obesity facts.* https://www.cdc.gov/healthyschools/ obesity/facts.htm.
5. Ferguson, M., Capra, S., Bauer, J., et al. (1999). Development of a valid and reliable malnutrition screening tool for adult acute care hospital patients. *Nutrition, 15,* 458–464.
6. Frantsve-Hawley, J., Bader, J. D., Welsh, J. A., et al. (2017). A systematic review of the association between consumption of sugar-containing beverages and excess weight gain among children under age 12. *J Public Health Dent, 77,* S43–S66.
7. Geller, A. I., Shehab, N., Weidle, N. J., et al. (2015). Emergency department visits for adverse events related to dietary supplements. *N Engl J Med, 373,* 1531–1540.
8. Gittner, L. S. (2014). Obesity prevention in children from birth to age 5. *Prim Prev Insights, 4,* 1–9.
9. Heymsfield, S. B., & Wadden, T. A. (2017). Mechanisms, pathophysiology, and management of obesity. *N Engl J Med, 376,* 254–266.
10. Lipek, T., Igel, U., Gausche, R., et al. (2015). Obesogenic environments: Environmental approaches to obesity prevention. *J Pediatr Endocrinol Metab, 28,* 485–495.
11. Mangels, S. R. (2018). Malnutrition in older adults: An evidence-based review of risk factors, assessment, and interventions. *Am J Nurs, 118*(3), 34–42.
12. Millar, L., Rowland, B., Nichols, M., et al. (2014). Relationship between raised BMI and sugar sweetened beverage and high fat food consumption among children. *Obesity (Silver Spring), 22*(5), E96–E103.
13. National Academy of Sciences, Committee to Reexamine IOM Pregnancy Weight Guidelines, Institute of Medicine, National Research Council, Rasmussen, K. M., & Yaktine, A. L. (Eds.). (2009). *Weight gain during pregnancy: Reexamining the guidelines.* Washington, DC: National Academies Press.
14. National Institute of Diabetes and Digestive and Kidney Diseases (NIDDK). (2017). *Overweight & Obesity Statistics.* https://www.niddk.nih.gov/health-information/health -statistics/overweight-obesity.
15. Nestle Nutrition Institute. *Nutrition Screening as Easy as MNA.* https://www.mna-elderly.com/forms/mna_guide _english_sf.pdf.
16. Qi, Q., Chu, A. Y., Kang, J. H., et al. (2012). Sugar-sweetened beverages and genetic risk of obesity. *N Engl J Med, 367,* 1387–1396.
17. Rivera, J., McPherson, A., Hamilton, J., et al. (2016). Mobile apps for weight management: A scoping review. *JMIR mHealth and uHealth, 4*(3), e87.
18. Sauer, A. C., Alish, C. J., Stausbaugh, K., et al. (2016). Nurses needed: Identifying malnutrition in hospitalized older adults. *NursingPlus Open, 2,* 21–25.
19. Shao, A., Campbell, W. W., Chen, C.-Y. O., et al. (2017). The emerging global phenomenon of sarcopenic obesity: Role of functional foods; a conference report. *J Funct Foods, 33,* 244–250.
20. Vellas, B., Villars, H., Abellan, G., et al. (2006). Overview of the MNA®: Its history and challenges. *J Nutr Health Aging, 10*(6), 456–465.

STRUCTURE AND FUNCTION

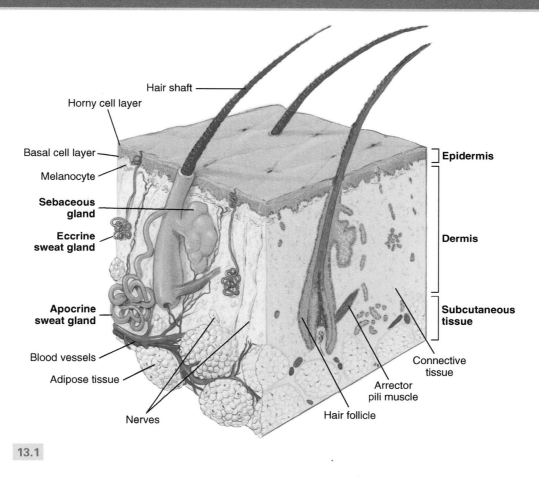

Hair shaft

Horny cell layer

Basal cell layer

Melanocyte

Sebaceous gland

Eccrine sweat gland

Apocrine sweat gland

Blood vessels

Adipose tissue

Nerves

Epidermis

Dermis

Subcutaneous tissue

Connective tissue

Arrector pili muscle

Hair follicle

13.1

SKIN

The skin is the largest organ system in the body—it covers 20 square feet of surface area in the average adult. The skin is the sentry that guards the body from environmental stresses (e.g., trauma, pathogens, dirt) and adapts it to other environmental influences (e.g., heat, cold). The skin has two layers: the outer, highly differentiated *epidermis* and the inner, supportive *dermis* (Fig. 13.1). Beneath these is the *subcutaneous* layer of adipose tissue.

Epidermis

The **epidermis** is thin but tough. Its cells are bound tightly together into sheets that form a rugged protective barrier.

It is stratified into several zones. The inner **basal cell layer** forms new skin cells. Their major ingredient is the tough, fibrous protein *keratin*. The melanocytes interspersed along this layer produce the pigment *melanin*, which gives brown tones to the skin and hair. People of all skin colors have the same number of melanocytes; however, the amount of melanin they produce varies with genetic, hormonal, and environmental influences.

From the basal layer the new cells migrate up and flatten into the outer **horny cell layer.** This consists of dead keratinized cells that are interwoven and closely packed. The cells are constantly being shed, or desquamated, and are replaced with new cells from below. The epidermis is completely replaced every 4 weeks.

On the palms and soles skin is thicker because of work and weight bearing. The epidermis is avascular; it is nourished by blood vessels in the dermis below.

Skin color is derived from three sources: (1) mainly from the brown pigment *melanin*, (2) from the yellow-orange tones of the pigment *carotene*, and (3) from the red-purple tones in the underlying vascular bed. All people have skin of varying shades of brown, yellow, and red; the relative proportion of these shades affects the prevailing color. Skin color is further modified by the thickness of the skin and the presence of edema.

Dermis

The **dermis** is the inner supportive layer consisting mostly of connective tissue, or *collagen*. This is the tough, fibrous protein that enables the skin to resist tearing. The dermis also has resilient elastic tissue that allows the skin to stretch with body movements. The nerves, sensory receptors, blood vessels, and lymphatics lie in the dermis. In addition, appendages from the epidermis such as the hair follicles, sebaceous glands, and sweat glands are embedded in the dermis.

Subcutaneous Layer

The *subcutaneous layer* is adipose tissue, which is lobules of fat cells. The subcutaneous tissue stores fat for energy, provides insulation for temperature control, and aids in protection by its soft cushioning effect. The loose subcutaneous layer also gives skin its increased mobility over structures underneath.

Hair

Hairs are threads of keratin. The hair *shaft* is the visible projecting part, and the *root* is below the surface embedded in the follicle. At the root the *bulb matrix* is the expanded area where new cells are produced at a high rate. Hair growth is cyclical, with active and resting phases. Each follicle functions independently; thus while some hairs are resting, others are growing. Around the hair follicle are the muscular *arrector pili*, which contract and elevate the hair so it resembles "goose flesh" when the skin is exposed to cold or in emotional states.

People have two types of hair. Fine, faint **vellus hair** covers most of the body (except the palms and soles, the dorsa of the distal parts of the fingers, the umbilicus, the glans penis, and inside the labia). The other type is **terminal hair,** the darker, thicker hair that grows on the scalp and eyebrows and, after puberty, on the axillae, the pubic area, and the face and chest in the male.

Sebaceous Glands

These glands produce a protective lipid substance, *sebum*, which is secreted through the hair follicles. Sebum oils and lubricates the skin and hair and forms an emulsion with water that retards water loss from the skin. (Dry skin results from loss of water, not directly from loss of oil.) Sebaceous glands are everywhere except on the palms and soles. They are most abundant in the scalp, forehead, face, and chin.

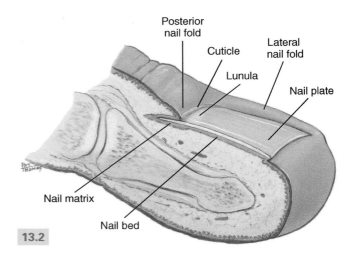

13.2

Sweat Glands

There are two types of sweat glands. The **eccrine** glands are coiled tubules that open directly onto the skin surface and produce a dilute saline solution called *sweat*. The evaporation of sweat reduces body temperature. Eccrine glands are widely distributed through the body and are mature in the 2-month-old infant.

The **apocrine** glands produce a thick, milky secretion and open into the hair follicles. They are located mainly in the axillae, anogenital area, nipples, and navel and are vestigial in humans. They become active during puberty, and secretion occurs with emotional and sexual stimulation. Bacterial flora residing on the skin surface react with apocrine sweat to produce a characteristic musky body odor. The functioning of apocrine glands decreases in the aging adult.

Nails

The nails are hard plates of keratin on the dorsal edges of the fingers and toes (Fig. 13.2). The nail plate is clear, with fine longitudinal ridges that become prominent in aging. Nails take their pink color from the underlying nail bed of highly vascular epithelial cells. The lunula is the white, opaque, semilunar area at the proximal end of the nail. It lies over the nail matrix where new keratinized cells are formed. The nail folds overlap the posterior and lateral borders. The cuticle works like a gasket to cover and protect the nail matrix.

FUNCTION OF THE SKIN

The skin is a waterproof, rugged covering that has protective and adaptive properties:

- **Protection.** Skin minimizes injury from physical, chemical, thermal, and light-wave sources.
- **Prevents penetration.** Skin is a barrier that stops invasion of microorganisms and loss of water and electrolytes from within the body.
- **Perception.** Skin is a vast sensory surface holding the neurosensory end-organs for touch, pain, temperature, and pressure.

- **Temperature regulation.** Skin allows heat dissipation through sweat glands and heat storage through subcutaneous insulation.
- **Identification.** People identify one another by unique combinations of facial characteristics, hair, skin color, and even fingerprints. Self-image is often enhanced or diminished by the way society's standards of beauty measure up to each person's perceived characteristics.
- **Communication.** Emotions are expressed in the sign language of the face and body posture. Vascular mechanisms such as blushing or blanching also signal emotional states.
- **Wound repair.** Skin allows cell replacement of surface wounds.
- **Absorption and excretion.** Skin allows limited excretion of some metabolic wastes, by-products of cellular decomposition such as minerals, sugars, amino acids, cholesterol, uric acid, and urea.
- **Production of vitamin D.** The skin is the surface on which ultraviolet (UV) light converts cholesterol into vitamin D.

❖ DEVELOPMENTAL COMPETENCE

Infants and Children

The hair follicles develop in the fetus at 3 months' gestation; by midgestation most of the skin is covered with **lanugo,** the fine downy hair of the newborn infant. In the first few months after birth, this is replaced by fine vellus hair. If terminal hair on the scalp is present at birth, it tends to be soft and suffer a patchy loss, especially at the temples and occiput. Also present at birth is **vernix caseosa,** the thick, cheesy substance made up of sebum and shed epithelial cells.

The newborn's skin is similar in structure to the adult's, but many of its functions are not fully developed. The newborn's skin is thin, smooth, and elastic and is relatively more permeable than that of the adult; thus the infant is at greater risk for fluid loss. Sebum, which holds water in the skin, is present for the first few weeks of life, producing milia (see p. 215) and cradle cap in some babies. Then sebaceous glands decrease in size and production and do not resume functioning until puberty. Temperature regulation is not effective. Eccrine sweat glands do not secrete in response to heat until the first few months of life and then only minimally throughout childhood. The skin cannot protect much against cold because it cannot contract and shiver and because the subcutaneous layer is inefficient. In addition, the pigment system is inefficient at birth.

As the child grows, the epidermis thickens, toughens, and darkens, and the skin becomes better lubricated. Hair growth accelerates. At puberty secretion from apocrine sweat glands increases in response to heat and emotional stimuli, producing body odor. Sebaceous glands become more active; the skin looks oily, and acne develops. Subcutaneous fat deposits increase, especially in females.

Secondary sex characteristics that appear during adolescence are evident in the skin. In the female the diameter of the areola enlarges and darkens, and breast tissue develops. Coarse pubic hair develops in males and females, then axillary hair, and then coarse facial hair in males.

The Pregnant Woman

Metabolism is increased in pregnancy; as a way to dissipate heat, the peripheral vasculature dilates, and the sweat and sebaceous glands increase secretion. Fat deposits are laid down, particularly in the buttocks and hips, as maternal reserves for the nursing baby. See p. 217 for expected skin color changes due to increased hormone levels.

The Aging Adult

The skin is a mirror that reflects aging changes that proceed in *all* our organ systems; it just happens to be the one organ that we can view directly. The aging process carries a slow atrophy of skin structures. The aging skin loses its elasticity; it folds and sags. By the 70s to 80s, it looks parchment thin, lax, dry, and wrinkled.

The outer layer of the epidermis thins and flattens. This allows chemicals easier access into the body. Wrinkling occurs because the underlying dermis thins and flattens. A loss of elastin, collagen, and subcutaneous fat and reduction in muscle tone occur. The loss of collagen increases the risk for shearing, tearing injuries.

Sweat and sebaceous glands decrease in number and function, leaving dry skin. Decreased response of the sweat glands to thermoregulatory demand also puts the aging person at greater risk for heat stroke. The vascularity of the skin diminishes while the vascular fragility increases; a minor trauma may produce dark red discolored areas, or **senile purpura.**

Sun exposure and cigarette smoking further accentuate aging changes in the skin. Coarse wrinkling, decreased elasticity, atrophy, speckled and uneven coloring, more pigment changes, and a yellowed, leathery texture occur. Chronic sun damage is even more prominent in light-skinned persons.

An accumulation of factors places the aging person at risk for skin disease and breakdown: the thinning of the skin, the decrease in vascularity and nutrients, the loss of protective cushioning of the subcutaneous layer, a lifetime of environmental trauma to skin, the social changes of aging (e.g., less nutrition, limited financial resources), the increasingly sedentary lifestyle, and the chance of immobility. When skin breakdown does occur, subsequent cell replacement is slower, and wound healing is delayed.

In the aging hair matrix, the number of functioning melanocytes decreases; therefore the hair looks gray or white and feels thin and fine. A person's genetic script determines the onset of graying and the number of gray hairs. Hair distribution changes. Males may have a symmetric W-shaped balding in the frontal areas. Some testosterone is present in both males and females; as it decreases with age, axillary and pubic hair decrease. As the female's estrogen also decreases, testosterone is unopposed, and the female may have some bristly facial hairs. Nails grow more slowly. Their surface is lusterless and characterized by longitudinal ridges resulting from local trauma at the nail matrix.

Because the aging changes in the skin and hair can be viewed directly, they carry a profound psychological impact. For many people self-esteem is linked to a youthful appearance. This view is compounded by media advertising in Western society. Although sagging and wrinkling skin and graying and thinning hair are normal processes of aging, they prompt a loss of self-esteem for many adults.

 ## CULTURE AND GENETICS

Melanin protects the skin against harmful UV rays, a genetic advantage accounting for the lower incidence of skin cancer among darkly pigmented African Americans and American Indians. Invasive melanoma makes up about 1% of all skin cancer cases but accounts for the vast majority of skin cancer deaths.[1] The incidence of melanoma is 21 times higher in whites than in Hispanics, and 26 times higher in whites than in blacks. Women outnumber men in melanoma cases before age 50 years, but by age 65 years men have double the rates of women and by age 80 years they are triple.[1] Risk factors are high exposure to UV radiation from sunlight or indoor tanning beds, family history of melanoma, and the presence of atypical or numerous ($\geq$50) moles. The risk is increased for persons who sunburn easily or who have natural blond or red hair. Advancing age is a risk because of the accumulation of DNA damage over time.[18] About 95% of skin melanoma cases are attributable to UV radiation exposure.[10]

Almost 300 genes are responsible for increased chromosomal sensitivity to sun damage. There is a succession of genetic mutation during the progression from benign through intermediate lesions to melanoma, with ultraviolet radiation a factor throughout.[14] This occurs from sunlight and from indoor tanning beds. Users of indoor tanning beds are overwhelmingly teenage girls and young women. Anyone who has ever used a tanning bed has a 23% increased risk of developing melanoma, and this risk increases for anyone who has used a tanning bed over 10 times in a lifetime or for users under age 25 years.[4] Four states in the United States have passed legislation restricting children from using tanning salons (Texas 16.5 years, New York 17 years, Vermont 18 years, California 18 years). However, evidence shows low compliance to the laws restricting access to tanning beds by teens because of lack of enforcement by regulatory agencies.[8] In addition, primary care pediatricians have low rates of counseling teens against tanning beds. Evidence shows that about one-third of pediatricians discussed indoor tanning at least once with their patients ages 10 to 13; about half discussed this with older teens.[2] Nurses and nurse practitioners should share the risks of tanning bed use with their patients.

Several skin conditions are common among blacks: **Keloids** are scars that form at the site of a wound and grow beyond the normal boundaries of the wound (see p. 229). African Americans have very compact collagen bundles just below the epidermis that form the keloid. Areas of postinflammatory **hypopigmentation** or **hyperpigmentation** appear as dark or light spots after acne has resolved. **Pseudofolliculitis**, also known as "razor bumps" or "ingrown hairs," is caused by shaving too closely with an electric or straight razor. **Melasma**, or the "mask of pregnancy," is a patchy tan-to–dark brown discoloration of the face.

SUBJECTIVE DATA

1. Past history of skin disease (allergies, hives, psoriasis, eczema)
2. Change in pigmentation
3. Change in mole (size or color)
4. Excessive dryness or moisture
5. Pruritus
6. Excessive bruising
7. Rash or lesion
8. Medications
9. Hair loss
10. Change in nails
11. Environmental or occupational hazards
12. Patient-centered care

Examiner Asks	Rationale
1. Past history of skin disease. Any past skin disease or problem? • How was this treated? • Any family history of allergies or allergic skin problem? • Any known allergies to drugs, plants, animals? • Any birthmarks, tattoos?	Significant familial predisposition: allergies, hay fever, psoriasis, atopic dermatitis (eczema), acne. Identify offending allergen. Although professional tattooing now uses aseptic conditions, non–TB mycobacterial infections still occur, as well as inflammatory and hypersensitivity reactions. Skin

Examiner Asks	Rationale
	cancers occur, but it is unclear whether these are coincidental or due to potential carcinogenic tattoo inks.[15]
2. **Change in pigmentation.** Any **change** in skin color or **pigmentation**?	Hypopigmentation (loss of color); hyperpigmentation (increase in color).
• A generalized color change (all over) or localized?	Generalized change suggests systemic illness: pallor, jaundice, cyanosis.
3. **Change in mole.** Any **change in a mole:** color, size, shape, sudden appearance of tenderness, bleeding, itching?	Signs suggest neoplasm in pigmented nevus. May be unaware of change in nevus on back or buttocks that he or she cannot see.
• Any "sores" that do not heal?	
4. **Excessive dryness or moisture.** Any change in the feel of your skin: temperature, **moisture**, texture?	Seborrhea—Oily.
• Any excess **dryness?** Is it seasonal or constant?	Xerosis—Dry.
5. **Pruritus.** Any skin itching? Is it mild (prickling, tingling) or intense (intolerable)?	Pruritus is the most common skin symptom; occurs with dry skin, aging, drug reactions, allergy, obstructive jaundice, uremia, lice.
• Does it awaken you from sleep?	
• Where is the itching? When did it start?	Presence or absence of pruritus helps diagnosis. Scratching causes excoriation of primary lesion.
• Any other skin pain or soreness? Where?	
6. **Excessive bruising.** Any excess **bruising?** Where on the body? • How did this happen? • How long have you had it?	Multiple cuts and bruises, bruises in various stages of healing, bruises above knees and elbows, and illogical explanation—consider physical abuse. Frequent falls may be caused by dizziness of neurologic or cardiovascular origin. Frequent minor trauma may be a side effect of alcoholism or other drug abuse.
7. **Rash or lesion.** Any skin **rash** or **lesion**? • Onset. When did you first notice it?	Rashes are a common cause of seeking health care. A careful history is important; it may predict the type of lesion you will see in the examination and its cause.
• Location. Where did it start?	Identify the primary site; it may give clue to cause.
• Where did it spread? • Character or quality. Describe the color. • Is it raised or flat? Any crust, odor? Does it feel tender, warm? • Duration. How long have you had it? • Setting. Anyone at home or work with a similar rash? Have you been camping, acquired a new pet, tried a new food, drug? Does the rash seem to come with stress?	Migration pattern, evolution. Identify new or relevant exposure, any household or social contacts with similar symptoms.
• Alleviating and aggravating factors. What home remedies have you tried? Bath, lotions, heat? Do they help or make it worse? • Associated symptoms. Any itching, fever? • What do you think rash/lesion means?	Myriad over-the-counter remedies are available. People try them and seek professional help only when they do not work. Assess person's perception of cause: fear of cancer, tickborne illnesses, or sexually transmitted infections.

Subjective Data

Examiner Asks	Rationale
• Coping strategies. How has rash/lesion affected your self-care, hygiene, ability to function at work/home/socially?	Assess effectiveness of coping strategies. Chronic skin diseases may increase risk for loss of self-esteem, social isolation, and anxiety.
• Any new or increased stress in your life?	Stress can exacerbate chronic skin illness.
8. Medications. Which **medications** do you take? • Prescription and over-the-counter? • Recent change?	Drugs, especially antibiotics, may cause allergic skin eruption. Drugs may increase sunlight sensitivity and give burn response: sulfonamides, thiazide diuretics, oral hypoglycemic agents, tetracycline. Drugs can cause hyperpigmentation: antimalarials, anticancer agents, hormones, metals, and tetracycline.
• How long on medication?	Even after a long time on medication, a person may develop sensitivity.
9. Hair loss. Any recent **hair loss?** • A gradual or sudden onset? Symmetric? Associated with fever, illness, increased stress?	**Alopecia** is a significant loss. A full head of hair equates with vitality in many cultures. If treated as a trivial problem, the person may seek alternative, unproven methods of treatment.
• Any unusual hair growth? • Any recent change in texture, appearance?	**Hirsutism** is shaggy or excessive hair.
10. Change in nails. Any **change in nails:** shape, color, brittleness? Do you tend to bite or chew nails?	
11. Environmental or occupational hazards. Any **environmental** or **occupational** hazards? • With your occupation such as dyes, toxic chemicals, radiation? • How about hobbies? Do you perform any household or furniture repair work? • How much sun exposure do you get from outdoor work, leisure activities, sunbathing, tanning salons?	Majority of skin cancers result from environmental or occupational agents. People at risk: outdoor sports enthusiasts, farmers, sailors, outdoor workers; also creosote workers, roofers, coal workers. Unprotected sun exposure accelerates aging and produces lesions. At more risk: light-skinned people, light eye and hair color, freckles, and those regularly in sun.
• Recently been bitten by insect: bee, tick, mosquito?	Identify contactants that produce lesions or contact dermatitis.
• Any recent exposure to plants, animals in yard work, camping?	Tell people with chronic recurrent urticaria (hives) to keep diary of meals and environment to identify triggers.
12. Patient-centered care. What do you do to care for your skin, hair, nails? Which cosmetics, soaps, chemicals do you use? • Clip cuticles on nails, use adhesive for false fingernails?	Assess **self-care** and influence on self-concept—may be important with the media emphasis in this society on high norms of beauty. Many over-the-counter remedies are costly and exacerbate skin problems.
• If you have allergies, how do you control your environment to minimize exposure? • Do you perform a skin self-examination?	See Patient Teaching, p. 220.

Additional History for Infants and Children

1. Does the child have any birthmarks?

Examiner Asks	Rationale

2. Was there any change in skin color as a newborn?
  - Any jaundice? Which day after birth?
  - Any cyanosis? What were the circumstances?

Physiologic jaundice, see p. 215.

3. Have you noted any rash or sores? What seems to bring it on?
  - Have you introduced a new food or formula? When? Does your child eat chocolate, cow's milk, eggs?

Generalized rash—consider allergic reaction to new food.

Irritability and general fussiness may indicate the presence of pruritus.

4. Does the child have any diaper rash? How do you care for this? How do you wash diapers? How often do you change diapers? How do you clean skin?

Occlusive diapers or infrequent changing may cause rash. Infant may be allergic to certain detergent or disposable wipes.

5. Does the child have any burns or bruises?
Where?
How did it happen?

A careful history can distinguish expected childhood bumps and bruises from any lesion that indicates child abuse or neglect: cigarette burns; excessive bruising, especially above knees or elbows; linear whip marks. With abuse the history often does not coincide with the physical appearance and location of lesion.

6. Has the child had any exposure to contagious skin conditions: scabies, impetigo, lice? Or to communicable diseases: measles, chickenpox, scarlet fever? Or to toxic plants: poison ivy?
  - Are the child's vaccinations up-to-date?

7. Does the child have any habits or habitual movements such as nail-biting, twisting hair, rubbing head on mattress?

8. Which steps are taken to protect the child from sun exposure? What about sunscreens and sunblocks? How do you treat sunburn?

Excessive sun, including severe or blistering sunburns in childhood, increases risk for melanoma in later life.[1]

Additional History for the Adolescent

1. Have you noticed any skin problems such as pimples, blackheads?
  - How long have you had them?
  - How do you treat them?
  - How do you feel about it?

Over 85% of teenagers have acne; the psychological effect is significant, with poor self-esteem, scarring, depression. Multifactorial causes include increased sebum production, microbes, inflammation.[19]

Additional History for the Aging Adult

1. Which changes have you noticed in your skin in the past few years?

Assess impact of aging on self-concept. Normal aging changes may cause distress. Many "aging" changes, including skin cancers, are the result of chronic sun damage.

2. Any delay in wound healing?
  - Any skin itching?

Pruritus with aging occurs with side effects of medicine or systemic disease (e.g., liver or kidney disease, cancer, lymphoma), but senile pruritus is usually caused by dry skin (**xerosis**), too-frequent bathing, or use of soap. Scratching with dirty, jagged fingernails produces excoriations.

Subjective Data

Examiner Asks	Rationale
3. Any other skin pain?	Some diseases such as herpes zoster (shingles) produce more intense sensations of pain, itching in aging people. Other diseases (e.g., diabetes) may reduce pain sensation in extremities. In addition, some aging people tolerate chronic pain as "part of growing old" and hesitate to "complain."
4. Any change in feet, toenails? Any bunions? Is it possible to wear shoes?	Some aging people cannot reach down to their feet to give self-care.
5. Have you had any falls this year? How many?	Multiple bruises, trauma from falls.
6. Any history of diabetes, peripheral vascular disease?	Risk for skin lesions in feet or ankles.
7. What do you do to care for your skin?	A bland lotion is important to retain moisture in aging skin. Dermatitis may ensue from certain cosmetics, creams, ointments, and dyes applied to achieve a youthful appearance. Aging skin has a delayed inflammatory response to irritants. If not alerted by warning signs (e.g., pruritus, redness), continued exposure may cause dermatitis.

Objective Data

OBJECTIVE DATA

PREPARATION

Try to control external variables that change skin color and confuse your findings (Table 13.1).

Learn to consciously attend to skin characteristics. You grow so accustomed to seeing the skin that you are likely to ignore it as you assess the organ systems underneath. Yet the skin holds information about body circulation, nutritional status, signs of systemic diseases, and topical data on the integument itself.

EQUIPMENT NEEDED

Strong direct lighting (natural daylight is ideal to evaluate skin characteristics, but halogen light will suffice)
Small centimeter ruler
Penlight
Gloves

TABLE 13.1 External Variables Influencing Skin Color

VARIABLE		CAUSES		MISLEADING OUTCOME
Emotions				
Fear, anger	→	Peripheral vasoconstriction	→	False pallor
Embarrassment	→	Flushing in face and neck	→	False erythema
Environment				
Hot room	→	Vasodilation	→	False erythema
Chilly or air-conditioned room	→	Vasoconstriction	→	False pallor, coolness
Cigarette smoking	→	Vasoconstriction	→	False pallor
Physical				
Prolonged elevation	→	Decreased arterial perfusion	→	Pallor, coolness
Dependent position	→	Venous pooling	→	Redness, warmth, distended veins
Immobilization, prolonged inactivity	→	Slowed circulation	→	Pallor, coolness, pale nail beds, prolonged capillary filling time

Know the person's normal skin coloring. Baseline knowledge is important to assess color or pigment changes. If this is the first time you are examining the person, ask about his or her usual skin color and any self-monitoring practices.

The Complete Physical Examination. Although it is presented alone in this chapter, skin assessment is integrated throughout the complete examination; it is not a separate step. At the beginning of the examination, assessing the person's hands and fingernails is a nonthreatening way to accustom him or her to your touch. As you move through the examination, scrutinize the outer skin surface first before you concentrate on the underlying structures. Separate intertriginous areas (areas with skinfolds) such as under large breasts, obese abdomen, and the groin and inspect them thoroughly. These areas are dark, warm, and moist and provide the perfect conditions for irritation or infection. Finally always remove the person's socks and inspect the feet, the toenails, and the folds between the toes.

The Regional Examination. Help the person remove clothing and assess the skin as one entity. Stand back at first to get an overall impression; this helps reveal distribution patterns. Then inspect lesions carefully. With a skin rash, check all areas of the body because the person cannot see some locations. Inspect mucous membranes, too, because some disorders have characteristic lesions here.

Needed for special procedures:
    Wood's light (filtered UV light)
    Lighted magnifier

Normal Range of Findings

Inspect and Palpate the Skin

Color

General Pigmentation. Observe the skin tone. Normally it is even and consistent with genetic background. It varies from pinkish tan to ruddy dark tan or from light to dark brown and may have yellow or olive overtones. Dark-skinned people normally have areas of lighter pigmentation on the palms, nail beds, and lips (Fig. 13.3, *A*).

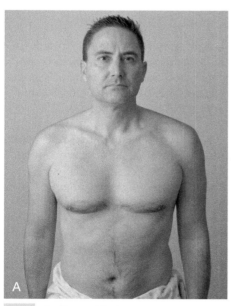

13.3 A, Even skin tone.

General pigmentation is darker in sun-exposed areas. Common (benign) pigmented areas also occur:

Abnormal Findings

An acquired condition is **vitiligo,** the complete absence of melanin pigment in patchy areas of white or light skin on the face, neck, hands, feet, and body folds and around orifices (Fig. 13.3, *B*). Vitiligo occurs in all people, although dark-skinned people are more severely affected and potentially suffer a greater threat to their body image.

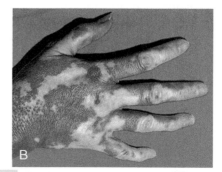

13.3 B, Vitiligo.   (Lookingbill, 1993.)

Objective Data

Normal Range of Findings

- **Freckles** (ephelides)—Small, flat macules of brown melanin pigment that occur on sun-exposed skin (Fig. 13.4, *A*).
- **Mole** (nevus)—A clump of melanocytes, tan-to-brown color, flat or raised. Acquired nevi have symmetry, small size (6 mm or less), smooth borders, and single uniform pigmentation. The **junctional nevus** (Fig. 13.4, *B*) is macular only and occurs in children and adolescents. In young adults it progresses to the **compound nevus** (Fig. 13.4, *C*), which is macular and papular. The intradermal nevus (mainly in older age) has nevus cells in only the dermis.

- **Birthmarks**—May be tan to brown in color.

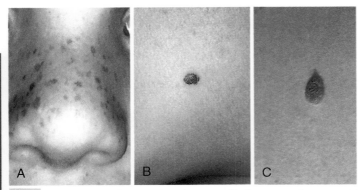

13.4 **A,** Freckles. **B,** Junctional nevus. **C,** Compound nevus. (Hurwitz, 1993.)

Widespread Color Change. Note any color change over the entire body. Normally there is no change. In dark-skinned people the amount of normal pigment may mask color changes. Lips and nail beds vary with the person's skin color and may not be accurate signs. The more reliable sites have the least pigmentation such as under the tongue, the buccal mucosa, the palpebral conjunctiva, and the sclera. See Table 13.2 for specific clues to assessment.

Pallor. When the red-pink tones from the oxygenated hemoglobin in the blood are lost, the skin takes on the color of connective tissue (collagen), which is mostly white. Pallor is common in acute high-stress states such as anxiety or fear because of the powerful peripheral vasoconstriction from sympathetic nervous system stimulation. The skin also looks pale with vasoconstriction from exposure to cold and from cigarette smoking and in the presence of edema.

Look for pallor in dark-skinned people by the absence of the luster of the underlying red tones. The brown-skinned individual shows yellowish-brown color, and the black-skinned person appears ashen or gray. Observe generalized pallor in the mucous membranes, lips, and nail beds. Look for the pallor of anemia in the palpebral conjunctiva and nail beds. Inspect the conjunctiva near the outer and inner canthi. The coloration is often lighter near the inner canthus.

Erythema. Intense redness of the skin is from excess blood (hyperemia) in the dilated superficial capillaries. This sign is *expected* with fever, local inflammation, or emotional reactions such as blushing in vascular flush areas (cheeks, neck, and upper chest).

The erythema with fever or localized inflammation has an increased skin temperature from the increased rate of blood flow. Because you cannot see inflammation in dark-skinned people, you must palpate the skin for increased warmth or taut or tightly pulled surfaces that may indicate edema and hardening of deep tissues or blood vessels.

Abnormal Findings

Danger signs: abnormal characteristics of pigmented lesions are summarized in the mnemonic **ABCDEF**:

Asymmetry (*not* regularly round or oval, two halves of lesion do not look the same)

Border irregularity (notching, scalloping, ragged edges, poorly defined margins)

Color variation (areas of brown, tan, black, blue, red, white, or combination)

Diameter greater than 6 mm (i.e., the size of a pencil eraser), although early melanomas may be diagnosed at a smaller size.

Elevation or **E**volution

Funny looking (refers to the "ugly duckling" sign, in which the suspicious lesion stands out as looking different compared with its neighboring nevi)[11] (see Table 13.10, Malignant Skin Lesions, p. 238).

Additional symptoms: rapidly changing lesion; a new pigmented lesion; development of itching, burning, or bleeding in a mole. All of these signs should raise suspicion of malignant melanoma and warrant referral.

These are: pallor (white), erythema (red), cyanosis (blue), and jaundice (yellow).

Ashen gray color in dark skin or marked pallor in light skin occurs with anemia, shock, and arterial insufficiency (see Table 13.2, Detecting Color Changes in Light and Dark Skin, p. 223).

The pallor of shock presents with rapid pulse rate, oliguria, apprehension, and restlessness.

Chronic iron deficiency anemia may show "spoon" nails, with a concave shape. Fatigue, exertional dyspnea, rapid pulse, dizziness, and impaired mental function accompany most severe anemias.

Erythema occurs with polycythemia, venous stasis, carbon monoxide poisoning, and the extravascular presence of red blood cells (petechiae, ecchymosis, hematoma) (see Table 13.2 and Table 13.7, Vascular Lesions, p. 231).

Normal Range of Findings

Cyanosis. This is a bluish mottled color from decreased perfusion (Fig. 13.5); the tissues have high levels of deoxygenated blood. This is best seen in the lips, nose, cheeks, ears, and oral mucous membranes and in artificial fluorescent light. Do not confuse cyanosis with the common and normal bluish tone on the lips of dark-skinned persons of Mediterranean origin.

Be aware that cyanosis can be a nonspecific sign. A person who is anemic could have hypoxemia without ever looking blue, because not enough hemoglobin is present (either oxygenated or reduced) to color the skin. On the other hand, a person with polycythemia (an increase in the number of red blood cells) looks ruddy blue at all times and may not necessarily be hypoxemic. This person just cannot fully oxygenate the massive numbers of red blood cells.

Cyanosis is difficult to observe in darkly pigmented people (see Table 13.2). Given that most conditions causing cyanosis also cause decreased oxygenation of the brain, other clinical signs such as changes in level of consciousness and signs of respiratory distress are evident.

Jaundice. A yellowish skin color indicates rising amounts of bilirubin in the blood. Except for physiologic jaundice in the newborn (p. 215), jaundice does not occur normally. It is *first* noted in the junction of the hard and soft palate in the mouth and in the sclera. Then the eyes appear yellow, but do not confuse scleral jaundice with the normal yellow subconjunctival fatty deposits that are common in the outer sclera of dark-skinned persons. The scleral yellow of jaundice extends up to the edge of the iris.

As levels of serum bilirubin rise, jaundice is evident in the skin over the rest of the body. This is best assessed in direct natural daylight. Common calluses on palms and soles often look yellow; do not interpret these as jaundice.

Temperature

Palpate the skin; it should be warm, and the temperature should be equal bilaterally; warmth suggests normal circulatory status (Fig. 13.6). Hands and feet may be slightly cooler in a cool environment.

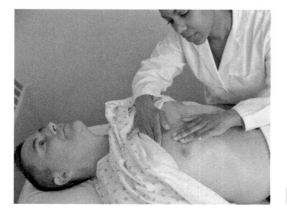

13.6

Abnormal Findings

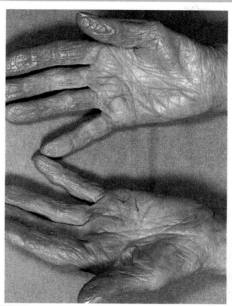

13.5   Cyanosis, especially in fingertips. (Patton, 2012.)

Cyanosis indicates hypoxemia and occurs with shock, cardiac arrest, heart failure, chronic bronchitis, and congenital heart disease.

Jaundice occurs with hepatitis, cirrhosis, sickle-cell disease, transfusion reaction, and hemolytic disease of the newborn.

Light or clay-colored stools and dark golden urine often accompany jaundice in both light- and dark-skinned people.

Objective Data

Normal Range of Findings	Abnormal Findings

Hypothermia. Generalized coolness may be induced such as in hypothermia used for surgery or high fever. Localized coolness is expected with an immobilized extremity, as when a limb is in a cast or with an intravenous infusion.

General hypothermia accompanies shock, cardiac arrest.

Localized hypothermia occurs in peripheral arterial insufficiency and Raynaud disease.

Hyperthermia. Generalized hyperthermia occurs with an increased metabolic rate such as in fever or after heavy exercise. A localized area feels hyperthermic with trauma, infection, or sunburn.

Hyperthyroidism has an increased metabolic rate, causing warm, moist skin.

Moisture

Perspiration appears normally on the face, hands, axillae, and skinfolds in response to activity, a warm environment, or anxiety. **Diaphoresis,** or profuse perspiration, accompanies an increased metabolic rate such as occurs in heavy activity or fever.

Diaphoresis occurs with thyrotoxicosis, heart attack, anxiety, or pain.

Look for **dehydration** in the oral mucous membranes. Normally there is none, and the mucous membranes look smooth and moist. Be aware that dark skin may normally look dry and flaky but this does not necessarily indicate systemic dehydration.

With dehydration, mucous membranes are dry, and lips look parched and cracked. With extreme dryness the skin is fissured, resembling cracks in a dry lake bed.

Texture

Normal skin feels smooth and firm, with an even surface.

Hyperthyroidism—skin feels smoother and softer, like velvet.

Hypothyroidism—skin feels rough, dry, and flaky.

Thickness

The epidermis is uniformly thin over most of the body, although thickened callus areas are normal on palms and soles. A callus is a circumscribed overgrowth of epidermis and is an adaptation to excessive pressure from the friction of work and weight bearing.

Very thin, shiny skin (atrophic) occurs with arterial insufficiency.

Edema

Edema is fluid accumulating in the interstitial spaces; it is not present normally. To check for edema, imprint your thumbs firmly for 3 to 4 seconds against the ankle malleolus or the tibia. Normally the skin surface stays smooth. If your pressure leaves a dent in the skin, "pitting" edema is present. See Chapter 21, p. 515, for a full explanation of assessing edema.

Edema masks normal skin color and obscures pathologic conditions such as jaundice or cyanosis because the fluid lies *between* the surface and the pigmented and vascular layers. It makes dark skin look lighter.

Edema shows in dependent body parts (feet, ankles, and sacral areas), where the skin looks puffy and tight.

Unilateral edema has a local or peripheral cause. Bilateral edema or edema that is generalized over the whole body **(anasarca)**—consider a central problem such as heart failure or kidney failure.

Mobility and Turgor

Pinch up a large fold of skin on the anterior chest under the clavicle (Fig. 13.7). Mobility is the ease of skin to rise, and turgor is its ability to return to place promptly when released. This reflects the elasticity of the skin.

Mobility is decreased with edema.

Poor turgor is evident in severe dehydration or extreme weight loss; the pinched skin recedes slowly or "tents" and stands by itself.

Scleroderma, literally "hard skin," is a chronic connective tissue disorder associated with decreased mobility.

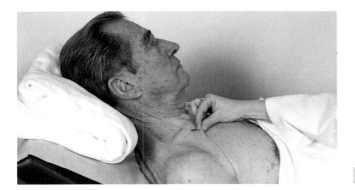

13.7

Normal Range of Findings	Abnormal Findings

Vascularity or Bruising

Cherry (senile) angiomas are small (1 to 5 mm), smooth, slightly raised bright red dots that commonly appear on the trunk in all adults older than 30 years (Fig. 13.8). They normally increase in size and number with aging and are not significant.

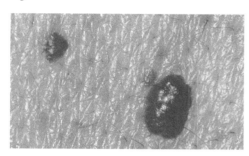

13.8 Cherry angioma.
(Lemmi & Lemmi, 2011.)

Any bruising (contusion) should be consistent with the expected trauma of life. Normally there are no venous dilations or varicosities.

> Multiple bruises at different stages of healing and excessive bruises above knees or elbows raise concern about physical abuse (see Chapter 7).

Document the presence of any tattoos (a permanent skin design from indelible pigment) on the person's chart. Inspect skin of tattoo for any infection or inflammation; normally there are no reactions.

> Needle marks from intravenous street drugs may be visible on the antecubital fossae, forearms, or on any available vein.

Lesions

If any lesions are present, note the:
1. Color.
2. Elevation: flat, raised, or pedunculated.
3. Pattern or shape: the grouping or distinctness of each lesion (e.g., annular, grouped, confluent, linear). The pattern may be characteristic of a certain disease.
4. Size, in centimeters: use a ruler to measure. Avoid household descriptions such as "quarter size" or "pea size."
5. Location and distribution on body: is it generalized or localized to area of a specific irritant; around jewelry, watchband, eyes?
6. Any exudate. Note its color and any odor.

> Lesions are traumatic or pathologic changes in previously normal structures. When a lesion develops on previously unaltered skin, it is **primary**. However, when a lesion changes over time or changes because of scratching or infection, it is **secondary**. Study Table 13.3 for the shapes and Tables 13.4 and 13.5 for the characteristics of primary and secondary skin lesions. The terms used (e.g., *macule, papule*) are helpful to describe any lesion you encounter.

Palpate lesions. Wear a glove if you anticipate contact with blood, mucosa, or any body fluid. Roll a nodule between the thumb and index finger to assess depth. Gently scrape a scale to see if it comes off. Note the nature of its base or whether it bleeds when the scale comes off. Note the surrounding skin temperature. However, the erythema associated with rashes is not always accompanied by noticeable increases in skin temperature (Fig. 13.9).

> Note the pattern and characteristics of common skin lesions (see Table 13.9, p. 236) and malignant skin lesions (Table 13.10, p. 238).

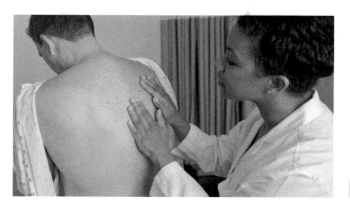

13.9

Objective Data

Normal Range of Findings	Abnormal Findings

Does the lesion blanch with pressure or stretch? Stretching the area of skin between your thumb and index finger decreases (blanches) the normal underlying red tones, thus providing more contrast and brightening the macules. Red macules from dilated blood vessels *will* blanch momentarily, whereas those from extravasated blood (petechiae) do not. Blanching also helps identify a macular rash in dark-skinned people.

Use a magnifier and light for closer inspection of the lesion (Fig. 13.10). Use a Wood's light (i.e., a UV light filtered through a special glass) to detect fluorescing lesions. With the room darkened, shine the Wood's light on the area.

Under the Wood's light, lesions with blue-green fluorescence indicate fungal infection (e.g., tinea capitis [scalp ringworm]).

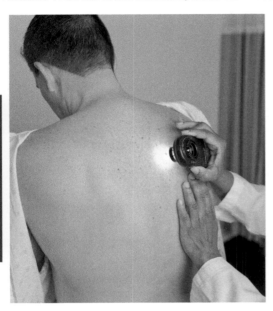

13.10

Inspect and Palpate the Hair

Color

Hair color comes from melanin production and may vary from pale blond to total black. Graying begins as early as the 30s because of reduced melanin production in the follicles. Genetic factors affect the onset of graying.

Texture

Scalp hair may be fine or thick and may look straight, curly, or kinky. It should look shiny, although this characteristic may be lost with the use of some beauty products such as dyes, rinses, or permanents (Fig. 13.11).

Note dull, coarse, or brittle scalp hair. Gray, scaly, well-defined areas with broken hairs accompany tinea capitis, a ringworm infection found mostly in school-age children (see Table 13.11, Abnormal Conditions of Hair, p. 239).

Loss of eyebrows and scalp hair is expected with chemotherapy, hypothyroidism.

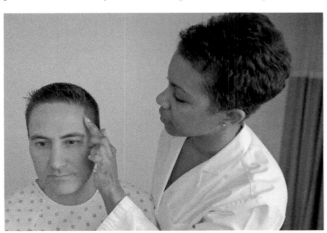

13.11

Objective Data

Normal Range of Findings	Abnormal Findings

Distribution

Fine vellus hair coats the body, whereas coarser terminal hairs grow at the eyebrows, eyelashes, and scalp. During puberty, distribution conforms to normal male and female patterns. At first coarse curly hairs develop in the pubic area, then in the axillae, and last in the facial area in boys. In the genital area the female pattern is an inverted triangle; the male pattern is an upright triangle with pubic hair extending up to the umbilicus. In Asians body hair may be diminished.

Absent or sparse genital hair suggests endocrine abnormalities.

Hirsutism—excess body hair. In females this forms a male pattern on the face and chest and indicates endocrine abnormalities (see Table 13.11).

Lesions

Separate the hair into sections and lift it, observing the scalp. With a history of itching, inspect the hair behind the ears and in the occipital area as well. All areas should be clean and free of any lesions or pest inhabitants. Many people normally have seborrhea (dandruff), which is indicated by loose white flakes.

Head or pubic lice. Distinguish dandruff from nits (eggs) of lice, which are oval and adherent to hair shaft and cause intense itching (see Table 13.11).

Inspect and Palpate the Nails

Shape and Contour

The nail surface is normally slightly curved or flat, and the posterior and lateral nail folds are smooth and rounded. Nail edges are smooth, rounded, and clean, suggesting adequate self-care (Fig. 13.12).

Jagged nails, bitten to the quick, or traumatized nail folds suggest nervous picking habits.

Chronically dirty nails suggest poor self-care or the chronic staining of some occupations and cigarette use.

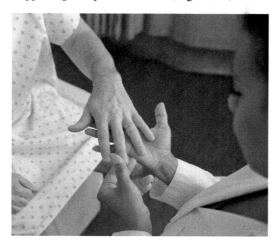

13.12

The Profile Sign. View the index finger at its profile and note the angle of the nail base; it should be about 160 degrees (Fig. 13.13). The nail base is firm to palpation. Curved nails are a variation of normal with a convex profile. They may look like clubbed nails, but notice that the angle between nail base and nail is normal (i.e., 160 degrees or less).

Clubbing of nails occurs with congenital cyanotic heart disease, lung cancer, and pulmonary diseases.

In early clubbing the angle straightens out to 180 degrees, and the nail base feels spongy to palpation. Then the nail becomes convex as the digit grows (see Late Clubbing, p. 242).

Objective Data

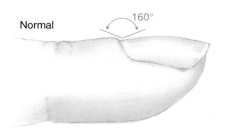

Normal   160°

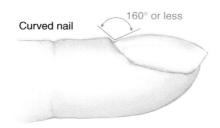

Curved nail   160° or less

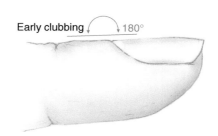

Early clubbing   180°

13.13

Normal Range of Findings	Abnormal Findings

Consistency

The surface is smooth and regular, not brittle or splitting.

Nail thickness is uniform.

The nail firmly adheres to the nail bed, and the nail base is firm to palpation.

Pits, transverse grooves, or lines may indicate a nutrient deficiency or accompany acute illness that disturbs nail growth (see Table 13.12, Abnormal Conditions of the Nails, p. 242).

Nails are thickened and ridged with arterial insufficiency.

A spongy nail base accompanies clubbing.

Color

The translucent nail plate is a window to the even, pink nail bed underneath.

Dark-skinned people may have brown-black pigmented areas or linear bands or streaks along the nail edge (Fig. 13.14). All people normally may have white hairline linear markings from trauma or picking at the cuticle called *leukonychia* (Fig. 13.15). Note any abnormal marking in the nail beds.

Cyanosis or marked pallor.

Brown linear streaks (especially sudden appearance) are abnormal in light-skinned people and may indicate melanoma.

Splinter hemorrhages, transverse ridges, or Beau lines (see Table 13.12).

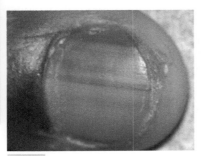

13.14 Linear pigmentation. (Lemmi & Lemmi, 2011.)

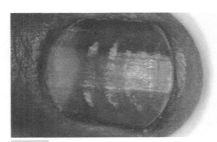

13.15 Leukonychia striata. (Lemmi & Lemmi, 2011.)

Capillary Refill. With the index or middle fingertip at heart level, depress the nail edge at least 5 seconds to blanch and then release, noting the return of color.[3] Normally color return is instant or at least within a few seconds in a cold environment. This indicates the status of the peripheral circulation. A healthy color return takes 1 or 2 seconds (see Fig. 13.12).

Inspect the toenails. Separate the toes and note the smooth skin in between.

Cyanotic nail beds or sluggish color return: consider cardiovascular or respiratory dysfunction, septic shock.

Athlete's foot scaling.

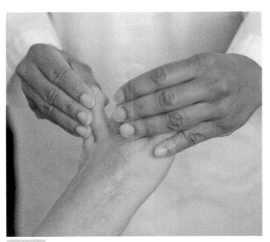

13.16

Normal Range of Findings	Abnormal Findings

❖ DEVELOPMENTAL COMPETENCE

Infants

Skin Color—General Pigmentation. Black newborns initially have lighter-toned skin than their parents because of immature pigment function. Their full melanotic color is evident in the nail beds and scrotal folds. The **mongolian spot** is a common variation of hyperpigmentation in African-American, Asian, American Indian, and Latino newborns (Fig. 13.17). It is a blue-black–to-purple macular area at the sacrum or buttocks but sometimes on the abdomen, thighs, shoulders, or arms. It is caused by deep dermal melanocytes. It gradually fades during the first year. By adulthood these spots are lighter but are frequently still visible. Mongolian spots are present in 90% of blacks, 80% of Asians and American Indians, and 9% of whites. If you are unfamiliar with mongolian spots, be careful not to confuse them with bruises. Recognition of this normal variation is particularly important when dealing with children who might be erroneously identified as victims of child abuse.

Bruising is a common soft-tissue injury that follows a rapid, traumatic, or breech birth.

Multiple bruises in various stages of healing or pattern injury suggests child abuse (see Chapter 7, p. 106).

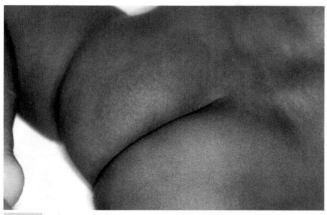

13.17 Mongolian spot.   (Lemmi & Lemmi, 2011.)

The **café au lait spot** is a large round or oval patch of light brown pigmentation (thus the name *coffee with milk*), which is usually present at birth (Fig. 13.18). Usually these patches are normal.

Six or more café au lait macules, each more than 1.5 cm in diameter, are diagnostic of neurofibromatosis, an inherited neurocutaneous disease.

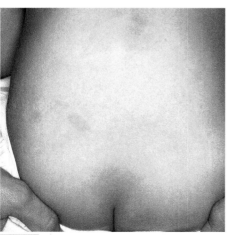

13.18 Café au lait spot. (Bowden, 1998.)

Objective Data

Normal Range of Findings

Abnormal Findings

Skin Color Change. Three erythematous states are common variations in the neonate:

1. The newborn's skin has a beefy red flush for the first 24 hours because of vasomotor instability; then the color fades to its normal color.
2. The **harlequin color change** occurs when the baby is in a side-lying position. The lower half of the body turns red, and the upper half blanches with a distinct demarcation line down the midline. The cause is unknown, and it is transient.
3. Finally, **erythema toxicum** is a common rash that appears in the first 3 to 4 days of life. Sometimes called the *flea bite* rash or newborn rash, it consists of tiny punctate red macules and papules on the cheeks, trunk, chest, back, and buttocks (Fig. 13.19). The cause is unknown; no treatment is needed.

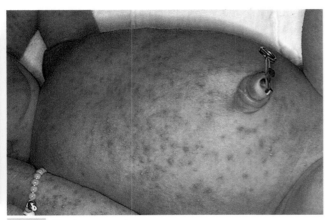

13.19 Erythema toxicum.   (Hurwitz, 1993.)

Two temporary cyanotic conditions may occur:

1. **Acrocyanosis** is a bluish color around the lips, hands and fingernails, and feet and toenails. This may last for a few hours and disappear with warming.

2. **Cutis marmorata** is a transient mottling in the trunk and extremities in response to cooler room temperatures (Fig. 13.20). It forms a reticulated red or blue pattern over the skin.

Persistent generalized cyanosis indicates distress such as cyanotic congenital heart disease.

Persistent or pronounced cutis marmorata occurs with Down syndrome or prematurity.

Green-brown discoloration of the skin, nails, and cord occurs with passing of meconium in utero, indicating fetal distress.

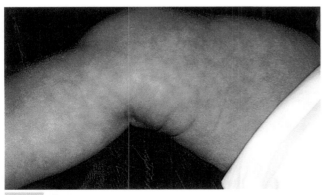

13.20 Cutis marmorata.   (Hurwitz, 1993.)

Normal Range of Findings

Physiologic jaundice is a normal variation in about half of all newborns. A yellowing of the skin, sclera, and mucous membranes develops **after the 3rd or 4th day** of life because of the increased numbers of red blood cells that hemolyze after birth. The hemoglobin in the red blood cells is metabolized by the liver and spleen; its pigment is converted into bilirubin.

Carotenemia also produces a yellow-orange color in light-skinned persons but no yellowing in the sclera or mucous membranes. It comes from ingesting large amounts of foods containing carotene, a vitamin A precursor. Carotene-rich foods are popular as prepared infant foods, and the absorption of carotene is enhanced by mashing, pureeing, and cooking. The color is best seen on the palms and soles, forehead, tip of the nose and nasolabial folds, chin, behind the ears, and over the knuckles; it fades to normal color within 2 to 6 weeks of withdrawing carotene-rich foods from the diet.

Moisture. The vernix caseosa is the moist, white, cream cheese–like substance that covers part of the skin in all newborns. Perspiration is present after 1 month of age.

Texture. **Milia** is a common variation (Fig. 13.21); you will note tiny white papules on the forehead and eyelids, also on cheeks, nose, and chin, caused by sebum that occludes the opening of the follicles. Tell parents not to squeeze the lesions; milia resolve spontaneously within a few weeks.

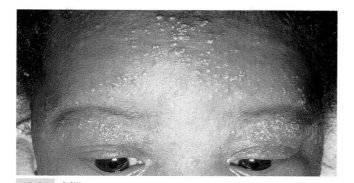

13.21 Milia.   (Cohen, 2013.)

Thickness. In the neonate the epidermis is normally thin, but you will also note well-defined areas of subcutaneous fat. The baby's skin dimples over joints, but there is no break in the skin. Check for any defect or break in the skin, especially over the length of the spine.

Mobility and Turgor. Test mobility and turgor over the abdomen in an infant.

Abnormal Findings

Jaundice on the 1st day of life may indicate hemolytic disease. Jaundice after 2 weeks of age may indicate biliary tract obstruction.

Green-tinged vernix occurs with meconium staining.

Excessive sweating in children may accompany hypoglycemia, heart disease, or hyperthyroidism.

Lack of subcutaneous fat occurs in prematurity and malnutrition.

A red sacrococcygeal dimple occurs with a pilonidal cyst or sinus (see Table 26.1 on p. 724).

Poor turgor, or "tenting," indicates dehydration, especially combined with delayed capillary refill and tachypnea. Also occurs with malnutrition.

Objective Data

Objective Data

Normal Range of Findings

Vascularity or Bruising. One common vascular birthmark is a **nevus simplex** (**stork bite**, or salmon patch); it is a flat, irregularly shaped red or pink patch found on the forehead, eyelid, or upper lip but most commonly at the back of the neck (nuchal area) (Fig. 13.22). It is present at birth and usually fades during the first year.

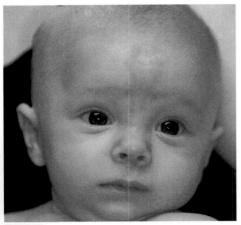

13.22 Nevus simplex (stork bite). (Eichenfield, 2015.)

Hair. A newborn's skin is covered with fine downy lanugo (Fig. 13.23), especially in a preterm infant. Dark-skinned newborns have more lanugo than lighter-skinned newborns. Scalp hair may be lost in the few weeks after birth, especially at the temples and occiput. It grows back slowly.

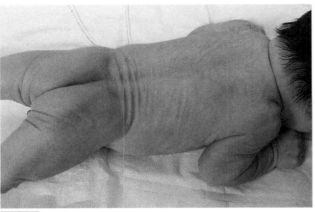

13.23 Lanugo.   (Murray, 2010.)

Nails. A newborn's nail beds may be blue (cyanotic) for the first few hours of life; then they turn pink.

Adolescents

The increase in sebaceous gland activity creates increased oiliness and **acne.** Acne is the most common skin problem of adolescence. Almost all teens have some acne, even in the milder form of open comedones (blackheads) (Fig. 13.24, *A*) and closed comedones (whiteheads). Severe acne includes papules, pustules, and nodules (Fig. 13.24, *B*). Acne lesions usually appear on the face and sometimes on the chest, back, and shoulders. Acne may appear in children as early as 7 to 8 years of age; then the lesions increase in number and severity and peak at 14 to 16 years in girls and at 16 to 19 years in boys.

Abnormal Findings

Port-wine stain, strawberry mark (immature hemangioma), cavernous hemangioma (see Table 13.7, Vascular Lesions).

Bruising may suggest abuse (see Table 13.7).

Scaly, crusted scalp occurs with seborrheic dermatitis, "cradle cap" (see Table 13.11).

In people with dark skin color, acne has the resulting effects of hyperpigmentation, keloids, and scarring.

Normal Range of Findings	Abnormal Findings

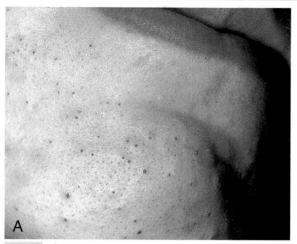

13.24   A, Open comedones.

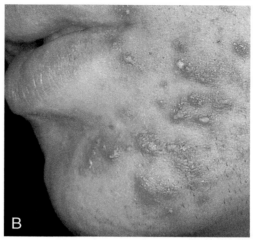

B, Severe acne.   (Habif, 2005.)

The Pregnant Woman

Striae are jagged linear "stretch marks" of silver-to-pink color that appear during the 2nd trimester on the abdomen, breasts, and sometimes thighs. They occur in half of all pregnancies. They fade after delivery but do not disappear. The change in hormone levels causes numerous color changes. On the abdomen is the **linea nigra,** a brownish-black line down the midline (see Fig. 31.5). **Chloasma** is an irregular brown patch of hyperpigmentation on the face. It may occur with pregnancy or in women taking oral contraceptive pills. Chloasma disappears after delivery or discontinuation of the pills. **Vascular spiders** (spider angioma) are common in pregnancy because of increased estrogen and may resolve after childbirth. These lesions have tiny red centers with radiating branches and occur on the face, neck, upper chest, and arms.

More than 5 spider angioma occur with significant liver disease when the liver cannot metabolize estrogen.

The Aging Adult

Skin Color and Pigmentation. **Senile lentigines** are common variations of hyperpigmentation. Commonly called *liver spots,* these are small, flat, brown macules (Fig. 13.25). These circumscribed areas are clusters of melanocytes that appear after extensive sun exposure. They appear on the forearms and dorsa of the hands. They are not malignant and require no treatment.

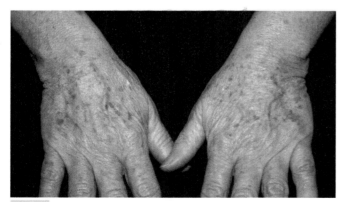

13.25   Lentigines.   (Marks, 2019.)

Objective Data

Normal Range of Findings	Abnormal Findings

Keratoses are raised, thickened areas of pigmentation that look crusted, scaly, and warty. One type, **seborrheic keratosis,** looks dark, greasy, and "stuck on" (Fig. 13.26). They develop mostly on the trunk but also on the face and hands and on both unexposed and sun-exposed areas. They do not become cancerous.

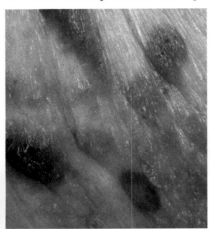

13.26 Seborrheic keratosis. (Lemmi & Lemmi, 2011.)

Another type, **actinic (senile** or **solar) keratosis,** is less common (Fig. 13.27). These lesions are red-tan scaly plaques that increase over the years to become raised and roughened. They may have a silvery-white scale adherent to the plaque. They occur on sun-exposed surfaces and are directly related to sun exposure. They are premalignant and may develop into squamous cell carcinoma.

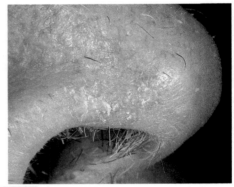

13.27 Actinic keratosis. (Habif, 2001.)

Moisture. Dry skin (xerosis) is common in the aging person because of a decline in the number and output of the sweat glands and sebaceous glands. The skin itches and looks flaky and loose.

Texture. **Acrochordons,** or "skin tags," are overgrowths of normal skin that form a stalk and are polyp-like (Fig. 13.28). They occur frequently on eyelids, cheeks and neck, and axillae and trunk.

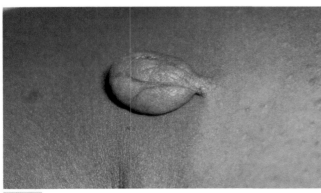

13.28 Skin tags. (Marks, 2019.)

Normal Range of Findings	Abnormal Findings

Sebaceous hyperplasia consists of raised yellow papules with a central depression. They are more common in men, occurring over the forehead, nose, or cheeks. They have a pebbly look (Fig. 13.29).

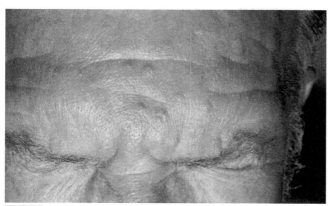

13.29 Sebaceous hyperplasia.   (Callen, 1993.)

Thickness. With aging, the skin looks as thin as parchment, and the subcutaneous fat diminishes. Thinner skin is evident over the dorsa of the hands, forearms, lower legs, dorsa of feet, and bony prominences. The skin may feel thicker over the abdomen and chest.

Aging skin increases risk for pressure ulcer development (see Table 13.6, Pressure Injuries [PI], p. 230).

Hair. With aging the amount of hair decreases in the axillae and pubic areas. After menopause white women may develop bristly hairs on the chin or upper lip resulting from unopposed androgens. In men coarse terminal hairs develop in the ears, nose, and eyebrows, although the beard is unchanged. Male-pattern balding, or alopecia, is a genetic trait. It is usually a gradual receding of the anterior hairline in a symmetric **W** shape. In men and women scalp hair gradually turns gray because of the decrease in melanocyte function.

Nails. With aging the nail growth rate decreases, and local injuries in the nail matrix may produce longitudinal ridges. The surface may be brittle or peeling and sometimes yellowed. Toenails also are thickened and may grow misshapen, almost grotesque. The thickening may be a process of aging, or it may be caused by chronic peripheral vascular disease.

Fungal infections are common in older adults, with thickened, crumbling toenails and erythematous scaling between the toes.

A healthy, capillary refill time is longer in aging adults, (1.5 to 2 seconds, with 4 seconds as the upper limit).[3]

Mobility and Turgor. The skin turgor is decreased (less elasticity), and the skin recedes slowly or "tents" and stands by itself (Fig. 13.30).

Loss of collagen with aging increases risk of skin tears (Fig. 13.31) from minor trauma or from moving or grabbing the person. Handle with care!

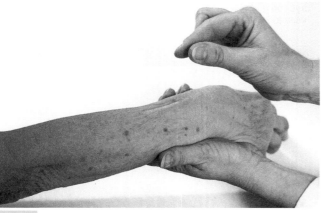

13.30

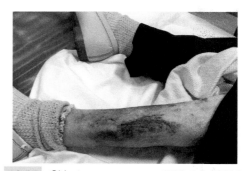

13.31 Skin tear.   (Williams, 2020.)

Objective Data

HEALTH PROMOTION AND PATIENT TEACHING

(To adolescents and adults) *I want to teach you to examine your skin, using the ABCDEF rule (see p. 206) to raise warning signals of any suspicious lesions. Use a well-lighted room that has a full-length mirror. It helps to have a small handheld mirror. Ask a family member to search skin areas difficult to see (e.g., behind ears, back of neck, back). Follow the sequence outlined in Fig. 13.32, and report any suspicious lesions promptly to a physician or nurse.*

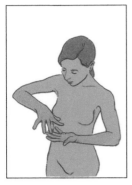

1. Undress completely. Check forearms, palms, space between fingers. Turn over hands and study the backs.

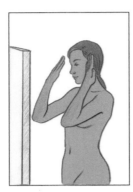

2. Face mirror; bend arms at elbow. Study arms in mirror.

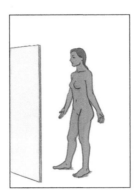

3. Face mirror and study entire front of body. Start at face, neck, torso, working down to lower legs.

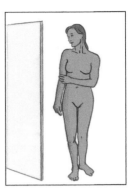

4. Pivot to right side facing mirror. Study sides of upper arms, working down to ankles. Repeat with left side.

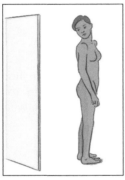

5. With back to mirror, study buttocks, thighs, lower legs.

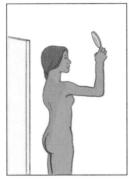

6. Use the handheld mirror to study upper back.

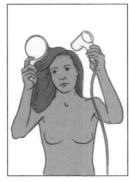

7. Use the handheld mirror to study scalp, lifting the hair. A blow-dryer on a cool setting helps to lift hair.

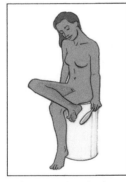

8. Sit on chair or bed. Study insides of each leg and soles of feet. Use the small mirror to help.

13.32   Skin self-examination.

DOCUMENTATION AND CRITICAL THINKING
Sample Charting

SUBJECTIVE

No history of skin disease; no present change in pigmentation or in nevi; no pruritus, bruising, rash, or lesions. On no medications. No work-related skin hazards. Uses SPF 30 sun-block cream when outdoors.

OBJECTIVE

Skin: Color tan-pink, even pigmentation, with no suspicious nevi. Warm to touch, dry, smooth, and even. Turgor good, no lesions.
Hair: Even distribution, thick texture, no lesions or pest inhabitants.
Nails: No clubbing or deformities. Nail beds pink with prompt capillary refill.

ASSESSMENT

Warm, dry, intact skin.

Focused Assessment: Clinical Case Study 1[a]

H.H. is a 3-year-old female who arrives with her mother. H.H.'s mother brought her in because of H.H.'s fever, fatigue, and rash of 3 days' duration.

SUBJECTIVE

2 weeks PTA (prior to arrival)—H.H. was playing with a preschool classmate who "became sick and is missing school because of some kind of rash."
3 days PTA—Mother reports fever 101°-102.4°F (38.3°-39°C) and states, "She's just so tired and cranky." That evening parents note "tiny blisters" on chest and back.
1 day PTA—Blisters on chest changed to white and now are scabbed. Mom reports new eruption of blisters on shoulders, thighs, and face that "just make her scratch so much."

OBJECTIVE

Vital signs: Temp 101°F (38.3°C). BP 100/63 mm Hg (sitting). Pulse 100 bpm. Resp 24/min.
General appearance: Appears fatigued and irritable.
Skin: Generalized vesiculopustular rash covering face, trunk, upper arms, and thighs. Small vesicles on face; pustules and red-honey–colored crusts and scabbing located on trunk; skin warm and otherwise dry w/good turgor.
HEENT: Tympanic membranes pearly gray w/landmarks visible and intact; no discharge; mucosa dark pink w/o lesions; tonsils 1+ w/o exudate; no lymphadenopathy.
Cardiovascular: No murmurs or other abnormal heart sounds.
Respiratory: Hyperresonant to percussion; breath sounds clear, no adventitious sounds.

ASSESSMENT

Varicella
Acute pain and pruritus
Potential for transmission of infection to others

[a]Please note that space does not allow a detailed plan for each sample clinical problem in the text. Please develop your own treatment plans as a critical-thinking exercise.

Focused Assessment: Clinical Case Study 2

B.G. is a 79-year-old retired widow, in good health until recent hospitalization after a fall.
Problem List 1 Fractured right hip—hip replacement on 11/24

SUBJECTIVE

11/27, Aching pain in left hip (nonoperative side).

OBJECTIVE

Erosion 2 × 2 cm with surrounding erythema covering L ischium. Erosion is moist; no active bleeding. Area very warm and tender to touch.

ASSESSMENT

Pressure injury, L hip
Acute pain
Decreased mobility

Focused Assessment: Clinical Case Study 3

M.G. is a 62-year-old retired female in good health with no chronic illnesses. She takes a multivitamin daily but has no prescription medications. She enters the clinic today with complaints of itching, tingling, and severe pain on her right flank.

SUBJECTIVE

Tingling, itching, and severe pain on right flank for 4 days. Pain does not radiate. Reports having a "weird rash" that developed this morning.

OBJECTIVE

Temperature 98.4° F (36.9° C). Pulse 89 bpm. Resp 18/min. BP 116/72 mm Hg.
Skin: Zosteriform rash on right flank, approximately 7 cm long. Some vesicles intact; others eroded likely from scratching. Surrounding skin red. Left flank has intact skin with no lesions.

ASSESSMENT

Herpes zoster, right flank
Acute pain
Potential for infection R/T broken vesicles on right flank

ABNORMAL FINDINGS

TABLE 13.2	Detecting Color Changes in Light and Dark Skin	
Etiology	Light Skin	Dark Skin
Pallor		
Anemia—Decreased hematocrit Shock—Decreased perfusion, vasoconstriction	Generalized pallor	Brown skin appears yellow-brown, dull; black skin appears ashen gray, dull; skin loses its healthy glow—Check areas with least pigmentation such as conjunctivae, mucous membranes
Local arterial insufficiency	Marked localized pallor (e.g., lower extremities, especially when elevated)	Ashen gray, dull; cool to palpation
Albinism—Total absence of pigment melanin throughout the integument	Whitish pink	Tan, cream, white
Vitiligo—Patchy depigmentation from destruction of melanocytes	Patchy milky-white spots, often symmetric bilaterally	Same
Cyanosis		
Increased amount of unoxygenated hemoglobin Central—Chronic heart and lung disease cause arterial desaturation	Dusky blue	Dark but dull, lifeless; only severe cyanosis is apparent in skin—Check conjunctivae, oral mucosa, nail beds
Peripheral—Exposure to cold, anxiety	Nail beds dusky	
Erythema		
Hyperemia—Increased blood in engorged arterioles (e.g., inflammation, fever, alcohol intake, blushing)	Red, bright pink	Purplish tinge but difficult to see; palpate for increased warmth with inflammation, taut skin, and hardening of deep tissues
Polycythemia—Increased red blood cells, capillary stasis	Ruddy blue in face, oral mucosa, conjunctiva, hands, and feet	Well concealed by pigment; check for redness in lips
Carbon monoxide poisoning	Bright cherry red in face and upper torso	Cherry-red color in nail beds, lips, and oral mucosa
Venous stasis—Decreased blood flow from area, engorged venules	Dusky rubor of dependent extremities; a prelude to necrosis with pressure sore	Easily masked; use palpation for warmth or edema
Jaundice		
Increased serum bilirubin from liver inflammation or hemolytic disease such as after severe burns, some infections	Yellow in sclera, hard palate, mucous membranes, then over skin	Check sclera for yellow near limbus; do not mistake normal yellowish fatty deposits in the scleral periphery for jaundice; jaundice best noted in junction of hard and soft palate, also palms

Continued

Abnormal Findings

TABLE 13.2	Detecting Color Changes in Light and Dark Skin—cont'd	
Etiology	Light Skin	Dark Skin
Carotenemia—Increased serum carotene from ingestion of large amounts of carotene-rich foods	Yellow-orange in forehead, palms and soles, nasolabial folds, but no yellowing in sclera or mucous membranes	Yellow-orange tinge in palms and soles
Uremia—Renal failure causes retained urochrome pigments in the blood	Orange-green or gray overlying pallor of anemia; may also have ecchymoses and purpura	Easily masked; rely on laboratory and clinical findings
Brown-Tan		
Addison disease—Cortisol deficiency stimulates increased melanin production	Bronzed appearance; an "eternal tan," most apparent around nipples, perineum, genitalia, and pressure points (inner thighs, buttocks, elbow, axillae)	Easily masked; rely on laboratory and clinical findings
Café au lait spots—Caused by increased melanin pigment in basal cell layer	Tan to light brown, irregularly shaped, oval patch with well-defined borders	

TABLE 13.3	Common Shapes and Configurations of Lesions

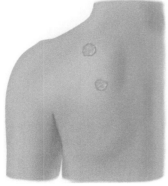

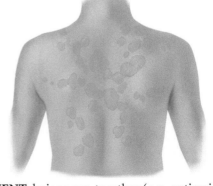

ANNULAR, or circular, begins in center and spreads to periphery (e.g., tinea corporis or ringworm, tinea versicolor, pityriasis rosea).

CONFLUENT, lesions run together (e.g., urticaria [hives]).

◀ **DISCRETE,** distinct, individual lesions that remain separate (e.g., acrochordon or skin tags, acne).

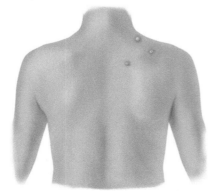

TABLE 13.3	Common Shapes and Configurations of Lesions—cont'd

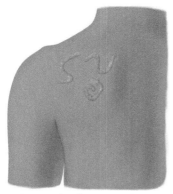

GYRATE, twisted, coiled spiral, snakelike

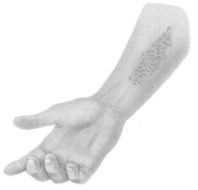

GROUPED, clusters of lesions (e.g., vesicles of contact dermatitis).

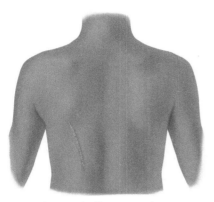

LINEAR, a scratch, streak, line, or stripe.

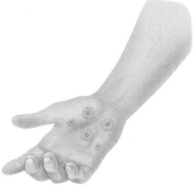

TARGET, or iris, resembles iris of eye, concentric rings of color in lesions (e.g., erythema multiforme).

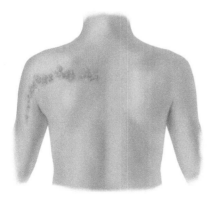

ZOSTERIFORM, linear arrangement along a unilateral nerve route (e.g., herpes zoster).

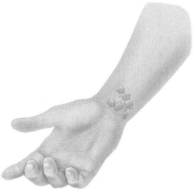

POLYCYCLIC, annular lesions grow together (e.g., lichen planus, psoriasis).

TABLE 13.4 | Primary Skin Lesions

The immediate result of a specific causative factor; primary lesions develop on previously unaltered skin.

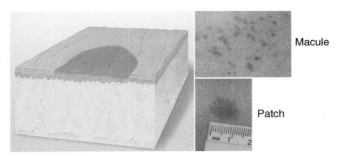

Macule

Patch

Macule

Solely a color change, flat and circumscribed, of less than 1 cm. Examples: freckles, flat nevi, hypopigmentation, petechiae, measles, scarlet fever.

Patch

Macules that are larger than 1 cm. Examples: mongolian spot, vitiligo, café au lait spot, chloasma, measles rash.

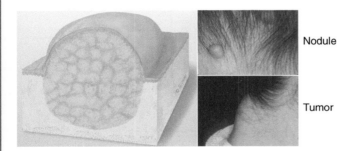

Nodule

Tumor

Nodule

Solid, elevated, hard or soft, larger than 1 cm. May extend deeper into dermis than papule. Examples: xanthoma, fibroma, intradermal nevi.

Tumor

Larger than a few centimeters in diameter, firm or soft, deeper into dermis; may be benign or malignant, although "tumor" implies "cancer" to most people. Examples: lipoma, hemangioma.

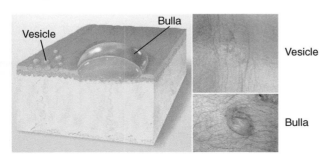

Vesicle

Bulla

Vesicle

Bulla

Papule

Something you can feel (i.e., solid, elevated, circumscribed, less than 1 cm diameter) caused by superficial thickening in epidermis. Examples: elevated nevus (mole), lichen planus, molluscum, wart (verruca).

Plaque

Papules coalesce to form surface elevation wider than 1 cm. A plateaulike, disk-shaped lesion. Examples: psoriasis, lichen planus.

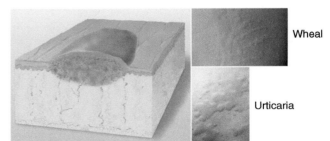

Wheal

Urticaria

Wheal

Superficial, raised, transient, and erythematous; slightly irregular shape from edema (fluid held diffusely in the tissues). Examples: mosquito bite, allergic reaction, dermographism.

Urticaria (Hives)

Wheals coalesce to form extensive reaction, intensely pruritic.

◀ Vesicle

Elevated cavity containing free fluid, up to 1 cm; a "blister." Clear serum flows if wall is ruptured. Examples: herpes simplex, early varicella (chickenpox), herpes zoster (shingles), contact dermatitis.

◀ Bulla

Larger than 1 cm diameter; usually single chambered (unilocular); superficial in epidermis; thin-walled and ruptures easily. Examples: friction blister, pemphigus, burns, contact dermatitis.

Continued

TABLE 13.4	Primary Skin Lesions—cont'd

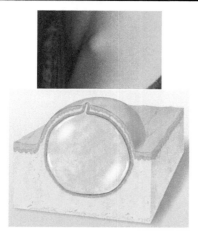

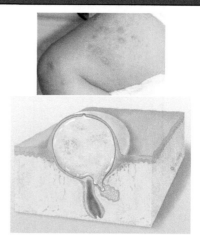

Cyst

Encapsulated fluid-filled cavity in dermis or subcutaneous layer, tensely elevating skin. Examples: sebaceous cyst, wen.

Pustule

Turbid fluid (pus) in the cavity. Circumscribed and elevated. Examples: impetigo, acne.

See Illustration Credits for source information.

Line drawings © Pat Thomas, 2010.

TABLE 13.5	Secondary Skin Lesions

Resulting from a change in a primary lesion from the passage of time; an evolutionary change.

NOTE: Combinations of primary and secondary lesions may coexist in the same person. Such combined designations may be termed *papulosquamous, maculopapular, vesiculopustular,* or *papulovesicular.*

Debris on Skin Surface

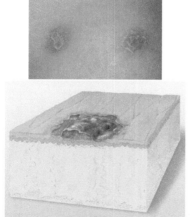

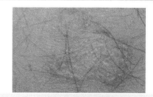

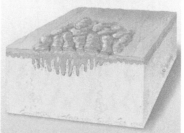

Crust

The thickened, dried-out exudate left when vesicles/pustules burst or dry up. Color can be red-brown, honey, or yellow, depending on fluid ingredients (blood, serum, pus). Examples: impetigo (dry, honey-colored), weeping eczematous dermatitis, scab after abrasion.

Scale

Compact, desiccated flakes of skin, dry or greasy, silvery or white, from shedding of dead excess keratin cells. Examples: after scarlet fever or drug reaction (laminated sheets), psoriasis (silver, micalike), seborrheic dermatitis (yellow, greasy), eczema, ichthyosis (large, adherent, laminated), dry skin.

Continued

Abnormal Findings

TABLE 13.5	Secondary Skin Lesions—cont'd

Break in Continuity of Surface

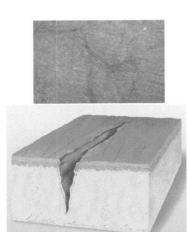

Fissure
Linear crack with abrupt edges; extends into dermis; dry or moist. Examples: cheilosis—at corners of mouth caused by excess moisture; athlete's foot.

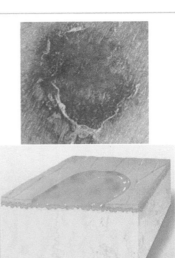

Erosion
Scooped out but shallow depression. Superficial; epidermis lost; moist but no bleeding; heals without scar because erosion does not extend into dermis.

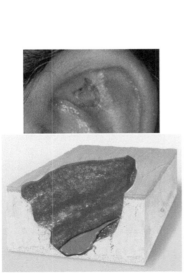

Ulcer
Deeper depression extending into dermis, irregular shape; may bleed; leaves scar when heals. Examples: stasis ulcer, pressure injury, chancre.

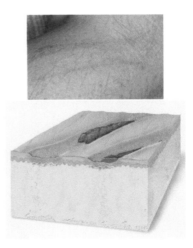

Excoriation
Self-inflicted abrasion; superficial; sometimes crusted; scratches from intense itching. Examples: insect bites, scabies, dermatitis, varicella.

Continued

TABLE 13.5 | **Secondary Skin Lesions—cont'd**

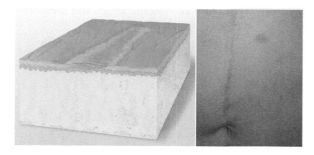

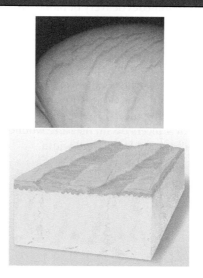

Scar

After a skin lesion is repaired, normal tissue is lost and replaced with connective tissue (collagen). This is a permanent fibrotic change. Examples: healed area of surgery or injury, acne.

Atrophic Scar

The resulting skin level is depressed with loss of tissue; a thinning of the epidermis. Example: striae.

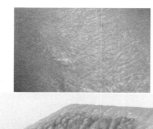

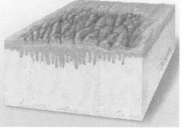

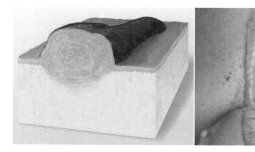

Lichenification

Prolonged, intense scratching eventually thickens skin and produces tightly packed sets of papules; looks like surface of moss (or lichen).

Keloid

A benign excess of scar tissue beyond sites of original injury: surgery, acne, ear piercing, tattoos, infections, burns.[16] Looks smooth, rubbery, shiny and "clawlike"; feels smooth and firm. Found in ear lobes, back of neck, scalp, chest, and back; may occur months to years after initial trauma. Most common ages are 10-30 years; higher incidence in blacks, Hispanics, and Asians.

Abnormal Findings

TABLE 13.6 **Pressure Injuries (PI) (Pressure Ulcer, Decubitus Ulcer)**

PIs appear on the skin over a bony prominence when circulation is impaired, e.g., when confined to bed or immobilized. Immobilization impedes delivery of blood carrying oxygen and nutrients to the skin, and it impedes venous drainage carrying metabolic wastes away from the skin. This results in ischemia and cell death. Common sites for PIs are on the back (heel, ischium, sacrum, elbow, scapula, vertebra) or the side (ankle, knee, hip, rib, shoulder).

Risk factors for PIs include impaired mobility, thin fragile skin of aging, decreased sensory perception (thus unable to respond to pain accompanying prolonged pressure), impaired level of consciousness (also unable to respond), moisture from urine or stool incontinence, excessive perspiration or wound drainage, shearing injury (being pulled down or across in bed), poor nutrition, and infection. Knowledge of risk factors and prevention of PIs is far more easily accomplished than is treatment of existing ulcers. However, once PIs occur, they are assessed by stage, depending on the pressure ulcer depth.[12] Once stage 3 or 4 ulcers occur, measure wound size daily. Use disposable rulers with mm and cm markings, and measure the greatest overall wound length and width.

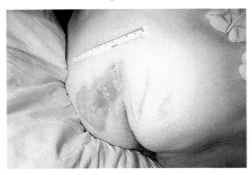

Stage 1—Non-Blanchable Erythema

Intact skin is red but unbroken. Localized redness in lightly pigmented skin does not blanch (turn light with fingertip pressure). Dark skin appears darker but does not blanch. May have changes in sensation, temperature, or firmness.

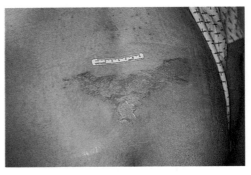

Stage 2—Partial-Thickness Skin Loss

Loss of epidermis and exposed dermis. Superficial ulcer looks shallow like an abrasion or open blister with a red-pink wound bed. No visible fat or deeper tissue.

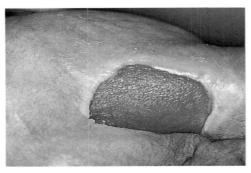

Stage 3—Full-Thickness Skin Loss

PI extends into subcutaneous tissue and resembles a crater. See subcutaneous fat, granulation tissue, and rolled edges, but not muscle, bone, or tendon.

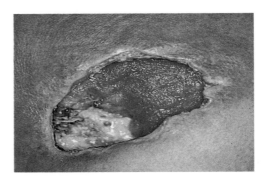

Stage 4—Full-Thickness Skin/Tissue Loss

PI involves all skin layers and extends into supporting tissue. Exposes muscle, tendon, or bone, and may show slough (stringy matter attached to wound bed) or eschar (black or brown necrotic tissue), rolled edges, and tunneling.

Deep Tissue Pressure Injury (DTPI)

Localized, non-blanchable color change to deep red, maroon, purple in intact or nonintact skin. Dark skin appears darker but does not blanch. Or, epidermis may separate, revealing dark wound or blood-filled blister.[12] Preceded by pain and temperature change. Begins in the muscle closest to the bone, in older adults and those with a lower BMI, commonly on skin over coccyx, sacrum, buttocks, heels.[13]

PI Caused by Medical Device

Skin or mucosa has PI that looks like pattern or shape of medical device, e.g., IV hub, endotracheal tube, cervical collar, anti-thromboembolism stocking.[7]

See Illustration Credits for source information.

ABNORMAL FINDINGS
FOR ADVANCED PRACTICE

TABLE 13.7	Vascular Lesions

Hemangiomas

Caused by a benign proliferation of blood vessels in the dermis.

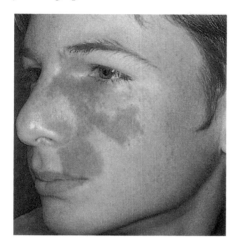

Port-Wine Stain (Nevus Flammeus)

A large, flat, macular patch covering the scalp or face, frequently along the distribution of cranial nerve V. The color is dark red, bluish, or purplish and intensifies with crying, exertion, or exposure to heat or cold. The marking consists of mature capillaries. It is present at birth and usually does not fade. The use of yellow light lasers now makes photoablation of the lesion possible, with minimal adverse effects.

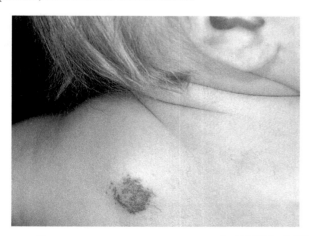

Strawberry Mark (Immature Hemangioma)

A raised bright red area with well-defined borders about 2 to 3 cm in diameter. It does not blanch with pressure. It consists of immature capillaries, is present at birth or develops in the first few months, and usually disappears by age 5 to 7 years. Requires no treatment, although parental and peer pressure may prompt treatment.

◀ Cavernous Hemangioma (Mature)

A reddish-blue, irregularly shaped, solid and spongy mass of blood vessels. It may be present at birth, may enlarge during the first 10 to 15 months, and does not involute spontaneously.

Continued

TABLE 13.7	Vascular Lesions—cont'd

Telangiectases

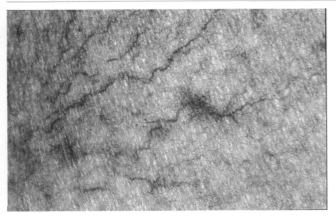

◀ Telangiectasia

Caused by vascular dilation; permanently enlarged and dilated blood vessels that are visible on the skin surface.

Spider or Star Angioma ▶

A fiery red, star-shaped marking with a solid circular center. Capillary radiations extend from the central arterial body. With pressure, note a central pulsating body and blanching of extended legs. Develops on face, neck, or chest; may be associated with pregnancy, chronic liver disease, or estrogen therapy or may be normal.

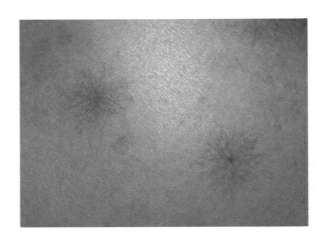

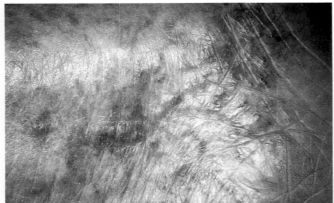

◀ Venous Lake

A blue-purple dilation of venules and capillaries in a star-shaped, linear, or flaring pattern. Pressure causes them to empty or disappear. Located on the legs near varicose veins and also on the face, lips, ears, and chest.

Continued

TABLE 13.7	Vascular Lesions—cont'd

Purpuric Lesions

Caused by blood flowing out of breaks in the vessels. Red blood cells and blood pigments are deposited in the tissues (extravascular). Difficult to see in dark-skinned people.

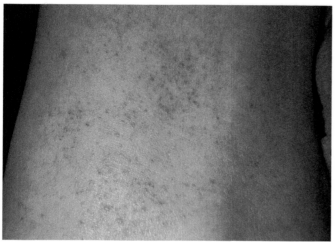

◀ Petechiae

Tiny punctate hemorrhages, 1 to 3 mm, round and discrete; dark red, purple, or brown in color. Caused by bleeding from superficial capillaries; will not blanch. May indicate abnormal clotting factors. In dark-skinned people petechiae are best visualized in the areas of lighter melanization (e.g., the abdomen, buttocks, and volar surface of the forearm). When the skin is black or very dark brown, petechiae cannot be seen in the skin.

Most of the diseases that cause bleeding and microembolism formation such as thrombocytopenia, subacute bacterial endocarditis, and other septicemias are characterized by petechiae in the mucous membranes and on the skin. Thus you should inspect for petechiae in the mouth, particularly the buccal mucosa, and in the conjunctivae.

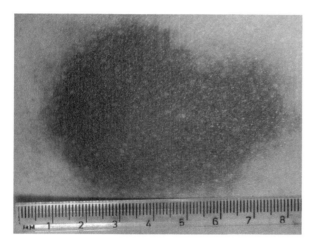

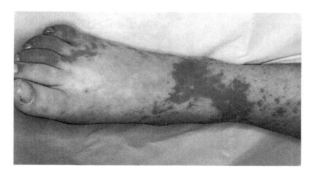

Purpura

Confluent and extensive patch of petechiae and ecchymoses; >3 mm, flat, red to purple, macular hemorrhage. Seen in generalized disorders such as thrombocytopenia and scurvy. Also occurs in old age as blood leaks from capillaries in response to minor trauma and diffuses through dermis.

Ecchymosis

A purplish patch resulting from extravasation of blood into the skin, >3 mm in diameter.

Contusion (Bruise) ▶

A mechanical injury (e.g., a blow) results in hemorrhage into tissues. Skin is intact. Color in a light-skinned person is usually (1) red-blue or purple immediately after or within 24 hours of trauma and generally progresses to (2) blue to purple, (3) blue-green, (4) yellow, and (5) brown to disappearing. A recent bruise in a dark-skinned person is deep, dark purple. Note that it is *not* possible to date the age of a bruise from its color. Pressure on a bruise will *not* cause it to blanch. A bruise usually occurs from trauma but can also result from bleeding disorders and liver dysfunction.

Note that a bruise is *different* from petechiae, ecchymosis, and purpura because these three are *not* caused by blunt force trauma.

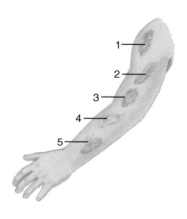

TABLE 13.8	Common Skin Lesions in Children

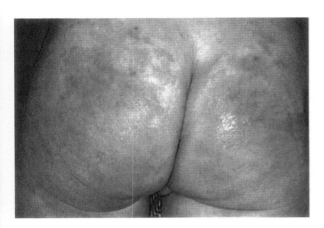

Diaper Dermatitis

Red, moist, maculopapular patch with poorly defined borders in diaper area, extending along inguinal and gluteal folds. History of infrequent diaper changes or occlusive coverings. Inflammatory disease caused by skin irritation from ammonia, heat, moisture, occlusive diapers.

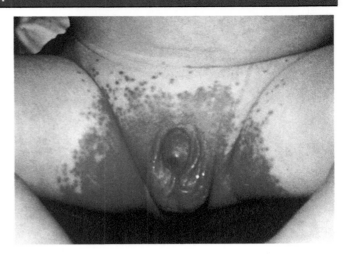

Intertrigo (Candidiasis)

Scalding red, moist patches with sharply demarcated borders, some loose scales. Usually in genital area extending along inguinal and gluteal folds. Aggravated by urine, feces, heat, and moisture; the *Candida* fungus infects the superficial skin layers.

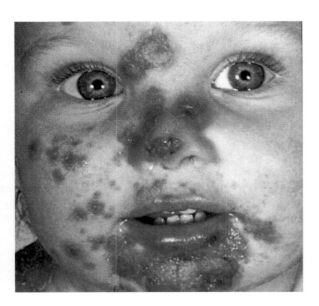

Impetigo

Moist, thin-roofed vesicles with thin, erythematous base. Rupture to form erosions and thick, honey-colored crusts. Highly contagious bacterial infection of skin; most common in infants and children. Infection can spread to other body areas and other children and adults by direct contact.[17]

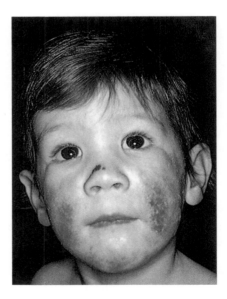

Atopic Dermatitis (Eczema)

A chronic inflammatory skin lesion caused by overstimulated immune system, genetic changes in skin, and environmental triggers.[16] Erythematous papules and vesicles, with weeping, oozing, flaking, fissures, crusts, and severe pruritus. Great effect on quality of life: sleep, behavior, mood, absences from school and work.

Continued

TABLE 13.8 | **Common Skin Lesions in Children—cont'd**

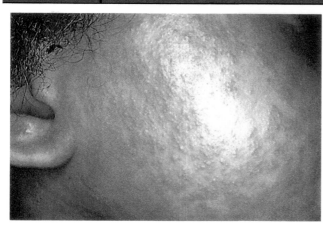

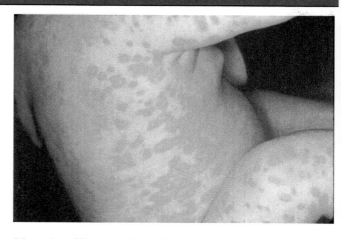

Measles (Rubeola) in Dark Skin

Measles (Rubeola) in Light Skin

Red-purple maculopapular blotchy rash in dark skin *(on left)* and light skin *(on right)* appears on 3rd or 4th day of illness. Rash appears first behind ears and spreads over face and then over neck, trunk, arms, and legs; looks "coppery" and does not blanch. Also characterized by Koplik spots in mouth—bluish white, red-based elevations of 1 to 3 mm (see Table 17.4, p. 372). Vaccine refusal has caused a decline in herd immunity and numerous outbreaks of infectious diseases.[6]

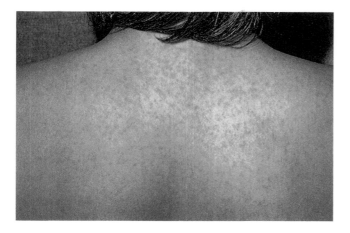

German Measles (Rubella)

Pink, papular rash (similar to measles but paler) first appears on face, then spreads. Distinguished from measles by presence of neck lymphadenopathy and absence of Koplik spots.

Chickenpox (Varicella)

Small, tight vesicles first appear on trunk and spread to face, arms, and legs (not palms or soles). Shiny vesicles on an erythematous base are commonly described as the "dewdrop on a rose petal." Vesicles erupt in succeeding crops over several days; they become pustules and then crusts. Intensely pruritic.

TABLE 13.9 | Common Skin Lesions

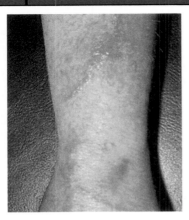

Primary Contact Dermatitis

Local inflammatory reaction to an irritant in the environment or an allergy. Characteristic location of lesions often gives clue. Often erythema shows first, followed by swelling, wheals (or urticaria), or maculopapular vesicles, scales. Frequently accompanied by intense pruritus. Example here: poison ivy.

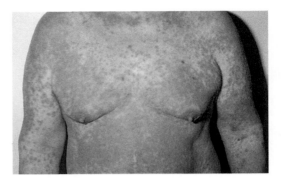

Allergic Drug Reaction

Erythematous and symmetric rash, usually generalized. Some drugs produce urticarial rash or vesicles and bullae. History of drug ingestion.

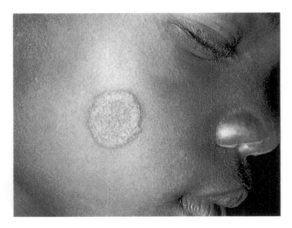

Tinea Corporis (Ringworm of the Body)

Scales—hyperpigmented in whites, depigmented in dark-skinned people; on chest, abdomen, back of arms forming multiple circular lesions with clear centers.

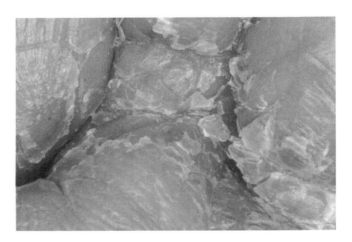

Tinea Pedis (Ringworm of the Foot)

"Athlete's foot," a fungal infection, first appears as small vesicles between toes, on sides of feet, and on soles; grows scaly and hard. Found in chronically warm, moist feet: children after gymnasium activities, athletes, aging adults who cannot dry their feet well.

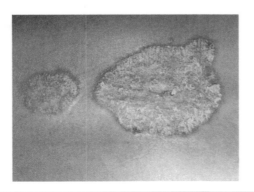

◀ Psoriasis

A hereditary chronic inflammatory skin disease with environmental triggers. Plaque psoriasis is a raised scaly, erythematous patch, with silvery scales, often pruritic and painful. Occurs on scalp, extensor surfaces of knees and elbows, lower back.[5] Accompanied by nail pitting, onycholysis (see Table 13.12, p. 242).

Continued

TABLE 13.9	**Common Skin Lesions—cont'd**

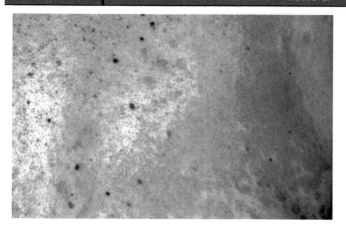

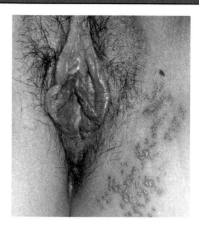

Tinea Versicolor

Fine, scaling, round patches of pink, tan, or white (thus the name) that do not tan in sunlight, caused by a superficial fungal infection. Usual distribution is on neck, trunk, and upper arms—a short-sleeved turtleneck sweater area. Most common in otherwise healthy young adults. Responds to oral antifungal medication.

Herpes Zoster (Shingles)

Small, grouped vesicles emerge along route of cutaneous sensory nerve, then pustules, then crusts. Caused by the varicella zoster virus (VZV), a reactivation of the dormant virus of chickenpox. Acute appearance, unilateral, does not cross midline. Commonly on trunk; can be anywhere. If on ophthalmic branch of cranial nerve V, it poses risk to eye. Most common in adults older than 50 years. Pain is often severe and long-lasting in aging adults, called *postherpetic neuralgia*.

NOTE: Be observant! The photo above is *not* genital herpes. This is herpes zoster with a linear lesion on only one side.

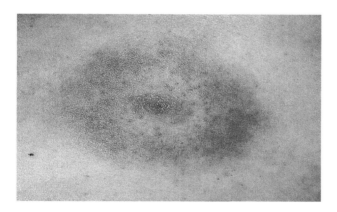

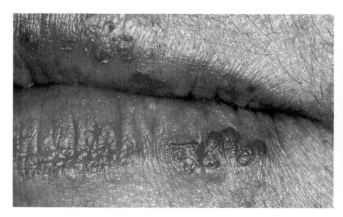

Erythema Migrans of Lyme Disease

Lyme disease (LD) is not fatal but may have serious arthritic, cardiac, or neurologic sequelae. It is caused by a spirochete bacterium carried by the black or dark brown deer tick, which is common in the Northeast and upper Midwest (with cases in people who spend time outdoors) in May through September.

The first stage (early localized LD) has the distinctive bull's-eye, red macular or papular rash (shown above) in only 50% of cases. The rash radiates from the site of the tick bite (5 cm or larger) with some central clearing; it is usually located in axillae, midriff, inguina, or behind knees, with regional lymphadenopathy. Rash fades in 4 weeks; untreated individual then may have disseminated disease with fatigue, anorexia, fever, chills, or joint or muscle aches. Antibiotic treatment shortens symptoms and decreases risk for sequelae.[12a]

Labial Herpes Simplex (Cold Sores)

Herpes simplex virus (HSV) infection has a prodrome of skin tingling and sensitivity. Lesion then erupts with tight vesicles followed by pustules and produces acute gingivostomatitis with many shallow, painful ulcers. Common location is upper lip; also in oral mucosa and tongue.

See Illustration Credits for source information.

TABLE 13.10 Malignant Skin Lesions

The link between ultraviolet (UV) radiation and skin cancer is well known; the UV radiation in sunlight and indoor tanning beds promotes all three forms of skin cancer shown below. More than half a person's lifetime sun damage occurs before adulthood.

Basal Cell Carcinoma ▶

Usually starts as a small, pink or red papule (may be deeply pigmented) with a pearly translucent top and overlying telangiectasia (broken blood vessel). Then develops rounded, pearly borders with central red ulcer or looks like large open pore with central yellowing. Most common form of skin cancer; slow but inexorable growth. Basal cell cancers occur on sun-exposed areas of face, ears, scalp, shoulders.

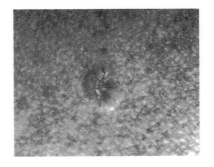

Squamous Cell Carcinoma ▶

Squamous cell cancers arise from actinic keratoses or de novo. Erythematous scaly patch with sharp margins, 1 cm or more. Develops central ulcer and surrounding erythema. Usually on hands or head, areas exposed to UV radiation; *at right*, on habitually sun-exposed bald scalp. Less common than basal cell carcinoma but grows rapidly.

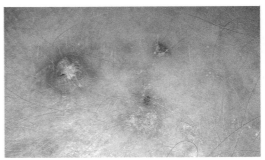

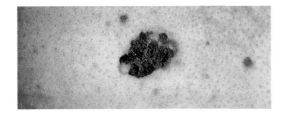

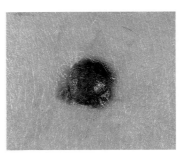

Malignant Melanoma

The malignant transformation of melanocytes may arise from preexisting nevus or de novo. Usually brown; can be tan, black, pink-red, purple, or mixed pigmentation. Often irregular or notched borders. May have scaling, flaking, oozing texture. Risk factors are UV radiation from sun exposure and indoor tanning, aging, and family history. In men, most melanomas are located on the trunk and back; in women most are on the legs and feet; in older adults, most are on the head and neck.[4] Of the major subtypes of early melanoma, the most common is superficial spreading melanoma *(on left)*; it begins as a brown to black macule with irregular borders and color variation. Nodular melanoma *(on right)* is the next most common, with quickly growing blue, black, pink or red nodules, possibly with ulceration or bleeding.

| TABLE 13.11 | Abnormal Conditions of Hair |

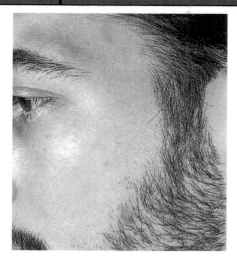

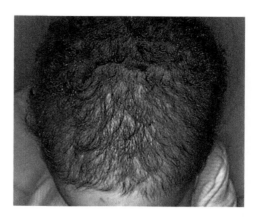

AIDS-Related Kaposi Sarcoma: Patch Stage

Kaposi sarcoma (KS) is a common vascular cancer in HIV-infected persons. Considered an AIDS-defining illness, KS can occur at any stage of HIV infection. Here multiple patch-stage early lesions are faint pink on the temple and beard area. They easily could be mistaken for bruises or nevi and be ignored. The use of highly active antiretroviral therapy has decreased the risk of this cancer.

Toxic Alopecia

Patchy, asymmetric balding that accompanies severe illness or use of chemotherapy in which growing hairs are lost and resting hairs are spared. Regrowth occurs after illness or discontinuation of toxin.

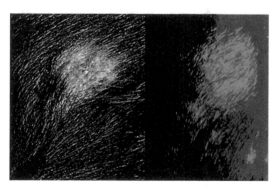

◄ Tinea Capitis (Scalp Ringworm)

Rounded, patchy hair loss on scalp, leaving broken-off hairs, pustules, and scales on skin. Caused by fungal infection; lesions may fluoresce blue-green under Wood's light. Usually seen in children and farmers; highly contagious; may be transmitted by another person, by domestic animals, or from soil.

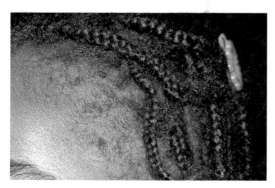

◄ Traction Alopecia

The cause is mechanical, not androgenic, and the hair loss is linear or oval along hairline, a part in hair, or scattered. The "fringe sign" is alopecia along the temporal hairline. Trauma is from tight braiding, tight ponytail, barrettes, cornrows, hair weaves. Black hair is intrinsically fragile and the continuous pulling in one direction can break hair and cause loss. Improves with loosening the braids, especially around the hairline, redoing braids after 2 to 3 months in a different direction, or using larger-diameter braids.[9]

Continued

TABLE 13.11	Abnormal Conditions of Hair—cont'd

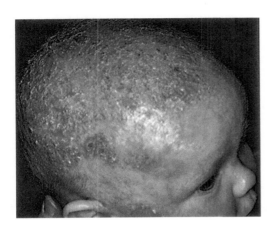

Seborrheic Dermatitis (Cradle Cap)

Thick, yellow-to-white, greasy, adherent scales with mild erythema on scalp and forehead; very common in early infancy. Resembles eczema lesions, except that cradle cap is distinguished by absence of pruritus, presence of "greasy" yellow-pink lesions, and negative family history of allergy.

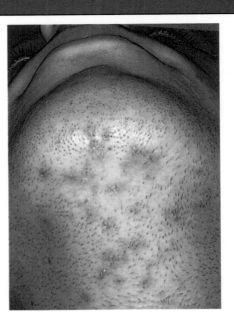

Folliculitis Barbae ("Razor Bumps")

Superficial inflammatory infection of hair follicles. Multiple pustules, "whiteheads," with hair visible at center and erythematous base. Usually involves face and neck and is common in black and Latino men if they have tight curly hair. Occurs after shaving when growing out hairs curl in on themselves and pierce the skin, making a foreign-body inflammatory reaction.

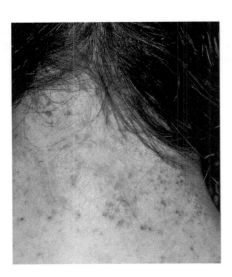

Pediculosis Capitis (Head Lice)

History includes intense itching of the scalp, especially the occiput. The nits (eggs) of lice are easier to see in the occipital area and around the ears, appearing as 2- to 3-mm oval translucent bodies, adherent to the hair shafts. Common among school-age children. Over-the-counter pediculicide shampoos are available; however, nit removal by daily combing of wet hair with a fine-tooth metal comb is especially important.

Continued

TABLE 13.11	Abnormal Conditions of Hair—cont'd

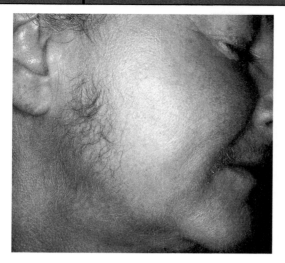

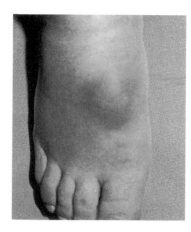

Hirsutism

Excess body hair in females forming a male sexual pattern (upper lip, face, chest, abdomen, arms, legs); caused by endocrine or metabolic dysfunction, or occasionally is idiopathic.

Furuncle and Abscess

Red, swollen, hard, tender, pus-filled lesion caused by acute, localized bacterial (usually staphylococcal) infection; usually on back of neck, buttocks, occasionally on wrists or ankles. Furuncles are caused by infected hair follicles, whereas abscesses are caused by traumatic introduction of bacteria into skin. Abscesses are usually larger and deeper than furuncles.

See Illustration Credits for source information.

TABLE 13.12	Abnormal Conditions of the Nails

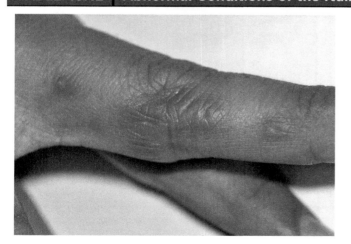

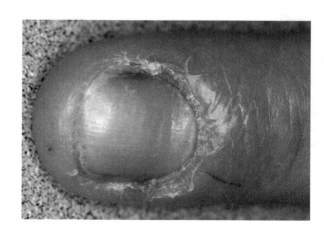

Scabies

An intensely pruritic contagion caused by the scabies mite. Mites form a linear or curved elevated burrow on the fingers, web spaces of hands, and wrists. Highly contagious. Severe itching causes sleep disturbance and bacterial skin infections. A common communicable disease in resource-poor countries.

Paronychia

Red, swollen, tender inflammation of the nail folds. Acute paronychia is usually a bacterial infection with pus in the proximal nail fold, pain, and throbbing. Chronic paronychia is most often a fungal infection from a break in the cuticle in those who perform "wet" work.

TABLE 13.12	Abnormal Conditions of the Nails—cont'd

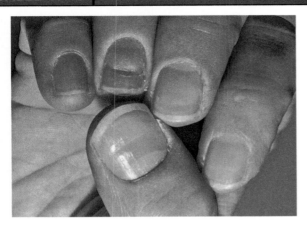

Beau Line

Transverse furrow or groove. A depression across the nail that extends down to the nail bed. Occurs with any trauma that temporarily impairs nail formation such as acute illness, toxic reaction, or local trauma. Dent appears first at cuticle and moves forward as nail grows.

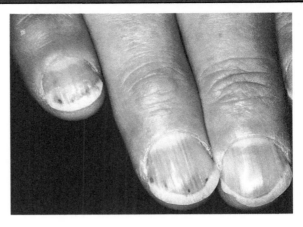

Splinter Hemorrhages

Red-brown linear streaks from damage to nail bed capillaries. They occur with systemic diseases (vasculitis), with trauma or sports-related injuries, and with endocarditis.

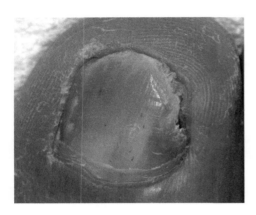

Onychomycosis

This is a slow, persistent fungal infection of fingernails and, more often, toenails, common in older adults. Fungus causes change in color (green where nail plate separated from bed), texture, and thickness, with nail crumbling or breaking and loosening of the nail plate, usually beginning at the distal edge and progressing proximally.

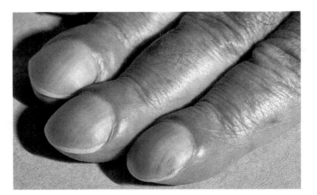

Late Clubbing

Inner edge of nail elevates; nail bed angle is greater than 180 degrees. Distal phalanx looks rounder, wider, and shiny.

Chronic lung inflammation, lung cancers, heart defects with right-to-left shunts may cause release of growth factors (e.g., platelet-derived growth factor) and promote growth of vessels. Clubbing usually develops slowly over years; if the primary disease is treated, clubbing can reverse.

Continued

TABLE 13.12	Abnormal Conditions of the Nails—cont'd

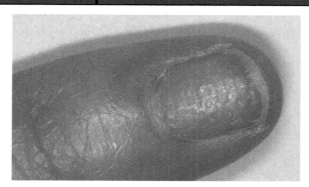

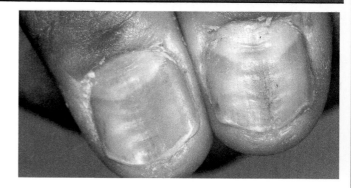

Pitting

Sharply defined pitting and crumbling of nails with distal detachment often occurs with psoriasis.

Habit-Tic Dystrophy

Depression down middle of nail or multiple horizontal ridges caused by continuous picking of cuticle by another finger of same hand, which causes injury to nail base and nail matrix.

See Illustration Credits for source information.

Summary Checklist: Skin, Hair, and Nails Examination

1. **Inspect the skin:**
   Color
   General pigmentation
   Areas of hypopigmentation or hyperpigmentation
   Abnormal color changes
2. **Palpate the skin:**
   Temperature
   Moisture
   Texture
   Thickness
   Edema
   Mobility and turgor
   Hygiene
   Vascularity or bruising
3. **Note any lesions:**
   Color
   Shape and configuration
   Size
   Location and distribution on body
4. **Inspect and palpate the hair:**
   Texture
   Distribution
   Any scalp lesions
5. **Inspect and palpate the nails:**
   Shape and contour
   Consistency
   Color
6. **Teach skin self-examination**

REFERENCES

1. American Cancer Society (ACS). (2017). *Cancer Facts & Figures 2017.* https://www.cancer.org/cancer-facts-and-figures-2017.pdf.
2. Balk, S. J., Gottschlich, A., Holman, D. M., et al. (2017). Counseling on sun protection and indoor tanning. *Pediatr, 140*(6), 1–10.
3. Bridges, E. (2017). Assessing patients during septic shock resuscitation. *Am J Nurs, 117*(10), 34–41.
4. Canavan, T., & Cantrell, W. (2016). Recognizing melanoma: Diagnosis and treatment options. *Nurse Pract, 41*(4), 24–29.
5. Cantrell, W. (2017). Psoriasis & psoriatic therapies. *Nurse Pract, 42*(7), 35–39.
6. Colgrove, J. (2016). Vaccine refusal revisited – The limits of public health persuasion and coercion. *N Engl J Med, 375*(14), 1316–1354.
7. Delmore, B. A., & Ayello, E. A. (2017). Pressure injuries caused by medical devices and other objects. *Am J Nurs, 117*(12), 36–46.
8. Driscoll, D. W., & Darcy, J. (2015). Indoor tanning legislation. *Pediat Nurs, 41*(2), 59–88.
9. Haskin, A., & Aguh, C. (2016). All hairstyles are not created equal: What the dermatologist needs to know about black hairstyling practices and the risk of traction alopecia (TA). (2016). *J Am Acad Dermatol, 75*(2), 606–611.
10. Islami, F., Sauer, A. G., Miller, K. D., et al. (2018). Proportion and number of cancer cases and deaths attributable to potentially modifiable risk factors in the United States. *CA Cancer J Clin, 68*(1), 31–54.
11. Jensen, J. D., & Elewski, B. E. (2015). The ABCDEF Rule: Combining the "ABCDE Rule" and the "Ugly duckling" sign in an effort to improve patient self-screening examinations. *J Clin Aesthet Dermatol, 8*(2), 15.
12. National Pressure Ulcer Advisory Panel (NPUAP). (2016). *NPUAP pressure injury stages.* http://www.npuap.org/resources/educational-and-clinical-resources/npuap-pressure-injury-stages/.
12a. Patton, S. K. (2018). Lyme disease: Diagnosis, treatment, and prevention. *Am J Nurs, 118*(4), 38–46.

13. Preston, A., Rao, A., Strauss, R., et al. (2017). Deep tissue pressure injury. *Am J Nurs, 117*(5), 50–57.

14. Shain, A. H., Kovalyshyn, I., Sriharan, A., et al. (2015). The genetic evolution of melanoma from precursor lesions. *N Engl J Med, 373*(20), 1926–1935.

15. Simunovic, C., & Shinohara, M. M. (2014). Complications of decorative tattoos. *Am J Clin Dermatol, 15*, 525–536.

16. Stein, S. L., & Cifu, A. S. (2016). Management of atopic dermatitis. *JAMA, 315*(14), 1510–1511.

17. VanRavenstein, K., Durham, C. O., Williams, T. H., et al. (2017). Diagnosis and management of impetigo. *Nurse Pract, 42*(3), 40–44.

18. Wellbrock, C. (2016). Melanoma and the microenvironment – age matters. *N Engl J Med, 375*(7), 696–698.

19. Zaenglein, A. L., Pathy, A. L., Schlosser, B. J., et al. (2016). Guidelines of care for the management of acne vulgaris. *J Am Acad Dermatol, 74*, 945–973.

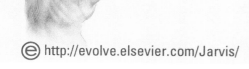

CHAPTER 14

Head, Face, Neck, and Regional Lymphatics

STRUCTURE AND FUNCTION

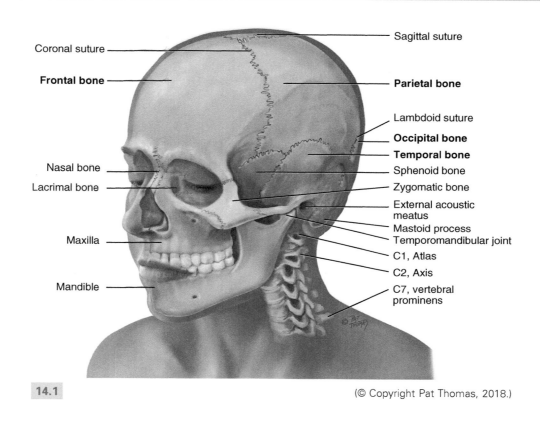

Coronal suture

Frontal bone

Nasal bone

Lacrimal bone

Maxilla

Mandible

Sagittal suture

Parietal bone

Lambdoid suture

Occipital bone

Temporal bone

Sphenoid bone

Zygomatic bone

External acoustic meatus

Mastoid process

Temporomandibular joint

C1, Atlas

C2, Axis

C7, vertebral prominens

14.1

(© Copyright Pat Thomas, 2018.)

THE HEAD

The **skull** is a rigid bony box that protects the brain and special sense organs, and it includes the bones of the cranium and the face (Fig. 14.1). Note the location of these **cranial bones:** frontal, parietal, occipital, and temporal. Use these names to describe any of your clinical findings in the corresponding areas.

The adjacent cranial bones unite at meshed immovable joints called the **sutures.** The bones are not firmly joined at birth; this allows for the mobility and change in shape needed for the birth process. The sutures gradually ossify during early childhood. The **coronal** suture *crowns* the head from ear to ear at the union of the frontal and parietal bones. The **sagittal** suture *separates* the head lengthwise between the two parietal bones. The **lambdoid** suture separates the parietal bones crosswise from the occipital bone.

The 14 **facial bones** also articulate at sutures (note the nasal bone, zygomatic bone, and maxilla), except for the mandible (the lower jaw). It moves up, down, and sideways from the temporomandibular joint, which is anterior to each ear.

The cranium is supported by the cervical vertebrae: C1, the "atlas"; C2, the "axis"; and down to C7. The C7 vertebra has a long spinous process that is palpable when the head is flexed. Feel this useful landmark, the **vertebra prominens,** on your own neck.

Inside the skull the brain is held by membranous meninges. These suspend and support the brain and are shock absorbers in case of trauma. Because of the rigid bone, a traumatic blow to the skull jostles the brain back and forth and may result in concussion (see p. 262).

245

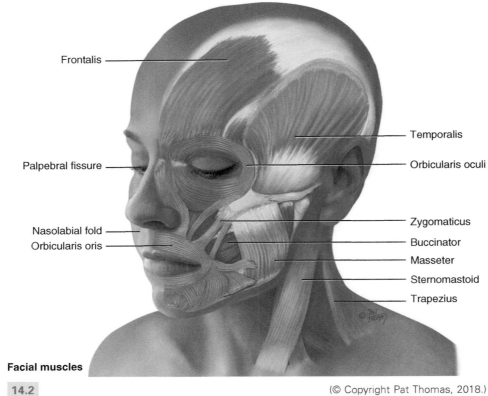

Facial muscles

14.2

(© Copyright Pat Thomas, 2018.)

The human **face** has many appearances and expressions that reflect mood. The expressions are formed by the facial muscles (Fig. 14.2), which are mediated by cranial nerve VII, the facial nerve. Facial muscle function is symmetric bilaterally, except for an occasional quirk or wry expression.

Facial structures are symmetric; the eyebrows, eyes, ears, nose, and mouth appear about the same on both sides. The

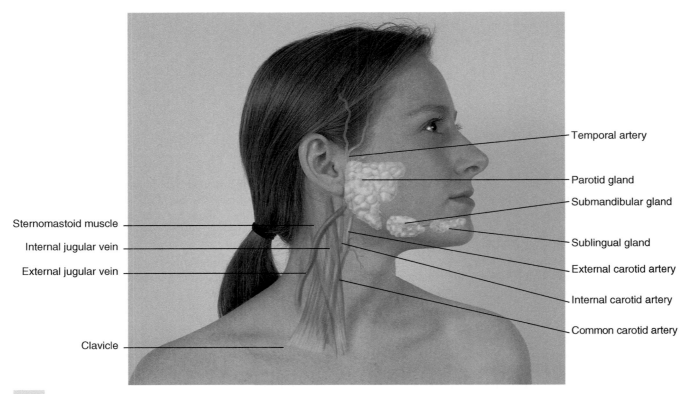

14.3

palpebral fissures—the openings between the eyelids—are equal bilaterally. Also the nasolabial folds—the creases extending from the nose to each corner of the mouth—should look symmetric. Facial sensations of pain or touch are mediated by the 3 sensory branches of cranial nerve V, the trigeminal nerve. (Testing for sensory function is described in Chapter 24.)

Two pairs of **salivary glands** are accessible to examination on the face (Fig. 14.3). The **parotid** glands are in the cheeks over the mandible, anterior to and below the ear. They are the largest of the salivary glands but are not normally palpable. The **submandibular** glands are beneath the mandible at the angle of the jaw. A third pair, the **sublingual** glands, lie in the floor of the mouth. (Salivary gland function follows in Chapter 17.) The **temporal artery** lies superior to the temporalis muscle; its pulsation is palpable anterior to the ear.

THE NECK

The **neck** is delimited by the base of the skull and inferior border of the mandible above and by the manubrium sterni, the clavicle, the first rib, and the first thoracic vertebra below. Think of the neck as a *conduit* for the passage of many structures that are lying in close proximity: blood vessels, muscles, nerves, lymphatics, and viscera of the respiratory and digestive systems. Blood vessels include the common and internal carotid arteries and their associated veins (see Fig. 14.3). The internal carotid artery branches off the common carotid and runs inward and upward to supply the brain; the external carotid artery supplies the face, salivary glands, and superficial temporal area. The carotid artery and internal jugular vein lie beneath the sternomastoid muscle. The external jugular vein runs diagonally across the sternomastoid muscle. (See assessment of the neck vessels in Chapter 20.)

The major **neck muscles** are the **sternomastoid** and the **trapezius** (Fig. 14.4); they are innervated by cranial nerve XI, the spinal accessory. The sternomastoid muscle arises from the sternum and the clavicle and extends diagonally across the neck to the mastoid process behind the ear. It accomplishes head rotation and flexion. The two trapezius muscles on the upper back arise from the occipital bone and the vertebrae and extend fanning out to the scapula and clavicle. The trapezius muscles move the shoulders and extend and turn the head.

The sternomastoid muscle divides each side of the neck into two triangles. The **anterior triangle** lies in front, between the sternomastoid and the midline of the body, with its base up along the lower border of the mandible and its apex down at the suprasternal notch. The **posterior triangle** is behind the sternomastoid muscle, with the trapezius muscle on the other side and its base along the clavicle below. It contains the posterior belly of the omohyoid muscle. These triangles are helpful guidelines when describing findings in the neck.

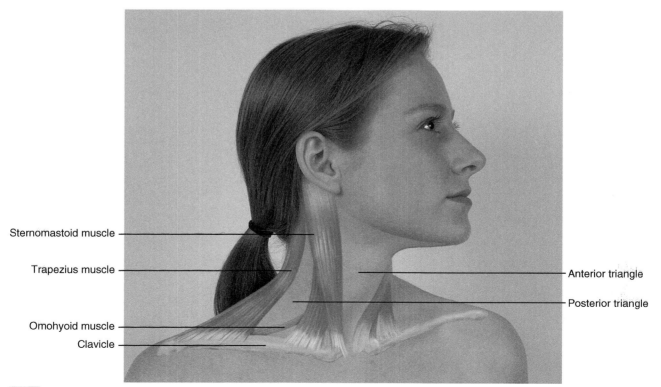

Sternomastoid muscle

Trapezius muscle

Omohyoid muscle

Clavicle

Anterior triangle

Posterior triangle

14.4

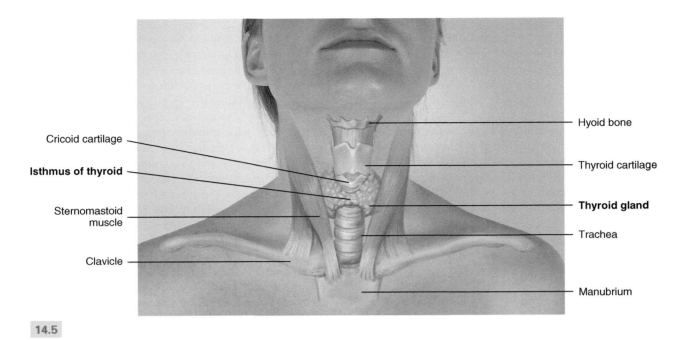

Cricoid cartilage

Isthmus of thyroid

Sternomastoid muscle

Clavicle

Hyoid bone

Thyroid cartilage

Thyroid gland

Trachea

Manubrium

14.5

The **thyroid gland** is an important endocrine gland with a rich blood supply. It straddles the trachea in the middle of the neck (Fig. 14.5). This highly vascular endocrine gland synthesizes and secretes thyroxine (T_4) and triiodothyronine (T_3), hormones that stimulate the rate of cellular metabolism.

The gland has two lobes, both conical in shape, each curving posteriorly between the trachea and the sternomastoid muscle. The lobes are connected by a thin isthmus.

The neck cartilages are important landmarks for locating the thyroid gland. The **thyroid** cartilage has a small, palpable

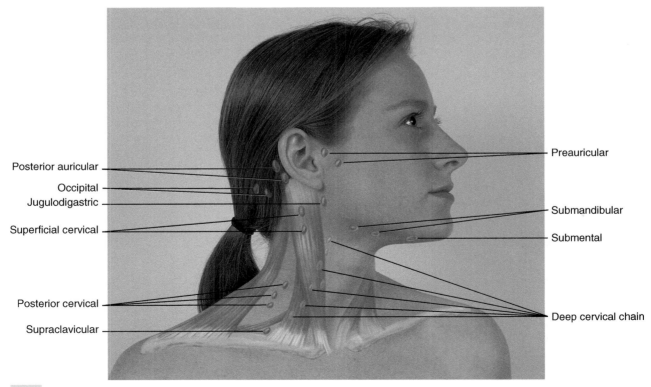

Posterior auricular

Occipital

Jugulodigastric

Superficial cervical

Posterior cervical

Supraclavicular

Preauricular

Submandibular

Submental

Deep cervical chain

14.6

V in its upper edge. This is the prominent "Adam's apple" in men. Beneath that is the **cricoid** cartilage, or upper tracheal ring. Beneath the cricoid cartilage, the isthmus of the thyroid gland hugs the 2nd and 3rd tracheal rings.

LYMPHATICS

The lymphatic system is developed more fully in Chapter 21. However, the head and neck have a rich supply of 60 to 70 **lymph nodes** (Fig. 14.6). Note that their labels correspond to adjacent structures.

- *Preauricular,* in front of the ear
- *Posterior auricular* (mastoid), superficial to the mastoid process
- *Occipital,* at the base of the skull
- *Submental,* midline, behind the tip of the mandible
- *Submandibular,* halfway between the angle and the tip of the mandible
- *Jugulodigastric (tonsillar),* under the angle of the mandible
- *Superficial cervical,* overlying the sternomastoid muscle
- *Deep cervical,* deep under the sternomastoid muscle
- *Posterior cervical,* in the posterior triangle along the edge of the trapezius muscle
- *Supraclavicular,* just above and behind the clavicle, at the sternomastoid muscle

You also should be familiar with the direction of the **drainage patterns** of the lymph nodes (Fig. 14.7). When nodes are enlarged, check the area they drain for the source of the problem. Explore the area proximal (upstream) to the enlarged node. All head and neck structures eventually drain into the deep cervical chain.

The **lymphatic system** is a separate vessel system from the cardiovascular system and a major part of the immune system, whose job it is to detect and eliminate foreign substances from the body. The vessels gather the clear, watery fluid (lymph) from the tissue spaces into the circulation.

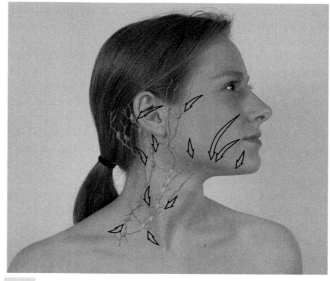

14.7

Lymph nodes are small, oval clusters of lymphatic tissue that are set at intervals along the lymph vessels like beads on a string. The nodes slowly filter the lymph and engulf pathogens, preventing harmful substances from entering the circulation. Nodes are located throughout the body but are accessible to examination only in four areas: head and neck, arms, axillae, and inguinal region. The greatest supply is in the head and neck.

❖ DEVELOPMENTAL COMPETENCE

Infants and Children

The bones of the neonatal skull are separated by sutures and **fontanels,** the spaces where the sutures intersect (Fig. 14.8). These membrane-covered "soft spots" allow for growth of the brain during the 1st year. They gradually ossify; the

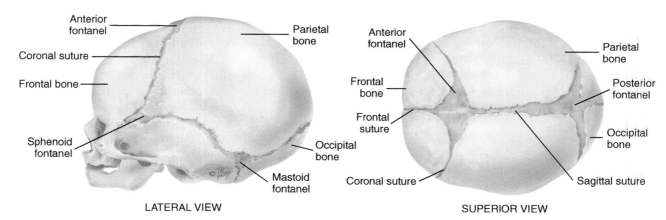

LATERAL VIEW   SUPERIOR VIEW

BONES OF THE NEONATAL SKULL

14.8

© Pat Thomas, 2006.

triangle-shaped posterior fontanel is closed by 1 to 2 months, and the diamond-shaped anterior fontanel closes between 9 months and 2 years.

During the fetal period head growth predominates. Head size is greater than chest circumference at birth. The head size grows during childhood, reaching 90% of its final size when the child is 6 years old. But during infancy, trunk growth predominates, so head size changes in proportion to body height. Facial bones grow at varying rates, especially nasal and jaw bones. In the toddler the mandible and maxilla are small, and the nasal bridge is low; thus the whole face seems small compared with the skull.

Lymphoid tissue is well developed at birth and grows to adult size when the child is 6 years old. The child's lymphatic tissue continues to grow rapidly until age 10 or 11 years, actually exceeding its adult size before puberty. Then the lymphatic tissue slowly atrophies.

In adolescence facial hair appears on boys, first above the lip, then on cheeks and below the lip, and last on the chin. A noticeable enlargement of the thyroid cartilage occurs, and with it the voice deepens.

The Pregnant Woman

The thyroid gland enlarges slightly during pregnancy as a result of hyperplasia of the tissue and increased vascularity.

The Aging Adult

The facial bones and orbits appear more prominent, and the facial skin sags as a result of decreased elasticity, decreased subcutaneous fat, and decreased moisture in the skin. The lower face may look smaller if teeth have been lost.

CULTURE AND GENETICS

Headache. Headache (HA) is a leading cause of acute pain and lost productivity, as well as a leading reason for seeking care in outpatient offices, urgent care centers, and emergency departments. Headaches are classified by etiology (see Table 14.1, p. 265) (tension, migraine, sinus); however, misdiagnosis is common, with migraine especially being misclassified as sinus or tension HA. Migraine HA is particularly disabling, affecting work productivity, routine household chores, and social relationships.[11] Chronic migraine (frequency ≥15 days/month) is more common in women than men, with peaks in midlife for both sexes. Chronic migraine is more prevalent among whites and Hispanics. The traditional etiologic explanation was spasm of cerebral vessels, causing vasodilation. Current theories include stimulation of cranial nerve V (trigeminal), with neurotransmitter changes in the central nervous system and changes in vessel tone.[4]

SUBJECTIVE DATA

1. Headache	3. Dizziness	5. Lumps or swelling
2. Head injury	4. Neck pain, limitation of motion	6. History of head or neck surgery

Examiner Asks	Rationale
1. Headache. Any unusually frequent or unusually severe **headaches?** • Onset. When did *this kind* of headache start? • Gradual, over hours or a day? • Or suddenly, over minutes or less than 1 hour? • Ever had *this kind* of headache before? • Location. Where do you feel it: frontal, temporal, behind your eyes, like a band around the head, in the sinus area, or in the occipital area? • Is pain localized on one side or all over? • Character. Throbbing (pounding, shooting) or aching (viselike, constant pressure, dull)?	This is a more meaningful question than "Do you ever have headaches?" because most people have had at least one HA. Because many conditions have a HA a detailed history is important. A red flag is a severe HA in an adult or child who has never had one before. Tension headaches are occipital, frontal, or with bandlike tightness; migraines are supraorbital, retro-orbital, or frontotemporal; sinus headaches produce pain around the eye or cheek. Unilateral or bilateral (e.g., with cluster headaches, pain is always unilateral and always on the same side of the head). Character is viselike with tension headache, throbbing with migraine or temporal arteritis (see Table 14.1, p. 265).

Examiner Asks	Rationale

- Is it mild, moderate, or severe?

- Course and duration. What time of day do the headaches occur: morning, evening, awaken you from sleep?
  How long do they last? Hours, days?
  Have you noted any daily headaches or several within a time period?
- Precipitating factors. What brings it on: activity or exercise, work environment, emotional upset, anxiety, alcohol? (Also note signs of depression.)
- Associated factors. Any relation to other symptoms: any nausea and vomiting? (Note which came first, headache or nausea.) Any vision changes, pain with bright lights, neck pain or stiffness, fever, weakness, moodiness, stomach problems?

- Do you have any other illness?

- Do you take any medications?

- What makes it worse: movement, coughing, straining, exercise?
- Pattern. Any family history of headache?
- What is the frequency of your headaches: once a week? Are your headaches occurring closer together?
- Are they getting worse? Or are they getting better?
- (For females) When do they occur in relation to your menstrual periods?
- Effort to treat. What seems to help: going to sleep, medications, positions, rubbing the area?

- Patient-centered care. How have these headaches affected your self-care or your ability to function at work, home, and socially? What do you need to help you cope?

2. Head Injury. Any **head injury** or blow to your head?

- Onset. When? Please describe exactly what happened.
- Setting. Any hazardous conditions? Were you wearing a helmet or hard hat?
- How did you feel just before injury: dizzy, light-headed, had a blackout, had a seizure?
- Lose consciousness and then fall? (Note which came first.)
- Knocked unconscious? Or did you fall and lose consciousness a few minutes later?
- Any history of illness (e.g., heart trouble, diabetes, epilepsy)?
- Location. Exactly where did you hit your head?

Rationale

Pain is often severe with migraine or excruciating with cluster headache.

Migraines occur ≥15 days/month if chronic or <15 days/month if episodic; each lasting 1 to 3 days.

Alcohol, stress, menstruation, and eating chocolate or cheese may precipitate migraines.

Nausea, vomiting, and visual disturbances are associated with migraines; anxiety and stress are associated with tension headaches; nuchal rigidity and fever are associated with meningitis or encephalitis.

Hypertension, fever, hypothyroidism, and vasculitis produce headaches.

Oral contraceptives, bronchodilators, alcohol, nitrates, and carbon monoxide inhalation produce headaches.

Migraines have a family history.

See Table 14.1, Primary Headaches, p. 265.

With migraines people lie down to feel better, whereas with cluster headaches they need to move—even to pace the floor—to feel better.

Concussion results after a direct blow to the skull causes the brain to shift rapidly back and forth inside (see Health Promotion and Patient Teaching, p. 262).

Evidence consistently shows that helmet use decreases the severity of injuries after a motorcycle crash and increases the chance of survival.[2]

Loss of consciousness *before* a fall may have a cardiac cause (e.g., heart block).

Examiner Asks	Rationale
• Duration. How long were you unconscious? Any symptoms afterward—headache, vomiting, projectile vomiting? Any change in level of consciousness *after* injury: dazed or sleepy?	A changing level of consciousness is most important in evaluating neurologic deficit.
• Associated symptoms. Any pain in the head or neck, vision change, discharge from ear or nose—is it bloody or watery? Are you able to move all extremities? Any tremors, staggered walk, numbness, and tingling? • Pattern. Are symptoms worse, better, unchanged since injury? • Effort to treat. Emergency department or hospitalized? Any medications?	
3. Dizziness. Experienced any **dizziness**? Tell me what you mean by dizziness. Describe it for me. ("Dizziness" is a vague, general term, related to multiple causes. Try not to prompt the person by suggesting descriptors such as "spinning," but note words offered. "I feel like I'm going to faint" suggests presyncope; "I feel like I'm spinning" suggests vertigo; "I feel like I'm going to fall down" suggests disequilibrium.[7])	Dizziness includes: **Presyncope**, a light-headed, swimming sensation or feeling of fainting or falling caused by decreased blood flow to brain or heart irregularity causing decreased cardiac output. **Vertigo** is true rotational spinning often from labyrinthine-vestibular disorder in inner ear. With *objective* vertigo the person feels like the room is spinning; with *subjective* vertigo the person feels like he or she is spinning. **Disequilibrium** is a shakiness or instability when walking related to musculoskeletal disorder or multisensory deficits.[7]
• Onset. Abrupt or gradual? After a change in position such as sudden standing? • Associated factors. Any nausea and vomiting, pallor, immobility, decreased hearing acuity, or tinnitus along with the dizziness? Any palpitations or shortness of breath?	Vertigo together with unilateral hearing loss suggests Meniere disease.[12]
4. Neck Pain. Any neck pain? • Onset. How did the pain start: injury, automobile accident, after lifting, from a fall? Or with fever? Or did it have a gradual onset? • Location. Does pain radiate? To the shoulders, arms? • Associated symptoms. Any **limitations to range of motion** (ROM), numbness or tingling in shoulders, arms, or hands? • Precipitating factors. Which movements cause pain? Do you need to lift or bend at work or home? • Does stress seem to bring it on? • Patient-centered care. Able to do your work, sleep? What do you need to help you cope?	Acute onset of neck stiffness, HA, fever occurs with meningitis. Pain creates a vicious circle. Tension increases pain and disability, which produces more anxiety.
5. Lumps or Swelling. Any **lumps** or **swelling** in the neck? Any recent infection? Any tenderness? For a lump that persists, how long have you had it? Has it changed in size?	Tenderness suggests acute infection. A persistent lump arouses suspicion of malignancy. For people older than 40 years, suspect malignancy until proven otherwise.
• Any history of prior irradiation of head, neck, upper chest?	Increased risk for salivary and thyroid tumors.
• Any difficulty swallowing? • Do you smoke? For how long? How many packs a day? Do you chew tobacco?	**Dysphagia.** Smoking and chewing tobacco increase risk for oral and respiratory cancer.

Examiner Asks	Rationale
• When was your last alcoholic drink? How much alcohol do you drink a day?	Smoking and moderate-to-heavy alcohol drinking increase the risk for cancer.
• Ever had a thyroid problem? Overfunctioning or underfunctioning? How was it treated: surgery, irradiation, any medication?	
6. History of Head or Neck Surgery. Ever had surgery of the head or neck? For what condition? When did the surgery occur? How do you feel about results?	Surgery for head and neck cancer often is disfiguring and increases risk for body image disturbance.

Additional History for Infants and Children

1. Did the mother use alcohol or street drugs during pregnancy? How often? How much was used per episode?	Alcohol increases the risk for fetal alcohol spectrum disorders, with distinctive facial features (see Table 14.2, p. 268). Cocaine use causes neurologic, developmental, and emotional problems.
2. Was delivery vaginal or by cesarean section? Any difficulty? Use of forceps?	Forceps may increase the risk for caput succedaneum, cephalhematoma, and Bell palsy.
3. What were you told about the baby's growth? Was it on schedule? Did the head seem to grow and fontanels close on schedule? Did the baby achieve head control? At about what age (in months)?	

Additional History for the Aging Adult

1. Patient-centered care. If dizziness is a problem, how does this affect your daily activities? Are you able to drive safely, maneuver about the house safely?	Assess self-care. Assess potential for injury.
2. If neck pain is a problem, how does this affect your daily activities? Are you able to turn head while driving, perform at work, do housework, sleep, look down when using stairs?	

OBJECTIVE DATA

Normal Range of Findings	Abnormal Findings

The Head

Inspect and Palpate the Skull

Size and Shape

Note the general size and shape. **Normocephalic** is the term that denotes a round symmetric skull that is appropriately related to body size. Be aware that "normal" includes a wide range of sizes.

To assess shape, place your fingers in the person's hair and palpate the scalp. The skull normally feels symmetric and smooth. Cranial bones that have normal protrusions are the forehead, the side of each parietal bone, the occipital bone, and the mastoid process behind each ear. There is no tenderness to palpation.

Microcephaly, abnormally small head; macrocephaly, abnormally large head (hydrocephaly, acromegaly). (See Table 14.2, p. 266).

Note lumps, depressions, or abnormal protrusions.

Temporal Area

Palpate the temporal artery above the zygomatic (cheek) bone between the eye and top of the ear.

The temporomandibular joint is just below the temporal artery and anterior to the tragus. Palpate the joint as the person opens the mouth and note normally smooth movement with no limitation or tenderness.

Tenderness and a hard band to palpation with temporal arteritis.

Crepitation, limited ROM, or tenderness.

Normal Range of Findings	Abnormal Findings

Inspect the Face

Facial Structures

Inspect the face, noting the facial expression and its appropriateness to behavior or reported mood. Anxiety is common in the hospitalized or ill person.

Although the shape of facial structures may vary somewhat depending on ancestry, features always should be symmetric. Expect symmetry of eyebrows, palpebral fissures, nasolabial folds, and sides of the mouth.

Note any abnormal facial structures (coarse facial features, exophthalmos, changes in skin color or pigmentation) or any abnormal swelling. Also note any involuntary movements (tics) in the facial muscles. Normally none occur.

Abnormal Findings:

Hostility or aggression.

Tense, rigid muscles may indicate anxiety or pain; a flat affect may indicate depression.

Marked asymmetry with central brain lesion (e.g., stroke) or peripheral cranial nerve VII damage (Bell palsy). See Table 14.5, Abnormal Facies With Chronic Illness, p. 272.

Edema in the face occurs first around the eyes (periorbital) and the cheeks, where the subcutaneous tissue is relatively loose.

Note grinding of jaws, tics, fasciculations, or excessive blinking.

Nystagmis accompanies a presenting concern of vertigo.

The Neck

Inspect and Palpate the Neck

Symmetry

Head position is centered in the midline, and the accessory neck muscles should be symmetric. The head should be held erect and still.

Abnormal Findings:

Head tilt occurs with muscle spasm. Rigid head and neck occur with arthritis.

Range of Motion (ROM)

Note any limitation of movement during active motion. Ask the person to touch the chin to the chest, turn the head to the right and left, try to touch each ear to the shoulder (without elevating shoulders), and extend the head backward. When the neck is supple, motion is smooth and controlled.

Abnormal Findings:

Note pain at any specific movement.

Note ratchety or limited movement from cervical arthritis or inflammation of neck muscles. The arthritic neck is rigid; the person turns at the shoulders rather than at the neck.

Test muscle strength and the status of cranial nerve XI by trying to resist the person's movements with your hands as the person shrugs the shoulders and turns the head to each side.

As the person moves the head, note enlargement of the salivary and lymph glands. Normally, no enlargement is present. Note a swollen parotid gland when the head is extended; look for swelling below the angle of the jaw. Also note thyroid gland enlargement. Normally, none is present.

Abnormal Findings:

Thyroid enlargement may be a unilateral lump, or it may be diffuse and look like a doughnut lying across the lower neck (see Table 14.3, Swellings on the Head or Neck, p. 269).

Also note any obvious pulsations. The carotid artery runs medial to the sternomastoid muscle, and it creates a brisk localized pulsation just below the angle of the jaw. Normally, there are no other pulsations while the person is in the sitting position (see Chapter 20).

Lymph Nodes

Using a gentle circular motion of your finger pads, palpate the lymph nodes (Fig. 14.9). (Normally, the salivary glands are not palpable. When symptoms warrant, check for parotid tenderness by palpating in a line from the outer corner of the eye to the lobule of the ear.) Beginning with the preauricular lymph nodes in front of the ear, palpate the 10 groups of lymph nodes in a routine order. Many nodes are closely packed, so you must be systematic and thorough in your examination. Once you establish your sequence, do not vary or you may miss some small nodes.

Abnormal Findings:

The parotid is swollen with mumps (see Table 14.3, p. 270).

Parotid enlargement has been found with AIDS. See discussion of enlarged lymph nodes, lymphadenopathy, p. 256.

Normal Range of Findings

Abnormal Findings

Posterior auricular — ② ①— Preauricular

Occipital — ③

Jugulodigastric — ⑥

Superficial cervical — ⑦

⑤ ④

Submandibular

Submental

⑨ ⑧

Posterior cervical

Supraclavicular — ⑩

Deep cervical chain

14.9

Use gentle pressure because strong pressure could push the nodes into the neck muscles. It is usually most efficient to palpate with both hands, comparing the two sides symmetrically. However, the submental gland under the tip of the chin is easier to explore with one hand. When you palpate with one hand, use your other hand to position the person's head. For the deep cervical chain, tip the person's head toward the side being examined to relax the ipsilateral muscle (Fig. 14.10). Then you can press your fingers under the muscle. Search for the supraclavicular node by having the person hunch the shoulders and elbows forward (Fig. 14.11); this relaxes the skin. The inferior belly of the omohyoid muscle crosses the posterior triangle here; do not mistake it for a lymph node.

Objective Data

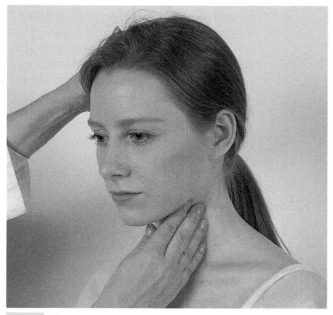

14.10   Palpate the deep cervical chain.

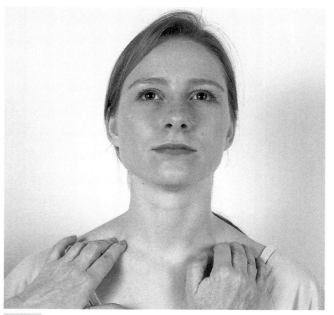

14.11   Palpate supraclavicular nodes.

Normal Range of Findings

If any nodes are palpable, note their location, size, shape, delimitation (discrete or matted together), mobility, consistency, and tenderness. Cervical nodes often are palpable in healthy persons, although this palpability decreases with age (Fig. 14.12, *A*). Normal nodes feel movable, discrete, soft, and nontender.

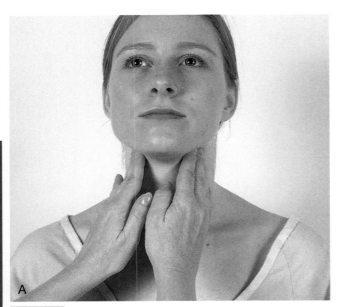

14.12, A

If nodes are enlarged or tender, check the area they drain for the source of the problem. For example, those in the upper cervical or submandibular area often relate to inflammation or a neoplasm in the head and neck. Follow up on or refer your findings. An enlarged lymph node, particularly when you cannot find the source of the problem, deserves prompt attention.

Abnormal Findings

Lymphadenopathy means enlargement of the lymph nodes (>1 cm) from infection, allergy, or neoplasm. (See Fig. 14.12, *B*, due to infectious mononucleosis.)

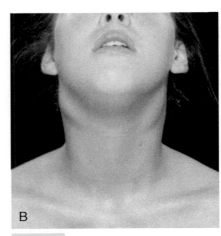

14.12, B   (Dean, Garrett, and Tyrrell, 2008.)

The following criteria are common clues but are not definitive in all cases:
- Acute infection—acute onset, <14 days' duration; nodes are bilateral, enlarged, warm, tender, and firm but freely movable.
- Chronic inflammation (e.g., in tuberculosis the nodes are clumped).
- Cancerous nodes are hard (feel like a rock), >3 cm, unilateral, nontender, matted, and fixed to adjacent structures.
- Nodes with HIV infection are enlarged, firm, nontender, and mobile. Occipital node enlargement is common with HIV infection.
- A single enlarged, nontender, hard left supraclavicular node may indicate neoplasm in thorax or abdomen (Virchow node).
- Painless, rubbery, discrete nodes that gradually appear occur with Hodgkin lymphoma, commonly in the cervical region.

Normal Range of Findings	Abnormal Findings

Trachea

Normally, the trachea is midline; palpate for any tracheal shift. Place your index finger on the trachea in the sternal notch and slip it off to each side (Fig. 14.13). The space should be symmetric on both sides. Note any deviation from the midline.

Conditions of tracheal shift:
- The trachea is *pushed to the unaffected* (or healthy) side with an aortic aneurysm, a tumor, unilateral thyroid lobe enlargement, and pneumothorax.
- The trachea is *pulled toward the affected* (diseased) side with large atelectasis, pleural adhesions, or fibrosis.
- Tracheal tug is a rhythmic downward pull that is synchronous with systole and occurs with aortic arch aneurysm.

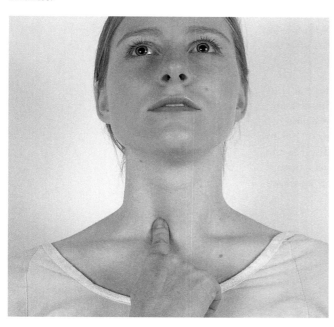

14.13

Thyroid Gland

The thyroid gland is difficult to palpate; arrange your setting to maximize your likelihood of success. Position a standing lamp to shine tangentially across the neck to highlight any possible swelling. Tilt the head back to stretch the skin against the thyroid. Supply the person with a glass of water and first inspect the neck as the person takes a sip and swallows. Thyroid tissue moves up with a swallow and then falls into its resting position.

Posterior Approach. To palpate, move behind the person (Fig. 14.14, *A*). Ask the person to sit up very straight and then to bend the head slightly forward and to the right. This relaxes the neck muscles on the right side. Use the fingers of your left hand to push the trachea slightly to the right.

Look for diffuse enlargement or a nodular lump.

Abnormalities: enlarged lobes that are easily palpated before swallowing or are tender to palpation (see large goiter in Fig. 14.14, *B*) or the presence of nodules or lumps. See Table 14.4, Thyroid Hormone Disorders, p. 271.

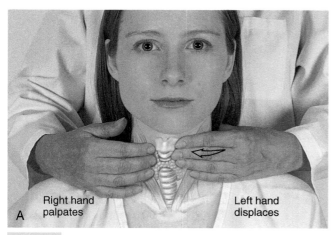

Right hand palpates · Left hand displaces

A

14.14, A

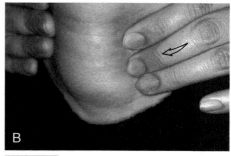

B

14.14, B

(Lemmi & Lemmi, 2011.)

Objective Data

Normal Range of Findings	Abnormal Findings

Curve your right fingers between the trachea and the sternomastoid muscle, retracting it slightly, and ask the person to take a sip of water. The thyroid moves up under your palpating fingers with the trachea and larynx as the person swallows. Reverse the procedure for the left side.

Often you cannot palpate the normal adult thyroid. If the person has a long, thin neck, you sometimes feel the isthmus over the tracheal rings. The lateral lobes usually are not palpable; palpable lobes feel rubbery but smooth. Check them for enlargement, consistency (soft, firm, or hard), symmetry, and the presence of nodules.

Anterior Approach. This is an alternate method of palpating the thyroid, but it is more awkward to perform, especially for a beginning examiner. Stand facing the person. Try to identify the isthmus by placing your thumb 3 cm below the thyroid cartilage prominence as the person swallows. Then, ask him or her to tip the head forward and to the right. Use your right thumb to displace the trachea slightly to the person's right. Hook your left thumb and fingers around the sternomastoid muscle. Feel for lobe enlargement as the person swallows (Fig. 14.15).

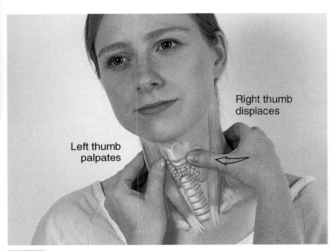

Left thumb palpates

Right thumb displaces

14.15

Auscultate the Thyroid

If the thyroid gland is enlarged, auscultate it for the presence of a **bruit**. This is a soft, pulsatile, whooshing, blowing sound heard best with the bell of the stethoscope. The bruit is not present normally.

A bruit occurs with accelerated or turbulent blood flow, indicating hyperplasia of the thyroid (e.g., hyperthyroidism).

DEVELOPMENTAL COMPETENCE

Infants and Children
Skull

Measure an infant's **head size** with measuring tape at each visit up to age 2 years, then annually up to age 6 years. (Measurement of head circumference is presented in detail in Chapter 9.)

The newborn's head measures about 32 to 38 cm (average around 34 cm) and is 2 cm larger than chest circumference. At age 2 years both measurements are the same. During childhood the chest circumference grows to exceed head circumference by 5 to 7 cm.

Note an abnormal increase in head size or failure to grow.

Microcephalic—head size less than norms for age. Macrocephalic—an enlarged head or head rapidly increasing in size (e.g., hydrocephalus [increased cerebrospinal fluid]).

Normal Range of Findings

Observe the infant's head from all angles, not just the front. The contour should be symmetric. Some racial variation occurs in normal head shapes.

Two common variations in the newborn cause the shape of the skull to look markedly asymmetric. A **caput succedaneum** is edematous swelling and ecchymosis of the presenting part of the head caused by birth trauma (Fig. 14.16). It feels soft, and it may extend across suture lines. It gradually resolves during the first few days of life and needs no treatment.

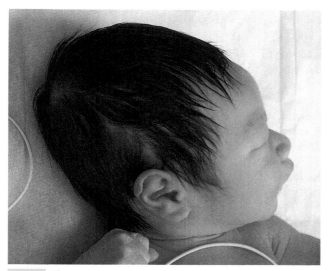

14.16   Caput succedaneum. (Murray and McKinney, 2014.)

A **cephalhematoma** is a subperiosteal hemorrhage, which is also a result of birth trauma (Fig. 14.17, *A*). It is soft, fluctuant, and well defined over one cranial bone because the periosteum (i.e., the covering over each bone) holds the bleeding in place. It appears several hours after birth and gradually increases in size. No discoloration is present, but it looks bizarre; parents need reassurance that it will be resorbed during the first few weeks of life without treatment. Rarely a large hematoma may persist to 3 months.

As you palpate the newborn's head, the suture lines feel like ridges. By 5 to 6 months they are smooth and not palpable.

Abnormal Findings

Frontal bulges, or "bossing," occur with prematurity or rickets.

An infant with cephalhematoma is at greater risk for jaundice as the red blood cells within the hematoma are broken down and reabsorbed (Fig. 14.17, *B*).

Sutures palpable when the child is older than 6 months.

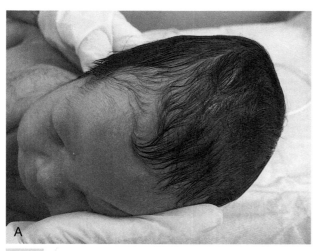

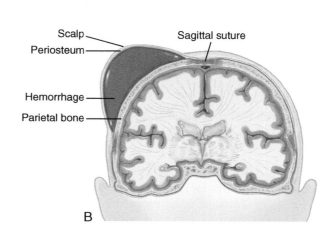

14.17   **A,** Cephalhematoma. (Murray and McKinney, 2014.)

Objective Data

Normal Range of Findings

A newborn's head may feel asymmetric, and the involved ridges more prominent because of *molding* of the cranial bones during engagement and passage through the birth canal. Molding is overriding of the cranial bones; usually the parietal bone overrides the frontal or occipital bone. Reassure parents that this lasts only a few days or a week. Babies delivered by cesarean section are noted for their evenly round heads.

Also, *positional molding* (**positional plagiocephaly**) may occur as the infant continually sleeps in the recommended position on the back to decrease the incidence of sudden infant death syndrome (SIDS). This is a flattening of the dependent cranial bone, the occiput, in an infant who did not have occipital flatness at birth. Inspection from behind shows a normal-appearing head shape with even horizontally placed ears. Inspection from the top shows a flat side of the occiput with the ear on that side displaced anteriorly, and the ear may fold forward. Head circumference is normal. (Note patient teaching on p. 262.)

Gently palpate the skull and **fontanels** while the infant is calm and somewhat in a sitting position (crying, lying down, or vomiting may cause the anterior fontanel to look full and bulging). The skull should feel smooth and fused except at the fontanels. The fontanels feel firm, slightly concave, and well defined against the edges of the cranial bones. You may see slight arterial pulsations in the anterior fontanel.

The posterior fontanel may not be palpable at birth. If it is, it measures 1 cm and closes by 1 to 2 months. The anterior fontanel may be small at birth and enlarge to 2.5 cm × 2.5 cm. A large diameter of 4 to 5 cm occasionally may be normal under 6 months. A small fontanel usually is normal. The anterior fontanel closes between 9 months and 2 years. Early closure may be insignificant if head growth proceeds normally.

Note the infant's **head posture** and **head control.** The infant can turn the head side to side by 2 weeks and shows the **tonic neck reflex** when supine and the head is turned to one side (extension of same arm and leg, flexion of opposite arm and leg) (Fig. 14.18). The tonic neck reflex disappears between 3 and 4 months, and then the head is maintained in the midline. Head control is achieved by 4 months, when the baby can hold the head erect and steady when pulled to a vertical position. (See Chapters 23 and 24 for further details.)

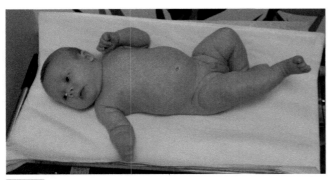

14.18 Tonic neck reflex.

Face

Check **facial features** for symmetry, appearance, and presence of swelling. Note symmetry of wrinkling when the infant cries or smiles (e.g., both sides of the lips rise, and both sides of forehead wrinkle). Children love to comply when you ask them to "make a face." Normally, no swelling is evident. Parotid gland

Abnormal Findings

Marked asymmetry, as in *craniosynostosis,* is a severe deformity caused by premature closure of the sutures. This causes a distinctive head shape (see Table 14.2, p. 267) that correlates with the specific closed suture.

Marked plagiocephaly (see Table 14.2) requires a custom-shaped helmet to afford room for brain growth in the flattened area while moderating growth in other areas. Used before sutures fuse.

Flattening also occurs with rickets.

A true tense or bulging fontanel occurs with acute increased intracranial pressure.

Depressed and sunken fontanels occur with dehydration or malnutrition.

Marked pulsations occur with increased intracranial pressure.

Delayed closure or larger-than-normal fontanel size occurs with hydrocephalus, Down syndrome, hypothyroidism, or rickets.

A small fontanel is a sign of microcephaly, as is early closure.

Tonic neck reflex beyond 5 months may indicate brain damage.

In children head tilt occurs with habit spasm, poor vision, and brain tumor.

Head lag after 4 months may indicate mental or motor retardation.

Unilateral immobility indicates nerve damage (central or peripheral) (e.g., note angle of mouth droop on paralyzed side).

Normal Range of Findings	**Abnormal Findings**

enlargement is seen best when the child sits and looks up at the ceiling; the swelling appears below the angle of the jaw.

Some facies are characteristic of congenital abnormalities or chronic allergy. See Table 14.2, p. 267.

Neck

An infant's neck looks short; it lengthens during the first 3 to 4 years. You can see the neck better by supporting the infant's shoulders and tilting the head back a little. This positioning also enhances palpation of the trachea, which is buried deep in the neck. Feel for the row of cartilaginous rings in the midline or just slightly to the right of midline.

A short neck or webbing (loose fanlike folds) may indicate congenital abnormality (e.g., Down or Turner syndrome), or it may occur alone.

Assess muscle development with gentle passive ROM. Cradle the infant's head with your hands and turn it side to side and test forward flexion, extension, and rotation. Note any resistance to movement, especially flexion. Ask a child to actively move through the ROM, as you would an adult.

Head tilt and limited ROM occur with torticollis (wryneck) or from sternomastoid muscle injury during birth or a congenital defect.
Resistance to flexion (nuchal rigidity) and pain on flexion suggest meningitis.

During infancy cervical lymph nodes are not palpable normally. But a child's lymph nodes are—they feel more prominent than an adult's until after puberty, when lymphoid tissue begins to atrophy. Palpable nodes less than 3 mm are normal. They may be up to 1 cm in size in the cervical and inguinal areas but are discrete, move easily, and are nontender. Children have a higher incidence of infection, so you can expect a greater incidence of inflammatory adenopathy. No other mass should occur in the neck.

Cervical nodes >1 cm are considered enlarged.
Thyroglossal duct cyst—cystic lump high up in midline, tense, nontender, freely movable, and rises up when swallowing.
Supraclavicular nodes enlarge with Hodgkin lymphoma.

The thyroid gland is difficult to palpate in an infant because of the short, thick neck. The child's thyroid may be palpable normally.

Special Procedures

Percussion. With an infant, you may directly percuss with your plexor finger against the head surface. This yields a resonant or "cracked pot" sound, which is normal before closure of the fontanels.

Auscultation. Bruits are common in the skull in children younger than 4 or 5 years or in children with anemia. They are systolic or continuous and are heard over the temporal area.

The sound occurs with hydrocephalus from separation of cranial sutures (Macewen sign).
After 5 years of age, bruits indicate increased intracranial pressure, aneurysm, or arteriovenous shunt.

The Pregnant Woman

During the second trimester chloasma may show on the face. This is a blotchy, hyperpigmented area over the cheeks and forehead that fades after delivery. The thyroid gland may be palpable normally during pregnancy.

The Aging Adult

The temporal arteries may look twisted and prominent. In some aging adults a mild rhythmic tremor of the head may be normal. **Isolated head tremors** are benign and include head nodding (as if saying yes or no) and tongue protrusion. If some teeth have been lost, the lower face looks unusually small, with the mouth sunken in.

Painful to palpation with giant cell arteritis, an inflammatory condition affecting older adults, with peak incidences between 70-90 years.[16]

The neck may show an increased anterior cervical (concave or inward) curve when the head and jaw are extended forward to compensate for kyphosis of the spine. During the examination, direct the older adult to perform ROM slowly; he or she may experience dizziness with side movements. An older adult may have prolapse of the submandibular glands, which could be mistaken for a tumor. But drooping submandibular glands feel soft and are present bilaterally.

Many older adults have low-lying thyroid glands that are impossible to palpate. The gland lies behind the sternomastoid muscles and clavicles.

Objective Data

HEALTH PROMOTION AND PATIENT TEACHING

(To the parents of a newborn.) *"Because your baby sleeps flat on the back, I would like to teach you about tummy time during the day; place the baby on his or her tummy while awake and supervised."* This helps prevent the development of flat spots (positional plagiocephaly) on the back of the head and helps strengthen head, neck, and shoulder muscles. A newborn can be prone on the parent's lap 2-3 times a day for a few minutes, with a gradual increase to 20 minutes a day on the floor for a 3- to 4-month-old.

(To young athletes and parents of athletes.) *"We want you to stay safe in your sport, and most athletes and parents do not know the signs of concussion. A concussion is a direct blow to the head, causing the brain inside to rattle back and forth on its attachments. Serious signs of concussion are forgetfulness of recent events, loss of consciousness, and mental cloudiness. Other signs are headache, nausea and vomiting, loss of balance, and blurred vision. Later signs include difficulty in concentrating, poor short-term memory, slow reaction time,* and *irritability."*[9] Young athletes are more susceptible to concussion because of thinner cranial bones, larger head-to-body ratio, immature central nervous system, and larger subarachnoid space in which the brain can rattle. A detailed history with evidence of direct impact helps with diagnosis. After a concussion a graduated return to play is best. Recovery is a stepwise progression with 24 hours or more in each step: complete physical and brain rest; light aerobic exercise (walking, swimming, stationary bike); sport-specific exercise that is nonimpact, such as running in soccer; noncontact training drills; full-contact "controlled" practice after medical clearance; and then return to normal game play.[9] The U.S. Centers for Disease Control and Prevention (CDC) has created online courses called **HEADS UP: Concussion in Youth Sports,** designed for health care professionals and youths, parents, and coaches. This material is easily accessed at https://www.cdc.gov/headsup/policy/index.html.

DOCUMENTATION AND CRITICAL THINKING

Sample Charting

SUBJECTIVE

Denies any unusually frequent or severe headache; no history of head injury, dizziness, or syncope; no neck pain, limitation of motion, lumps, or swelling.

OBJECTIVE

Head: Normocephalic, no lumps, no lesions, no tenderness, no trauma.
Face: Symmetric, no drooping, no weakness, no involuntary movements.
Neck: Supple with full ROM, no pain. Symmetric, no cervical lymphadenopathy or masses. Trachea midline, thyroid not palpable. No bruits.

ASSESSMENT

Normocephalic, atraumatic, and symmetric head and neck

Clinical Case Study 1

F.V. is a 57-year-old insurance executive who is in his 4th postoperative day after a transurethral resection of the prostate gland. He also has chronic hypertension, managed by oral hydrochlorothiazide, exercise, and a low-salt diet.

SUBJECTIVE

Complaining of dizziness, a light-headed feeling that occurred on standing and cleared on sitting. States, "I'm afraid of falling." No previous episodes of dizziness. Denies palpitations, nausea, or vomiting. States urine pink-tinged as it was yesterday, with no red blood. No pain medications today. On 2nd day of same antihypertensive medication he took before surgery.

OBJECTIVE

Vital signs: BP 142/88 mm Hg RA sitting, 94/58 mm Hg RA standing. Pulse 94 bpm sitting and standing, regular rhythm, no skipped beats. Temp 98.6° F (37° C). Color tannish-pink, no pallor, skin warm and dry.

Neuro: Alert and oriented to person, place, and time. Speech clear and fluent. Moving all extremities, no weakness. No nystagmus, no ataxia, past-pointing test normal. Romberg sign negative (normal). Intake/output in balance. Urine faint pink-tinged, no clots.

Lab: Hematocrit 45%, serum chemistries normal.

ASSESSMENT

Orthostatic hypotension
Presyncope
Potential for falls

Clinical Case Study 2

A.B. is a 33-year-old female civil engineer with no known health problems, on no medication, taking a multivitamin daily.

SUBJECTIVE

Delivered a healthy baby girl 13 months PTA, not breastfeeding, baby sleeps through the night. A.B.'s menses regular since delivery but reports that the flow is heavy. A.B. reports that she feels depressed, is unable to lose weight despite efforts, has severe fatigue, reporting "some days I feel like I can't even lift my arms," weakness (hard to open a jar). She also reports brittle nails, constipation, and an increased sensitivity to cold.

OBJECTIVE

Vital signs: BP 118/88 mm Hg. Temp 96.9° F (36.1° C); Pulse 62 bpm regular. Resp 12/min.
General appearance: Skin cool, pale, and dry. Nails appear brittle but kempt.
Neck: Thyroid enlarged on palpation but no nodules. No lymphadenopathy.
Lungs: Clear and equal bilaterally.
Heart: S_1 S_2 regular, no murmurs or extra heart sounds.
Lab: TSH 6.29 MIU/mL (range 0.47-4.68 MIU/mL), free T_4: 0.9 ng/dL (range 0.8-2.2 ng/dL)

ASSESSMENT

Hypothyroidism by lab results
Fatigue R/T hypothyroidism

Clinical Case Study 3

L.M. is a 36-year-old female auto plant worker here today for mild abdominal pain, hot flashes, palpitations, and anxiety, reporting, "I'm going to jump out of my skin."

SUBJECTIVE

Has been experiencing the previous symptoms for 3 months along with mild hand tremors, increased appetite, weight loss, heat intolerance, poor concentration, and difficulty sleeping. For the past month, L.M. has noticed that her eyes feel dry and irritated. She reports menstrual periods that are "not regular anymore." Last menstrual period 2 weeks PTA, scant flow.

OBJECTIVE

Vital signs: BP 90/60 mm Hg. Temp: 99.5° F (37.5° C). Pulse 145 bpm and irregular. Resp 24/min. Cardiac monitor located in office shows atrial fibrillation.

Documentation and Critical Thinking

Eyes: White sclera shows between iris and upper/lower lids when L.M. looks down. Staring, unblinking appearance.
Skin: Warm, moist, smooth. Perspiration evident.
Neck: Moderately enlarged thyroid with no nodules. No lymphadenopathy.
Heart: S_1 S_2 irregularly irregular with midsystolic murmur grade 2/6 at left lower sternal border.
Lungs: Clear and equal bilaterally.
Abdomen: Soft, no masses or tenderness. Active bowel sounds.
DTRs: Brisk ankle jerk. Other DTRs 2+ and = bilaterally.
Lab: Serum T_4 18.5 mcg/dL; TSH undetectable.

ASSESSMENT

Hyperthyroidism—Graves disease

Clinical Case Study 4

A.M. is a 5-year-old boy who presents to the clinic with his father. The family adopted a dog from the animal shelter 8 months PTA.

SUBJECTIVE

A.M.'s father reports that A.M. has had "sneezing fits," a runny nose, and coughing for the past few months and that it seems better when A.M. is at school. Father states, "He just won't stop rubbing his nose and eyes."

OBJECTIVE

Vital signs: Temp 98.6° F (37° C). BP 93/60 mm Hg (sitting). Pulse 90 bpm. Resp 24/min (at rest, open-mouthed).
General appearance: Alert and active child who is smiling and talkative.
HEENT: Normocephalic, no lumps, no lesions. Palpable anterior cervical lymph nodes (1 mm), discrete, move easily, nontender. Light-blue areas in skin under eyes, creasing present on palpebrae inferior and superior to the tip of nose. Minimal fluid in middle ear, denies tenderness to palpation of sinus cavities; swollen turbinates bilat, and consistently sniffles and clears throat. Reddened posterior pharynx c̄ exudate present.
Cardiovascular: No murmurs or abnormal heart sounds.
Respiratory: Breath sounds = bilat, expiratory wheezing present bilat that clears with cough.

ASSESSMENT

Allergic rhinitis R/T newly obtained household pet
Needs health teaching regarding allergies

ABNORMAL FINDINGS

TABLE 14.1	Primary Headaches (Diagnosed by Patient History With No Abnormal Findings in Physical Examination or Laboratory Testing)		
	Tension	**Migraine**	**Cluster**
	Tension	Migraine*	Cluster
Definition	Headache (HA) of musculoskeletal origin; may be a mild-to-moderate, less disabling form of migraine	HA of genetically transmitted vascular and trigeminal nerve origin; HA plus prodrome, aura, other symptoms; 2-3 times as common in women as in men[3]	Rare HA that is intermittent, excruciating, unilateral, with autonomic signs
Location	Usually both sides, across frontal, temporal, and/or occipital region of head: forehead, sides, and back of head	Commonly one-sided but may occur on both sides Pain is often behind the eyes, the temples, or forehead	Always one-sided Often behind or around the eye, temple, forehead, cheek
Character	Bandlike tightness, viselike Nonthrobbing, nonpulsatile	Throbbing, pulsating	Continuous, burning, piercing, excruciating
Duration	Gradual onset, lasts 30 minutes to days	Rapid onset, peaks 1-2 hr, lasts 4-72 hr, sometimes longer	Abrupt onset, peaks in minutes, lasts 45-90 min
Quantity and severity	Diffuse, dull aching pain Mild-to-moderate pain	Moderate-to-severe pain	Can occur multiple times a day, in "clusters," lasting weeks Severe, stabbing pain
Timing	Situational, in response to overwork, posture	≈2 per month, last 1-3 days ≈1 in 10 patients have weekly headaches	1-2/day, each lasting $\frac{1}{2}$ to 2 hr for 1 to 2 months; then remission for months or years
Aggravating symptoms or triggers	Stress, anxiety, depression, poor posture Not worsened by physical activity	Hormonal fluctuations (premenstrual) Foods (e.g., alcohol, caffeine, MSG, nitrates, chocolate, cheese) Hunger Letdown after stress Sleep deprivation Sensory stimuli (e.g., flashing lights or perfumes) Changes in weather Physical activity	Exacerbated by alcohol, stress, daytime napping, wind or heat exposure

*For a comparison with sinusitis, see Table 17.1, p. 367.

Continued

TABLE 14.1	Primary Headaches (Diagnosed by Patient History With No Abnormal Findings in Physical Examination or Laboratory Testing)—cont'd		
	Tension	**Migraine**	**Cluster**
Associated symptoms	Fatigue, anxiety, stress Sensation of a band tightening around head, of being gripped like a vise Sometimes photophobia or phonophobia	Aura (visual changes such as blind spots or flashes of light, tingling in an arm or leg, vertigo) Prodrome (change in mood, behavior, hunger, cravings, yawning) Nausea, vomiting, photophobia, phonophobia, abdominal pain Person looks sick Family history of migraine	Ipsilateral autonomic signs: Nasal congestion or runny nose, watery or reddened eye, eyelid drooping, miosis Feelings of agitation
Relieving factors, efforts to treat	Rest, massaging muscles in area, NSAID medication	Lie down, darken room, use eyeshade, sleep, take NSAID early, try to avoid opioid	Need to move, pace floor

Images © Pat Thomas, 2014.

TABLE 14.2	Pediatric Abnormalities

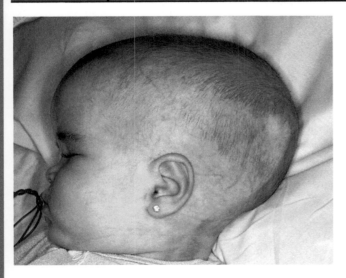

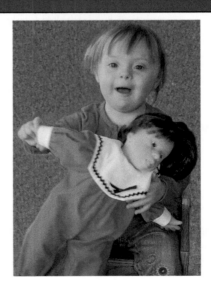

Hydrocephalus

Obstruction of drainage of cerebrospinal fluid results in excessive accumulation, increasing intracranial pressure, and enlargement of the head. The face looks small compared with the enlarged cranium. The increasing pressure also produces dilated scalp veins, frontal bossing, and downcast or "setting sun" eyes (sclera visible above iris). The cranial bones thin, sutures separate, and percussion yields a "cracked pot" sound (Macewen sign).

Down Syndrome

This is the most common chromosomal aberration (trisomy 21). Head and face characteristics may include upslanting eyes with inner epicanthal folds; flat nasal bridge; small, broad, flat nose; protruding, thick tongue; ear dysplasia; short, broad neck with webbing; and small hands with single palmar crease. Child also has mental disability, often congenital heart deformities. Educational services in many U.S. areas will maximize child's potential.

Continued

TABLE 14.2	**Pediatric Abnormalities—cont'd**

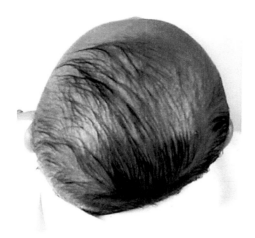

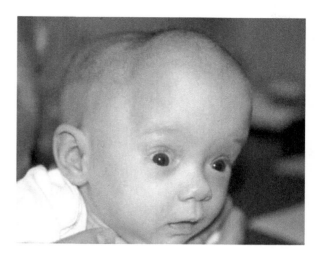

Plagiocephaly

Positional or deformational plagiocephaly has increased dramatically since the "Back to Sleep" campaign started in 1992 to prevent SIDS. It is asymmetry of the cranium when seen from the top caused by a positional preference. It is not associated with premature closing of cranial sutures, and growth of the brain proceeds normally. This can be mitigated by "tummy time," when the parent places the infant prone for awake playing. Physical therapy and corrective headbands are further treatments.

Craniosynostosis

Premature closing of one or multiple cranial sutures (shown above) results in a malformed head and a cosmetic deformity. Mechanisms involve genetic mutations coding structural proteins or growth factor receptors. Severe deformities cannot contain the brain, eyes, and optic nerves inside the cranial vault, and hypoplasia of the face results, warranting surgery.

Atopic (Allergic) Facies

Children with chronic allergies often develop characteristic facial features. These include exhausted face, blue shadows below the eyes ("allergic shiners") from sluggish venous return; a double or single crease on the lower eyelids (Morgan lines); central facial pallor; and open-mouth breathing (allergic gaping), which can lead to malocclusion of the teeth and malformed jaw because the child's bones are still forming.

▶

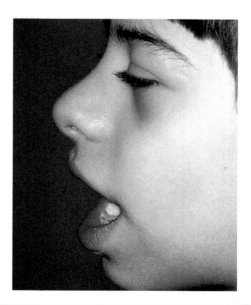

Continued

TABLE 14.2	Pediatric Abnormalities—cont'd

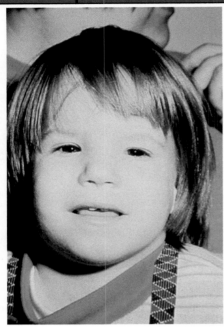

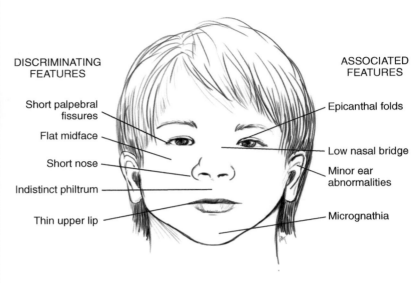

DISCRIMINATING FEATURES

- Short palpebral fissures
- Flat midface
- Short nose
- Indistinct philtrum
- Thin upper lip

ASSOCIATED FEATURES

- Epicanthal folds
- Low nasal bridge
- Minor ear abnormalities
- Micrognathia

Fetal Alcohol Spectrum Disorders (FASD)

Alcohol is teratogenic to the developing fetus, resulting in severe cognitive and psychosocial impairment and changes in facial and brain structure. The incidence is increasing in the United States, even with public warnings to avoid alcohol during pregnancy. Characteristic facies include narrow palpebral fissures, epicanthal folds, thin upper lip, and midfacial hypoplasia. These malformations may be recognizable at birth but more so during childhood. FASDs include a wide range of neurologic and behavioral deficits,[8] even without facial malformations. Infants often have smaller head circumference, decreased birth weight and length, feeding problems, and irritability. Children may exhibit intrusive talking, inattention, poor abstract reasoning, and problems with independent activities of daily living.[15] The severity of FASDs increases with the amount of alcohol consumed during pregnancy. This is now the leading preventable cause of intellectual disability, learning disability, and birth defects.[13]

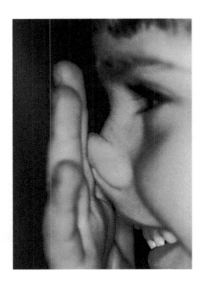

◀ Allergic Salute and Crease

The transverse line on the nose is also a feature of chronic allergies. It is formed when the child chronically uses the hand to push the nose up and back (the "allergic salute") to relieve itching and free swollen turbinates, which allow air passage.

TABLE 14.3	Swellings on the Head or Neck

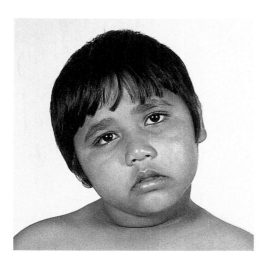

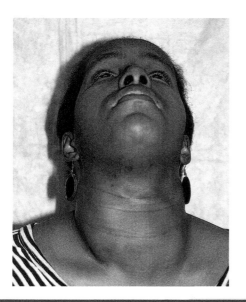

Congenital Torticollis

A hematoma in one sternomastoid muscle, probably injured by intrauterine malposition, results in head tilt to one side and limited neck ROM to the opposite side. You feel a firm, discrete, nontender mass in mid-muscle on the involved side. This requires treatment, or the muscle can become fibrotic and permanently shortened with permanent limitation of ROM, asymmetry of the head and face, and visual problems from a nonhorizontal position of the eyes.

Simple Diffuse Goiter (SDG)

Endemic goiter, a chronic enlargement of the thyroid gland, is common in wide regions of the world (especially mountainous regions) where the soil is low in iodine. Iodine is an essential element in the formation of thyroid hormones.

◄ Thyroid—Multinodular Goiter (MNG)

Multiple nodules usually indicate inflammation or a multinodular goiter rather than a neoplasm. However, suspect any rapidly enlarging or firm nodule. Refer all patients with a nodule for ultrasonography.

Single Nodule (not illustrated): Thyroid nodules are palpable in 1% to 5% of ambulatory care patients but can be identified in 50% of ultrasound studies.[10] Over 95% of these are benign. Suspect any painless, rapidly growing nodule, especially a single nodule in a young person. Cancerous nodules usually are hard and fixed to surrounding structures. At increased risk are females; persons with a history of goiter or nodules, or family history of thyroid cancer[1]; size >4 cm; and persons with a history of radiation exposure, especially in childhood.[5]

Continued

TABLE 14.3   Swellings on the Head or Neck—cont'd

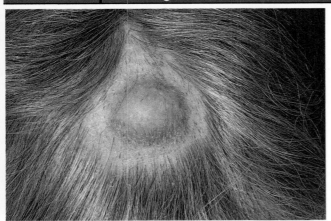

◀ Pilar Cyst (Wen)

This is a smooth, firm, fluctuant swelling on the scalp that contains sebum and keratin. Tense pressure of the contents causes overlying skin to be shiny and taut. It is a benign growth.

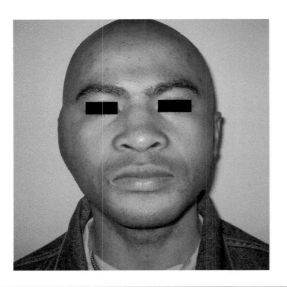

◀ Parotid Gland Enlargement

Rapid painful inflammation of the parotid occurs with mumps. Mumps is a contagious viral infection of the salivary glands preventable by a vaccine. Parotid swelling also occurs with blockage of a duct, abscess, or tumor. Note swelling anterior to lower ear lobe. Stensen duct obstruction can occur in aging adults dehydrated from diuretics or anticholinergics.

ROM, Range of motion.
See Illustration Credits for source information.

TABLE 14.4	Thyroid Hormone Disorders

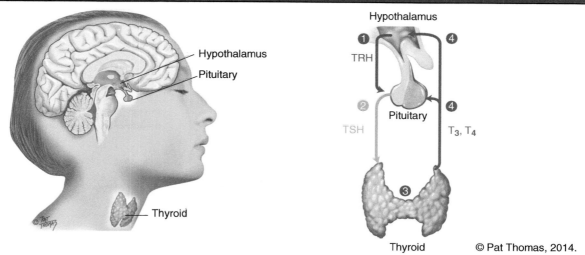

© Pat Thomas, 2014.

The hypothalamic-pituitary-thyroid axis regulates the production of thyroid hormones by a negative feedback system, much like the thermostat that guides your household furnace. (1) The hypothalamus secretes thyrotropin-releasing hormone (TRH), which (2) acts on the anterior pituitary to secrete thyroid-stimulating hormone (TSH), which (3) directs the thyroid gland to produce T_3 and T_4 hormones. When T_3 and T_4 hormones are high in the bloodstream ("hot" like a furnace), they (4) direct the pituitary and hypothalamus to shut off their signaling hormones. That is the negative feedback. When T_3 and T_4 hormone levels are low (thyroid is like a cold furnace), the pituitary sends out increasing TSH to stimulate new production of T_3 and T_4 hormones. Your body metabolism is most comfortable in a healthy balance of hormone levels.

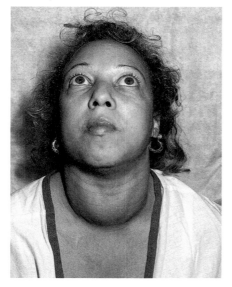

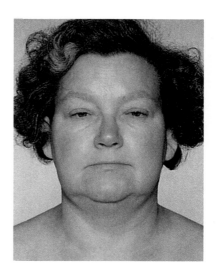

Graves Disease (Hyperthyroidism)

An autoimmune disease with increased production of thyroid hormones causes an increased metabolic rate, just like ramping up the furnace. This is manifested by goiter, eyelid retraction, and exophthalmos (bulging eyeballs). Symptoms include nervousness, fatigue, weight loss, muscle cramps, and heat intolerance. Signs include forceful tachycardia; shortness of breath; excessive sweating; fine muscle tremor[14]; thin silky hair; warm, moist skin; infrequent blinking; a staring appearance; and brisk ankle jerks.

Myxedema (Hypothyroidism)

A deficiency of thyroid hormone means that the thyroid furnace is cold. This reduces the metabolic rate and, when severe, causes a nonpitting edema or myxedema. Usual cause is Hashimoto thyroiditis. Symptoms include fatigue and cold intolerance. Signs include puffy, edematous face, especially around eyes (periorbital edema); puffy hands and feet; coarse facial features; cool, dry skin; dry, coarse hair and eyebrows; slow reflexes; and sometimes thick speech.

See Illustration Credits for source information.

Abnormal Findings

TABLE 14.5 Abnormal Facies With Chronic Illness

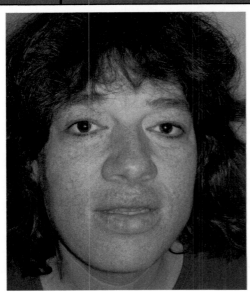

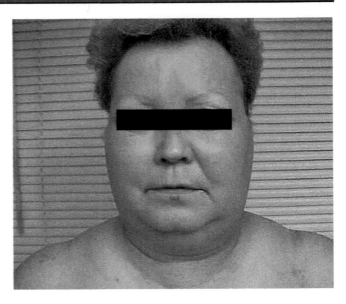

Acromegaly

Excessive secretion of growth hormone from the pituitary gland after puberty creates an enlarged skull and thickened cranial bones. Note the elongated head, massive face, overgrowth of nose and lower jaw, heavy eyebrow ridge, and coarse facial features.

Cushing Syndrome

With excessive secretion of adrenocorticotropic hormone (ACTH) and chronic steroid use, the person develops a rounded, "moonlike" face; prominent jowls; red cheeks; hirsutism on the upper lip, lower cheeks, and chin; and acneiform rash on the chest.

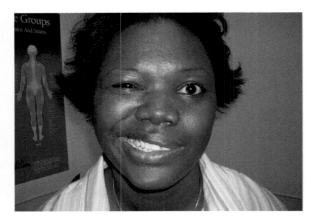

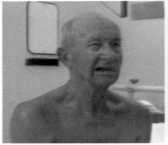 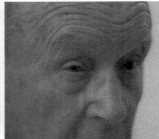

Bell Palsy (Left Side)

A **lower motor neuron** lesion (**peripheral**), producing rapid onset of cranial nerve VII paralysis of facial muscles; almost always unilateral. This may be a reactivation of herpes simplex virus (HSV-1) latent since childhood. Note complete paralysis of one-half of the face; person cannot wrinkle forehead, raise eyebrow, close eyelid, whistle, or show teeth on the left side. Usually presents with smooth forehead, wide palpebral fissure, flat nasolabial fold, drooling, and pain behind the ear. This is greatly improved if corticosteroids and antivirals are given within 72 hours of onset.[6]

Stroke or "Brain Attack"

An **upper motor neuron** lesion (**central**). A stroke is an acute neurologic deficit caused by blood clot of a cerebral vessel, as in atherosclerosis (ischemic stroke), or a rupture in a cerebral vessel (hemorrhagic stroke). If you suspect a stroke, ask if the person can smile. Note paralysis of the lower facial muscles but also note that the upper half of face is not affected because of the intact nerve from the unaffected hemisphere. The person is still able to wrinkle the forehead and close the eyes. (Compare this with Bell palsy.) However, stroke requires emergency 9-1-1 treatment. See the F.A.S.T plan in Chapter 24.

TABLE 14.5	Abnormal Facies With Chronic Illness—cont'd

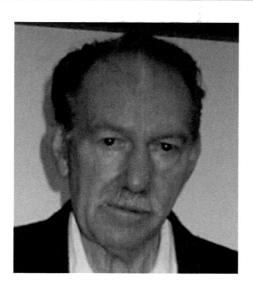

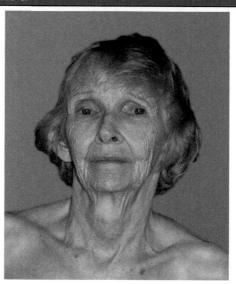

Parkinson Syndrome

A deficiency of the neurotransmitter *dopamine* and degeneration of the substantia nigra of the basal ganglia in the brain. The immobility of features produces a face that is flat and expressionless, "masklike," with elevated eyebrows, staring gaze, oily skin, and drooling.

Cachectic Appearance

Accompanies chronic wasting diseases such as cancer, dehydration, and starvation. Features include sunken eyes; hollow cheeks; and exhausted, defeated expression.

See Illustration Credits for source information.

Abnormal Findings

Summary Checklist: Head, Face, and Neck, Including Regional Lymphatics Examination

1. **Inspect and palpate the skull**
   General size and contour
   Note any deformities, lumps, tenderness
   Palpate temporal artery, temporomandibular joint

2. **Inspect the face**
   Facial expression
   Symmetry of movement (cranial nerve VII)
   Any involuntary movements, edema, lesions

3. **Inspect and palpate the neck**
   Active ROM
   Enlargement of salivary glands, lymph nodes, thyroid gland
   Position of trachea

4. **Auscultate thyroid (if enlarged) for bruit**

REFERENCES

1. American Cancer Society (ACS). (2017). *Cancer facts & figures 2017*. https://www.cancer.org/content/dam/cancer-org/research/cancer-facts-and-statistics/2017/.pdf.
2. Busko, A., Hubbard, Z., & Zakrison, T. (2017). Motorcycle-helmet laws and public health. *N Engl J Med, 376*(13), 1208–1209.
3. Charles, A. (2017). Migraine. *N Engl J Med, 377*(6), 553–560.
4. Copstead, L., & Banasik, J. (2019). *Pathophysiology* (6th ed.). St. Louis: Elsevier.
5. Fagin, J. A., & Wells, S. A. (2016). Biologic and clinical perspectives on thyroid cancer. *N Engl J Med, 375*(11), 1054–1067.
6. Hernandez, J. M., & Sherbino, J. (2017). Do antiviral medications improve symptoms in the treatment of Bell's palsy? *Ann Emerg Med, 69*(3), 364–365.
7. Hogue, J. D. (2015). Office evaluation of dizziness. *Prim Care Clin Office Pract, 42*(2), 249–258.
8. Hoyme, H. E., Kalberg, W. O., Elliott, A. J., et al. (2016). Updated clinical guidelines for diagnosing fetal alcohol spectrum disorders. *Pediatrics, 138*(2), 1–18.

9. Jamault, V., & Duff, E. (2013). Adolescent concussions; when to return to play. *Nurse Pract, 38*(2), 17–21.

10. McGee, S. (2018). *Evidence-based physical diagnosis* (4th ed.). St. Louis: Elsevier.

11. Moriarty, M., & Mallick-Searle, T. (2016). Diagnosis and treatment for chronic migraine. *Nurse Pract, 41*(6), 18–32.

12. Muncie, H. L., Sirmans, S. M., & James, E. (2017). Dizziness: Approach to evaluation and management. *Am Fam Phys, 95*(3), 154–162.

13. Roszel, E. L. (2015). Central nervous system deficits in fetal alcohol spectrum disorder. *Nurse Pract, 40*(4), 24–33.

14. Smith, T. J., & Hegedus, L. (2016). Graves' disease. *N Engl J Med, 375*(16), 1552–1564.

15. Walker, D. S., Edwards, W., & Herrington, C. (2016). Fetal alcohol spectrum disorders. *Nurse Pract, 41*(8), 28–35.

16. Weyand, C. M., & Goronzy, J. J. (2014). Giant-cell arteritis and polymyalgia rheumatic. *N Engl J Med, 371*(1), 50–56.

STRUCTURE AND FUNCTION

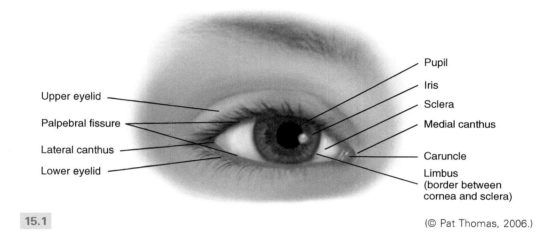

Upper eyelid

Palpebral fissure

Lateral canthus

Lower eyelid

Pupil

Iris

Sclera

Medial canthus

Caruncle

Limbus
(border between
cornea and sclera)

15.1

(© Pat Thomas, 2006.)

EXTERNAL ANATOMY

About 1 inch in diameter, the eye is the sensory organ of vision. Humans are very visual beings. The eyes carry visual data that are crucial for our survival, education, and pleasure. More than half of our neocortex is involved with processing visual information.

Because this sense is so important to humans, the eye is well protected by the bony orbital cavity, surrounded with a cushion of fat. The **eyelids** are like two rapid window shades that further protect the eye from injury, strong light, and dust. The upper eyelid is the larger and more mobile one. The eyelashes are short hairs in double or triple rows that curve outward from the lid margins, filtering out dust and dirt.

The **palpebral fissure** is the elliptical open space between the eyelids (Fig. 15.1). When closed, the lid margins approximate completely. When open, the upper lid covers part of the iris. The lower lid margin is just at the **limbus,** the border between the cornea and sclera. The **canthus** is the corner of the eye, the angle where the lids meet. At the inner canthus the **caruncle** is a small, fleshy mass containing sebaceous glands.

Within the upper lid, **tarsal plates** are strips of connective tissue that give it shape (Fig. 15.2). The tarsal plates contain the **meibomian glands,** modified sebaceous glands that

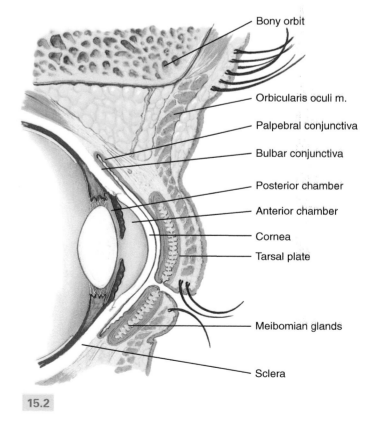

Bony orbit

Orbicularis oculi m.

Palpebral conjunctiva

Bulbar conjunctiva

Posterior chamber

Anterior chamber

Cornea

Tarsal plate

Meibomian glands

Sclera

15.2

Structure and Function

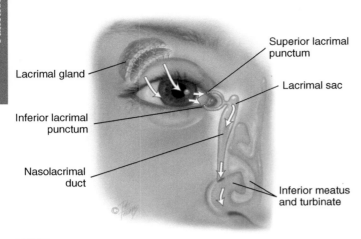

15.3 Lacrimal apparatus.   (© Pat Thomas, 2006.)

membrane folded like an envelope between the eyelids and the eyeball. The *palpebral* conjunctiva lines the lids and is clear, with many small blood vessels. It forms a deep recess and then folds back over the eye. The *bulbar* conjunctiva overlays the eyeball, with the white sclera showing through. At the limbus, the conjunctiva merges with the cornea. The cornea covers and protects the iris and pupil.

The **lacrimal apparatus** provides constant irrigation to keep the conjunctiva and cornea moist and lubricated (Fig. 15.3). The lacrimal gland, in the upper outer corner over the eye, secretes tears. The tears wash across the eye and are drawn up evenly as the lid blinks. They drain into the **puncta,** visible on the upper and lower lids at the inner canthus. They then drain into the nasolacrimal sac, through the ½-inch–long nasolacrimal duct, and empty into the inferior meatus inside the nose. A tiny fold of mucous membrane prevents air from being forced up the nasolacrimal duct when the nose is blown.

secrete an oily lubricating material onto the lids. This stops the tears from overflowing and helps form an airtight seal when the lids are closed.

The exposed part of the eye has a transparent protective covering, the **conjunctiva.** The conjunctiva is a thin mucous

Extraocular Muscles

Six muscles attach the eyeball to its orbit (Fig. 15.4, *A*) and serve to direct our eyes to points of our interest. These

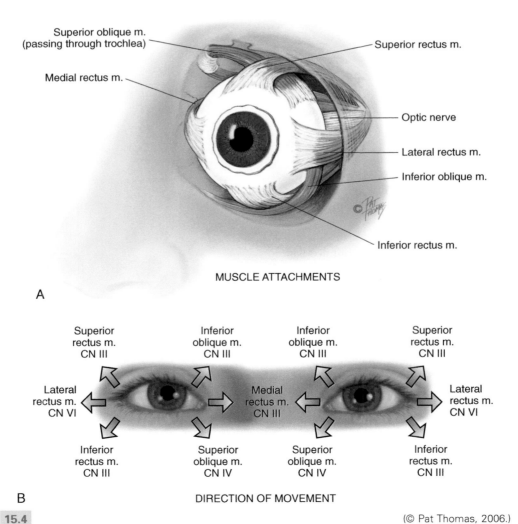

MUSCLE ATTACHMENTS

A

DIRECTION OF MOVEMENT

B

15.4

(© Pat Thomas, 2006.)

extraocular muscles (EOMs) give the eye both straight and rotary movement. The four straight, or *rectus,* muscles are the superior, inferior, lateral, and medial rectus muscles. The two slanting, or *oblique,* muscles are the superior and inferior muscles.

Each muscle is coordinated, or yoked, with one in the other eye. This ensures that when the two eyes move, their axes always remain parallel (called *conjugate movement).* Parallel axes are important because the human brain can tolerate seeing only one image. Although some animals can perceive two different pictures through each eye, humans have a binocular, single-image visual system. This occurs because our eyes move as a pair. For example, the two yoked muscles that allow looking to the far right are the right lateral rectus and the left medial rectus.

Movement of the EOMs (Fig. 15.4, *B*) is stimulated by three **cranial nerves** (CNs). The abducens nerve (CN VI) innervates the lateral rectus muscle (which abducts the eye); the trochlear nerve (CN IV) innervates the superior oblique muscle; and the oculomotor nerve (CN III) innervates all the rest—the superior, inferior, and medial rectus and the inferior oblique muscles. Note that the superior oblique muscle is located on the superior aspect of the eyeball; but, when it contracts, it enables the person to look downward and inward.

INTERNAL ANATOMY

The eye is an asymmetric sphere composed of three concentric coats: (1) the outer fibrous **sclera,** (2) the middle vascular **choroid,** and (3) the inner nervous **retina** (Fig. 15.5). Inside the retina is the transparent vitreous body. The only parts accessible to examination are the sclera anteriorly and the retina through the ophthalmoscope.

The Outer Layer. The **sclera** is a tough, protective white covering. It is continuous anteriorly with the smooth, transparent cornea, which covers the iris and pupil. The cornea is part of the refracting media of the eye, bending incoming light rays to focus them on the inner retina.

The **cornea** is thin, transparent, and very sensitive to touch; contact with a wisp of cotton stimulates a blink in both eyes, called the *corneal reflex.* The trigeminal nerve (CN V) carries the afferent sensation into the brain, and the facial nerve (CN VII) carries the efferent message that stimulates the blink.

The Middle Layer. The **choroid** has dark pigmentation to prevent light from reflecting internally and is heavily vascularized to deliver blood to the retina. Anteriorly the choroid is continuous with the ciliary body and the iris. The muscles of the ciliary body control the thickness of the lens. The iris functions as a diaphragm, varying the opening at its center, the pupil. This controls the amount of light admitted into the retina. The muscle fibers of the iris contract the pupil in bright light and accommodate for near vision; they dilate the pupil in dim light and accommodate for far vision. The color of the iris varies from person to person.

The **pupil** is round and regular. Its size is determined by a balance between the parasympathetic and sympathetic chains of the autonomic nervous system. Stimulation of the parasympathetic branch, through CN III, causes constriction of the pupil. Stimulation of the sympathetic branch dilates

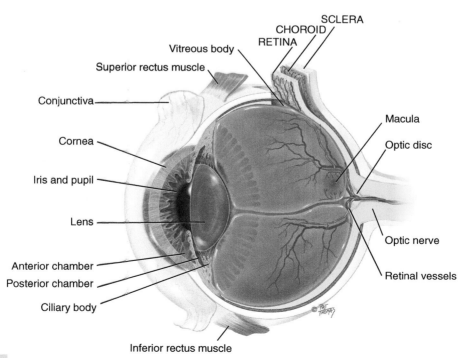

Conjunctiva

Cornea

Iris and pupil

Lens

Anterior chamber

Posterior chamber

Ciliary body

Superior rectus muscle

Vitreous body

RETINA

CHOROID

SCLERA

Macula

Optic disc

Optic nerve

Retinal vessels

Inferior rectus muscle

15.5

(© Pat Thomas, 2018.)

the pupil and elevates the eyelid. As mentioned earlier, the pupil size also reacts to the amount of ambient light and accommodation, or focusing an object on the retina.

The **lens** is a biconvex disc located just posterior to the pupil. The transparent lens serves as a refracting medium, keeping a viewed object in continual focus on the retina. Its thickness is controlled by the ciliary body; the lens bulges for focusing on near objects and flattens for far objects.

The **anterior chamber** is posterior to the cornea and in front of the iris and lens. The **posterior chamber** lies behind the iris to the sides of the lens. These contain the clear, watery aqueous humor that is produced continually by the ciliary body. The continuous flow of fluid serves to deliver nutrients to the surrounding tissues and drain metabolic wastes. Intraocular pressure is determined by a balance between the amount of aqueous produced and resistance to its outflow at the angle of the anterior chamber.

The Inner Layer. The **retina** is the visual receptive layer of the eye in which light waves are changed into nerve impulses. It surrounds the soft, gelatinous vitreous body. The retinal structures viewed through the ophthalmoscope are the optic disc, the retinal vessels, the general background, and the macula (Fig. 15.6).

The **optic disc** (or optic papilla) is the area in which fibers from the retina converge to form the optic nerve. Located toward the nasal side of the retina, it has these characteristics: a color that varies from creamy yellow-orange to pink; a round or oval shape; margins that are distinct and sharply demarcated, especially on the temporal side; and a physiologic cup, the smaller circular area inside the disc where the blood vessels exit and enter.

The **retinal vessels** normally include a paired artery and vein extending to each quadrant, growing progressively smaller in caliber as they reach the periphery. The arteries appear brighter red and narrower than the veins, and they have a thin sliver of light on them (the arterial light reflex). The general background of the fundus varies in color, depending on the person's skin color. The **macula** is located on the temporal side of the fundus. It is a slightly darker pigmented region surrounding the **fovea centralis,** the area of sharpest and keenest vision. The macula receives and transduces light from the center of the visual field.

VISUAL PATHWAYS AND VISUAL FIELDS

Objects reflect light. The light rays are refracted through the transparent media (cornea, aqueous humor, lens, and vitreous body) and strike the retina. The retina transforms the light stimulus into nerve impulses that are conducted through the optic nerve and the optic tract to the visual cortex of the occipital lobe.

The image formed on the retina is upside down and reversed from its actual appearance in the outside world (Fig. 15.7) (i.e., an object in the upper temporal visual field of the right eye reflects its image onto the lower nasal area of the retina). All retinal fibers collect to form the optic nerve, but they maintain this same spatial arrangement, with nasal fibers running medially and temporal fibers running laterally.

At the optic chiasm, nasal fibers (from both temporal visual fields) cross over. The left optic tract now has fibers from the left half of each retina, and the right optic tract contains fibers only from the right. Thus the right side of the brain looks at the left side of the world.

VISUAL REFLEXES

Pupillary Light Reflex. The pupillary light reflex is the normal constriction of the pupils when bright light shines on

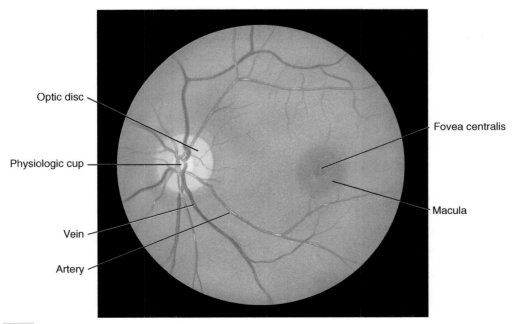

Optic disc

Physiologic cup

Vein

Artery

Fovea centralis

Macula

15.6

LEFT VISUAL FIELD   RIGHT VISUAL FIELD

Temporal   Nasal   Nasal   Temporal

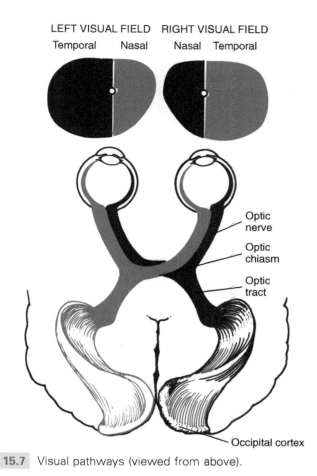

Optic
nerve

Optic
chiasm

Optic
tract

Occipital cortex

15.7 Visual pathways (viewed from above).

the retina (Fig. 15.8). It is a subcortical reflex arc (i.e., we have no conscious control over it); the sensory afferent link is CN II (the optic nerve), and the motor efferent path is CN III (the oculomotor nerve).

When one eye is exposed to bright light, a *direct light reflex* (constriction of that pupil) and a *consensual light reflex* (simultaneous constriction of the other pupil) occur. This happens because the optic nerve carries the sensory afferent message in and then synapses with both sides of the brain. For example, consider the light reflex in a person who is blind in one eye. Stimulation of the normal eye produces both a direct and a consensual light reflex. Stimulation of the blind eye causes no response because the sensory afferent in CN II is destroyed.

Fixation. Fixation is a reflex direction of the eye toward an object attracting our attention. The image is fixed in the center of the visual field, the fovea centralis. This consists of very rapid ocular movements to put the target back on the fovea and somewhat slower (smooth pursuit) movements to track the target and keep its image on the fovea. These ocular movements are impaired by drugs, alcohol, fatigue, and inattention.

Accommodation. Accommodation is adaptation of the eye for near vision. It is accomplished by increasing the curvature of the lens through the muscles of the ciliary body. Although the lens cannot be observed directly, the components of accommodation that can be observed are convergence (motion toward) of the axes of the eyeballs and pupillary constriction.

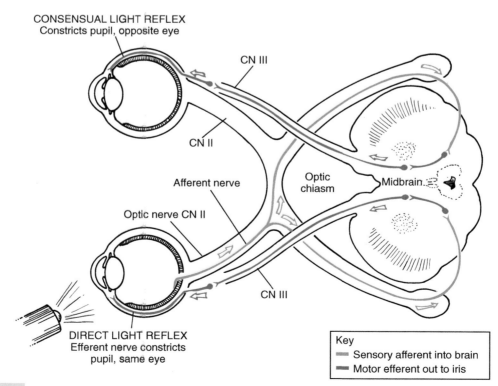

CONSENSUAL LIGHT REFLEX
Constricts pupil, opposite eye

CN III

CN II

Afferent nerve

Optic
chiasm

Midbrain

Optic nerve CN II

CN III

DIRECT LIGHT REFLEX
Efferent nerve constricts
pupil, same eye

Key

Sensory afferent into brain

Motor efferent out to iris

15.8

Structure and Function

◆ DEVELOPMENTAL COMPETENCE

Infants and Children

At birth eye function is limited, but it matures fully during the early years. Peripheral vision is intact in the newborn infant. The macula, the area of keenest vision, is absent at birth but is developing by 4 months and is mature by 8 months. Eye movements may be poorly coordinated at birth. By 3 to 4 months of age the infant establishes binocularity and can fixate on a single image with both eyes simultaneously.

In structure the eyeball reaches adult size by 8 years. At birth the iris shows little pigment, and the pupils are small. The lens is nearly spherical at birth, growing flatter throughout life. Its consistency changes from that of soft plastic at birth to rigid glass in old age.

The Aging Adult

Changes in eye structure cause distinct facial changes in aging. Loss of skin elasticity causes wrinkling and drooping; fat tissues and muscles atrophy; and the external eye structures appear as on p. 300. Lacrimal glands involute, causing decreased tear production and a feeling of dryness and burning.

On the globe itself an infiltration of degenerative lipid material shows around the limbus (see discussion of *arcus senilis*, p. 300). Pupil size decreases. The lens loses elasticity, becoming hard and glasslike. This glasslike quality decreases the ability of the lens to change shape to accommodate for near vision, a condition termed **presbyopia.** By 40 years of age 50% of people have presbyopia and need printed images magnified[6]; the prevalence is 83% in later years.[3] By 70 years of age the normally transparent fibers of the lens begin to thicken and yellow; this is the beginning of a cataract.

Inside the globe the vitreous humor is not renewed continuously. Thus *floaters* appear from debris that accumulates. Visual acuity diminishes gradually after 50 years and even more so after 70 years. Near vision is commonly affected because of the decreased power of accommodation in the lens (presbyopia). In the early 40s a person may have blurred vision and difficulty reading. The aging person also needs more light to see because of a decreased adaptation to darkness, and this condition may affect the function of night driving. All of these changes affect **safety,** increase the risk of falls and other accidental injuries, and challenge the ability to live independently.

Aging itself brings an increased risk of vision-robbing diseases. The prevalence of decreased vision in each disease will increase even more in the coming years as the U.S. population ages. In older adults the most common causes of decreased visual functioning are:

1. **Cataract** formation—a clouding of the crystalline lens partly due to ultraviolet radiation. This is curable with lens replacement surgery, which the older person can consider when vision changes interfere with daily activities.[6] Cataract prevalence increases with age, affecting 24.4 million Americans by age 40 years and older, and affecting half of Americans by age 75 years.[1]

2. **Glaucoma**—an optic nerve neuropathy characterized by loss of peripheral vision, caused by increased intraocular pressure. Age is the primary risk; over 2.7 million adults over 40 years of age have the disease, and another 2 million do not know that they have it.[1] Because women have a longer life expectancy than men in the United States, women account for greater numbers of age-related eye diseases. In this case, women account for 61% of those with glaucoma.[11]

3. **Age-related macular degeneration (AMD)**—a loss of central vision caused by yellow deposits (drusen) and neovascularity in the macula. AMD prevalence rises sharply with older age; by age 80 years, 1 in 10 Americans suffer from late-stage AMD, with more women than men afflicted.[1]

    With AMD the person is unable to read books or papers, sew, or do fine work and has difficulty distinguishing faces. When the lifestyle is oriented around these activities, loss of central vision causes great distress. Peripheral vision is not affected; for a while the person can manage self-care and not become completely disabled.

4. **Diabetic retinopathy**—the leading cause of blindness in adults 25 to 74 years of age.[9] This vision impairment results in difficulty driving, reading, managing diabetes treatment, and other self-care. The prevalence has decreased slightly as a result of intensified prevention measures and newer treatments, such as the injection of steroids into the vitreous and anti-growth factor drugs.[8] However, this progress could be offset by increasing obesity rates, increased numbers of older adults, and improved detection of diabetes (see Table 15.10, Retinal Vessel and Background Abnormalities, p. 315).

🌐 CULTURE AND GENETICS

Culturally based variability exists in the color of the iris and retinal pigmentation, with darker irides having darker retinas behind them. Individuals with light retinas generally have better night vision but can have pain in an environment that has too much light.

Cataracts are a leading cause of blindness worldwide, and experts estimate that 80% of cataracts are preventable or curable with surgery.[10] In the United States, African-American men and women were more likely to have cataracts in every age category.[6] Cataract surgery is cost-effective, and it also may help reduce poverty by returning people to work and increasing social mobility. Barriers to cataract surgery include low socioeconomic status, transportation issues, lack of insurance, and poor surveillance methods.[10]

Glaucoma prevalence increases with age, and African Americans are 3 to 6 times more likely to develop the condition than are Caucasians. Primary open-angle glaucoma is the leading cause of blindness in African Americans and Hispanics.[5,6] Family history of glaucoma in a first-degree relative increases the risk for developing the disease. Measurement of intraocular pressure alone is not sufficient to detect glaucoma; visual field testing using special equipment in an ophthalmology office increases detection.[5]

Age-related macular degeneration is present in 19.7% of U.S. adults over age 75 years; the disease is more prevalent in Caucasians. Additional risk factors include positive family history, cigarette smoking, hyperopia, light iris color, hypertension, hypercholesterolemia, and female gender.[6]

Visual impairment (VI) is not being able to see letters on the eye chart at line 20/50 or below. By 2050, the number of people with VI or blindness is expected to double because of the aging population and shifting demographics.[13] In 2015 the highest numbers of these conditions were found in Caucasians, women, and older adults, and that will be true in 2050. In 2015 African Americans were the minority group with the highest prevalence of VI and blindness; this will shift to Hispanic people in 2050 as they are the fastest-growing minority group and have a longer life expectancy. VI and blindness have a huge impact on physical and mental health, increasing the risk for lost productivity, chronic health conditions, accidents and injuries, social isolation, depression, and mortality.[13] VI is largely due to uncorrected refractive error and could so easily be improved through glasses, contact lenses, and refractive surgery. Vision screening is low in cost and yields huge relief from the health problems listed above.

Vision screening is crucial in preschool children to detect strabismus ("cross-eye") and amblyopia ("lazy eye"). Data show identical screening rates (80.7%) among black and white children but a rate of 69.8% in Hispanic children. The U.S. Preventive Services Task Force recommends screening at least once in *all* children ages 3 to 5 years to detect amblyopia or its risk factors.[4]

SUBJECTIVE DATA

1. Vision difficulty (decreased acuity, blurring, blind spots)
2. Pain
3. Strabismus, diplopia
4. Redness, swelling
5. Watering, discharge
6. History of ocular problems
7. Glaucoma
8. Use of glasses or contact lenses
9. Patient-centered care

Examiner Asks	Rationale
1. Vision difficulty. Any **difficulty seeing** or any blurring? Any blind spots? Come on suddenly or progress slowly? In one eye or both? • Constant or does it come and go? • Do objects appear out of focus, or does it feel like a clouding over objects? Does it feel like "grayness" of vision? • Do spots move in front of your eyes? One or many? In one or both eyes? • Any halos/rainbows around objects? Or rings around lights? • Any blind spot? Does it move as you shift your gaze? Any loss of peripheral vision? • Any night blindness? **2. Pain.** Any eye pain? Please describe. • Come on suddenly? • Quality—Burning or itching? Or sharp, stabbing pain? Pain with bright light? • A foreign body sensation? Or deep aching? Or headache in brow area?	Floaters are common with myopia or after middle age as a result of condensed vitreous fibers. Usually not significant, but acute onset of floaters ("shade" or "cobwebs") occurs with retinal detachment. Halos around lights occur with acute narrow-angle glaucoma. **Scotoma,** a blind spot inside an area of normal or decreased vision, occurs with glaucoma and optic nerve disorders. Night blindness occurs with optic atrophy, glaucoma, vitamin A deficiency. *Sudden onset* of eye symptoms (pain, floaters, blind spot, loss of peripheral vision) requires emergency referral. Quality is valuable in diagnosis. **Photophobia** is the inability to tolerate light. **NOTE:** Some common eye diseases do not cause pain (e.g., cataract, glaucoma).

Subjective Data

3. **Strabismus, diplopia.** Any history of crossed eyes? Now or in the past? Does this occur with eye fatigue?
   • Ever see double? Constant, or does it come and go? Does your double vision go away if you cover one eye or the other?

Strabismus is a deviation in the parallel axes of the two eyes.

Diplopia is the perception of two images of a single object. Diplopia in one eye is caused by dry eyes, uncorrected refractive error, cataract. Binocular diplopia, seen only when both eyes are open, occurs with misalignment of axes of eyes.

4. **Redness, swelling.** Any **redness** or **swelling** in the eyes?
   • Any infections? Now or in the past? When do these occur? In a particular time of year? Anyone else in home with same condition?

Redness occurs with conjunctivitis and other "red-eye" conditions (see Table 15.6, p. 311).

5. **Watering, discharge.** Any **watering** or excessive tearing?

Lacrimation (tearing) and epiphora (excessive tearing) are caused by irritants or obstruction in drainage of tears.

   • Any **discharge?** Any matter in the eyes? Is it hard to open your eyes in the morning? What color is the discharge?
   • How do you remove matter from your eyes?

Purulent discharge is thick and yellow. Crusts form at night. Assess hygiene practices and how to avoid cross-contamination.

6. **History of ocular problems.** Any **history** of injury or surgery to eye? Or any history of allergies?

Allergens (e.g., makeup, contact lens solution) cause irritation of conjunctiva or cornea.

7. **Glaucoma.** Ever been tested for **glaucoma?** Results?
   • Any family history of glaucoma?

Glaucoma is characterized by increased intraocular pressure.

8. **Use of glasses or contact lenses.** Do you wear **glasses** or **contact lenses?** How do they work for you?
   • Last time your prescription was checked? Was it changed?
   • If you wear contact lenses, are there any problems such as pain, photophobia, watering, or swelling?

Adults with glasses or contacts need an annual check to keep prescription current; adults without correction need a check every 2 or 3 years. An examination after age 40 should screen for age-related eye diseases.
Assess self-care behaviors.

   • How do you care for contacts? How long do you wear them? How do you clean them? Do you remove them for certain activities?

9. **Patient-centered care.** Last vision test? Ever tested for color vision?
   • Any environmental conditions at home or at work that may affect your eyes? For example, flying sparks, metal bits, smoke, dust, chemical fumes? If so, do you wear goggles to protect your eyes?
   • Which medications are you taking? Systemic or topical? Do you take any medication specifically for the eyes?

Self-care behaviors for eyes and vision.
Work-related eye disease (e.g., an auto mechanic with a foreign body from metal working or radiation damage from welding).
Medication side effects (e.g., prednisone may cause cataracts or increased intraocular pressure).

   • How about smoking—Do you smoke?
   • If you have experienced a vision loss, how do you cope? Do you have books with large print, books on audio tape or CD, braille?
   • Do you maintain your living environment the same?
   • Do you sometimes fear complete loss of vision?

Cigarette smoking is associated with AMD, cataract, diabetic retinopathy, and eye inflammation.
A constant spatial layout eases navigation through the home.

Additional History for Infants and Children

1. Any vaginal infections in the mother at time of delivery?

Genital herpes and gonorrhea have risk of eye disease for the newborn.

2. Considering age of child, which developmental milestones of vision have you (parent) noted?

The parent is most often the one to detect vision problems.

Examiner Asks	Rationale

3. Does the child have routine vision testing at school?

4. Are you (parent) aware of safety measures to protect child's eyes from trauma? Do you inspect toys?
  - Have you taught the child safe care of sharp objects and how to carry and use them?

Additional History for the Aging Adult

1. Have you noticed any visual difficulty with climbing stairs or driving? Any problem with night vision?

Loss of depth perception, contrast sensitivity, peripheral or central vision may occur.

2. When was the last time you were tested for glaucoma?

At age 60 or 65 years people need annual examination to screen for vision changes and age-related eye diseases.

  - Any aching pain around eyes? Any loss of peripheral vision?
  - If you have glaucoma, how do you manage your eyedrops?

Compliance may be a problem if symptoms are absent. Assess ability to administer eyedrops.

3. Is there a history of cataracts? Any loss or progressive blurring of vision?

4. Do your eyes ever feel dry? Burning? What do you do for this?

Decreased tear production may occur.

5. Any decrease in usual activities such as reading or sewing? Driving?

AMD is a loss of central vision that impairs daily pleasures and activities.

OBJECTIVE DATA

PREPARATION
Position the person standing for vision screening; then sitting up with the head at your eye level.

EQUIPMENT NEEDED
Snellen eye chart
Handheld visual screener
Opaque card or occluder
Penlight
Ophthalmoscope
Applicator stick (occasionally)

Normal Range of Findings	Abnormal Findings

Test Central Visual Acuity

Snellen Eye Chart
The Snellen alphabet chart is the most commonly used and accurate measure of visual acuity. It has lines of letters arranged in decreasing size (Fig. 15.9).

Place the Snellen alphabet chart in a well-lit spot at eye level. Position the person on a mark exactly 20 feet from the chart. Use an opaque card to shield one eye at a time during the test; inadvertent peeking may result when shielding the eye with the person's own fingers. If the person wears glasses or contact lenses, leave them on. Remove only reading glasses because they blur distance vision. Ask the person to read to the smallest line of letters possible. Encourage trying the next smallest line also. (NOTE: Use a Snellen picture chart for people who cannot read letters. See p. 296.)

Note hesitancy, squinting, leaning forward, misreading letters.

Objective Data

Normal Range of Findings	Abnormal Findings

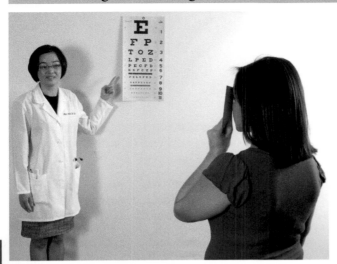

15.9

Record the result using the numeric fraction at the end of the last successful line read. Indicate whether the person missed any letters or if corrective lenses were worn (e.g., "Right 20/30 −1, with glasses") (i.e., the right eye scored 20/30, missing one letter).

Normal visual acuity is 20/20. Contrary to some people's impression, the numeric fraction is *not* a percentage of normal vision. Instead, the top number (numerator) indicates the distance the person is standing from the chart, and the denominator gives the distance at which a normal eye could have read that particular line. Thus "20/30" means, "You can read at 20 feet what the normal eye can see from 30 feet away."

The larger the denominator, the poorer the vision. If vision is poorer than 20/30, refer to an ophthalmologist or optometrist. Impaired vision results from refractive error, opacity in the media (cornea, lens, vitreous), or disorder in the retina or optic pathway.

If the person is unable to see even the largest letters, shorten the distance to the chart until it is seen and record that distance (e.g., "10/200"). If visual acuity is even lower, assess whether the person can count your fingers when they are spread in front of the eyes or distinguish light perception from your penlight.

Schedule a prompt referral to ophthalmologist.

Near Vision

At the hospital bedside or for people older than 40 years, test near vision with a handheld vision screener with various sizes of print (e.g., a Jaeger card) (Fig. 15.10). Hold the card in good light about 35 cm (14 inches) from the eye—this distance equals the print size on the 20-foot chart. Test each eye separately with the person wearing glasses. A normal result is "14/14" in each eye, read without hesitancy and without moving the card closer or farther away. When no vision screening card is available, ask the person to read from a magazine or newspaper.

Presbyopia, the decrease in power of accommodation with aging, is suggested when the person moves the card farther away.

Normal Range of Findings	Abnormal Findings

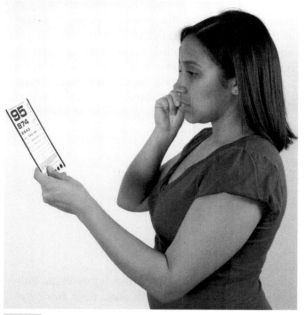

15.10

Objective Data

Test Visual Fields

Confrontation Test

This test screens for loss of peripheral vision. It compares the person's peripheral vision with your own, assuming that yours is normal. Position yourself at eye level about 2 feet away. Looking straight at you, the person covers one eye with an opaque card (here the right eye) as you cover the opposite eye (here the left) (Fig. 15.11, *A* and *B*). You are testing the uncovered eye. Hold a wiggling finger as a target midline between you and the person and slowly advance it in from the periphery in several directions.

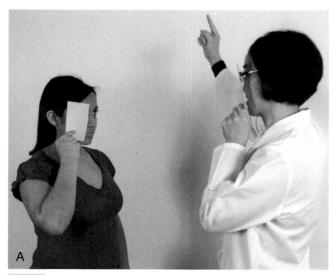
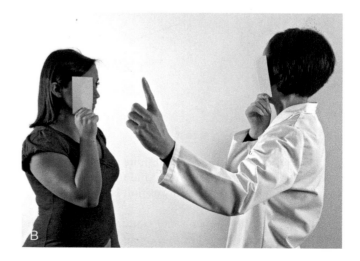

A   B

15.11

Normal Range of Findings

Ask the person to say "now" as the target is first seen; this should be just as you also see the object. For the temporal direction, start your finger somewhat behind the person. Estimate the angle between the anteroposterior axis of the eye and the peripheral axis where the object is first seen. Normal results are about 50 degrees upward, 90 degrees temporally, 70 degrees inferiorly, and 60 degrees nasally.

The sensitivity of confrontation testing can be increased by combining the wiggling finger test with a moving red target.[7] Hold a 5-mm red-topped pin beyond the boundary of each quadrant between the horizontal and vertical axes. Move it inward and ask the person to state when the pin first appears as red.

Inspect Extraocular Muscle Function

Corneal Light Reflex (Hirschberg Test)
Assess the parallel alignment of the eye axes by shining a light toward the person's eyes. Direct the person to stare straight ahead as you hold the light about 30 cm (12 inches) away. Note the reflection of the light on the two corneas; it should be in exactly the same spot on each eye. See the bright white dots in Fig. 15.27 for symmetry of the corneal light reflex.

Diagnostic Positions Test
Leading the eyes through the six cardinal positions of gaze elicits any muscle weakness during movement (Fig. 15.12). Ask the person to hold the head steady and follow the movement of your finger only with the eyes. Hold the target back about 30 cm (12 inches) so the person can focus on it comfortably, move it to each of the six positions, hold it momentarily, then back to center. Progress clockwise. A normal response is parallel tracking of the object with both eyes.

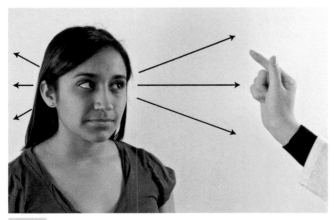

15.12 Diagnostic positions test.

In addition to parallel movement, note any **nystagmus**—a fine, oscillating movement best seen around the iris. Mild nystagmus at an extreme lateral gaze is normal; nystagmus at any other position is not.

Finally note that the upper eyelid continues to overlap the superior part of the iris, even during downward movement. You should not see a white rim of sclera between the lid and the iris. If noted, this is termed *lid lag*.

Abnormal Findings

If the person is unable to see the object as the examiner does, the test suggests peripheral field loss. In an older adult this screens for glaucoma. Promptly refer to a specialist for more precise testing (see Table 15.5, Visual Field Loss). Acutely diminished visual fields occur with diseases of the retina and with stroke.

Asymmetry of the light reflex indicates deviation in alignment from eye muscle weakness or paralysis. If you see this, perform the cover test described on p. 298.

Eye movement is not parallel. Failure to follow in a certain direction indicates weakness of an EOM or dysfunction of the cranial nerve innervating it.

Nystagmus occurs with disease of the semicircular canals in the ears, a paretic eye muscle, multiple sclerosis, or brain lesions.

Lid lag occurs with hyperthyroidism.

Normal Range of Findings	Abnormal Findings

Inspect External Ocular Structures

Begin with the most external points and logically work your way inward.

General

Already you will have noted the person's ability to move around the room, with vision functioning well enough to avoid obstacles and to respond to your directions. Also note the facial expression; a relaxed expression accompanies adequate vision.

Groping with hands.

Squinting or craning forward.

Eyebrows

Look for symmetry between the two eyes. Normally the eyebrows are present bilaterally, move symmetrically as the facial expression changes, and have no scaling or lesions (Fig. 15.13).

Unequal or absent movement with nerve damage.
Scaling with seborrhea.

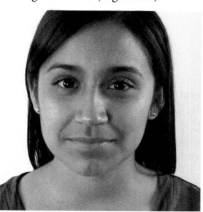

15.13

Eyelids and Lashes

The upper lids normally overlap the superior part of the iris and approximate completely with the lower lids when closed. The skin is intact without redness, swelling, discharge, or lesions.

The palpebral fissures are horizontal in non-Asians, whereas Asians normally have an upward slant.

Note that the eyelashes are distributed evenly along the lid margins and curve outward.

Lid lag with hyperthyroidism.
Incomplete closure creates risk for corneal damage.
Ptosis, drooping of upper lid.
Periorbital edema, lesions (see Tables 15.2, Eyelid Abnormalities, and 15.3, Lesions on the Eyelids).
Ectropion and entropion (see Table 15.2, p. 307).

Eyeballs

The eyeballs are aligned normally in their sockets with no protrusion or sunken appearance. Blacks normally may have a slight protrusion of the eyeball beyond the supraorbital ridge.

Exophthalmos (protruding eyes) and enophthalmos (sunken eyes) (see Table 15.2).

Conjunctiva and Sclera

Ask the person to look up. Using your thumbs, slide the lower lids down along the bony orbital rim. Take care not to push against the eyeball. Inspect the exposed area (Fig. 15.14). The eyeball looks moist and glossy. Numerous small blood vessels normally show through the transparent conjunctiva. Otherwise the conjunctivae are clear and show the normal color of the structure below—pink over the lower lids and white over the sclera. Note any color change, swelling, or lesions.

General reddening (see Table 15.6, Red Eye—Vascular Disorders, p. 311).
Cyanosis of the lower lids.
Pallor near the outer canthus of the lower lid may indicate anemia (the inner canthus normally contains less pigment).

Objective Data

Normal Range of Findings	Abnormal Findings

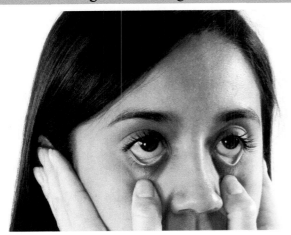

15.14

The sclera is china white, although blacks occasionally have a gray-blue or "muddy" color to the sclera. Also in dark-skinned people you normally may see small brown macules (like freckles) on the sclera, which should not be confused with foreign bodies or petechiae. Finally, blacks may have yellowish fatty deposits beneath the lids away from the cornea. Do not confuse these yellow spots with the overall scleral yellowing that accompanies jaundice.

Scleral icterus is an even yellowing of the sclera extending up to the cornea, indicating jaundice.

Tenderness, foreign body, discharge, or lesions.

Lacrimal Apparatus

Ask the person to look down. With your thumbs, slide the outer part of the upper lid up along the bony orbit to expose under the lid. Inspect for any redness or swelling.

Normally the puncta drain the tears into the lacrimal sac. Presence of excessive tearing may indicate blockage of the nasolacrimal duct. Check this by pressing the index finger against the sac, just inside the lower orbital rim, not against the side of the nose (Fig. 15.15). Pressure slightly everts the lower lid, but there should be no other response to pressure.

Swelling of the lacrimal gland may show as a visible bulge in the outer part of the upper lid.

Puncta red, swollen, tender to pressure.

Watch for any regurgitation of fluid out of the puncta, which confirms duct blockage.

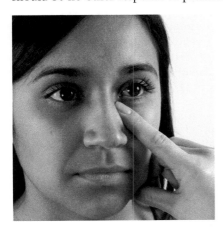

15.15

Inspect Anterior Eyeball Structures

Cornea and Lens

Shine a light from the side across the cornea and check for smoothness and clarity. This oblique view highlights any abnormal irregularities in the corneal surface. There should be no opacities (cloudiness) in the cornea, the anterior

A corneal abrasion causes irregular ridges in reflected light, producing a

Objective Data

Normal Range of Findings

chamber, or the lens behind the pupil. Do not confuse an **arcus senilis** with opacity. The arcus senilis is a normal finding in older adults and is illustrated on p. 301.

Iris and Pupil

The iris normally appears flat, with a round regular shape and even coloration. Note the size, shape, and equality of the pupils. Normally the pupils appear round, regular, and of equal size in both eyes. In the adult, resting pupil size is from 3 to 5 mm. A small number of people (5%) normally have pupils of two different sizes, which is termed **anisocoria.**

To test the **pupillary light reflex,** darken the room and ask the person to gaze into the distance. (This dilates the pupils.) Advance a light in from the side* and note the response. Normally you will see (1) constriction of the same-sided pupil (a *direct light reflex*), and (2) simultaneous constriction of the other pupil (a *consensual light reflex*).

In the acute-care setting, gauge the pupil size in millimeters, both before and after the light reflex (Fig. 15.16). Recording the pupil size in millimeters is more accurate when many nurses and physicians care for the same person or when small changes may be significant signs of increasing intracranial pressure. Normally the resting size is 3, 4, or 5 mm and decreases equally in response to light. The size is measured using this gauge:

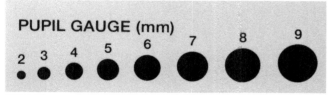

15.16

Test for **accommodation** by asking the person to focus on a distant object (Fig. 15.17). This process dilates the pupils. Then have the person shift the gaze to a near object such as your finger held about 7 to 8 cm (3 inches) from the person's nose. A normal response includes (1) pupillary constriction, and (2) convergence of the axes of the eyes.

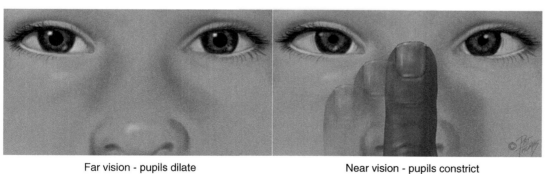

Far vision - pupils dilate   Near vision - pupils constrict

15.17   (© Pat Thomas, 2006.)

Record the normal response to all these maneuvers as PERRLA, or **P**upils **E**qual, **R**ound, **R**eact to **L**ight, and **A**ccommodation.

Abnormal Findings

shattered look to light rays (see Table 15.7, Abnormalities on Cornea and Iris, p. 312).

Irregular shape.

Although they may be normal, all unequal-size pupils call for a consideration of central nervous system injury.

Dilated pupils.

Dilated and fixed pupils.

Constricted pupils.

Unequal or no response to light (see Table 15.4, Pupil Abnormalities, p. 309).

Absence of constriction or convergence. Asymmetric response.

*Always advance the light in from the *side* to test the light reflex. If you advance from the front, the pupils constrict to accommodate for near vision. Thus you do not know what the pure response to the light would have been.

Normal Range of Findings	Abnormal Findings

Advanced Practice Techniques

Inspection of the Ocular Fundus

The ophthalmoscope enlarges your view of the eye so that you can inspect the **media** (anterior chamber, lens, vitreous) and the **ocular fundus** (the internal surface of the retina). It accomplishes this by directing a beam of light through the pupil to illuminate the inner structures. Thus using the ophthalmoscope is like peering through a keyhole (the pupil) into an interesting room beyond.

The ophthalmoscope should function as an appendage of your own eye. This takes some practice. Practice holding the instrument and focusing at objects around the room before you approach a "real" person. Hold the ophthalmoscope right up to your eye, braced firmly against the cheek and brow. Extend your index finger onto the lens selector dial so that you can refocus as needed during the procedure without taking your head away from the ophthalmoscope to look. Now look about the room, moving your head and the instrument together as one unit. Keep both your eyes open; just view the field through the ophthalmoscope.

Recall that the ophthalmoscope contains a set of lenses that control the focus (Fig. 15.18). The unit of strength of each lens is the *diopter*. The black numbers indicate a positive diopter; they focus on objects nearer in space to the ophthalmoscope. The red numbers show a negative diopter and are for focusing on objects farther away.

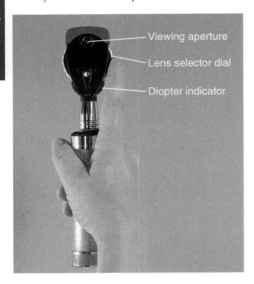

Viewing aperture
Lens selector dial
Diopter indicator

15.18

To examine a person, darken the room to help dilate the pupils. (Dilating eyedrops are not needed during a screening examination. When indicated, they dilate the pupils for a wider look at the fundus background and macular area. Eyedrops are used only when glaucoma can be ruled out completely because dilating the pupils in the presence of glaucoma can precipitate an acute episode.)

Remove your eyeglasses and those of the other person; they obstruct close movement and you can compensate for their correction by using the diopter setting. Contact lenses may be left in; they pose no problem as long as they are clean.

Select the large round aperture with the white light for the routine examination. If the pupils are small, use the smaller white light. (Although the instrument has other shape and color apertures, these are rarely used in a screening examination.) The light must have maximum brightness; replace old or dim batteries.

Tell the person, "Please keep looking at that light switch (or mark) on the wall across the room, even though my head will get in the way." Staring at a distant fixed object helps to dilate the pupils and hold the retinal structures still.

Normal Range of Findings

Match sides with the person. That is, hold the ophthalmoscope in your *right* hand up to your *right* eye to view the person's *right* eye. You must do this to avoid bumping noses during the procedure. Place your free hand on the person's shoulder or forehead (Fig. 15.19, *A*). This helps orient you in space because, once you have the ophthalmoscope in position, you have only a very narrow range of vision. In addition, your thumb can anchor the upper lid and help prevent blinking.

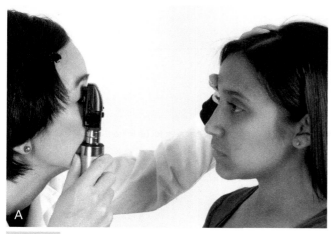

15.19, A

Begin about 25 cm (10 inches) away from the person at an angle about 15 degrees lateral to the person's line of vision. Note the red glow filling the person's pupil. This is the **red reflex,** caused by the reflection of your ophthalmoscope light off the inner retina. Keep sight of the red reflex and steadily move closer to the eye. If you lose the red reflex, the light has wandered off the pupil and onto the iris or sclera. Adjust your angle to find it again.

As you advance, adjust the lens to +6 and note any opacities in the media. These appear as dark shadows or black dots interrupting the red reflex. Normally none are present. Progress toward the person until your foreheads almost touch (Fig. 15.19, *B*).

Cataracts appear as opaque black areas against the red reflex (see Table 15.8, Lens Opacities, p. 314).

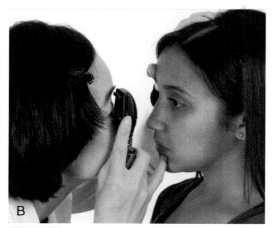

15.19, B

Adjust the diopter setting to bring the ocular fundus into sharp focus. If you and the person have normal vision, this should be at 0. Moving the diopters compensates for nearsightedness or farsightedness. Use the red lenses for nearsighted eyes and the black for farsighted eyes (Fig. 15.20).

Objective Data

Normal Range of Findings	Abnormal Findings

NORMAL EYE

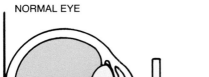

The person's eye and your eye are normal. The 0 diopter (clear glass) will focus sharply on the retina

0 Diopter

MYOPIA (nearsighted)

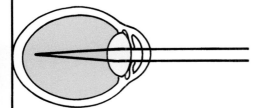

In myopia, the globe is longer than normal and light rays focus in *front* of the retina

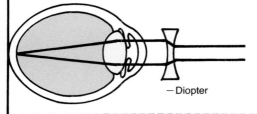

Compensate for myopia in yourself or the other person by using a negative diopter (red number or concave lens). This corrects the focal point onto the retina

— Diopter

HYPEROPIA (farsighted)

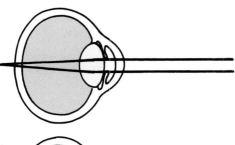

In hyperopia, the globe is shorter than normal. Light rays would focus behind the retina (if they could pass through)

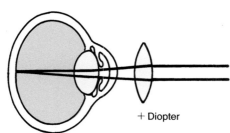

Compensate for hyperopia by using a positive diopter (black number or convex lens). This bends the light rays so the focal point is on the retina

+ Diopter

15.20

Normal Range of Findings	Abnormal Findings

Moving in on the 15-degree lateral line should bring your view just to the optic disc. If the disc is not in sight, track a blood vessel as it grows larger, and it will lead you to the disc. Systematically inspect the structures in the ocular fundus: (1) optic disc, (2) retinal vessels, (3) general background, and (4) macula (Fig. 15.21). (NOTE: The illustration here shows a large area of the fundus. Your actual view through the ophthalmoscope is much smaller—slightly larger than 1 disc diameter.)

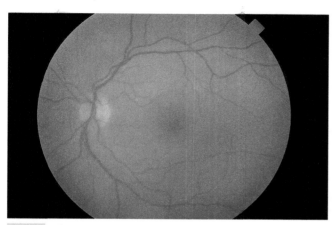

15.21   Normal ocular fundus. (Heather Boyd-Monk and Wills Eye Hospital.)

Optic Disc

The most prominent landmark is the optic disc, located on the nasal side of the retina. Explore these characteristics:

1. **Color**	Creamy yellow-orange to pink.
2. **Shape**	Round or oval.
3. **Margins**	Distinct and sharply demarcated, although the nasal edge may be slightly fuzzy.
4. **Cup-disc ratio**	Distinctness varies. When visible, physiologic cup is a brighter yellow-white than rest of the disc. Its width is not more than one-half the disc diameter (Fig. 15.22).

Abnormal Findings:

Pallor. Hyperemia.
Irregular shape.
Blurred margins.

Cup extending to the disc border (see Table 15.9, Optic Disc Abnormalities, p. 314).

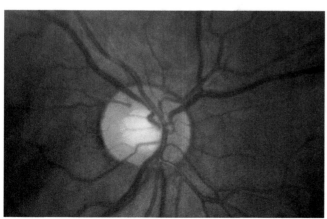

15.22   Normal optic disc.   (Lemmi & Lemmi, 2011.)

Two normal variations may ring around the disc margins. A **scleral crescent** is a gray-white, new-moon shape. It occurs when pigment is absent in the choroid layer and you are looking directly at the sclera. A **pigment crescent** is black; it is caused by accumulation of pigment in the choroid.

Normal Range of Findings	Abnormal Findings

The diameter of the disc, or DD, is a standard of measure for other fundus structures (Fig. 15.23). To describe a finding, note its clock-face position and its relationship to the disc in size and distance (e.g., "... macula at 3:00, 2 DD from the disc").

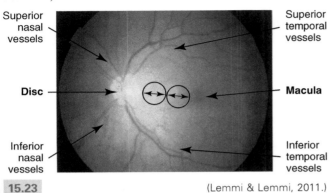

Superior nasal vessels
Superior temporal vessels
Disc
Macula
Inferior nasal vessels
Inferior temporal vessels

15.23 (Lemmi & Lemmi, 2011.)

Retinal Vessels

This is the only place in the body where you can view blood vessels directly. Many systemic diseases that affect the vascular system show signs in the retinal vessels. Follow a paired artery and vein out to the periphery in the four quadrants (see Fig. 15.22), noting these points:

1. **Number**	A paired artery and vein pass to each quadrant. Vessels look straighter at the nasal side.	Absence of major vessels.
2. **Color**	Arteries are brighter red than veins. They also have the arterial light reflex, with a thin stripe of light down the middle.	
3. **A : V ratio**	The ratio comparing the artery-to-vein width is 2:3 or 4:5.	Arteries too constricted. Veins dilated.
4. **Caliber**	Arteries and veins show a regular decrease in caliber as they extend to the periphery.	Focal constriction. Neovascularization (proliferation of new vessels).
5. **A-V (arteriovenous) crossing**	An artery and vein may cross paths. This is not significant if within 2 DD of disc and if no sign of interruption in blood flow is seen. There should be no indenting or displacing of vessel.	Crossings more than 2 DD away from disc. Nicking or pinching of underlying vessel. Vessel engorged peripheral to crossing (see Table 15.10).
6. **Tortuosity**	Tortuosity is mild vessel twisting; when present in both eyes is usually congenital and not significant.	Extreme tortuosity or marked asymmetry in two eyes.
7. **Pulsations**	Pulsations are present in veins near the disc as their drainage meets the intermittent pressure of arterial systole (often hard to see).	Absent pulsations.

General Background of the Fundus

The color normally varies from light red to dark brown–red, generally corresponding with the person's skin color. Your view of the fundus should be clear; no lesions should obstruct the retinal structures.

Abnormal lesions: hemorrhages, exudates, microaneurysms.

Macula

The macula is 1 DD in size and located 2 DD temporal to the disc (Fig. 15.23). Inspect this area last in the funduscopic examination. A bright light on this area of central vision causes some watering and discomfort and pupillary constriction. Note that the normal color of the area is somewhat darker than the rest of the fundus but is even and homogeneous. Clumped pigment may occur with aging.

Clumped pigment occurs with trauma or retinal detachment.

Objective Data

Normal Range of Findings	Abnormal Findings

Within the macula you may note the foveal light reflex. This is a tiny white glistening dot reflecting your ophthalmoscope light.

Hemorrhage or exudate in the macula occurs with senile macular degeneration.

Eversion of the Upper Lid

This maneuver is not part of the normal examination, but it is useful when you must inspect the conjunctiva of the upper lid, as with eye pain or suspicion of a foreign body. Most people are apprehensive of any eye manipulation. Enhance their cooperation by using a calm and gentle, yet deliberate, approach.

1. Ask the person to keep both eyes open and look down. This relaxes the eyelid, whereas closing it would tense the orbicularis muscle.
2. Slide the upper lid up along the bony orbit to lift up the eyelashes.
3. Grasp the lashes between your thumb and forefinger and gently pull down and outward.
4. With your other hand, place the tip of an applicator stick on the upper lid above the level of the internal tarsal plates (Fig. 15.24, *A*).
5. Gently push down with the stick as you lift the lashes. This uses the edge of the tarsal plate as a fulcrum and flips the lid inside out. Take special care not to push in on the eyeball.
6. Secure the everted position by holding the lashes against the bony orbital rim (Fig. 15.24, *B*).
7. Inspect for any color change, swelling, lesion, or foreign body.
8. To return to normal position, gently pull the lashes outward as the person looks up.

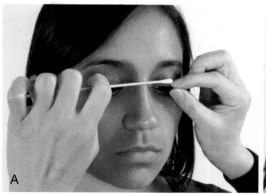 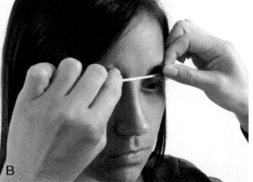

15.24

❖ DEVELOPMENTAL COMPETENCE

Infants and Children

The eye examination is often deferred at birth because of transient edema of the lids from birth trauma or instillation of silver nitrate at birth. The eyes should be examined within a few days and at every well-child visit thereafter.

Visual Acuity. The child's age determines the screening measures used. With a newborn, test visual reflexes and attending behaviors. Test **light perception** using the blink reflex; the neonate blinks in response to bright light (Fig. 15.25). The pupillary light reflex also shows that the pupils constrict in response to light. These reflexes indicate that the lower portion of the visual apparatus is intact. But you cannot infer that the infant can *see*; this requires later observation to show that the brain has received images and can interpret them.

Absent blinking.
Absent pupillary light reflex, especially after 3 weeks, indicates blindness.

Normal Range of Findings

Abnormal Findings

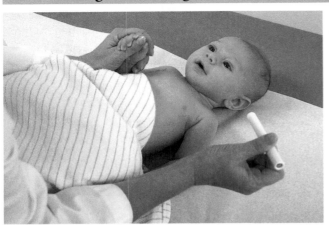

15.25

As you introduce an object to the infant's line of vision, note these attending behaviors:

- **Birth to 2 weeks**—Refusal to reopen eyes after exposure to bright light; increasing alertness to object; infant may fixate on an object.
- **By 2 to 4 weeks**—Infant can fixate on an object.
- **By 1 month**—Infant can fixate and follow a light or bright toy.
- **By 6 weeks**—Infant makes some visual response to your face.

Decreased vision may occur in premature infants or infants with neurologic deficits.

- **By 3 to 4 months**—Infant can fixate, follow, and reach for the toy.
- **By 6 to 10 months**—Infant can fixate and follow the toy in all directions.

Use a picture chart or the Snellen E chart for the preschooler from 3 to 6 years of age. The E chart shows the capital letter E in varying sizes pointing in different directions. The child points his or her fingers in the direction the "table legs" are pointing. By 7 to 8 years of age, when the child is familiar with reading letters, begin to use the standard Snellen alphabet chart. Normally a child achieves 20/20 acuity by 6 to 7 years of age (Fig. 15.26).

Myopia is the most common visual disorder during childhood. Criteria for referral are:

1. Age 3 years—Vision 20/50 or less in either eye.
2. Age 4 years and older—20/40 or less in either eye.
3. Difference between two eyes is one line or more.
4. Child shows other signs of vision impairment, regardless of acuity.

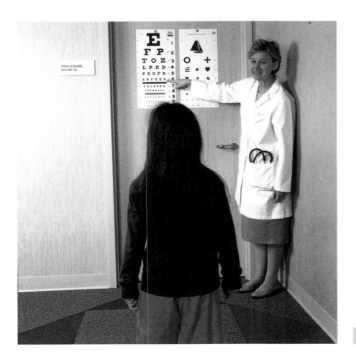

15.26

Objective Data

Normal Range of Findings

Visual Fields. Assess peripheral vision with the confrontation test in children older than 3 years when the preschooler is able to stay in position. As with the adult, the child should see the moving target at the same time your normal eyes do. Use a small toy and make the test a game. Often a young child forgets to say "now" or "stop" as the moving toy is seen. Rather, note the instant the child's eyes deviate or head shifts position to gaze at the moving toy. Match this nearly automatic response with your own sighting.

Color Vision. Color deficient is an inherited recessive X-linked trait affecting about 8% of white males and 4% of black males. It is rare in females (0.4%); the condition is relative and not disabling, although it may affect the person's ability to discern traffic lights or school performance in which color is a learning tool.

Test children once between the ages of 4 and 8 years, or adults for preemployment examinations. Use the Ishihara test, in which each card has a pattern of dots printed against a background of many colored dots. Ask the child to identify each pattern. A person with normal color vision can see each pattern.

Extraocular Muscle Function. Testing for **strabismus** (squint, crossed eye) is an important screening measure between ages 3 and 5 years. Strabismus causes disconjugate vision because one eye deviates off the fixation point. To avoid diplopia or unclear images, the brain begins to suppress data from the weak eye (a suppression scotoma), causing visual acuity in this otherwise normal eye to begin to deteriorate from disuse. Early recognition and treatment are essential to restore binocular vision. Diagnosis after 6 years of age has a poor prognosis. Test malalignment by the corneal light reflex and the cover test.

Check the **corneal light reflex** by shining a light toward the child's eyes. The light should be reflected at exactly the same spot in the two corneas (Fig. 15.27).

Some asymmetry (where one light falls off center) under 6 months of age is normal.

Abnormal Findings

A color-deficient person cannot see the letter against the field color.

Untreated strabismus can lead to permanent visual damage. The resulting loss of vision from disuse is amblyopia ex anopsia. About 1% to 6% of children under 6 years of age have amblyopia or its risk factors. Untreated vision problems may cause accidents, injuries, depression and anxiety, problems at school, and poor self-esteem. Also, these children may be targets of bullying behaviors.[4]

Asymmetry in the corneal light reflex after 6 months is abnormal and must be referred.

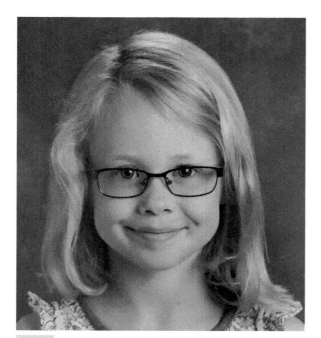

15.27

Normal Range of Findings	Abnormal Findings

Objective Data

Normal Range of Findings

Cover Test. Perform the **cover test** on all children. This test detects small degrees of deviated alignment by interrupting the fusion reflex that normally keeps the two eyes parallel. Ask the child to stare straight ahead at your nose or at a familiar puppet.

With an opaque card, cover one eye. As it is covered, note the uncovered eye. A normal response is a steady, fixed gaze.

Meanwhile the macular image has been suppressed on the covered eye. If muscle weakness exists, the covered eye drifts into a relaxed position.

Now uncover the eye and observe it for movement. It should stare straight ahead. If it jumps to re-establish fixation, eye muscle weakness exists. Repeat with the other eye.

Function of the extraocular muscles during movement can be assessed during the early weeks by the child's following a brightly colored toy as a target. An older infant can sit on the parent's lap as you move the toy in all directions. After 2 years of age, direct the child's gaze through the six cardinal positions of gaze. You may stabilize the child's chin with your hand to prevent him or her from moving the entire head.

External Eye Structures. Inspect the ocular structures as described in the earlier section. A neonate usually holds the eyes tightly shut. Do not attempt to pry them open; that just increases contraction of the orbicularis oculi muscle. Hold the newborn supine and gently lower the head; the eyes will open. The eyes will also open when you hold the infant at arm's length and slowly turn him or her in one direction (Fig. 15.28). In addition to inspecting the ocular structures, this also tests the vestibular function reflex. The baby's eyes look in the same direction as the body is being turned. When the turning stops, the eyes shift to the opposite direction after a few quick beats of nystagmus. Also termed *doll's eyes,* this reflex disappears by 2 months of age.

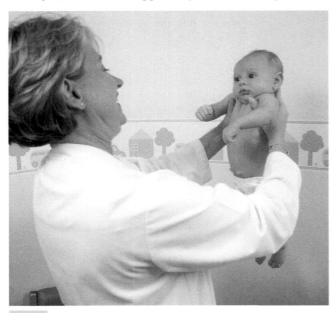

15.28

Eyelids and Lashes. Normally the upper lids overlie the superior part of the iris. In newborns the *setting-sun sign* is common. The eyes appear to deviate

Abnormal Findings

If the eye jumps to fixate on the designated point, it was out of alignment before.

A **phoria** is a mild weakness noted only when fusion is blocked. **Tropia** is more severe—a constant malalignment of the eyes (see Table 15.1, Extraocular Muscle Dysfunction, p. 305)

The setting-sun sign also occurs with hydrocephalus as the globes protrude.

Normal Range of Findings

down, and you see a white rim of sclera over the iris. It may show as you rapidly change the neonate from a sitting to a supine position.

Many infants have an *epicanthal fold,* an excess skinfold extending over the inner corner of the eye, partly or totally overlapping the inner canthus. It occurs frequently in Asian children and in 20% of whites. In non-Asians, it disappears as the child grows, usually by 10 years of age. While they are present, epicanthal folds give a false appearance of malalignment, termed **pseudostrabismus** (Fig. 15.29). Yet the corneal light reflex is normal.

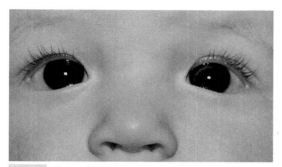

15.29   Pseudostrabismus.   (Zitelli, 2007.)

Asian infants normally have an upward slant of the palpebral fissures. Entropion, a turning inward of the eyelid, is found normally in some Asian children. If the lashes do not abrade the corneas, it is not significant.

Conjunctiva and Sclera. A newborn may have a transient chemical conjunctivitis from the instillation of silver nitrate. This appears within 1 hour and lasts not more than 24 hours after birth. The sclera should be white and clear, although it may have a blue tint as a result of thinness at birth. The lacrimal glands are not functional at birth.

Iris and Pupils. The iris normally is blue or slate gray in light-skinned newborns and brown in dark-skinned infants. By 6 to 9 months the permanent color is differentiated. Brushfield spots, or white specks around the edge of the iris, occasionally may be normal.

A searching nystagmus is common just after birth. The pupils are small but constrict to light.

The Ocular Fundus. The amount of data gathered during the funduscopic examination depends on the child's ability to hold the eyes still and on your ability to glean as much data as possible in a brief period of time.

A complete funduscopic examination is difficult to perform on an infant, but at least check the red reflex when the infant fixates at the bright light for a few seconds. Note any interruption.

Perform a funduscopic examination on an infant between 2 and 6 months of age. Position the infant (up to 18 months) lying on the table. The fundus appears pale, and the vessels are not fully developed. There is no foveal light reflection because the macula area will not be mature until 1 year.

Inspect the fundus of the young child and school-age child as described in the preceding section on the adult. Allow the child to handle the equipment. Explain why you are darkening the room and that you will leave a small light on. Assure the child that the procedure will not hurt. Direct the young child to look at an appealing picture, perhaps a toy or an animal, during the examination.

Abnormal Findings

Blank sunken eyes accompany malnutrition, dehydration, and a severe illness.

An upward lateral slope together with epicanthal folds and hypertelorism (large spacing between eyes) occurs with Down syndrome.

Ophthalmia neonatorum (conjunctivitis of the newborn) is a purulent discharge caused by a chemical irritant or a bacterial or viral agent from the birth canal.

Absence of iris color occurs with albinism.

Brushfield spots usually suggest Down syndrome.

Constant nystagmus, prolonged setting-sun sign, marked strabismus, and slow lateral movements suggest vision loss.

An interruption in the red reflex indicates opacity in the cornea or lens. An absent red reflex occurs with congenital cataracts or retinal disorders.

Papilledema is rare in the infant because the fontanels and open sutures absorb any increased intracranial pressure if it occurs.

Normal Range of Findings	Abnormal Findings

The Aging Adult

Visual Acuity. Perform the same examination as described in the adult section. Central acuity may decrease, particularly after 70 years of age. Peripheral vision may be diminished.

Ocular Structures. The eyebrows may show a loss of the outer 1/3 to 1/2 of hair because of a decrease in hair follicles. The remaining brow hair is coarse (Fig. 15.30). As a result of atrophy of elastic tissues, the skin around the eyes may show wrinkles or crow's feet. The upper lid may be so elongated as to rest on the lashes, resulting in a pseudoptosis.

In older adults with severe vision impairment, 46.7% reported having fallen in the previous year.[2]

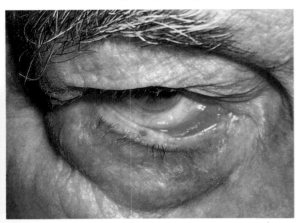

15.30 Pseudoptosis.   (Albert and Jakobiec, 1994.)

The eyes may appear sunken from atrophy of the orbital fat. In addition, the orbital fat may herniate, causing bulging at the lower lids and inner third of the upper lids.

The lacrimal apparatus may decrease tear production, causing the eyes to look dry and lusterless and the person to report a burning sensation. **Pingueculae** commonly show on the sclera (Fig. 15.31). These yellowish elevated nodules are caused by a thickening of the bulbar conjunctiva from prolonged exposure to sun, wind, and dust. Pingueculae appear at the 3 and 9 o'clock positions—first on the nasal side and then on the temporal side.

Ectropion (lower lid dropping away) and entropion (lower lid turning in) (see Table 15.2).

Distinguish pinguecula from the abnormal **pterygium,** also an opacity on the bulbar conjunctiva, but one that grows over the cornea (see Table 15.7).

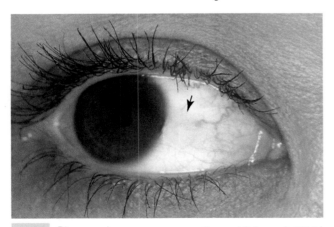

15.31 Pinguecula.   (Lemmi & Lemmi, 2011.)

The cornea may look cloudy with age. An **arcus senilis** is commonly seen around the cornea (Fig. 15.32). This is a gray-white arc or circle around the limbus; it is caused by deposition of lipid material. As more lipid accumulates, the cornea may look thickened and raised, but the arcus has no effect on vision.

Normal Range of Findings	Abnormal Findings

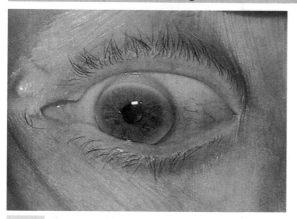

15.32   Arcus senilis.   (Swartz, 2015.)

Xanthelasma are soft, raised yellow lipid-laden plaques occurring on the lids at the inner canthus (Fig. 15.33). They commonly occur around the 50s and more frequently in women. They occur with both high and normal blood levels of cholesterol and have no pathologic significance.

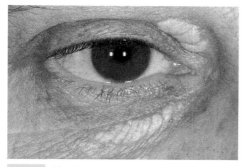

15.33   Xanthelasma.   (Mannis, 2017.)

Pupils are small in old age, and the pupillary light reflex may be slowed. The lens loses transparency and looks opaque.

The Ocular Fundus. Retinal structures generally have less shine. The blood vessels look paler, narrower, and attenuated. Arterioles appear paler and straighter, with a narrower light reflex. More arteriovenous crossing defects occur.

A normal development on the retinal surface are **drusen,** or benign degenerative hyaline deposits (Fig. 15.34). They are small, round, yellow dots that are scattered haphazardly on the retina. Although they do not occur in a pattern, they are usually symmetrically placed in the two eyes. They have no effect on vision.

Drusen are easily confused with the abnormal finding *hard exudates,* which occur with a more circular or linear pattern (see Table 15.10, p. 315). Also, drusen in the macular area occur with macular degeneration.

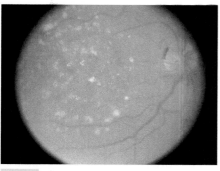

15.34   Drusen. (Friedman, N., & Pineda, R., 1998.)

Objective Data

HEALTH PROMOTION AND PATIENT TEACHING

(To all adults over 40 years) *I want to refer you to an eye specialist for screening for glaucoma. This is a progressive eye disease that affects over 2 million Americans and robs them of peripheral (side) vision. Most people with glaucoma have no symptoms and do not know they have the disease, but it can be treated. An eye specialist can screen you with specific equipment that we do not have in the hospital or in the primary care office.*

Glaucoma is a set of progressive eye neuropathies that can lead to severe visual field loss and blindness. It is the leading cause of irreversible blindness among blacks and Hispanics.[5] Glaucoma can reduce peripheral vision without yet harming central vision. Those who have glaucoma who are not blind still may have limited function, e.g., less able to drive a car or to read. The two most common forms of glaucoma are primary open-angle glaucoma (POAG) and primary angle-closure glaucoma (PACG). POAG is 7 times more common than PACG. Unrecognized and untreated, glaucoma is chronic, progressive, and causes irreversible visual field loss.[5] This progresses to tunnel vision and then to loss of central vision.

Risk factors include older age, black or Hispanic heritage, diabetes mellitus, and a family history of glaucoma. The American Academy of Ophthalmology recommends regular screening at age 40 years by an eye professional, and earlier for those with risk factors. Eye specialist screening uses measurement of the thickness of the optic nerve fibers, formal visual field testing, measurement of intraocular pressure, and stereoscopic optic nerve examination. Treatment may include eye drop medication, laser trabeculoplasty, and/or surgery to slow or prevent further vision loss. Unfortunately, treatments do not recover vision already lost from glaucoma. Therefore, early detection is critical to stop the progress of the disease.

DOCUMENTATION AND CRITICAL THINKING

Sample Charting

SUBJECTIVE

Vision reported "good" with no recent change. No eye pain, no inflammation, no discharge, no lesions. Wears no corrective lenses, vision last tested 1 year PTA; test for glaucoma at that time was normal.

OBJECTIVE

Snellen chart: Right 20/20, Left 20/20 −1. Fields normal by confrontation. Corneal light reflex symmetric bilaterally. Diagnostic positions test shows EOMs intact. Brows and lashes present. No ptosis. Conjunctiva clear. Sclera white. No lesions. PERRLA.
Fundi: Red reflex present bilaterally. Discs flat with sharp margins. Vessels present in all quadrants without crossing defects. Retinal background has even color with no hemorrhages or exudates. Macula has even color.

ASSESSMENT

Healthy vision function
Healthy eye structures

Clinical Case Study 1

E.K. is a 34-year-old married female homemaker brought to the emergency department by police after a reported domestic quarrel.

SUBJECTIVE

States husband struck her about the face and eyes with his fists about 1 hour PTA. "When he's drunk, he goes crazy." Pain in L cheek and both eyes felt immediately and continues. Alarmed at "bright red blood on eyeball." No bleeding from eye area or cheek. Vision intact just after trauma. Now reports difficulty opening lids.

OBJECTIVE

Sitting quietly and hunched over, hands over eyes. Voice tired and flat. L cheek swollen and discolored; no laceration. Lids edematous and discolored both eyes. No skin laceration. L lid swollen almost shut. L eye—Round 1-mm bright red patch over lateral aspect of globe. No active bleeding out of eye, iris intact, anterior chamber clear. R eye—Conjunctiva clear, sclera white, cornea and iris intact, anterior chamber clear. PERRLA. Pupils: RE resting 4 mm, constricted 1 mm; LE resting 4 mm, constricted 1 mm. Vision 14/14 both eyes by Jaeger card.

ASSESSMENT

Ecchymoses L cheek and both eyes
Subconjunctival hemorrhage L eye
Pain and inflammation
Decreased self-esteem

Clinical Case Study 2

S.T. is a 63-year-old married male postal carrier admitted to the medical center for surgery for suspected brain tumor. After postanesthesia recovery, S.T. is admitted to the neurology ICU, awake, lethargic with slowed but correct verbal responses, oriented × 3, moving all four extremities, vital signs stable. Pupils: RE resting 4 mm, constricted 2 mm = LE resting 4 mm, constricted 2 mm with sluggish response. Assessments are made q 15 minutes.

SUBJECTIVE

No response now to verbal stimuli.

OBJECTIVE

Semicomatose—No response to verbal stimuli, does withdraw R arm and leg purposefully to painful stimuli. No movement L arm or leg. Pupils: RE fixed and dilated 5 mm; LE resting 4 mm, constricted 2 mm. Vitals remain stable as noted on graphic sheet.

ASSESSMENT

Unilateral dilated and fixed R pupil
Decreased level of consciousness
Decreased mobility—No movement L side

Clinical Case Study 3

N.T. is a 14-year-old teen who presents to your office with "eye pain × 1 day."

SUBJECTIVE

"My eyes itch so bad. It feels like something is in there; and this morning when I woke up, I couldn't open my eyes. They were matted shut." Reports that yesterday his left eye felt "dry and itchy even though it kept watering," but now reports same symptoms in both eyes.

OBJECTIVE

Vital signs: Temp 97.8° F (36.6° C). BP 100/68 mm Hg (sitting). Pulse 78 bpm. Resp 14/min.
Vision: 20/20 both eyes without correction by Snellen chart.
General appearance: Anxious, consistently rubbing eyes and dabbing with the sleeve of his shirt.
HEENT: Normocephalic, preauricular nodes palpable (1 mm); purulent yellow discharge from both eyes, conjunctivae bright red bilat.; external canals clear w/o redness, bilat tympanic membranes pearly gray with visible landmarks; no exudate to throat.
Respiratory: Breath sounds clear in all fields; no adventitious sounds.

Documentation and Critical Thinking

ASSESSMENT

Conjunctivitis, both eyes
Acute pain and inflammation

Clinical Case Study 4

V.K. is an 87-year-old widowed female homemaker, living independently, who is admitted to hospital for observation and adjustment of digitalis medication. Cardiac status has been stable during hospital stay.

SUBJECTIVE

Reports desire to monitor own medication at home but fears problems because of blurred vision. First noted distant vision blurred 5 years ago, but near vision seemed to improve at that time. "I started to read better without my glasses!" Since then, blurring at distant vision has increased; near vision now blurred also.

    Able to navigate home environment without difficulty. Fixes simple meals with cold foods. Receives hot meal from "Meals on Wheels" at lunch. Enjoys TV, though it looks somewhat blurred. Unable to write letters, sew, or read paper, which she regrets.

OBJECTIVE

Vision by Jaeger card Right 20/200, Left 20/400 −1, with glasses on. Fields intact by confrontation. EOMs intact. Brow hair absent lateral third. Upper lids have folds of redundant skin, but lids do not droop. Lower lids and lashes intact. Xanthelasma present both inner canthi. Conjunctiva clear, sclera white, iris intact, L pupil looks cloudy, PERRLA, RE resting 3 mm, constricted 2 mm = LE resting 3 mm, constricted 2 mm.

Fundi: Red reflex has central dark spot both eyes. Discs flat, with sharp margins. Observed vessels normal. Unable to see in all four quadrants or macular area because of small pupils.

ASSESSMENT

Central opacity, both eyes
Central visual acuity deficit, both eyes
Loss of diversional activity

TABLE 15.1	Extraocular Muscle Dysfunction

NOTE: **Pseudostrabismus** has the appearance of strabismus because of epicanthic fold but is normal for a young child (see Fig. 15.29 on p. 299).

Asymmetric Corneal Light Reflex

Strabismus is true disparity of the eye axes. This constant malalignment is also termed *tropia* and is likely to cause amblyopia.
A. Esotropia—Inward turning of the eye.
B. Exotropia—Outward turning of the eyes.

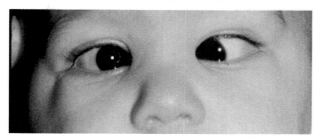

A, Left esotropia.

B, Exotropia.

Cover Test

C. Uncovered eye—If it jumps to fixate on designated point, it was out of alignment before (i.e., when you cover the stronger eye [C1], the weaker eye now tries to fixate [C2]).

Phoria—Mild weakness, apparent only with the cover test and less likely to cause amblyopia than a tropia but still possible.

D. Covered eye—If this is the weaker eye, once macular image is suppressed, it will drift to relaxed position (D1).

As eye is uncovered—If it jumps to reestablish fixation (D2), weakness exists.
Esophoria—Nasal (inward) drift.
Exophoria—Temporal (outward) drift.

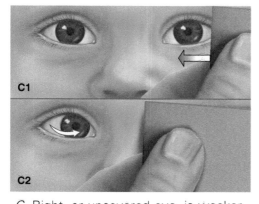

C, Right, or uncovered eye, is weaker.

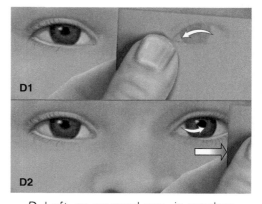

D, Left, or covered eye, is weaker.

Diagnostic Positions Test

(Paralysis apparent during movement through six cardinal positions of gaze.)

If eye will not turn:	Indicates dysfunction in cranial nerve
Straight nasal	III
Up and nasal	III
Up and temporal	III
Straight temporal	VI
Down and temporal	III
Down and nasal	IV

▶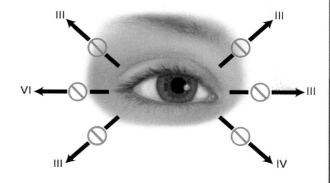

See Illustration Credits for source information.

TABLE 15.2	Eyelid Abnormalities

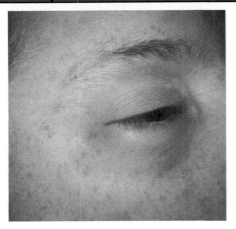

Periorbital Edema

Lids are swollen and puffy. Lid tissues are loosely connected, so excess fluid is easily apparent. This occurs with local infections; crying; trauma; and systemic conditions such as congestive heart failure, renal failure, allergy, hypothyroidism (myxedema).

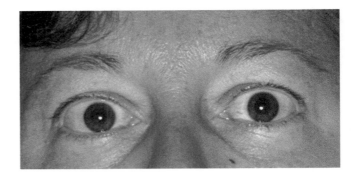

Exophthalmos (Protruding Eyes)

Exophthalmos is a forward displacement of the eyeballs and widened palpebral fissures. Note "lid lag," in which the upper lid rests well above the limbus and white sclera is visible. Acquired bilateral exophthalmos is associated with thyrotoxicosis.

Enophthalmos (Sunken Eyes) (Not Illustrated)

A look of narrowed palpebral fissures shows with enophthalmos, in which the eyeballs are recessed. Bilateral enophthalmos is caused by loss of fat in the orbits and occurs with dehydration and chronic wasting illnesses. For illustration, see Cachectic Appearance in Table 14.5, p. 273.

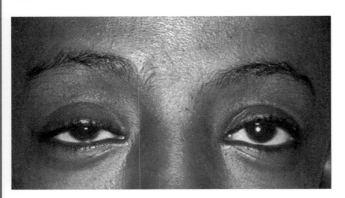

Ptosis (Drooping Upper Lid)

Ptosis occurs from neuromuscular weakness (e.g., myasthenia gravis with bilateral fatigue as the day progresses), oculomotor cranial nerve III damage, or sympathetic nerve damage (e.g., Horner syndrome) or is congenital as in this example. It is a positional defect that gives the person a sleepy appearance and impairs vision.

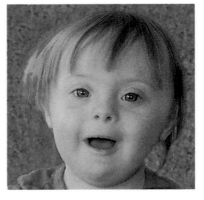

Upward Palpebral Slant

Although normal in many children, when combined with epicanthal folds, hypertelorism (large spacing between the eyes), and Brushfield spots (light-colored areas in outer iris), it indicates Down syndrome.

Continued

| TABLE 15.2 | Eyelid Abnormalities—cont'd |

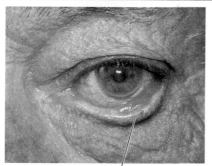

Ectropion

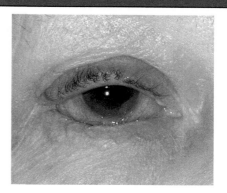

Ectropion

The lower lid is loose and rolling out (eversion), does not approximate to eyeball. Puncta cannot siphon tears effectively; thus excess tearing results. The eyes feel dry and itchy because the tears do not drain correctly. Exposed palpebral conjunctiva increases risk for inflammation. It occurs in aging from atrophy of elastic and fibrous tissues but may result from trauma, chronic inflammation, or Bell palsy.

Entropion

The lower lid rolls in (inversion) because of spasm of lids or scar tissue contracting. Constant rubbing of lashes may irritate cornea, leading to tearing and red eye. The person feels a "foreign body" sensation.

| TABLE 15.3 | Lesions on the Eyelids |

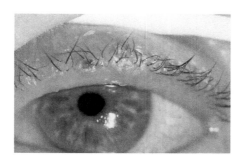

Blepharitis (Inflammation of the Eyelids)

Red, scaly, greasy flakes and thickened, crusted lid margins occur with staphylococcal infection or seborrheic dermatitis of the lid edge. Symptoms include burning, itching, tearing, foreign body sensation, and some pain.

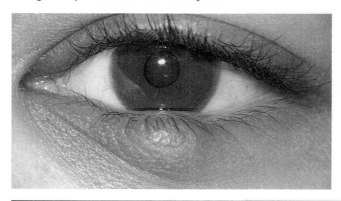

Dacryocystitis (Inflammation of the Lacrimal Sac)

Dacryocystitis is infection and blockage of sac and duct. Pain, warmth, redness, and swelling occur below the inner canthus toward the nose. Tearing is present. Pressure on sac yields purulent discharge from puncta.

Dacryoadenitis is an infection of the lacrimal gland (not illustrated). Pain, swelling, and redness occur in the outer third of the upper lid. It occurs with mumps, measles, and infectious mononucleosis or from trauma.

◀ Chalazion

A beady nodule protruding on the lid, chalazion is an obstruction and inflammation of a meibomian gland. If chronic, it is a nontender, firm, discrete swelling with freely movable skin overlying the nodule. If acutely inflamed, it is tender, warm, and red and points inside and not on lid margin (in contrast with stye).

Continued

TABLE 15.3	Lesions on the Eyelids—cont'd

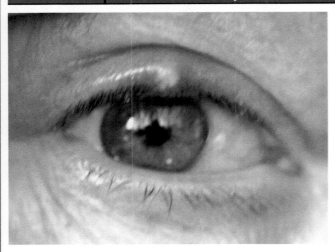

◀ Hordeolum (Stye)

Hordeolum is an acute localized staphylococcal infection of the hair follicles at the lid margin. It is painful, red, and swollen—a superficial, elevated pustule at the lid margin. Rubbing the eyes can cause cross-contamination and development of another stye. Managed with warm compresses, topical antibiotic ointment, may be combined with steroid ointment.[6]

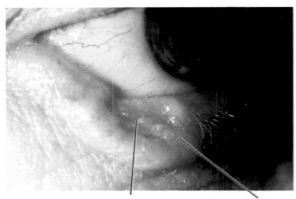

Central ulceration   Basal cell carcinoma

◀ Basal Cell Carcinoma

It is most often on the lower lid and presents as a small, painless nodule with central ulceration and sharp, rolled-out pearly edges. It occurs in older adults; associated with ultraviolet exposure and light skin. It is locally invasive, but metastasis is rare.

See Illustration Credits for source information.

TABLE 15.4	Pupil Abnormalities

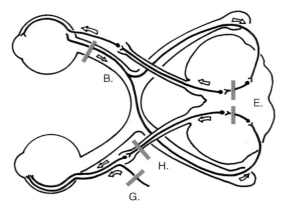

Red lines indicate the location of a lesion that stops the transmission of vision.

Continued

TABLE 15.4 | **Pupil Abnormalities—cont'd**

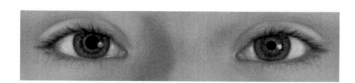

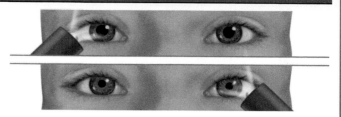

A. Unequal Pupil Size—Anisocoria

Although this exists normally in 5% of the population, consider central nervous system disease.

B. Monocular Blindness

When light is directed to the blind eye, no response occurs in either eye. When light is directed to the normal eye, both pupils constrict (direct and consensual response to light) as long as the oculomotor nerve is intact.

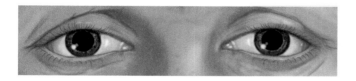

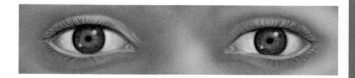

C. Dilated and Fixed Pupils—Mydriasis

Enlarged pupils occur with stimulation of the sympathetic nervous system, reaction to sympathomimetic drugs, use of dilating drops, acute glaucoma, or past or recent trauma. They also herald central nervous system injury, circulatory arrest, or deep anesthesia.

D. Constricted and Fixed Pupils—Miosis

Miosis occurs with the use of pilocarpine drops for glaucoma treatment, the use of narcotics, with iritis, and with brain damage of pons.

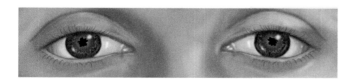

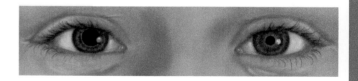

E. Argyll Robertson Pupil

There is no reaction to light; pupil does constrict with accommodation. Small and irregular bilaterally. Argyll Robertson pupil occurs with central nervous system syphilis, brain tumor, meningitis, and chronic alcoholism.

F. Tonic Pupil (Adie's Pupil)

Reaction to light and accommodation is sluggish. Tonic pupil is usually unilateral, a large regular pupil that does react, but sluggishly after long latent time. There is no pathologic significance.

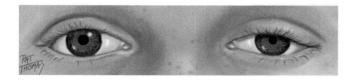

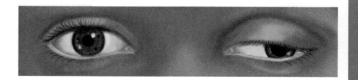

G. Horner Syndrome

A unilateral small, regular pupil does react to light and accommodation. Occurs with Horner syndrome, a lesion of the sympathetic nerve. Also note ptosis and absence of sweat (anhidrosis) on same side.

H. Cranial Nerve III Damage

Unilateral dilated pupil has no reaction to light or accommodation and occurs with oculomotor nerve damage. Ptosis with eye deviating down and laterally may be present.

TABLE 15.5 | **Visual Field Loss**

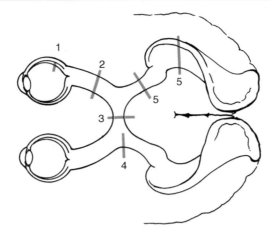

Red lines indicate the location of a lesion that interrupts the transmission of vision.

1. Retinal damage
   - Macula—Central blind area (e.g., diabetes):

   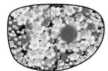

   - Localized damage—Blind spot (scotoma) corresponding to particular area:

   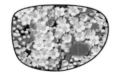

   - Increasing intraocular pressure—Decrease in peripheral vision (e.g., glaucoma). Starts with paracentral scotoma in early stage:

   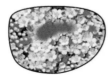

   - Retinal detachment—A shadow or diminished vision in one quadrant or one-half of visual field:

   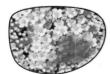

2. Lesion in globe or optic nerve—Injury here yields one blind eye, or unilateral blindness:

   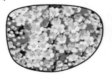

3. Lesion at optic chiasm (e.g., pituitary tumor)—Injury to crossing fibers only yields loss of nasal part of each retina and loss of both temporal visual fields. Bitemporal (heteronymous) hemianopsia:

   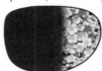

4. Lesion of outer uncrossed fibers at optic chiasm (e.g., aneurysm of left internal carotid artery exerts pressure on uncrossed fibers). Injury yields left nasal hemianopsia:

   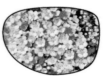

5. Lesion R optic tract or R optic radiation
   Visual field loss in R nasal and L temporal fields
   Loss of same half of visual field in both eyes is homonymous hemianopsia:

   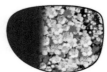

TABLE 15.6 | Red Eye—Vascular Disorders

NOTE: Always check visual acuity with any eye disorder. The following warrant emergency referral to ophthalmologist: sudden vision loss, trauma, herpes zoster infection (shingles) on face, corneal damage, distorted pupil, and severe pain.[12]

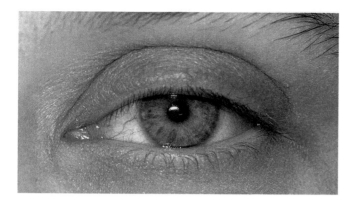

Conjunctivitis

Infection of the conjunctiva, "pink eye," has red, beefy-looking vessels at periphery but is usually clearer around iris, commonly from viral or bacterial infection, allergy, or chemical irritation. Purulent discharge accompanies bacterial infection. Preauricular lymph node is often swollen and painful, with a history of upper respiratory infection. Symptoms include itching, burning, foreign body sensation, and eyelids stuck together on awakening. Person has normal vision, normal pupil size, and reaction to light.

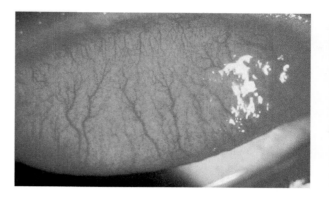

Allergic Conjunctivitis

Note the upper lid, conjunctiva, and cornea are inflamed from seasonal allergen (e.g., pollen, spores) or persistent allergen (e.g., house dust mite, animal dander). Symptoms include eye itching (not present in nonallergic conditions), redness, watering, discomfort. It does not obscure vision. Signs are diffuse redness of conjunctivae, lid swelling, upper tarsal surface that shows velvety thickening, redness, small papillae (shown above).

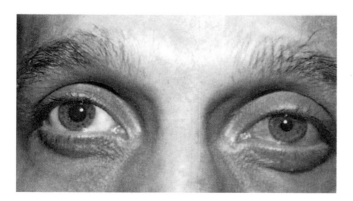

Iritis (Circumcorneal Redness)

There is a deep, dull red halo around the iris and cornea. Note that redness is around the iris, in contrast with conjunctivitis, in which redness is more prominent at the periphery. Pupil shape may be irregular from swelling of iris. Person also has marked photophobia, constricted pupil, blurred vision, and throbbing pain. Warrants immediate referral.

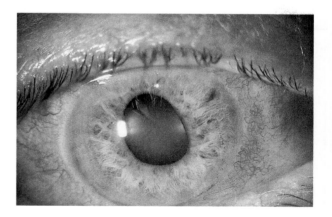

Primary Angle-Closure Glaucoma (PACG)

Acute narrow-angle glaucoma shows circumcorneal redness around the iris, with a dilated pupil. Pupil is oval, dilated; cornea looks "steamy"; and anterior chamber is shallow. Acute glaucoma occurs with sudden increase in intraocular pressure from blocked outflow from anterior chamber. The person experiences a sudden clouding of vision, sudden eye pain, and halos around lights. This requires emergency treatment to avoid permanent vision loss.[12]

Continued

TABLE 15.6 Red Eye—Vascular Disorders—cont'd

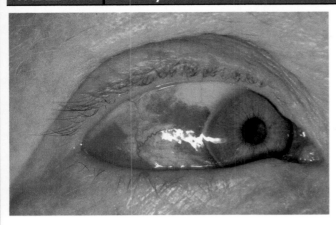

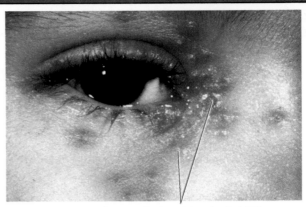

Seropurulent vesicles due to HSV

Subconjunctival Hemorrhage

A red patch on the sclera, subconjunctival hemorrhage looks alarming but is usually not serious. The red patch has sharp edges like a spot of paint, although here it is extensive. It occurs from increased intraocular pressure from coughing, vomiting, weight lifting, labor during childbirth, straining at stool, or trauma.

Herpes Simplex Virus (HSV)

Lid vesicles from primary HSV, associated with fever, preauricular lymphadenopathy. **Herpes zoster ophthalmicus** is a serious presentation of "shingles" involving the ophthalmic nerve. May have prodrome: numbness and tingling or burning along nerve route, fever, headache, malaise. Signs are acute, painful reddened conjunctivae; unilateral maculopapular rash with vesicles and ulcers; and ocular signs that threaten vision. Severity increases with older age.

See Illustration Credits for source information.

TABLE 15.7 Abnormalities on Cornea and Iris

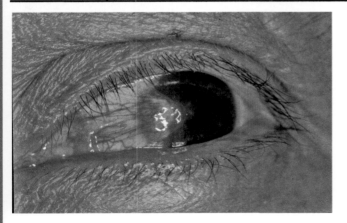

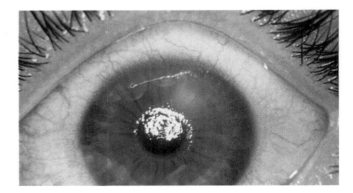

Pterygium

A triangular opaque wing of bulbar conjunctiva overgrows toward the center of the cornea. It looks membranous, translucent, and yellow to white; usually invades from nasal side; and may obstruct vision as it covers pupil. It occurs usually from chronic exposure to a hot, dry, sandy climate, which stimulates the growth of a pinguecula (see p. 300) into a pterygium.

Corneal Abrasion

This is the most common result of a blunt eye injury, but irregular ridges are usually visible only when fluorescein stain reveals yellow-green branching. Top layer of corneal epithelium is removed due to scratches or poorly fitting or overworn contact lenses. Because the area is rich in nerve endings, the person feels intense pain; a foreign body sensation; and lacrimation, redness, and photophobia.

Continued

TABLE 15.7 | **Abnormalities on Cornea and Iris—cont'd**

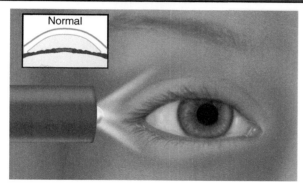

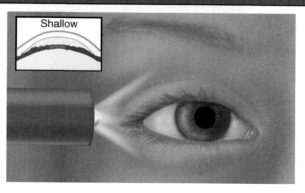

Normal Anterior Chamber (for Contrast)

A light directed across the eye from the temporal side illuminates the entire iris evenly because the normal iris is flat and creates no shadow.

Shallow Anterior Chamber

The iris is pushed anteriorly because of increased intraocular pressure. Because direct light is received from the temporal side, only the temporal part of the iris is illuminated; the nasal side is shadowed, the "shadow sign." This may be a sign of acute angle-closure glaucoma; the iris looks bulging because aqueous humor cannot circulate.

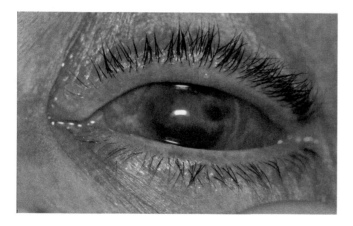

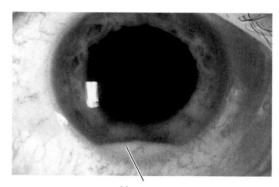

Hypopyon

Hyphema

Blood in the anterior chamber is a serious result of herpes zoster infection. Also occurs with blunt trauma (a fist or a baseball) or spontaneous hemorrhage. Suspect scleral rupture or major intraocular trauma. Note that gravity settles blood in front of iris.

Hypopyon

Layer of white blood cells in anterior chamber occurs with iritis and with inflammation in the anterior chamber. Symptons are pain, red eye, and possibly decreased vision.

See Illustration Credits for source information.

TABLE 15.8 | Lens Opacities

Cataracts

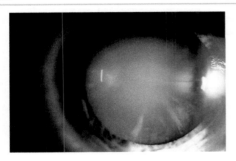

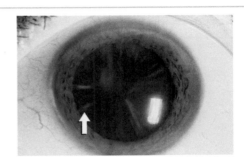

Central Gray Opacity—Nuclear Cataract

Nuclear cataract shows as an opaque gray surrounded by a black background as it forms in the center of lens nucleus. Through the ophthalmoscope it looks like a black center against the red reflex. It begins after age 40 years and develops slowly, gradually obstructing vision.

Star-Shaped Opacity—Cortical Cataract

Cortical cataract shows as asymmetric, radial, white spokes with black center. Through ophthalmoscope, black spokes are evident against the red reflex (not shown here). This forms in the outer cortex of lens, progressing faster than nuclear cataract.

See Illustration Credits for source information.

TABLE 15.9 | Optic Disc Abnormalities

Papilledema   Retinal hemorrhages

Optic Atrophy (Disc Pallor)

Optic atrophy is a white or gray color of the disc as a result of partial or complete death of the optic nerve. This results in decreased visual acuity, decreased color vision, and decreased contrast sensitivity.

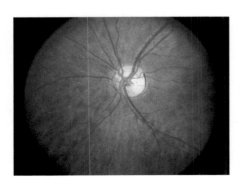

Papilledema (Choked Disc)

Increased intracranial pressure causes venous stasis in the globe, showing redness, congestion, and elevation of the disc; blurred margins; hemorrhages; and absent venous pulsations. This is a serious sign of intracranial pressure, usually caused by a space-occupying mass (e.g., a brain tumor or hematoma). Visual acuity is not affected.

◀ Excessive Cup-Disc Ratio

With primary open-angle glaucoma, the increased intraocular pressure decreases blood supply to retinal structures. The physiologic cup enlarges to more than half of the disc diameter, vessels appear to plunge over edge of cup, and vessels are displaced nasally. This is asymptomatic, although the person may have decreased vision or visual field defects in the late stages of glaucoma.

See Illustration Credits for source information.

TABLE 15.10 | **Retinal Vessel and Background Abnormalities**

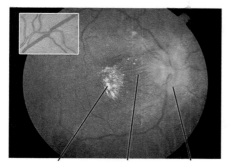

Macular star   Retinal folds   Disc edema

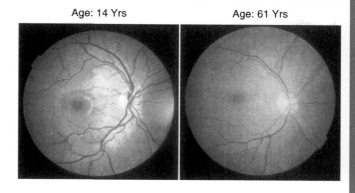

Age: 14 Yrs   Age: 61 Yrs

Arteriovenous Crossing (Nicking)

Inset shows arteriovenous crossing with interruption of blood flow. When vein is occluded, it dilates distal to crossing. This person also has disc edema and hard exudates in a macular star pattern that occur with acutely elevated (malignant) hypertension. With hypertension, the arteriole wall thickens and becomes opaque so that no blood is seen inside it (silver-wire arteries).

Narrowed (Attenuated) Arteries

This is a generalized decrease in arteriole diameter. The light reflex also narrows. It occurs with severe hypertension (shown above on the right) and with occlusion of the central retinal artery and retinitis pigmentosa.

Diabetic Retinopathy

Findings are nonproliferative changes that occur *within* the retina (microaneurysms, dot hemorrhages, blot hemorrhages, lipid exudates), and proliferative changes that occur on the inner surface of the retina or vitreous. Proliferative changes are new vessel formations, or neovascularization, that increase risk of retinal detachment or vitreous hemorrhage.[9]

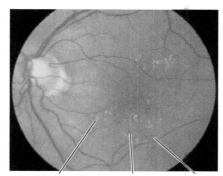

Lipid   Dot hemorrhage   Micro-
exudate   aneurysm

◀ **Moderate nonproliferative diabetic retinopathy.** Microaneurysms are round, punctate red dots that are localized dilations of a small vessel. Their edges are smooth and discrete. The vessel itself is too small to view with the ophthalmoscope; only the isolated red dots are seen. Dot hemorrhages are deep intraretinal hemorrhages that look splattered on. They are distinguished from microaneurysms by the blurred irregular edges. Lipid (hard) exudates are small yellow-white spots with distinct edges and a smooth, solid-looking surface. They often form a circular or linear pattern. (This is in contrast with drusen, which have a scattered haphazard location [see Fig. 15.34]).

◀ **Severe nonproliferative diabetic retinopathy.** Note lipid exudates as described and larger flame-shaped hemorrhages that look linear or spindle shaped.

Proliferative diabetic retinopathy (not shown). Neovascularization is new vessel formation that looks like radiating spokes.

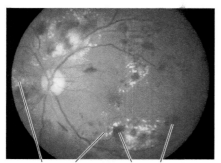

Lipid exudate   Intraretinal hemorrhages

See Illustration Credits for source information.

Summary Checklist: Eye Examination

1. **Test visual acuity**
   Snellen eye chart
   Near vision (those older than 40 years or having difficulty reading)
2. **Test visual fields—Confrontation test**
3. **Inspect extraocular muscle function**
   Corneal light reflex (Hirschberg test)
   Cover test (if indicated)
   Diagnostics positions test

4. **Inspect external eye structures**
   General
   Eyebrows
   Eyelids and lashes
   Eyeball alignment
   Conjunctiva and sclera
   Lacrimal apparatus
5. **Inspect anterior eyeball structures**
   Cornea and lens
   Iris and pupil
   Size, shape, and equality
   Pupillary light reflex
   Accommodation

6. **Inspect ocular fundus**
   Optic disc (color, shape, margins, cup-disc ratio)
   Retinal vessels (number, color, artery-vein [A : V] ratio, caliber, arteriovenous crossings, tortuosity, pulsations)
   General background (color, integrity)
   Macula

REFERENCES

1. American Academy of Ophthalmology. (n.d.). *Eye health statistics.* www.aao.org/newsroom/eye-health-statistics.
2. Crews, J. E., Chou, C., Stevens, J. A., et al. (2016). Falls among persons aged ≥65 years with and without severe vision impairment. Centers for Disease Control and Prevention. *MMWR Morb Mortal Wkly Rep, 65*(17), 433–437.
3. Frick, K. D., Joy, S. M., Wilson, D. A., et al. (2015). The global burden of potential productivity loss from uncorrected presbyopia. *Ophthalmology, 122,* 1706–1710.
4. Grossman, D. C., Curry, S. J., Owens, D. K., et al. (2017). Vision screening in children aged 6 months to 5 years: US Preventive Services Task Force. *JAMA, 318*(9), 836–844.
5. Gupta, D., & Chen, P. P. (2016). Glaucoma. *Am Fam Physician, 93*(8), 668–674.
6. Kaiser, P. K., Friedman, N. J., & Pineda, R. (2014). *The Massachusetts eye and ear infirmary illustrated manual of ophthalmology* (4th ed.). Philadelphia: Saunders.
7. Kerr, N. M., Chew, S. S., Eady, E. K., et al. (2010). Diagnostic accuracy of confrontation visual field tests. *Neurology, 74,* 1184–1190.
8. Leasher, J. L., Bourne, R., Flaxman, S. R., et al. (2016). Global estimates on the number of people blind or visually impaired by diabetic retinopathy. *Diabetes Care, 39,* 1643–1649.
9. McGee, S. (2018). *Evidence-based physical diagnosis* (4th ed.). St. Louis: Elsevier.
10. Mundy, K. M., Nichols, E., & Londsey, J. (2016). Socioeconomic disparities in cataract prevalence, characteristics, and management. *Semin Ophthalmol, 31*(4), 358–363.
11. National Eye Institute. (2017). *Glaucoma, open-angle.* https://www.nei.nih.gov/eyedata/glaucoma.
12. Ossorio, A. (2015). Red eye emergencies in primary care. *Nurse Pract, 40*(12), 45–53.
13. Varma, R., Vajaranant, T., Burkemper, B., et al. (2016). Visual impairment and blindness in adults in the United States from 2015 to 2050. *JAMA Ophthalmol, 134*(7), 802–809.

Ears

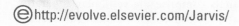

STRUCTURE AND FUNCTION

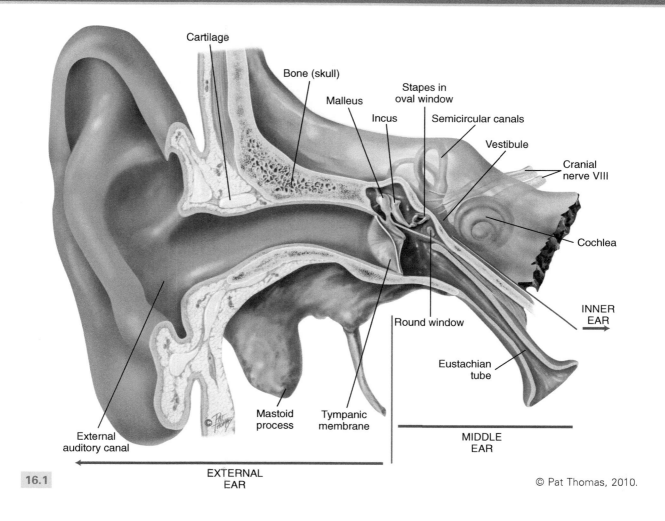

Cartilage

Bone (skull)

Malleus

Incus

Stapes in oval window

Semicircular canals

Vestibule

Cranial nerve VIII

Cochlea

Round window

INNER EAR

Eustachian tube

Mastoid process

Tympanic membrane

MIDDLE EAR

External auditory canal

16.1

EXTERNAL EAR

© Pat Thomas, 2010.

EXTERNAL EAR

The ear is the sensory organ for hearing and maintaining equilibrium. It has three parts: the external ear, the middle ear, and the inner ear. The external ear is called the **auricle** or **pinna** and consists of movable cartilage and skin (Fig. 16.1).

Its characteristic shape serves to funnel sound waves into its opening, the **external auditory canal**. The canal is a cul-de-sac 2.5 to 3 cm long in the adult and terminates at the **eardrum**, or **tympanic membrane (TM)**. The canal is lined with glands that secrete cerumen, a yellow, waxy material that lubricates and protects the ear. The wax forms a sticky barrier that helps keep foreign bodies from entering and reaching the sensitive tympanic membrane. Cerumen migrates out to the meatus by the movements of chewing and talking.

The outer one third of the canal is cartilage; the inner two thirds tunnels through the temporal bone and is covered by thin, sensitive skin. The canal has a slight S-curve in the adult. The outer one third curves up and toward the back of the head, whereas the inner two thirds angles down and forward toward the nose.

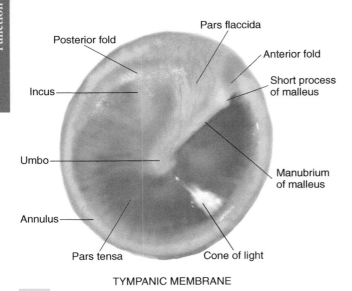

TYMPANIC MEMBRANE

16.2

The TM separates the external and middle ear and is tilted obliquely to the ear canal, facing downward and somewhat forward. It is translucent with a pearly gray color and a prominent cone of light in the anteroinferior quadrant, which is the reflection of the otoscope light (Fig. 16.2). The drum is oval and slightly concave, pulled in at its center by one of the middle ear ossicles, the **malleus.** The parts of the malleus show through the translucent drum; these are the **umbo,** the **manubrium** (handle), and the **short process.** The small, slack, superior section of the TM is called the **pars flaccida.** The remainder of the drum, which is thicker and more taut, is the **pars tensa.** The **annulus** is the outer fibrous rim of the drum.

Lymphatic drainage of the external ear flows to the parotid, mastoid, and superficial cervical nodes.

MIDDLE EAR

The middle ear is a tiny air-filled cavity inside the temporal bone (see Fig. 16.1). It contains tiny ear bones, or auditory ossicles: the **malleus, incus,** and **stapes.** It has several openings. Its opening to the outer ear is covered by the tympanic membrane. The openings to the inner ear are the oval window at the end of the stapes and the round window. Another opening is the **eustachian tube,** which connects the middle ear with the nasopharynx and allows passage of air. The tube is normally closed, but it opens with swallowing or yawning.

The middle ear has three functions: (1) it conducts sound vibrations from the outer ear to the central hearing apparatus in the inner ear; (2) it protects the inner ear by reducing the amplitude of loud sounds; and (3) its eustachian tube allows equalization of air pressure on each side of the tympanic membrane so the membrane does not rupture (e.g., during altitude changes in an airplane).

INNER EAR

The inner ear is embedded in bone. It contains the **bony labyrinth,** which holds the sensory organs for equilibrium and hearing. Within the bony labyrinth, the **vestibule** and the **semicircular canals** comprise the vestibular apparatus, and the **cochlea** (Latin for "snail shell") contains the central hearing apparatus. Although the inner ear is not accessible to direct examination, you can assess its functions.

HEARING

Note the landmarks of the auricle, and use these terms to describe your findings (Fig. 16.3). The mastoid process, the bony prominence behind the lobule, is not part of the ear but is an important landmark.

The function of hearing involves the auditory system at three levels: peripheral, brainstem, and cerebral cortex. At the peripheral level the ear transmits sound and converts its vibrations into electrical impulses, which can be analyzed by the brain. For example, you hear an alarm bell ringing in the hall. Its sound waves travel instantly to your ears. The *amplitude* is how loud the alarm is; its *frequency* is the pitch (in this case, high) or the number of cycles per second. The sound waves produce vibrations on your tympanic membrane. These vibrations are carried by the middle ear ossicles to your oval window. Then the sound waves travel through your cochlea, which is coiled like a snail shell, and are dissipated against the round window. Along the way the **basilar membrane** vibrates at a point specific to the frequency of the sound. In this case the high frequency of the alarm stimulates the basilar membrane at its base near the stapes (Fig. 16.4). The numerous fibers along the basilar membrane

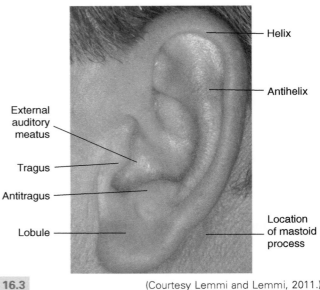

16.3 (Courtesy Lemmi and Lemmi, 2011.)

are the receptor hair cells of the **organ of Corti,** the sensory organ of hearing. As the hair cells bend, they mediate the vibrations into electric impulses. The electrical impulses are conducted by the auditory portion of cranial nerve VIII to the brainstem.

The function at the brainstem level is *binaural interaction,* which permits locating the direction of a sound in space and identifying the sound. How does this work? Each ear is actually one half of the total sensory organ. The ears are located on each side of a movable head. Cranial nerve VIII from each ear sends signals to both sides of the brainstem. Areas in the brainstem are sensitive to differences in intensity and timing of the messages from the two ears, depending on the way the head is turned.

Finally the function of the cortex is to interpret the meaning of the sound and begin the appropriate response. All this happens in the split second that it takes you to react to the alarm.

Pathways of Hearing. The normal pathway of hearing is air conduction (AC), described earlier; it is the most efficient. An alternate route of hearing is by bone conduction (BC). Here the bones of the skull vibrate. These vibrations are transmitted directly to the inner ear and to cranial nerve VIII (see Fig. 16.4).

Hearing Loss. Anything that obstructs the transmission of sound impairs hearing. A **conductive** hearing loss involves a mechanical dysfunction of the external or middle ear. It is a partial loss because the person is able to hear if the sound amplitude is increased enough to reach normal nerve elements in the inner ear. Conductive hearing loss may be caused by impacted cerumen, foreign bodies, a perforated tympanic membrane, pus or serum in the middle ear, and otosclerosis (a decrease in mobility of the ossicles). (See Table 16.1 on p. 335.)

Sensorineural (or perceptive) loss signifies pathology of the inner ear, cranial nerve VIII, or the auditory areas of the cerebral cortex.[4] A simple increase in amplitude may not enable the person to understand words. Sensorineural hearing loss may be caused by *presbycusis,* a gradual nerve degeneration that occurs with aging, and by ototoxic drugs, which affect the hair cells in the cochlea. A **mixed** loss is a combination of conductive and sensorineural types in the same ear. (See Table 16.1 on p. 335.)

Equilibrium. The 3 semicircular canals, or labyrinth, in the inner ear constantly feed information to your brain about the position of your body in space (see Fig. 16.1). They work like plumb lines to determine verticality or depth. The plumb lines of the ear register the angle of your head in relation to gravity. If the labyrinth ever becomes inflamed, it feeds the

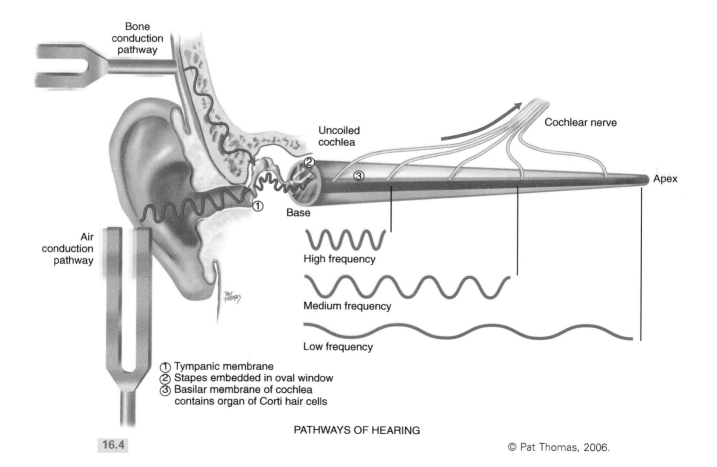

Bone conduction pathway

Uncoiled cochlea

Cochlear nerve

Apex

Base

Air conduction pathway

High frequency

Medium frequency

Low frequency

① Tympanic membrane
② Stapes embedded in oval window
③ Basilar membrane of cochlea
  contains organ of Corti hair cells

PATHWAYS OF HEARING

16.4

© Pat Thomas, 2006.

wrong information to the brain, creating a staggering gait and a strong spinning, whirling sensation called *vertigo*.

❖ DEVELOPMENTAL COMPETENCE

Infants and Children

The inner ear starts to develop early in the 5th week of gestation. In early development the ear is posteriorly rotated and low set; later it ascends to its normal placement around eye level. If maternal rubella infection occurs during the 1st trimester, it can damage the organ of Corti and impair hearing.

The infant's eustachian tube is relatively shorter and wider, and its position is more horizontal than the adult's; thus it is easier for pathogens from the nasopharynx to migrate through to the middle ear (Fig. 16.5). The lumen is surrounded by lymphoid tissue, which increases during childhood; thus the lumen is easily occluded. These factors place the infant at greater risk for middle ear infections than the adult. The infant's and the young child's external ear canals are shorter and have a slope opposite to that of the adult's.

The Adult

Otosclerosis is a cause of conductive hearing loss in young adults between the ages of 20 and 40 years. It is a gradual bone formation that causes the footplate of the stapes to become fixed in the oval window, impeding the transmission of sound and causing progressive deafness.

The Aging Adult

In the older adult, cilia lining the ear canal become coarse and stiff. This may cause cerumen to accumulate and oxidize, which greatly reduces hearing. The cerumen itself is drier because of atrophy of the apocrine glands. A life history of frequent ear infections may result in scarring on the drum.

Impacted cerumen is common in aging adults and other at-risk groups (e.g., institutionalized and mentally disabled), who may underreport the associated hearing loss. Cerumen impaction also blocks conduction in those wearing hearing aids. Cerumen should be removed when it leads to conductive hearing loss or interferes with full assessment of the ear. Ceruminolytics are wax-softening agents that expedite removal with electric or manual irrigators.

Age-related hearing loss (presbycusis) is documented in ⅔ of adults over 70 years of age and is associated with communication problems, a decrease in health-related quality of life, and a loss of physical and cognitive function, as well as depression, dementia, an increase in falls, an increase in hospitalizations, social isolation and loneliness, and even increased mortality[1,3]! It is a sensorineural loss that affects the middle ear structures or causes damage to nerve cells in the inner ear or to cranial nerve VIII. The person first notices a high-frequency tone loss, such as difficulty hearing a phone ringing or a microwave beeping. Also it is harder to hear consonants than vowels, and words sound garbled. The ability to localize sound is impaired. This hearing loss is accentuated with competing background noise (e.g., with music, with dishes clattering, or at a large, noisy party).

🌐 CULTURE AND GENETICS

Presbycusis affects men more than women of the same age, and there is a lower prevalence among African Americans compared with whites or Hispanics.[1] Reasons for this are unknown, but current theories relate to melanin pigment protection in the cochlea or other environmental factors. There is a socioeconomic gradient of hearing loss, too, with adults of lower income or education level at greater risk.[1]

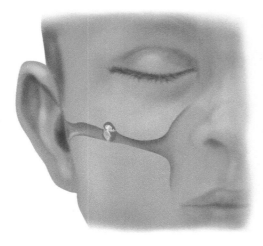

INFANT
Horizontal eustachian tube

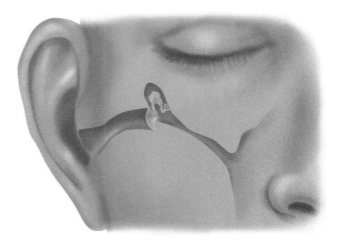

ADULT
Sloped eustachian tube

16.5

Otitis media, or OM (middle ear infection), occurs because of obstruction of the eustachian tube or passage of nasopharyngeal secretions into the middle ear. This creates a ripe environment for bacteria to grow. Acute OM is so common that up to 60% of children experience an episode during the 1st year of life, and by age 3 years up to 83% have suffered an episode.[9]

Besides the anatomy of the infant eustachian tube, the following risk factors predispose to acute OM: absence of breastfeeding in the first 3 months of age, preterm birth, exposure to secondhand tobacco smoke (SHS), daycare attendance, male sex, pacifier use, seasonality (fall and winter), and bottle-feeding.[9] Ambulatory visits for acute OM have decreased in the past 20 years, a decrease best explained by a concurrent increase in the number of smoke-free households. Public awareness of the dangers of SHS on child health together with the surge in no-smoking rules in households and vehicles may be responsible. Also, hospital admissions for acute OM have decreased since the addition of pneumococcal and influenza vaccinations to the early childhood immunization schedule.[10]

The most important side effect of acute OM is the persistence of fluid in the middle ear after treatment. This middle ear effusion can impair hearing, placing the child at risk for delayed cognitive development.

Cerumen is genetically determined, with two distinct types. Wet, honey-brown wax occurs in Caucasians and African Americans, and a dry, flaky white wax is found in East Asians and American Indians. The presence and composition of cerumen are not related to poor hygiene. Cerumen is supposed to be present—to lubricate, waterproof, and clean the external auditory canal.[8] Cerumen also is antibacterial, and it traps foreign bodies. Take care to avoid mistaking the flaky, dry cerumen for eczematous lesions.

Subjective Data

SUBJECTIVE DATA

1. Earache
2. Infections
3. Discharge
4. Hearing loss
5. Environmental noise
6. Tinnitus
7. Vertigo
8. Patient-centered care

Examiner Asks/	Rationale
1. Earache. Any **earache** or other pain in ears? • Location—Feel close to the surface or deep in the head? • Does it hurt when you push on the ear? • Character—Dull, aching or sharp, stabbing? Constant or come and go? Is it affected by changing position of head? • Any accompanying cold symptoms or sore throat? Any problems with sinuses or teeth? • Ever been hit on the ear or the side of the head or had any sport injury? Ever had any trauma from a foreign body? • What have you tried to relieve pain?	**Otalgia** occurs directly from ear disease or is referred pain from a problem in teeth or oropharynx. Virus/bacteria from upper respiratory infection (URI) may migrate up the eustachian tube to inflame the middle ear. Trauma may rupture the TM. Assess effect of coping strategies.
2. Infections. Any ear **infections?** As an adult or in childhood? • How frequent were they? How were they treated?	A history of chronic ear problems alerts you to possible hearing loss.
3. Discharge. Any **discharge** from your ears? • Does it look like pus, or is it bloody? • Any odor to the discharge? • Any relation between the discharge and the ear pain?	**Otorrhea** suggests infected canal or perforated eardrum such as: *External otitis*—Purulent, sanguineous, or watery discharge. *Acute OM with perforation*—Purulent discharge. *Cholesteatoma*—Dirty yellow-gray discharge, foul odor. Typically with perforation—Ear pain occurs first, stops with a popping sensation; then drainage occurs.

Subjective Data

Examiner Asks	Rationale
4. Hearing loss. Do you have any trouble hearing? • Onset—Did the loss come on slowly or all at once? Trouble understanding speech?	**Presbycusis** is gradual onset over years, bilateral, mostly high-frequency loss, worse in noisy environments, whereas a trauma hearing loss is often sudden. Refer any sudden loss in one or both ears *not* associated with URI.
• Character—Has all your hearing decreased or just on hearing certain sounds? • In which situations do you notice the loss: conversations, using the telephone, listening to TV, at a party? • Do people seem to shout at you?	Loss shows with competition from background noise, as at a party. *Recruitment*—A hearing loss with low-intensity speech, but sound actually becomes painful when speaker repeats in a loud voice.
• Do ordinary sounds seem hollow, as if you are hearing in a barrel or under water? • Recently traveled by airplane? • Any family history of hearing loss? • Effort to treat—Any hearing aid or other device? Anything to help hearing? • Coping strategies—How does the loss affect your daily life? Any job problems? Feel embarrassed? Frustrated? How do your family, friends react?	This happens when cerumen expands and becomes impacted, as after swimming or showering. Hearing loss can cause social isolation, decreased quality of life, functional decline, cognitive decline, depression.[3]

Note to examiner—During history note these clues from normal conversation that indicate unreported hearing loss.
1. Person lip-reads or watches your face and lips closely rather than your eyes
2. Frowns or strains forward to hear
3. Postures head to catch sounds with better ear
4. Misunderstands your questions or frequently asks you to repeat
5. Acts irritable or shows startle reflex when you raise your voice (recruitment)
6. Person's speech sounds garbled, possibly vowel sounds distorted
7. Inappropriately loud voice
8. Flat, monotonous tone of voice

Examiner Asks	Rationale
5. Environmental noise. Do you consider the noise level where you are working now to be high? What about your leisure time? Are you regularly exposed to sounds so loud that you have to shout to make yourself heard by someone standing more than one yard away? Regularly exposed to gunfire noise? • Noise protection—Any steps to protect your ears such as headphones or ear plugs?	Old trauma to hearing initially goes unnoticed but results in further decibel loss in later years.
6. Tinnitus. Ever felt ringing, roaring, or buzzing in your ears? When did this occur? How long have you had it? (**NOTE:** Tinnitus is bothersome and persistent when it lasts 6 months or longer.[11]) • Seem louder at night?	**Tinnitus** is the perception of sound without an external source[1a]; it occurs with sensorineural hearing loss, cerumen impaction, middle ear infection, and other ear disorders. Tinnitus seems louder with no competition from environmental noise.

Examiner Asks	Rationale
• Are you taking any medication?	The main ototoxic drugs in clinical use: aminoglycoside antibiotics (loss develops in 20% of patients) and the anticancer drug cisplatin (loss in 60% to 65% of patients).[2] Also possibly ototoxic are furosemide, vancomycin, and chronic use of aspirin.
• How does tinnitus affect your everyday life? Difficulty concentrating, sleeping, at work, leisure time, time with others?	Tinnitus can cause sleep disturbance, depression, or anxiety and be so debilitating that person cannot lead a normal life.[11]
7. Vertigo. Ever felt **vertigo;** that is, the room spinning around or yourself spinning? (Vertigo is a true twirling motion.) Is the feeling worse with a change in head position, getting in or out of bed, rolling over in bed, bending forward, or tilting the head back?[5]	Benign paroxysmal positional vertigo is the most common type of vertigo, with brief (<1 minute) spinning sensations. Occurs with dysfunction of labyrinth. Increases risk for falls and doing daily activities.[5] Feeling of spinning of person (**subjective vertigo**) or of objects around person (**objective vertigo**).
• Ever felt dizzy, as if you are not quite steady, like falling or losing your balance? Giddy, light-headed?	Distinguish true vertigo from dizziness or light-headedness.
8. Patient-centered care. How do you clean your ears?	Potential trauma from invasive instruments. Cotton-tipped applicators can impact cerumen, causing hearing loss.
• Last time you had your hearing checked? • If a hearing loss was noted, did you obtain a hearing aid? How long have you had it? Do you wear it? How does it work? Any trouble with upkeep, cleaning, changing batteries?	Prescribe frequency of hearing assessment according to person's age or risk factors.

Additional History for Infants and Children

1. Ear infections. At what age was the child's first episode? How many ear infections in the past 6 months? How many total? How were these treated? • Has the child had any surgery such as insertion of ear tubes or removal of tonsils? • Are infections increasing in frequency or severity or staying the same? • Does anyone in the home smoke cigarettes?	A first episode within 3 months of life increases risk for recurrent OM. Recurrent OM is 3 episodes in past 3 months or 4 within past year. Passive and parental smoke are risk factors for OM.
• Does your child receive child care outside your home? In a daycare center or someone else's home? How many children are in the group?	Daycare attendance and bottle-feeding (as opposed to breastfeeding) are risk factors for OM.
2. Does the child seem to be hearing well? • Have you noticed that the infant startles with loud noise? Did the infant babble around 6 months? Does he or she talk? At what age did he or she start talking? Was the speech intelligible? • Ever had the child's hearing tested? If there was a hearing loss, did it follow any diseases in the child or mother during pregnancy? (**NOTE:** It is important to catch any problem early, because a child with hearing loss is at risk for delayed speech and social development and learning deficit.)	Children at risk for hearing deficit: those exposed to maternal rubella or maternal ototoxic drugs in utero; premature infants; low-birth-weight infants; trauma or hypoxia at birth; and infants with congenital liver or kidney disease. In children the incidence of meningitis, measles, mumps, OM, and any illness with persistent high fever may increase risk for hearing deficit.
3. Does the child tend to put objects in the ears? Is the older child or adolescent active in contact sports?	These children are at increased risk for trauma.

Subjective Data

OBJECTIVE DATA

PREPARATION

Position the adult sitting up straight with his or her head at your eye level. Occasionally the ear canal is partially filled with cerumen, which obstructs your view of the TM. If the eardrum is intact and no current infection is present, a preferred method of cleaning the adult canal is to soften the cerumen with a warmed solution of mineral oil and hydrogen peroxide. Then the canal is irrigated with warm water (body temperature) with a bulb syringe or a low-pulsatile dental irrigator (Water-Pik). Direct fluid to the posterior wall. Leave space around the irrigator tip for water to escape. Do not irrigate if the history or examination suggests perforation or infection.

EQUIPMENT NEEDED

Otoscope with bright light (fresh batteries give off white—not yellow—light).
Pneumatic bulb attachment, sometimes used with infant or young child.

Normal Range of Findings	Abnormal Findings

Inspect and Palpate the External Ear

Size and Shape

The ears are of equal size bilaterally with no swelling or thickening. Ears of unusual size and shape may be a normal familial trait with no clinical significance.

Microtia—ears smaller than 4 cm vertically; *macrotia*—ears larger than 10 cm.
Edema with infection or trauma.

Skin Condition

The skin color is consistent with the person's facial skin color. The skin is intact, with no lumps or lesions. On some people you may note **Darwin tubercle,** a small, painless nodule at the helix. This is a congenital variation and is not significant (Fig. 16.6).

Reddened, excessively warm skin with inflammation (see Table 16.2, External Ear Abnormalities, p. 335).
Crusts and scaling occur with otitis externa, eczema, contact dermatitis, seborrhea.
Enlarged, tender lymph nodes in the region indicate inflammation of the pinna or mastoid process.
Red-blue discoloration with frostbite.
Tophi, sebaceous cyst, chondrodermatitis, keloid, carcinoma (see Table 16.3, Lumps and Lesions on the Ear, p. 336).

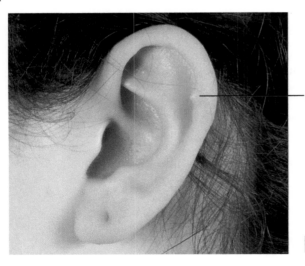

Darwin tubercle

16.6

Tenderness

Move the pinna and push on the tragus. They should feel firm, and movement should produce no pain. Palpating the mastoid process should also produce no pain.

Pain with movement occurs with otitis externa and furuncle.
Pain at the mastoid process may indicate mastoiditis or enlarged posterior auricular node.

The External Auditory Meatus

Note the size of the opening to direct your choice of speculum for the otoscope. No swelling, redness, or discharge should be present.

A sticky, yellow discharge accompanies otitis externa or may indicate OM if the drum has ruptured.

Normal Range of Findings	**Abnormal Findings**

Some cerumen is usually present. The color varies from gray-yellow to light brown and black, and the texture varies from moist and waxy to dry and desiccated. A large amount of cerumen obscures visualization of the canal and drum.

Inspect with the Otoscope

As you inspect the external ear, note the size of the auditory meatus. Choose the largest speculum that fits comfortably in the ear canal, and attach it to the otoscope. Tilt the person's head slightly away from you toward the opposite shoulder. This method brings the obliquely sloping eardrum into better view.

Pull the pinna up and back on an adult or older child; this helps straighten the S-shape of the canal (Fig. 16.7). (Pull the pinna down on an infant and a child younger than 3 years [see Fig. 16.13]). Hold the pinna gently but firmly. Do not release traction on the ear until you have finished the examination and the otoscope is removed.

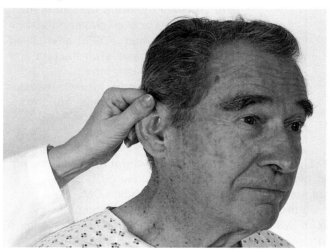

16.7

Hold the otoscope "upside down" along your fingers and have the dorsa (back) of your hand touching the person's cheek braced to steady the otoscope (Fig. 16.8). This position feels awkward to you only at first. It soon will feel natural, and you will find it useful to prevent forceful insertion. Your stabilizing hand also acts as a protecting lever if the person suddenly moves the head.

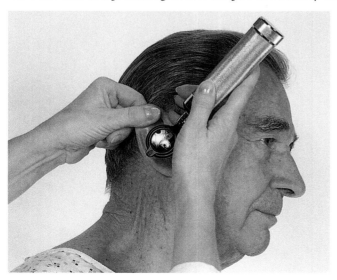

16.8

Objective Data

Normal Range of Findings	Abnormal Findings

Insert the speculum slowly and carefully along the axis of the canal. Watch the insertion; then put your eye up to the otoscope. Avoid touching the inner "bony" section of the canal wall, which is covered by a thin epithelial layer and is sensitive to pain. Sometimes you cannot see anything but canal wall. If so, try to reposition the person's head, apply more traction on the pinna, and re-angle the otoscope to look forward toward the person's nose.

Once it is in place, you may need to rotate the otoscope slightly to visualize the entire eardrum; do this gently. A final note—perform the otoscopic examination before you test hearing; ear canals with impacted cerumen give the erroneous impression of pathologic hearing loss.

The External Canal

Note any redness and swelling, lesions, foreign bodies, or discharge. If any discharge is present, note the color and odor. (Clean any discharge from the speculum before examining the other ear to avoid contamination with possibly infectious material.) For a person with a hearing aid, note any irritation on the canal wall from poorly fitting ear molds.

Redness and swelling occur with otitis externa; canal may be completely closed with swelling.

Purulent otorrhea suggests otitis externa or OM if the drum has ruptured.

Frank blood or clear, watery drainage (cerebrospinal fluid [CSF]) after head injury suggests basal skull fracture and warrants immediate referral.

Foreign body, polyp, furuncle, exostosis (see Table 16.4, Ear Canal Abnormalities, p. 338).

The Tympanic Membrane

Color and Characteristics. Systematically explore its landmarks (Fig. 16.9). The normal eardrum is shiny and translucent, with a pearl gray color. The cone-shaped light reflex is prominent in the anteroinferior quadrant (at the 5 o'clock position in the right drum and the 7 o'clock position in the left drum). This is the reflection of your otoscope light. Sections of the malleus are visible through the translucent drum: the umbo, manubrium, and short process. (Infrequently you also may see the incus behind the drum; it shows as a whitish haze in the upper posterior area.) At the periphery the annulus looks whiter and denser.

Yellow-amber drum color occurs with OM with effusion (serous).

Red color with acute OM.

Absent or distorted landmarks.

Air/fluid level or air bubbles behind drum indicate OM with effusion (see Tables 16.5, Abnormal Views Seen on Otoscopy, and 16.6, Abnormal Tympanic Membranes, pp. 335 to 337).

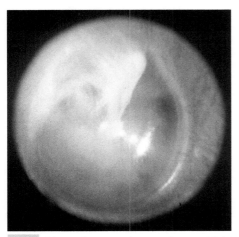

16.9 Normal tympanic membrane *(right ear).*
(Courtesy Lemmi and Lemmi, 2011.)

Normal Range of Findings	Abnormal Findings

Position. The eardrum is flat and slightly pulled in at the center.

Retracted drum due to vacuum in middle ear with obstructed eustachian tube.

Bulging drum due to increased pressure in OM.

Integrity of Membrane. Inspect the eardrum and the entire circumference of the annulus for perforations. The normal TM is intact. Some adults may show scarring, which is a dense white patch on the drum. This is a sequela of repeated ear infections.

Examine the other ear but switch otoscope hands so the hand holding the otoscope braces against the person's cheek.

Perforation shows as a dark oval area or as a larger opening on the drum.

Vesicles on drum (see Table 16.6).

Test Hearing Acuity

Your screening for a hearing deficit begins during the history; "Do you have difficulty hearing now?" If the answer is *yes,* perform audiometric testing or refer for audiometric testing. If the answer is *no,* screen using the whispered voice test described as follows.

A pure tone audiometer gives a precise quantitative measure of hearing by assessing the person's ability to hear sounds of varying frequency. This is a battery-powered, lightweight, handheld instrument that is available in most outpatient settings. With the patient sitting, prop his or her elbow on the armrest of the chair with the hand making a gentle fist. Tell the patient, "You will hear faint tones of different pitches. Please raise your finger as soon as you hear the tone; then lower your finger as soon as you no longer hear the tone." Choose tones of random loudness in decibels on the audioscope. Each tone is on for 1.5 seconds and off for 1.5 seconds. Test each ear separately and record the results. An audiometer gives a precise quantitative measure of hearing by assessing the person's ability to hear sounds of varying frequency.

This single question in people over 50 years has up to 90% agreement with hearing loss documented by audiometric testing.

Conductive and sensorineural loss (see Table 16.1, Hearing Loss, p. 335).

Whispered Voice Test

Stand arm's length (2 feet) behind the person. Test one ear at a time while masking hearing in the other ear to prevent sound transmission around the head. This is done by placing one finger on the tragus and pushing it in and out of the auditory meatus. Move your head to 1 to 2 feet from the person's ear. Exhale fully and whisper slowly a set of 3 random numbers and letters, such as "5, B, 6." Normally the person repeats each number/letter correctly after you say it. If the response is not correct, repeat the whispered test using a different combination of 3 numbers and letters. A passing score is correct repetition of 4 of a possible 6 numbers/letters. Assess the other ear using yet another set of whispered items "4, K, 2."

The person is unable to hear whispered items. A whisper is a high-frequency sound and is used to detect high-tone loss.

Tuning Fork Tests

Tuning fork tests measure hearing by air conduction (AC) or bone conduction (BC), in which the sound vibrates through the cranial bones to the inner ear. The AC route through the ear canal and middle ear is usually the more sensitive route. If hearing loss is identified by history or whispered voice test, tuning fork tests traditionally were used to distinguish conductive loss from sensorineural loss. However, up to 40% of normal hearing people lateralize the Weber test, i.e., hear the tone louder in one ear. The Rinne (pronounced RIN-neh) test is more accurate in detecting conductive hearing loss. (Technique is described in Table 16.7.) Be aware that neither test can distinguish normal hearing from a sensorineural loss in both ears[5a]—you should rely on audiometry.

With documented hearing loss, these tests may help distinguish conductive loss from sensorineural loss (see Table 16.7, Tuning Fork Tests, p. 342). But they cannot screen a conductive loss from a mixed conductive/sensorineural loss.[5a]

Objective Data

Objective Data

| Normal Range of Findings | Abnormal Findings |

The Vestibular Apparatus

The **Romberg test** assesses the ability of the vestibular apparatus in the inner ear to help maintain standing balance. Because the Romberg test also assesses intactness of the cerebellum and proprioception, it is discussed in Chapter 24 (see Fig. 24.21).

❖ DEVELOPMENTAL COMPETENCE

Infants and Young Children

Examination of the external ear is similar to that described for the adult, with the addition of examination of position and alignment on head. Note the ear position. The top of the pinna should match an imaginary line extending from the corner of the eye to the occiput. The ear should also be positioned within 10 degrees of vertical (Fig. 16.10).

Low-set ears are found with genetic disorders, including trisomy 21 (Down syndrome). Large prominent ears, misshapen ears, and creases on earlobes are nonspecific.

Preauricular skin tags may occur alone or with other facial anomalies.

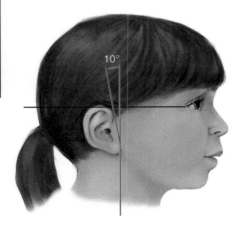

Normal alignment

16.10

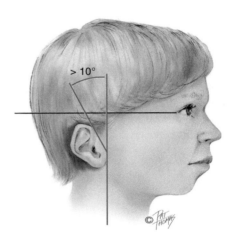

Low-set ears and deviation in alignment

© Pat Thomas, 2006.

Otoscopic Examination. In addition to its place in the complete examination, eardrum assessment is mandatory for any infant or child requiring care for illness or fever. For the infant or young child, the timing of the otoscopic examination is best toward the end of the complete examination. Many young children protest vigorously during this procedure no matter how well you prepare, and it is difficult to re-establish cooperation afterward. Save the otoscopic examination until last.

Ear pain and ear rubbing are associated with acute OM, as are a bulging red eardrum and middle ear effusion. Fever is usually present but not always (see Table 16.6).

Normal Range of Findings

To help prepare the child, let him or her hold your funny-looking "flashlight." You may wish to have the child look in the parent's or a toy puppet's ear as you hold the otoscope (Fig. 16.11).

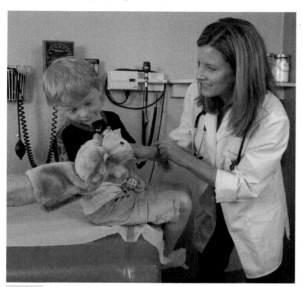

16.11

Positioning of the child is important. You need a clear view of the canal. Avoid harsh restraint, but you must protect the eardrum from injury in case of sudden head movement (Fig. 16.12). Enlist the aid of a cooperative parent. Prop an infant upright against the parent's chest or shoulder, with the parent's arm around the upper part of the head. A toddler can be held in the parent's lap with his or her arms gently secured. As you pull down on the pinna, gently push in on the child's tragus as a lead-in to inserting the speculum tip. This sometimes helps avoid the startling poke of the speculum tip.

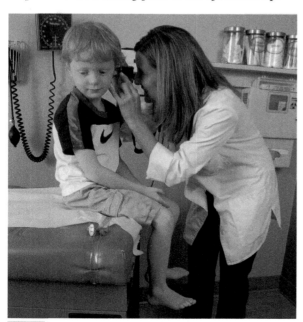

16.12

Objective Data

Normal Range of Findings	Abnormal Findings

Remember to pull the pinna straight down on an infant or a child younger than 3 years. This method matches the slope of the ear canal (Fig. 16.13).

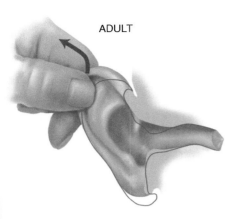

ADULT

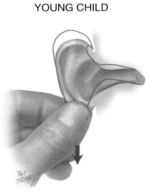

YOUNG CHILD

16.13

Adult—pull
pinna up and back

Infant/child under 3—pull
pinna straight down

At birth the patency of the ear canal is determined, but the otoscopic examination is not performed because the canal is filled with amniotic fluid and vernix caseosa. After a few days the TM is examined. During the first few days it often looks thickened and opaque. It may look "injected," meaning having a mild redness from increased vascularity. The eardrum also looks injected in infants after crying.

The position of the eardrum is more horizontal in the neonate, making it more difficult to see completely and harder to differentiate from the canal wall. By 1 month of age the drum is in the oblique (more vertical) position as in the older child, and examination is a bit easier.

When examining an infant or young child, a pneumatic bulb attachment enables you to direct a light puff of air toward the drum to assess **vibratility** (Fig. 16.14). For a secure seal, choose the largest speculum that fits in the ear canal without causing pain. A rubber tip on the end of the speculum gives a better seal. Give a small pump to the bulb (positive pressure) and release the bulb (negative pressure). Normally the TM moves inward with a slight puff and outward with a slight release.

Atresia—Absence or closure of the ear canal.

An abnormal response is no movement. Drum hypomobility indicates effusion or a high vacuum in the middle ear. For the newborn's first 6 weeks, drum immobility is the best indicator of middle ear infection.

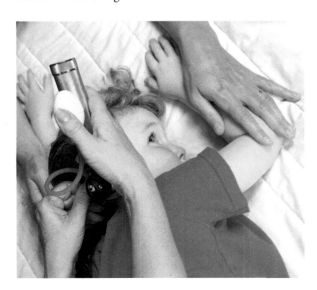

16.14

Normal Range of Findings	Abnormal Findings

Normally the tympanic membrane is intact. In a child being treated for chronic OM, you may note the presence of a tympanostomy tube in the central part of the eardrum. This is inserted surgically to equalize pressure and drain secretions. Finally, although the condition is not normal, it is not uncommon to note a foreign body in a child's canal such as a small stone or a bead.

> Chronic OM relieved by tympanostomy tubes (see Table 16.6).
> Foreign body must be removed (see Table 16.4).

Test Hearing Acuity. Use the developmental milestones listed here to assess hearing in an infant. Also attend to the parents' concern over the infant's inability to hear; their assessment is usually well founded.

The room should be silent and the baby contented. Make a loud, sudden noise (hand clap or squeeze toy) out of the baby's peripheral range of vision of about 30 cm (12 in). You may need to repeat a few times, but you should note these responses:

- Newborn—Startle (Moro) reflex, acoustic blink reflex
- 3 to 4 months—Acoustic blink reflex, infant stops movement and appears to "listen," stops sucking, quiets if crying, cries if quiet
- 6 to 8 months—Infant turns head to localize sound, responds to own name
- Preschool and school-age child—Child must be screened with audiometry

> Absence of alerting behavior may indicate congenital deafness.
>
> Failure to localize sound.
>
> No intelligible speech by age 2 years.

Note that a young child may be unaware of a hearing loss because the child does not know how one "ought" to hear. Note these behavioral manifestations of hearing loss:
1. The child is inattentive in casual conversation.
2. The child reacts more to movement and facial expression than to sound.
3. The child's facial expression is strained or puzzled.
4. The child frequently asks to have statements repeated.
5. The child confuses words that sound alike.
6. The child has an accompanying speech problem: speech is monotonous or garbled; the child mispronounces or omits sounds.
7. The child appears shy and withdrawn and "lives in a world of his or her own."
8. The child frequently complains of earaches.
9. The child hears better at times when the environment is more conducive.

The Aging Adult

An aging adult may have pendulous earlobes with linear wrinkling because of loss of elasticity of the pinna. Coarse, wiry hairs may be present at the opening of the ear canal. During otoscopy the eardrum normally may be whiter in color and more opaque, duller than in the younger adult. It also may look thickened.

A high-tone frequency hearing loss is apparent for those affected with **presbycusis**, the hearing loss that occurs with aging. Note any difficulty hearing in the whispered voice test and hearing consonants during conversational speech. The aging adult thinks that "people are mumbling" and feels isolated in family or friendship groups.

Objective Data

HEALTH PROMOTION AND PATIENT TEACHING

"Your newborn baby's hearing will be checked before the baby leaves the hospital or during the first month of life. This is important because the crucial time to learn language is in the first 3 years of life as the brain develops and matures. Hearing loss is not common but if there is a loss, research shows children develop better language skills if they get help early than those who do not get help."

The 1-3-6 program of universal newborn hearing screening operates in all states in the United States, resulting in screenings for 96% of babies within their 1st month of life.[6]

1 = All newborns are screened for hearing loss before they leave the hospital or within 1 month of life.

3 = All infants who do not pass the hearing screening should be scheduled immediately for a follow-up appointment with a pediatric audiologist. This examination must happen by age 3 months.

6 = If the follow-up examination confirms that the baby has hearing loss, the baby must receive appropriate interventions by 6 months of age, including hearing devices and early communication intervention (e.g., lipreading, signed English, American Sign Language, or others).

Two different tests are used for newborn hearing screening: (1) otoacoustic emissions (OAE) test—for this test a soft probe is placed just inside the baby's ear canal to measure the response (echo) when clicks or tones are played into the baby's ears, and (2) auditory brainstem response (ABR)—clicks or tones are played through soft earphones placed over the baby's ears while electrodes placed on the baby's head measure how the auditory nerve and brainstem carry sound from the ear to the brain. The electrodes come off like stickers and are painless.[6] The baby can rest or sleep during both tests; each test takes 5 to10 minutes.

Two to three of every 1,000 children in the United States are born with detectable hearing loss in one or both ears, and more lose some hearing later in childhood. Because the 1st 3 years of life represent the most intensive period for speech and language development, identifying hearing loss as early as possible is a high priority. Evidence shows that children with hearing loss who receive early intervention and amplification before 6 months of age do better than those receiving services after 6 months of age; by the 1st grade children identified earlier are 1 to 2 years ahead of their later-identified peers in language, cognitive, and social skills.[7]

DOCUMENTATION AND CRITICAL THINKING

Sample Charting

SUBJECTIVE

States hearing is good, no earaches, infections, discharge, hearing loss, tinnitus, or vertigo.

OBJECTIVE

Pinna: Skin intact with no masses, lesions, tenderness, or discharge.
Otoscope: External canals are clear with no redness, swelling, lesions, foreign body, or discharge. Both TMs are pearly gray in color, with light reflex and landmarks intact; no perforations.
Hearing: Responds appropriately to conversation. Whispered sounds heard bilaterally.

ASSESSMENT

Healthy ear structures
Hearing accurate

Clinical Case Study 1

A 2-month-old male (T.W.) is brought to the clinic by his foster mother because he "won't stop crying and just can't seem to stay asleep."

SUBJECTIVE

Foster mom reports that T.W. has had a cold for the past 7 days but the crying and inability to sleep just started yesterday. Foster mom reports, "He seems to be happier when he's sitting up, which makes it hard to feed him his bottle." She states that she usually lays the child down for naps with a bottle elevated on a blanket so she can "get some work done." Reports giving T.W. infant acetaminophen 2 hours PTA for his apparent discomfort.

OBJECTIVE

Vital signs: Temp 100° F (37.8° C) (rectal). Unable to obtain BP because of infant motion. Pulse 180 bpm. Resp 40/min.
General appearance: Infant appears fussy and unable to get comfortable, even in mother's arms.
HEENT: Anterior fontanel open and flat w/ minimal overriding sutures, posterior fontanel closed; conjunctivae clear, sclerae white, visibly tearing; bilat TMs dull red and bulging, no light reflex, no mobility on pneumatic otoscopy; oral mucosa pink, tonsils 1+; no lymphadenopathy.
Cardiovascular: Regular rate and rhythm, no murmurs.
Respiratory: Breath sounds equal with coarseness that clears with cough; unlabored.

ASSESSMENT

Acute otitis media (bilat)
Acute pain R/T inflammation in tympanic membranes
Deficient knowledge (parents) R/T risk factors for otitis media

Clinical Case Study 2

T.R. is a 15-year-old male high school student who comes to the health center to seek care for "cough off and on all winter and earache since last night."

SUBJECTIVE

6 weeks PTA—Nonproductive cough throughout day, no fever, no nasal congestion, no chest soreness. T.R.'s father gave him an over-the-counter decongestant, which helped, but cough continued off/on since. Does not smoke.
1 day PTA—Intermittent cough continues, nasal congestion and thick white mucus. Also earache R ear; treated self with heating pad, pain unrelieved. Pain is moderate, not deep and throbbing. Says R ear feels full, "hollow headed," voices sound muffled and far away, switches telephone to L ear to talk. No sore throat, no fever, no chest congestion or soreness.

OBJECTIVE

Vital signs: Temp 98.6° F (37° C) (oral). Pulse 76 bpm. BP 106/72 mm Hg.
Ears: L ear, canal, TM normal. R ear and canal normal, R TM retracted, with multiple air bubbles; drum color is yellow/amber. No sinus tenderness.
Nose: Turbinates bright red and swollen, mucopurulent discharge.
Throat: Not reddened, tonsils 1+.
Neck: One R anterior cervical node enlarged, firm, movable, tender. All others not palpable.
Lungs: Breath sounds clear to auscultation, resonant to percussion throughout.

ASSESSMENT

Otitis media with effusion, R ear, with mild URI
Transient conductive hearing loss
Pain R/T middle ear pressure

Documentation and Critical Thinking

Clinical Case Study 3

E.S. is a 78-year-old retired woman with a medical diagnosis of angina pectoris, which has responded to nitroglycerin PRN and periods of rest between activity. She has been independent in her own home and is coping well with activity restrictions through help from neighbors and family. Now hospitalized for evaluation of acute chest pain episode; MI has been ruled out, pain diagnosed as anginal; to be released to own home with a beta-blocking medication and nitroglycerin PRN.

Just before this hospitalization, Mrs. S. received a hearing aid after evaluation by an audiologist at senior center. Mrs. S. was born in Germany, immigrated to United States at age 5 years; considers English her primary language.

SUBJECTIVE

Since this hospitalization, feels "irritable and nervous." Relates this to worry about heart and also, "I get so mixed up in here, this room is so strange, and I just can't hear the nurses. They talk like cavemen, 'oo-i-ee-uou.'" Tried using her new hearing aid but no relief. "It just kept screeching in my ear, and it made the monitor beep so loud it drove me crazy." States no tinnitus, no vertigo.

OBJECTIVE

Ears: Pinna with elongated lobes, but no tenderness to palpation, no discharge, no masses or lesions. Both canals clear of cerumen. Both TM appear gray-white, slightly opaque and dull, although all landmarks visible. No perforation.
Hearing: Difficulty hearing room conversation. Unable to hear whispered voice bilaterally.

ASSESSMENT

Chest pain/angina pectoris
Deficient knowledge R/T lack of teaching on hearing aid
Age-related hearing loss
Anxiety R/T change in heart health and communication problems

TABLE 16.1 | Hearing Loss

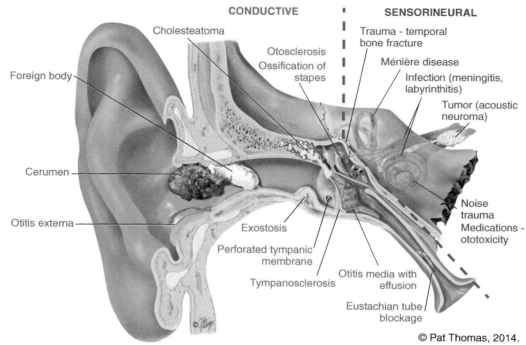

© Pat Thomas, 2014.

Hearing loss may be sensorineural, conductive, or mixed. Age-related sensorineural loss (presbycusis) affects half of those over 60 years and 80% of those over 85 years[2]; the incidence will increase as current baby boomers age. Despite its prevalence, loss is underscreened and undertreated. This leads to social isolation, diminished quality of life, even cognitive impairment and depression. Hearing aids can improve this loss. Note other causes of sensorineural loss in the figure. Conductive hearing loss blocks sound transmission somewhere in the external auditory canal, tympanic membrane, or middle ear.

TABLE 16.2 | External Ear Abnormalities

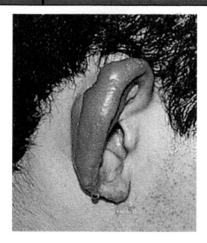

Frostbite

Reddish-blue discoloration and swelling of auricle after exposure to extreme cold. Vesicles or bullae may develop, the person feels pain and tenderness, and ear necrosis may ensue.

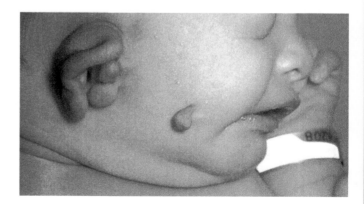

Branchial Remnant and Ear Deformity

A facial remnant or leftover of the embryologic branchial arch usually appears as a skin tag; in this case, one containing cartilage. Occurs most often in the preauricular area, in front of the tragus. When bilateral, there is increased risk for renal anomalies.

Continued

TABLE 16.2 | **External Ear Abnormalities—cont'd**

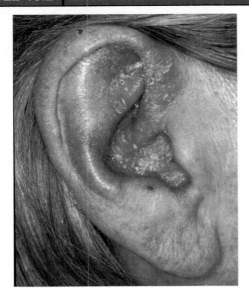

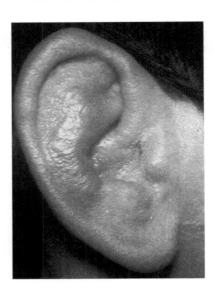

Otitis Externa (Swimmer's Ear)

An infection of the outer ear, with severe painful movement of the pinna and tragus, redness and swelling of pinna and canal, scanty purulent discharge, scaling, itching, fever, and enlarged tender regional lymph nodes. Hearing normal or slightly diminished. More common in hot, humid weather. Swimming causes canal to become waterlogged and swell; skinfolds set up for infection. Prevent by using rubbing alcohol or 2% acetic acid eardrops after every swim.

Cellulitis

Inflammation of loose, subcutaneous connective tissue. Shows as thickening and induration of auricle with distorted contours.

See Illustration Credits for source information.

TABLE 16.3 | **Lumps and Lesions on the Ear**

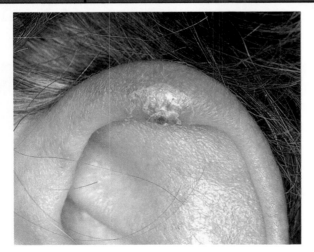

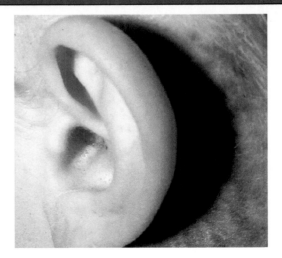

Chondrodermatitis Nodularis Helicus

Painful nodules develop on rim of helix (where there is no cushioning subcutaneous tissue) as a result of repetitive mechanical pressure or environmental trauma (sunlight). They are small, indurated, dull red, poorly defined, and very painful.

Battle Sign

Trauma to the side of the head may lead to a basilar skull fracture involving the temporal bone. This shows as ecchymotic discoloration just posterior to the pinna and over the mastoid process. A look inside the ear canal may show hemotympanum as well (see Table 16.6, p. 342).

Continued

TABLE 16.3 | Lumps and Lesions on the Ear—cont'd

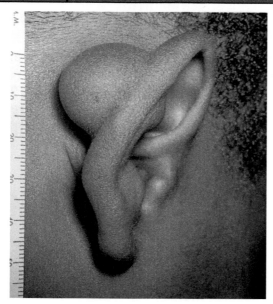

Sebaceous Cyst

Location is commonly behind lobule in the postauricular fold. A nodule with central black punctum indicates blocked sebaceous gland. It is filled with waxy sebaceous material and painful if it becomes infected. Often are multiple.

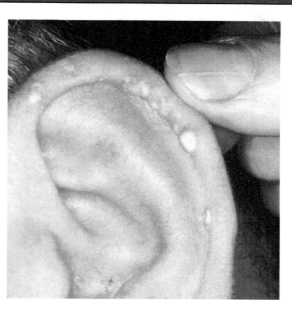

Tophi

Small, whitish yellow, hard, nontender nodules in or near helix or antihelix; contain greasy, chalky material of uric acid crystals and are a sign of gout.

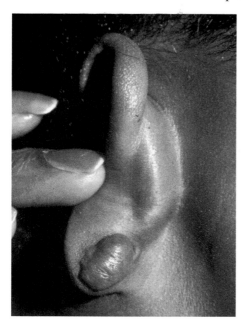

Keloid

Overgrowth of scar tissue, which invades original site of trauma. It is more common in darkly pigmented people, although it also occurs in whites. In the ear it is most common at lobule at site of a pierced ear. Overgrowth shown here is unusually large.

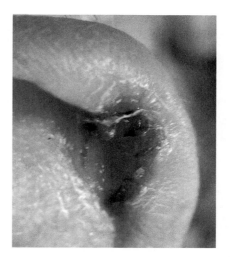

Carcinoma

Ulcerated, crusted nodule with indurated base that fails to heal. Bleeds intermittently. Must refer for biopsy. Usually occurs on the superior rim of the pinna, which has the most sun exposure. May occur also in ear canal and show chronic discharge that is either serosanguineous or bloody.

See Illustration Credits for source information.

ABNORMAL FINDINGS
FOR ADVANCED PRACTICE

TABLE 16.4	Ear Canal Abnormalities

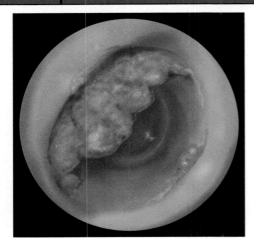

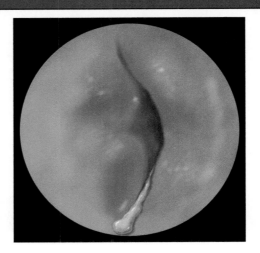

Excessive Cerumen

Produced or is impacted because of narrow, tortuous canal or poor cleaning method. May show as round ball partially obscuring drum or totally occluding canal. Even when canal is 90% to 95% blocked, hearing stays normal. But when last 5% to 10% is totally occluded (when cerumen expands after swimming or showering), person has ear fullness and sudden hearing loss.

Otitis Externa

Severe swelling of canal, inflammation, tenderness. In the figure above, canal lumen is narrowed to one-fourth normal size. (See complete description in Table 16.2.)

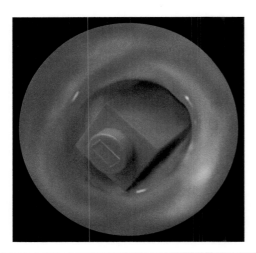

◀ Foreign Body

Usually it is children who place a foreign body in the ear (in the figure at left, a toy completely occludes the canal), which is later noted on routine examination. Common objects are beans, corn, breakfast cereals, jewelry beads, small stones, sponge rubber. Cotton is most common in adults and becomes impacted from cotton-tipped applicators. A trapped live insect is rare but makes the person especially frantic.

Continued

TABLE 16.4	Ear Canal Abnormalities—cont'd

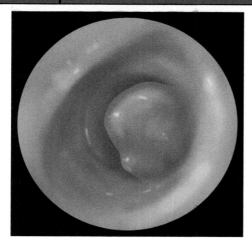

Osteoma

Single, stony hard, rounded nodule that obscures the drum; nontender; overlying skin appears normal. Attached to inner third, the bony part, of canal. Benign, but refer for removal.

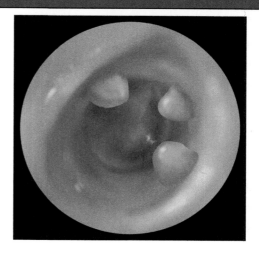

Exostosis

More common than osteoma. Small, bony hard, rounded nodules of hypertrophic bone, covered with normal epithelium. Arise near the drum but usually do not obstruct the view of the drum. Usually multiple and bilateral, occur more frequently in cold-water swimmers. Needs no treatment, although may cause accumulation of cerumen, which blocks the canal.

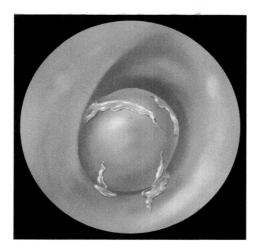

Polyp

Arises in canal from granulomatous or mucosal tissue; redder than surrounding skin and bleeds easily; bathed in foul, purulent discharge; indicates chronic ear disease. Benign but refer for excision.

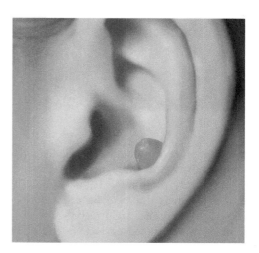

Furuncle

Exquisitely painful, reddened, infected hair follicle. It may occur on tragus on cartilaginous part of ear canal. Regional lymphadenopathy often accompanies a furuncle.

Images © Pat Thomas, 2010.

TABLE 16.5	Abnormal Views Seen on Otoscopy	
Appearance of Eardrum	Indicates	Suggested Condition
Yellow-amber color	Serum or pus	Otitis media with effusion (OME) or chronic otitis media
Prominent landmarks	Retraction of drum	Vacuum in middle ear from obstructed eustachian tube
Air/fluid level or air bubbles	Serous fluid	Otitis media with effusion
Absent or distorted light reflex	Bulging of eardrum	Acute otitis media
Bright red color	Infection in middle ear	Acute otitis media
Blue or dark red color	Blood behind drum	Trauma, skull fracture
Dark, round or oval areas	Perforation	Drum rupture
White dense areas	Scarring	Sequelae of infections
Diminished or absent landmarks	Thickened drum	Chronic otitis media
Black or white dots on drum or canal	Colony of growth	Fungal infection

TABLE 16.6	Abnormal Tympanic Membranes

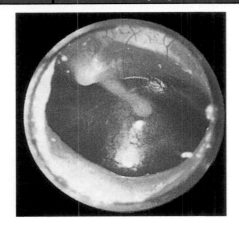

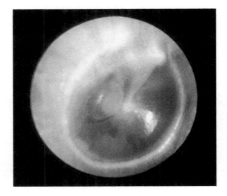

Retracted Drum

Landmarks look more prominent and well defined. Malleus handle looks shorter and more horizontal than normal. Short process is very prominent. Light reflex is absent or distorted. The drum is dull and lusterless and does not move. These signs indicate negative pressure and middle ear vacuum from obstructed eustachian tube and serous otitis media.

Otitis Media With Effusion (OME)

An amber-yellow drum suggests serum in middle ear that transudes to relieve negative pressure from the blocked eustachian tube. You may note an air/fluid level with a fine black dividing line or air bubbles visible behind drum. Symptoms are feeling of fullness, transient hearing loss, popping sound with swallowing. Also called *serous otitis media, glue ear.*

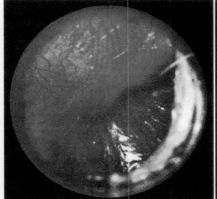

Early stage

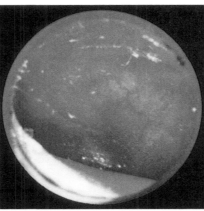

Later stage

◄ Acute Otitis Media

This results when the middle ear fluid is infected. An absent light reflex from increasing middle ear pressure is an early sign. Redness and bulging are first noted in superior part of drum (pars flaccida), along with earache and fever. Then fiery red bulging of entire drum occurs along with deep throbbing pain. Accompanied by possible fever and transient hearing loss. Pneumatic otoscopy reveals drum hypomobility.

Continued

| TABLE 16.6 | Abnormal Tympanic Membranes—cont'd |

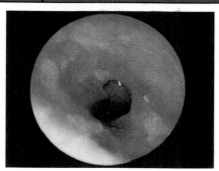

◀ Perforation

If the acute otitis media is not treated, the drum may rupture from increased pressure. Perforations also occur from trauma (e.g., a slap on the ear). Usually the perforation appears as a round or oval darkened area on the drum. *Central* perforations occur in the pars tensa. *Marginal* perforations occur at the annulus. Marginal perforations are called *attic perforations* when they occur in the superior part of the drum, the pars flaccida.

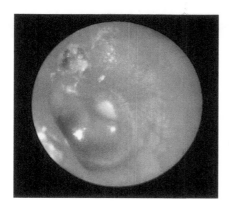

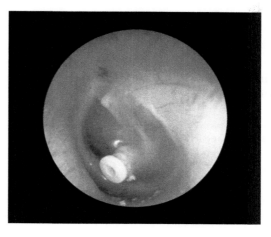

Cholesteatoma ▲

An overgrowth of epidermal tissue in the middle ear or temporal bone may result over the years after a marginal TM perforation. It has a pearly white, cheesy appearance. Growth of cholesteatoma can erode bone and produce hearing loss. Early signs include otorrhea, otalgia, unilateral conductive hearing loss, tinnitus.

Insertion of Tympanostomy Tubes

Polyethylene tubes are inserted surgically into the eardrum to relieve middle ear pressure and promote drainage of chronic or recurrent middle ear infections. Number of acute infections tends to decrease because of improved aeration. Tubes extrude spontaneously in 12 to 18 months.

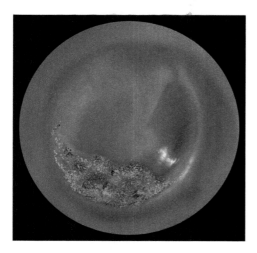

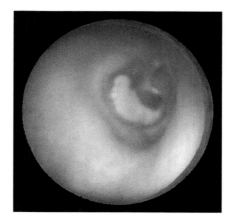

Fungal Infection (Otomycosis)

Colony of black or white dots on drum or canal wall suggests a yeast or fungal infection.

Scarred Drum

Dense white patches on the eardrum are sequelae of repeated ear infections. They do not necessarily affect hearing.

Continued

TABLE 16.6 | Abnormal Tympanic Membranes—cont'd

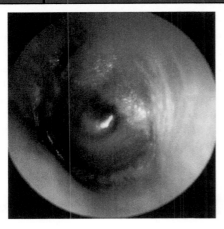

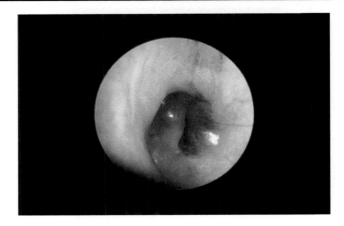

Blue Drum (Hemotympanum)

This indicates blood in the middle ear, as in trauma resulting in skull fracture.

Bullous Myringitis

Small vesicles containing blood are on the eardrum; it accompanies mycoplasma pneumonia and viral infections. Blood-tinged discharge and severe otalgia may be present.

See Illustration Credits for source information.

TABLE 16.7 | Tuning Fork Tests

Weber Test

Rinne Test

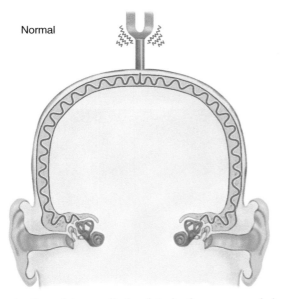

Normal

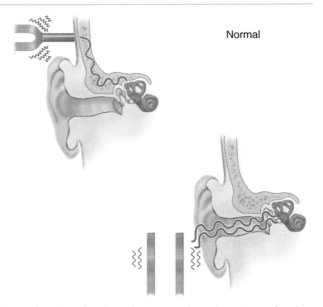

Normal

Normal—Sound is equally loud in both ears; sound does not lateralize.

Normal—Sound is heard twice as long by air conduction (AC) as by bone conduction (BC); a "positive" Rinne, or AC > BC.

Continued

TABLE 16.7 | **Tuning Fork Tests—cont'd**

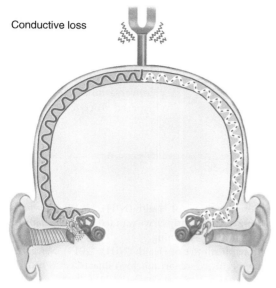

Conductive loss

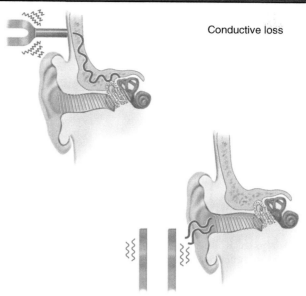

Conductive loss

Conductive loss—Sound lateralizes to "poorer" ear from background room noise, which masks hearing in normal ear. "Poorer" ear (the one with conductive loss) is not distracted by background noise and thus has a better chance to hear bone-conducted sound. Examples: transient conductive loss with serous or purulent otitis media.

Conductive loss—Person hears equally long by bone conduction as by air conduction (AC = BC) or even longer (AC < BC). The Rinne test may be accurate to detect conductive loss, and loss can be confirmed by audiometry.[5a]

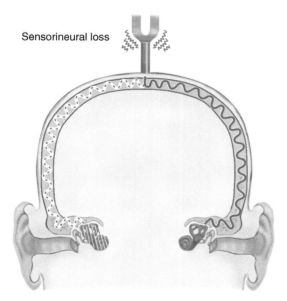

Sensorineural loss

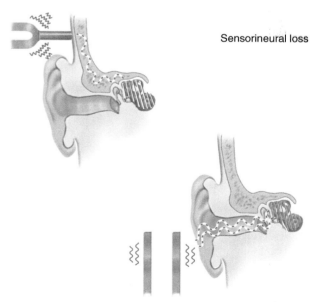

Sensorineural loss

Sensorineural loss—Sound lateralizes to "better" ear or unaffected ear. Poor ear (the one with nerve loss) is unable to perceive the sound. However, many people with unilateral loss (conductive or sensorineural) still localize the sound in the midline.[7b] Confirm with audiometry.

Sensorineural loss—Normal ratio of AC > BC is intact but is reduced overall. That is, person hears poorly both ways. Confirm with audiometry.

Summary Checklist: Ear Examination

1. **Inspect external ear:**
   Size and shape of auricle
   Position and alignment on head
   Note skin condition—Color, lumps, lesions
   Check movement of auricle and tragus for tenderness
   Evaluate external auditory meatus—Note size, swelling, redness, discharge, cerumen, lesions, foreign bodies
2. **Otoscopic examination:**
   External canal
   Cerumen, discharge, foreign bodies, lesions
   Redness or swelling of canal wall
3. **Inspect tympanic membrane:**
   Color and characteristics
   Note position (flat, bulging, retracted)
   Integrity of membrane
4. **Test hearing acuity:**
   Note behavioral response to conversational speech
   Whispered voice test

REFERENCES

1. Bainbridge, K. E., & Wallhagen, M. I. (2014). Hearing loss in an aging American population. *Annu Rev Public Health*, *35*, 139–152.
1a. Bauer, C. A. (2018). Tinnitus. *N Engl J Med*, *378*(13), 1224–1230.
2. Cunningham, L. L., & Tucci, D. L. (2017). Hearing loss in adults. *N Engl J Med*, *377*(25), 2465–2473.
3. Genther, D. J., Betz, J., & Pratt, S. (2015). Association of hearing impairment and mortality in older adults. *J Gerontol A Biol Sci Med Sci*, *70*(1), 85–90.
4. Jensen, E. A., Harmon, E. D., & Smith, W. (2017). Early identification of idiopathic sudden sensorineural hearing loss. *Nurse Pract*, *42*(9), 10–16.
5. Kim, J., & Zee, D. S. (2014). Benign paroxysmal positional vertigo. *N Engl J Med*, *370*(12), 1138–1147.
5a. McGee, S. (2018). *Evidence-based physical diagnosis* (4th ed.). Philadelphia: Elsevier.
6. National Institutes of Health (NIH). (2017). *Your baby's hearing screening.* https://www.nided.nih.gov/health/your-babys-hearing-screening.
7. National Institutes of Health (NIH). (2010). *Newborn hearing screening.* https://report.nih.gov/nihfactsheets/Pdfs/NewbornHearingScreening(NIDCD).pdf.
8. Prokop-Prigge, K. A., Thaler, E., Wysocki, C. J., et al. (2014). Identification of volatile organic compounds in human cerumen. *J Chromatogr B Analyt Technol Biomed Life Sci*, *953–954*, 48–52.
9. Rosa-Olivares, J., Porro, A., Rodriguez-Varela, M., et al. (2015). Otitis media. *Pediatr Rev*, *36*(11), 480–488.
10. Tawfik, K. O., Ishman, S. L., Altaye, M., et al. (2017). Pediatric acute otitis media in the era of pneumococcal vaccination. *Otolaryngology*, *156*(5), 938–945.
11. Tunkel, D. E., Bauer, C. A., Sun, G. H., et al. (2014). Clinical practice guideline: Tinnitus. *Otolaryngology*, *151*(2), S1–S40.

Nose, Mouth, and Throat

STRUCTURE AND FUNCTION

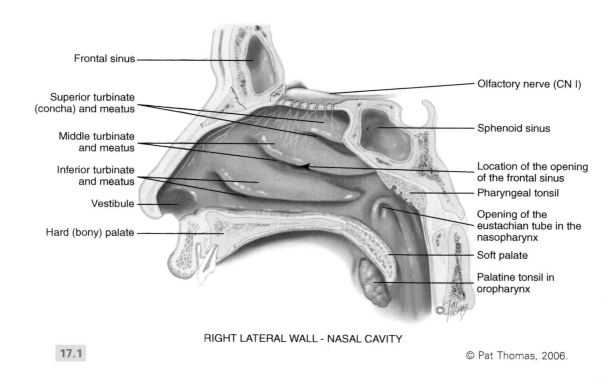

Frontal sinus

Superior turbinate (concha) and meatus

Middle turbinate and meatus

Inferior turbinate and meatus

Vestibule

Hard (bony) palate

Olfactory nerve (CN I)

Sphenoid sinus

Location of the opening of the frontal sinus

Pharyngeal tonsil

Opening of the eustachian tube in the nasopharynx

Soft palate

Palatine tonsil in oropharynx

RIGHT LATERAL WALL - NASAL CAVITY

17.1

© Pat Thomas, 2006.

NOSE

The **nose** is the first segment of the respiratory system. It warms, moistens, and filters the inhaled air, and it is the sensory organ for smell. Inside, the **nasal cavity** is much larger than the external nose would indicate (Fig. 17.1). It extends back over the roof of the mouth. The anterior edge of the cavity is lined with numerous coarse nasal hairs, or vibrissae. The rest of the cavity is lined with a blanket of ciliated mucous membrane. The nasal hairs filter the coarsest matter from inhaled air, whereas the mucous blanket filters out dust and bacteria. Nasal mucosa appears redder than oral mucosa because of the rich blood supply present to warm the inhaled air.

The nasal cavity is divided medially by the **septum** into two slitlike air passages. The anterior part of the septum holds a rich vascular network, *Kiesselbach plexus,* the most common site of nosebleeds. In many people the nasal septum is not absolutely straight and may deviate toward one passage.

The lateral walls of each nasal cavity contain three parallel bony projections—the superior, middle, and inferior **turbinates.** They increase the surface area so more blood vessels and mucous membranes are available to warm, humidify, and filter the inhaled air. Underlying each turbinate is a cleft, the **meatus,** which is named for the turbinate above. The sinuses drain into the middle meatus, and tears from the nasolacrimal duct drain into the inferior meatus.

The olfactory receptors (hair cells) lie at the roof of the nasal cavity and in the upper one-third of the septum. These receptors for smell merge into the olfactory nerve, cranial nerve I, which transmits to the temporal lobe of the brain. Although it is not necessary for human survival, the sense of smell adds to nutrition by enhancing the pleasure and taste of food.

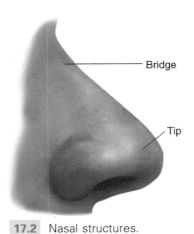

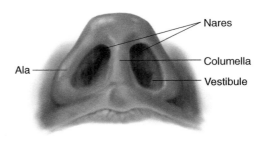

17.2 Nasal structures.

© Pat Thomas, 2006.

The external nose is shaped like a triangle with one side attached to the face (Fig. 17.2). On its leading edge the superior part is the *bridge,* and the free corner is the *tip.* The oval openings at the base of the triangle are the *nares;* just inside, each naris widens into the *vestibule.* The *columella* divides the two nares and is continuous inside with the nasal septum. The *ala* is the lateral outside wing of the nose on either side.

The upper third of the external nose is made up of bone; the lower part is cartilage.

The **paranasal sinuses** are air-filled pockets within the cranium (Fig. 17.3). They communicate with the nasal cavity and are lined with the same type of ciliated mucous membrane. They lighten the weight of the skull bones; serve as resonators for sound production; and provide mucus,

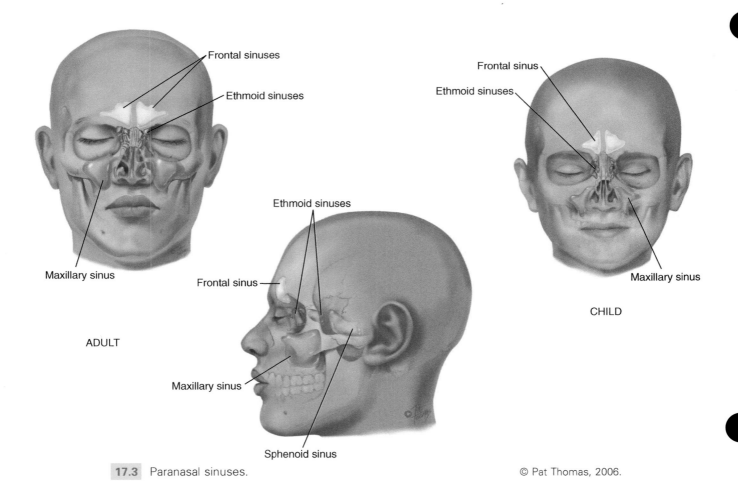

17.3 Paranasal sinuses.

© Pat Thomas, 2006.

which drains into the nasal cavity. The sinus openings are narrow and easily occluded, which may cause inflammation or sinusitis.

Two pairs of sinuses are accessible to examination: the **frontal** sinuses in the frontal bone above and medial to the orbits, and the **maxillary** sinuses in the maxilla (cheekbone) along the side walls of the nasal cavity. The other two sets are smaller and deeper: the **ethmoid** sinuses between the orbits, and the **sphenoid** sinuses deep within the skull in the sphenoid bone.

Only the maxillary and ethmoid sinuses are present at birth. The maxillary sinuses reach full size after all permanent teeth have erupted. The ethmoid sinuses grow rapidly between 6 and 8 years of age and after puberty. The frontal sinuses are absent at birth, are fairly well developed between 7 and 8 years of age, and reach full size after puberty. The sphenoid sinuses are minute at birth and develop after puberty.

MOUTH

The mouth is the first segment of the digestive system and an airway for the respiratory system. The **oral cavity** is a short passage bordered by the lips, palate, cheeks, and tongue. It contains the teeth and gums, tongue, and salivary glands (Fig. 17.4).

The lips are the anterior border of the oral cavity (i.e., the transition zone from the outer skin to the inner mucous membrane lining the oral cavity). The arching roof of the mouth is the palate; it is divided into two parts. The anterior **hard palate** is made up of bone and is a whitish color. Posterior to this is the **soft palate,** an arch of muscle that is pinker in color and mobile. The **uvula** is the free projection hanging down from the middle of the soft palate. The cheeks are the side walls of the oral cavity.

The floor of the mouth consists of the horseshoe-shaped mandible bone, the tongue, and underlying muscles. The **tongue** is a mass of striated muscle arranged in a crosswise pattern so it can change shape and position. The papillae are the rough, bumpy elevations on its dorsal surface. Note the larger vallate papillae in an inverted V shape across the posterior base of the tongue, and do not confuse them with abnormal growths. Underneath, the ventral surface of the tongue is smooth and shiny and has prominent veins. The **frenulum** is a midline fold of tissue that connects the tongue to the floor of the mouth.

The ability of the tongue to change shape and position enhances its functions in mastication, swallowing, teeth cleansing, and speech formation. The tongue also functions in taste sensation. Microscopic taste buds are in the papillae at the back and along the sides of the tongue and on the soft palate.

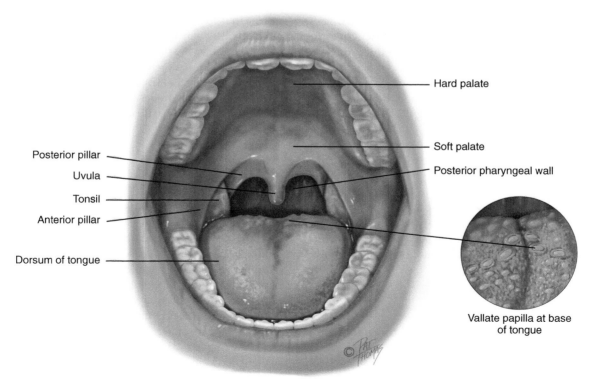

Hard palate

Soft palate

Posterior pharyngeal wall

Posterior pillar

Uvula

Tonsil

Anterior pillar

Dorsum of tongue

Vallate papilla at base of tongue

ORAL CAVITY

17.4

© Pat Thomas, 2010.

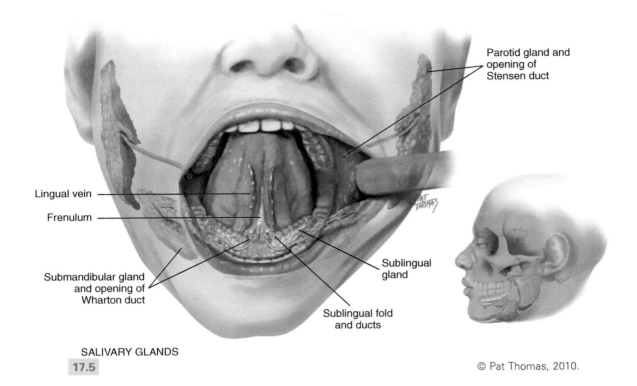

Parotid gland and
opening of
Stensen duct

Lingual vein

Frenulum

Submandibular gland
and opening of
Wharton duct

Sublingual
gland

Sublingual fold
and ducts

SALIVARY GLANDS
17.5

© Pat Thomas, 2010.

The mouth contains three pairs of salivary glands (Fig. 17.5). The largest, the **parotid** gland, lies within the cheeks in front of the ear, extending from the zygomatic arch down to the angle of the jaw. Its duct, Stensen duct, runs forward to open on the buccal mucosa opposite the second molar. The **submandibular** gland is the size of a walnut. It lies beneath the mandible at the angle of the jaw. Wharton duct runs up and forward to the floor of the mouth and opens at either side of the frenulum. The smallest, the almond-shaped **sublingual** gland, lies within the floor of the mouth under the tongue. It has many small openings along the sublingual fold under the tongue.

The glands secrete saliva, the clear fluid that moistens and lubricates the food bolus, starts digestion, and cleans and protects the mucosa.

Adults have 32 **permanent** teeth—16 in each arch. Each tooth has three parts: the crown, the neck, and the root. The gums (gingivae) collar the teeth. They are thick, fibrous tissues covered with mucous membrane. They are different from the rest of the oral mucosa because of their pale pink color and stippled surface.

THROAT

The throat, or pharynx, is the area behind the mouth and nose. The **oropharynx** is separated from the mouth by a fold of tissue on each side, the anterior tonsillar pillar (see Fig. 17.4). Behind the folds are the **tonsils,** each a mass of lymphoid tissue. The tonsils are the same color as the surrounding mucous membrane, although they look more

granular and their surface shows deep crypts. Tonsillar tissue enlarges during childhood until puberty and then involutes. The posterior pharyngeal wall is seen behind these structures. Some small blood vessels may show on it.

The **nasopharynx** is continuous with the oropharynx, although it is above the oropharynx and behind the nasal cavity. The pharyngeal tonsils (adenoids) and eustachian tube openings are located here (see Fig. 17.1).

The oral cavity and throat have a rich lymphatic network. Review the lymph nodes and their drainage patterns in Chapter 14, and keep this in mind when evaluating the mouth.

✦ DEVELOPMENTAL COMPETENCE

Infants and Children

In the infant salivation starts at 3 months. The baby drools for a few months before learning to swallow the saliva. This drooling does not herald the eruption of the first tooth, although many parents think it does.

Both sets of teeth begin development in utero. Children have 20 **deciduous,** or temporary, teeth. These erupt between 6 and 24 months of age. All 20 teeth should appear by 2½ years of age. The deciduous teeth are lost beginning at 6 years through 12 years of age. They are replaced by the permanent teeth, starting with the central incisors (Fig. 17.6). The permanent teeth appear earlier in girls than in boys, and they erupt earlier in black children than in white children.

The nose develops its shape during adolescence, along with secondary sex characteristics. This growth starts at age

12 or 13 years, reaching full growth at age 16 years in females and age 18 years in males.

The Pregnant Woman

Nasal stuffiness and epistaxis may occur during pregnancy as a result of increased vascularity in the upper respiratory tract. The gums also may be hyperemic and softened and may bleed with normal toothbrushing. Contrary to superstitious folklore, pregnancy does not cause tooth decay or loss.

The Aging Adult

A gradual loss of subcutaneous fat starts during later adult years, making the nose appear more prominent. The nasal hairs grow coarser and stiffer and may not filter the air as well. The hairs protrude and may cause itching and sneezing. The sense of smell may diminish after age 60 years because of a decrease in the number of olfactory nerve fibers.

In the oral cavity, the soft tissues atrophy, and the epithelium thins, especially in the cheeks and tongue. This results in loss of taste buds, with about an 80% reduction in taste functioning. Further impairments to taste include a decrease in salivary secretion that is needed to dissolve flavoring agents. Atrophic tissues ulcerate easily, which increases risk for infections such as oral candidiasis. The risk for malignant oral lesions also increases.

Many dental changes occur with aging. The tooth surface is abraded. The gums begin to recede, and the teeth begin to erode at the gum line. A smooth V-shaped cavity forms around the neck of the tooth, exposing the nerve and making the tooth hypersensitive. Some tooth loss may occur from bone resorption (osteoporosis), which decreases the inner tooth structure and its outer support. Natural tooth loss is exacerbated by years of inadequate dental care, decay, poor oral hygiene, and tobacco use.

If tooth loss occurs, the remaining teeth drift, causing **malocclusion.** The stress of chewing with maloccluding teeth causes: (1) further tooth loss; (2) muscle imbalance from a mandible and maxilla now out of alignment, which produces muscle spasms, tenderness, and chronic headaches; and (3) stress on the temporomandibular joint, leading to osteoarthritis, pain, and inability to fully open the mouth.

A diminished sense of taste and smell decreases the older adult's interest in food and may contribute to malnutrition. Saliva production decreases; saliva acts as a solvent for food flavors and helps move food around the mouth. Decreased saliva flow also occurs with the use of medications that have anticholinergic effects. More than 250 medications have a side effect of dry mouth.

The absence of some teeth and trouble with mastication encourage the older person to eat soft foods (usually high in

UPPER DECIDUOUS

	Erupt (months)	Shed (years)
Central incisor	6 to 8	6 to 7
Lateral incisior	8 to 11	8 to 9
Canine (cuspid)	16 to 20	11 to 12
First molar	10 to 16	10 to 11
Second molar	20 to 30	10 to 12

UPPER PERMANENT

	Erupt (years)
Central incisor	7 to 8
Lateral incisior	8 to 9
Canine (cuspid)	11 to 12
First premolar	10 to 11
Second premolar	10 to 12
First molar	6 to 7
Second molar	12 to 13
Third molar	17 to 25

LOWER DECIDUOUS

	Erupt (months)	Shed (years)
Second molar	20 to 30	11 to 13
First molar	10 to 16	10 to 12
Canine	16 to 20	9 to 11
Lateral incisior	7 to 10	7 to 8
Central incisor	5 to 7	5 to 6

LOWER PERMANENT

	Erupt (years)
Third molar	17 to 25
Second molar	12 to 13
First molar	6 to 7
Second premolar	11 to 13
First premolar	10 to 12
Canine	9 to 11
Lateral incisior	7 to 8
Central incisor	6 to 7

DECIDUOUS AND PERMANENT TEETH

17.6

© Pat Thomas, 2006.

Subjective Data

carbohydrates) and decrease meat and fresh vegetable intake. This produces a risk for nutritional deficit for protein, vitamins, and minerals.

CULTURE AND GENETICS

Bifid uvula shows the uvula split either completely or partially (see Table 17.6, p. 374) and occurs in about 2% of the general population and up to 10% in some American Indian groups. The incidence of **cleft lip** with or without **cleft palate** is one in every 940 births in the United States; isolated cleft palate is less common.[1] Rates are higher in Asians and American Indians (1:500 births) and lower in African heritage births (1:2500). Males have a 2:1 ratio over females for cleft lip with or without cleft palate.[1] **Torus palatinus** is a benign bony ridge running in the middle of the hard palate (see Fig. 17.17) and occurs in 20% to 35% of the U.S. population, more commonly in females. **Leukoedema** is a benign, milky, bluish-white opaque appearance of the buccal mucosa that occurs commonly in African Americans.

Dental caries (tooth decay) is an infectious process that occurs when bacteria (*Streptococcus mutans*) interact with carbohydrates in juice, sweet drinks, or food and then soften and demineralize the tooth enamel.[2] There has been a significant increase in decay in the United States: 42% of children ages 2 to 11 years have dental caries in their primary teeth; 23% of children ages 2 to 11 years have untreated dental caries; and 21% of children ages 6 to 11 years have dental caries in their permanent teeth.[13] In all groups, black and Hispanic children and children in lower-income families have more decay. Other groups at risk for dental disease and lack of access to dental care are rural residents, minorities, older adults, pregnant women, the homeless, those with low income, people with developmental disabilities, and people who are institutionalized.[6] These trends are significant because poor oral health is associated with diabetes, coronary artery and peripheral vascular disease, and metabolic syndrome, possibly through a mechanism of chronic inflammation.[6]

Periodontal disease affects the structures surrounding the tooth, including the gingiva and alveolar bone. This condition is caused by chronic inflammation, which is a key factor linking type 2 diabetes and periodontitis.[20] This connection is a concern because rates of obesity are increasing in children, along with an increasing incidence of type 2 diabetes. The chronic elevated blood glucose levels result in gingival inflammation, which leads to gingivitis and periodontal disease.[20]

Among middle-aged and older adults, the incidence of oral and pharyngeal cancers had declined over the past 30 years, possibly due to a reduction in smoking rates (although tobacco and alcohol use still account for about 75% of oral cancers).[7] However, the decline is reversing, with a rise in oropharyngeal cancer now linked to infection with human papillomavirus (HPV). These cancers occur in younger adults too, more often in men than in women, and are associated with changes in sexual norms.[9] These sexual factors include oral sex (especially >5 oral sexual partners), multiple sexual partners, and having oral sex at a younger age (possibly perceived as less risky than genital sex).[9,12] The HPV vaccine offers the most effective protection from the oncogenic HPV 16 strain. Patient education is crucial.

SUBJECTIVE DATA

Nose
1. Discharge
2. Frequent colds (upper respiratory infections)
3. Sinus pain
4. Trauma
5. Epistaxis (nosebleeds)
6. Allergies
7. Altered smell

Mouth and Throat
1. Sores or lesions
2. Sore throat
3. Bleeding gums
4. Toothache
5. Hoarseness
6. Dysphagia
7. Altered taste
8. Smoking, alcohol consumption

9. Patient-centered care
Dental care pattern
Dentures or appliances

Examiner Asks	Rationale
Nose	
1. **Discharge.** Any **nasal discharge** or runny nose? Continuous? • Is the discharge watery, purulent, mucoid, bloody?	**Rhinorrhea** occurs with colds, allergies, sinus infection, trauma.
2. **Frequent colds.** Any unusually frequent or severe colds (upper respiratory infections [URIs])? How often do these occur?	Most people have occasional colds; thus asking this more precise question yields more meaningful data.

Examiner Asks	Rationale
3. Sinus pain. Any **sinus pain** or sinusitis? How is this treated? • Do you have chronic postnasal drip?	Up to 90% of patients with viral URI also have viral sinusitis, which resolves without antibiotics.[15]
4. Trauma. Ever had any **trauma** or a blow to the nose? • Can you breathe through your nose? Are both sides obstructed or one?	Trauma may cause deviated septum, which may cause nares to be obstructed.
5. Epistaxis (nosebleeds) Any nosebleeds? How often? • How much bleeding—a teaspoonful or does it pour out? • Color of the blood—red or brown? Clots? • From one nostril or both? • Aggravated by nose-picking or scratching? • How do you treat the nosebleeds? Are they difficult to stop?	**Epistaxis** occurs with trauma, vigorous nose blowing, foreign body. Person should sit with head tilted forward, pinch soft part of nose above nostrils for 10 to 15 minutes.
6. Allergies. Any **allergies** or hay fever? To what are you allergic (e.g., pollen, dust, pets)? • How was this determined? • Which type of environment makes it worse? Can you avoid exposure? • Use inhalers, nasal spray, nose drops? How often? Which type? • How long have you used them?	"Seasonal" rhinitis if caused by pollen; "perennial" if allergen is dust.[11] Misuse of nasal medications irritates the mucosa, causing rebound swelling, a common problem.
7. Altered smell. Experienced any change in sense of smell?	Sense of smell diminishes with cigarette smoking, chronic allergies, aging.

Mouth and Throat

Examiner Asks	Rationale
1. Sores or lesions. Noticed any **sores** or **lesions** in the mouth, tongue, or gums? • How long have you had them? Ever had this lesion before? • Is it single or multiple? • Does it seem to be associated with stress, season change, food? • How have you treated the sore? Applied any local medication?	History helps determine whether oral lesions have infectious, traumatic, immunologic, or malignant etiology.
2. Sore throat. How about **sore throats**? How frequently do you get them? Have a sore throat now? When did it start? • Is it associated with cough, fever, fatigue, decreased appetite, headache, postnasal drip, or hoarseness? • Is it worse when arising? What is the humidity level in the room where you sleep? Any dust or smoke inhaled at work? • Usually get a throat culture for the sore throats? Were any documented as streptococcal? • How have you treated this sore throat: medication, gargling? How effective are these? Have your tonsils or adenoids been removed?	Most sore throats are viral and resolve in 3-5 days without antibiotics. However, *group A streptococcal* (GAS) pharyngitis is more likely with fever over 100.4° F, absence of cough, tonsillar exudates, and cervical adenopathy.[8] Confirm with rapid antigen test and backup throat culture. Untreated GAS can cause peritonsillar abscess, rheumatic fever, and glomerulonephritis (though rare in the United States).
3. Bleeding gums. Any **bleeding gums**? How long have you had them?	
4. Toothache. Any **toothache**? Do your teeth seem sensitive to hot, cold? Have you lost any teeth?	
5. Hoarseness. Any **hoarseness**, voice change? For how long? • Feel like having to clear your throat? Or like a "lump in your throat"? • Use your voice a lot at work, recreation? • Does the hoarseness seem associated with a cold, sore throat?	Hoarseness of the larynx has many causes: overuse of the voice, URI, chronic inflammation, lesions, or a neoplasm.

Examiner Asks	Rationale

6. Dysphagia. Any difficulty swallowing? How long have you had it?
- Feel as if food gets stopped at a certain point?
- Any pain with this?

Dysphagia occurs with pharyngitis, gastroesophageal reflux disease, stroke and other neurologic diseases, esophageal cancer.

7. Altered taste. Any change in sense of taste?

8. Smoking, alcohol consumption. Do you smoke? Pipe or cigarettes? Smokeless tobacco? How many packs per day? For how many years?

- When was your last alcoholic drink? How much alcohol did you drink that time? How much alcohol do you usually drink?

Chronic tobacco use leads to tooth loss, coronal and root caries, and periodontal disease in older adults.

Chronic use of tobacco, alcohol, and both together highly increases risk for oral and pharyngeal cancers.

9. Patient-centered care. Tell me about your daily dental care. How often do you use a toothbrush and floss?
- Last dental examination? Do dental problems affect which foods you eat?
- Do you have a dental appliance: braces, bridge, head gear?
- Wear dentures? All the time? How long have you had this set? How do they fit?
- Any sores or irritation on the palate or gums?

Assess self-care behaviors for oral hygiene.

Periodic dental screening is necessary to note caries.

Lesions may arise from ill-fitting dentures, or the presence of dentures may mask the eruption of new lesions.

Additional History for Infants and Children

1. Does the child have any mouth infections or sores such as thrush or canker sores? How frequently do these occur?

2. Does the child have frequent sore throat or tonsillitis? How often? How are these treated? Have they ever been documented as streptococcal infections?

Children ages 5 to 15 years have a higher incidence of GAS pharyngitis than adults do (37% vs. 10%). Must confirm with rapid antigen test and backup throat culture.[8]

3. Did the child's teeth erupt about on time?

- Do the teeth seem straight to you?
- Is the child using a bottle? How often during the day? Does the child go to sleep with a bottle at night?
- Have you noticed any thumb sucking after the child's secondary teeth came in?
- Have you noticed the child grinding his or her teeth? Does this happen at night?

Eruption is delayed with Down syndrome, cretinism, rickets.

Malocclusion.

Prolonged bottle use increases risk for tooth decay and middle ear infections.

Prolonged thumb sucking (after ages 6 to 7 years) may affect occlusion.

Bruxism usually occurs in sleep or from dental problems or nervous tension.

4. Patient-centered care. How are the child's dental habits? Use a toothbrush regularly? How often does the child see a dentist?
- Do you use fluoridated water or fluoride supplement?

- Are vaccinations up to date? We recommend a one-time Tdap (tetanus-diphtheria-pertussis) booster for all adults >19 years.

Evaluate child's self-care. Early self-care has best compliance.

Pertussis (whooping cough) is on the rise because of lack of adherence to recommended vaccination schedule and waning immunity in adolescents and adults, who become carriers to unvaccinated infants.[14]

Additional History for the Aging Adult

1. Any dryness in the mouth? Are you taking any medications? (Note prescribed and over-the-counter medications.)

Xerostomia (dry mouth) is a side effect of many drugs: antidepressants, anticholinergics, antispasmodics, antihypertensives, antipsychotics, bronchodilators.

Examiner Asks	Rationale
2. Have you lost any teeth? Can you chew all types of food?	Note a decrease in eating meat, fresh vegetables, and cleansing foods such as apples.
3. Are you able to care for your own teeth or dentures?	Self-care may be decreased by physical disability (arthritis), loss or access and/or income, vision loss, confusion, or depression.
4. Noticed a change in your sense of taste or smell?	Some people add extra salt and sugar to enhance food when taste begins to wane. Diminished smell also may decrease the person's ability to detect food spoilage, natural gas leaks, or smoke from a fire.

OBJECTIVE DATA

PREPARATION

Position the person sitting up straight with his or her head at your eye level. If the person wears dentures, offer a paper towel and ask the person to remove them.

EQUIPMENT NEEDED

Otoscope with short, wide-tipped nasal speculum attachment
Penlight
Two tongue blades
Cotton gauze pad (4 × 4 inches)
Gloves

Normal Range of Findings	Abnormal Findings
Inspect and Palpate the Nose	

External Nose

Normally the nose is symmetric, in the midline, and in proportion to other facial features (Fig. 17.7). Inspect for any deformity, asymmetry, inflammation, or skin lesions. If an injury is reported or suspected, palpate gently for any pain or break in contour.

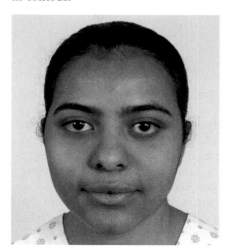

17.7

Normal Range of Findings

Test the patency of the nostrils by pushing each nasal wing shut with your finger while asking the person to sniff inward through the other naris. This reveals any obstruction, which later is explored with the nasal speculum. The sense of smell, mediated by cranial nerve I, is not tested in a routine examination. (See cranial nerve testing in Chapter 24.)

Nasal Cavity

Attach the short, wide-tipped speculum to the otoscope head, and insert this combined apparatus into the nasal vestibule, avoiding pressure on the nasal septum. Gently lift up the tip of the nose with your finger before inserting.

View each nasal cavity with the person's head erect and then with the head tilted back. Inspect the nasal mucosa, noting its normal red color and smooth, moist surface (Fig. 17.8). Note any swelling, discharge, bleeding, or foreign body.

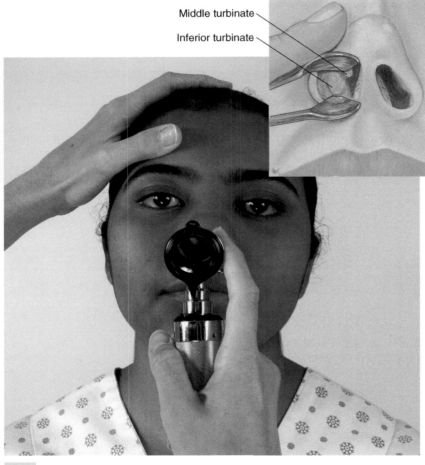

Middle turbinate
Inferior turbinate

17.8

Observe the nasal septum for deviation (Fig. 17.9). A deviated septum is common and is not significant unless air flow is obstructed. (If present in a hospitalized patient, document the deviated septum in the event that the person needs nasal suctioning or a nasogastric tube.) Also note any perforation or bleeding in the septum.

Abnormal Findings

Absence of sniff indicates obstruction (e.g., common cold, nasal polyps, rhinitis).

Rhinitis—Nasal mucosa is swollen and bright red with URI.

Discharge is common with rhinitis and sinusitis, varying from watery and copious to thick, purulent, and green-yellow.

With chronic allergy mucosa looks swollen, boggy, pale, and gray.

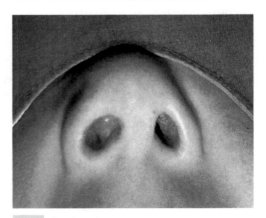

17.9 Deviated septum. (Fireman, 1996.)

A deviated septum looks like a hump or shelf in one nasal cavity.

Perforation is seen as a spot of light from a penlight shining in the other naris and occurs with cocaine use.

Epistaxis commonly comes from the anterior septum (see Table 17.1, Nose Abnormalities, p. 367).

Normal Range of Findings	Abnormal Findings

Inspect the turbinates (the bony ridges curving down from the lateral walls). The superior turbinate will not be in your view, but the middle and inferior turbinates appear the same light red color as the nasal mucosa. Note any swelling but do not try to push the speculum past it. Turbinates are quite vascular and tender if touched.

Note any polyps (benign growths that accompany chronic allergy), and distinguish them from the normal turbinates.

Polyps are smooth, pale gray, avascular, mobile, nontender (see Table 17.1).

Palpate the Sinus Areas

Using your thumbs, press the frontal sinuses by pressing firmly up and *under* the eyebrows (Fig. 17.10, *A*) and over the maxillary sinuses *below* (not over) the cheekbones (Fig. 17.10, *B*). Take care not to press directly on the eyeballs.

The person should feel firm pressure but no pain.

Sinus areas are tender to palpation in people with chronic allergies and acute infection (sinusitis).

Another sign of sinusitis is to check for focal pain when the person bends over (if able).

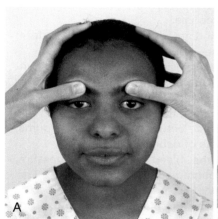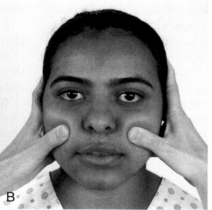

17.10

Transillumination

There is no evidence to support the practice of transillumination of the frontal or maxillary sinuses when you suspect sinus inflammation. The diagnosis requires distinct differences in the illumination of one of the sinus pair. Thus the technique would not help in chronic sinusitis that has diffuse swelling of all sinus mucosa. Although there is more fluid collection with acute sinusitis, the asymmetry of light illumination still is not valid because many healthy sinuses normally do not transilluminate.

Inspect the Mouth

Begin with anterior structures and move posteriorly. Use a tongue blade to retract structures and a bright light for optimal visualization.

Lips

Inspect the lips for color, moisture, cracking, or lesions. Retract the lips and note their inner surface as well (Fig. 17.11). All racial groups have lips that are deeper or pinker than facial skin. However, some African Americans normally may have bluish lips and a dark line on the gingival margin.

In light-skinned people: circumoral pallor occurs with shock and anemia; cyanosis with hypoxemia and chilling; cherry red lips with carbon monoxide poisoning, acidosis from aspirin poisoning, or ketoacidosis.

Objective Data

Normal Range of Findings	Abnormal Findings

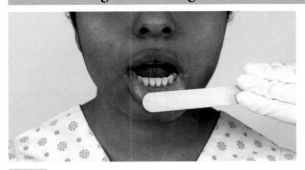

17.11

Cheilitis (perlèche)—Cracking at the corners.

Herpes simplex, other lesions (see Table 17.2, Lip Abnormalities, p. 369).

Teeth and Gums

The condition of the teeth is an index of the person's general health. Your examination should not replace the regular dental examination; but you should note any diseased, absent, loose, or abnormally positioned teeth. The teeth normally look white, straight, evenly spaced, and clean and free of debris or decay.

Compare the number of teeth with the number expected for the person's age. Ask the person to bite as if chewing something and note alignment of upper and lower jaw. Normal occlusion in the back is the upper teeth resting directly on the lower teeth; in the front the upper incisors slightly override the lower incisors.

Normally the gums look pink or coral with a stippled (dotted) surface. The gum margins at the teeth are tight and well defined (Fig. 17.12). Check for swelling; retraction of gingival margins; and spongy, bleeding, or discolored gums. Some African Americans normally may have a dark melanotic line along the gingival margin.

Discolored teeth appear brown with excessive fluoride use, yellow with tobacco use.

Grinding down of tooth surface; plaque—soft debris; caries—decay.

Malocclusion (poor biting relationship), protrusion of upper or lower incisors.

Gingival hyperplasia (see Table 17.3), crevices between teeth and gums, pockets of debris.

Gums bleed with slight pressure, indicating gingivitis.

Dark line on gingival margins occurs with lead and bismuth poisoning.

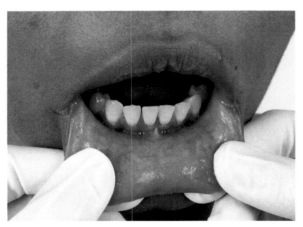

17.12

Tongue

Check the tongue for color, surface characteristics, and moisture. The color is pink and even. The dorsal surface is normally roughened from the papillae. A thin white coating may be present (Fig. 17.13, *A*). Ask the person to touch the tongue to the roof of the mouth. Its ventral surface looks smooth and glistening and shows veins (Fig. 17.13, *B*). Saliva is present.

Beefy red, swollen tongue. Smooth glossy areas (see Table 17.5, Tongue Abnormalities, p. 373).

Enlarged tongue occurs with hypothyroidism, acromegaly; a small tongue accompanies malnutrition.

Dry mouth occurs with dehydration, fever; tongue has deep vertical fissures.

Normal Range of Findings

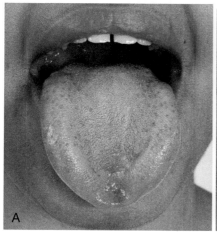 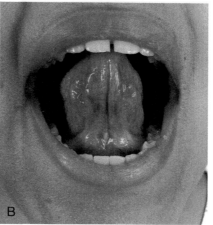

17.13

With a glove,[a] hold the tongue with a cotton gauze pad for traction and swing it out and to each side (Fig. 17.14). Inspect for any white patches or lesions; normally none are present. If any occur, palpate them for induration.

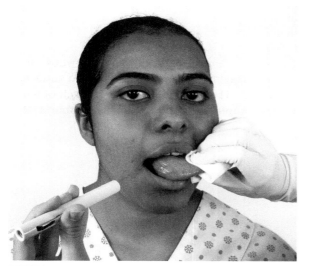

17.14

Inspect carefully the entire U-shaped area under the tongue behind the teeth. Note any white patches, nodules, or ulcerations. If lesions are present or for any person older than 50 years or with a positive history of smoking or alcohol use, use your gloved hand to palpate the area and the rest of the oral mucosa. Place your other hand under the jaw to stabilize the tissue and to "capture" any abnormality (Fig. 17.15). Note any induration.

Abnormal Findings

Saliva is decreased when taking anticholinergic and other medications.

Excess saliva and drooling occur with gingivostomatitis and Parkinson disease.

Oral precancerous and cancerous lesions (see Table 17.5). The lateral and ventral tongue and the floor of the mouth are high-risk sites for oral squamous cell cancer.[7]

Any lesion or ulcer persisting for more than 2 weeks must be investigated.

An indurated area may be a mass or lymphadenopathy, and it must be investigated.

[a]Always wear gloves to examine mucous membranes. This follows Standard Precautions to prevent the spread of communicable disease.

Objective Data

Normal Range of Findings	Abnormal Findings

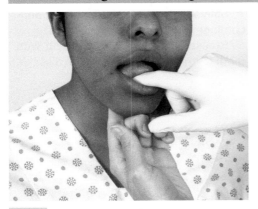

17.15   Bimanual palpation.

Buccal Mucosa

Hold the cheek open with a wooden tongue blade and check the buccal mucosa for color, nodules, or lesions. It looks pink, smooth, and moist, although patchy hyperpigmentation is common and normal in dark-skinned people.

Expect to find **Stensen duct,** the opening of the parotid salivary gland. It looks like a small dimple opposite the upper second molar. You also may see a raised occlusion line on the buccal mucosa parallel with the level the teeth meet. This is caused by the teeth closing against the cheek.

A larger patch also may be present along the buccal mucosa. This is **leukoedema,** a benign, milky, bluish-white, opaque area, more common in blacks and East Indians. When it is mild, the patch disappears as you stretch the cheeks. It is always bilateral. With age it looks grayish-white and thickened. The cause is unknown. Do not mistake leukoedema for oral infections such as candidiasis (thrush).

Fordyce granules are small, isolated white or yellow papules on the mucosa of cheek, tongue, and lips (Fig. 17.16). These little sebaceous cysts are painless and not significant.

Dappled brown patches are present with Addison disease (chronic adrenal insufficiency).

Orifice of Stensen duct looks red with mumps.

Koplik spots—Early prodromal (early warning) sign of measles.

Candida infection usually rubs off, leaving a clear or raw denuded surface.

The chalky white raised patch of **leukoplakia** is abnormal (see Table 17.4, Buccal Mucosa Abnormalities).

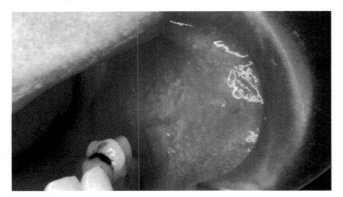

17.16   Fordyce granules.   (Ibsen & Phelan, 1996.)

Palate

Shine your light up to the roof of the mouth. The more anterior hard palate is white with irregular transverse rugae. The posterior soft palate is pinker, smooth, and upwardly movable. A normal variation is a nodular bony ridge down the middle of the hard palate, a **torus palatinus** (Fig. 17.17). This benign growth arises after puberty; is more common in American Indians, Inuits, and Asians; and is more common in females than in males.

The hard palate appears yellow with jaundice. In blacks with jaundice it may look yellow, muddy yellow, or green-brown.

Normal Range of Findings

Oral Kaposi sarcoma is the most common early lesion in people with AIDS (see Table 17.6, Oropharynx Abnormalities, p. 375).

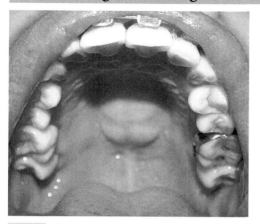

17.17   Torus palatinus.   (Flint, 2015.)

Observe the uvula; it normally looks like a fleshy pendant hanging in the midline (Fig. 17.18). Ask the person to say "ahhh," and note the soft palate and uvula rise in the midline. This tests one function of cranial nerve X, the vagus nerve.

A *bifid* uvula looks as if it is split in two; more common in American Indians (see Table 17.6).

Any deviation to the side or absent movement indicates nerve damage, which also occurs with poliomyelitis and diphtheria.

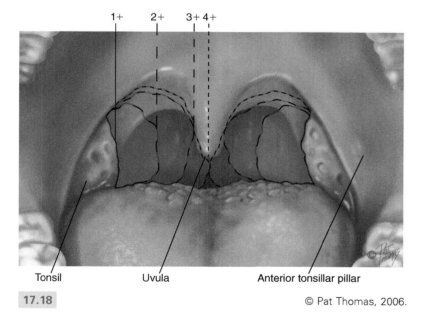

1+   2+   3+ 4+

Tonsil   Uvula   Anterior tonsillar pillar

17.18   © Pat Thomas, 2006.

Inspect the Throat

With your light observe the oval, rough-surfaced **tonsils** behind the anterior tonsillar pillar (see Fig. 17.18). Their color is the same pink as the oral mucosa, and their surface is peppered with indentations, or crypts. In some people the crypts collect small plugs of whitish cellular debris. This does not indicate infection. However, there should be no exudate on the tonsils. Tonsils are graded in size as follows:

1+ Visible
2+ Halfway between tonsillar pillars and uvula
3+ Touching the uvula
4+ Touching one another

With an acute infection tonsils are bright red and swollen and may have exudate or large white spots.

A white membrane covering the tonsils may accompany infectious mononucleosis, leukemia, and diphtheria.

Objective Data

Normal Range of Findings

You may normally see 1+ or 2+ tonsils in healthy people, especially in children, because lymphoid tissue is proportionately enlarged until puberty.

Enlarge your view of the posterior pharyngeal wall by depressing the tongue with a tongue blade (Fig. 17.19). Push down halfway back on the tongue; if you push on its tip, the tongue humps up in back. Press slightly off center to avoid eliciting the gag reflex. You can help the person whose gag reflex is easily triggered by offering a tongue blade to depress his or her own tongue. (Some people can lower their own tongue so the tongue blade is not needed.) Scan the posterior wall for color, exudate, and lesions. When finished, discard the tongue blade.

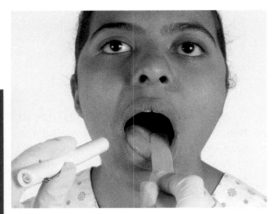

17.19

Although usually it is not done in the screening examination, touching the posterior wall with the tongue blade elicits the gag reflex. This tests cranial nerves IX and X, the glossopharyngeal and vagus.

Test cranial nerve XII, the hypoglossal nerve, by asking the person to stick out the tongue. It should protrude in the midline. Children enjoy this request! Note any tremor, loss of movement, or deviation to the side.

During the examination notice any breath odor, *halitosis*. This is common and usually has a local cause such as poor oral hygiene and decaying food debris between the teeth. Other common smells are caused by odoriferous foods, alcohol consumption, heavy smoking, or dental infection. Occasionally it may indicate a systemic disease.

❖ DEVELOPMENTAL COMPETENCE

Infants and Children

Because the oral examination is intrusive for the infant or young child, the timing is best toward the end of the complete examination, along with the ear examination. But if any crying episodes occur earlier, seize the opportunity to examine the open mouth and oropharynx.

Abnormal Findings

Tonsils are enlarged to 2+, 3+, or 4+ with an acute infection.

Clinical features help but are not sufficient in determining the cause of pharyngitis. **Viral** pharyngitis shows erythematous tonsils with no hypertrophy or exudates. When accompanied by cough, hoarseness, and rhinorrhea, a rapid antigen test and/or culture may not be needed in low risk groups. **Streptococcal** pharyngitis shows with erythematous, enlarged tonsils with exudates. Four features suggest streptococcal cause: absence of cough; swollen, tender anterior cervical nodes; fever >100.4° F (38° C); tonsillar exudate. With these features and in children 3 to 14 years, rapid antigen testing is warranted.[8,16] (See Table 17.6.)

Infectious mononucleosis shows erythematous, exudative enlarged tonsils[10] that "kiss" the uvula.

With CN XII damage, the tongue deviates *toward* the paralyzed side.

A fine tremor of the tongue occurs with hyperthyroidism; a coarse tremor occurs with cerebral palsy and alcoholism.

Diabetic ketoacidosis has a sweet, fruity breath odor; this acetone smell also occurs in children with malnutrition or dehydration. Others are an ammonia breath odor with uremia; a musty odor with liver disease; a foul, fetid odor with dental or respiratory infections; an alcohol odor with alcohol ingestion; a mouselike smell of the breath with diphtheria.

Normal Range of Findings	Abnormal Findings

As with the ear examination, let the parent help position the child. Place the infant supine on the examining table with the arms restrained (Fig. 17.20). The older infant and toddler may be held on the parent's lap with one of the parent's hands gently holding the arms down. Only if necessary, direct the parent's other hand to hold the child's head against the parent's chest.

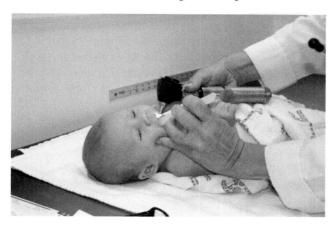

17.20

Use a game to help prepare the young child. Encourage the preschool child to use a tongue blade to look into a puppet's mouth. Or place a mirror so the child can look into his or her mouth just as you look. The school-age child is usually cooperative and loves to show off missing or new teeth (Fig. 17.21).

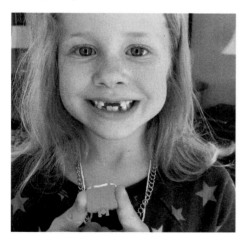

17.21

Be discriminating in your use of the tongue blade. It may be necessary for a full view of oral structures, but it produces a strong gag reflex in the infant. You may avoid the tongue blade completely with a cooperative preschooler and school-age child. Try asking the young child to "Open your mouth as big as a LION." Or say, "Can you stick out your WHOLE TONGUE?" Then ask the child to move the tongue in different directions. To enlarge your view of the oropharynx, ask the child to stick out the tongue and "pant like a dog."

At some point you will encounter an uncooperative young child who clenches the teeth and refuses to open the mouth. If all your other efforts have failed, slide the tongue blade along the buccal mucosa and turn it between the back teeth. Push down to depress the tongue. This stimulates the gag reflex, and the child opens the mouth wide for a few seconds. You will have a *brief* look at the throat. Make the most of it.

Objective Data

Normal Range of Findings	Abnormal Findings

Normal Range of Findings

Nose. The newborn may have milia across the nose. The nasal bridge may be flat in black and Asian children. There should be no nasal flaring or narrowing with breathing.

It is essential to determine the patency of the nares in the immediate newborn period because most newborns are obligate nose breathers. Nares blocked with amniotic fluid are suctioned gently with a bulb syringe. If obstruction is suspected, a small-lumen (5 to 10 Fr) catheter is passed down each naris to confirm patency.

Avoid the nasal speculum when examining the infant and young child. Instead gently push up the tip of the nose with your thumb while using your other hand to shine the light into the naris. With a toddler be alert for the possible foreign body lodged in the nasal cavity (see Table 17.1, p. 368).

Only in children older than 8 years of age do you need to palpate the sinus areas. In younger children sinus areas are too small for palpation.

Mouth and Throat. A normal finding in infants is the **sucking tubercle,** a small pad in the middle of the upper lip from friction of breastfeeding or bottle-feeding. Note the number of teeth and whether it is appropriate for the child's age. Also note pattern of eruption, position, condition, and hygiene. Use this guide for children younger than 2 years of age: the child's age in months minus the number 6 should equal the expected number of deciduous teeth. Normally all 20 deciduous teeth are in by 2½ years. Saliva is present after 3 months of age and shows in excess with teething children.

Mobility should allow the tongue to extend at least as far as the alveolar ridge.

Note any bruising or laceration on the buccal mucosa or gums of the infant or young child.

On the palate, **Epstein pearls** are a normal finding in newborns and infants (Fig. 17.22). They are small, whitish, glistening, pearly papules along the median raphe of the hard palate and on the gums, where they look like teeth. They are small retention cysts and disappear in the first few weeks.

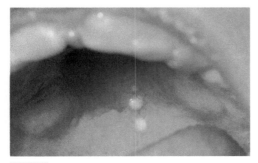

17.22 Epstein pearls.   (Zitelli, 2007.)

Bednar aphthae are traumatic areas or ulcers on the posterior hard palate on either side of the midline. They result from abrasions while sucking.

Abnormal Findings

Nasal flaring in the infant indicates respiratory distress.

A transverse ridge across the nose occurs in a child with chronic allergy from wiping the nose upward with the palm (see Table 14.2, p. 268). Nasal narrowing on inhalation is seen with chronic nasal obstruction and mouth breathing.

Inability to pass catheter through nasal cavity indicates choanal atresia, which needs immediate intervention (see Table 17.1).

No teeth by age 1 year.

Discolored teeth appear yellow or yellow-brown with infants taking tetracycline or who were exposed during the last trimester; appear green or black with excessive iron ingestion (this reverses when the iron is stopped).

Malocclusion: upper or lower dental arches are out of alignment.

Ankyloglossia, a short lingual frenulum, can limit protrusion and impair speech development (see Table 17.5).

Trauma may indicate child abuse from forced feeding of bottle or spoon.

A high-arched palate is usually normal in the newborn, but a very narrow or high arch also occurs with Turner syndrome, Ehlers-Danlos syndrome, Marfan syndrome, and Treacher Collins syndrome or develops in the mouth-breather in chronic allergies.

Objective Data

Normal Range of Findings	Abnormal Findings

The tonsils are not visible in the newborn. They gradually enlarge during childhood, remaining proportionately larger until puberty. Tonsils appear still larger if the infant is crying or gagging. Normally the newborn can produce a strong, lusty cry.

Insert your gloved finger into the baby's mouth and palpate the hard and soft palate as the baby sucks. The sucking reflex can be elicited in infants up to 12 months old.

As teeth begin to erupt in the older infant and child, check age at eruption, sequence, and condition. Teeth should emerge straight up or down from the gums, and enamel should be clear white and smooth. Lift the upper lip to check for dental caries (tooth decay); normally there are none.

Nursing bottle caries are brown discolorations on upper front teeth (see Table 17.3).

The Pregnant Woman

Gum hypertrophy (surface looks smooth, and stippling disappears) may occur normally at puberty or during pregnancy (pregnancy gingivitis) (Fig. 17.23).

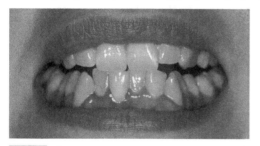

17.23   Early gingivitis. (Lemmi & Lemmi, 2011.)

The Aging Adult

The nose may appear more prominent on the face from a loss of subcutaneous fat. In the edentulous person the mouth and lips fold in, giving a "purse-string" appearance. The teeth may look slightly yellowed, although the color is uniform. Yellowing results from the dentin visible through worn enamel. The surface of the incisors may show vertical cracks from a lifetime of exposure to extreme temperatures. The teeth may look longer as the gum margins recede (Fig. 17.24).

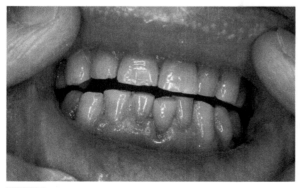

17.24   Receded gums.   (Lemmi & Lemmi, 2011.)

The surfaces look worn down or abraded. Old dental work deteriorates, especially at the gum margins. The teeth loosen with bone resorption and may move with palpation.

The tongue looks smoother as a result of papillary atrophy. The aging adult's buccal mucosa is thinned and may look shinier, as though it were "varnished."

Objective Data

HEALTH PROMOTION AND PATIENT TEACHING

"The most helpful thing we can do today is to talk about your smoking and tobacco dependence. Probably you know that smoking leads to many heart and lung diseases and to many cancers. But the good news is that tobacco dependence is very treatable. Also, you will see benefits within 24 hours as your lungs clear themselves of mucus and other smoking leftovers. Have you ever tried to quit? What worked? What didn't work? As we start, it is important to know that smoking is a form of addiction and that most people cannot quit without help from a counselor, a nurse, or a doctor."

Your time and resources in your clinical setting will determine how many smoking-cessation efforts you can take on yourself. Smoking is the world's leading cause of early death and disability; smoking cigarettes leads to at least 21 diseases, including 12 types of cancer, 6 types of heart and blood vessel disease, and to diabetes, chronic obstructive lung disease, pneumonia, and influenza."[3] So it is imperative that you make an effort to teach at every patient encounter. At the very least, consider the Very Brief Advice on Smoking, which you can adapt to your work situation. [Ask] *"Do you smoke or use tobacco products? At what age did you start smoking? How many packs of cigarettes per day do you smoke? How many years have you smoked this amount?"* [Advise] *"Smoking cigarettes leads to many heart and lung diseases and to many types of cancer. Stopping smoking is the very best thing you can do to improve your health. The best way to quit is a combination of behavioral support and medication. We have a local, friendly stop-smoking service. The people there are experts, and I can send you to them if you'd like?"*[17] [Act] Refer the person to the stop-smoking service, or make a note in the person's record that you have advised and the person is not ready to quit. Make sure that your communication is nonjudgmental, and focus on the person—help him or her to understand attitudes about smoking and quitting and to make an independent decision. Note the more detailed recommendations in Fig. 17.25,[17] and adapt them to your setting.

When people smoke over 10 cigarettes per day or smoke within 30 to 60 minutes of waking up, it is likely that they will experience withdrawal symptoms when quitting. These people have greater success if pharmacotherapy is included in the cessation program. Make sure that medications are available and affordable before prescriptions are written.

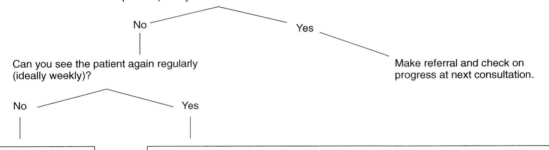

17.25 Deciding what smoking cessation interventions you can deliver. (Van Schayck, Williams, & Barchilon, 2017.)

Medications include nicotine-replacement therapy by skin patch and gum,[5] varenicline (a nicotinic receptor partial agonist), and bupropion (to reduce the craving). Measuring expired carbon monoxide (CO) via a CO monitor is a strong motivational tool that is available in many settings.[17] Your confidence in tackling this communication is important. Tobacco addiction is a chronic condition. Relapses are unfortunate but expected, and a buildup in smoke-free days eventually will lead to successful quitting.[18]

DOCUMENTATION AND CRITICAL THINKING

Sample Charting

SUBJECTIVE

Nose: No history of discharge, sinus problems, obstruction, epistaxis, or allergy. Colds 1-2/yr, mild. Fractured nose during high school sports, treated by MD.

Mouth and throat: No pain, lesions, bleeding gums, toothache, dysphagia, or hoarseness. Occasional sore throat with colds. Tonsillectomy, age 8. Smokes cigarettes 1 PPD × 9 years. Alcohol, 1-2 drinks socially about 2×/month. Visits dentist annually, dental hygienist 2×/year, flosses daily. No dental appliance.

OBJECTIVE

Nose: Symmetric, no deformity or skin lesions. Nares patent. Mucosa pink; no discharge, lesions, or polyps; no septal deviation or perforation. Sinuses—no tenderness to palpation.

Mouth: Can clench teeth. Mucosa and gingivae pink, no masses or lesions. Teeth all present, straight, and in good repair. Tongue smooth, pink, no lesions, protrudes in midline, no tremor.

Throat: Mucosa pink, no lesions or exudate. Uvula rises in midline on phonation. Tonsils out. Gag reflex present.

ASSESSMENT

Nose and oral structures intact and appear healthy
Needs teaching about risks of cigarette smoking

Clinical Case Study 1

B.D., a 34-year-old electrician, seeks care for "sore throat for 2 days."

SUBJECTIVE

2 days PTA—Experienced sudden onset of sore throat, swollen glands, fever 101° F, occasional shaking chills, extreme fatigue.

Today—Symptoms remain. Cough productive of yellow sputum. Treated self with aspirin for minimal relief. Unable to eat past 2 days because "throat on fire." Taking adequate fluids, on bed rest. Not aware of exposure to other sick people. Does not smoke.

OBJECTIVE

Ears: Tympanic membranes pearly gray with landmarks intact.
Nose: No discharge. Mucosa pink, no swelling.
Mouth: Mucosa and gingivae pink, no lesions.
Throat: Tonsils 3+. Pharyngeal wall bright red with yellow-white exudate; exudate also on tonsils.
Neck: Enlarged anterior cervical nodes bilaterally, painful to palpation. No other lymphadenopathy.
Chest: Resonant to percussion throughout. Breath sounds clear anterior and posterior. No adventitious sounds.

ASSESSMENT

Pharyngitis
Throat pain

Documentation and Critical Thinking

Clinical Case Study 2

D.C. is a 67-year-old homeless man who is brought to the emergency department (ED) after being found intoxicated in a local park. After 6 hours in the ED, D.C. is awake and cooperative. The nurses notice grimacing as he eats.

SUBJECTIVE

D.C. reports sensitivity when eating and drinking. Does not have medical or dental insurance. Has never been to the dentist. Encouraged to have his teeth cleaned "years ago," but did not have the money.

OBJECTIVE

Vital signs: Temp 98.4° F (36.7° C). Pulse 68 bpm. Resp 14/min, unlabored, in no distress.
Rates pain at 6/10, but only when eating or drinking.
Ears: Pinna intact. TMs pearly gray with landmarks intact. Hearing is good.
Mouth: Oral mucosa pink; uvula rises midline on phonation; tonsils absent. Gums appear red and swollen. Receding gingival margins noted. Brown and black spots noted on all molars bilaterally. All teeth appear yellow.
Chest: Thorax symmetric AP < transverse diameter. Resonant to percussion. Breath sounds clear and = bilat. No adventitious sounds.
Heart: S_1 and S_2 not accentuated or diminished; no murmurs.

ASSESSMENT

Severe gingivitis
Dental caries
Potential for malnutrition and weight loss
Acute pain
Lack of social support

Clinical Case Study 3

E.V. is a 61-year-old professor who has been admitted to the hospital for chemotherapy for carcinoma of the breast. This is her 5th day in the hospital. She now is worried about "soreness and a white coating" in the mouth.

SUBJECTIVE

Felt soreness on tongue and cheeks during night. Now pain persists, and E.V. can see a "white coating" on tongue and cheeks. "I'm worried. Is this more cancer?"

OBJECTIVE

General appearance: E.V. generally appears restless and overly aware.
Mouth: Oral mucosa pink. Large white, cheesy patches covering most of dorsal surface of tongue and buccal mucosa. Will scrape off with tongue blade, revealing red eroded area beneath.
Bleeds with slight contact. Posterior pharyngeal wall pink, no lesions. Patches soft to palpation. No palpable lymph nodes.

ASSESSMENT

Oral lesion, candidiasis
Anxiety

Documentation and Critical Thinking

TABLE 17.1 | **Nose Abnormalities**

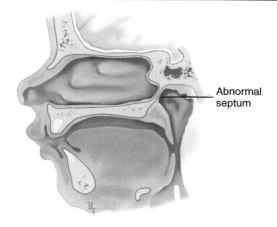

Abnormal septum

Choanal Atresia

Congenital bony septum between the nasal cavity and the pharynx is not common in the newborn; but when bilateral, it is an airway emergency because newborns are obligate nose breathers. Note airway obstruction, stridor, and cyclical cyanosis that improves with crying because baby then breathes through the mouth. When unilateral, the infant may be asymptomatic until the first respiratory infection.

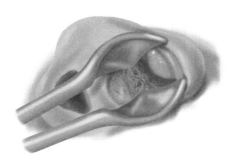

Epistaxis

The most common site of a nosebleed is Kiesselbach plexus in the anterior septum. Peak incidence is bimodal, <18 years and >50 years. Causes include nose picking, forceful coughing or sneezing, fracture, foreign body, illicit drug use (cocaine), topical nasal drugs, warfarin (Coumadin), aspirin, or a coagulation disorder. Bleeding from the anterior septum is easily controlled and rarely severe. A posterior hemorrhage is less common (<10%) but more profuse, harder to manage, and more serious.

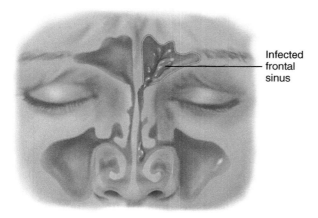

Infected frontal sinus

Sinusitis

Acute inflamed infected sinus areas following URI are over 90% viral in origin and do not need antibiotics. Consider bacterial infection when signs last over 10 days without improvement.[15] Major signs are mucopurulent drainage, nasal obstruction, facial pain or pressure. May also have fever, chills, malaise. Maxillary sinusitis has dull, throbbing pain in cheek and teeth and pain with palpation and when bending over. Frontal sinusitis has pain above supraorbital ridge.

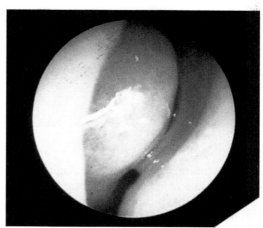

Seasonal Allergic Rhinitis (AR or Hay Fever)

AR is an abnormal immune response from repeated exposure to antigens, with rhinorrhea, itching of nose and eyes, lacrimation, nasal congestion, and sneezing. Note serous edema and swelling of turbinates to fill the air space. Turbinates are usually pale (although they may appear violet), and their surface looks smooth and glistening. Common allergens are dust mite, animal dander, mold, pollen. AR produces disordered sleep, obstructive sleep apnea, sinusitis, avoidance of outdoor activities, and poor work performance.[19]

Continued

TABLE 17.1 | Nose Abnormalities—cont'd

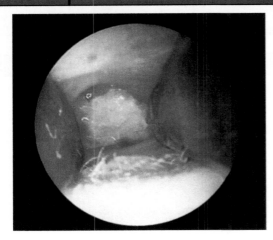

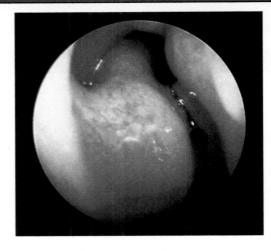

Foreign Body

Children particularly are apt to put an object up the nose (here, yellow plastic foam), producing unilateral mucopurulent drainage and foul odor. Because some risk for aspiration exists, removal should be prompt. Watch out for impaction from a small button battery from an electronic device (watch, video game). Once occluding the nostril, the battery can release voltage or chemicals that cause burns, necrosis, or perforation.

Acute Rhinitis (Nonallergic)

The first sign is a clear, watery discharge, rhinorrhea, which later becomes purulent, with sneezing, nasal itching, stimulation of cough reflex, and inflamed mucosa, which causes nasal obstruction. Turbinates are dark red and swollen.

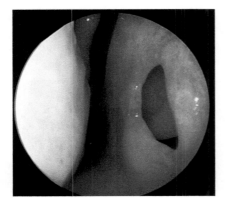

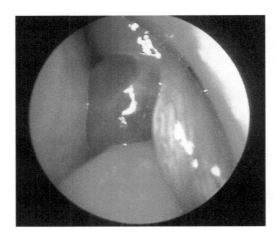

Perforated Septum

A hole in the septum, usually in the cartilaginous part, caused by snorting cocaine or methamphetamine, chronic infection, trauma from continual picking of crusts, or nasal surgery. It is seen directly or as a spot of light when the penlight is directed into the other naris.

Nasal Polyps

Smooth, pale gray nodules, which are overgrowths of mucosa, are most commonly caused by chronic allergic rhinitis. May be stalked. A common site is protrusion from the middle meatus. Often multiple, they are mobile and nontender in contrast to turbinates. They may obstruct air passageways as they get larger. Symptoms are absence of sense of smell and a "valve that moves" in the nose as the person breathes.

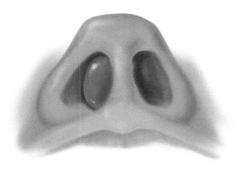

◄ Furuncle

A small boil located in the skin or mucous membrane; appears red and swollen and is quite painful. Avoid any manipulation or trauma that may spread the infection.

See Illustration Credits for source information.

TABLE 17.2 | **Lip Abnormalities**

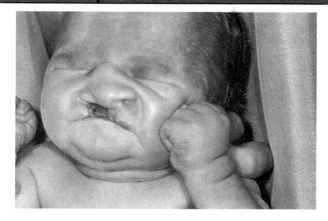

Cleft Lip

Maxillofacial clefts are common congenital deformities and occur with strong family history; maternal use of phenytoin (Dilantin), alcohol, and certain drugs; and maternal diabetes. Early treatment preserves the functions of speech and language formation and deglutition (swallowing).

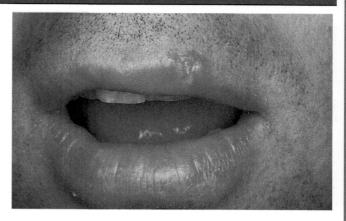

Herpes Simplex 1 (HSV-1)

The common cold sores are groups of clear vesicles with a surrounding indurated erythematous base. These evolve into pustules, which rupture, weep, and crust and heal in 4 to 10 days. The most likely site is the lip-skin junction; infection often recurs in the same site. HSV-1 lesion is highly contagious and spread by direct contact. Recurrent infections may be precipitated by sunlight, fever, colds, and allergy.

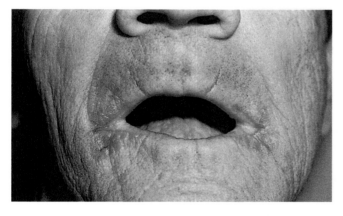

Angular Cheilitis (Stomatitis, Perlèche)

Erythema, scaling, and shallow and painful fissures at the corners of the mouth occur with excess salivation and *Candida* infection. It is often seen in edentulous persons and those with poorly fitting dentures, causing folding in of corners of mouth, which creates a warm, moist environment favoring growth of yeast.

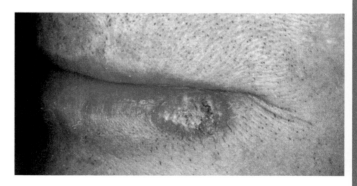

Carcinoma

The initial lesion is round and indurated; it becomes crusted and ulcerated with an elevated border. Most occur between the outer and middle thirds of the lip. Any lesion that is still unhealed after 2 weeks should be referred.

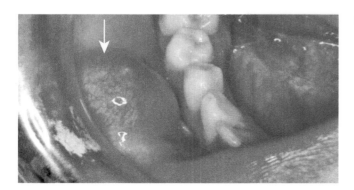

◀ Retention "Cyst" (Mucocele)

A round, well-defined, translucent nodule that may be very small or up to 1 to 2 cm. It is a pocket of mucus that forms when a duct of a minor salivary gland ruptures. The benign lesion also may occur on the buccal mucosa, on the floor of the mouth, or under the tip of the tongue.

ABNORMAL FINDINGS
FOR ADVANCED PRACTICE

TABLE 17.3	Teeth and Gum Abnormalities

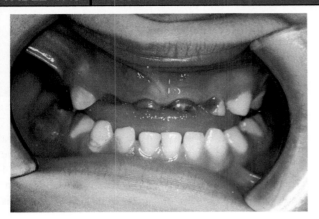

Baby Bottle Tooth Decay

Destruction of numerous deciduous teeth may occur in infants and toddlers who take a bottle of milk, juice, or sweetened drink to bed and prolong bottle-feeding past the age of 1 year. Liquid pools around the upper front teeth. Mouth bacteria act on carbohydrates in the liquid, especially sucrose, forming metabolic acids. Acids break down tooth enamel and destroy its protein.

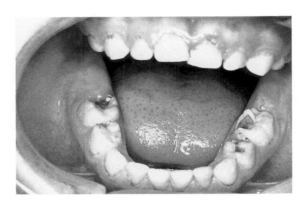

Dental Caries

Progressive destruction of tooth. Decay initially looks chalky white. Later it turns brown or black and forms a cavity. Early decay shows only on x-ray image. Susceptible sites are tooth surfaces where food debris, bacterial plaque, and saliva collect.

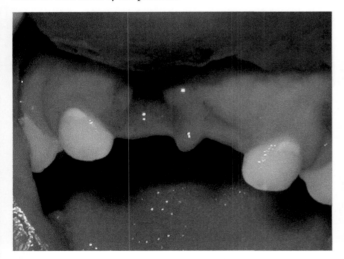

Tooth Avulsion

A traumatic injury may dislodge a primary (deciduous) or a permanent tooth from its alveolar socket. Trauma is often the result of falls or sports collision. The time to reimplantation is crucial for viability. During this time, the tooth must be stored in an appropriate solution (milk is acceptable and at hand) because dry storage of >15 minutes increases the risk of necrosis. Do not touch root; ask patient about tetanus vaccine and need for bacterial endocarditis prophylaxis.[4]

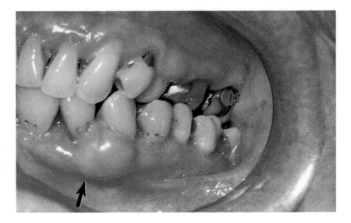

Epulis

A benign nontender, fibrous nodule of the gum seen emerging between the teeth; an overgrowth of vascular granulation tissue.

TABLE 17.3 | **Teeth and Gum Abnormalities—cont'd**

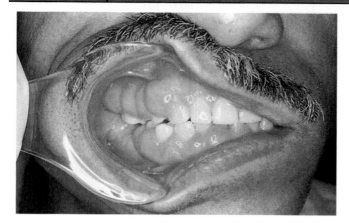

Gingival Hyperplasia

Painless enlargement of the gums, sometimes overreaching the teeth. This occurs with puberty, pregnancy, and leukemia and with long therapeutic use of phenytoin (Dilantin).

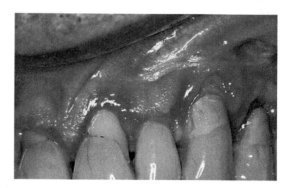

Gingivitis

Gum margins are red and swollen and bleed easily. This case is severe; gingival tissue has desquamated, exposing roots of teeth. Inflammation is usually caused by poor dental hygiene or vitamin C deficiency. The condition may occur in pregnancy and puberty because of changing hormonal balance.

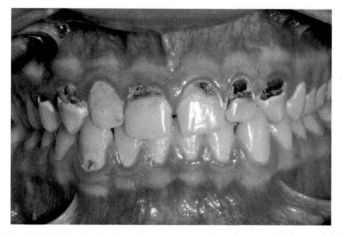

◀ Meth Mouth

Illicit methamphetamine abuse (crystal meth, meth ice) leads to extensive dental caries, gingivitis, tooth cracking, and edentulism. Methamphetamine causes vasoconstriction and decreased saliva, and its use increases the urge to consume sugars and starches and give up oral hygiene. Absence of the buffering saliva leads to increased acidity, and the increased plaque encourages bacterial growth. These conditions and carbohydrate presence produce caries, cracking of enamel, and the damage seen here.

See Illustration Credits for source information.

TABLE 17.4 | **Buccal Mucosa Abnormalities**

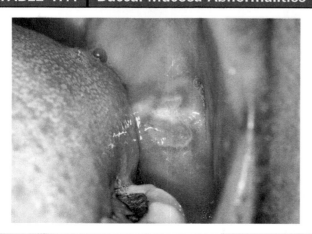

◀ Aphthous Ulcers

A common "canker sore" is a vesicle at first and then a small, round, "punched-out" ulcer with a white base surrounded by a red halo. It is quite painful and lasts for 1 to 2 weeks. The cause is unknown, although it is associated with stress, fatigue, and food allergy.

Continued

Abnormal Findings

TABLE 17.4 | Buccal Mucosa Abnormalities—cont'd

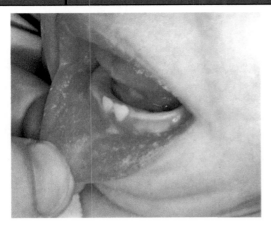

Koplik Spots in Measles

Small blue-white spots with irregular red halo scattered over mucosa opposite the molars. An early sign, and pathognomonic, of measles.

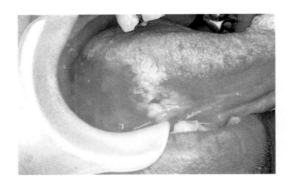

Leukoplakia

Chalky white, thick, raised patch with well-defined borders. The lesion is firmly attached and does not scrape off. It may occur on the lateral edges of tongue. It is caused by chronic irritation of smoking and alcohol use. Lesions are precancerous; must refer to specialist. (Here the lesion is associated with squamous carcinoma.)

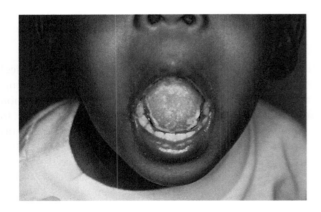

◄ Candidiasis or Monilial Infection

A white, cheesy, curdlike patch on the buccal mucosa and tongue. It scrapes off, leaving a raw, red surface that bleeds easily. Termed *thrush* in the newborn. It is an opportunistic infection that occurs after the use of antibiotics and corticosteroids and in immunosuppressed people.

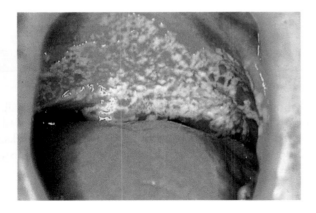

Candidiasis in Adult

The *Candida* species as normal oral flora is present in 60% of healthy adults. Overgrowth of *Candida* occurs with steroid inhaler use, HIV infection, use of broad-spectrum antibiotics or corticosteroids, leukemia, malnutrition, or reduced immunity.

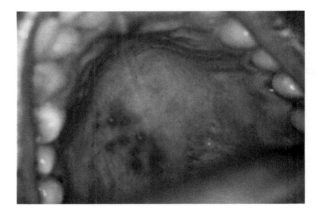

Herpes Simplex 1

HSV-1 infection on the hard palate (see discussion in Table 17.2).

See Illustration Credits for source information.

TABLE 17.5 | Tongue Abnormalities

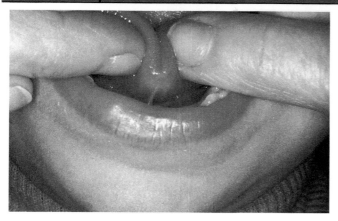

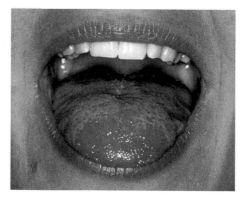

Ankyloglossia

A short lingual frenulum, here fixing the tongue tip to the floor of the mouth and gums (tongue-tie). This limits mobility and affects speech (pronunciation of *a, d, n)* if the tongue tip cannot be elevated to the alveolar ridge. A congenital defect.

Geographic Tongue (Migratory Glossitis)

Pattern of normal coating interspersed with bright red, shiny, circular bald areas caused by atrophy of the filiform papillae, with raised pearly borders. Pattern resembles a map and changes with time. Not significant, and its cause is not known.

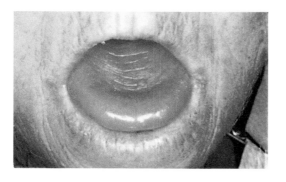

◄ Smooth, Glossy Tongue (Atrophic Glossitis)

The surface is slick and shiny; the mucosa thins and looks red from decreased papillae. Accompanied by dryness of tongue and burning. Occurs with vitamin B_{12} deficiency (pernicious anemia), folic acid deficiency, and iron deficiency anemia. Here also note angular cheilitis.

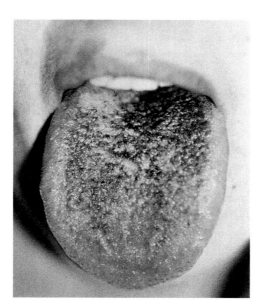

◄ Black Hairy Tongue

This is not really hair but rather the elongation of filiform papillae and painless overgrowth of mycelial threads of fungus infection on the tongue. Color varies from black-brown to yellow. It occurs after use of antibiotics, which inhibit normal bacteria and allow proliferation of fungus, and with heavy smoking.

Continued

TABLE 17.5	Tongue Abnormalities—cont'd

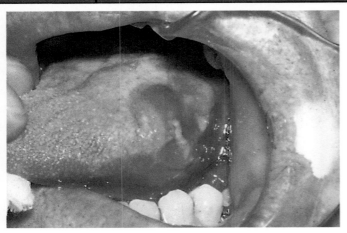

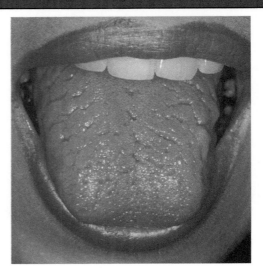

Carcinoma

An ulcer with rolled edges; indurated. Occurs particularly at sides, base, and under the tongue. It grows insidiously and may go unnoticed for months. It may have associated leukoplakia. Rich lymphatic drainage increases risk for early metastasis. Smoking and alcohol use account for most cases of oral cancer. HPV-related oral pharyngeal cancers also are increased.[9]

Fissured or Scrotal Tongue

Deep furrows divide the papillae into small irregular rows. The condition occurs in 5% of the general population and in Down syndrome. The incidence increases with age. (Vertical, or longitudinal, fissures also occur with dehydration because of reduced tongue volume.)

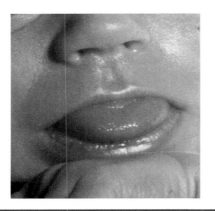

◀ Enlarged Tongue (Macroglossia)

The tongue is enlarged and may protrude from the mouth. The condition is not painful but may impair speech development. Here it occurs with Down syndrome; it also occurs with cretinism, myxedema, and acromegaly. A transient swelling also occurs with local infections.

See Illustration Credits for source information.

TABLE 17.6	Oropharynx Abnormalities

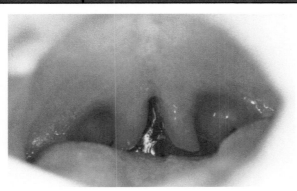

◀ Bifid Uvula

The uvula looks partly severed and may indicate a submucous cleft palate, which feels like a notch at the junction of the hard and soft palates. This may affect speech development because it prevents necessary air trapping. The incidence is more common in American Indians.

Continued

TABLE 17.6 | Oropharynx Abnormalities—cont'd

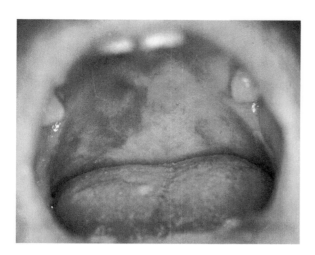

Oral Kaposi Sarcoma

Bruiselike, dark red or violet, confluent macule, usually on the hard palate, may be on soft palate or gingival margin. Oral lesions may be among the earliest lesions to develop with AIDS.

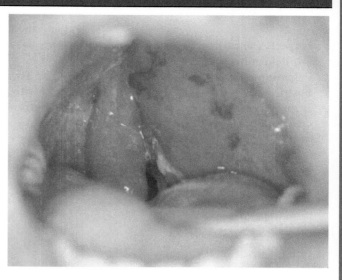

Peritonsillar Abscess

Untreated acute streptococcal pharyngitis may cause suppurative complications, peritonsillar abscess, or suppurative thrombophlebitis. Thrombophlebitis is Lemierre syndrome, a rare but life-threatening condition caused by the gram-negative *F. necrophorum*, leading to sepsis. The two major red flags are worsening symptoms or neck swelling, along with fever and decreased range of motion.[16]

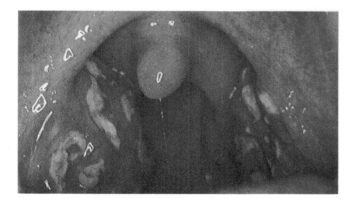

Acute Tonsillitis and Pharyngitis

Bright red throat; swollen tonsils; white or yellow exudate on tonsils and pharynx; swollen uvula; and enlarged, tender anterior cervical and tonsillar nodes. Accompanied by severe sore throat, painful swallowing, fever >101° F of sudden onset. Bacterial infections may have absence of cough.

With severe symptoms (listed above) or sore throat lasting >3-5 days, consider streptococcal infection and confirm with rapid antigen testing or throat culture. Treat positive tests with antibiotics. Untreated GAS pharyngitis may produce peritonsillar abscess, lymphadenitis, or acute rheumatic fever (although this is now rare in the United States).

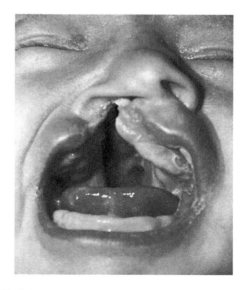

Cleft Palate

A congenital defect, the failure of fusion of the maxillary processes. Wide variation occurs in the extent of cleft formation, from upper lip only, palate only, uvula only, to cleft of the nostril and the hard and soft palates.

See Illustration Credits for source information.

Summary Checklist: Nose, Mouth, and Throat Examination

Nose
1. **Inspect external nose for symmetry, any deformity, or lesions**
2. **Palpation**—Test patency of each nostril
3. **Inspect with nasal speculum:**
   Color and integrity of nasal mucosa
   Septum—Note any deviation, perforation, or bleeding
   Turbinates—Note color, any exudate, swelling, or polyps

4. **Palpate the sinus areas**—Note any tenderness

Mouth and Throat
1. **Inspect with penlight:**
   Lips, teeth and gums, tongue, buccal mucosa—Note color; whether structures are intact; any lesions
   Palate and uvula—Note integrity and mobility as person phonates
   Grade tonsils

   Pharyngeal wall—Note color, any exudate, or lesions
2. **Palpation:**
   When indicated in adults, bimanual palpation of mouth
   In the neonate, palpate for integrity of palate and to assess sucking reflex

REFERENCES

1. American Speech Language Hearing Association (ASHA). (2017). *Cleft lip and palate: Incidence and prevalence.* http://www.asha.org/PRPSpecificTopic.aspx?folderid=8589942918&section=Incidence_and_Prevalence.
2. Berger, C., Bachman, J., Casalone, G., et al. (2014). An oral health program for children. *Nurse Pract, 39*(2), 48–53.
3. Carter, B. D., Abnet, C. C., & Feskanich, D. (2015). Smoking and mortality—beyond established causes. *N Engl J Med, 372*(7), 631–640.
4. Hicks, R. W., Green, R., & Van Wicklin, S. A. (2016). Dental avulsions. *Nurse Pract, 41*(6), 58–62.
5. Hsia, S., Myers, M. G., & Chen, T. C. (2017). Combination nicotine replacement therapy: Strategies for initiation and tapering. *Prevent Med, 97*, 45–49.
6. Jablonski, R., Mertz, E., Featherstone, J., et al. (2014). Maintaining oral health across the life span. *Nurse Pract, 39*(6), 39–48.
7. Janotha, B. L., & Tamari, K. (2017). Oral squamous cell carcinoma. *Nurse Pract, 42*(4), 26–30.
8. Kalra, M. G., Higgins, K. E., & Perez, E. D. (2016). Common questions about Streptococcal pharyngitis. *Am Fam Physician, 94*(1), 24–31.
9. Katz, A. (2017). Human papillomavirus-related oral cancers. *Am J Nurs, 117*(1), 34–40.
10. Kessenich, C. R., & Flanagan, M. (2015). Diagnosis of infectious mononucleosis. *Nurse Pract, 40*(8), 13–15.
11. Krouse, H. U., & Krouse, J. H. (2014). Allergic rhinitis. *Nurse Pract, 39*(4), 20–29.
12. McKiernan, J., & Thom, B. (2016). Human papillomavirus-related oropharyngeal cancer. *Am J Nurs, 116*(8), 34–44.
13. National Institutes of Health (NIH). (2014). *Dental caries (tooth decay) in children (age 2 to 11).* https://www.nidcr.nih.gov/DataStatistics/FindDataByTopic/DentalCaries/DentalCariesChildren2to11.htm.
14. Rivard, G., & Viera, A. (2014). Staying ahead of pertussis. *J Fam Practice, 63*(11), 658–669.
15. Rosenfeld, R. M. (2016). Acute sinusitis in adults. *N Engl J Med, 375*(10), 962–970.
16. Ruppert, S. D., & Fay, V. P. (2015). Pharyngitis. *Nurse Pract, 40*(7), 18–25.
17. Van Schayck, O. C. P., Williams, S., & Barchilon, V. (2017). Treating tobacco dependence: Guidance for primary care on life-saving interventions. *Npj Primary Care Resp Med, 27*(38), 1–12.
18. Verbiest, M., Brakema, E., Van der Kleij, R., et al. (2017). National guidelines for smoking cessation in primary care. *NPJ Prim Care Resp Med, 27*(92), 1–11.
19. Wheatley, L. M., & Togias, A. (2015). Allergic rhinitis. *N Engl J Med, 372*(5), 456–463.
20. Wooton, A. K., Melchior, L. M., Coan, L. L., et al. (2018). Periodontal disease in children with type 2 diabetes mellitus. *Nurse Pract, 43*(2), 30–36.

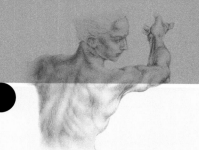
Breasts, Axillae, and Regional Lymphatics

STRUCTURE AND FUNCTION

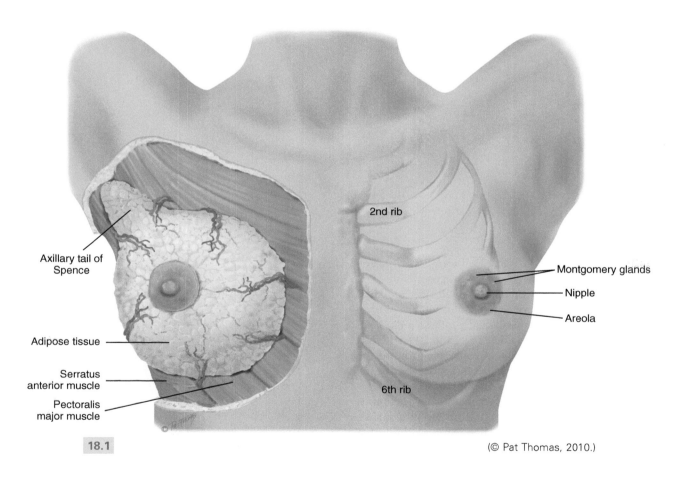

2nd rib

Axillary tail of
Spence

Montgomery glands

Nipple

Areola

Adipose tissue

Serratus
anterior muscle

Pectoralis
major muscle

6th rib

18.1

(© Pat Thomas, 2010.)

The female breasts, or mammary glands, are accessory reproductive organs, and the function is to produce milk for nourishing the newborn. The **breasts** lie anterior to the pectoralis major and serratus anterior muscles (Fig. 18.1). They are located between the 2nd and 6th ribs, extending from the side of the sternum to the midaxillary line. The superior lateral corner of breast tissue, called the axillary **tail of Spence,** projects up and laterally into the axilla.

The **nipple** is just below the center of the breast. It is rough, round, and usually protuberant; its surface looks wrinkled and indented with tiny milk duct openings. The **areola** surrounds the nipple for a 1- to 2-cm radius. In the areola are small elevated sebaceous glands, called *Montgomery glands.* These secrete a protective lipid material during lactation. The areola also has smooth muscle fibers that cause nipple erection when stimulated. Both the nipple and areola are more darkly pigmented than the rest of the breast surface; the color varies from pink to brown, depending on the person's skin color and parity (condition of giving birth). Breasts are present in men too, although rudimentary throughout life.

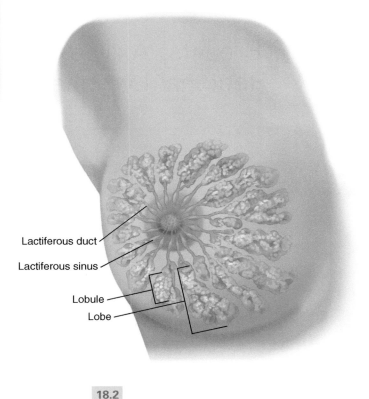

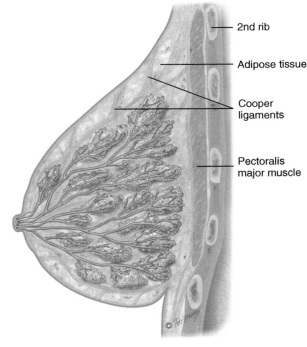

18.2

(© Pat Thomas, 2010.)

INTERNAL ANATOMY

The breast has (1) glandular tissue; (2) fibrous tissue, including the suspensory ligaments; and (3) adipose tissue (Fig. 18.2). The **glandular tissue** contains 15 to 20 lobes radiating from the nipple, and these are composed of lobules. Within each lobule are clusters of alveoli that produce milk. Each lobe empties into a lactiferous duct. The 15 to 20 lactiferous ducts form a collecting duct system converging toward the nipple. There the ducts form ampullae, or lactiferous sinuses, behind the nipple, which are reservoirs for storing milk.

The suspensory ligaments (**Cooper ligaments**) are fibrous connective tissue extending vertically from the skin surface to attach on chest wall muscles. These support the breast tissue. The lobes are embedded in **adipose tissue.** These layers of subcutaneous and retromammary fat actually provide most of the bulk of the breast. The relative proportion of glandular, fibrous, and fatty tissue varies, depending on age, cycle, pregnancy, lactation, and general nutritional state.

The breast may be divided into four quadrants by imaginary horizontal and vertical lines intersecting at the nipple (Fig. 18.3). This makes a convenient map to describe clinical findings. In the upper outer quadrant note the axillary **tail of Spence,** the cone-shaped breast tissue that projects up into the axilla, close to the pectoral group of axillary lymph nodes. The upper outer quadrant is the site of most breast tumors.

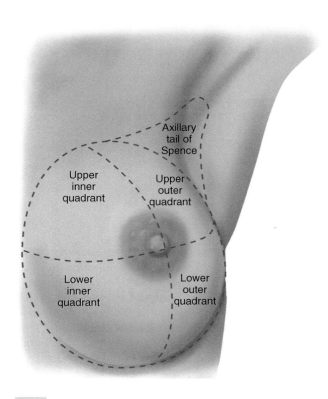

18.3

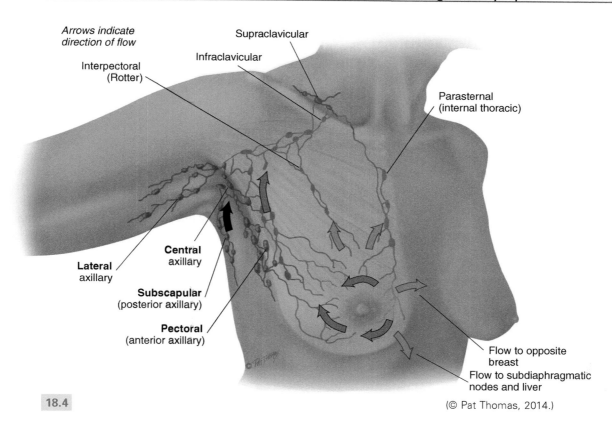

18.4

(© Pat Thomas, 2014.)

LYMPHATICS

The breast has extensive lymphatic drainage. Most of the lymph, more than 75%, drains into the ipsilateral (same side) axillary nodes. Four groups of axillary nodes are present (Fig. 18.4):

1. **Central axillary nodes**—High up in the middle of the axilla, over the ribs and serratus anterior muscle. These receive lymph from the other three groups of nodes.
2. **Pectoral** (anterior)—Along the lateral edge of the pectoralis major muscle, just inside the anterior axillary fold.
3. **Subscapular** (posterior)—Along the lateral edge of the scapula, deep in the posterior axillary fold.
4. **Lateral**—Along the humerus, inside the upper arm.

From the central axillary nodes, drainage flows up to the infraclavicular and supraclavicular nodes.

A smaller amount of lymphatic drainage does not take these channels but instead flows directly up to the infraclavicular group, or deep into the chest, or into the abdomen, or directly across to the opposite breast.

❖ DEVELOPMENTAL COMPETENCE

During embryonic life ventral epidermal ridges, or "milk lines," are present and curve down from the axilla to the groin bilaterally (Fig. 18.5). The breast develops along the ridge over the thorax, and the rest of the ridge atrophies. Occasionally a **supernumerary nipple** (i.e., an extra nipple) persists

and is visible somewhere along the track of the mammary ridge (see Fig. 18.7). At birth the only breast structures present are the lactiferous ducts within the nipple. The nipple is inverted, flat, and rises above the skin during childhood. No alveoli have developed. Little change occurs until puberty.

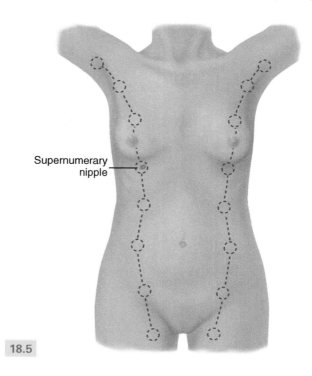

18.5

Supernumerary
nipple

The Adolescent

At puberty the estrogen hormones stimulate breast changes. The breasts enlarge, mostly as a result of extensive fat deposition. The duct system also grows and branches; and masses of small, solid cells develop at the duct endings. These are potential alveoli.

The mean onset of breast development was between 8 and 9 years for African-American girls and 10 years for white girls.[8] These data reflected a trend toward earlier breast development in the second half of the 20th century. Now into the 21st century the ages have dropped still more, and both sets of data have been linked to increases in body mass index (BMI) and the epidemic of obesity. Fat cells' aromatase secretes a form of estrogen, which may account for the changes.[7] Current ages for onset of breast budding (Tanner stage 2) vary by race, ethnicity, and BMI: mean age of onset is 8.8 years for African-American girls; 9.2 years for Hispanic girls, 9.6 years for Caucasian girls; and 9.9 years for Asian girls. Overall, girls with greater BMIs achieved breast budding at younger ages.[4] The obesity epidemic may be a "prime driver" in achieving early breast budding and then early menarche. Evidence suggests that girls with earlier sexual maturation are at risk for low self-esteem and higher rates of depression, as well as are more likely to be influenced by older or deviant peers or to start intercourse and substance use.[4]

Occasionally one breast may grow faster than the other, producing a temporary asymmetry. This may cause some

TABLE 18.1	Sexual Maturity Rating in Girls
Stage	
1. **Preadolescent:** There is only a small elevated nipple.	
2. **Breast bud stage:** A small mound of breast and nipple develops; the areola widens.	
3. The breast and areola enlarge; the nipple is flush with the breast surface.	
4. The areola and nipple form a secondary mound over the breast.	
5. **Mature breast:** Only the nipple protrudes; the areola is flush with the breast contour (the areola may continue as a secondary mound in some normal women).[15]	

distress; reassurance is necessary. Tenderness is common also. Although the age of onset varies widely, the five stages of breast development follow this classic description of sexual maturity rating, or **Tanner staging** (Table 18.1).

Full development from stage 2 to stage 5 takes an average of 3 years, although the range is 1.5 to 6 years. During this time pubic hair develops, and axillary hair appears 2 years after the onset of pubic hair. The beginning of breast development, termed **thelarche,** precedes the beginning of menstruation, or **menarche,** by about 2 years. Menarche occurs in Tanner stage 3 or 4, usually just after the peak of the adolescent growth spurt around 12 years of age. This helps to assess the development of adolescent girls and increases their knowledge about their own development.

Breasts of the nonpregnant woman change with the ebb and flow of hormones during the monthly menstrual cycle. Nodularity increases from midcycle up to menstruation. During the 3 to 4 days before menstruation, the breasts feel full, tight, heavy, and occasionally sore. The breast volume is smallest on days 4 to 7 of the menstrual cycle.

The Pregnant Woman

During pregnancy breast changes start during the second month and are a common early sign of pregnancy. Pregnancy stimulates the expansion of the ductal system and supporting fatty tissue and development of the true secretory alveoli. Thus the breasts enlarge and feel more nodular. The nipples grow larger, darker, and more erectile. The areolae become larger and a darker brown as pregnancy progresses, and the tubercles become more prominent. (The brown color fades after lactation, but the areolae never return to the original color.) A venous pattern is prominent over the skin surface (see Fig. 31.6, p. 812).

After the fourth month **colostrum** may be expressed. This thick, yellow fluid is the precursor for milk, containing the same amount of protein and lactose but practically no fat. The breasts produce colostrum for the first few days after delivery. It is rich with antibodies that protect the newborn against infection; thus breastfeeding is important. Milk production (lactation) begins 1 to 3 days after delivery. The whitish color is from emulsified fat and calcium caseinate.

The Aging Woman

After menopause ovarian secretion of estrogen and progesterone decreases, which causes the breast glandular tissue to atrophy. This is replaced with fibrous connective tissue. The fat envelope atrophies also, beginning in the middle years and becoming marked in the woman's 70s and 80s. These changes decrease breast size and elasticity so the breasts droop and sag, looking flattened and flabby. Drooping is accentuated by kyphosis in some older women.

The decreased breast size makes inner structures more prominent. A breast lump may have been present for years but is suddenly palpable. Around the nipple the lactiferous ducts are more palpable and feel firm and stringy because of fibrosis and calcification. The axillary hair decreases.

THE MALE BREAST

The male breast is a rudimentary structure consisting of a thin disk of undeveloped tissue underlying the nipple. The areola is well developed, although the nipple is relatively very small. During adolescence it is common for the breast tissue to enlarge temporarily, producing **gynecomastia** (see Fig. 18.20, p. 394). This condition is usually temporary, but reassurance is necessary for the adolescent male, whose attention is riveted on his body image. Gynecomastia may reappear in the aging male and may be the result of testosterone deficiency.

 ## CULTURE AND GENETICS

Breast Cancer

Today a woman with breast cancer is *half* as likely to die from cancer as she was 30 years ago, partly because of treatments that target expression of the estrogen receptor and HER2, the cell-surface receptor.[16] Also, cancer-specific mutations in our DNA can be measured if family history suggests increased risk. We all have certain tumor suppressor genes termed *BRCA1* and *BRCA2*; women who inherit a mutation on one or both have a higher risk of developing breast or ovarian cancer compared with women in the general population, who have a 10% risk of breast cancer.[2] The cumulative breast cancer risk up to 80 years was 72% for *BRCA1* mutation carriers and 69% for *BRCA2* carriers. The cumulative risk of ovarian cancer to age 80 years was 44% for *BRCA1* carriers and 17% for *BRCA2* carriers.[9] Ashkenazi Jewish women had a significantly higher prevalence of these gene mutations compared with other Caucasians.[3] These findings endorse the importance of family history and possible testing for gene mutation in risk assessment.

The relative 5-year survival rate has increased significantly for both black and white women since 1975; the most recent findings are 83% for black women and 92% for white women.[2] Breast cancer survival varies by stage when diagnosed (localized, regional, or distant), with overall 99% survival for localized disease, 85% for regional disease, and 27% for distant-stage disease. The racial disparity in survival is because of a later stage at diagnosis in black women and higher rates of the aggressive, triple negative breast cancer.[2] Also for every stage of breast cancer, Asian-Pacific Islander women have the highest survival rate and non-Hispanic black women have the lowest rate of survival; associated factors are poverty, lower education levels, and a lack of health insurance.[2] These findings endorse the importance of breast cancer screening and early detection.

Screening mammography can discover small, potentially curable breast cancers, and the American Cancer Society recommends beginning optional annual screening for those at average risk at ages 40 to 44 years and definite annual mammography beginning at age 45 years.[2] However, racial disparities exist in screening mammography rates. Black and Hispanic women had lower screening utilization when compared with the white population. For blacks, the lower screening rates were present in the age group of 40 to 65 years and the >65 age group; for Hispanics, lower screening rates were present only in the age group of 40 to 65 years. Asian/Pacific Islanders and whites had no difference in mammography utilization.[1] Lower rates are associated with failure to have a regular primary physician who repeatedly recommends screening mammography. Other important though less vital factors are lower income, lower educational levels, unemployment, pain, embarrassment, lack of health insurance, and residence in low-income and inner-city neighborhoods.[1,10]

Lifestyle factors, especially alcohol drinking, affect breast cancer risk. A review of 14 meta-analyses shows an association between even light drinking (3 to 6 drinks/week) and an increased risk of breast cancer.[12] There is a dose-response relationship between alcohol drinking of all levels and risk of breast cancer. Alcohol drinking between menarche and the first pregnancy may be more important than alcohol exposure in later life. This is because undifferentiated nulliparous breast tissue may be more susceptible to the metabolism of alcohol that yields carcinogens.[12] Postmenopausal breast cancer is 1.5 times higher in overweight women and 2 times higher in obese women than in women of healthy weights, likely because of higher estrogen levels in fat tissue. Adulthood weight gain increases risk; each 11 pounds gained increases the risk of postmenopausal breast cancer by 11%.[2] Regular physical activity yields a 10% to 20% lower risk of breast cancer compared with those who are inactive. There is no evidence linking fat intake and breast cancer, but consuming high levels of fruit and vegetables may lower the risk of breast cancer. Evidence shows that smoking may slightly increase the risk of breast cancer, especially long-term heavy usage and for those who start smoking before their first pregnancy.[2]

SUBJECTIVE DATA

Breast

1. Pain
2. Lump
3. Discharge
4. Rash
5. Swelling
6. Trauma
7. History of breast disease
8. Surgery or radiation
9. Medications
10. Patient-centered care
    Perform breast self-examination
    Last mammogram

Axilla

1. Tenderness, lump, or swelling
2. Rash

In many cultures the female breasts signify more than their primary purpose of lactation. Women are surrounded by excessive media influence that feminine norms of beauty and desirability are enhanced by and depend on the size of the breasts and their appearance. Women leaders have tried to refocus this attitude, stressing women's self-worth as individual human beings, not as stereotyped sexual objects. The intense cultural emphasis shows that the breasts are crucial to a woman's self-concept and her perception of her femininity. Matters pertaining to the breast affect the body image and generate deep emotional responses.

This emotionality may take strong forms that you observe as you discuss the woman's history. Some women may be embarrassed talking about their breasts, as evidenced by lack of eye contact, minimal response, nervous gestures, or inappropriate humor. A young adolescent is acutely aware of her own development in relation to her peers. Or a woman who has found a breast lump may come to you with fear, high anxiety, and even panic. Although many breast lumps are benign, women initially assume the worst possible outcome (i.e., cancer, disfigurement, and death). While you are collecting the subjective data, tune in to cues for these behaviors that call for a straightforward and reasoned attitude.

Examiner Asks	Rationale
Breast	
1. **Pain.** Any **pain** or tenderness in the breasts? When did you first notice it? • Where is the pain? Localized or all over? • Is the painful spot sore to touch? Do you feel a burning or pulling sensation?	**Mastalgia** occurs with trauma, inflammation, infection, and benign breast disease.
• Is the pain cyclic? Any relation to your menstrual period?	Cyclic pain is common with normal breasts, oral contraceptives, and benign breast (fibrocystic) disease.

Examiner Asks	Rationale

• Is the pain brought on by strenuous activity, especially involving one arm; a change in activity; manipulation during sex; part of underwire bra; exercise?

Is pain related to specific cause?

2. **Lump.** Ever noticed a **lump** or **thickening** in the breast? Where?
   • When did you first notice it? Changed at all since then?
   • Does the lump have any relation to your menstrual period?
   • Noticed any change in the overlying skin: redness, warmth, dimpling, swelling?

Carefully explore the presence of any lump. A lump present for many years and exhibiting no change may not be serious but still should be explored. Approach any recent change or new lump with suspicion.

3. **Discharge.** Any **discharge** from the nipple?
   • When did you first notice this?
   • What color is the discharge?
   • Consistency—thick or runny?
   • Odor?

Galactorrhea. Note medications that may cause clear nipple discharge: oral contraceptives, phenothiazines, diuretics, digitalis, steroids, methyldopa, calcium channel blockers.

Bloody or blood-tinged discharge always is significant. Any discharge with a lump is significant.

4. **Rash.** Any **rash** on the breast?
   • When did you first notice this?
   • Where did it start? On the nipple, areola, or surrounding skin?

Paget disease starts with a small crust on the nipple apex and spreads to areola (see Table 18.6, Abnormal Nipple Discharge, p. 401).

Eczema or other dermatitis rarely starts at the nipple unless it is caused by breastfeeding. It usually starts on the areola or surrounding skin and then spreads to the nipple.

5. **Swelling.** Any **swelling** in the breasts? In one spot or all over?
   • Related to your menstrual period, pregnancy, or breastfeeding?
   • Any change in bra size?

6. **Trauma.** Any **trauma** or injury to the breasts?
   • Did it result in any swelling, lump, or break in skin?

A lump from an injury (seat belt injury, direct blow) is caused by local hematoma or edema and resolves shortly.

7. **History of breast disease.** Any history of breast disease yourself?
   • What type? How was it diagnosed?
   • When did it occur?
   • How is it being treated?

Past breast cancer (CA) increases the risk for recurrent CA (see Table 18.2, Breast CA Risk Factors in Women, p. 385).

The presence of benign breast disease makes the breasts harder to examine; the general lumpiness conceals a new lump.

   • Any breast cancer in your family? Who? Sister, mother, maternal grandmother, maternal aunts, daughter? How about your father's side?
   • At what age did this relative have breast cancer?

Breast CA occurring before menopause in certain family members increases risk for this woman (see Table 18.2).

8. **Surgery or radiation.** Ever had **surgery** on the breasts? Was it a biopsy? What were the biopsy results?
   • Mastectomy? Mammoplasty—augmentation or reduction?
   • Ever had radiation to chest? What was it for? At what age?

Biopsy-confirmed atypical hyperplasia increases breast cancer risk.

Female lymphoma survivors treated with chest or axillary radiation between 10 and 30 years of age are at high risk of breast CA; screen with mammography and imaging annually beginning 8 to 10 years after diagnosis.[17]

Subjective Data

Examiner Asks	Rationale
9. **Medications.** Have you taken oral contraceptives? For how long?	Oral contraceptives are effective for birth control and may benefit dysmenorrhea or menorrhagia. A recent large study observed a 20% higher risk of breast CA among women under 50 who were current or recent users than among women who had never used oral contraceptives. Risk increased with longer use.[11] However, the 20% higher risk is in the context of low rates of breast CA among younger women, so the absolute risk is still low.
• Hormone replacement therapy? Estrogen and progestin? Estrogen only? For how long?	Combined hormone therapy (HT) after menopause increases risk of breast CA; risk is greater with starting HT soon after menopause. Higher risk is associated with longer use. Breast CA risk in relation to estrogen-alone therapy is unclear.[2]
• Do you drink alcohol? How many days per week? How many standard drinks per occasion?	Much evidence states that drinking alcohol increases breast CA risk in women by 7% to 10% for 1 drink per day, with a 20% higher risk for 2 to 3 drinks per day. Evidence shows alcohol drinking before the 1st pregnancy may particularly affect risk.[2]
10. **Patient-centered care** • Have you ever been taught **breast self-examination** (BSE)? • How often do you perform it? What helps you remember? • Ever had **mammography,** a screening x-ray image of the breasts? When was the last mammogram? • The American Cancer Society does not recommend clinical breast examination (CBE) for screening among average-risk women at any age. It *does recommend* screening mammography with the opportunity to begin at ages 40 to 44 years; annual mammography from ages 45 to 54 years; and a transition to biennial mammography over age 55 years or a continuation of annual mammography. The ACS states that early detection of breast CA leads to less extensive surgery, the use of chemotherapy with fewer serious side effects, and possibly the option to forgo chemotherapy.[2]	Awareness that BSE, CBE, and mammograms are complementary screening measures. With good BSE practice, a woman knows how her breasts normally feel and can detect any change more easily. Mammography can reveal cancers too small to be detected by the woman or by the most experienced examiner. However, interval lumps may become palpable between mammograms.

Axilla

1. **Tenderness, lump, or swelling.** Any **tenderness** or **lump** in the underarm area? Where? When did you first notice it?

Breast tissue extends up into the axilla. The axilla also contains many lymph nodes.

2. **Rash.** Any axillary **rash?** Please describe it. Seem to be a reaction to deodorant?

Additional History for the Preadolescent

1. Have you noticed your breasts changing?
   • How long has this been happening?
2. Many girls also notice other changes in their bodies that come with growing up. What have you noticed?
   • What do you think about all this?

Developing breasts are the most obvious sign of puberty and the focus of attention for most girls, especially in comparison with peers. Assess each girl's perception of her own development, and provide teaching and reassurance as indicated.

Examiner Asks	Rationale

Additional History for the Pregnant Woman

1. Have you noticed any enlargement or fullness in the breasts?
   - Is there any tenderness or tingling?
   - Do you have a history of inverted nipples?

2. Are you planning to breastfeed your baby?

Breast changes are expected and normal during pregnancy. Assess the woman's knowledge and provide reassurance.

Inverted nipples may need special care in preparation for breastfeeding.

Breastfeeding alone for 6 months provides the perfect food and antibodies for the baby, decreases risk for ear infections, promotes bonding, provides relaxation, is protective against breast and ovarian CA, and places less burden on the environment.

Additional History for the Menopausal Woman

1. Have you noticed any change in the breast contour, size, or firmness? (NOTE: Change may not be as apparent to obese women or to women whose earlier pregnancies already have produced breast changes.)

Decreased estrogen level causes decreased firmness. Rapid decrease in estrogen level causes actual shrinkage.

Risk Factor Profile for Breast Cancer

Breast CA is the second major cause of death from cancer in women. However, early detection and improved treatment have increased survival rates. The 5-year survival rate for localized breast CA has increased from 78% in the 1940s to 99% today. If the cancer has spread regionally, the survival rate is 85%.[2] Note the risk factors listed in Table 18.2.

The best way to detect a person's risk for breast CA is by asking the right history questions. Table 18.2 highlights risk factors for breast CA; from these, you can fashion your questions. Be aware that most breast cancers occur in women with no identifiable risk factors except sex and age. Just because a woman does not report the cited risk factors does not mean that you or she should fail to consider breast CA seriously.

Subjective Data

TABLE 18.2   Breast Cancer Risk Factors in Women*

Relative Risk	Factor	Relative Risk	Factor
>4.0	• Age (65+ vs. <65 years, although risk increases across all ages until age 80) • Biopsy-confirmed atypical hyperplasia • Certain inherited genetic mutations for breast cancer (*BRCA1* and/or *BRCA2*) • Ductal carcinoma in situ • Lobular carcinoma in situ • Mammographically dense breasts • Personal history of early-onset (<40 years) breast cancer • Two or more first-degree relatives with breast cancer diagnosed at an early age	1.1-2.0	• Alcohol consumption • Ashkenazi Jewish heritage • Diethylstilbestrol (DES) exposure • Early menarche (<12 years) • Height (tall) • High socioeconomic status • Late age at first full-term pregnancy (>30 years) • Late menopause (>55 years) • Never breastfed a child • No full-term pregnancies • Obesity (postmenopausal)/adult weight gain • Personal history of endometrial, ovarian, or colon cancer • Proliferative breast disease without atypia (ductal hyperplasia and fibroadenoma) • Recent and long-term use of menopausal HT containing estrogen and progestin • Recent oral contraceptive use
2.1-4.0	• Personal history of breast cancer (40+ years) • High endogenous estrogen or testosterone levels (postmenopausal) • High-dose radiation to chest • One first-degree relative with breast cancer		

From American Cancer Society (2018). *Breast Cancer Facts & Figures 2017-2018.* Atlanta: American Cancer Society.
*Relative risk compares the risk of disease among people with a particular exposure to the risk to the risk among people without that exposure. If the relative risk is above 1.0, risk is higher among exposed than unexposed persons.[2]

OBJECTIVE DATA

PREPARATION

The CBE screens for breast masses and abnormalities, evaluates any presenting symptoms, and presents an opportunity for you to teach breast self-awareness and examination. The American Cancer Society no longer recommends CBE for average-risk women; the ACS states there is clear evidence of the benefits of screening but less clear evidence about the balance of benefits and harms (false positives).[2] However, you must perform CBE at the initial patient encounter to determine risk.[5] CBE also is warranted with high-risk women, in those with breast pain or nipple discharge, or when a palpable mass is found by the woman. Counsel lifestyle recommendations to decrease risk. Plan to spend a few minutes on each breast for a careful examination.

Begin with the woman sitting up and facing you. You may use a short gown, open at the back, and lift it up to the woman's shoulders during inspection. During palpation when the woman is supine, cover one breast with the gown while examining the other. Be aware that many women are embarrassed to have their breasts examined; use a sensitive but matter-of-fact approach.

After your examination be prepared to teach the woman BSE.

EQUIPMENT NEEDED

Small pillow
Ruler marked in centimeters
Pamphlet or teaching aid for BSE

Normal Range of Findings	Abnormal Findings

Inspect the Breasts

General Appearance

Note symmetry of size and shape (Fig. 18.6). It is common to have a slight asymmetry in size; often the left breast is slightly larger than the right.

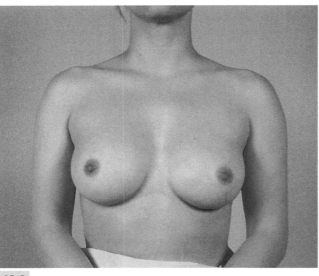

18.6

A sudden increase in the size of one breast signifies inflammation or new growth.

Skin

The skin normally is smooth and of even color. Note any localized areas of redness, bulging, or dimpling. Also note any skin lesions or focal vascular pattern. A fine blue vascular network is visible normally during pregnancy. Pale linear striae, or stretch marks, often follow pregnancy.

Normally no edema is present. Edema exaggerates the hair follicles, giving a "pigskin" or "orange-peel" look (also called *peau d'orange*).

Hyperpigmentation.
Redness and heat with inflammation.
Unilateral dilated superficial veins in a nonpregnant woman.
Edema (see Table 18.3, Signs of Retraction and Inflammation, p. 398).

Normal Range of Findings	Abnormal Findings

Lymphatic Drainage Areas

Observe the axillary and supraclavicular regions. Note any bulging, discoloration, or edema.

Nipple

The nipples should be placed symmetrically on the same plane on the two breasts. Nipples usually protrude, although some are flat and some are inverted. They tend to stay in their original condition. Distinguish a recently retracted nipple from one that has been inverted for many years or since puberty. Normal nipple inversion may be unilateral or bilateral and usually can be pulled out (i.e., it is not fixed).

Note any dry scaling, fissure or ulceration, and bleeding or other discharge.

A **supernumerary nipple** is a normal and common variation (Fig. 18.7). An extra nipple along the embryonic "milk line" on the thorax or abdomen is a congenital finding. Usually it is 5 to 6 cm below the breast near the midline and has no associated glandular tissue. It looks like a mole, although a close look reveals a tiny nipple and areola. It is not significant; merely distinguish it from a mole.

Deviation in pointing (see Table 18.3).

Recent nipple retraction signifies acquired disease (see Table 18.3).

Explore any discharge, especially in the presence of a breast mass.

Rarely additional glandular tissue, called a *supernumerary breast,* is present.

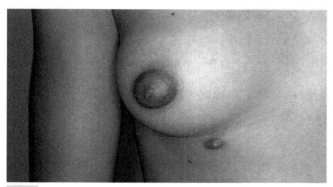

18.7 Supernumerary nipple and areolar complex. (Callen, 1993.)

Maneuvers to Screen for Retraction

Direct the woman to change position while you check the breasts for skin retraction signs. First ask her to lift her arms slowly over her head. Both breasts should move up symmetrically (Fig. 18.8).

Retraction signs are caused by fibrosis in the breast tissue, usually caused by growing neoplasms. The fibrosis shortens with time, causing contrasting signs with the normally loose breast tissue.

Note a lag in the movement of one breast.

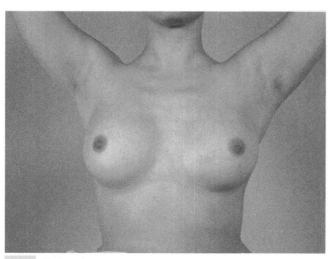

18.8 Retraction maneuver.

Normal Range of Findings

Next ask her to push her hands onto her hips (Fig. 18.9) and to push her two palms together (Fig. 18.10). These maneuvers contract the pectoralis major muscle. A slight lifting of both breasts occurs.

Abnormal Findings

Note a dimpling or a pucker, which indicates skin retraction (see Table 18.3).

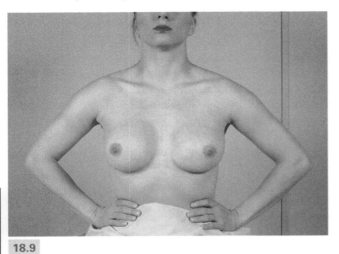

18.9

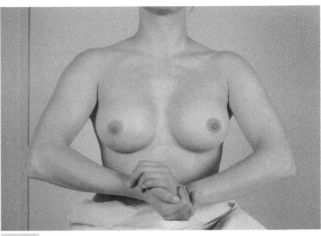

18.10

Ask the woman with large, pendulous breasts to lean forward while you support her forearms. Note the symmetric free-forward movement of both breasts (Fig. 18.11).

Note fixation to chest wall or skin retraction (see Table 18.3).

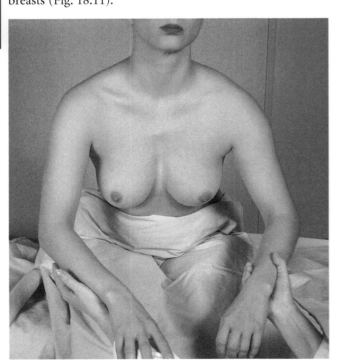

18.11

Inspect and Palpate the Axillae

Examine the axillae while the woman is sitting. Inspect the skin, noting any rash or infection. Lift the woman's arm and support it yourself so her muscles are loose and relaxed. Use your right hand to palpate the left axilla (Fig. 18.12). Reach your fingers high into the axilla. Move them firmly down in four directions:

Normal Range of Findings

Abnormal Findings

(1) down the chest wall in a line from the middle of the axilla, (2) along the anterior border of the axilla, (3) along the posterior border, and (4) along the inner aspect of the upper arm. Move the woman's arm through range of motion to increase the surface area that you can reach.

Usually nodes are not palpable, although you may feel a small, soft, nontender node in the central group. Expect some tenderness when palpating high in the axilla. Note any enlarged and tender lymph nodes.

Nodes enlarge with any local infection of the breast, arm, or hand and with breast cancer metastases.

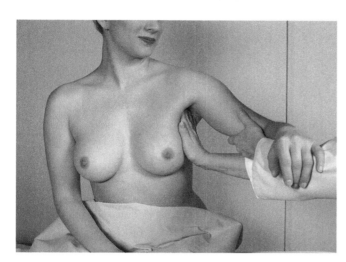

18.12

Palpate the Breasts

Help the woman to a supine position. Tuck a small pad under the side to be palpated and raise her arm over her head. These maneuvers flatten the breast tissue and displace it medially. Any significant lumps then feel more distinct (Fig. 18.13). For pendulous breasts, to distribute the tissue medially across the chest wall, ask the woman to rotate her hips opposite to the side you are palpating.

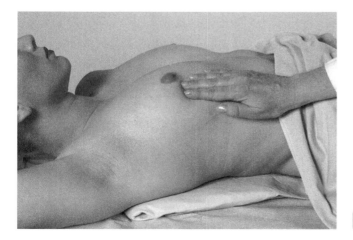

18.13

Use the pads of your first 3 fingers and make a gentle rotary motion on the breast. Vary your pressure so you are palpating light, medium, and deep tissue in each location. The vertical strip pattern (Fig. 18.14) is the best way to detect a breast mass, but two other patterns are in common use: from the nipple palpating out to the periphery as if following spokes on a wheel and palpating in concentric circles out to the periphery.

Normal Range of Findings

Abnormal Findings

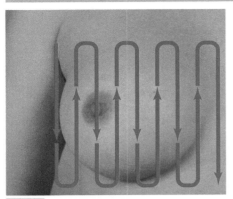

18.14 Vertical strip pattern of palpation.

For the vertical strip pattern, start high in the axilla and palpate down the midaxillary line just lateral to the breast down to the bra line. Proceed medially in overlapping vertical lines ending at the sternal edge. Take care to palpate every square inch of the breast and examine the tail of Spence high into the axilla. This should take a few minutes with each breast. Be consistent and thorough in your approach to each woman.

In nulliparous women normal breast tissue feels firm, smooth, and elastic. After pregnancy the tissue feels softer and looser. Premenstrual engorgement is normal from increasing progesterone. This consists of slight enlargement, tenderness to palpation, and generalized nodularity; the lobes feel prominent, and their margins more distinct.

In addition, normally you may feel a firm transverse ridge of compressed tissue in the lower quadrants (see Fig. 18.13). This is the **inframammary ridge,** and it is especially noticeable in large breasts. Do not confuse it with an abnormal lump.

What about the occasional woman with breast implants? Correctly placed implants are located behind the breast tissue. Therefore follow the same steps for CBE as shown for the woman without implants.

After palpating over the four breast quadrants, palpate the nipple (Fig. 18.15). Note any induration or subareolar mass. With your thumb and forefinger gently depress the nipple tissue into the well behind the areola. The tissue should move inward easily. If the woman reports spontaneous nipple discharge, press the areola inward with your index finger; repeat from a few different directions. If any discharge appears, note its color and consistency. *Physiologic (benign) discharge* is usually bilateral. This **galactorrhea** is white, milky, present during pregnancy, breastfeeding, and up to 1 year after weaning.

Heat, redness, and swelling in nonlactating and nonpostpartum breasts indicate inflammation.

Pathologic discharge is spontaneous, unilateral, has blood, or is clear, serous; it is sometimes associated with a mass[13] (see Table 18.6). Note the number of discharge droplets and the quadrant(s) producing them. Blot the discharge on a white gauze pad to ascertain its color. Test any abnormal discharge for the presence of blood.

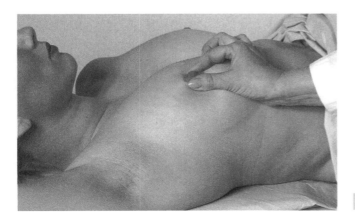

18.15

Objective Data

Normal Range of Findings	Abnormal Findings

For the woman with large, pendulous breasts, you may palpate by using a bimanual technique (Fig. 18.16). The woman is in a sitting position, leaning forward. Support the inferior part of the breast with one hand. Use your other hand to palpate the breast tissue against your supporting hand.

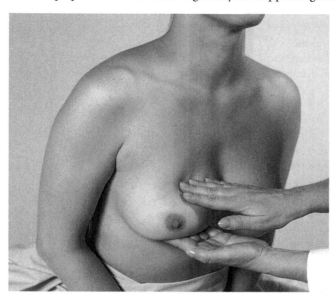

18.16

If the woman mentions a breast lump that she has discovered herself, examine the unaffected breast first to learn a baseline of normal consistency for this woman. If you do feel a lump or mass, note the following characteristics (Fig. 18.17):

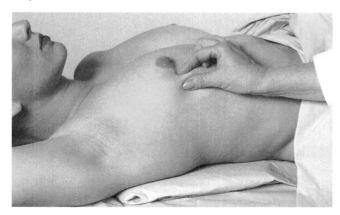

18.17

1. **Location**—Using the breast as a clock face, describe the distance in centimeters from the nipple (e.g., "7:00, 2 cm from the nipple"). Or diagram the breast in the woman's record and mark in the location of the lump.
2. **Size**—Judge in centimeters in 3 dimensions: width × length × thickness.
3. **Shape**—State whether the lump is oval, round, lobulated, or indistinct.
4. **Consistency**—State whether the lump is soft, firm, or hard.
5. **Movable**—Is the lump freely movable, or is it fixed when you try to slide it over the chest wall?
6. **Distinctness**—Is the lump solitary or multiple?
7. **Nipple**—Is it displaced or retracted?
8. **Note the skin over the lump**—Is it erythematous, dimpled, or retracted?
9. **Tenderness**—Is the lump tender to palpation?
10. **Lymphadenopathy**—Are any regional lymph nodes palpable?

Abnormal Findings

See Table 18.4, Breast Lumps, and Table 18.5, Differentiating Breast Lumps, for a description of common breast lumps with these characteristics.

Screening measures aim to detect breast lumps when small and potentially curable. The acronym BREAST lists physical signs associated with more advanced cancer: *B*reast mass, *R*etraction, *E*dema, *A*xillary mass, *S*caly nipple, *T*ender breast.

Objective Data

Objective Data

Normal Range of Findings	Abnormal Findings

Premenopausal women at midcycle often have tissue edema and mastalgia (pain) that make it hard to detect a lesion. If your findings are in question, consider asking this woman to return for a follow-up examination the first week after her menses, when hormone levels are lower and edema is not present.

The woman with a healing or healed **mastectomy** needs special consideration. She may be very concerned about a recurrence of cancer and be anxious for your findings. Inspect and palpate as described previously. Be gentle around the scar area because these tissues are quite sensitive. There should be no inflammation or infection. Lymphedema of the upper arms is a common sequela because of interruption of lymphatic drainage and removal of nodes.

Teach Breast Self-Examination

Finish your own assessment first and then teach breast self-awareness. The goal is that the woman becomes familiar with the look and feel of her breasts so she can detect any change and report it promptly. The American Cancer Society no longer recommends a structured monthly BSE[2] because many women with breast cancer have detected their lumps by chance as when bathing or dressing. Still, use this opportunity to teach the proper technique of BSE, knowing that some women will choose to perform it regularly and some occasionally (Fig. 18.18).

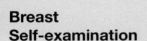

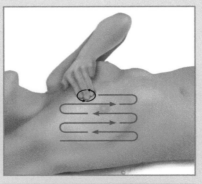

Breast Self-examination

Lie down. Press the 3 middle fingers in a circular motion and use 3 levels of pressure. Follow an up and down pattern.

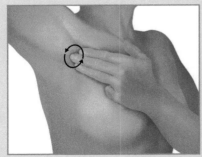

Sit up. Examine underarm with arm slightly raised.

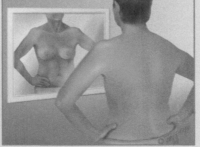

Note surface changes with hands pushed on hips, shoulders hunched.

18.18   (© Pat Thomas, 2014.)

The best time to perform BSE is right after the menstrual period (day 4 to 7 of the cycle), when the breasts are the smallest and least congested. Instruct the woman not having menstrual periods (pregnant or menopausal) to choose a familiar date as a reminder, such as the first of the month. Keep your teaching simple, and give her a pamphlet to reinforce the steps. Tell her what to look for

Normal Range of Findings	Abnormal Findings

as she inspects her breasts in front of a mirror disrobed to the waist. At home she can palpate while in the shower, where soap and water assist palpation. Or she can lie supine. Watch her palpate her own breasts while you are there to monitor her technique. Correct and encourage her return demonstration.

What are the potential harms of CBE and BSE? Concern exists that these procedures may result in more false-positives, creating anxiety and unnecessary biopsies. However, the value of early detection of breast cancer is clear. Screening mammography is available for many groups of women in developed countries, and BSE is available to virtually all women. BSE is valuable to women who are younger or older than the ages recommended for screening mammography or who have barriers to access mammography. BSE is cheap and noninvasive, can be accomplished without visits to expert professionals, and enhances patient-centered care.

The Male Breast

Your examination of the male breast can be abbreviated, but do not omit it. Combine the breast examination with that of the anterior thorax. Inspect the chest wall, noting the skin surface and any lumps or swelling. Palpate the nipple area for any lump or tissue enlargement (Fig. 18.19). It should feel even, with no nodules. Palpate the axillary lymph nodes.

Male breast CA is rare (see Table 18.8, Male Breast Abnormalities, p. 403) but usually presents with painless, firm, retroareolar lump. Also note less frequent signs: nipple discharge (clear or bloody), ulceration, retraction, axillary lymphadenopathy. Nipple discharge is rare but strongly associated with CA; thus it demands detailed evaluation.

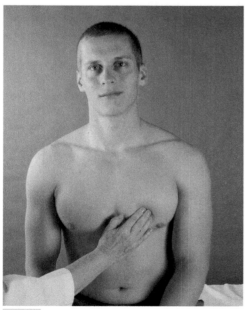

18.19

The normal male breast has a flat disk of undeveloped breast tissue beneath the nipple. **Gynecomastia** is a benign growth of this breast tissue, making it distinguishable from the other tissues in the chest wall (Fig. 18.20). It feels like a smooth, firm, movable subareolar fibrous mass. This occurs in about one half of adolescent boys at 13 or 14 years of age. It can be unilateral or bilateral and usually is temporary. The adolescent is acutely aware of his body image and feels distressed. Reassure him that this change is normal, common, and temporary.

Gynecomastia also occurs with use of anabolic steroids, some medications, cirrhosis, and other diseases. See Table 18.8.

Objective Data

Normal Range of Findings	Abnormal Findings

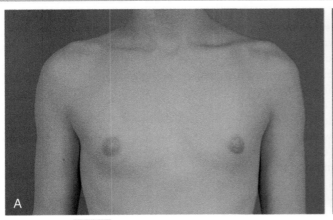

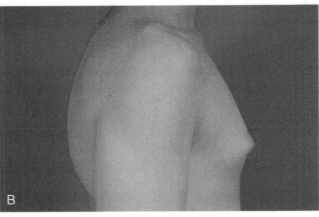

18.20 Adolescent gynecomastia.

(Hammond, 2009)

✦ DEVELOPMENTAL COMPETENCE

Infants and Children

In the neonate the breasts may be enlarged and visible from maternal estrogen crossing the placenta. They may secrete a clear or white fluid, called *witch's milk*. This is not significant and is resolved within a few days to a few weeks.

Note the position of the nipples on the prepubertal child. They should be symmetric, just lateral to the midclavicular line between the 4th and 5th ribs. The nipple is flat, and the areola is darker pigmented.

Premature thelarche is early breast development with no other hormone-dependent signs (pubic hair, menses).

The Adolescent

Adolescent breast development begins on an average between 8 and 10 years of age. Expect some asymmetry during growth. Record the stage of development using the Tanner staging described on p. 380. Use the chart to teach the adolescent normal developmental stages and to assure her of her own normal progress.

You should consider BMI (derived from weight and height) when evaluating breast budding. The trend toward earlier breast budding is now well established. When this occurs without an accompanying earlier age of menarche, it raises the question of cause—is it truly hormonal, or is it obesity, exogenous estrogen exposure, or other cause?[6] Note that it is difficult to distinguish breast budding from excess adipose tissue.

With maturing adolescents, palpate the breasts as you would with the adult. The breasts normally feel firm and uniform. Note any mass.

Note precocious development before age 8 years. It is usually normal but also occurs with thyroid dysfunction, stilbestrol ingestion, or ovarian or adrenal tumor.

Note delayed development with hormonal failure, anorexia nervosa, or severe malnutrition.

At this age a mass is almost always a benign fibroadenoma or a cyst (see Table 18.4).

The Pregnant Woman

A delicate blue vascular pattern is visible over the breasts. The breasts increase in size, as do the nipples. Jagged linear stretch marks, or striae, may develop if the breasts have a large increase. The nipples also become darker and more erectile. The areolae widen, grow darker, and contain the small, scattered, elevated Montgomery glands. On palpation the breasts feel more nodular, and thick yellow colostrum can be expressed after the first trimester.

The Lactating Woman

Colostrum changes to milk production around the 3rd postpartum day. At this time the breasts may become engorged, appearing enlarged, reddened, and shiny and feeling warm and hard. Frequent nursing helps drain the ducts and sinuses and stimulate milk production. Nipple soreness is normal, appearing around the

Normal Range of Findings	Abnormal Findings

20th nursing, lasting 24 to 48 hours and then disappearing rapidly. The nipples may look red and irritated. They may even crack but heal rapidly if kept dry and exposed to air. Again, frequent nursing is the best treatment for nipple soreness.

One section of the breast surface appearing red and tender indicates a plugged duct (see Table 18.7, Disorders Occurring During Lactation, p. 402).

The Aging Woman

Increasing age is the primary risk factor for developing breast CA; therefore an annual CBE is important.

On inspection the breasts look pendulous, flattened, and sagging. Nipples may be retracted but can be pulled outward. On palpation the breasts feel more granular, and the terminal ducts around the nipple feel more prominent and stringy. Thickening of the inframammary ridge at the lower breast is normal, and it feels more prominent with age.

Reinforce the value of the BSE. Women older than 50 years have an increased risk for breast CA. Older women may have problems with arthritis, limited range of motion, or decreased vision that may inhibit self-care. Suggest aids to the self-examination (e.g., talcum powder helps fingers glide over skin).

Because atrophy causes shrinkage of normal glandular tissue, cancer detection is somewhat easier. Any palpable lump that cannot be positively identified as a normal structure should be referred.

HEALTH PROMOTION AND PATIENT TEACHING

(To the person who asks you about her/his own breast cancer risk.) *I hear you asking about your own chances of getting breast cancer. Let's review your health history to see how many risk factors you have, and let's talk about how much these factors increase the risk.*

Many women will come to you well read and well informed about breast cancer. Perhaps they have a relative or friend who is a breast cancer survivor. Some factors increase breast cancer risk significantly (e.g., having a *BRCA1* gene mutation), and other factors have a small effect on risk. You may choose to use the *Breast Cancer Risk Assessment Tool* found at https://www.cancer.gov/bcrisktool/. It is important to stress that the tool can estimate the woman's risk, but it cannot predict whether *this woman* will get breast cancer.[14] The tool has recently been updated for (1) African-American women, following the findings from the Contraceptive and Reproductive Experiences (CARE) study; and (2) Asian-American and Pacific Islander women following findings from the Asian-American Breast Cancer Study (AABCS).

The tool uses 7 key risk factors for calculating a woman's risk of developing breast cancer within the next 5 years: age; age at first period; age at time of birth of first child (or has not given birth); family history of breast cancer (mother, sister, or daughter); number of past breast biopsies; number of breast biopsies showing atypical hyperplasia; and race/ethnicity. Please stress that this tool does not predict cancer risk for *this person*; instead it gives the average risk for a group of women with similar risk factors. It has limitations; it does not give a good estimate for some women of invasive breast cancer, ductal carcinoma in situ, or lobular carcinoma in situ. Further, it is limited in predicting risk in those with a strong family history of breast cancer or who may have an inherited gene mutation. For more information about hereditary breast cancer syndromes go to the National Cancer Institute (NCI) website at http://www.cancer.gov/types/breast/hp/breast_ovarian_genetics_pdg/.

DOCUMENTATION AND CRITICAL THINKING

Sample Charting

FEMALE

SUBJECTIVE

States no breast pain, lump, discharge, rash, swelling, or trauma. No history of breast disease herself or in mother, sister, daughter. No history of breast surgery. Never been pregnant. Performs BSE occasionally.

OBJECTIVE

Inspection: Breasts symmetric. Skin smooth with even color and no rash or lesions. Arm movement shows no dimpling or retractions. No nipple discharge, no lesions.

Palpation: Breast contour and consistency firm and homogeneous. No masses or tenderness. No lymphadenopathy.

ASSESSMENT

Healthy breast structure

Has knowledge of breast self-examination

MALE

SUBJECTIVE

No pain, lump, rash, or swelling.

OBJECTIVE

No masses or tenderness. No lymphadenopathy.

Clinical Case Study 1

L.B. is a 32-year-old female, married with a 3-week-old son. Uneventful pregnancy and immediate postpartum period. Successfully breastfeeding. Reports feeding her son every 3 hours during the day and every 4 to 5 hours at night. Alternating breasts as instructed by lactation consultant.

SUBJECTIVE

L.B. reports flulike symptoms for the past 2 days, including extreme fatigue, fever, and chills. Reports "my right breast is hot and really hurts when I nurse. I think maybe I'm doing something wrong." No personal or family history of breast disease.

OBJECTIVE

Vital signs: Temperature 102° F (38.9° C). Pulse 114 bpm. Resp 18/min. BP 110/76 mm Hg.

General appearance: Appears anxious. Grimacing with movement. Dark circles under eyes. Wearing coat over hospital gown.

Breasts: Nipples flat. No lesions. Breast milk discharge from bilateral nipples. Breast movement symmetric bilaterally. No retractions. Upper inner quadrant of right breast red, swollen.

Palpation: Left breast consistency firm and homogenous. No masses or tenderness. Right breast upper inner quadrant warm, hard, and tender. Remainder of breast firm and homogenous. No lymphadenopathy.

Thorax: Symmetric, no lumps or lesions, breath sounds clear and = bilat.

Cardiovascular: S_1 S_2 not accentuated or diminished; no murmurs or extra sounds.

ASSESSMENT

Acute mastitis

Acute pain

Potential for infection

Potential for ineffective breastfeeding

Clinical Case Study 2

D.B. is a 62-year-old female bank comptroller, married, with no children. History of hypertension, managed by diuretic medication and diet. No other health problems until annual company physical exam 3 days PTA, when MD "found a lump in my right breast."

SUBJECTIVE

3 days PTA—MD noted lump in R breast during annual physical exam. MD did not describe lump but told D.B. it was "serious" and needed immediate biopsy. D.B. has not felt it herself. States has noted no skin changes, no nipple discharge. No previous history of breast disease. Mother died at age 54 years of breast cancer; no other relative with breast disease. D.B. has had no term pregnancies; two spontaneous abortions, ages 28, 31 years. Menopause completed at age 52 years.

Aware of BSE but has never performed it. "I feel so bad. If only I had been doing it. I should have found this myself." Married 43 years. States husband supportive, but "I just can't talk to him about this. I can't even go near him now."

OBJECTIVE

Inspection—Breasts symmetric when sitting, arms down. Nipples flat. No lesions, no discharge. As lifts arms, left breast elevates, right breast stays fixed. Dimple in right breast, 9 o'clock position, apparent at rest and with muscle contraction. Leaning forward reveals left breast falls free, right breast flattens.

Palpation—Left breast feels soft and granular throughout, no mass. Right breast soft and granular, with large, stony hard mass in outer quadrant. Lump is 5 cm × 4 cm × 2 cm, at 9 o'clock position, 3 cm from nipple. Borders irregular, mass fixed to tissues, no pain with palpation.

One firm, palpable lymph node in center of right axilla. No palpable nodes on the left.

ASSESSMENT

Lump in R breast
Anxiety

Clinical Case Study 3

Father brings his 9-year-old African-American daughter (B.K.) to the clinic because of complaints of "chest pain." Father has raised her since her mother's death from cancer 7 years ago. He wrings his hands, asks many questions, and at times is tearful during B.K.'s history intake and physical examination.

SUBJECTIVE

B.K.'s father states, "She's been complaining of her chest hurting for over 3 weeks now. I think it's her breasts, but she's too young for puberty, isn't she? I'm worried something's really wrong. You know, like with what happened to her mother." B.K. doesn't appear concerned but "wonders why it (her breasts) feels this way." Rates pain at a "2" on a 1-to-10 pain scale and describes it as a consistent, dull, aching pain to general breast and nipple area.

OBJECTIVE

Vital signs: Temp 97°.9 F (36.6° C) (orally). BP 96/68 mm Hg (sitting, legs uncrossed). Pulse 70 bpm. Resp 22/min.

General appearance: Good hygiene, dressed appropriate for weather, developmentally appropriate in relation to age, talkative, and appears comfortable except during breast examination.

HEENT: Normocephalic; no lymphadenopathy.

Cardiovascular: No murmurs or other abnormal heart sounds.

Respiratory: Breath sounds clear; no adventitious sounds.

Chest: Visible and palpable elevation of the breast to the left nipple (2.1 cm in width × 0.2 cm in depth) and papillae w/o separation of contour of the breast and areola. Right breast flat w/o detectable elevation. Skin smooth w/even brown color; no rash, lesions or nipple discharge. States tenderness during palpation of breasts. No lymphadenopathy.

Genitourinary: No swelling, lesions, or discharge to genitalia and/or urethra. Scant, coarse, pigmented hair to labia.

ASSESSMENT

Age-appropriate breast budding, Tanner stage 2
Acute pain
Parental anxiety

Documentation and
Critical Thinking

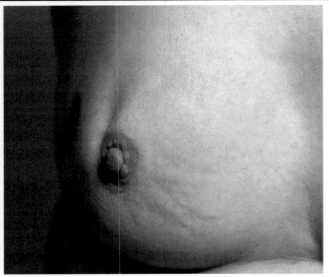

◀ Dimpling

The shallow dimple (also called a *skin tether*) shown here is a sign of skin retraction. Cancer causes fibrosis, which contracts the suspensory ligaments. The dimple may be apparent at rest, with compression, or with lifting of the arms. Also note the distortion of the areola here as the fibrosis pulls the nipple toward it.

Nipple Retraction. The retracted nipple looks flatter and broader, like an underlying crater. A recent retraction suggests cancer, which causes fibrosis of the whole duct system and pulls in the nipple. It also may occur with benign lesions such as ectasia of the ducts. Do not confuse retraction with the normal long-standing type of nipple inversion, which has no broadening and is not fixed.

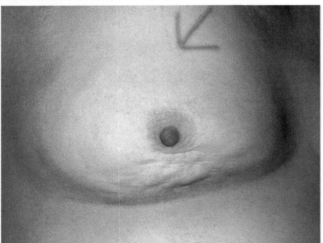

◀ Edema (Peau d'Orange)

Widespread peau d'orange results from skin infiltration of cancer and skin edema. Lymphatic obstruction produces edema. This thickens the skin and exaggerates the hair follicles, giving a pigskin or orange-peel look. Edema usually begins in the skin around and beneath the areola, the most dependent area of the breast.

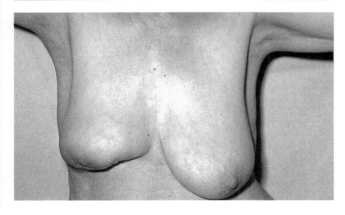

Fixation

Asymmetry, distortion, or decreased mobility with the elevated arm maneuver. As cancer becomes invasive, the fibrosis fixes the breast to the underlying pectoral muscles. Here note that the right breast is held against the chest wall.

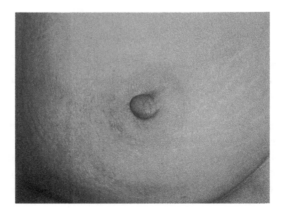

Deviation in Nipple Pointing

An underlying cancer causes fibrosis in the mammary ducts, which pulls the nipple angle toward it. Here note the swelling behind the right nipple and that the nipple tilts laterally.

See Illustration Credits for source information.

TABLE 18.4	Breast Lumps

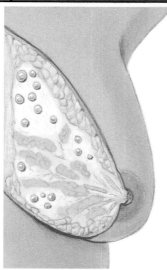

◄ Benign ("Fibrocystic") Breast Disease

Multiple tender masses that occur with numerous symptoms and physical findings: (1) swelling and tenderness (cyclic discomfort), (2) nodularity (significant lumpiness, both cyclic and noncyclic), (3) dominant lumps (including cysts and fibroadenomas), (4) nipple discharge (including intraductal papilloma and duct ectasia), and (5) infections and inflammations (including subareolar abscess, lactational mastitis, breast abscess, and Mondor disease).

Many women have some form of benign breast disease. Nodularity occurs bilaterally; regular, firm nodules are mobile, well demarcated, and feel rubbery like small water balloons. Pain may be dull, heavy, and cyclic as nodules enlarge. Some women have nodularity but no pain. Cysts are discrete, fluid-filled sacs. Dominant lumps and nipple discharge must be investigated carefully. Nodularity itself is not premalignant but produces difficulty in detecting other cancerous lumps.

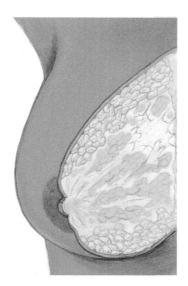

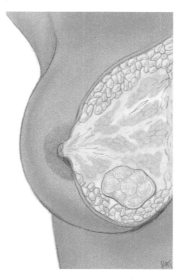

Cancer

Solitary, unilateral, 3-dimensional, usually nontender mass. Solid, hard, dense, and fixed to underlying tissues or skin as cancer becomes invasive. Borders are irregular and poorly delineated. Grows constantly. Requires diagnostic mammogram for those over age 30 years and at average risk.[13] Most common in upper outer quadrant. Found in women 30 to 80 years of age; increased risk across all ages until age 80 years. As cancer advances, signs include firm or hard irregular axillary nodes; skin dimpling; nipple retraction, elevation, and discharge.

Fibroadenoma

Benign mass, most commonly self-detected in late adolescence and early adulthood. Solitary nontender mass that is solid, firm, rubbery, and elastic. Round, oval, or lobulated; 1 to 5 cm. Freely movable, slippery; fingers slide it easily through tissue. Usually no axillary lymphadenopathy but frequently painful. Diagnose by palpation, ultrasound, and needle biopsy. Because of risk of deformity of surgery to a growing breast, excisional surgery is reserved for masses >5 cm; for continuously enlarging, well-circumscribed, multiple masses; or with suspicious ultrasound findings.

TABLE 18.5	Differentiating Breast Lumps		
	Fibroadenoma	Benign Breast Disease	Cancer
Likely age	15-30 years, can occur up to 55 years	30-55 years; decreases after menopause	30-80 years, risk increases after 50 years
Shape	Round, lobular	Round, lobular	Irregular, star-shaped
Consistency	Usually firm, rubbery	Firm to soft, rubbery	Firm to stony hard
Demarcation	Well demarcated, clear margins	Well demarcated	Poorly defined
Number	Usually single	Usually multiple; may be single	Single
Mobility	Very mobile, slippery	Mobile	Fixed
Tenderness	Usually none	Tender; usually increases before menses; may be noncyclic	Usually none, can be tender
Skin retraction	None	None	Usually
Pattern of growth	Grows quickly and constantly	Size may increase or decrease rapidly; cyclic with menstrual periods	Grows constantly
Risk to health	Benign—Diagnose by ultrasound and biopsy; may spontaneously resolve in women <20 years.	Benign, although general lumpiness may mask other cancerous lump	Serious, needs early treatment

ABNORMAL FINDINGS
FOR ADVANCED PRACTICE

TABLE 18.6	Abnormal Nipple Discharge

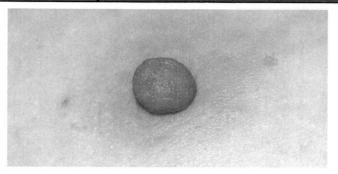

Mammary Duct Ectasia

Pastelike matter in subareolar ducts produces sticky, purulent discharge that may be cream-colored, green, or bloody. A single duct discharge is shown here. Caused by stagnation of cellular debris and secretions in the ducts, leading to obstruction, inflammation, and infection. Itching, burning, or drawing pain occurs around nipple. May have subareolar redness and swelling. Ducts are palpable as rubbery, twisted tubules under areola. May have palpable mass, soft or firm, poorly delineated. Not malignant but needs biopsy.

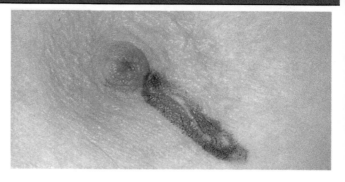

Intraductal Papilloma

These are discrete benign tumors that arise in a single or multiple papillary duct(s). May have serous or serosanguineous discharge. Often there is a palpable nodule in underlying duct (highlighted here). Most common in women ages 40 to 60 years. Most are benign, although multiple papillomas have a higher risk of subsequent cancer than do solitary ones. Requires core needle biopsy and possible excision.

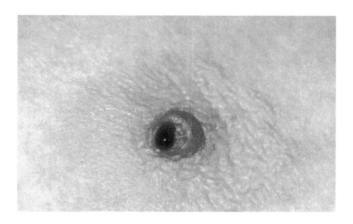

Carcinoma

Bloody nipple discharge that is unilateral and from a single duct requires further investigation. Although there was no palpable lump associated with the discharge shown here, mammography revealed a 1-cm, centrally located, ill-defined mass.

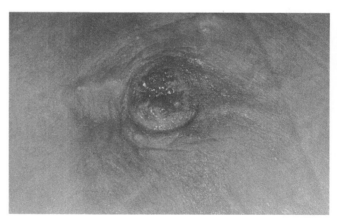

Paget Disease (Intraductal Carcinoma)

Early lesion has unilateral, clear yellow discharge and dry, scaling crusts, friable at nipple apex. Spreads outward to areola with erythematous halo on areola and crusted, eczematous, retracted nipple. Later lesion shows nipple reddened, ulcerated with bloody discharge, and an erythematous plaque surrounding the nipple. Symptoms include tingling, burning, itching. Except for the expected redness and occasional cracking from initial breastfeeding, any other dermatitis of the nipple area must be explored carefully and referred immediately.

See Illustration Credits for source information.

TABLE 18.7	Disorders Occurring During Lactation

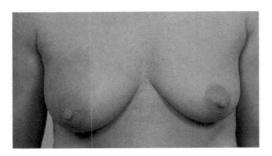

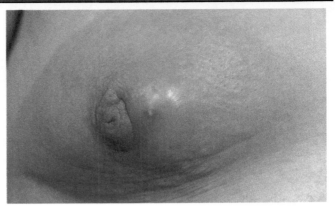

Mastitis

This is uncommon; an inflammatory mass before abscess formation. Usually occurs in single quadrant. Area is red, swollen, tender, very hot, and hard, here forming outward from areola upper edge in right breast. The woman also has a headache, malaise, fever, chills, sweating, increased pulse, flulike symptoms. May occur during first 4 months of lactation from infection or from stasis from plugged duct. Treat with rest, local heat to area, antibiotics, and frequent nursing to keep breast as empty as possible. Must not wean now, or the breast will become engorged, and the pain will increase. Mother's antibiotic not harmful to infant. Usually resolves in 2 to 3 days.

Breast Abscess

A rare complication of generalized infection (e.g., mastitis) if untreated. A pocket of pus that feels hard, looks red, and is quite tender accumulates in one local area. Here there is extensive nipple edema, and abscess is "pointing" at 3 o'clock position on areolar margin. May breastfeed depending on location of abscess, associated pain, and type of medicine. Continue to nurse on unaffected side. Treat with antibiotics, surgical incision, and drainage.

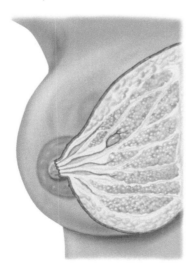

◄ Plugged Duct

This is common when milk is not removed completely because of poor latching, ineffective suckling, infrequent nursing, or switching to second breast too soon. There is a tender lump that may be reddened and warm to touch. No infection. It is important to keep breast as empty as possible and milk flowing. The woman should nurse her baby frequently on affected side first to ensure complete emptying and manually express any remaining milk. A plugged duct usually resolves in less than 1 day.

See Illustration Credits for source information.

TABLE 18.8	Male Breast Abnormalities

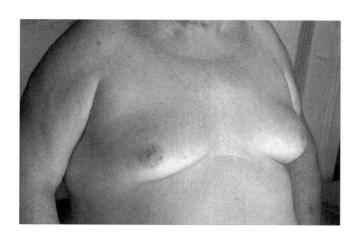

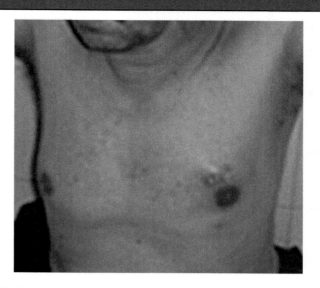

Gynecomastia

Benign enlargement of male breast that occurs when estrogen concentration exceeds testosterone levels. It is a mobile disk of tissue located centrally under the nipple-areola. At puberty it is usually mild and transient. In older men it is bilateral, tender, and firm but not as hard as breast cancer. Gynecomastia occurs with Cushing syndrome, liver cirrhosis (because estrogens cannot be metabolized), adrenal disease, hyperthyroidism, and numerous drugs: alcohol and marijuana; estrogen treatment for prostate cancer; antibiotics (metronidazole, isoniazid); spironolactone.

Male Breast Cancer

Less than 1% of breast cancers occur in men.[2] It presents as a painless palpable mass—hard, irregular, nontender, fixed to the area; may have nipple retraction. Nipple discharge, is a significant warning of early breast cancer. Note retraction and ulceration shown here. Early spread to axillary lymph nodes occurs because of minimal breast tissue. Because of lack of screening and general awareness, men are diagnosed 5 years later than women and at later stages, with the mean age at 67 years.[7a]

See Illustration Credits for source information.

Abnormal Findings

Summary Checklist: Breasts and Regional Lymphatics Examination

1. **Inspect breasts** as the woman sits, raises arms overhead, pushes hands on hips, leans forward.

2. **Inspect** the supraclavicular and infraclavicular areas.
3. **Palpate the axillae** and regional lymph nodes.

4. With woman supine, **palpate the breast tissue,** including tail of Spence, the nipples, and areolae.
5. **Teach BSE.**

REFERENCES

1. Ahmed, A. T., Welch, B. T., Brinjkji, W., et al. (2017). Racial disparities in screening mammography in the United States. *J Am Coll Radiol, 14,* 157–165.
2. American Cancer Society. (2018). *Breast cancer facts & figures 2017-2018.* www.cancer.org.
2a. Baron, R., Drucker, K., Lagdamen, L., et al. (2018). Breast cancer screening: a review of current guidelines. *Am J Nurs, 118*(7), 34–42.
3. Bayraktar, S., Jackson, M., Gutierrez-Barrera, A. M., et al. (2015). Genotype-phenotype correlations by ethnicity and mutation location in BRCA mutation carriers. *Breast J, 21*(3), 260–267.
4. Biro, F. M., Greenspan, L. C., Galvez, M. P., et al. (2013). Onset of breast development in a longitudinal cohort. *Pediatrics, 132,* 1019–1027.
5. Bryan, T., & Snyder, E. (2013). The clinical breast exam: a skill that should not be abandoned. *J Gen Intern Med,* 1–4.
6. Cabrera, S. M., Bright, G. M., Frane, J. W., et al. (2014). Age of thelarche and menarche in contemporary US females. *J Pediatr Endocrinol Metab, 27*(0), 47–51.
7. Crocker, M. K., Stern, E. A., Sedaka, N. M., et al. (2014). Sexual dimorphisms in the associations of BMI and body fat

with indices of pubertal development in girls and boys. *J Clin Endocrinol Metab, 99,* e1519–e1529.

7a. Giordano, S. H. (2018). Breast cancer in men. *N Engl J Med, 378*(24), 2311–2320.

8. Herman-Giddens, M. E., Slora, E. J., Wasserman, R. C., et al. (1997). Secondary sexual characteristics and menses in young girls seen in office practice. *Pediatrics, 99,* 505–512.

9. Kuchenbaecker, K. B., Hopper, J. L., Barnes, D. R., et al. (2017). Risks of breast, ovarian, and contralateral breast cancer for *BRCA1* and *BRCA2* mutation carriers. *JAMA, 317*(23), 2402–2406.

10. Million-Underwood, S., & Kelber, S. T. (2015). Exploratory study of breast cancer screening practices of urban women: A closer look at who is and is not getting screened. *ABNF J, 26*(2), 30–38.

11. Morch, L. S., Skovlund, C. W., Hannaford, P. C., et al. (2017). Contemporary hormonal contraception and the risk of breast cancer. *N Engl J Med, 377*(23), 2228–2239.

12. Shield, K. D., Soejomataram, I., & Rehm, J. (2016). Alcohol use and breast cancer: a critical review. *Alcohol Clin Exp Res, 40*(6), 1166–1181.

13. Smania, M. A. (2017). Evaluation of common breast complaints in primary care. *Nurse Pract, 42*(10), 9–16.

14. Susan, G. Komen©. (2018). *Estimating breast cancer risk.* https://ww5.komen.org/BreastCancer/GailAssessmentModel .html.

15. Tanner, J. M. (1962). *Growth at adolescence* (2nd ed.). Oxford, UK: Blackwell Scientific.

16. Turner, N. C. (2017). Signatures of DNA-repair deficiencies in breast cancer. *N Engl J Med, 377*(25), 2490–2492.

17. Wilbur, J. (2015). Surveillance of the adult cancer survivor. *Am Fam Physician, 91*(1), 29–36.

STRUCTURE AND FUNCTION

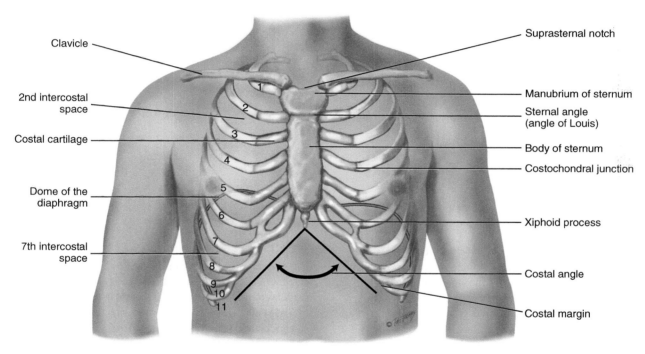

19.1

ANTERIOR THORACIC CAGE

(© Pat Thomas, 2010.)

Labels (clockwise from top left): Clavicle, 2nd intercostal space, Costal cartilage, Dome of the diaphragm, 7th intercostal space, Suprasternal notch, Manubrium of sternum, Sternal angle (angle of Louis), Body of sternum, Costochondral junction, Xiphoid process, Costal angle, Costal margin

POSITION AND SURFACE LANDMARKS

The **thoracic cage** is a bony structure with a conical shape, which is narrower at the top (Fig. 19.1). It is defined by the **sternum,** 12 pairs of **ribs,** and 12 thoracic **vertebrae.** Its "floor" is the **diaphragm,** a musculotendinous septum that separates the thoracic cavity from the abdomen. The first seven ribs attach directly to the sternum via their costal cartilages; ribs 8, 9, and 10 attach to the costal cartilage above, and ribs 11 and 12 are "floating," with free palpable tips. The **costochondral junctions** are the points at which the ribs join their cartilages. They are not palpable.

Anterior Thoracic Landmarks

Surface landmarks on the thorax are signposts for underlying respiratory structures. Knowing landmarks helps you localize

a finding and facilitates communication of your findings to others.

   Suprasternal Notch. Feel this hollow U-shaped depression just above the sternum, between the clavicles.

   Sternum. The "breastbone" has three parts: the manubrium, the body, and the xiphoid process. Walk your fingers down the manubrium a few centimeters until you feel a distinct bony ridge, the sternal angle.

   Sternal Angle. Often called the *angle of Louis,* this is the articulation of the manubrium and body of the sternum, and it is continuous with the 2nd rib. The angle of Louis is a useful place to start counting ribs, which helps localize a respiratory finding horizontally. Identify the angle of Louis, palpate lightly to the 2nd rib, and slide down to the 2nd intercostal space. Each intercostal space is numbered by the rib above it. Continue counting down the ribs in the middle

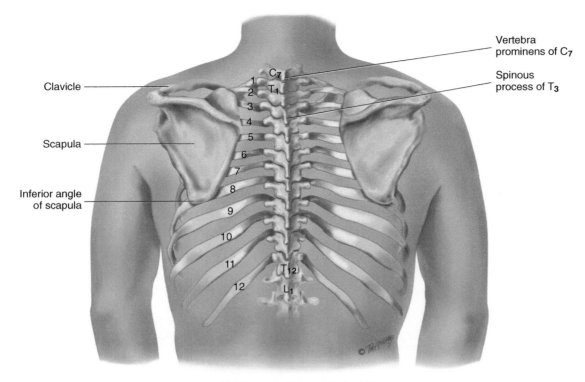

Clavicle

Scapula

Inferior angle of scapula

C7
1
2   T1
3
4
5
6
7
8
9
10
11   T12
12   L1

Vertebra prominens of C7

Spinous process of T3

POSTERIOR THORACIC CAGE

19.2

(© Pat Thomas, 2010.)

of the hemithorax, not close to the sternum where the costal cartilages lie too close together to count. You can palpate easily down to the 10th rib.

The angle of Louis also marks the site of tracheal bifurcation into the right and left main bronchi; it corresponds with the upper border of the atria of the heart, and it lies above the 4th thoracic vertebra on the back.

Costal Angle. The right and left costal margins form an angle where they meet at the xiphoid process. Usually 90 degrees or less, this angle increases when the rib cage is chronically overinflated, as in emphysema.

Posterior Thoracic Landmarks

Counting ribs and intercostal spaces on the back is a bit harder because of the muscles and soft tissue surrounding the ribs and spinal column (Fig. 19.2).

Vertebra Prominens. Start here. Flex your head and feel for the most prominent bony spur protruding at the base of the neck. This is the spinous process of C7. If two bumps seem equally prominent, the upper one is C7, and the lower one is T1.

Spinous Processes. Count down these knobs on the vertebrae, which stack together to form the spinal column. Note that the spinous processes align with their same numbered ribs only down to T_4. After T_4 the spinous processes angle downward from their vertebral body and overlie the vertebral body and rib below.

Inferior Border of the Scapula. The scapulae are located symmetrically in each hemithorax. The lower tip is usually at the 7th or 8th rib.

Twelfth Rib. Palpate midway between the spine and the person's side to identify its free tip.

Reference Lines

Use the reference lines to pinpoint a finding vertically on the chest. On the anterior chest note the **midsternal** line and the **midclavicular** line. The midclavicular line bisects the center of each clavicle at a point halfway between the palpated sternoclavicular and acromioclavicular joints (Fig. 19.3).

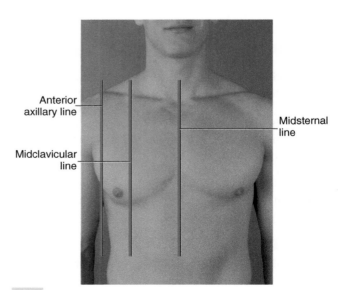

Anterior axillary line

Midclavicular line

Midsternal line

19.3

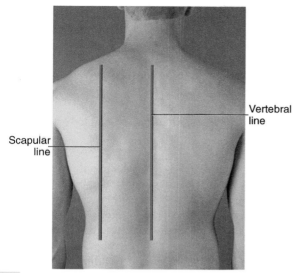

19.4

The posterior chest wall has the **vertebral** (or midspinal) line and the **scapular** line, which extends through the inferior angle of the scapula when the arms are at the sides of the body (Fig. 19.4).

Lift up the person's arm 90 degrees and divide the lateral chest by three lines: the **anterior axillary** line extends down from the anterior axillary fold where the pectoralis major muscle inserts; the **posterior axillary** line continues down from the posterior axillary fold where the latissimus dorsi muscle inserts; and the **midaxillary** line runs down from the apex of the axilla and lies between and parallel to the other two (Fig. 19.5).

THE THORACIC CAVITY

The **mediastinum** is the middle section of the thoracic cavity containing the esophagus, trachea, heart, and great vessels.

The right and left **pleural cavities,** on either side of the mediastinum, contain the lungs.

Lung Borders. In the anterior chest the **apex,** or highest point, of lung tissue is 3 to 4 cm above the inner third of the clavicles. The **base,** or lower border, rests on the diaphragm at about the 6th rib in the midclavicular line. Laterally lung tissue extends from the apex of the axilla down to the 7th or 8th rib. Posteriorly the location of C7 marks the apex of lung tissue, and T10 usually corresponds to the base. Deep inspiration expands the lungs, and their lower border drops to the level of T_{12}.

Lobes of the Lungs

The lungs are paired but not precisely symmetric structures (Fig. 19.6). The right lung is shorter than the left lung because of the underlying liver. The left lung is narrower than the right lung because the heart bulges to the left. The right lung has three lobes, and the left lung has two lobes. These lobes are not arranged in horizontal bands like dessert layers in a parfait glass. Rather they stack in diagonal sloping segments and are separated by **fissures** that run obliquely through the chest.

Anterior. On the anterior chest the **oblique** (the major or diagonal) fissure crosses the 5th rib in the midaxillary line and terminates at the 6th rib in the midclavicular line. The right lung also contains the **horizontal** (minor) fissure, which divides the right upper and middle lobes. This fissure extends from the 5th rib in the right midaxillary line to the 3rd intercostal space or 4th rib at the right sternal border.

Posterior. The most remarkable point about the posterior chest is that it is almost all lower lobe (Fig. 19.7). The upper lobes occupy a smaller band of tissue from their apices at T_1 down to T_3 or T_4. At this level the lower lobes begin, and their inferior border reaches down to the level of T_{10} on expiration and T_{12} on inspiration. Note that the right middle lobe does not project onto the posterior chest at all. If the person abducts the arms and places the hands

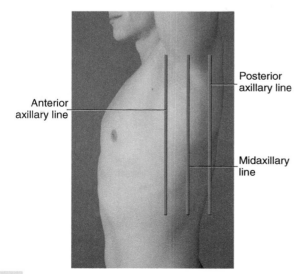

19.5

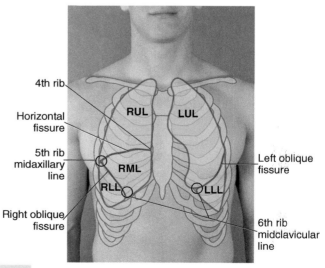

19.6

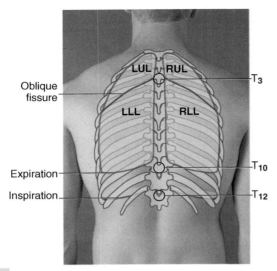

19.7

on the back of the head, the division between the upper and lower lobes corresponds to the medial border of the scapulae.

Lateral. Laterally lung tissue extends from the apex of the axilla down to the 7th or 8th rib. The right upper lobe extends from the apex of the axilla down to the horizontal fissure at the 5th rib (Fig. 19.8). The right middle lobe extends from the horizontal fissure down and forward to the 6th rib at the midclavicular line. The right lower lobe continues from the 5th rib to the 8th rib in the midaxillary line.

The left lung contains only two lobes, upper and lower (Fig. 19.9). These are seen laterally as two triangular areas separated by the oblique fissure. The left upper lobe extends from the apex of the axilla down to the 5th rib at the midaxillary line. The left lower lobe continues down to the 8th rib in the midaxillary line.

Using these landmarks, with a marker try to trace the outline of each lobe on a willing partner. Take special note of the three points that commonly confuse beginning examiners:

1. The left lung has no middle lobe.
2. The anterior chest contains mostly upper and middle lobe with very little lower lobe.
3. The posterior chest contains almost all lower lobe.

Pleurae

The thin, slippery **pleurae** are serous membranes that form an envelope between the lungs and the chest wall (Fig. 19.10). The **visceral** pleura lines the outside of the lungs, dipping down into the fissures. It is continuous with the **parietal** pleura lining the inside of the chest wall and diaphragm.

The inside of the envelope, the pleural cavity, is a potential space filled only with a few milliliters of lubricating fluid. It normally has a vacuum, or negative pressure, which holds the lungs tightly against the chest wall. The lungs slide smoothly and noiselessly up and down during respiration, lubricated by a few milliliters of fluid. Think of this as similar to two glass slides with a drop of water between them; although it is difficult to pull apart the slides, they slide smoothly back and forth. The pleurae extend approximately 3 cm below the level of the lungs, forming the **costodiaphragmatic recess.** This is a potential space; when it abnormally fills with air or fluid, it compromises lung expansion.

Trachea and Bronchial Tree

The **trachea** lies anterior to the esophagus and is 10 to 11 cm long in the adult. It begins at the level of the cricoid cartilage in the neck and bifurcates just below the sternal angle into the right and left main bronchi (Fig. 19.11). Posteriorly tracheal bifurcation is at the level of T_4 or T_5. The right main bronchus is shorter, wider, and more vertical than the left main bronchus.

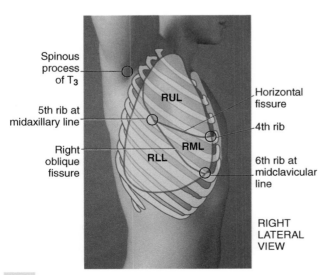

19.8

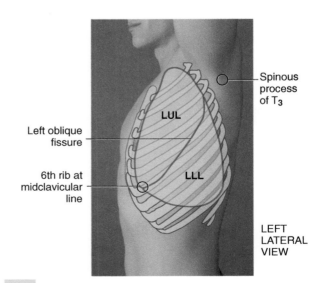

19.9

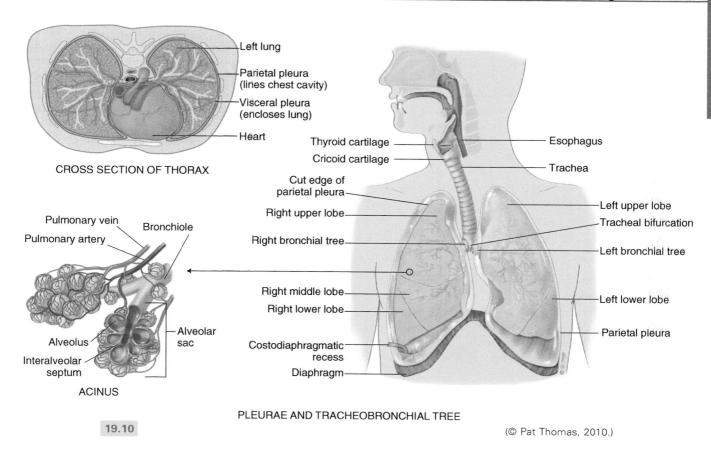

CROSS SECTION OF THORAX

- Left lung
- Parietal pleura (lines chest cavity)
- Visceral pleura (encloses lung)
- Heart

ACINUS

- Pulmonary vein
- Pulmonary artery
- Bronchiole
- Alveolar sac
- Alveolus
- Interalveolar septum

PLEURAE AND TRACHEOBRONCHIAL TREE

- Thyroid cartilage
- Cricoid cartilage
- Cut edge of parietal pleura
- Right upper lobe
- Right bronchial tree
- Right middle lobe
- Right lower lobe
- Costodiaphragmatic recess
- Diaphragm
- Esophagus
- Trachea
- Left upper lobe
- Tracheal bifurcation
- Left bronchial tree
- Left lower lobe
- Parietal pleura

19.10   (© Pat Thomas, 2010.)

The **trachea** and **bronchi** transport gases between the environment and the lung parenchyma. They constitute the *dead space,* or space that is filled with air but is not available for gaseous exchange. This is about 150 mL in the adult. The bronchial tree also protects alveoli from small particulate matter in the inhaled air. The bronchi are lined with goblet cells, which secrete mucus that entraps the particles, and cilia, which sweep particles upward where they can be swallowed or expelled.

An **acinus** is a functional respiratory unit that consists of the bronchioles, alveolar ducts, alveolar sacs, and the alveoli. Gaseous exchange occurs across the respiratory membrane in the alveolar duct and in the millions of alveoli. Note how the alveoli are clustered like grapes around each alveolar duct. This creates millions of interalveolar septa (walls) that increase tremendously the working space available for gas exchange. This bunched arrangement creates a surface area for gas exchange that is as large as a tennis court.

MECHANICS OF RESPIRATION

There are four major functions of the respiratory system: (1) supplying oxygen to the body for energy production; (2) removing carbon dioxide as a waste product of energy reactions; (3) maintaining homeostasis (acid-base balance) of arterial blood; and (4) maintaining heat exchange (less important in humans).

By supplying oxygen to the blood and eliminating excess carbon dioxide, respiration maintains the pH or the acid-base balance of the blood. The body tissues are bathed by blood that normally has a narrow acceptable range of pH. Although a number of compensatory mechanisms regulate the pH, the lungs help maintain the balance by adjusting the level of carbon dioxide through respiration. Hypoventilation (slow, shallow breathing) causes carbon dioxide to build up in the blood, and hyperventilation (rapid, deep breathing) causes carbon dioxide to be blown off.

- Thyroid cartilage
- Tracheal bifurcation
- Right main bronchus
- Cricoid cartilage
- Trachea
- Sternal angle
- Left main bronchus

19.11   (© Pat Thomas, 2010.)

Control of Respirations

Normally our breathing pattern changes without our awareness in response to cellular demands. This involuntary control of respirations is mediated by the respiratory center in the brainstem (pons and medulla). The major feedback loop is humoral regulation, or the change in carbon dioxide and oxygen levels in the blood and, less important, the hydrogen ion level. The *normal stimulus to breathe* for most of us is an increase of carbon dioxide in the blood, or **hypercapnia.** A decrease of oxygen in the blood (**hypoxemia**) also increases respirations but is less effective than hypercapnia.

Changing Chest Size

Respiration is the physical act of breathing; air rushes into the lungs as the chest size increases (inspiration) and is expelled from the lungs as the chest recoils (expiration). The mechanical expansion and contraction of the chest cavity alters the size of the thoracic container in two dimensions: (1) the vertical diameter lengthens or shortens, which is accomplished by downward or upward movement of the diaphragm; and (2) the anteroposterior (AP) diameter increases or decreases, which is accomplished by elevation or depression of the ribs (Fig. 19.12).

In inspiration increasing the size of the thoracic container creates a slightly negative pressure in relation to the atmosphere; therefore air rushes in to fill the partial vacuum. The major muscle responsible for this increase is the diaphragm. During inspiration contraction of the bell-shaped diaphragm causes it to descend and flatten. This lengthens the vertical diameter. Intercostal muscles lift the sternum and elevate the ribs, making them more horizontal. This increases the AP diameter.

Expiration is primarily passive. As the diaphragm relaxes, elastic forces within the lung, chest cage, and abdomen cause it to dome up. All this squeezing creates a relatively positive pressure within the alveoli, and the air flows out.

Forced inspiration such as that after heavy exercise or occurring pathologically with respiratory distress commands the use of the accessory neck muscles to heave up the sternum and rib cage. These neck muscles are the sternomastoids, the scaleni, and the trapezii. In forced expiration the abdominal muscles contract powerfully to push the abdominal viscera forcefully in and up against the diaphragm, making it dome upward and squeeze against the lungs.

❖ DEVELOPMENTAL COMPETENCE

Infants and Children

During the first 5 weeks of fetal life the primitive lung bud emerges; by 16 weeks the conducting airways reach the same

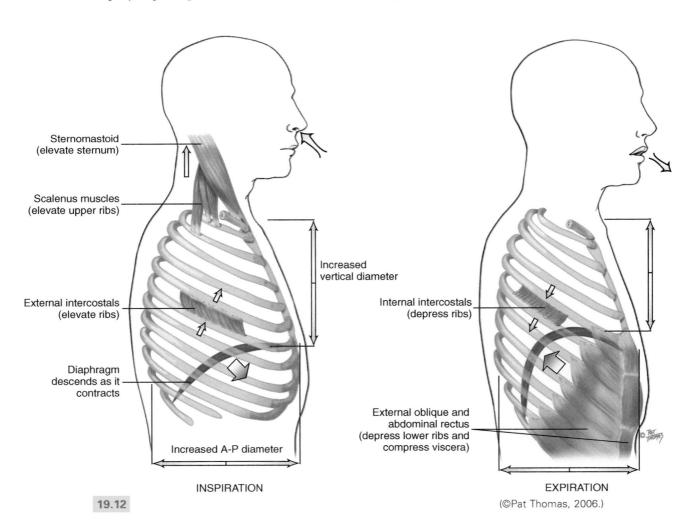

Sternomastoid
(elevate sternum)

Scalenus muscles
(elevate upper ribs)

External intercostals
(elevate ribs)

Diaphragm
descends as it
contracts

Increased
vertical diameter

Increased A-P diameter

INSPIRATION

Internal intercostals
(depress ribs)

External oblique and
abdominal rectus
(depress lower ribs and
compress viscera)

EXPIRATION

19.12

(©Pat Thomas, 2006.)

number as in the adult; at 32 weeks **surfactant,** the complex lipid substance needed for sustained inflation of the air sacs, is present in adequate amounts; and by birth the lungs have 70 million primitive alveoli ready to start the job of respiration.

Breath is life. When the newborn inhales the first breath, the lusty cry that follows reassures straining parents that their baby is all right (Fig. 19.13). The baby's body systems all develop in utero, but the respiratory system alone does not function until birth. Birth demands its instant performance.

When the cord is cut, blood is cut off from the placenta, and it gushes into the pulmonary circulation. Respiratory development continues throughout childhood, with increases in diameter and length of airways and in size and number of alveoli, reaching the adult range of 300 million by adolescence.

The relatively smaller size and immaturity of children's pulmonary systems and the presence of parents and caregivers who smoke result in enormous vulnerability and increased risks to child health. There is a long list of adverse effects on infants and children because of exposure to secondhand smoke (SHS). If the mother smokes during pregnancy, the baby has an increased risk of lower birth weight, decreased head growth, and sudden infant death syndrome (SIDS).[6] After birth, SHS exposure increases the infant's risk of upper and lower respiratory tract infections, otitis media, asthma, tooth decay, hearing loss, and metabolic syndrome, as well as later risks for attention-deficit/hyperactivity disorder, behavioral disorders, learning disabilities, cognitive disabilities, and problems at school.[6] It is crucial for pregnant women and infants and children to avoid SHS (see p. 430 for Patient Teaching).

The Pregnant Woman

The enlarging uterus elevates the diaphragm 4 cm during pregnancy. This decreases the vertical diameter of the thoracic cage, but this decrease is compensated for by an increase in the horizontal diameter. The increase in estrogen level relaxes the chest cage ligaments. This allows an increase in the transverse diameter of the chest cage by 2 cm, and the costal angle widens. The total circumference of the chest cage increases by 6 cm. Although the diaphragm is elevated, it is not fixed. It moves with breathing even more during pregnancy, which results in a 40% increase in tidal volume.[11]

The growing fetus increases the oxygen demand on the mother's body. This is met easily by the increasing tidal volume (deeper breathing). Little change occurs in the respiratory rate. An increased awareness of the need to breathe develops early in pregnancy. This **physiologic dyspnea** affects close to 75% of women; does not alter activities of daily living; and is not associated with cough, wheezing, or exercise.[11]

The Aging Adult

The costal cartilages become calcified; thus the thorax is less mobile. Respiratory muscle strength declines after age 50 years and continues to decrease into the 70s. A more significant change is the decrease in elastic properties within the

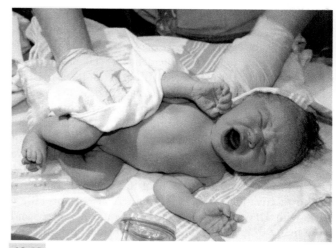

19.13

lungs, making them less distensible and lessening their tendency to collapse and recoil. In all, the aging lung is a more rigid structure that is harder to inflate.

These changes result in an increase in small airway closure, which yields a *decreased vital capacity* (the maximum amount of air that a person can expel from the lungs after first filling the lungs to maximum) and an *increased residual volume* (the amount of air remaining in the lungs even after the most forceful expiration).

With aging, histologic changes (i.e., a gradual loss of intraalveolar septa and a decreased number of alveoli) also occur; therefore less surface area is available for gas exchange. In addition, the lung bases become less ventilated as a result of closing off of a number of airways. This increases the older person's risk for dyspnea with exertion beyond his or her usual workload.

The histologic changes also increase the older person's risk for postoperative pulmonary complications. He or she has a greater risk for postoperative atelectasis and infection from a decreased ability to cough, a loss of protective airway reflexes, and increased secretions.

CULTURE AND GENETICS

Lung cancer is the 2nd most commonly diagnosed cancer in both men and women, but it is the leading cause of cancer death in the United States.[1] Tobacco smoking causes almost 90% of lung cancers, and smoking causes a high mutational burden.[18] This means that there are many mutations in the DNA genome of smokers compared with the very low mutation rate in nonsmokers. The complexity of this high mutation rate is what makes it so difficult to identify targeted drug treatments against lung cancer.

Tuberculosis (TB) is an airborne lung disease that has infected one-third of the world's population. Because of increased globalization and air travel, TB has been termed a "social and migratory" disease.[10] TB is rampant in crowded living conditions with scant physical space between persons. In addition, TB is spread in countries with armed conflict, because thousands of civilians are on the run from their homes, living in crowded refugee camps, and receiving insufficient, if any, health care services.[10]

In the United States, the incidence of TB has declined slightly each year through 2016. Among U.S.-born persons, TB incidence is stable among Caucasians and Asians, and has decreased in all other racial/ethnic groups, including Hispanics, African Americans, American Indian/Alaska Natives, and Native Hawaiian/Pacific Islanders.[16] However, almost 68% of U.S. cases occur among foreign-born persons, the top five countries of origin being Mexico, the Philippines, India, Vietnam, and China. About 90% of these cases are attributable to reactivation of latent TB. Others at risk for TB are those with HIV coinfection, those who are homeless, and those living in group settings such as shelters, prisons, and long-term-care facilities.[16] Because of the slow decline in incidence, the goal of U.S. TB elimination will not occur in this century. Thus it is imperative to increase efforts to identify and treat active TB cases and to increase target testing and treatment of latent TB in high-risk populations.

The prevalence of **asthma** is 8.4% in children ages <18 years, making it the most common chronic disease in childhood. The highest burden of asthma is among those living at or below the federal poverty level. By race/ethnicity, as of 2015 asthma prevalence has remained at 7.8% in white non-Hispanics and has decreased somewhat in black non-Hispanics (10.3%) and among Hispanics (6.6%).[5] Children living in the inner city are disproportionately at risk for asthma, although evidence about environmental (viral respiratory infections, air pollution) versus genetic risk factors is difficult to distinguish. It is known, however, that some children with persistent asthma have reduced growth of lung function. These children are at increased risk of chronic airflow obstruction and possibly COPD by early adulthood.[13] Adult asthma is a chronic lung condition of airflow obstruction and airway inflammation. This obstruction usually is reversible and is managed by avoidance of known triggers (smoking, pets, chemicals, household allergens) and with drug therapy.[7,20] For both children and adults with asthma, these interventions are difficult to attain for families living at or below the federal poverty level.

Extrinsic/allergic (or pediatric-onset) asthma involves a complex interaction between genetic susceptibility (bronchial hyperresponsiveness, atopy, elevated immunoglobulin E) and environmental factors (viral respiratory infections, air pollution). Long-term exposure to traffic-related air pollution increases risk for allergic disease in children, as shown from global evidence in Asia and India.[3a]

SUBJECTIVE DATA

1. Cough
2. Shortness of breath
3. Chest pain with breathing
4. History of respiratory infections
5. Smoking history
6. Environmental exposure
7. Patient-centered care

Examiner Asks	Rationale
1. Cough. Do you have a **cough?** When did it start? Gradual or sudden? • How long have you had it? • How often do you cough? At any special time of day or just on arising? Cough wake you up at night?	Acute cough lasts less than 2 or 3 weeks; chronic cough lasts over 2 months. Conditions with characteristic timing of cough: (1) continuous throughout day—acute illness (e.g., respiratory infection); (2) afternoon/evening—may be exposure to irritants at work; (3) night—postnasal drip, sinusitis; (4) early morning—chronic bronchial inflammation of smokers.
• Do you cough up any phlegm or sputum? How much? What color is it?	Chronic bronchitis has a history of productive cough for 3 months of the year for 2 years in a row.
• Cough up any blood? Does it look like streaks or frank blood? Does the sputum have a foul odor?	**Hemoptysis.** Some other conditions have characteristic sputum production: (1) white or clear mucoid—colds, bronchitis, viral infections; (2) yellow or green—bacterial infections; (3) rust colored—TB, pneumococcal pneumonia; (4) pink, frothy—pulmonary edema, some sympathomimetic medications have a side effect of pink-tinged mucus.

Examiner Asks	Rationale
• How would you describe your cough: hacking, dry, barking, hoarse, congested, bubbling?	Some conditions have a characteristic cough: mycoplasma pneumonia—hacking; early heart failure—dry; croup—barking; colds, bronchitis, pneumonia—congested.
• Does the cough seem to come with anything: activity, position (lying down), fever, congestion, talking, anxiety? • Does activity make it better or worse? • Which treatment have you tried? Prescription or over-the-counter medications, vaporizer, rest, position change? • Does the cough bring on anything: chest pain, ear pain? Is it tiring? Are you concerned about it?	Assess effectiveness of coping strategies. Note severity.
2. Shortness of breath. Are you having any **shortness of breath** now? Within the last day, have you been short of breath?	In hospitalized patients **dyspnea** is a common burdensome symptom and a predictor of negative outcomes.[17]
• Ever had any shortness of breath or hard-breathing spells? When did it start? What brings it on? How severe is it? How long does it last?	Determine how much activity precipitates the shortness of breath (SOB)—state specific number of blocks walked, number of stairs. Chronic dyspnea is SOB lasting >1 month and may have neurogenic, respiratory, or cardiac origin. It also occurs with anemia, anxiety, and deconditioning[21] (see Table 19.7, p. 439, for the differential diagnosis of dyspnea and its findings).
• Is it affected by position such as lying down?	**Orthopnea** is difficulty breathing when supine. State number of pillows needed to achieve comfort (e.g., "two-pillow orthopnea").
• Occur at any specific time of day or night?	**Paroxysmal nocturnal dyspnea** is awakening from sleep with SOB and needing to be upright to achieve comfort. Diaphoresis.
• SOB episodes associated with night sweats? • Cough, chest pain, or bluish color around lips or nails? Wheezing sound? • Episodes seem to be related to food, pollen, dust, animals, season, emotion, or exercise?	Cyanosis signals hypoxia. Asthma attacks may occur with a specific allergen or extreme cold, anxiety. Asthma often described as "chest tightness."
• What do you do in a hard-breathing attack? Take a special position or use pursed-lip breathing? Use any oxygen, inhalers, or medications? • How does the SOB affect your work or home activities? Getting better or worse or staying about the same? Note to examiner: For people with a smoking history, dyspnea, and cough, you can use the short 5-item Lung Function Questionnaire to identify who should be assessed with spirometry for chronic obstructive pulmonary disease (COPD) (see p. 416).	Assess effect of coping strategies and the need for more teaching. Assess effect on activities of daily living.
3. Chest pain with breathing. Any **chest pain with breathing?** Please point to the exact location. • When did it start? Constant, or does it come and go? • Describe the pain: burning, stabbing? • Brought on by respiratory infection, coughing, or trauma? Is it associated with fever, deep breathing, unequal chest inflation? • What have you done to treat it? Medication or heat application?	Chest pain of thoracic origin occurs with muscle soreness from coughing or from inflammation of pleura overlying pneumonia. Distinguish this from chest pain of cardiac origin (see Chapter 20) or heartburn of stomach acid.

Subjective Data

Examiner Asks	Rationale

4. **History of respiratory infections.** Any **past history** of breathing trouble or lung diseases such as bronchitis, emphysema, asthma, pneumonia?
   - Any unusually frequent or unusually severe colds?

   - Any family history of allergies, tuberculosis, or asthma?

Consider sequelae after these conditions.

Because most people have had some colds, it is more meaningful to ask about excess number or severity.
Assess possible risk factors.

5. **Smoking history.** Do you **smoke** cigarettes or cigars? At what age did you start? How many packs per day do you smoke now? For how long?

   - Have you ever tried to quit? What helped? Why do you think it did not work? What activities do you associate with smoking?
   - Live with someone who smokes?

   Note to examiner: Depending on the person's stage of readiness to quit smoking, you can offer counseling and encouragement using the five *As*:[19]

   Ask about his or her tobacco use status at every visit and record the person's response.
   Advise Give clear, nonjudgmental, and personalized suggestions for quitting. "I understand that quitting is difficult and challenging, but it is the most important thing you can do for your own health and for your family."
   Assess each person's readiness for and interest in quitting. The response will affect the next step. If he or she is willing to quit, you'll offer resources and assistance. If not, you'll help the person determine the barriers to cessation.
   Assist each person with a specific cessation plan that includes medications, behavioral modification, exercise programs, or referrals. Encourage to pick a quit date and give support and feedback.
   Arrange follow-up visits. If relapse occurs, state that you are there to help start over again. Remind that quitting takes practice and often does not happen in the first attempt.[19]

State number of packs per day and number of years smoked.

Most people already know they should quit smoking. Instead of admonishing, assess smoking behavior and ways to modify daily smoking activities, identify triggers, and how to manage withdrawal.

6. **Environmental exposure.** Are there any **environmental conditions** that may affect your breathing? Where do you work? At a factory, chemical plant, coal mine, farming, outdoors in a heavy traffic area?

   - Do you do anything to protect your lungs such as wear a mask or have the ventilatory system checked at work? Do you do anything to monitor your exposure? Do you have periodic examinations, pulmonary function tests, x-ray image?
   - Do you know which specific symptoms to note that may signal breathing problems?

Traffic-related air pollution increases risk of allergic rhinitis and asthma.
Farmers may be at risk for grain or pesticide inhalation. People in rural Midwest have risk for histoplasmosis exposure; those in Southwest and Mexico have risk for coccidioidomycosis. Coal miners have risk for pneumoconiosis. Stone cutters, miners, and potters have risk for silicosis. Other irritants: asbestos, radon.
Assess **self-care** measures.

General symptoms: cough, SOB. Some gases produce specific symptoms: carbon monoxide—dizziness, headache, fatigue; sulfur dioxide—cough, congestion.

Examiner Asks	Rationale
7. Patient-centered care. Last TB skin test, chest x-ray study, pneumonia vaccine, or influenza immunization?	"Flu" vaccine is modified annually. The CDC recommends annual flu vaccine for everyone age 6 months or older, especially important for those at high risk of flu complications, including pregnant women, older adults and young children, those with chronic medical conditions, residents of nursing homes and group care, health care workers, and those who are immunosuppressed.

Subjective Data

Additional History for Infants and Children

1. Has the child had any frequent or very severe colds?	Limit of 4 to 6 uncomplicated upper respiratory infections per year is expected in early childhood.
2. Is there any history of allergy in the family? • For child younger than 2 years: At what age were new foods introduced? Was the child breastfed or bottle-fed?	Consider new foods or formula as possible allergens. Exclusive breastfeeding ≥6 months protects against ear, throat, and sinus infections; this protection lasts well beyond infancy and up to 6 years of age.[12]
3. Does the child have a cough? Seem congested? Have noisy breathing or wheezing? (Further questions similar to those listed in the section on adults.)	Screen for onset and follow course of childhood chronic asthma, bronchitis.
4. Which measures have you taken to child-proof your home? Yard? Is there any possibility of the child inhaling or swallowing toxic substances? Has anyone reviewed with you the small things that are choking hazards (e.g., nuts, pins, seed, beans, corn, pen cover, toy pieces, hard candy, paper clip)? • Has anyone taught you emergency care measures in case of accidental choking or a hard-breathing spell?	Young children, especially <3 years, are at risk for foreign body aspiration, poisoning, and injury. Assess knowledge level of parent and caregivers.
5. Any smokers in the home or in the car with child? If so, insist that they not smoke in the house or car or anywhere near the child. Do not go to restaurants or other indoor places where there is smoking.	Postnatal SHS exposure increases risk for acute and chronic ear and respiratory infections in children.[6]

Additional History for the Aging Adult

1. Have you noticed any shortness of breath or fatigue with your daily activities?	Older adults have a less efficient respiratory system (decreased vital capacity, less surface area for gas exchange); thus they have less tolerance for activity.
2. Tell me about your usual amount of physical activity.	May have reduced exercise capacity because of pulmonary function deficits. Sedentary or bedridden people are at risk for respiratory dysfunction.
3. For those with a history of COPD, lung cancer, or TB: How are you getting along each day? Any weight change in the past 3 months? How much? • How about energy level? Do you tire more easily? How does your illness affect you at home? At work?	Assess coping strategies. Activities may decrease because of increasing shortness of breath or pain.

Examiner Asks	Rationale
4. Do you have any chest pain with breathing? • Any chest pain after a bout of coughing? After a fall?	Some older adults feel pleuritic pain less intensely than younger adults. Precisely localized sharp pain (points to it with one finger)—consider fractured rib or muscle injury.

For people with a frequent productive cough and/or a long smoking history, use the following questionnaire. This is a simple, short tool to identify persons who will need spirometry testing to confirm the diagnosis of COPD.[9]

Lung Function Questionnaire

Do you suffer from breathing problems and/or frequent cough?

These questions ask about your breathing problems and/or frequent cough. As you answer these questions, think about how you feel physically when you experience these symptoms. For each question, choose the one answer that best describes your symptoms. Share the answers with your healthcare provider.

Step 1: Answer each question and write the score in the box next to it.
Step 2: Add together the scores in each box to get your total score.
Step 3: Take the test to your provider to talk about your score.

1. How often do you cough up mucus?

   Never (5)   Rarely (4)   Sometimes (3)   Often (2)   Very often (1)   SCORE ☐

2. How often does your chest sound noisy (wheezy, whistling, rattling) when you breathe?

   Never (5)   Rarely (4)   Sometimes (3)   Often (2)   Very often (1)   ☐

3. How often do you experience shortness of breath during physical activity (walking up a flight of stairs or walking up an incline without stopping to rest)?

   Never (5)   Rarely (4)   Sometimes (3)   Often (2)   Very often (1)   ☐

4. How many years have you smoked?

   Never smoked (5)   10 years or less (4)   11-20 years (3)   21-30 years (2)   More than 30 years (1)   ☐

5. What is your age?

   Less than 40 years (5)   40-49 years (4)   50-59 years (3)   60-69 years (2)   70 years or older (1)   ☐

Step 4: If your score is <u>18 or less</u>, you may be at risk for Chronic Obstructive Pulmonary Disease (COPD). COPD includes chronic bronchitis, emphysema, or both.   TOTAL ☐

(© Copyright 2013 GSK. All rights reserved.)

OBJECTIVE DATA

PREPARATION

Ask the person to sit upright. Ask a man to disrobe to the waist. Ask a woman to leave the gown on and open at the back; when examining the anterior chest, lift up the gown and drape it on her shoulders rather than removing it completely. Ensure further comfort by: a warm room, a warm diaphragm endpiece, and a private examination time with no interruptions.

For smooth choreography in a complete examination, begin the respiratory examination just after palpating the thyroid gland when you are standing behind the person. Perform the inspection, palpation, percussion, and auscultation on the posterior and lateral thorax. Then move to face the person and repeat the four maneuvers on the anterior chest. This avoids repetitiously moving front to back around the person.

Finally, clean your stethoscope endpiece with an alcohol wipe. Because your stethoscope touches many people, it is a vector for bacteria and viruses. Cleaning with an alcohol wipe is very effective.

EQUIPMENT NEEDED

Stethoscope
Alcohol wipe

Normal Range of Findings	Abnormal Findings

Inspect the Posterior Chest

Thoracic Cage

Note the **shape and configuration** of the chest wall. The spinous processes should appear in a straight line. The thorax is symmetric, in an elliptical shape, with downward sloping ribs, about 45 degrees relative to the spine. The scapulae are placed symmetrically in each hemithorax.

The anteroposterior (AP) diameter should be less than the transverse diameter. The ratio of AP to transverse diameter is about 0.70 to 0.75 in adults, and it increases with age.

The neck and trapezius muscles should be developed normally for age and occupation.

Note the **position** the person takes to breathe. This includes a relaxed posture and the ability to support one's own weight with arms comfortably at the sides or in the lap.

Assess the **skin color** and **condition.** Color should be consistent with person's genetic background, with allowance for sun-exposed areas on the chest and the back. No cyanosis or pallor should be present. Note any lesions. Inquire about any change in a nevus on the back (e.g., where the person may have difficulty monitoring) (see Chapter 13).

Skeletal deformities may limit thoracic cage excursion: scoliosis, kyphosis (see Table 19.3, Configurations of the Thorax, p. 433).

AP = transverse diameter, or "barrel chest." Ribs are horizontal, chest appears as if held in continuous inspiration. This occurs in COPD from hyperinflation of the lungs (see Table 19.3).

Neck muscles are hypertrophied in COPD from aiding in forced respirations across the obstructed airways.

People with COPD often sit in a tripod position, leaning forward with arms braced against their knees, chair, or bed. This gives them leverage so the abdominal, intercostal, and neck muscles all can aid in expiration.

Cyanosis occurs with tissue hypoxia.

Palpate the Posterior Chest

Symmetric Expansion

Confirm **symmetric chest expansion** by placing your warmed hands sideways on the posterolateral chest wall with thumbs pointing together at the level of T_9 or T_{10}. Slide your hands medially to pinch up a small fold of skin between your thumbs (Fig. 19.14).

Ask the person to take a deep breath. Your hands serve as mechanical amplifiers; as the person inhales deeply, your thumbs should move apart symmetrically. Note any lag in expansion.

Unequal chest expansion occurs with marked atelectasis, lobar pneumonia, pleural effusion, thoracic trauma such as fractured ribs, or pneumothorax.

Pain accompanies deep breathing when the pleurae are inflamed.

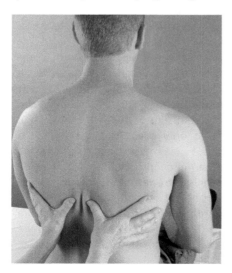

19.14

Objective Data

Normal Range of Findings	Abnormal Findings

Tactile Fremitus

Assess **tactile** (or **vocal**) **fremitus.** Fremitus is a palpable vibration. Sounds generated from the larynx are transmitted through patent bronchi and the lung parenchyma to the chest wall, where you feel them as vibrations.

Use either the palmar base (the ball) of the fingers or the ulnar edge of one hand and touch the person's chest while he or she repeats the words "ninety-nine" or "blue moon." These are resonant phrases that generate strong vibrations. Start over the lung apices and palpate from one side to the other (Fig. 19.15).

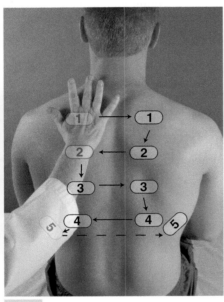

19.15

Symmetry is most important; the vibrations should feel the same in the corresponding area on each side. Avoid palpating over the scapulae because bone damps out sound transmission.

The following factors affect the intensity of tactile fremitus:

- Fremitus is most prominent between the scapulae and around the sternum, sites where the major bronchi are closest to the chest wall. It normally decreases as you progress down because more and more tissue impedes sound transmission.
- Fremitus feels greater over a thin chest wall than over an obese or heavily muscular one where thick tissue damps the vibration.
- A loud, low-pitched voice generates more fremitus than a soft, high-pitched one.

Note any areas of abnormal fremitus. Sound is conducted better through a uniformly dense structure than through a porous one, which changes in shape and solidity (as does the lung tissue during normal respiration). Thus conditions that increase the density of lung tissue make a better conducting medium for sound vibrations and increase tactile fremitus.

Asymmetric findings suggest dysfunction that you can assess further with the stethoscope.

Decreased fremitus occurs with obstructed bronchus, pleural effusion or thickening, pneumothorax, or emphysema. Any barrier that comes between the sound and your palpating hand decreases fremitus.

Increased fremitus occurs with compression or consolidation of lung tissue (e.g., lobar pneumonia). This is present only when the bronchus is patent and the consolidation extends to the lung surface. Note that only gross changes increase fremitus. Small areas of early pneumonia do not significantly affect it.

Rhonchal fremitus is palpable with thick bronchial secretions.

Pleural friction fremitus is palpable with inflammation of the pleura (see Table 19.5, Abnormal Tactile Fremitus, p. 436).

Normal Range of Findings	Abnormal Findings

Using the fingers, gently **palpate the entire chest wall.** This enables you to note any areas of tenderness, to note skin temperature and moisture, to detect any superficial lumps or masses, and to explore any skin lesions noted on inspection.

Crepitus is a coarse, crackling sensation palpable over the skin surface. It occurs in subcutaneous emphysema when air escapes from the lung and enters the subcutaneous tissue, as after open thoracic injury or surgery.

Percuss the Posterior Chest

Lung Fields

Determine the **predominant note over the lung fields.** Start at the apices and percuss the band of normally resonant tissue across the tops of both shoulders (Fig. 19.16). Then, percussing in the interspaces, make a side-to-side comparison all the way down the lung region. Percuss at 5-cm intervals. Avoid the damping effect of the scapulae and ribs.

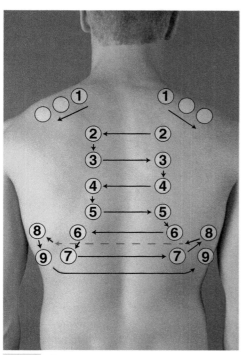

19.16 Sequence for percussion.

Resonance is the low-pitched, clear, hollow sound that predominates in healthy lung tissue in the adult (Fig. 19.17). However, resonance is a relative term and has no constant standard. The resonant note may be duller in the athlete with a heavily muscular chest wall and in the heavily obese adult in whom subcutaneous fat produces scattered dullness.

Asymmetry is important: one side with prominent dullness or marked hyperresonance indicates underlying disease. **Hyperresonance** is a lower-pitched, booming sound found when too much air is present such as in emphysema or pneumothorax.

A **dull** note (soft, muffled thud) signals abnormal density in the lungs, as with pneumonia, pleural effusion, atelectasis, or tumor.

Objective Data

Normal Range of Findings	Abnormal Findings

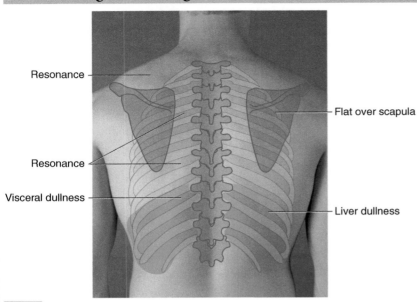

Resonance

Flat over scapula

Resonance

Visceral dullness

Liver dullness

19.17 Expected percussion notes.

The depth of penetration of percussion has limits. Percussion sets into motion only the outer 5 to 7 cm of tissue. It does not penetrate to reveal any change in density deeper than that. In addition, an abnormal finding must be 2 to 3 cm wide to yield an abnormal percussion note. Lesions smaller than that are not detectable by percussion.

The technique of measuring **diaphragmatic excursion** using percussion is no longer recommended for two reasons: (1) in persons with lung disease, evidence shows that clinicians usually overestimate diaphragmatic movement and that their results differ from chest image by 1 to 3 cm; and (2) evidence shows that diaphragmatic excursion of <2 cm is an unreliable and infrequent sign of COPD.[14] You should attend to other physical examination signs of COPD as shown throughout this chapter.

Auscultate the Posterior Chest

The passage of air through the tracheobronchial tree creates a characteristic set of sounds that are audible through the chest wall.

Breath sounds are changed by obstruction in the passageways or by disease in the lung parenchyma, the pleura, or the chest wall.

Breath Sounds

Evaluate the presence and quality of **normal breath sounds.** The person is sitting, leaning forward slightly, with arms resting comfortably across the lap. Instruct the person to breathe through the mouth, a little bit deeper than usual, but to stop if he or she begins to feel dizzy. Be careful to monitor the breathing throughout the examination, and offer times for the person to rest and breathe normally. The person is usually willing to comply with your instructions in an effort to please you and be a "good patient." Watch that he or she does not hyperventilate to the point of fainting.

Clean the flat diaphragm endpiece of the stethoscope and hold it firmly on the person's chest wall. Listen to at least one full respiration in each location. Side-to-side comparison is most important.

Do not confuse background noise with lung sounds. Become familiar with these extraneous noises that may be confused with lung pathology if not recognized:

Normal Range of Findings	Abnormal Findings

1. Examiner's breathing on stethoscope tubing
2. Stethoscope tubing bumping together
3. Patient shivering
4. Patient's hairy chest: movement of hairs under stethoscope sounds like crackles (rales)—minimize this by pressing harder or by wetting the hair with a damp cloth
5. Rustling of paper gown or paper drapes

Crackles are abnormal lung sounds (see Table 19.6, Adventitious Lung Sounds, p. 437).

While standing behind the person, listen to the following lung areas: posterior from the apices at C7 to the bases (around T10) and laterally from the axilla down to the 7th or 8th rib. Use the sequence illustrated in Fig. 19.18.

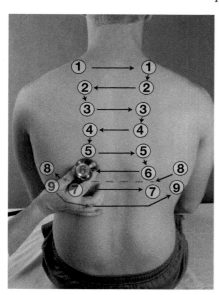

19.18

Continue to visualize approximate locations of the lobes of each lung so you correlate your findings to anatomic areas. As you listen, think (1) what AM I hearing over this spot? and (2) what should I EXPECT to be hearing? You should expect to hear three types of normal breath sounds in the adult and older child: **bronchial** (sometimes called *tracheal* or *tubular*), **bronchovesicular,** and **vesicular.** Study the description of the characteristics of these normal breath sounds in Table 19.1.

Objective Data

TABLE 19.1   Characteristics of Normal Breath Sounds

	PITCH	AMPLITUDE	DURATION	QUALITY	NORMAL LOCATION
BRONCHIAL (TRACHEAL)	High	Loud	Inspiration < expiration	Harsh, hollow tubular	Trachea and larynx
BRONCHOVESICULAR	Moderate	Moderate	Inspiration = expiration	Mixed	Over major bronchi where fewer alveoli are located: posterior, between scapulae especially on right; anterior, around upper sternum in 1st and 2nd intercostal spaces
VESICULAR	Low	Soft	Inspiration > expiration	Rustling, like the sound of the wind in the trees	Over peripheral lung fields where air flows through smaller bronchioles and alveoli

Normal Range of Findings

Note the normal location of the three types of breath sounds on the chest wall of the adult and older child (Figs. 19.19 and 19.20).

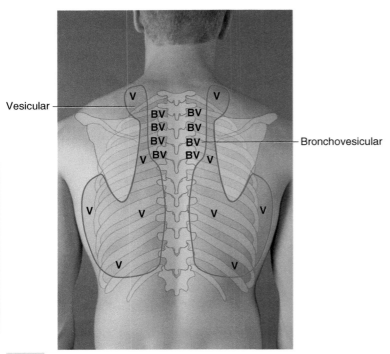

Vesicular

BV — Bronchovesicular

19.19

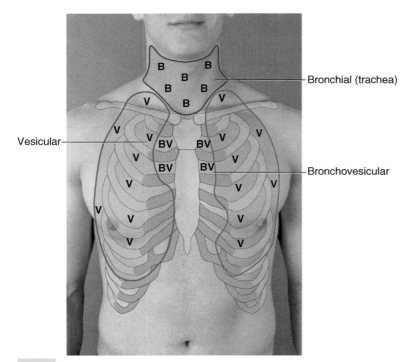

Bronchial (trachea)

Vesicular

Bronchovesicular

19.20

Abnormal Findings

Decreased or **absent breath sounds** occur:
1. When the bronchial tree is obstructed at some point by secretions, mucus plug, or a foreign body
2. In emphysema as a result of loss of elasticity in the lung fibers and decreased force of inspired air; the lungs also are already hyperinflated, so the inhaled air does not make as much noise
3. When anything obstructs transmission of sound between the lung and your stethoscope such as pleurisy or pleural thickening or air (pneumothorax) or fluid (pleural effusion) in the pleural space

A silent chest means that no air is moving in or out; an ominous sign.

Increased breath sounds mean that sounds are louder than they should be (e.g., bronchial sounds are abnormal when they are heard over an abnormal location, the peripheral lung fields). They have a high-pitched, tubular quality, with a prolonged expiratory phase and a distinct pause between inspiration and expiration. They sound very close to your stethoscope, as if they were right *in* the tubing close to your ear. They occur when consolidation (e.g., pneumonia) or compression (e.g., fluid in the intrapleural space) yields a dense lung area that enhances the transmission of sound from the bronchi. When the inspired air reaches the alveoli, it hits solid lung tissue that conducts sound more efficiently to the surface.

Normal Range of Findings	Abnormal Findings

Adventitious Sounds

Note the presence of any **adventitious sounds.** These are added sounds that are *not* normally heard in the lungs. If present, they are heard as being superimposed on the breath sounds. They are caused by moving air colliding with secretions in the tracheobronchial passageways or by the popping open of previously deflated airways. Sources differ as to the classification and nomenclature of these sounds (see Table 19.6, p. 437), but **crackles** (or rales) and **wheeze** (or rhonchi) are terms commonly used by most examiners. If you hear adventitious sounds, describe them as inspiratory versus expiratory, loudness, pitch, and location on the chest wall.

Crackles are discontinuous popping sounds heard over inspiration; **wheezes** are continuous musical sounds heard mainly over expiration. Study Table 19.6 for a complete description of these and other abnormal adventitious breath sounds.

One type of adventitious sound, **atelectatic crackles,** is not pathologic. Atelectatic crackles are short, popping, crackling sounds that last only a few breaths. When sections of alveoli are not fully aerated (as in sleepers or in older adults), they deflate slightly and accumulate secretions. Crackles are heard when these sections are expanded by a few deep breaths. Atelectatic crackles are heard only in the periphery, usually in dependent portions of the lungs, and disappear after the first few breaths or after a cough.

Voice Sounds

The spoken voice can be auscultated over the chest wall just as it can be felt in tactile fremitus described earlier. Normal voice transmission is soft, muffled, and indistinct; you can hear sound through the stethoscope but cannot distinguish exactly what is being said. Pathology that increases lung density enhances transmission of voice sounds.

Consolidation or compression of lung tissue will enhance the voice sounds, making the words more distinct.

Voice sounds are not elicited routinely. Rather these are supplemental maneuvers performed if you suspect lung pathology on the basis of earlier data. When they are performed, you are testing for the possible presence of **bronchophony, egophony,** and **whispered pectoriloquy** (see Table 19.8, p. 441).

Inspect the Anterior Chest

Note the **shape and configuration** of the chest wall. The ribs are sloping downward with symmetric interspaces. The costal angle is within 90 degrees. Development of abdominal muscles is as expected for the person's age, weight, and athletic condition.

Note the person's **facial expression.** The facial expression should be relaxed and benign, indicating an unconscious effort of breathing.

Barrel chest has horizontal ribs and costal angle >90 degrees.

Hypertrophy of abdominal muscles occurs in chronic emphysema.

Tense, strained, tired facies and purse-lipped breathing (the lips in a whistling position) accompany COPD. By exhaling slowly and against a narrow opening, the pressure in the bronchial tree remains positive, and fewer airways collapse.

Assess the **level of consciousness.** The level of consciousness should be alert and cooperative.

Cerebral hypoxia may be reflected by excessive drowsiness or anxiety, restlessness, and irritability.

Note skin **color and condition.** The lips and nail beds are free of cyanosis or unusual pallor. The nails are of normal configuration. Explore any skin lesions.

Clubbing of distal phalanx occurs with COPD because of growth of vascular connective tissue.

Cutaneous angiomas (spider nevi) associated with liver disease or portal hypertension may be evident on the chest.

Objective Data

Objective Data

Normal Range of Findings

Assess the quality of **respirations.** Normal relaxed breathing is automatic and effortless, regular and even, and produces no noise. The chest expands symmetrically with each inspiration. Note any localized lag on inspiration.

No retraction or bulging of the interspaces should occur on inspiration.

Normally accessory muscles are not used to augment respiratory effort. However, with very heavy exercise the accessory neck muscles (scalene, sternomastoid, trapezius) are used momentarily to enhance inspiration.

The respiratory rate is within normal limits for the person's age (see Table 10.2, p. 143), and the pattern of breathing is regular. Occasional sighs normally punctuate breathing.

Palpate the Anterior Chest

Palpate **symmetric chest expansion.** Place your hands on the anterolateral wall with the thumbs along the costal margins and pointing toward the xiphoid process (Fig. 19.21).

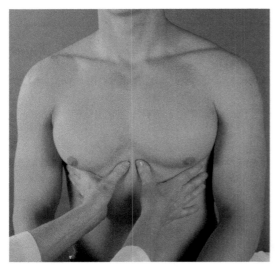

19.21

Ask the person to take a deep breath. Watch your thumbs move apart symmetrically and note smooth chest expansion with your fingers. Any limitation in thoracic expansion is easier to detect on the anterior chest because greater range of motion exists with breathing here.

Assess **tactile (vocal) fremitus.** Begin palpating over the lung apices in the supraclavicular areas (Fig. 19.22). Compare vibrations from one side to the other as the person repeats "ninety-nine." Avoid palpating over female breast tissue because breast tissue normally damps the sound.

Abnormal Findings

Noisy breathing occurs with severe asthma or chronic bronchitis.

Unequal chest expansion occurs when part of the lung is obstructed (pneumonia) or collapsed or when guarding to avoid postoperative or pleurisy pain.

Retraction suggests obstruction of respiratory tract or that increased inspiratory effort is needed, as with atelectasis. Bulging indicates trapped air as in the forced expiration associated with emphysema or asthma.

Accessory muscles are used in acute airway obstruction and massive atelectasis.

Rectus abdominis and internal intercostal muscles are used to force expiration in COPD.

Tachypnea and hyperventilation, bradypnea and hypoventilation, periodic breathing (see Table 19.4, Respiratory Patterns, p. 435).

Abnormally wide costal angle with little inspiratory variation occurs with emphysema.

A lag in expansion occurs with atelectasis, pneumonia, and postoperative guarding.

A palpable grating sensation with breathing indicates pleural friction fremitus (see Table 19.5, p. 436).

Normal Range of Findings	Abnormal Findings

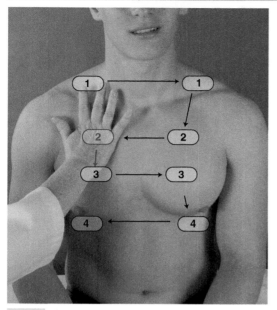

19.22   Assess tactile fremitus.

Palpate the anterior chest wall to note any tenderness (normally none is present) and detect any superficial lumps or masses (again, normally none are present). Note skin mobility and turgor and skin temperature and moisture.

If any lumps are found in the breast tissue, refer the patient to a specialist.

Percuss the Anterior Chest

Begin percussing the apices in the supraclavicular areas. Then, percussing the interspaces and comparing one side with the other, move down the anterior chest.

Interspaces are easier to palpate on the anterior chest than on the back. Do not percuss directly over female breast tissue because this would produce a dull note. Shift the breast tissue over slightly, using the edge of your stationary hand. In females with large breasts, percussion may yield little useful data. With all people use the sequence illustrated in Fig. 19.23.

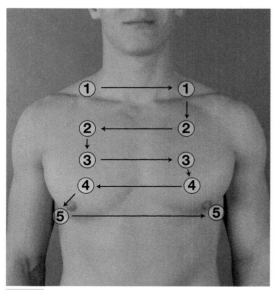

19.23   Sequence for percussion and auscultation.

Normal Range of Findings	Abnormal Findings

Note the borders of cardiac dullness normally found on the anterior chest, and do not confuse these with suspected lung pathology (Fig. 19.24). In the right hemithorax, the upper border of liver dullness is located in the 5th intercostal space in the right midclavicular line. On the left, tympany is evident over the gastric space.

Lungs are hyperinflated with chronic emphysema, which results in hyperresonance where you would expect cardiac dullness.

Dullness behind the right breast occurs with right middle lobe pneumonia.

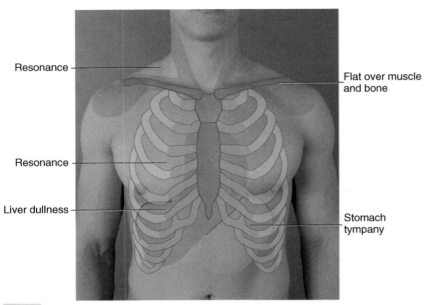

Resonance

Flat over muscle and bone

Resonance

Liver dullness

Stomach tympany

19.24 Expected percussion notes.

Auscultate the Anterior Chest

Breath Sounds

Auscultate the lung fields over the anterior chest from the apices in the supraclavicular areas down to the 6th rib. Progress from side to side as you move downward and listen to one full respiration in each location. Use the sequence indicated for percussion. Do not place your stethoscope directly over the female breast. Displace the breast and listen directly over the chest wall.

Evaluate normal breath sounds, noting any abnormal breath sounds and adventitious sounds. If the situation warrants, assess the voice sounds on the anterior chest.

Study Table 19.9, p. 442, for a complete description of abnormal respiratory conditions.

Measurement of Pulmonary Function Status

The **forced expiratory time** is the number of seconds it takes for the person to exhale from total lung capacity to residual volume. It is a screening measure of airflow obstruction. Although the test usually is not performed in the respiratory assessment, it is useful when you wish to screen for pulmonary function.

Ask the person to inhale as deeply as possible and then to blow all out hard, as quickly as possible, with the mouth open. Listen with your stethoscope over the sternum. The normal time for full expiration is 4 seconds or less.

A forced expiration of 6 seconds or more occurs with obstructive lung disease. Refer this person for more precise pulmonary function studies.

In an ambulatory care setting, a handheld **spirometer** measures lung health in chronic conditions such as asthma. Ask the patient to inhale deeply and then to exhale into the spirometer as fast as possible until the most air possible is exhaled. The *forced vital capacity (FVC)* is the total volume of air exhaled. The *forced expiratory volume in 1 second (FEV1)* is the volume exhaled in the first measured second. A normal outcome is a FEV1/FVC ratio of 75% or greater, meaning that no significant obstruction of airflow is present.

Mild obstruction of airflow is an FEV1/FCV ratio of 60% to 70%; moderate obstruction is a measure of 50% to 60%; severe obstruction is a ratio of less than 50%.

Normal Range of Findings	Abnormal Findings

The **pulse oximeter** is a noninvasive method to assess arterial oxygen saturation (SpO_2) and is described in Chapter 10. A healthy person with no lung disease and no anemia normally has an SpO_2 of 97% to 99%. However, every SpO_2 result must be evaluated in the context of the person's hemoglobin level, acid-base balance, and ventilatory status.

The **6-minute walk test** (6 MWT) is a safer, simple, inexpensive, clinical measure of functional status in aging adults. The 6 MWT is used as an outcome measure for people in pulmonary rehabilitation because it mirrors conditions that are used in everyday life.[8] Locate a flat-surfaced corridor that has little foot traffic, is wide enough to permit comfortable turns, and has a controlled environment. Ensure that the person is wearing comfortable shoes and equip him or her with a pulse oximeter to monitor oxygen saturation. Ask the person to set his or her own pace to cover as much ground as possible in 6 minutes, and assure the person it is all right to slow down or to stop to rest at any time. Use a stopwatch to time the walk. A person who walks >300 meters in 6 minutes is more likely to engage in activities of daily living.

Ask the person to stop the walk if you measure an SpO_2 below 85% to 88% or if extreme breathlessness occurs.

❖◉ DEVELOPMENTAL COMPETENCE

Infants and Children

To prepare, let the parent hold an infant supported against the chest or shoulder (Fig. 19.25). Ignore the usual sequence of the physical examination; seize the opportunity with a sleeping infant to inspect and then to listen to lung sounds next. This way you can concentrate on the breath sounds before the baby wakes up and possibly cries. However, infant crying does not have to be a problem for you because it actually enhances palpation of tactile fremitus and auscultation of breath sounds.

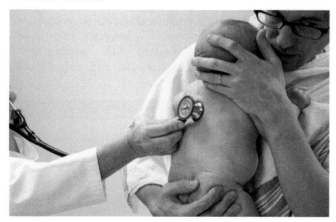

19.25

A child may sit upright on the parent's lap. Offer the stethoscope and let the child handle it. This reduces any fear of the equipment. Promote the child's participation; school-age children usually are delighted to hear their own breath sounds when you place the stethoscope properly. While listening to breath sounds, ask the young child to take a deep breath and "blow out" your penlight while you hold the stethoscope with your other hand. Time your letting go of the penlight button so the light goes off after the child blows. Or ask the child to "pant like a dog" while you auscultate.

Inspection. The infant has a rounded thorax with an equal AP–to-transverse chest diameter (Fig. 19.26). By age 6 years the thorax reaches the adult ratio of 1:2 (AP–to-transverse diameter). The newborn's chest circumference is 30 to 36 cm and is 2 cm smaller than the head circumference until 2 years of age. The chest wall is thin with little musculature. The ribs and the xiphoid are prominent; you can both see and feel the sharp tip of the xiphoid process. The thoracic cage is soft and flexible.

Note a barrel shape persisting after age 6 years, which may develop with chronic asthma or cystic fibrosis.

Normal Range of Findings	Abnormal Findings

19.26 Round thorax in an infant.

The newborn's first respiratory assessment is part of the **Apgar scoring system** to measure the successful transition to extrauterine life (Table 19.2). The five standard parameters are scored at 1 minute and 5 minutes after birth. A 1-minute Apgar with a total score of 7 to 10 indicates a newborn in good condition, needing only suctioning of the nose and mouth and otherwise routine care.

In the immediate newborn period, depressed respirations are caused by maternal drugs, interruption of the uterine blood supply, or obstruction of the tracheobronchial tree with mucus or fluid.

A 1-minute Apgar with a total score of 3 to 6 indicates a moderately depressed newborn needing more resuscitation and subsequent close observation. A score of 0 to 2 indicates a severely depressed newborn needing full resuscitation, ventilatory assistance, and subsequent intensive care.

TABLE 19.2	Apgar Scoring System			
	2	**1**	**0**	
Heart rate	Over 100	Slow (below 100)	Absent	_____
Respiratory effort	Good, sustained cry; regular respirations	Slow, irregular, shallow	Absent	_____
Muscle tone	Active motion, spontaneous flexion	Some flexion of extremities; some resistance to extension	Limp, flaccid	_____
Reflex irritability (response to catheter in nares)	Sneeze, cough, cry	Grimace, frown	No response	_____
Color	Completely pink	Body pink, extremities pale	Cyanotic, pale	_____
			Total score	_____

The infant breathes through the nose rather than the mouth and is an obligate nose breather until 3 months. Slight flaring of the lower costal margins may occur with respirations, but normally no flaring of the nostrils and no sternal retractions or intercostal retractions occur. The diaphragm is the newborn's major respiratory muscle. Intercostal muscles are not well developed. Thus you observe the abdomen bulge with each inspiration but see little thoracic expansion.

Count the respiratory rate for 1 full minute. Normal rates for the newborn are 30 to 40 breaths/min but may spike up to 60 breaths/minute. Obtain the most accurate respiratory rate by counting when the infant is asleep because infants

Marked retractions of sternum and intercostal muscles indicate increased inspiratory effort, as in atelectasis, pneumonia, asthma, and acute airway obstruction.

Rapid respiratory rates accompany pneumonia, fever, pain, heart disease, and anemia.

Normal Range of Findings

reach rapid rates with very little excitation when awake. The respiratory pattern may be irregular when extremes in room temperature occur or with feeding or sleeping. Brief periods of apnea less than 10 to 15 seconds are common. This periodic breathing is more common in premature infants.

Palpation. Palpate symmetric chest expansion by encircling the infant's thorax with both hands. Further palpation should yield no lumps, masses, or crepitus, although you may feel the costochondral junctions in some normal infants.

Auscultation. Auscultation normally yields bronchovesicular breath sounds in the peripheral lung fields of the infant and young child up to age 5 to 6 years. Their relatively thin chest walls with underdeveloped musculature do not damp off the sound as do the thicker walls of adults; thus breath sounds are louder and harsher.

Fine crackles are the adventitious sounds commonly heard in the immediate newborn period from opening of the airways and clearing of fluid. Because the newborn's chest wall is so thin, transmission of sounds is enhanced; and sound is heard easily all over the chest, making localization of breath sounds a problem. Even bowel sounds are easily heard in the chest. Try using the smaller pediatric diaphragm endpiece or place the bell over the infant's interspaces and not over the ribs. Use the pediatric diaphragm on an older infant or toddler (Fig. 19.27).

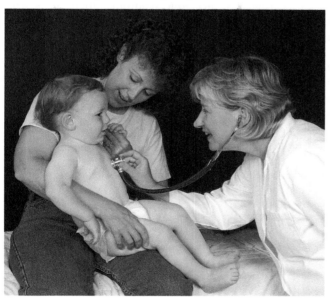

19.27

The Pregnant Woman

The thoracic cage appears wider, and the costal angle widens by about 50%. Respirations are deeper, with a 40% increase in tidal volume.

The Aging Adult

The chest cage commonly shows an increased AP diameter, giving a round barrel shape and **kyphosis** or an outward curvature of the thoracic spine (see Table 19.3, p. 434). The person compensates by holding the head extended and tilted back. You may palpate marked bony prominences because of decreased subcutaneous fat. Chest expansion may be somewhat decreased with the older person, although it still should be symmetric. The costal cartilages become calcified with aging, resulting in a less mobile thorax.

The older person may tire easily, especially during auscultation when deep mouth breathing is required. Take care that this person does not hyperventilate

Abnormal Findings

In an infant tachypnea of 50 to 100 breaths/min during sleep may be an early sign of heart failure.

Asymmetric expansion occurs with diaphragmatic hernia or pneumothorax.

Crepitus is palpable around a fractured clavicle, which may occur with difficult forceps delivery.

Diminished breath sounds occur with pneumonia, atelectasis, pleural effusion, or pneumothorax.

Persistent fine crackles that are scattered over the chest occur with pneumonia, bronchiolitis, or atelectasis.

Crackles only in upper lung fields occur with cystic fibrosis; crackles only in lower lung fields occur with heart failure.

Expiratory wheezing occurs with lower airway obstruction (e.g., asthma or bronchiolitis). When unilateral, it may be foreign body aspiration.

Persistent peristaltic sounds with diminished breath sounds on the same side may indicate diaphragmatic hernia.

Stridor is a high-pitched inspiratory crowing sound heard without the stethoscope, occurring with upper airway obstruction (e.g., croup, foreign body aspiration, or acute epiglottitis).

Objective Data

Normal Range of Findings	Abnormal Findings

and become dizzy. Allow brief rest periods or quiet breathing. If the person does feel faint, holding the breath for a few seconds restores equilibrium.

The Acutely Ill Person

Ask a second examiner to hold the person's arms and support him or her in the upright position. If no one else is available, you need to roll the person from side to side, examining the uppermost half of the thorax. This obviously prevents you from comparing findings from one side to another. In addition, side flexion of the trunk alters percussion findings because the ribs of the upward side may flex closer together.

HEALTH PROMOTION AND PATIENT TEACHING

"Now let's talk about protecting yourself and your children from secondhand smoke. You've mentioned that your father lives close to you and that he smokes. Breathing secondhand smoke hurts the normal function of your heart, blood, and blood vessels, increasing the risk of heart attack. It is dangerous for children and increases the risk of ear and chest infections. There are some ways to help yourself and your family."

Secondhand smoke (SHS) is a mixture of sidestream and mainstream smoke and contains over 7000 chemicals, of which hundreds are toxic and 70 can cause cancer.[4] Sidestream smoke is the smoke seen from the burning end of a tobacco product, whereas mainstream smoke is the smoke exhaled from the person smoking. There is no safe level of SHS for nonsmokers, pregnant women, babies, or children. Nonsmokers exposed to SHS at home or work increase their risk of heart disease by 25% to 30% and their risk for stroke by 20% to 30%.[4] Pregnant women exposed to SHS increase their risk of low-birth-weight infants, as well as the risk of sudden infant death syndrome (SIDS). Babies and children exposed to SHS are at increased risk for upper and lower respiratory tract infections, otitis media, asthma, dental caries, hearing loss, metabolic syndrome, attention-deficit/hyperactivity disorder, behavioral disorders, learning disabilities, and school difficulties.[6]

"Ways to help yourself and your family: Do not allow anyone to smoke near your children; do not allow anyone to smoke in the home or car with you or your children, even with the window rolled down; make sure your children's daycare and schools are tobacco-free; do not go to a restaurant, mall, or public place that allows smoking; talk to your teenagers about these same methods."

DOCUMENTATION AND CRITICAL THINKING

Sample Charting

SUBJECTIVE

No cough, shortness of breath, or chest pain with breathing. No history of respiratory diseases. Has "one or no" colds per year. Has never smoked. Works in well-ventilated office on a smoke-free campus. Last TB skin test 4 years PTA, negative. Never had chest x-ray.

OBJECTIVE

Inspection: AP < transverse diameter. Resp 16/min, relaxed and even.
Palpation: Chest expansion symmetric. Tactile fremitus equal bilaterally. No tenderness to palpation. No lumps or lesions.
Percussion: Resonant to percussion over lung fields.
Auscultation: Vesicular breath sounds clear over lung fields and = bilaterally. No adventitious sounds.

ASSESSMENT

Intact thoracic structures
Lung sounds clear and equal

R.B. is a 37-year-old male exercise trainer who teaches 10 to 12 clients per day in a small gym and comes to clinic, saying, "I'm really sick." Last visit to care provider was 10 years PTA for ankle sprain. Runs and works out 1 hour most days. Has never smoked. Drinks occasionally on weekends, 1 or 2 beers per occasion. No history of allergies, hospitalizations. No family history of TB, asthma, heart disease, or cancer. No vaccines since childhood.

SUBJECTIVE

2 days PTA—Client in R.B.'s gym was coughing productive mucus and dripping on hands and equipment. R.B. cleaned equipment but next day felt sudden-onset overwhelming fatigue and fever. Unable to sleep because of fever of 102° to 104° F (38.9° to 40° C), headache, severe joint and muscle pain, and stuffy nose that completely obstructs when lying down.

Now—Headache, stuffy nose, sneezing, sore throat, severe cough, chest pain in sternum with coughing, severe muscle aches and pains. No nausea, vomiting, or diarrhea.

OBJECTIVE

Vital signs: Temp 102.8° F (39.3° C). Pulse 88 bpm. Resp 20/min. BP 108/74 mm Hg, L arm sitting.

Ears—TMs clear with landmarks intact.

Nose—Turbinates red and swollen with yellow purulent mucus.

Throat—Tonsils out, throat red, R & L anterior cervical nodes enlarged and tender.

Chest—Respirations not labored, chest expansion symmetric, no tenderness to palpation. Resonant to percussion and = bilaterally. Vesicular breath sounds clear over peripheral lung fields. Loud, low-pitched, gurgling crackles over anterior sternum at 4th and 5th interspace.

Abdomen—Bowel sounds present, soft, no tenderness.

ASSESSMENT

Influenza
Insomnia

E.S. is 53-year-old male line worker at urban automobile plant. Concerned with increasing shortness of breath for past 3 to 4 years. Reports 5 to 6 "colds" per year. Smokes cigarettes starting age 18, 1 PPD × 30 years, 1½ PPD × 5 years. Does not drink alcohol. Takes HCTZ 25 mg for hypertension, no other meds. No allergies. No hospitalizations or injuries. No family history of TB, allergies, heart disease, asthma, cancer.

SUBJECTIVE

Short of breath now after walking 1 flight of stairs or 1 block. Chest tightness. Early morning cough daily, with small amount white sputum × 2-3 years. Fatigue and SOB at work. Has 2-pillow orthopnea at night. Wakes 2-3 times/night to urinate or "catch breath." States thinking of quitting smoking, but previous attempts have not worked.

OBJECTIVE

Vital signs: BP 148/88 mm Hg. Temp 98° F (36.7° C). Pulse 88 bpm. Resp 24/min. Weight 134 lbs.

Inspection: Sitting on side of bed with arms propped on bedside table. Respirations: resting 24/min, regular, shallow with prolonged expiration; resp. ambulating 34/min. Increased use of accessory muscles, AP = transverse diameter with widening of costal angle, tense expression.

Palpation: Minimal but symmetric chest expansion. Tactile fremitus = bilaterally. No lumps, masses, or tenderness to palpation.

Percussion: Hyperresonance over lung fields.

Auscultation: Breath sounds diminished. Expiratory wheeze throughout posterior chest, R > L. No crackles.

ASSESSMENT

Potential chronic obstructive pulmonary disease
Hypertension
Decreased gas exchange

Decreased mobility
Insomnia

Clinical Case Study 3

A.G. is a 67-year-old female retired secretary who is admitted to a surgical unit following uncomplicated cholecystectomy. She has resisted interventions to walk in halls because of incisional pain and obesity (weight is 245 lbs). On 2nd postop day nurse answers call light and finds A.G. sitting bolt upright in bed gasping for breath and clutching bedsheets.

SUBJECTIVE

"I can't breathe, I can't breathe." (Nurse asks when this started.) "Few minutes ago and my chest hurts too, worse when I breathe in."

OBJECTIVE

Vital signs: Temp 99.2°F (37.3°C). Pulse 124 bpm. Resp 32/min, labored. BP 100/70 mm Hg. Pulse oximetry 78% on room air. (Nurse now calls for help, administers O_2 15 L/min via Venturi mask, continues with assessment.)
Mental status: Alert, apprehensive.
Skin: Pale, ashen, cool, diaphoretic, delayed capillary refill.
Chest: Labored breathing, symmetrical expansion, breath sounds labored though present in both lungs, decreased in posterior right base, crackles over posterior right base.

ASSESSMENT

Acute respiratory distress

Clinical Case Study 4

C.T. is a 9-month-old girl who comes to the clinic with her father because of "a bad cold." C.T. attends daycare and lives at home with two school-age siblings, parents, and paternal grandmother. The adults smoke in the home.

SUBJECTIVE

6 days PTA: C.T.'s 4-year-old brother came home from preschool "with a cold that he gave to our whole family."
2 days PTA: C.T. has "cold" with cough, fever (temp unknown because of not having a thermometer at home), and decreased intake of formula.
Now: C.T. "looks and sounds worse. I don't think she's breathing right." Reported last bottle and wet diaper was 6 hours ago.
Birth history: Born at 36 weeks' gestation, spontaneous rupture of membranes (SROM), vaginal birth w/o complications; weight 5 lbs 1 oz (2.3 kg); birth length 19 in (48.2 cm); head circumference 32.5 cm.

OBJECTIVE

Vital signs: Temp 102°F (38.9°C) (axillary). BP 80/56 mm Hg (sitting on exam table). Pulse 192 bpm. Resp 70/min. Weight 13 lbs (5.9 kg). Height 27.5 in. (69.8 cm). Head circumference 41.5 cm.
General appearance: Labored breathing w/ nasal flaring while sitting upright on dad's lap. Attempts to suck from a bottle but gives up, gasping, after latching on for a few seconds.
HEENT: Normocephalic; eyes clear; TM pearly gray bilat; thick, copious amounts of mucus to bilat nares and pharynx.
Cardiovascular: Tachycardic; no abnormal heart sounds.
Respiratory: Tachypneic, crackles at bases, wheezes bilat, and harsh, productive cough; moderate intercostal and subcostal retractions.

ASSESSMENT

Respiratory syncytial virus (RSV) bronchiolitis
Dyspnea
Decreased gas exchange
Potential for fluid volume deficit
Need for health teaching on dangers of secondhand smoke

ABNORMAL FINDINGS

TABLE 19.3	Configurations of the Thorax

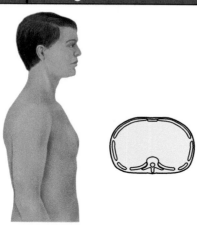

Normal Adult (for Comparison)

The thorax has an elliptical shape with an anteroposterior-to-transverse diameter documented as 1:2 or 0.70.

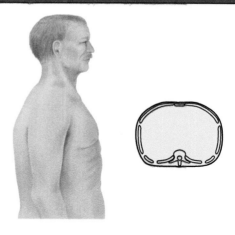

Barrel Chest

Note equal AP-to-transverse diameter and that ribs are horizontal instead of the normal downward slope. This is associated with normal aging and also with chronic emphysema and asthma as a result of hyperinflation of lungs.

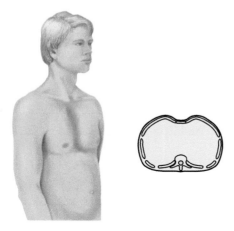

Pectus Excavatum

A markedly sunken sternum and adjacent cartilages (also called *funnel breast*). Depression begins at second intercostal space, becoming depressed most at junction of xiphoid with body of sternum. More noticeable on inspiration. Congenital, usually not symptomatic. When severe, sternal depression may cause embarrassment and a negative self-concept. Surgery may be indicated.

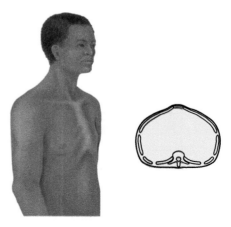

Pectus Carinatum

A forward protrusion of the sternum, with ribs sloping back at either side and vertical depressions along costochondral junctions (pigeon breast). Less common than pectus excavatum, this minor deformity requires no treatment. If severe, surgery may be indicated.

Continued

TABLE 19.3	Configurations of the Thorax—cont'd

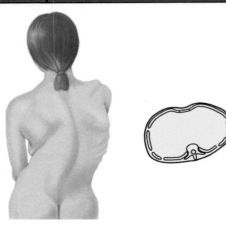 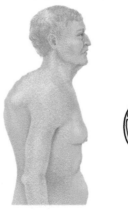 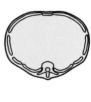

Scoliosis

A lateral S-shaped curvature of the thoracic and lumbar spine, usually with involved vertebrae rotation. Note unequal shoulder and scapular height and unequal hip levels, rib interspaces flared on convex side. More prevalent in adolescent age-groups, especially girls. Mild deformities are asymptomatic. If severe (>45 degrees) deviation is present, scoliosis may reduce lung volume, and person is at risk for impaired cardiopulmonary function. Primary impairment is cosmetic deformity, negatively affecting self-image.

Kyphosis

An exaggerated posterior curvature of the thoracic spine (humpback) that causes significant back pain and limited mobility. Severe deformities impair cardiopulmonary function. If the neck muscles are strong, compensation occurs by hyperextension of head to maintain level of vision.

Kyphosis is associated with aging, especially the "dowager's hump" of postmenopausal osteoporotic women. However, it is common well before menopause. Women with adequate exercise habits are less likely to have kyphosis.

TABLE 19.4	Respiratory Patterns[a]

Inspiration Expiration

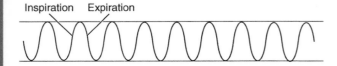 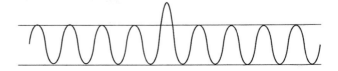

Normal Adult (for Comparison)

Rate—10 to 20 breaths/min
  Depth—500 to 800 mL
  Pattern—Even
  The ratio of pulse to respirations is fairly constant, about 4:1. Both values increase as a normal response to exercise, fear, or fever.
  Depth—Air moving in and out with each respiration.

Sigh

Occasional sighs punctuate the normal breathing pattern and are purposeful to expand alveoli. Frequent sighs may indicate emotional dysfunction and also may lead to hyperventilation and dizziness.

[a]Assess the (1) rate, (2) depth (tidal volume), and (3) pattern.

Continued

TABLE 19.4	Respiratory Patterns[a]—cont'd

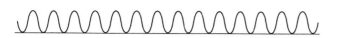

Tachypnea

Rapid, shallow breathing. Increased rate, >24 per minute. This is a normal response to fever, fear, or exercise. Rate also increases with respiratory insufficiency, pneumonia, alkalosis, pleurisy, and lesions in the pons.

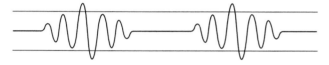

Bradypnea

Slow breathing. A decreased but regular rate (<10 per minute), as in drug-induced depression of the respiratory center in the medulla, increased intracranial pressure, and diabetic coma.

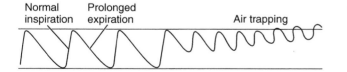

Cheyne-Stokes Respiration

A cycle in which respirations gradually wax and wane in a regular pattern, increasing in rate and depth and then decreasing. The breathing periods last 30 to 45 seconds, with periods of apnea (20 seconds) alternating the cycle. The most common cause is severe heart failure; other causes are renal failure, meningitis, drug overdose, and increased intracranial pressure. Occurs normally in infants and older adults during sleep.

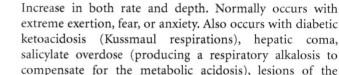

Hyperventilation

Increase in both rate and depth. Normally occurs with extreme exertion, fear, or anxiety. Also occurs with diabetic ketoacidosis (Kussmaul respirations), hepatic coma, salicylate overdose (producing a respiratory alkalosis to compensate for the metabolic acidosis), lesions of the midbrain, and alteration in blood gas concentration (either an increase in CO_2 or a decrease in oxygen). Hyperventilation blows off CO_2, causing a decreased level in the blood (alkalosis).

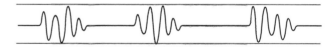

Hypoventilation

An irregular shallow pattern caused by an overdose of narcotics or anesthetics. May also occur with prolonged bed rest or conscious splinting of the chest to avoid respiratory pain.

Biot Respiration

Similar to Cheyne-Stokes respiration, except that the pattern is irregular. A series of normal respirations (3 to 4) is followed by a period of apnea. The cycle length is variable, lasting anywhere from 10 seconds to 1 minute. Seen with head trauma, brain abscess, heat stroke, spinal meningitis, and encephalitis.

◄ **Chronic Obstructive Breathing**

Normal inspiration and prolonged expiration to overcome increased airway resistance. In a person with chronic obstructive lung disease, any situation calling for increased heart rate (exercise) may lead to dyspneic episode (air trapping) because the person does not have enough time for full expiration.

TABLE 19.5	Abnormal Tactile Fremitus

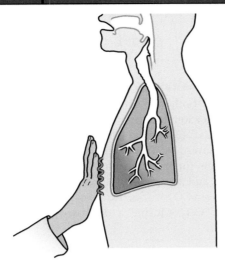

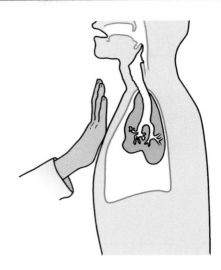

Increased Tactile Fremitus

Occurs with conditions that increase the density of lung tissue, thereby making a better conducting medium for vibrations (e.g., compression or consolidation [pneumonia]). There must be a patent bronchus, and consolidation must extend to lung surface for increased fremitus to be apparent.

Decreased Tactile Fremitus

Occurs when anything obstructs transmission of vibrations (e.g., an obstructed bronchus, pleural effusion or thickening, pneumothorax, and emphysema). Any barrier that gets in the way of the sound and your palpating hand decreases fremitus.

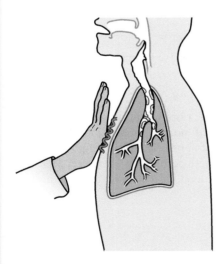

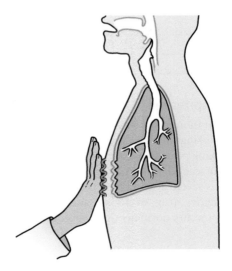

Rhonchal Fremitus

Vibration felt when inhaled air passes through thick secretions in the larger bronchi. This may decrease somewhat by coughing.

Pleural Friction Fremitus

Produced when inflammation of the parietal or visceral pleura causes a decrease in the normal lubricating fluid. The opposing surfaces make a coarse grating sound when rubbed together during breathing. This sound is best detected by auscultation, but it may be palpable and feels like two pieces of leather grating together. It is synchronous with respiratory excursion. Also called a *palpable friction rub.*

TABLE 19.6	Adventitious Lung Sounds		
Sound	**Description**	**Mechanism**	**Clinical Example**

Discontinuous Sounds

These are discrete, crackling sounds.

Crackles—Fine (formerly called *rales*)[3] Inspiration — Expiration	Discontinuous, high-pitched, short crackling, popping sounds heard during inspiration that are not cleared by coughing; you can simulate this sound by rolling a strand of hair between your fingers near your ear or by moistening your thumb and index finger and separating them near your ear	Inspiratory crackles: inhaled air collides with previously deflated airways; airways suddenly pop open, creating explosive crackling sound Expiratory crackles: sudden airway closing	*Late inspiratory crackles* occur with restrictive disease: pneumonia, heart failure, and interstitial fibrosis *Early inspiratory crackles* occur with obstructive disease: chronic bronchitis, asthma, and emphysema *Posturally induced crackles* (PICs) are fine crackles that appear with a change from sitting to the supine position or with a change from supine to supine with legs elevated
Crackles——Coarse	Loud, low-pitched bubbling and gurgling sounds that start in early inspiration and may be present in expiration; may decrease somewhat by suctioning or coughing but reappear shortly—sounds like opening a Velcro fastener	Inhaled air collides with secretions in the trachea and large bronchi	Pulmonary edema, pneumonia, pulmonary fibrosis, and the terminally ill who have a depressed cough reflex
Atelectatic crackles	Sound like fine crackles but do not last and are not pathologic; disappear after the first few breaths; heard in axillae and bases (usually dependent) of lungs	When sections of alveoli are not fully aerated, they deflate and accumulate secretions; crackles are heard when these sections reexpand with a few deep breaths	In aging adults, in bedridden persons, or in persons just aroused from sleep
Pleural friction rub	A very superficial sound that is coarse and low pitched; it has a grating quality as if two pieces of leather are being rubbed together; sounds just like crackles, but *close* to the ear; sounds louder if you push the stethoscope harder onto the chest wall; sound is inspiratory and expiratory	Caused when pleurae become inflamed and lose their normal lubricating fluid; their opposing roughened pleural surfaces rub together during respiration; heard best in anterolateral wall where greatest lung mobility exists	Pleuritis, accompanied by pain with breathing (rub disappears after a few days if pleural fluid accumulates and separates pleurae)

Continued

TABLE 19.6 | Adventitious Lung Sounds—cont'd

Sound	Description	Mechanism	Clinical Example

Continuous Sounds

These are connected, musical sounds.

Sound	Description	Mechanism	Clinical Example
Wheeze—High-pitched (sibilant)	High-pitched, musical squeaking sounds that sound polyphonic (multiple notes as in a musical chord); predominate in expiration but may occur in both expiration and inspiration	Air squeezed or compressed through passageways narrowed almost to closure by collapsing, swelling, secretions, or tumors; the passageway walls oscillate in apposition between the closed and barely open positions; the resulting sound is similar to that of a vibrating reed	Diffuse airway obstruction from acute asthma or chronic emphysema
Wheeze—Low-pitched (sonorous rhonchi)	Low-pitched; monophonic, single note, musical snoring, moaning sounds; they are heard throughout the cycle, although they are more prominent on expiration; may clear somewhat by coughing[3]	Airflow obstruction as described earlier by the vibrating reed mechanism; the pitch of the wheeze cannot be correlated to the size of the passageway that generates it	Bronchitis, single bronchus obstruction from airway tumor
Stridor	High-pitched, monophonic, inspiratory, crowing sound; louder in neck than over chest wall	Originating in larynx or trachea, upper airway obstruction from swollen, inflamed tissues or lodged foreign body	Croup and acute epiglottitis in children and foreign inhalation; obstructed airway may be life-threatening

ABNORMAL FINDINGS
FOR ADVANCED PRACTICE

TABLE 19.7	Diagnostic Clues to Chronic Dyspnea and Associated Systems			
System/Physiology	Example	History	Examination	Diagnostic Study
Pulmonary				
Alveolar	Chronic pneumonia	Fever, productive cough, shortness of breath	Fever, crackles, increased fremitus, bronchophony	Chest radiography, chest CT, bronchoscopy/ bronchoalveolar lavage, culture or biopsy
Interstitial	Idiopathic fibrosis	Exertional dyspnea, dry cough, malignancy, prescription or illicit drug use, chemical exposures	Hypoxia, clubbing, persistent inspiratory crackles	Chest radiography (fibrosis, interstitial markings), chest CT, bronchoscopy/biopsy
Obstruction of air flow	Chronic obstructive pulmonary disease	Tobacco use, cough, relief with bronchodilator, increased sputum production, hemoptysis and weight loss with malignancy	Wheezing, barrel chest, decreased breath sounds, accessory muscle use, clubbing, paradoxical pulse	Peak flow, spirometry, chest radiography (hyperinflation), pulmonary function testing (PFT)
Restrictive	Pleural effusion	Pleuritic chest pain, dyspnea not improved with oxygen	Decreased breath sounds, chest morphology, pleural rub, basal dullness	Chest radiography (effusion, anatomic abnormality), spirometry, PFT
Vascular	Chronic pulmonary emboli	Fatigue, pleuritic chest pain, prior emboli/deep venous thrombosis, syncope	Wheezing, lower extremity swelling, pleural rub, prominent P_2, murmur, right ventricular heave, jugular venous distention (JVD)	D-dimer, ventilation/ perfusion scan, CT angiography, echocardiography, right heart catheterization
Cardiac				
Arrhythmia	Atrial fibrillation	Palpitations, syncope	Irregular rhythm, pauses	ECG, event recorder, Holter monitor, stress testing
Heart failure	Ischemic cardiomyopathy	Dyspnea on exertion, paroxysmal nocturnal dyspnea, orthopnea, chest pain or tightness, prior coronary artery disease or atrial fibrillation	Edema, JVD, S_3, displaced cardiac apical impulse, hepatojugular reflex, murmur, crackles, wheezing, tachycardia, S_4	ECG, brain natriuretic peptide, echocardiography, stress testing, coronary angiography

Continued

TABLE 19.7 Diagnostic Clues to Chronic Dyspnea and Associated Systems—cont'd

System/Physiology	Example	History	Examination	Diagnostic Study
Cardiac—cont'd				
Restrictive or constrictive pericardial disease	Metastatic tumor	Viral infection, malignancy, chest radiation, inflammatory diseases	Decreased heart sounds	Echocardiography
Valvular	Aortic stenosis	Dyspnea on exertion	Murmur, JVD	Echocardiography
Gastrointestinal				
Aspiration	Gastroesophageal reflux disease	Postprandial, night cough	Intermittent crackles, wheezes	Chest radiography, esophagography, esophageal pH
Neuromuscular				
Respiratory muscle weakness	Phrenic nerve palsy	Known neuromuscular disorders, weakness	Atrophy	Maximal inspiratory and expiratory pressures
Psychological				
—	Anxiety	Anxiety, depression, history of trauma or abuse	Sighing	Normal

From Wahls, S.A. (2012). Causes and evaluation of chronic dyspnea. *Am Fam Phys* 86(2), 173-180.
CT, Computed tomography; *ECG,* electrocardiography; *JVD,* jugular venous distention; *PFT,* pulmonary function testing.

TABLE 19.8 | Voice Sounds

Technique	Normal Finding	Abnormal Finding
Bronchophony Ask the person to repeat "ninety-nine" while you listen with the stethoscope over the chest wall; listen especially if you suspect pathology	Normal voice transmission is soft, muffled, and indistinct; you can hear sound through the stethoscope but cannot distinguish exactly what is being said	Pathology that increases lung density enhances transmission of voice sounds; you auscultate a clear "ninety-nine" The words are more distinct than normal and sound close to your ear

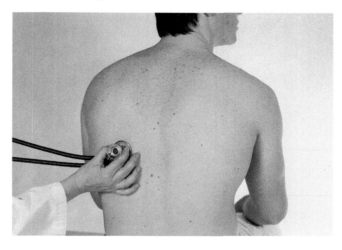

Technique	Normal Finding	Abnormal Finding
Egophony (Greek: "the voice of a goat") Auscultate the chest while the person phonates a long "ee-ee-ee-ee" sound	Normally you should hear "eeeeeeee" through your stethoscope	Over area of consolidation or compression the spoken "eeee" sound changes to a bleating long "aaaaa" sound
Whispered Pectoriloquy Ask the person to whisper a phrase such as "one-two-three" as you auscultate	The normal response is faint, muffled, and almost inaudible	With only small amounts of consolidation, the whispered voice is transmitted very clearly and distinctly, although still somewhat faint; it sounds as if the person is whispering right into your stethoscope, "one-two-three"

TABLE 19.9	Assessment of Common Respiratory Conditions

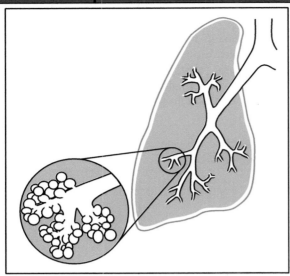

◀ **Normal Lung (for Comparison)**

Inspection AP < transverse diameter, relaxed posture, normal musculature; rate 10 to 18 breaths/min, regular; no cyanosis or pallor.

Palpation Symmetric chest expansion. Tactile fremitus present and equal bilaterally, diminishing toward periphery. No lumps, masses, or tenderness.

Percussion Resonant.

Auscultation Vesicular over peripheral fields. Bronchovesicular parasternally (anterior) and between scapulae (posterior). Infant and young child—bronchovesicular throughout.

Adventitious Sounds None.

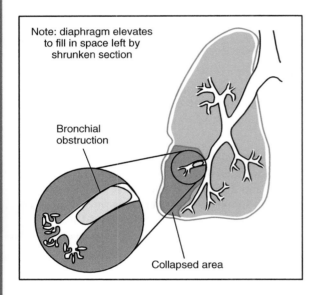

Note: diaphragm elevates to fill in space left by shrunken section

Bronchial obstruction

Collapsed area

◀ **Atelectasis (Collapse)**

Condition Collapsed shrunken section of alveoli or an entire lung as a result of (1) airway obstruction (e.g., the bronchus is completely blocked by thick exudate, aspirated foreign body, or tumor); the alveolar air beyond the obstruction is gradually absorbed by the pulmonary capillaries, and the alveolar walls cave in); (2) compression on the lung; and (3) lack of surfactant (hyaline membrane disease).

Inspection Cough. Lag on expansion on affected side. Increased respiratory rate and pulse. Possible cyanosis.

Palpation Chest expansion decreased on affected side. Tactile fremitus decreased or absent over area. With large collapse, tracheal shift toward affected side.

Percussion Dull over area (remainder of thorax sometimes may have hyperresonant note).

Auscultation Breath sounds decreased vesicular or absent over area. Voice sounds variable, usually decreased or absent over affected area.

Adventitious Sounds None if bronchus is obstructed. Occasional fine crackles if bronchus is patent.

Continued

TABLE 19.9	Assessment of Common Respiratory Conditions—cont'd

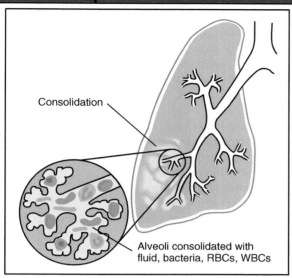

Consolidation

Alveoli consolidated with fluid, bacteria, RBCs, WBCs

◀ Lobar Pneumonia

Condition Infection in lung parenchyma leaves alveolar membrane edematous and porous; thus red blood cells (RBCs) and white blood cells (WBCs) pass from blood to alveoli. Alveoli progressively fill up (become consolidated) with bacteria, solid cellular debris, fluid, and blood cells, which replace alveolar air. This decreases surface area of the respiratory membrane, causing hypoxemia.

History Fever, cough with pleuritic chest pain, blood-tinged sputum, chills, SOB, fatigue.

Inspection Increased respirations >24/min. Guarding and lag on expansion on affected side. Children—Sternal retraction, nasal flaring.

Palpation Pulse >100 bpm, chest expansion decreased on affected side. Tactile fremitus increased if bronchus patent, decreased if bronchus obstructed.

Percussion Dull over lobar pneumonia.

Auscultation Tachycardia. Loud bronchial breathing with patent bronchus. Voice sounds have increased clarity; bronchophony, egophony, whispered pectoriloquy present. Children—Diminished breath sounds may occur early.

Adventitious Sounds Crackles, fine to medium.

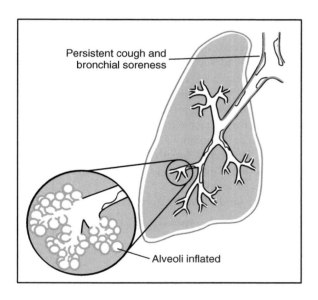

Persistent cough and bronchial soreness

Alveoli inflated

◀ Acute Bronchitis

Condition An acute infection of the trachea and larger bronchi characterized by cough, lasting up to 3 weeks. Over 90% of cases are viral and do not require antibiotics. Epithelium of bronchi are inflamed and damaged, releasing proinflammatory mediators. Large airways are narrowed from capillary dilation, increased mucus production, loss of cilia function, and swelling of epithelium. More cases occur with smokers, aging adults, children, and in winter months.

Inspection Cough is productive or nonproductive. Also sore throat, low-grade fever, postnasal drip, fatigue, substernal aching.

Palpation No pain, no increased fremitus.

Percussion Resonance predominates.

Auscultation May be clear and equal bilaterally. No egophony.

Adventitious Sounds No crackles (distinguishes the consolidation of pneumonia, no wheeze).

Continued

TABLE 19.9	Assessment of Common Respiratory Conditions—cont'd

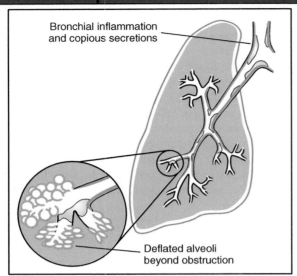

Bronchial inflammation and copious secretions

Deflated alveoli beyond obstruction

◀ **Chronic Bronchitis**

Condition Proliferation of mucus glands in the passageways, resulting in excessive mucus secretion. Inflammation of bronchi with partial obstruction of bronchi by secretions or constrictions. Sections of lung distal to obstruction may be deflated. Bronchitis may be acute or chronic with recurrent productive cough. Chronic bronchitis is usually caused by cigarette smoking.

Inspection Hacking, rasping cough productive of thick mucoid sputum. Chronic—Dyspnea, fatigue, cyanosis, possible clubbing of fingers.

Palpation Tactile fremitus normal.

Percussion Resonant.

Auscultation Normal vesicular. Voice sounds normal. Chronic—Prolonged expiration.

Adventitious Sounds Crackles over deflated areas. May have wheeze.

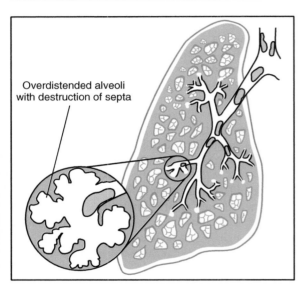

Overdistended alveoli with destruction of septa

◀ **Emphysema**

Condition Caused by destruction of pulmonary connective tissue (elastin, collagen); characterized by permanent enlargement of air sacs distal to terminal bronchioles and rupture of interalveolar walls. This increases airway resistance, especially on expiration, producing a hyperinflated lung and an increase in lung volume. Cigarette smoking accounts for 80% to 90% of cases of emphysema.

Inspection Increased AP diameter. Barrel chest. Accessory muscles used to aid respiration. Tripod position. SOB, especially on exertion. Respiratory distress. Tachypnea.

Palpation Decreased tactile fremitus and chest expansion.

Percussion Hyperresonant.

Auscultation Decreased breath sounds. May have prolonged expiration. Muffled heart sounds resulting from overdistention of lungs.

Adventitious Sounds Usually none; occasionally, wheeze.

Continued

TABLE 19.9 | Assessment of Common Respiratory Conditions—cont'd

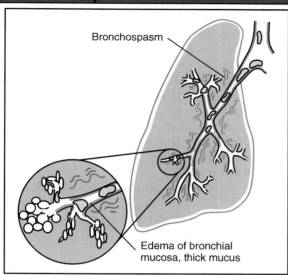

Bronchospasm

Edema of bronchial mucosa, thick mucus

◀ **Asthma (Reactive Airway Disease)**

Condition An allergic hypersensitivity to certain inhaled allergens (pollen), irritants (tobacco, ozone), microbes, stress, or exercise that produces a complex bronchospasm and inflammation, edema in walls of bronchioles, and secretion of highly viscous mucus. These factors greatly increase airway resistance, especially during expiration, and produce the wheezing, dyspnea, and chest tightness.

Inspection During severe attack: increased respiratory rate, SOB with audible wheeze, use of accessory neck muscles, cyanosis, apprehension, retraction of intercostal spaces. Expiration labored, prolonged. When chronic, may have barrel chest.

Palpation Tactile fremitus decreased, tachycardia.

Percussion Resonant. May be hyperresonant if chronic.

Auscultation Diminished air movement. Breath sounds decreased, with prolonged expiration. Voice sounds decreased.

Adventitious Sounds Bilateral wheezing on expiration, sometimes inspiratory and expiratory wheezing.

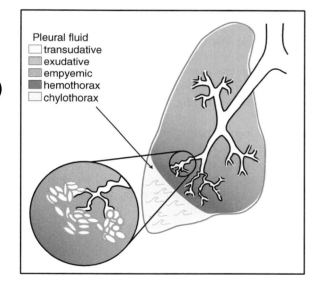

Pleural fluid
☐ transudative
☐ exudative
☐ empyemic
■ hemothorax
☐ chylothorax

◀ **Pleural Effusion (Fluid) or Thickening**

Condition Collection of excess fluid in intrapleural space, with compression of overlying lung tissue. Effusion may contain watery capillary fluid (transudative), protein (exudative), purulent matter (empyemic), blood (hemothorax), or milky lymphatic fluid (chylothorax). Gravity settles fluid in dependent areas of thorax. Presence of fluid subdues all lung sounds. Most common cause is heart failure; also infection and cancer.[15]

Inspection Increased respirations, dyspnea; may have dry cough, tachycardia, cyanosis, asymmetric expansion, abdominal distention.

Palpation Tactile fremitus decreased or absent. Tracheal shift away from affected side. Chest expansion decreased on affected side.

Percussion Dull percussion over affected area.

Auscultation Breath sounds decreased or absent. Voice sounds decreased or absent. When remainder of lung is compressed, may have bronchial breath sounds over the compression along with bronchophony, egophony, whispered pectoriloquy.

Adventitious Sounds Crackles, pleural rub.

Continued

TABLE 19.9 Assessment of Common Respiratory Conditions—cont'd

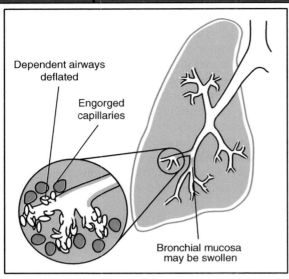

Dependent airways deflated
Engorged capillaries
Bronchial mucosa may be swollen

◀ **Heart Failure**

Condition Pump failure with increasing pressure of cardiac overload causes pulmonary congestion or an increased amount of blood present in pulmonary capillaries. Dependent air sacs deflated. Pulmonary capillaries engorged. Bronchial mucosa may be swollen.

Inspection Increased respiratory rate, SOB on exertion, orthopnea, paroxysmal nocturnal dyspnea, nocturia, ankle edema, pallor in light-skinned people.

Palpation Skin moist, clammy. Tactile fremitus normal.

Percussion Resonant.

Auscultation Normal vesicular. Heart sounds include S_3 gallop.

Adventitious Sounds Crackles at lung bases.

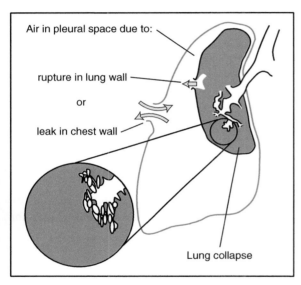

Air in pleural space due to:
rupture in lung wall
or
leak in chest wall
Lung collapse

◀ **Pneumothorax**

Condition Free air in pleural space causes partial or complete lung collapse. Air in pleural space neutralizes the usual negative pressure present; thus lung collapses. Usually unilateral. Pneumothorax can be (1) **spontaneous** (air enters pleural space through rupture in lung wall, (2) **traumatic** (air enters through opening or injury in chest wall), or (3) **tension** (trapped air in pleural space increases, compressing lung and shifting mediastinum to the unaffected side).

Inspection Unequal chest expansion. If large, tachypnea, cyanosis, apprehension, bulging in interspaces.

Palpation Tactile fremitus decreased or absent. Tracheal shift to opposite side (unaffected side). Chest expansion decreased on affected side. Tachycardia, decreased BP.

Percussion Hyperresonant.

Auscultation Breath sounds decreased or absent. Voice sounds decreased or absent.

Adventitious Sounds None.

Continued

TABLE 19.9   Assessment of Common Respiratory Conditions—cont'd

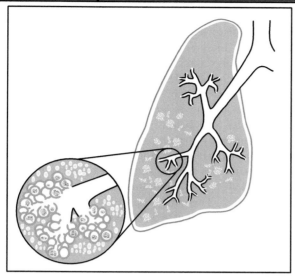

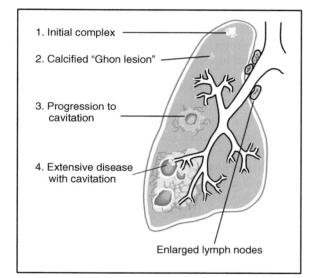

1. Initial complex
2. Calcified "Ghon lesion"
3. Progression to cavitation
4. Extensive disease with cavitation

Enlarged lymph nodes

◄ *Pneumocystis jiroveci (P. carinii)* Pneumonia

Condition This virulent form of pneumonia is a protozoal infection associated with AIDS. The parasite *P. jiroveci (P. carinii)* is common in the United States and harmless to most people, except to the immunocompromised, in whom a diffuse interstitial pneumonitis ensues. Cysts containing the organism and macrophages form in alveolar spaces, alveolar walls thicken, and the disease spreads to bilateral interstitial infiltrates of foamy, protein-rich fluid.

Inspection Anxiety, SOB, dyspnea on exertion, malaise are common; also tachypnea; fever; a dry, nonproductive cough; intercostal retractions in children; cyanosis.

Palpation Decreased chest expansion.

Percussion Dull over areas of diffuse infiltrate.

Auscultation Breath sounds may be diminished.

Adventitious Sounds Crackles may be present but often are absent.

◄ Tuberculosis

Condition Inhalation of tubercle bacilli into the alveolar wall starts: (1) Initial complex is acute inflammatory response—macrophages engulf bacilli but do not kill them. Tubercle forms around bacilli. (2) Scar tissue forms; lesion calcifies and shows on x-ray. (3) Reactivation of previously healed lesion. Dormant bacilli now multiply, producing necrosis, cavitation, and caseous lung tissue (cheeselike). (4) Extensive destruction as lesion erodes into bronchus, forming air-filled cavity. Apex usually has the most damage.

Subjective Initially asymptomatic, showing as positive skin test or on x-ray study. Progressive TB involves weight loss, anorexia, easy fatigability, low-grade afternoon fevers, night sweats. May have pleural effusion, recurrent lower respiratory infections.

Inspection Cough initially nonproductive, later productive of purulent, yellow-green sputum; may be blood tinged. Dyspnea, orthopnea, fatigue, weakness.

Palpation Skin moist at night from night sweats.

Percussion Resonant initially. Dull over any effusion.

Auscultation Normal or decreased vesicular breath sounds.

Adventitious Sounds Crackles over upper lobes common, persist following full expiration and cough.

Continued

TABLE 19.9 | Assessment of Common Respiratory Conditions—cont'd

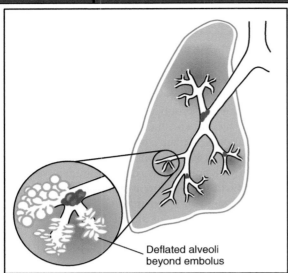

Deflated alveoli beyond embolus

◄ **Pulmonary Embolism**

Condition Undissolved materials (e.g., thrombus or air bubbles, fat globules) originating in legs or pelvis detach and travel through venous system, returning blood to right heart, and lodge to occlude pulmonary vessels. Over 95% arise from deep vein thrombi in lower legs as a result of stasis of blood, vessel injury, or hypercoagulability. Pulmonary occlusion results in ischemia of downstream lung tissue, increased pulmonary artery pressure, decreased cardiac output, and hypoxia. Rarely, a saddle embolus in bifurcation of pulmonary arteries leads to sudden death from hypoxia. More often small-to-medium pulmonary branches occlude, leading to dyspnea. These may resolve by fibrolytic activity.

Subjective Chest pain, worse on deep inspiration, dyspnea.

Inspection Apprehensive, restless, anxiety, mental status changes, cyanosis, tachypnea, cough, hemoptysis, PaO_2 <80% on pulse oximetry. Arterial blood gases show respiratory alkalosis.

Palpation Diaphoresis, hypotension.

Auscultation Tachycardia, accentuated pulmonic component of S_2 heart sound.

Adventitious Sounds Crackles, wheezes.

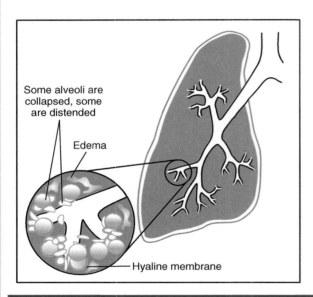

Some alveoli are collapsed, some are distended

Edema

Hyaline membrane

◄ **Acute Respiratory Distress Syndrome (ARDS)**

Condition An acute pulmonary insult (trauma, gastric acid aspiration, shock, sepsis) damages alveolar capillary membrane, leading to increased permeability of pulmonary capillaries and alveolar epithelium and to pulmonary edema. Gross examination (autopsy) would show dark red, firm, airless tissue, with some alveoli collapsed and hyaline membranes lining the distended alveoli.

Subjective Acute onset of dyspnea, apprehension.

Inspection Restlessness; disorientation; rapid, shallow breathing; productive cough; thin, frothy sputum; retractions of intercostal spaces and sternum. Decreased PaO_2, blood gases show respiratory alkalosis, x-ray films show diffuse pulmonary infiltrates; a late sign is cyanosis.

Palpation Hypotension.

Auscultation Tachycardia.

Adventitious Sounds Crackles, rhonchi.

Continued

TABLE 19.9	Assessment of Common Respiratory Conditions—cont'd

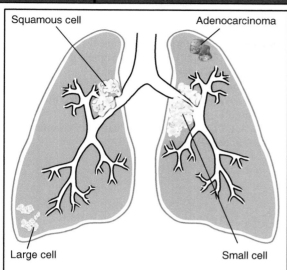

◀ **Lung Cancer**

Condition This is the most fatal of malignancies, claiming as many lives per year as breast, colorectal, and prostate cancers combined.[2] The major cause is tobacco smoking (90%), followed by exposure to secondhand smoke and asbestos exposure. Four types: squamous cell usually starts in central bronchi near the hilus; adenocarcinoma usually starts in periphery and escapes early detection; large cell also starts in periphery with tumors arranged as clusters; small cell (oat cell) compresses and narrows central bronchi.

Subjective Fatigue, nausea and vomiting, change in taste perception, anorexia. Persistent cough may also be productive; dyspnea; dull poorly localized chest pain. 10% to 25% are asymptomatic.

Inspection Weight loss, clubbing, hoarseness, anemia, hemoptysis, decreased O_2 saturation on oximetry

Auscultation May have wheezing, atelectasis, pleural effusion, pneumonia distal to obstruction.

Summary Checklist: Thorax and Lung Examination

1. **Inspection**
   Thoracic cage
   Respirations
   Skin color and condition
   Person's position
   Facial expression
   Level of consciousness

2. **Palpation**
   Confirm symmetric expansion
   Tactile fremitus
   Detect any lumps, masses, tenderness

3. **Percussion**
   Percuss over lung fields

4. **Auscultation**
   Assess normal breath sounds
   Note any abnormal breath sounds
   If abnormal breath sounds present, perform bronchophony, whispered pectoriloquy, egophony
   Note any adventitious sounds

REFERENCES

1. American Cancer Society (ACS). (2017). *Cancer Facts & Figures 2017.* https://www.cancer.org/cancer-facts-and-figures-2017.pdf.
2. Banisik, J. L., & Copstead, L. C. (2019). *Pathophysiology* (6th ed.). St. Louis: Elsevier.
3. Bohadana, A., Izbicki, G., & Kraman, S. S. (2014). Fundamentals of lung auscultation. *N Engl J Med, 370*(8), 744–751.
3a. Carlsten, C., & Rider, C. F. (2017). Traffic-related air pollution and allergic disease: an update in the context of global urbanization. *Curr Opin Allergy Clin Immunol, 17*(2), 85–89.
4. Centers for Disease Control and Prevention (CDC). (2017). *Health effects of secondhand smoke.* https://www.cdc.gov/tobacco/data_statistics/fact_sheets/secondhand_smoke/health_effects/index.htm.
5. Centers for Disease Control and Prevention (CDC). (2017). *Most recent asthma data.* https://www.cdc.gov/asthma/most_recent_data.htm.
6. Duby, J. C., & Langkamp, D. L. (2015). Another reason to avoid second-hand smoke. *J Pediatr, 167*(2), 224–225.
7. Durham, C. O., Fowler, T., Smith, W., et al. (2017). Adult asthma: Diagnosis and treatment. *Nurse Pract, 42*(11), 16–25.
8. Fujimoto, Y., Oki, Y., Kaneko, M., et al. (2017). Usefulness of the desaturation–distance ratio from the six-minute walk test for patients with COPD. *Int J Chron Obstruct Pulmon Dis, 12,* 2669–2675.
9. Hanania, N. A., Mannino, D. M., Yawn, B. P., et al. (2010). Predicting risk of airflow obstruction in primary care: Validation of the lung function questionnaire (LFQ). *Respir Med, 104*(8), 1160–1170.
10. Johnson, C., Moore, A., & Patterson-Johnson, J. (2017). Tuberculosis: Still an emerging threat. *Nurse Pract, 42*(7), 46–51.
11. Leveno, K. L., Corton, M. M., Dashe, J. S., et al. (2018). *Williams obstetrics* (25th ed.). New York: McGraw-Hill Education.
12. Li, R., Dee, D., Li, C., et al. (2014). Breastfeeding and risk of infections at 6 years. *Pediatrics, 134*(Suppl. 1), S13–S20.

13. McGeachie, J. J., Yates, K. P., Zhou, X., et al. (2016). Patterns of growth and decline in lung function in persistent childhood asthma. *N Engl J Med, 374*(19), 1842–1851.

14. McGee, S. (2018). *Evidence-based physical diagnosis* (4th ed.). St. Louis: Elsevier.

15. Ray, A., Masch, W. R., Saukkonen, K., et al. (2016). Case 18-2016: A 52-year-old-woman with a pleural effusion. *N Engl J Med, 374*, 24, 2378–2387.

16. Schmit, K. M., Wansaula, Z., Pratt, R., et al. (2017). Tuberculosis – United States, 2016. *MMWR Morb Mortal Wkly Rep, 66*, 289–294.

17. Stevens, J. P., Baker, K., Howell, M. D., et al. (2016). Prevalence and predictive value of dyspnea ratings in hospitalized patients: Pilot studies. *PLoS ONE, 11*(4), e0152601, 1–11.

18. Swanton, C., & Govindan, R. (2016). Clinical implications of genomic discoveries in lung cancer. *N Engl J Med, 374*, 19, 1864–1873.

19. U.S. Department of Health and Human Services. (2013). *Five A's of counseling patients to quit smoking.* https://www.ahrq .gov/professionals/clinicians-providers/guidelines_ recommendations/tobacco/5steps.html.

20. U.S. Environmental Protection Agency. (2017). *Asthma facts.* https://www.epa.gov/sites/production/files/2017-08/ documents/2017_asthma_fact_sheet.pdf.

21. Wahls, S. A. (2012). Causes and evaluation of chronic dyspnea. *Am Fam Physician, 86*(2), 173–180.

CHAPTER 20

Heart and Neck Vessels

http://evolve.elsevier.com/Jarvis/

STRUCTURE AND FUNCTION

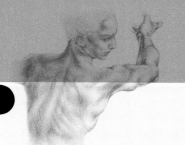

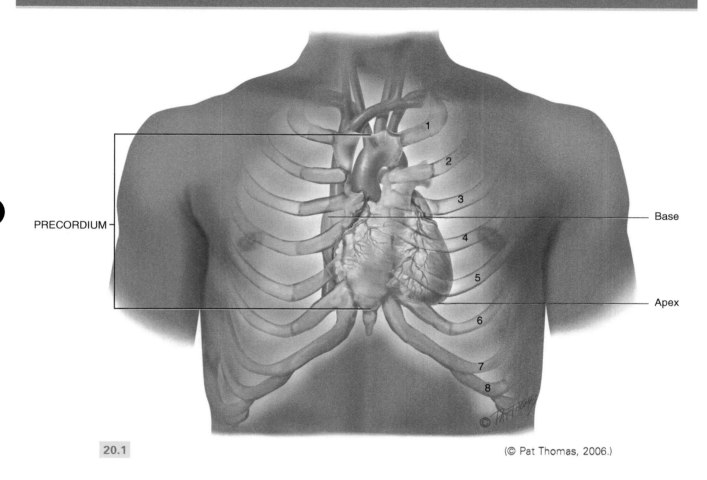

PRECORDIUM

1
2
3
Base
4
5
Apex
6
7
8

20.1

(© Pat Thomas, 2006.)

POSITION AND SURFACE LANDMARKS

The cardiovascular (CV) system consists of the **heart** (a muscular pump) and the **blood vessels.** The **precordium** is the area on the anterior chest directly overlying the heart and great vessels (Fig. 20.1). The great vessels are the major arteries and veins connected to the heart. The heart and great vessels are located between the lungs in the middle third of the thoracic cage **(mediastinum).** The heart extends from the 2nd to the 5th intercostal space and from the right border of the sternum to the left midclavicular line.

Inside the body the heart is rotated so its right side is anterior and its left side is mostly posterior. Of the heart's four chambers, the right ventricle is immediately behind the sternum and forms the greatest area of anterior cardiac surface. The left ventricle lies behind the right ventricle and forms the apex and slender area of the left border. The right atrium lies to the right and above the right ventricle and forms the right border. The left atrium is located posteriorly, with only a small portion, the left atrial appendage, showing anteriorly.

451

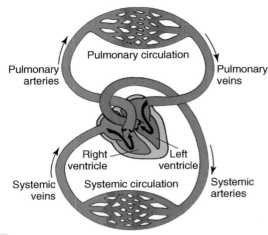

20.2   Two loops—separate but interdependent.

The blood vessels are arranged in two continuous loops, the *pulmonary circulation* and the *systemic circulation* (Fig. 20.2). When the heart contracts, it pumps blood simultaneously into both loops.

Think of the heart as an upside-down triangle in the chest. The "top" of the heart is the broader *base,* and the "bottom" is the *apex,* which points down and to the left (Fig. 20.3). During contraction the apex beats against the chest wall, producing an apical impulse. This is palpable in most people, normally at the fifth intercostal space, 7 to 9 cm from the midsternal line.

The **great vessels** lie bunched above the base of the heart. The **superior** and **inferior vena cava** return unoxygenated venous blood to the right side of the heart. The **pulmonary artery** leaves the right ventricle, bifurcates, and carries the venous blood to the lungs. The **pulmonary veins** return the freshly oxygenated blood to the left side of the heart, and the **aorta** carries it out to the body. The aorta ascends from the left ventricle, arches back at the level of the sternal angle, and descends behind the heart.

HEART WALL, CHAMBERS, AND VALVES

The **heart wall** has numerous layers. The **pericardium** is a tough, fibrous, double-walled sac that surrounds and protects the heart (see its cut edge in Fig. 20.4). It has two layers that contain a few milliliters of serous *pericardial fluid.* This ensures smooth, friction-free movement of the heart muscle. The pericardium is adherent to the great vessels, esophagus, sternum, and pleurae and is anchored to the diaphragm. The **myocardium** is the muscular wall of the heart; it does the pumping. The **endocardium** is the thin layer of endothelial tissue that lines the inner surface of the heart chambers and valves.

The common metaphor is to think of the heart as a pump. But consider that the heart is actually *two* pumps; the right side of the heart pumps blood into the lungs, and the left side simultaneously pumps blood into the body. The two pumps are separated by an impermeable wall, the septum. Each side has an **atrium** and a **ventricle.** The atrium (Latin for "anteroom") is a thin-walled reservoir for holding blood, and the thick-walled ventricle is the muscular pumping chamber. (It is common to use the following abbreviations to refer to the chambers: *RA,* right atrium; *RV,* right ventricle; *LA,* left atrium; and *LV,* left ventricle.)

The four **chambers** are separated by swinging-door–like structures, called *valves,* whose main purpose is to prevent backflow of blood. The valves are unidirectional; they can open only one way. They open and close *passively* in response to pressure gradients in the moving blood.

There are four **valves** in the heart (see Fig. 20.4). The two **atrioventricular** (AV) valves separate the atria and the ventricles. The right AV valve is the **tricuspid,** and the left AV valve is the bicuspid or **mitral** valve. The valves' thin leaflets are anchored by collagenous fibers (**chordae tendineae**) to papillary muscles embedded in the ventricle floor. The AV valves open during the heart's filling phase, or **diastole,** to allow the ventricles to fill with blood. During the pumping phase, or **systole,** the AV valves close to prevent regurgitation

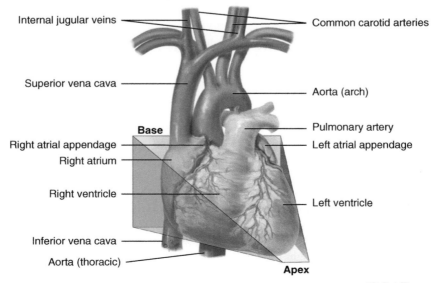

20.3

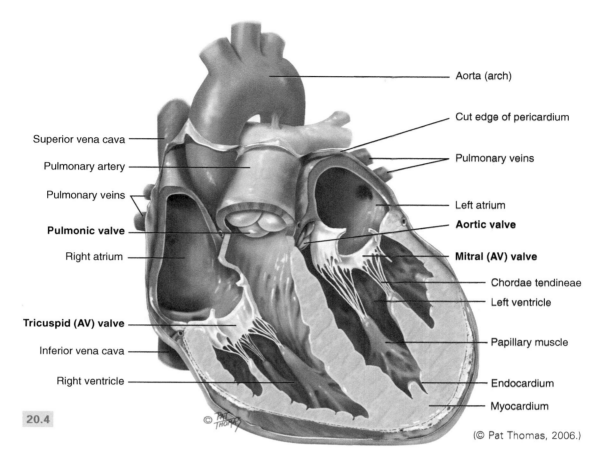

Aorta (arch)

Cut edge of pericardium

Superior vena cava

Pulmonary veins

Pulmonary artery

Pulmonary veins

Left atrium

Aortic valve

Pulmonic valve

Right atrium

Mitral (AV) valve

Chordae tendineae

Left ventricle

Tricuspid (AV) valve

Papillary muscle

Inferior vena cava

Right ventricle

Endocardium

Myocardium

20.4

(© Pat Thomas, 2006.)

of blood back up into the atria. The papillary muscles contract at this time so the valve leaflets meet and unite to form a perfect seal without turning themselves inside out.

The **semilunar** (SL) valves are set between the ventricles and the arteries. Each valve has three cusps that look like half moons. The SL valves are the **pulmonic** valve in the right side of the heart and the **aortic** valve in the left side of the heart. They open during pumping (**systole),** when blood ejects from the heart.

NOTE: There are no valves between the vena cava and the right atrium or between the pulmonary veins and the left atrium. For this reason abnormally high pressure in the left side of the heart gives a person symptoms of pulmonary congestion, and abnormally high pressure in the right side of the heart shows in the distended neck veins and abdomen.

DIRECTION OF BLOOD FLOW

Think of an unoxygenated red blood cell being drained downstream into the vena cava. It is swept along with the flow of venous blood and follows the route illustrated in Fig. 20.5.
1. From liver to RA through inferior vena cava.
   Superior vena cava drains venous blood from the head and
   upper extremities.
   From RA venous blood travels through tricuspid valve
   to RV.
2. From RV venous blood flows through pulmonic valve to
   pulmonary artery.
   Pulmonary artery delivers unoxygenated blood to lungs.

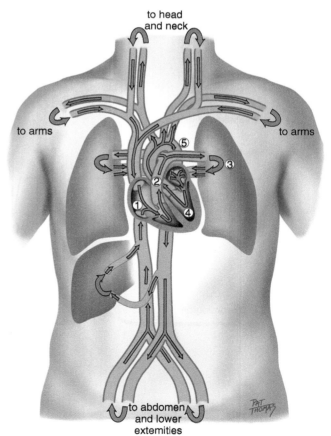

to head
and neck

to arms

to arms

to abdomen
and lower
extremities

20.5

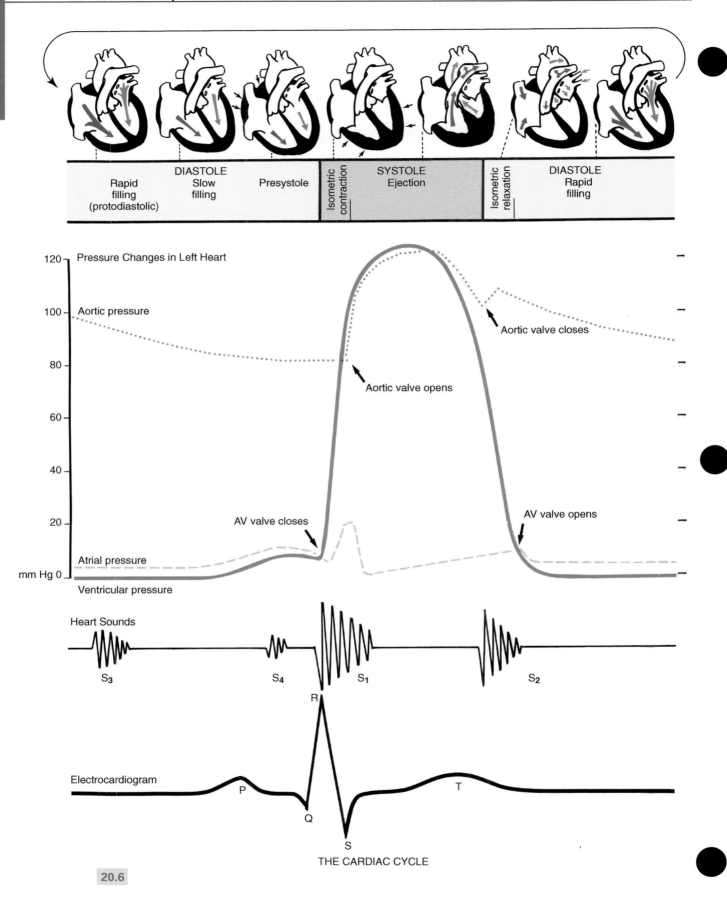

Rapid filling (protodiastolic)

DIASTOLE Slow filling

Presystole

Isometric contraction

SYSTOLE Ejection

Isometric relaxation

DIASTOLE Rapid filling

120

Pressure Changes in Left Heart

100

Aortic pressure

Aortic valve closes

80

Aortic valve opens

60

40

AV valve opens

20

AV valve closes

Atrial pressure

mm Hg 0

Ventricular pressure

Heart Sounds

S₃

S₄

S₁

S₂

R

Electrocardiogram

P

Q

S

T

THE CARDIAC CYCLE

20.6

3. Lungs oxygenate blood.
   Pulmonary veins return fresh blood to LA.
4. From LA arterial blood travels through mitral valve to LV.
   LV ejects blood through aortic valve into aorta.
5. Aorta delivers oxygenated blood to body.

Remember that the circulation is a continuous loop. The blood is kept moving by continually shifting pressure gradients. It flows from an area of higher pressure to one of lower pressure.

CARDIAC CYCLE

The rhythmic movement of blood through the heart is the **cardiac cycle.** It has two phases, **diastole** and **systole.** In **diastole** the ventricles relax and fill with blood. This takes up two-thirds of the cardiac cycle. Heart contraction is **systole.** During systole blood is pumped from the ventricles and fills the pulmonary and systemic arteries. This is one-third of the cardiac cycle.

Diastole. In diastole the ventricles are relaxed, and the AV valves (i.e., the tricuspid and mitral) are open (Fig. 20.6). (Opening of the normal valve is acoustically silent.) The pressure in the atria is higher than that in the ventricles; therefore blood pours rapidly into the ventricles. This first passive filling phase is called **early** or **protodiastolic filling.**

Toward the end of diastole the atria contract and push the last amount of blood (about 25% of stroke volume) into the ventricles. This active filling phase is called **presystole,** or **atrial systole,** or sometimes the *atrial kick*. It causes a small rise in left ventricular pressure. (Note that atrial systole occurs during ventricular diastole, a confusing but important point.)

Systole. Now so much blood has been pumped into the ventricles that ventricular pressure is finally higher than that in the atria; thus the mitral and tricuspid valves swing shut. The closure of the AV valves contributes to the first heart sound (**S₁**) and signals the beginning of systole. The AV valves close to prevent any regurgitation of blood back up into the atria during contraction.

For a very brief moment all four valves are closed. The ventricular walls contract. This contraction against a closed system works to build pressure inside the ventricles to a high level (**isometric contraction**). Consider first the left side of the heart. When the pressure in the ventricle finally exceeds pressure in the aorta, the aortic valve opens, and blood is ejected rapidly.

After the ventricle's contents are ejected, its pressure falls. When pressure falls below pressure in the aorta, some blood flows backward toward the ventricle, causing the aortic valve to swing shut. This closure of the semilunar valves causes the second heart sound (**S₂**) and signals the end of systole.

Diastole Again. Now all four valves are closed, and the ventricles relax (called **isometric** or **isovolumic relaxation**). Meanwhile the atria have been filling with blood delivered from the lungs. Atrial pressure is now higher than the relaxed ventricular pressure. The mitral valve drifts open, and diastolic filling begins again.

Events in the Right and Left Sides. The same events are happening at the same time in the right side of the heart, but pressures in the right side of the heart are much lower than those of the left side because less energy is needed to pump blood to its destination, the pulmonary circulation. Also, events occur just slightly later in the right side of the heart because of the route of myocardial depolarization. As a result, two distinct components to each of the heart sounds exist, and sometimes you can hear them separately. In the first heart sound the mitral component (**M₁**) closes just before the tricuspid component (**T₁**). And with **S₂**, aortic closure (**A₂**) occurs slightly before pulmonic closure (**P₂**).

HEART SOUNDS

Events in the cardiac cycle generate sounds that can be heard through a stethoscope over the chest wall. These include normal heart sounds and occasionally extra heart sounds and murmurs (Fig. 20.7).

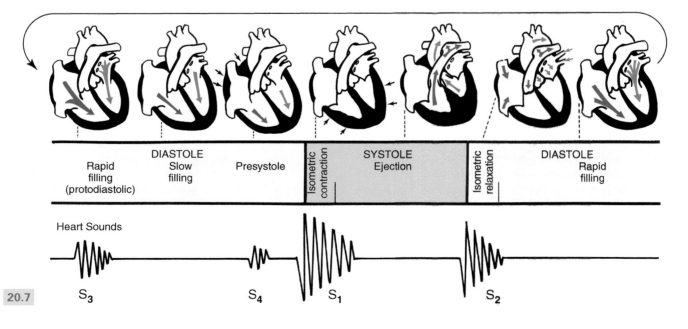

	DIASTOLE			Isometric contraction	SYSTOLE Ejection	Isometric relaxation	DIASTOLE
Rapid filling (protodiastolic)	Slow filling	Presystole					Rapid filling

Heart Sounds

S₃   S₄   S₁   S₂

Normal Heart Sounds

The **first heart sound** (**S₁**) occurs with closure of the AV valves and thus signals the beginning of systole. The mitral component of the first sound (M_1) slightly precedes the tricuspid component (T_1), but you usually hear these two components fused as one sound. You can hear S_1 over all the precordium, but usually it is loudest at the apex.

The **second heart sound** (**S₂**) occurs with closure of the semilunar valves and signals the end of systole. The aortic component of the second sound (A_2) slightly precedes the pulmonic component (P_2). Although it is heard over all the precordium, S_2 is loudest at the base.

Effect of Respiration. The volume of right and left ventricular systole is just about equal, but this can be affected by respiration. To learn this, consider the phrase:

> Mo**R**e to the **R**ight heart,
> **L**ess to the **L**eft

That means that during inspiration, intrathoracic pressure is decreased. This pushes more blood into the vena cava, increasing venous return to the right side of the heart, which increases right ventricular stroke volume. The increased volume prolongs right ventricular systole and delays pulmonic valve closure.

Meanwhile on the left side, a greater amount of blood is sequestered in the lungs during inspiration. This momentarily decreases the amount returned to the left side of the heart, decreasing left ventricular stroke volume. The decreased volume shortens left ventricular systole and allows the aortic valve to close a bit earlier. When the aortic valve closes significantly earlier than the pulmonic valve, you can hear the two components separately. This is a *split* S_2.

Extra Heart Sounds

Third Heart Sound (S₃). Normally diastole is a silent event. However, in some conditions ventricular filling creates vibrations that can be heard over the chest. These vibrations are S_3. S_3 occurs when the ventricles are resistant to filling during the early rapid filling phase (protodiastole). This occurs immediately after S_2, when the AV valves open and atrial blood first pours into the ventricles. (See a complete discussion of S_3 in Table 20.8, p. 491.)

Fourth Heart Sound (S₄). S_4 occurs at the end of diastole, at presystole, when the ventricle is resistant to filling. The atria contract and push blood into a noncompliant ventricle. This creates vibrations that are heard as S_4. S_4 occurs just before S_1.

Murmurs

Blood circulating through normal cardiac chambers and valves usually makes no noise. However, some conditions create turbulent blood flow and collision currents. These result in a murmur, much like a pile of stones or a sharp turn in a stream creates a noisy water flow. A murmur is a gentle, blowing, swooshing sound that can be heard on the chest wall. Conditions resulting in a murmur are as follows:

1. Velocity of blood increases (flow murmur) (e.g., in exercise, thyrotoxicosis)
2. Viscosity of blood decreases (e.g., in anemia)
3. Structural defects in the valves (a stenotic or narrowed valve, an incompetent or regurgitant valve) or unusual openings occur in the chambers (dilated chamber, septal defect)

Characteristics of Sound

All heart sounds are described by:

1. Frequency (pitch)—Heart sounds are described as high pitched or low pitched, although these terms are relative because all are low-frequency sounds, and you need a good stethoscope to hear them.
2. Intensity (loudness)—Loud or soft
3. Duration—Very short for heart sounds; silent periods are longer
4. Timing—Systole or diastole

CONDUCTION

Of all organs, the heart has a unique ability—automaticity. The heart can contract by itself, independent of any signals or stimulation from the body. It contracts in response to an electrical current conveyed by a conduction system (Fig. 20.8). Specialized cells in the sinoatrial (SA) node near the superior vena cava initiate an electrical impulse. (Because the SA node has an intrinsic rhythm, it is the "pacemaker.") The current flows in an orderly sequence, first across the atria to the AV node low in the atrial septum. There it is delayed slightly so the atria have time to contract before the ventricles are stimulated. Then the impulse travels to the bundle of His, the right and left bundle branches, and then through the ventricles.

The electrical impulse stimulates the heart to do its work, which is to contract. A small amount of electricity spreads to the body surface, where it can be measured and recorded on the electrocardiograph (ECG). The ECG waves are arbitrarily labeled *PQRST*, which stand for the following elements:

P wave—Depolarization of the atria
PR interval—From the beginning of the P wave to the beginning of the QRS complex (the time necessary for atrial depolarization plus time for the impulse to travel through the AV node to the ventricles)
QRS complex—Depolarization of the ventricles
T wave—Repolarization of the ventricles

Electrical events slightly *precede* the mechanical events in the heart. The ECG juxtaposed on the cardiac cycle is illustrated in Fig. 20.6.

PUMPING ABILITY

In the resting adult, the heart normally pumps between 4 and 6 L of blood per minute throughout the body. This **cardiac output** equals the volume of blood in each systole (called the *stroke volume)* times the number of beats per minute (rate). This is described as:

$$CO = SV \times R$$

The heart can alter its cardiac output to adapt to the

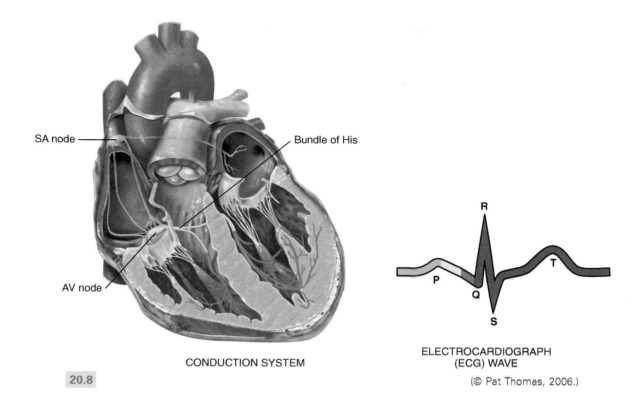

SA node	Bundle of His
AV node	

CONDUCTION SYSTEM

R

P   T

Q

S

ELECTROCARDIOGRAPH (ECG) WAVE

20.8

(© Pat Thomas, 2006.)

metabolic needs of the body. Preload and afterload affect the heart's ability to increase cardiac output.

Preload is volume—it is the venous return that builds during diastole. It is the length to which the ventricular muscle is stretched at the end of diastole just before contraction (Fig. 20.9).

When the volume of blood returned to the ventricles is increased (as when exercise stimulates skeletal muscles to contract and force more blood back to the heart), the muscle bundles are stretched beyond their normal resting state to accommodate. The force of this stretch is the preload. According to the Frank-Starling law, the greater the stretch, the stronger is the contraction of the heart. This increased contractility results in an increased volume of blood ejected (increased stroke volume).

Afterload is pressure—it is the opposing pressure the ventricle must generate to open the aortic valve against the higher aortic pressure. It is the resistance against which the ventricle must pump its blood. Once the ventricle is filled with blood, the ventricular end diastolic pressure is 5 to 10 mm Hg, whereas that in the aorta is 70 to 80 mm Hg. To overcome this difference, the ventricular muscle *tenses* (isovolumic contraction). After the aortic valve opens, rapid ejection occurs.

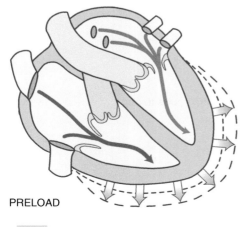

PRELOAD

20.9

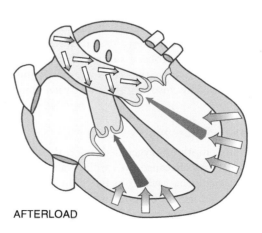

AFTERLOAD

(© Pat Thomas, 2006.)

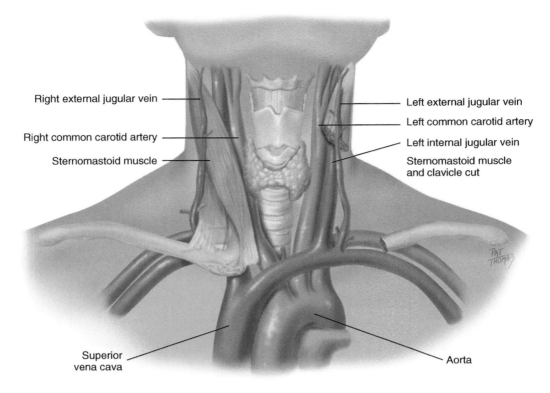

NECK VESSELS

20.10

THE NECK VESSELS

CV assessment includes the survey of vascular structures in the neck—the carotid artery and the jugular veins (Fig. 20.10). These vessels reflect the efficiency of cardiac function.

The Carotid Artery Pulse

Chapter 10 describes the pulse as a pressure wave generated by each systole pumping blood into the aorta. The carotid artery is a central artery (i.e., it is close to the heart). Its timing closely coincides with ventricular systole. (Assessment of the peripheral pulses follows in Chapter 21.)

The **carotid artery** is located in the groove between the trachea and the sternomastoid muscle, medial to and alongside that muscle. Note the characteristics of its waveform (Fig. 20.11): a smooth rapid upstroke, a summit that is rounded and smooth, and a downstroke that is more gradual and has a dicrotic notch caused by closure of the aortic valve (marked *D* in the figure).

Jugular Venous Pulse and Pressure

The **jugular veins** empty unoxygenated blood directly into the superior vena cava. Because no cardiac valve exists to separate the superior vena cava from the right atrium, the jugular veins give information about activity on the right side of the heart. Specifically they reflect filling pressure and volume changes. Because volume and pressure increase when

the right side of the heart fails to pump efficiently, the jugular veins reveal this.

Two jugular veins are present in each side of the neck (see Fig. 20.10). The larger **internal jugular** lies deep and medial to the sternomastoid muscle. It is usually not visible,

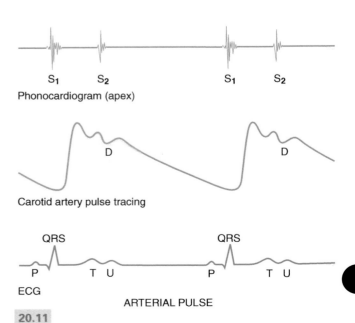

Phonocardiogram (apex)

Carotid artery pulse tracing

ECG

ARTERIAL PULSE

20.11

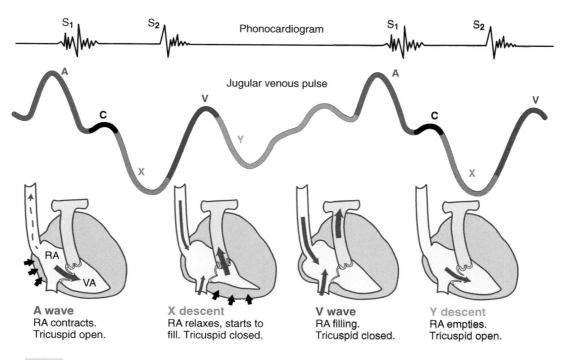

A wave
RA contracts.
Tricuspid open.

X descent
RA relaxes, starts to
fill. Tricuspid closed.

V wave
RA filling.
Tricuspid closed.

Y descent
RA empties.
Tricuspid open.

20.12   **Note:** Match color on waveform with its description.

although its diffuse pulsations may be seen in the sternal notch when the person is supine. The **external jugular** vein is more superficial; it lies lateral to the sternomastoid muscle, above the clavicle.

Although an arterial pulse is caused by a forward propulsion of blood, the jugular venous pulse is different. The jugular pulse results from a backwash, a waveform moving backward caused by events upstream. The jugular pulse has 5 components, as shown in Fig. 20.12.

The 5 components of the jugular venous pulse occur because of events in the right side of the heart. The A wave reflects atrial contraction because some blood flows backward to the vena cava during right atrial contraction. The C wave, or ventricular contraction, is backflow from the bulging upward of the tricuspid valve when it closes at the beginning of ventricular systole (not from the neighboring carotid artery pulsation). Next the X descent shows atrial relaxation when the right ventricle contracts during systole and pulls the bottom of the atria downward. The V wave occurs with passive atrial filling because of the increasing volume in the right atria and increased pressure. Finally the Y descent reflects passive ventricular filling when the tricuspid valve opens and blood flows from the RA to the RV.

✦ DEVELOPMENTAL COMPETENCE

The Pregnant Woman

The CV system adapts to ensure adequate blood supply to the uterus and placenta, to deliver oxygen and nutrients to the fetus, and to allow the mother to function normally during this altered state. Blood volume increases by 30% to 50% during pregnancy, with the most rapid expansion occurring during the second trimester. This creates an increase in stroke volume and cardiac output and an increased pulse rate of 10 to 20 beats/min. The pulse rate rises in the first trimester, peaks in the third trimester, and returns to baseline within the first 10 postpartum days.[11] Despite the increased cardiac output, arterial BP decreases in pregnancy as a result of peripheral vasodilation. The BP drops to its lowest point during the second trimester and rises after that.

Infants and Children

The fetal heart functions early; it begins to beat at the end of 3 weeks' gestation. The lungs are nonfunctional, but the fetal circulation compensates for this (Fig. 20.13). Oxygenation takes place at the placenta, and the arterial blood is returned to the right side of the fetal heart. There is no point in pumping all this freshly oxygenated blood through the lungs; therefore it is rerouted in two ways. First, about two-thirds of it is shunted through an opening in the atrial septum, the **foramen ovale,** into the left side of the heart, where it is pumped out through the aorta. Second, the rest of the oxygenated blood is pumped by the right side of the heart out through the pulmonary artery, but it is detoured through the **ductus arteriosus** to the aorta. Because they are both pumping into the systemic circulation, the right and left ventricles are equal in weight and muscle wall thickness.

Inflation and aeration of the lungs at birth produces circulatory changes. Now the blood is oxygenated through the

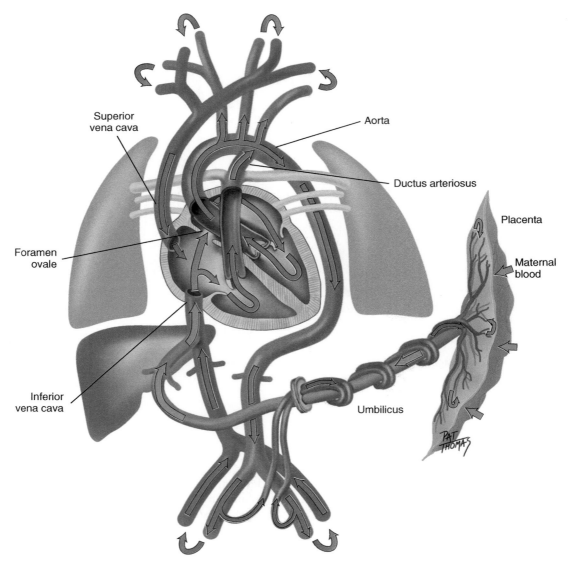

FETAL CIRCULATION
20.13

lungs rather than through the placenta. The foramen ovale closes within the first hour because of the new lower pressure in the right side of the heart than in the left side. The ductus arteriosus closes later, usually within 10 to 15 hours of birth. Now the left ventricle has the greater workload of pumping into the systemic circulation. So by the time the baby has reached 1 year of age, the mass of the left ventricle will have increased to reach the adult ratio of 2 : 1, left ventricle to right ventricle.

The heart's position in the chest is more horizontal in the infant than in the adult; thus the apex is higher, located at the fourth left intercostal space (Fig. 20.14). It reaches the adult position when the child reaches age 7 years.

The Aging Adult

It is difficult to isolate the "aging process" of the CV system *per se* because it is so closely interrelated with lifestyle, habits, and diseases. We know that lifestyle modifies the development of CV disease; smoking, diet, alcohol use, exercise patterns, and stress have an immense influence. Lifestyle also affects the aging process; cardiac changes once thought to be caused by aging are partially the result of the sedentary lifestyle accompanying aging (Fig. 20.15). What is left to be attributed to the aging process alone?

Hemodynamic Changes With Aging

With aging there is an increase in systolic BP, termed isolated systolic hypertension.[1] This is caused by thickening and stiffening of the large arteries, which in turn are caused by collagen and calcium deposits in vessel walls and loss of elastic fibers. This stiffening (arteriosclerosis) creates an increase in pulse wave velocity because the less compliant arteries cannot store the volume ejected.

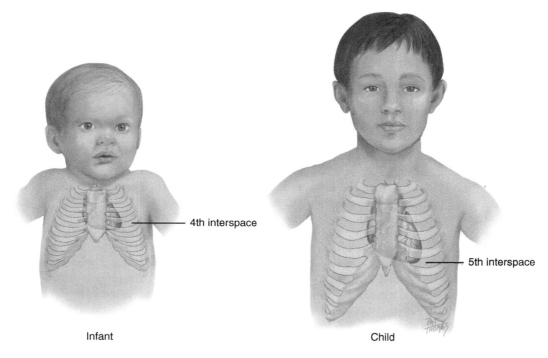

4th interspace

5th interspace

Infant

Child

HEART'S POSITION IN THE CHEST

20.14

The overall size of the heart does not increase with age, but left ventricular wall thickness increases. This is an adaptive mechanism to accommodate the vascular stiffening mentioned earlier that creates an increased workload on the heart.

Diastolic BP may decrease after the fifth decade.[1] Together with a rising systolic pressure, this increases the pulse pressure (the difference between the two).

No change in resting heart rate occurs with aging.

Cardiac output at rest is not changed with aging.

There is a decreased ability of the heart to augment cardiac output with exercise. This is shown by a decreased maximum heart rate with exercise and diminished sympathetic response. Noncardiac factors also cause a decrease in maximum work performance with aging: decrease in skeletal muscle performance, increase in muscle fatigue, increased sense of dyspnea. However, aerobic exercise conditioning modifies many of the aging changes in CV function.

Dysrhythmias. The presence of supraventricular and ventricular dysrhythmias increases with age. Ectopic beats are common in aging people; although these are usually asymptomatic in healthy older people, they may compromise cardiac output and BP when disease is present.

Tachydysrhythmias may not be tolerated as well in older people. The myocardium is thicker and less compliant, and early diastolic filling is impaired at rest. Thus it may not tolerate a tachycardia as well because of shortened diastole. Also, tachydysrhythmias may further compromise a vital organ whose function has already been affected by aging or disease.

Electrocardiograph. Age-related changes in the ECG occur as a result of histologic changes in the conduction system. These changes include:

- Prolonged P-R interval (first-degree AV block) and prolonged Q-T interval, but the QRS interval is unchanged.
- Left axis deviation from age-related mild LV hypertrophy and fibrosis in left bundle branch.
- Increased incidence of bundle branch block.

Although the hemodynamic changes associated with aging alone do not seem severe or portentous, the fact remains that the incidence of CV disease (CVD) increases with age. CVD is the leading cause of death in those ages 65 years and older. Certainly, lifestyle habits (smoking, chronic

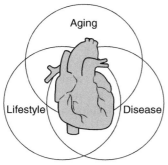

Aging

Lifestyle

Disease

20.15

(Lakatta, 1985.)

Structure and Function

alcohol use, obesity, lack of exercise, diet) play a significant role in the acquisition of heart disease. Also, increasing the physical activity of older adults—even at a moderate level—shows a reduced risk of death from CVDs and respiratory illnesses. Thus health teaching is a crucial treatment parameter.

 CULTURE AND GENETICS

Cardiovascular disease (CVD) is the most common underlying cause of death in the world, causing 31.5% of all global deaths.[3] About 80% of CVD deaths occur in low- and middle-income countries and occur almost equally in males and females.[2] There are cost-effective medications (aspirin, statins, and BP-lowering agents) to mitigate CVD burden, but these remain unaffordable for much of the world. In the United States, the projections are that by 2030, 43.9% of the adult population will have some form of CVD.[3]

However, between 2004 and 2014, death rates attributable to CVD declined 25.3%.[3] This may be due to early and sophisticated cardiac interventions and to stepped-up health teaching (such as smoking cessation), but these measures are not shared equally by all income groups in the United States. Also, CVD data have a geographic difference. Recent national data show a lessening in the decline in heart disease mortality, especially in younger adults.[22] Over 50% of U.S. counties showed increases in heart disease mortality among adults ages 35 to 64 years. These increases occurred in rural counties and in counties in medium and small cities. Further, these mortality increases occurred at the same time as increases in obesity and diabetes prevalence.

Inherited DNA variation and lifestyle factors each contribute independently to the development of a major form of CVD, that of coronary artery disease (CAD).[12] In our genetic code, there are 50 different DNA locations associated with the risk of CAD, and a high polygenic risk score is significant for the risk of CAD events (myocardial infarction, coronary revascularization, and death). However, among persons with a high genetic risk, adopting a favorable lifestyle is associated with a 46% lower risk of CAD events than is an unfavorable lifestyle.[12] A favorable lifestyle includes four healthful factors—no current smoking, no obesity (i.e., BMI <30), physical activity at least once per week, and a healthy diet (i.e., fruits, nuts, vegetables, whole grains, fish, and dairy products, with lesser amounts of refined grains, processed meats, red meats, sugary drinks, trans fats, and sodium).[12] This evidence quantifies the interaction between genetics and lifestyle risk factors and shows that at every level of genetic risk, adopting a healthy lifestyle is associated with a significant drop in the risk of CAD events.

High Blood Pressure. Untreated hypertension causes direct damage to the arterial system. Further, hypertension contributes to CAD because it accelerates the process of atherosclerosis; it increases the workload on the heart, and it increases the oxygen demand on the heart already compromised by atherosclerosis. More men than women have hypertension up to age 64 years; those ≥65 years show a higher percentage of women than men with hypertension.[3] The prevalence of hypertension in black Americans is among the highest in the world. The most recent prevalence statistics show hypertension in 45.0% and 46.3% of non-Hispanic black men and women; 34.5% and 32.3% among non-Hispanic white men and women; 28.8% and 25.7% among Asian men and women; and 28.9% and 30.7% among Hispanic men and women.[3] Compared with whites, African Americans develop high BP earlier in life, and their average BPs are much higher. This results in a greater rate of stroke, death from heart disease, and end-stage kidney disease for African Americans.

Smoking. Smoking increases the risk of CVD by increasing the oxygen demand on the heart while causing a concomitant decrease in oxygen supply, by an activation of platelets and fibrinogen, and by an adverse change in the lipid profile. Since the U.S. surgeon general's first report on the health risks of smoking, rates of smoking among adults have decreased—from 51% of men and 34% of women in 1965 to 16.5% of men and 13.7% of women in 2015.[3] This sharp decrease in smoking is in great measure one reason for the sharp decline in the CVD death rate during the same time period. One problem is that smoking rates increase as family income declines. Among adults ≥18 years of age living below the poverty level, 26.3% are current smokers, whereas among those living at or above the poverty level, 15.2% are current smokers.[3] There are many reasons for this, and none have simple answers.

Serum Cholesterol. High levels of low-density lipoprotein (LDL, or the "bad" cholesterol) add to the lipid core of plaque formation in coronary and carotid arteries, which results in MI and stroke. The U.S. prevalence of high levels of LDL cholesterol decreased from 43% in 2000 to 28.5% in 2014; in the same time period we saw the use of cholesterol-lowering statin drugs increase from 7% to 17%.[3]

Physical Activity (PA). PA has beneficial effects on high-density lipoprotein (HDL, or the "good" cholesterol), vitamin D, apolipoprotein B, and hemoglobin A1c. The PA guidelines for adults show that about 150 min/week of moderate-intensity aerobic activity, compared with none, can reduce the risk of CVD.[3] PA does not need to be vigorous. Evidence involving 1.1 million females without prior vascular disease and followed about 9 years showed that those who reported moderate activity had a lower risk of CVD, whereas strenuous PA was not as beneficial.[3]

Sex and Gender Differences. The leading cause of death in women is CVD, claiming more lives than cancer, chronic lower respiratory disease, and diabetes mellitus combined.[3] Sex differences are the biologic result of one chromosome difference between men (XY) and women (XX); e.g., women tend to have smaller coronary arteries than men.[16] Gender differences involve ethnicity, culture, and socioeconomic status, and these factors are closely involved in cardiac risk factors and cardiac risk lifestyle behaviors, e.g., obesity, smoking, physical activity, cardiac rehabilitation participation, delay in seeking treatment.[5,16] Because 80% of heart disease is preventable, gender differences have a greater influence in women's outcomes than do sex differences.

One reason women tend to delay seeking care for CVD is that their symptom cluster is different from men's. Women may not experience the crushing chest pain that is the most widely publicized symptom of heart disease. Women are more likely to experience prodromal symptoms for weeks or months before an acute cardiac syndrome (ACS). Prodromal symptoms are those that are intermittent and resolve spontaneously.[16] The most common prodromal symptom linked with ACS is fatigue.[4] Four prodromal symptoms linked with ACS are discomfort in the jaw or teeth, unusual fatigue, arm pain, and shortness of breath. At the time of having ACS, women are more likely to report fatigue, nausea, neck pain,

right arm pain, jaw pain, dizziness, and syncope than are men.[16] Providers are less likely to consider the women's symptoms as cardiac-related and may not take them seriously; this may shake women's confidence in their ability to link their symptoms as cardiac-related, which further delays women in seeking prompt treatment later when the symptoms grow more severe.[10] An ongoing prospective study that includes over a thousand patients currently reports that women with ACS were less likely to list chest pain as their primary symptom and likely to report more nausea, shoulder pain, and upper back pain.[8] Further, women with ACS report more symptoms when compared with men. These findings should increase awareness in patients and in clinicians that ACS is not always hallmarked by chest pain and that multiple symptoms may be present at the same time.

SUBJECTIVE DATA

1. Chest pain
2. Dyspnea
3. Orthopnea
4. Cough

5. Fatigue
6. Cyanosis or pallor
7. Edema
8. Nocturia

9. Past cardiac history
10. Family cardiac history
11. Patient-centered care (cardiac risk factors)

Examiner Asks	Rationale
1. Chest pain. Any **chest pain** or tightness? • Onset: When did it start? How long have you had it *this* time? Had this type of pain before? How often? • Location: Where did the pain start? Does the pain radiate to any other spot? • Character: How would you describe it? Crushing, stabbing, burning, viselike? Or aching, heaviness? (Allow the person to offer adjectives before you suggest them.) (Note if uses clenched fist to describe pain.) • Pain brought on by: activity—what type; rest; emotional upset; after eating; during sexual intercourse; with cold weather? • Any associated symptoms: sweating, ashen gray or pale skin, heart skips beat, shortness of breath, nausea or vomiting, racing of heart? • Pain made worse by moving the arms or neck, breathing, lying flat? • Pain relieved by rest or nitroglycerin? How many tablets?	Angina, an important cardiac symptom, occurs when the heart's own blood supply cannot keep up with metabolic demand. Chest pain also may have pulmonary, musculoskeletal, or gastrointestinal (GI) origin; important to differentiate! See Table 20.2, Differential Diagnosis of Chest Pain. A squeezing "clenched fist" sign is characteristic of angina, but the symptoms below may be anginal equivalents in the absence of chest pain.[6] Diaphoresis, cold sweats, pallor, grayness. Palpitations, dyspnea, nausea, tachycardia, fatigue. Try to differentiate pain of cardiac versus noncardiac origin.
2. Dyspnea. Any shortness of breath? • Which type of activity and how much brings on shortness of breath? How much activity brought it on 6 months ago?	**Dyspnea** on exertion (DOE)—Quantify exactly (e.g., DOE after walking two level blocks).

Examiner Asks	Rationale
• Onset: Does the shortness of breath come on unexpectedly? • Duration: Constant or does it come and go? • Seem to be affected by position? Lying down? • Awaken you from sleep at night?	Paroxysmal. Constant or intermittent. Recumbent. Paroxysmal nocturnal dyspnea (PND) occurs with heart failure. Lying down increases volume of intrathoracic blood, and the weakened heart cannot accommodate the increased load. Typically the person awakens after 2 hours of sleep with the perception of needing fresh air.
• Does the shortness of breath interfere with activities of daily living?	See Table 20.3, Clinical Portrait of Heart Failure, p. 487.
3. Orthopnea. How many pillows do you use when sleeping or lying down?	**Orthopnea** is the need to assume a more upright position to breathe. Note the exact number of pillows used.
4. Cough. Do you have a **cough?** • Duration: How long have you had it? • Frequency: Is it related to time of day? • Type: Dry, hacking, barky, hoarse, or congested? • Do you cough up mucus? Color? Any odor? Blood tinged?	Sputum production, mucoid or purulent. Hemoptysis is often a pulmonary disorder but also occurs with mitral stenosis.
• Associated with: activity, position (lying down), anxiety, talking? • Does activity make it better or worse (sit, walk, exercise)? • Relieved by rest or medication?	
5. Fatigue. Do you seem to tire easily? Able to keep up with your family and co-workers? • Onset: When did fatigue start? Sudden or gradual? Has any *recent* change occurred in energy level? • Fatigue related to time of day: all day, morning, evening?	Unusual fatigue is a top prodromal MI symptom for women.[4] Fatigue from decreased cardiac output is worse in the evening, whereas fatigue from anxiety or depression occurs all day or is worse in the morning.
6. Cyanosis or pallor. Ever noted your facial skin turning blue or ashen?	**Cyanosis** or **pallor** occurs with MI or low cardiac output states as a result of decreased tissue perfusion.
7. Edema. Any swelling of your feet and legs? • Onset: When did you first notice this? • Any recent change? • What time of day does the swelling occur? Do your shoes feel tight at the end of day? • How much swelling would you say there is? Are both legs equally swollen? • Does the swelling go away with: rest, elevation, after a night's sleep? • Any associated symptoms such as shortness of breath? If so, does the shortness of breath occur before leg swelling or after?	**Edema** is dependent when caused by heart failure. Cardiac edema is worse at evening and better in morning after elevating legs all night. Cardiac edema is bilateral; unilateral swelling has a local vein cause.

Examiner Asks	Rationale

8. Nocturia. Do you awaken at night with an urgent need to urinate? How long has this been occurring? Any recent change?

Nocturia—Recumbency at night promotes fluid resorption and excretion; this occurs with heart failure in the person who is ambulatory during the day.

9. Past cardiac history. Any **history** of: hypertension, elevated cholesterol or triglycerides, heart murmur, congenital heart disease, rheumatic fever or unexplained joint pains as child or youth, recurrent tonsillitis, anemia?
- Ever had heart disease? When was this? Treated by medication or heart surgery?
- Last ECG, stress ECG, serum cholesterol measurement, other heart tests?

10. Family cardiac history. Any **family history** of: hypertension, obesity, diabetes, CAD, sudden death at younger age?

11. Patient-centered care (cardiac risk factors).
- Nutrition: Please describe your usual daily diet. (Note if this diet is representative of the basic food groups, the amount of calories, cholesterol, and any additives such as salt.) What is your usual weight? Has there been any recent change?
- Smoking: Do you smoke cigarettes or other tobacco? At what age did you start? How many packs per day? For how many years have you smoked this amount? Have you ever tried to quit? If so, how did this go?
- Alcohol: How much alcohol do you usually drink each week, or each day? When was your last drink? How many drinks during that episode? Have you ever been told you had a drinking problem?
- Exercise: What is your usual amount of exercise each day or week? What type of exercise (state type or sport)? If a sport, what is your usual amount (light, moderate, heavy)?
- Drugs: Do you take any antihypertensives, beta-blockers, calcium channel blockers, digoxin, diuretics, aspirin/anticoagulants, over-the-counter or street drugs?

Risk factors for CAD—Collect data regarding elevated cholesterol, elevated BP, blood sugar levels above 100 mg/dL or known DM, obesity, cigarette smoking, low activity level, and length of any hormone replacement therapy for postmenopausal women.

Encourage men ages 45 to 79 years and women age 55 to 79 years to use low-dose aspirin if the potential benefit of preventing MI outweighs the potential risk of GI bleeding.[17] Vitamin D replacement is important; vitamin D deficiency increases risk of CVD and is associated with hypertension.[23]

Additional History for Infants

1. How was the mother's health during pregnancy? Any unexplained fever, rubella first trimester, other infection, hypertension, drugs taken?

2. Have you noted any cyanosis while nursing, crying? Is the baby able to eat, nurse, or finish bottle without tiring?

To screen for heart disease in infant, note fatigue during feeding. Infant with heart failure takes fewer ounces each feeding; becomes dyspneic with sucking; may be diaphoretic, then falls into exhausted sleep; awakens after a short time hungry again.

3. **Growth:** Has this baby grown as expected by growth charts and about the same as siblings or peers?

Poor weight gain.

4. **Activity:** Were this baby's motor milestones achieved as expected? Is the baby able to play without tiring? How many naps does the baby take each day? How long does a nap last?

Examiner Asks	Rationale

Additional History for Children

1. **Growth:** Has this child grown as expected by growth charts?

Poor weight gain.

2. **Activity:** Is this child able to keep up with siblings or age mates? Is the child willing or reluctant to go out to play? Is the child able to climb stairs, ride a bike, walk a few blocks? Does the child squat to rest during play or to watch television or assume a knee-chest position while sleeping? Have you noted "blue spells" during exercise?

Fatigue. Record specific limitations.

Cyanosis occurs in some congenital defects: tetralogy of Fallot or transposition of the great arteries.

3. Has the child had any chest pain?

Serious causes of chest pain are not common. Most causes are musculoskeletal pain and respiratory causes, including asthma. However, you should refer any acute onset of chest pain, or refer any concern about a potentially serious cardiac cause.[25]

4. Does the child have frequent respiratory infections? How many per year? How are they treated? Have any of these proved to be streptococcal infections?

5. **Family history:** Does the child have a sibling with heart defect? Is anyone in the child's family known to have chromosomal abnormalities such as Down syndrome?

Additional History for the Pregnant Woman

1. Have you had any high BP during this or earlier pregnancies?
   - What was your usual BP level before pregnancy? How has your BP been monitored during the pregnancy?
   - If high BP, what treatment has been started?
   - Any associated symptoms: weight gain; protein in urine; swelling in feet, legs, or face?

Gestational hypertension, see p. 480.

See Table 31.1, Preeclampsia, p. 821.

2. Have you had any faintness or dizziness with this pregnancy?

Additional History for the Aging Adult

1. Do you have any known heart or lung disease: hypertension, CAD, chronic emphysema, or bronchitis?
   - What efforts to treat this have been started?
   - Usual symptoms changed recently? Does your illness interfere with activities of daily living?

Risk of CVD increases with advancing age.

2. Do you take any medications for your illness such as digitalis? Aware of side effects? Have you recently stopped taking your medication? Why?

Noncompliance may be related to side effects or lack of finances.

3. **Environment:** Does your home have any stairs? How often do you need to climb them? Does this have any effect on activities of daily living?

OBJECTIVE DATA

PREPARATION

To evaluate the carotid arteries, the person can be sitting up. To assess the jugular veins and the precordium, the person should be supine with the head and chest elevated between 30 and 45 degrees.

Stand on the person's right side; this facilitates your hand placement, viewing of the neck veins, and auscultation of the precordium.

The room must be warm—Chilling makes the person uncomfortable, and shivering interferes with heart sounds. Take scrupulous care to ensure *quiet;* heart sounds are very soft, and any ambient room noise masks them.

Ensure the female's privacy by keeping her breasts draped. The female's left breast overrides part of the area you will need to examine. Gently displace the breast upward, or ask the woman to hold it out of the way.

When performing a regional CV assessment, use this order:

1. Pulse and BP (see Chapter 10)
2. Extremities (see Chapter 21)
3. Neck vessels
4. Precordium

The logic of this order is that you begin observations peripherally and move in toward the heart. For choreography of these steps in the complete physical examination, see Chapter 28.

EQUIPMENT NEEDED

Stethoscope with diaphragm and bell endpieces
Alcohol wipe (to clean endpiece)
Small centimeter ruler

Normal Range of Findings	Abnormal Findings

The Neck Vessels

Palpate the Carotid Artery

Located central to the heart, the carotid artery yields important information on cardiac function.

Palpate each carotid artery medial to the sternomastoid muscle in the neck (Fig. 20.16). Avoid excessive pressure on the carotid sinus area higher in the neck; excessive vagal stimulation here could slow down the heart rate, especially in older adults. Take care to palpate gently. Palpate only one carotid artery at a time to avoid compromising arterial blood to the brain.

Carotid sinus hypersensitivity is the condition in which pressure over the carotid sinus leads to a decreased heart rate, decreased BP, and cerebral ischemia with syncope. This may occur in older adults with hypertension or occlusion of the carotid artery.

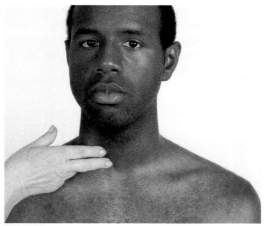

20.16

Normal Range of Findings	Abnormal Findings

Feel the contour and amplitude of the pulse. Normally the contour is smooth with a brisk upstroke and slower downstroke, and the normal strength is moderate. Your findings should be the same bilaterally.

Diminished pulse feels small and weak (decreased stroke volume as in cardiogenic shock).

Increased pulse feels full and strong in hyperkinetic states (see Table 21.1, Variations in Pulse Contour, p. 522).

Auscultate the Carotid Artery

For people middle-age or older or who show symptoms or signs of CVD, auscultate each carotid artery for the presence of a **bruit** (pronounced brú-ee) (Fig. 20.17). This is a blowing, swishing sound indicating blood flow turbulence; normally none is present.

A bruit indicates turbulence from a local vascular cause and is a marker for atherosclerotic disease. This increases the risk of transient ischemic attack (TIA) and ischemic stroke.[19] However, a bruit also occurs in 5% of those age 45 to 80 years who have no significant carotid disease.[9]

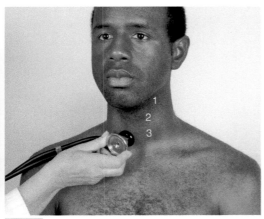

20.17

Keep the neck in a neutral position. Lightly apply the bell of the stethoscope over the carotid artery at three levels: (1) the angle of the jaw, (2) the midcervical area, and (3) the base of the neck (see Fig. 20.17). Avoid compressing the artery because this could create an artificial bruit, and it could compromise circulation if the carotid artery is already narrowed by atherosclerosis. Ask the person to take a breath, exhale, and hold it briefly while you listen so tracheal breath sounds do not mask or mimic a carotid artery bruit. (Holding the breath on inhalation also tenses the levator scapulae muscles, which makes it hard to hear the carotids.) Sometimes you can hear normal heart sounds transmitted to the neck; do not confuse these with a bruit.

A carotid bruit is audible when the lumen is occluded by ½ to ⅔. Bruit loudness increases as the atherosclerosis worsens until the lumen is occluded by ⅔. After that, bruit loudness decreases. When the lumen is completely occluded, the bruit disappears. Thus absence of a bruit does not ensure absence of a carotid lesion.

A murmur sounds much the same but is caused by a cardiac disorder. Some aortic valve murmurs (aortic stenosis) radiate to the neck and must be distinguished from a local bruit.

Inspect the Jugular Venous Pulse

From the jugular veins you can assess the **central venous pressure (CVP)** and thus judge the heart's efficiency as a pump and the intravascular volume status. Stand on the person's right side because the veins there have a direct route to the heart. You may use either the external or the internal jugular veins because measurements in both are similar.[15] You can see the top of the external jugular vein distention overlying the sternomastoid muscle or the pulsation of the internal jugular vein in the sternal notch. The latter is harder to see because of its deep position.

| **Normal Range of Findings** | **Abnormal Findings** |

Position the person supine anywhere from a 30- to a 45-degree angle, wherever you can best see the top of the vein or pulsations. In general the higher the venous pressure is, the higher the position you need. Remove the pillow to avoid flexing the neck; the head should be in the same plane as the trunk. Turn the person's head slightly away from the examined side and direct a strong light tangentially onto the neck to highlight pulsations and shadows.

Note the external jugular veins overlying the sternomastoid muscle. In some people the veins are not visible at all, whereas in others they are full in the supine position. As the person is raised to a sitting position, these external jugulars flatten and disappear, usually at 45 degrees.

Now look for pulsations of the internal jugular veins in the area of the suprasternal notch or around the origin of the sternomastoid muscle around the clavicle. You must be able to distinguish internal jugular vein pulsation from that of the carotid artery. It is easy to confuse them because they lie close together. Use the guidelines shown in Table 20.1.

> Unilateral distention of external jugular veins is caused by local cause (kinking or aneurysm).
>
> Full distended external jugular veins above 45 degrees signify increased CVP as with heart failure.

TABLE 20.1 Characteristics of Jugular Versus Carotid Pulsations

	INTERNAL JUGULAR PULSE	**CAROTID PULSE**
1. Location	Lower, more lateral, under or behind the sternomastoid muscle	Higher and medial to this muscle
2. Quality	Undulant and diffuse; two visible waves per cycle	Brisk and localized; one wave per cycle
3. Respiration	Varies with respiration; its level descends during inspiration when intrathoracic pressure is decreased	Does not vary
4. Palpable	No	Yes
5. Pressure	Light pressure at the base of the neck easily obliterates	No change
6. Position of person	Level of pulse drops and disappears as the person is brought to a sitting position	Unaffected

The Precordium

Inspect the Anterior Chest

Arrange tangential lighting to accentuate any flicker of movement.

Pulsations. You may or may not see the **apical impulse,** the pulsation created as the left ventricle rotates against the chest wall during systole. When visible, it occupies the 4th or 5th intercostal space, at or inside the midclavicular line. It is easier to see in children and in those with thinner chest walls.

> A **heave** or **lift** is a sustained forceful thrusting of the ventricle during systole. It occurs with ventricular hypertrophy as a result of increased workload. A right ventricular heave is seen at the sternal border; a left ventricular heave is seen at the apex (see Table 20.9, Abnormal Pulsations on the Precordium, p. 493).

Palpate the Apical Impulse

Localize the **apical impulse** precisely by using one finger pad (Fig. 20.18, *A*). Asking the person to "exhale and then hold it" helps the examiner locate the pulsation. You may need to roll the person midway to the left to find it; note that this also displaces the apical impulse farther to the left (Fig. 20.18, *B*). You feel it best at the end of expiration when the heart is closest to the chest wall; then it moves quickly away from your finger.

Normal Range of Findings	Abnormal Findings

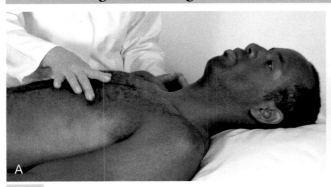
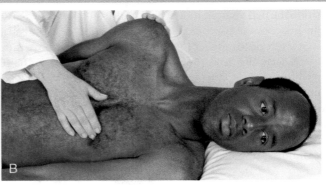

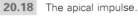

20.18   The apical impulse.

NOTE:

- *Location*—The apical impulse should occupy only one interspace, the 4th or 5th, and be at or medial to the midclavicular line
- *Size*—Normally 1 × 2 cm
- *Amplitude*—Normally a short, gentle tap
- *Duration*—Short; normally occupies only first half of systole

The apical impulse is palpable in the supine position in 25% to 40% of adults and in the left lateral position in 50% to 73% of adults.[15] It is not palpable in obese persons or in people with thick chest walls. With high cardiac output states (anxiety, fever, hyperthyroidism, anemia) the apical impulse increases in amplitude and duration.

Palpate Across the Precordium

Using the palmar aspects of your four fingers, gently palpate the apex, the left sternal border, and the base, searching for any other pulsations (Fig. 20.19). Normally none occur. If any are present, note the timing. Use the carotid artery pulsation as a guide, or auscultate as you palpate.

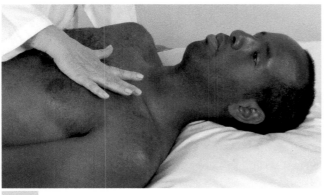

20.19

Cardiac enlargement:

Left ventricular dilation (volume overload) displaces impulse down and to left and increases size more than one space. A diameter of ≥4 cm is likely a dilated heart.[15] This occurs with heart failure and cardiomyopathy.

A **sustained** impulse with increased force and duration but no change in location occurs with left ventricular hypertrophy and no dilation (pressure overload) (see Table 20.9).

Not palpable with pulmonary emphysema because of overriding lungs.

A **thrill** is a palpable vibration. It feels like the throat of a purring cat. The thrill signifies turbulent blood flow and directs you to locate the origin of loud murmurs. However, absence of a thrill does not rule out the presence of a murmur.

Accentuated first and second heart sounds and extra heart sounds also may cause abnormal pulsations.

Normal Range of Findings	Abnormal Findings

Percussion[a]

Auscultation

Identify the auscultatory areas where you will listen. These include the four traditional valve "areas" (Fig. 20.20). The valve areas are not over the actual anatomic locations of the valves but are the sites on the chest wall where sounds produced by the valves are best heard. The sound radiates with the direction of blood flow.

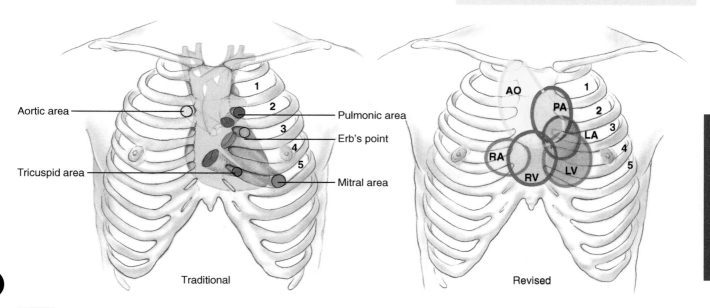

Aortic area — Pulmonic area

Erb's point

Tricuspid area — Mitral area

Traditional   Revised

AO   PA   LA   RA   RV   LV

20.20   AUSCULTATORY AREAS

The valve areas are:
- Second right interspace—Aortic valve area
- Second left interspace—Pulmonic valve area
- Left lower sternal border—Tricuspid valve area
- Fifth interspace at around left midclavicular line—Mitral valve area

Do not limit your auscultation to only four locations. Sounds produced by the valves may be heard all over the precordium. (For this reason many experts even discourage the naming of the valve areas.) Thus learn to inch your stethoscope in a rough **Z** pattern, from the base of the heart across and down and over to the apex. Or start at the apex and work your way up. Include the sites shown in Fig. 20.20.

Recall the characteristics of a good stethoscope (see Chapter 8). Clean the endpieces with an alcohol wipe; you will use both endpieces. Although all heart sounds are low frequency, the diaphragm detects relatively higher-pitched sounds, and the bell detects relatively lower-pitched ones. Make sure that your earpieces fit snugly and are aimed forward, toward your nose, to avoid air leak. These heart sounds are soft; enhance your success with a completely quiet room—no television, no radio, no talking, please.

---

[a]Percussion to outline the borders of the heart has been replaced by the chest x-ray image or echocardiogram. Evidence shows that these are more accurate in detecting heart enlargement. When the right ventricle enlarges, it does so in the anteroposterior diameter, which is better seen on x-ray image. Evidence from numerous comparison studies shows that the percussed cardiac border correlates "only moderately" with the true cardiac border.[15] In addition, percussion is of limited usefulness with the female breast tissue or in an obese person or a person with a muscular chest wall.

Objective Data

Normal Range of Findings	Abnormal Findings

Before you begin, alert the person: "I always listen to the heart in a number of places on the chest. Just because I'm listening for a long time, it does not necessarily mean that something is wrong."

After you place the stethoscope, try closing your eyes briefly to tune out any distractions. Concentrate and listen selectively to *one sound at a time.* Consider that at least 2, and perhaps 3 or 4, sounds may be happening in less than 1 second. You cannot process everything at once. Begin with the diaphragm endpiece and use the following routine: (1) note the rate and rhythm, (2) identify S_1 and S_2, (3) assess S_1 and S_2 separately, (4) listen for extra heart sounds, and (5) listen for murmurs.

Note the Rate and Rhythm. The rate ranges normally from 50 to 95 beats/min. (Review the full discussion of the pulse in Chapter 10 and the normal rates across age-groups.) The rhythm should be regular, although **sinus arrhythmia** occurs normally in young adults and children. With sinus arrhythmia, the rhythm varies with the person's breathing, increasing at the peak of inspiration and slowing with expiration. Note any other irregular rhythm. If one occurs, check if it has any pattern or if it is totally irregular.

When you notice any irregularity, check for a **pulse deficit** by auscultating the apical beat while simultaneously palpating the radial pulse. Count a serial measurement (one after the other) of apical beat and radial pulse. Normally every beat you hear at the apex should perfuse to the periphery and be palpable. The two counts should be identical. When different, subtract the radial rate from the apical, and record the remainder as the pulse deficit.

Identify S_1 and S_2. This is important because S_1 is the start of systole and thus serves as the reference point for the timing of all other cardiac sounds. You must learn to distinguish systole from diastole before you can attach meaning to all other sounds. Usually you can identify S_1 instantly because you hear a pair of sounds close together (lub-dup) and S_1 is the first of the pair. This guideline works, except in the cases of the tachydysrhythmias (rates >100 beats/min). Then the diastolic filling time is shortened, and the beats are too close together to distinguish.

Premature beat—An isolated beat is early, or a pattern occurs in which every third or fourth beat sounds early.

Irregularly irregular—No pattern to the sounds; beats come rapidly and at random intervals as in atrial fibrillation.

A **pulse deficit** signals a weak contraction of the ventricles; it occurs with atrial fibrillation, premature beats, and heart failure.

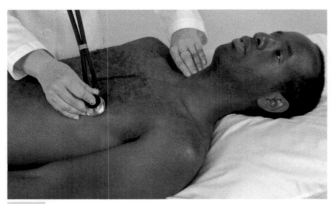

20.21

Other guidelines to distinguish S_1 from S_2 are:
- S_1 is louder than S_2 at the apex; S_2 is louder than S_1 at the base.
- S_1 coincides with the carotid artery pulse. Feel the carotid gently as you auscultate at the apex; the sound you hear as you feel each pulse is S_1 (Fig. 20.21).
- S_1 coincides with the R wave (the upstroke of the QRS complex) if the person is on an ECG monitor.

Objective Data

Normal Range of Findings

Listen to S₁ and S₂ Separately. Note whether each heart sound is normal, accentuated, diminished, or split. Inch your diaphragm across the chest as you do this.

First Heart Sound (S₁). Caused by closure of the AV valves, S_1 signals the beginning of systole. You can hear it over the entire precordium, although it is loudest at the apex (Fig. 20.22). (Sometimes the two sounds are equally loud at the apex because S_1 is lower pitched than S_2.)

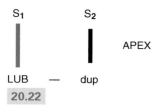

20.22

You can hear S_1 with the diaphragm with the person in any position and equally well in inspiration and expiration. A split S_1 is normal, but it occurs rarely. A split S_1 means that you are hearing the mitral and tricuspid components separately. It is audible in the tricuspid valve area, the left lower sternal border. The split is very rapid, with the two components only 0.03 second apart.

Second Heart Sound (S₂). The S_2 is associated with closure of the semilunar valves. You can hear it with the diaphragm over the entire precordium, although S_2 is loudest at the base (Fig. 20.23).

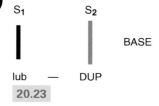

20.23

Splitting of S₂. A split S_2 is a normal phenomenon that occurs toward the end of inspiration in some people. Recall that closure of the aortic and pulmonic valves is nearly synchronous. Because of the effects of respiration on the heart described earlier, inspiration separates the timing of the two valves' closure, and the aortic valve closes 0.06 second before the pulmonic valve. Instead of one DUP, you hear a split sound—T-DUP (Fig. 20.24). During expiration, synchrony returns and the aortic and pulmonic components fuse together. A split S_2 is heard only in the pulmonic valve area, the second left interspace.

SPLITTING OF THE SECOND HEART SOUND

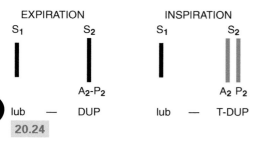

20.24

Abnormal Findings

Causes of accentuated or diminished S_1 (see Table 20.4, Variations in S_1, p. 488).

Both heart sounds are diminished with conditions that place an increased amount of tissue between the heart and your stethoscope: emphysema (hyperinflated lungs), obesity, pericardial fluid.

Accentuated or diminished S_2 (see Table 20.5, Variations in S_2, p. 489).

Objective Data

Normal Range of Findings	Abnormal Findings

Normal Range of Findings

When you first hear the split S_2, do *not* be tempted to ask the person to hold his or her breath so you can concentrate on the sounds. Breath holding only equalizes ejection times in the right and left sides of the heart and causes the split to go away. Instead, concentrate on the split as you watch the person's chest rise up and down with breathing. The split S_2 occurs about every 4th heartbeat, fading in with inhalation and fading out with exhalation.

Focus on Systole, Then on Diastole, and Listen for Any Extra Heart Sounds.
Listen with the diaphragm; then switch to the bell, covering all auscultatory areas (Fig. 20.25). Usually these are silent periods. When you do detect an extra heart sound, listen carefully to note its timing and characteristics. During systole the **midsystolic click** (which is associated with mitral valve prolapse) is the most common extra sound (see Table 20.7). The third and fourth heart sounds occur in diastole; either may be normal or abnormal (see Table 20.8).

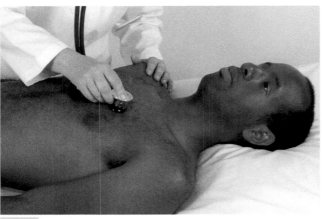

20.25

Listen for Murmurs. A murmur is a blowing, swooshing sound that occurs with turbulent blood flow in the heart or great vessels. Except for the innocent murmurs described, murmurs are abnormal. If you hear a murmur, describe it by indicating these following characteristics.

Timing. It is crucial to define the murmur by its occurrence in systole or diastole. You must be able to identify S_1 and S_2 accurately to do this. Try to further describe the murmur as being in early, mid, or late systole or diastole; throughout the cardiac event (termed *pansystolic, holosystolic/pandiastolic,* or *holodiastolic);* and whether it obscures or muffles the heart sounds.

Abnormal Findings

A **fixed split** is unaffected by respiration; the split is always there.

A **paradoxical split** is the opposite of what you would expect; the sounds fuse on inspiration and split on expiration (see Table 20.6, Variations in Split S_2, p. 489).

A pathologic S_3 (ventricular gallop) occurs with heart failure and volume overload; a pathologic S_4 (atrial gallop) occurs with CAD (see Table 20.8, p. 492, for a full description).

Murmurs may be caused by congenital and acquired valvular defects. Study Tables 20.10 and 20.11, pp. 494–499, for a complete description.

A systolic murmur may occur with a healthy heart or with heart disease; a diastolic murmur always indicates heart disease.

Normal heart tones[14]	**Lub**	**Dup**	**Lub**	**Dup**
	S_1	S_2	S_1	S_2
Early systolic murmur	**LSHSHSH**	**Dup**	**LSHSHSH**	**Dup**
	S_1	S_2	S_1	S_2
Midsystolic murmur	**LubSHSH Dup**		**LubSHSH Dup**	
	S_1 $\quad$ S_2		S_1 $\quad$ S_2	
Late systolic murmur	**Lub**	**SHSH P**	**Lub**	**SHSH P**
	S_1	S_2	S_1	S_2
Late systolic murmur and click (C) of mitral valve prolapse	**Lub** S_1	**KSHSH P** C $\quad$ S_2	**Lub** S_1	**KSHSH P** C $\quad$ S_2
Holosystolic murmur	**SHSHSHSHSH**		**SHSHSHSHSH**	
	S_1 $\quad$ S_2		S_1 $\quad$ S_2	

Objective Data

Normal Range of Findings	Abnormal Findings

Loudness. Describe the intensity in terms of six "grades." For example, record a grade 2 murmur as "2/6."

Grade 1—Barely audible; heard only in a quiet room and then with difficulty

Grade 2—Clearly audible but faint

Grade 3—Moderately loud; easy to hear

Grade 4—Loud; associated with a thrill palpable on the chest wall

Grade 5—Very loud; heard with one corner of the stethoscope lifted off the chest wall; associated thrill

Grade 6—Loudest; still heard with entire stethoscope lifted just off the chest wall; associated thrill

Pitch. Describe the pitch as high, medium, or low. The pitch depends on the pressure and rate of blood flow producing the murmur.

Pattern. The intensity may follow a pattern during the cardiac phase, growing louder (crescendo), tapering off (decrescendo) or increasing to a peak, and then decreasing (crescendo-decrescendo or diamond shaped). Because the whole murmur is just milliseconds long, it takes practice to diagnose any pattern.

Quality. Describe the quality as musical, blowing, harsh, or rumbling.

> The murmur of mitral stenosis is low-pitched and rumbling, whereas that of aortic stenosis is harsh (see Table 20.11).

Location. Describe the area of maximum intensity of the murmur (where it is best heard) by noting the valve area or intercostal spaces.

Radiation. The murmur may be transmitted downstream in the direction of blood flow and may be heard in another place on the precordium, the neck, the back, or the axilla.

Posture. Some murmurs disappear or are enhanced by a change in position.

Some murmurs are common in healthy children or adolescents and are termed *innocent* or *functional.* **Innocent** indicates having no valvular or other pathologic cause; **functional** is caused by increased blood flow in the heart (e.g., in anemia, fever, pregnancy, hyperthyroidism). The contractile force of the heart is greater in children. This increases blood flow velocity. The increased velocity plus a smaller chest measurement makes an audible murmur.

The innocent murmur is generally soft (grade 2), midsystolic, short, crescendo-decrescendo, and with a vibratory or musical quality ("vooot" sound like fiddle strings). It is heard at the 2nd or 3rd left intercostal space and disappears with sitting, and the young person has no associated signs of cardiac dysfunction. It is important to distinguish innocent murmurs from pathologic ones. Diagnostic tests such as ECG and echocardiogram will establish an accurate diagnosis.

Change Position. After auscultating in the supine position, roll the person toward his or her left side. Listen with the bell at the apex for the presence of any diastolic filling sounds (i.e., the S_3 or S_4) (Fig. 20.26).

> S_3 and S_4 and the murmur of mitral stenosis sometimes may be heard only when on the left side.

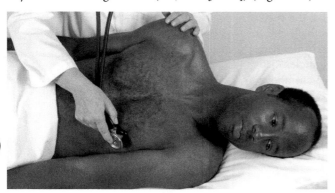

20.26

Objective Data

Normal Range of Findings

Ask the person to sit up, lean forward slightly, and exhale. Listen with the diaphragm firmly pressed at the base, right, and left sides. Check for the soft, high-pitched, early diastolic murmur of aortic or pulmonic regurgitation (Fig. 20.27).

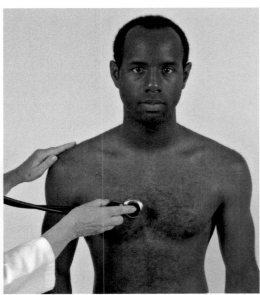

20.27

Standing to Squatting. A screening measure to detect hypertrophic cardiomyopathy in children, adolescents, and young adults is to change position, which changes the venous return to the heart. If the person has a systolic murmur, listen to the murmur while the person changes from standing to squatting, and then squatting to standing. Note any change in loudness of the murmur.

Procedures for Advanced Practice

Estimate the Jugular Venous Pressure

Think of the jugular veins as a CVP manometer attached directly to the right atrium. You can "read" the CVP at the highest level of pulsations. Use the angle of Louis (sternal angle) as an arbitrary reference point, and compare it with the highest level of the distended vein or venous pulsation.

Hold a vertical ruler on the sternal angle. Align a straightedge on the ruler like a T-square and adjust the level of the horizontal straightedge to the level of pulsation (Fig. 20.28, *A*). Read the level of intersection on the vertical ruler; normal jugular venous pulsation is 2 cm or less above the sternal angle. Also state the person's position (e.g., "internal jugular vein pulsations 3 cm above sternal angle when elevated 30 degrees").

Abnormal Findings

The soft diastolic murmur of aortic regurgitation may be heard only when the person is leaning forward in the sitting position.

The murmur of hypertrophic cardiomyopathy (HCM) grows *softer* with standing-to-squatting, and it grows *louder* with squatting-to-standing.[15] HCM is an inherited thickening of the myocardium, affecting 1 in 500 persons, men and women equally.

| **Normal Range of Findings** | **Abnormal Findings** |

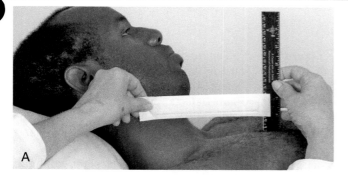

A

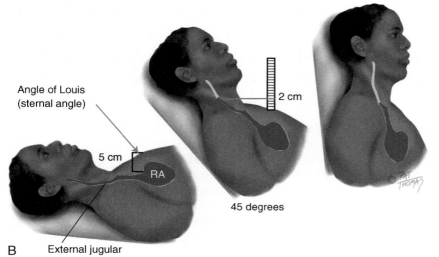

Angle of Louis
(sternal angle)

5 cm

RA

2 cm

45 degrees

B   External jugular

20.28

(B, © Pat Thomas, 2014.)

If you cannot find the internal jugular veins, use the external jugular veins and note the point where they look collapsed. Be aware that the technique of estimating venous pressure is difficult and is not always a reliable predictor of CVP. Consistency in grading among examiners is difficult to achieve.

If venous pressure is elevated or if you suspect heart failure, perform the **abdominojugular test** (formerly **hepatojugular reflux**) (Fig. 20.29). Position the person comfortably supine, and instruct him or her to breathe quietly through an open mouth. Hold your right hand over the midabdomen and watch the level of jugular pulsation as you push in with your hand. Exert firm sustained pressure for 10 seconds. This displaces venous blood out of the splanchnic vessels and adds its volume to the venous system. If the heart is able to pump this additional volume (i.e., if no elevated CVP is present), the jugular veins will rise for a few seconds and then recede back to the previous level.

Elevated pressure is a level of pulsation that is >3 cm above the sternal angle while at 45 degrees (Fig. 20.28, *B*). This occurs with heart failure, cardiac tamponade, and constrictive pericarditis.

Also, try to estimate a CVP for the patient with ascites or edema: when elevated, it suggests heart or lung disease; if normal, the problem may be something else, such as liver disease.[15]

If heart failure is present, the jugular veins will elevate more than 4 cm and stay elevated as long as you push (a positive test).

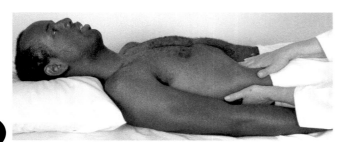

20.29   Abdominojugular test.

Objective Data

Normal Range of Findings	Abnormal Findings

❖ DEVELOPMENTAL COMPETENCE

Infants

The transition from fetal to pulmonic circulation occurs in the immediate newborn period. Fetal shunts normally close within 10 to 15 hours but may take up to 48 hours. Thus you should assess the CV system during the first 24 hours and again in 2 to 3 days.

Note any extracardiac signs that may reflect heart status (particularly in the skin), liver size, and respiratory status. The skin color should be pink to pinkish brown, depending on the infant's genetic heritage. If cyanosis occurs, determine its first appearance—at or shortly after birth versus after the neonatal period. Normally the liver is not enlarged, and the respirations are not labored. In addition, note the expected parameters of weight gain throughout infancy.

Palpate the apical impulse to determine the size and position of the heart. Because the infant's heart has a more horizontal placement, expect to palpate the apical impulse at the 4th intercostal space just lateral to the midclavicular line. It may or may not be visible.

The heart rate is best auscultated because radial pulses are hard to count accurately. Use the small (pediatric size) diaphragm and bell (Fig. 20.30). The heart rate may range from 100 to 180 beats/min immediately after birth and stabilize to an average of 120 to 140 beats/min. Infants normally have wide fluctuations with activity, from 170 beats/min or more with crying or being active to 70 to 90 beats/min with sleeping. Variations are greatest at birth and are even more so with premature babies.

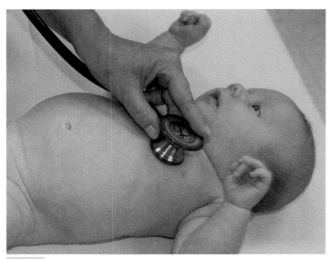

20.30

Abnormal Findings

Failure of shunts to close (e.g., patent ductus arteriosus [PDA], atrial septal defect [ASD]); see Table 20.10, Congenital Heart Defects.

Cyanosis at or just after birth signals oxygen desaturation of congenital heart disease (see Table 20.10).

The most important signs of heart failure in an infant are persistent tachycardia, tachypnea, and liver enlargement. Engorged veins, gallop rhythm, and pulsus alternans also are signs. Respiratory crackles (rales) are an important sign in adults but not in infants.

Failure to thrive occurs with cardiac disease.

The apex is displaced with:
- Cardiac enlargement, shifts to the left.
- Pneumothorax, shifts away from the affected side.
- Diaphragmatic hernia, shifts usually to right because this hernia occurs more often on the left.
- Dextrocardia, a rare anomaly in which the heart is located on right side of chest.

Persistent tachycardia is >200 beats/min in newborns or >150 beats/min in infants.

Bradycardia is <90 beats/min in newborns or <60 beats/min in older infants or children. This causes a serious drop in cardiac output because the small muscle mass of their hearts cannot increase stroke volume significantly.

Normal Range of Findings	Abnormal Findings

Expect the heart rhythm to have sinus arrhythmia, the phasic speeding up or slowing down with the respiratory cycle.

Investigate any irregularity except sinus arrhythmia.

Rapid rates make it more challenging to evaluate heart sounds. Expect heart sounds to be louder in infants than in adults because of the infant's thinner chest wall. Also, S_2 has a higher pitch and is sharper than S_1. Splitting of S_2 just after the height of inspiration is common, not at birth but beginning a few hours after birth.

Fixed split S_2 indicates atrial septal defect (see Table 20.10).

Murmurs in the immediate newborn period do not necessarily indicate congenital heart disease. They are relatively common in the first 2 to 3 days because of fetal shunt closure. These murmurs are usually grade 1 or 2, are systolic, accompany no other signs of cardiac disease, and disappear in 2 to 3 days. The murmur of PDA is a continuous machinery murmur, which disappears by 2 to 3 days. On the other hand, absence of a murmur in the immediate newborn period does not ensure a healthy heart; congenital defects can be present that are not signaled by an early murmur. It is best to listen frequently and to note and describe any murmur according to the characteristics listed on pp. 474–475.

Congenital defects are associated with: harsh murmur quality, location (right upper sternal border, left lower sternal border, apex), and timing (pansystolic, diastolic, or continuous).[24]

Children

Note any extracardiac or cardiac signs that may indicate heart disease: poor weight gain, developmental delay, persistent tachycardia, tachypnea, DOE, cyanosis, and clubbing. Note that clubbing of fingers and toes usually does not appear until late in the first year, even with severe cyanotic defects.

The apical impulse is sometimes visible in children with thin chest walls. Note any obvious bulge or any heave—these are not normal.

A precordial bulge to the left of the sternum with a hyperdynamic precordium signals cardiac enlargement. The bulge occurs because the cartilaginous rib cage is more compliant.

A substernal heave occurs with right ventricular enlargement; an apical heave occurs with left ventricular hypertrophy.

Palpate the apical impulse in the fourth intercostal space to the left of the midclavicular line until age 4 years; at the fourth interspace at the midclavicular line from ages 4 to 6 years, and in the fifth interspace to the right of the midclavicular line at age 7 years (Fig. 20.31).

The apical impulse moves laterally with cardiac enlargement.
Thrill (palpable vibration).

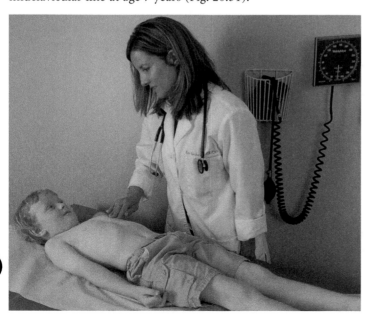

20.31

Normal Range of Findings	Abnormal Findings

The average heart rate slows as the child grows older, although it is still variable with rest or activity.

The heart rhythm remains characterized by sinus arrhythmia. Physiologic S_3 is common in children (see Table 20.8). It occurs in early diastole, just after S_2, and is a dull soft sound that is best heard at the apex.

A **venous hum**—caused by turbulence of blood flow in the jugular venous system—is common in healthy children and has no pathologic significance. It is a continuous, low-pitched, soft hum that is heard throughout the cycle, although it is loudest in diastole. Listen with the bell over the supraclavicular fossa at the medial third of the clavicle, especially on the right, or over the upper anterior chest.

The venous hum is usually not affected by respiration, may sound louder when the child stands, and is easily obliterated by occluding the jugular veins in the neck with your fingers.

> This latter maneuver helps differentiate the venous hum from other cardiac murmurs (e.g., PDA).

A **carotid bruit** is a benign murmur heard just above the clavicles. It is slightly harsh, early or midsystolic, often louder on the left, and will disappear completely by carotid artery compression.

Heart murmurs that are innocent (or functional) in origin are very common through childhood (often termed *Still's murmur*). They may have a 30% occurrence, although some authors say that nearly all children may demonstrate a murmur at some time. Most innocent murmurs have these characteristics: soft, relatively short, early or midsystolic ejection murmur; medium pitch; vibratory; best heard at the left lower sternal or midsternal border, with no radiation to the apex, base, or back.

> Distinguish innocent murmurs from pathologic ones. This may involve referral to another examiner or performing diagnostic tests (e.g., ECG or echocardiography).

For the child whose murmur has been shown to be innocent, it is very important that the parents understand this completely. They need to believe that this murmur is just a "noise" and has no pathologic significance. Otherwise the parents may become overprotective and limit activity for the child, which may result in the child developing a negative self-concept.

The Pregnant Woman

The vital signs usually yield an increase in resting pulse rate of 10 to 20 beats/min and a drop in BP from the normal prepregnancy level. The BP decreases to its lowest point during the second trimester and then slowly rises during the third trimester. It varies with position. It is usually lowest in the left lateral recumbent position, a bit higher when supine, and highest when sitting.[13]

> Gestational hypertension is BP ≥140/90 mm Hg on two separate measures without proteinuria, starting after 20th week of pregnancy. This returns to baseline by 12 weeks after delivery.[14]

Inspection of the skin often shows a mild hyperemia in light-skinned women because the increased cutaneous blood flow tries to eliminate the excess heat generated by the increased metabolism. Palpation of the apical impulse is higher and lateral compared with the normal position because the enlarging uterus elevates the diaphragm and displaces the heart up and to the left and rotates it on its long axis.

Auscultation of the heart sounds shows changes caused by the increased blood volume and workload. An exaggerated splitting of S_1 and increased loudness of S_1 are common, as is a loud, easily heard S_3. An ejection systolic murmur is common; heard at left sternal border; grade 1, 2 or 3 in intensity.[11]

A continuous murmur from breast vasculature is termed a **mammary souffle** (pronounced soof' f'l), which occurs near term or when the mother is lactating; it is caused by increased blood flow through the internal mammary artery. The murmur is heard in the 2nd, 3rd, or 4th intercostal space; it is continuous, although it is accented in systole. You can obliterate it by pressure with the stethoscope or one finger lateral to the murmur.

> Murmurs of aortic valve disease cannot be obliterated.

Normal Range of Findings	Abnormal Findings

The ECG has no changes except for a slight left axis deviation caused by the change in the heart's position.

The Aging Adult

A gradual rise in SBP is common with aging; the DBP stays fairly constant with a resulting widening of pulse pressure. Some older adults experience **orthostatic hypotension,** a sudden drop in BP when rising to sit or stand.

Use caution in palpating and auscultating the carotid artery. Avoid pressure in the carotid sinus area, which could cause a reflex slowing of the heart rate. Also, pressure on the carotid artery could compromise circulation if the artery is already narrowed by atherosclerosis.

The chest often increases in anteroposterior diameter with aging. This makes it more difficult to palpate the apical impulse and hear the splitting of S_2. The S_4 often occurs in older people with no known cardiac disease. Systolic murmurs are common, occurring in over 50% of aging people.

Occasional premature ectopic beats are common and do not necessarily indicate underlying heart disease. When in doubt, obtain an ECG. However, consider that the ECG records for only one isolated minute in time and may need to be supplemented by a test of 24-hour ambulatory heart monitoring.

The S_3 is associated with heart failure and is always abnormal over age 35 years (see Table 20.8).

HEALTH PROMOTION AND PATIENT TEACHING

*Let's spend some time talking about the **ABCS**[17] of heart health. In some areas of the country, we are seeing troubling increases in heart disease, especially among adults ages 35 to 64 years. There are health-promoting steps you can take now to keep your heart healthy.*

Appropriate aspirin therapy. Men ages 45 to 79 years may take a low-dose aspirin daily when the potential benefit of preventing a heart attack outweighs the potential harm of an increase in stomach bleeding. Women ages 55 to 79 years may choose to take low-dose aspirin when the potential benefit of preventing a stroke due to blood clot outweighs the potential harm of an increase in bleeding in the stomach. Let's take a look at whether you can tolerate aspirin and whether the low-dose aspirin is right for you.[21]

BP control. As of today you do not have hypertension. Because there are no symptoms you can feel if your blood pressure increases, I would like you to stop here every 3 months for a BP check with the nurses. No appointment necessary. If you ever do need medication to keep your BP at recommended levels, we will help you take the best medicine for you. There are changes in your daily life you can do to keep your BP low—more about those changes in a few minutes.

Cholesterol control. As of today you do not have worrisome cholesterol levels. We screen every year for men beginning at age 35 years and for women at age 45 years. An elevation in one type of cholesterol can damage the blood vessels that feed your heart. This is the low-density lipoprotein,

or LDL, and if it ever becomes elevated, we can help you control it through statin medications.

Smoking cessation. You have said today that you are willing to quit. This is probably the biggest thing you can do to protect your heart. I will give you advice on how to quit and make certain you are connected with our nurse telephone quit lines before you leave. We will get you started on quitting today. Then a nurse will call you every few days to talk about how you are doing. We will support you all the way until you are smoke free.

Small changes in your lifestyle. There are three modifications to your current lifestyle we can start to work on today. (1) A heart-healthy diet. I will give you 2 pamphlets on foods to increase (fruits and vegetables) and foods to avoid (such as trans fats and too much salt) to keep your heart healthy. (2) Physical activity. Let's look at finding time for you to be active. Aim for 30 minutes for 5 days of the week. You can set up a walking buddy for a daily stroll or try an exercise class or join a pickup sport such as soccer.[7] However, any exercise is better than none. We also have evidence that exercising on the weekend in the "weekend warrior" mode for just 1 or 2 times helps your heart.[18] These people tend to use sports or walking briskly and spend more workout time at the vigorous level. (3) Keep your weight in the healthy range. Actually, if you adopt a heart-healthy diet and increase your physical activity, your weight will naturally follow into a healthy range. However, we will check your weight range for your height and measure weight at each visit.

Health Promotion and Patient Teaching

DOCUMENTATION AND CRITICAL THINKING

Sample Charting

SUBJECTIVE

No chest pain, dyspnea, orthopnea, cough, fatigue, or edema. No history of hypertension, abnormal blood tests, heart murmur, or rheumatic fever in self. Last ECG 2 yrs PTA, result normal. No stress ECG or other heart tests.

Family history: Father with obesity, smoking, and hypertension, treated c̄ diuretic medication. No other family history significant for CV disease.

Personal habits: Diet balanced in 4 food groups, 2 to 3 c. regular coffee/day; no smoking; alcohol, 1 to 2 beers occasionally on weekend; exercise, runs 2 miles, 3 to 4 ×/week; no prescription or OTC medications or street drugs.

OBJECTIVE

Neck: Carotids' upstrokes are brisk and = bilaterally. No bruit. Internal jugular vein pulsations present when supine and disappear when elevated to a 45-degree position.

Precordium: Inspection. No visible pulsations; no heave or lift.

Palpation: Apical impulse in 5th ICS at left midclavicular line; no thrill.

Auscultation: Rate 68 bpm, rhythm regular, S_1-S_2 are crisp, not diminished or accentuated, no S_3, no S_4 or other extra sounds, no murmurs.

ASSESSMENT

Neck vessels healthy by inspection and auscultation
Heart sounds normal, no murmurs

Clinical Case Study 1

H.J. is a 56-year-old obese male with a past medical history of MI 6 months PTA, hypertension × 30 years, 50–pack/year history of smoking, type 2 diabetes × 1 year. Current medications include a beta-blocker, ACE-inhibitor, aspirin, oral antidiabetic medication, and a platelet inhibitor. H.J. is at the clinic for a 6-month follow-up with his cardiologist. Reports taking all medication except that he ran out of the beta-blocker last week.

SUBJECTIVE

H.J. reports increased breathlessness, nocturia, and fatigue 2 weeks PTA. For the past week, "my ankles look like melons after a day at work," and reports dizziness and palpitations ×2 days.

Family history includes father with MI resulting in death at age 50. Mother died in childbirth at age 21. Brother with hypertension and "some type of heart thing."

Personal habits: Smokes 2 ppd, drinks 1 to 2 beers at least 2 days per week. Caffeine intake of 1 to 2 cups of coffee each morning. "I try to eat healthy." Unable to provide 24-hour diet recall, but reports "salting everything, even my watermelon."

OBJECTIVE

Vital signs: Temperature 98.6° F (37° C). Pulse 130 bpm. Resp 22/min. BP 96/60 mm Hg, right arm, sitting.

Extremities: Skin cool, tan, no cyanosis. Bilateral upper extremities—no clubbing, no edema, capillary refill <3 seconds. Bilateral lower extremities—2+ pitting edema, no hair growth 10 cm below knees.

Cardiovascular, pulses: Carotid 2+, brachial 2+, radial 2+, femoral 2+, popliteal 0, PT 1+, DP 1+ (all pulses equal bilaterally).

Neck: Internal jugular vein pulsations 5 cm above sternal angle when elevated 30 degrees.

Heart Inspection: Apical impulse not visible. No heave. Palpation: Apical impulse not palpable. No thrill. Auscultation: Apical rate 120 bpm, irregularly irregular. S_1-S_2 present. S_1 varying intensity. S_3 gallop at apex and left lower sternal border. No murmur.

ASSESSMENT

Systolic heart failure
Atrial fibrillation
Decreased tissue perfusion
Need for health teaching on effects of smoking, extra salt, alcohol on heart, recommended dosing of beta blocker

Clinical Case Study 2

M.B. is a 35-year-old male originally from Northern India. Past medical history of rheumatic fever at age 10 years. Not treated. On no medications. All immunizations up to date.

SUBJECTIVE

M.B. reports worsening fatigue and dyspnea on exertion. "I've never had the same endurance as my friends, but my doctors in India told me that was normal." Substernal chest pain rated at 4/10 with exertion or stress. Relieved by rest. No family history of heart disease. No stress ECG or other heart tests. Nonsmoker. Reports no alcohol use. Denies use of illicit drugs. Eats a "balanced" diet in all food groups. 1 to 2 caffeinated beverages per day.

OBJECTIVE

Vital signs: Temperature 98.6° F (37° C). Pulse 74 bpm. Resp 14/min. BP 102/70 mm Hg, right arm, sitting.
Neck: Carotids 2+, equal bilaterally. Internal jugular vein pulsation present when supine, disappears when elevated 45 degrees.

Heart: Inspection: Lift at apex. Apical impulse visible 5th intercostal space, 4 cm left of midclavicular line. Palpation: Apical impulse 5th intercostal space, 4 cm left of midclavicular line, 2 cm × 2 cm. No thrills. Auscultation: S_1-S_2 present. S_1 accentuated. No S_3 or S_4. Low-pitched diastolic murmur grade 2/6 heard best at apex.

ASSESSMENT

Diastolic murmur, possibly mitral stenosis R/T childhood rheumatic fever
Fatigue
Decreased tissue perfusion

Clinical Case Study 3

N.V. is a 53-year-old male crane operator admitted to the CCU at University Medical Center (UMC) with chest pain.

SUBJECTIVE

1 year PTA—N.V. admitted to UMC with crushing substernal chest pain radiating to L shoulder, accompanied by nausea, vomiting, diaphoresis. Diagnosed as MI, hospitalized 7 days, discharged with nitroglycerin prn for anginal pain. Did not return to work. Activity included walking 1 mile/day, hunting. Had occasional episodes of chest pain with exercise, relieved by rest.

1 day PTA—Had increasing frequency of chest pain, about every 2 hours, lasting few minutes. Saw pain as warning to go to MD.
Day of admission—Severe substernal chest pain ("like someone sitting on my chest") unrelieved by rest. Saw personal MD; while in office had episode of chest pain similar to last year's, accompanied by diaphoresis; no N&V or SOB, relieved by 1 nitroglycerin. Transferred to UMC by paramedics. No further pain since admission 2 hours ago.
Family hx—Mother died of MI at age 57.
Personal habits—Smokes 1½ packs cigarettes daily × 34 years; no alcohol; diet—trying to limit fat and fried food, still high in added salt.

Documentation and
Critical Thinking

OBJECTIVE

Extremities: Skin tan pink, no cyanosis. Upper extrem.—capillary refill sluggish, no clubbing. Lower extrem.—no edema, no hair growth 10 cm below knee bilaterally.

Pulses:

Carotid	Brachial	Radial	Femoral	Popliteal	P.T.	D.P.	
2+	2+	2+	2+	0	0	1+	All = Bilaterally

BP R arm 104/66 mm Hg

Neck: External jugulars flat. Internal jugular pulsations present when supine and absent when elevated to 45 degrees.

Precordium: Inspection. Apical impulse visible 5th ICS, 7 cm left of midsternal line; no heave.

Palpation: Apical impulse palpable in 5th and 6th ICS; no thrill.

Auscultation: Apical rate 92 bpm, regular; S_1-S_2 are normal, not diminished or accentuated; no S_3 or S_4; grade 3/6 systolic murmur present at left lower sternal border.

ASSESSMENT

Substernal chest pain
Systolic murmur
Decreased tissue perfusion
Need for health teaching on effects of smoking

Clinical Case Study 4

L.B. is a 7-week-old female who is being admitted to the hospital for observation due to failure to thrive (FTT). The C-R monitor alarms, so you enter the room to find mom holding a sleeping baby. The monitor indicates a narrow QRS tachycardia.

SUBJECTIVE

Mom reports, "L.B. has always been a poor eater," vomits often with feeds, and is "overall less active and alert than my other kids were as babies." **Birth history:** Born at 40 weeks' gestation, SROM, vaginal birth w/o complications; weight 9 lbs (4.08 kg); birth length 21.5 in (56.6 cm); head circumference 34.5 cm.

OBJECTIVE

Vital signs: Temp 97.4° F (36.3° C, axillary). BP (unable to obtain). Pulse 236 bpm (sleeping). Resp 48/min. Weight 9 lbs 7 oz (4.3 kg). Head circumference 38 cm.

General appearance: Sleeping and pale w/labored breathing.

HEENT: Anterior and posterior fontanels flat; eyes clear; TM pearly gray bilat; nares patent bilat.

Cardiovascular: Tachycardia.

Respiratory: Tachypneic w/sternal and intercostal retractions; crackles to bilat lung bases.

Extremities: Mottled and cool to touch; 1+ pulses bilat.

ASSESSMENT

Supraventricular tachycardia (SVT)
Potential for weight loss
Decreased tissue perfusion: cerebral

ABNORMAL FINDINGS

TABLE 20.2	Differential Diagnosis of Chest Pain		
	Common Pain Description	Location/Radiation	Possible Associated Symptoms
Cardiovascular (Ischemic)			
Angina pectoris: stable (no change in pain pattern within last 60 days)	Pressurelike pain (e.g., tightness, squeezing, burning, heaviness that lasts 3-5 minutes precipitated by activity and often resolves with rest and/or nitroglycerin)	Generalized substernal or retrosternal: can radiate to teeth, jaw, neck, one or both arms or shoulders; or there may be no pain and only associated symptoms	Diaphoresis, nausea, vomiting, dyspnea, fatigue
Prinzmetal or variant angina	Pressurelike discomfort often occurring at rest, unrelated to physical or emotional stress	Retrosternal: can radiate to jaw, neck, left arm, or shoulder	Palpitations, syncope, or feelings of syncope
Acute coronary syndrome (ACS) (unstable angina, myocardial infarction)	Heaviness; viselike, squeezing, crushing, tightness; vague, burning, constricting, or pressure; poorly localized pain lasting 20-30 minutes to hours and does not resolve with rest or nitroglycerin	Generalized substernal or retrosternal: can radiate to teeth, jaw, neck, one or both arms or shoulders; or there may be no pain and only associated symptoms	Indigestion-like feeling, nausea, vomiting, dizziness, flushing, perspiration, palpitations, dyspnea, fatigue
Cardiovascular (Nonischemic)			
Pericarditis	Sudden sharp and stabbing pain relieved often by sitting or leaning forward and worsens by lying down or with inspiration	Substernal, which can radiate to trapezius muscle region	Dry cough, muscle and joint aches, fever
Mitral valve prolapse	Sharp pain not associated with activity	Chest pain without radiation	Fatigue, light-headedness, dyspnea, irregular heartbeat, palpitations, exercise intolerance
Aortic dissection	Sudden severe pain with change in location and/or tearing sensation lasting for hours	Anterior chest pain with radiation to the neck, jaw, or intrascapular region of the back	Mental status changes, limb pain and weakness, dyspnea
Pulmonary hypertension (secondary)	Cardiac-like chest pain with exertion	Chest region	Dyspnea, lower-extremity edema, fatigue
Pulmonary			
Pulmonary embolism	Sharp, stabbing pain worsening with deep breaths	Pain can be experienced in chest, back, shoulder, or upper abdomen	Dyspnea, hemoptysis, cough
Pneumonia	Sharp or stabbing pain associated with cough	Mostly generalized to one side of chest but can have upper abdominal pain	Cough, fever, dyspnea, chills, sputum, myalgia, malaise
Pneumothorax	Acute/sudden and sharp	Lateral region of the chest but can have referred pain to shoulder	Acute dyspnea, cough

Continued

TABLE 20.2	Differential Diagnosis of Chest Pain—cont'd		
	Common Pain Description	Location/Radiation	Possible Associated Symptoms
Gastrointestinal			
Gastroesophageal reflux	May be angina-like; however, usually burning sensation with eating large meals reproduced by lying down and relieved by sitting up	Retrosternal region	Cough, regurgitation of food, abdominal pain
Esophageal spasm	Crushing chest pain	Substernal	Dysphagia, sensation of object in throat or esophagus
Cholecystitis	Sudden onset of pain that crescendos and can last for up to 20 minutes, usually after eating a fatty meal	Epigastrium or right upper abdomen that can radiate to right intrascapular region, shoulder, or back	Nausea, vomiting, anorexia, fever
Pancreatitis	Sudden dull, boring, steady pain unrelieved by lying supine; leaning forward or the fetal position may ease pain	Epigastrium or periumbilical pain radiating to back	Nausea, vomiting, anorexia, and sometimes diarrhea
Dermatologic			
Herpes zoster	Unilateral, burning, borelike pain	Chest region in dermatome distribution	Tingling, itching, burning
Musculoskeletal/Neurologic			
Costochondritis	Sharp, pleuritic-type pain worsens with deep breathing, palpation, or movement	Area from 2nd through 5th intercostal spaces; can radiate to arm, depending on where initial inflammation occurs	Chest tightness, warmth at area of pain
Chest wall muscle strain	Sharp pain with moving, stretching, or pushing movements of the arms; palpation of area reproduces the pain	Area around the strained muscle, sternum, or ribs	Muscle spasm, crepitation, swelling, loss of strength
Psychogenic			
Depression	Heaviness	Chest region	Fatigue, restlessness, withdrawal, weight gain or loss, depressed mood
Anxiety	Sharp pain	Chest region	Palpitations, dizziness, sweating, shaking, restlessness, fatigue, irritability

Adapted from Zitkus, B. S. (2010). Take chest pain to heart. *Nurse Pract, 35*(9), 41-47.

TABLE 20.3 | Clinical Portrait of Heart Failure

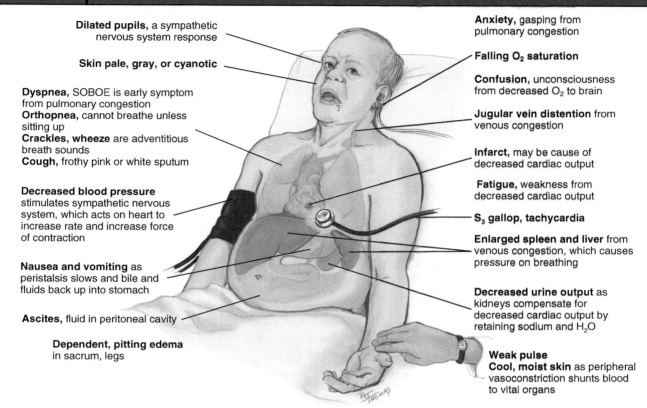

Dilated pupils, a sympathetic nervous system response

Skin pale, gray, or cyanotic

Dyspnea, SOBOE is early symptom from pulmonary congestion
Orthopnea, cannot breathe unless sitting up
Crackles, wheeze are adventitious breath sounds
Cough, frothy pink or white sputum

Decreased blood pressure stimulates sympathetic nervous system, which acts on heart to increase rate and increase force of contraction

Nausea and vomiting as peristalsis slows and bile and fluids back up into stomach

Ascites, fluid in peritoneal cavity

Dependent, pitting edema in sacrum, legs

Anxiety, gasping from pulmonary congestion

Falling O₂ saturation

Confusion, unconsciousness from decreased O_2 to brain

Jugular vein distention from venous congestion

Infarct, may be cause of decreased cardiac output

Fatigue, weakness from decreased cardiac output

S₃ gallop, tachycardia

Enlarged spleen and liver from venous congestion, which causes pressure on breathing

Decreased urine output as kidneys compensate for decreased cardiac output by retaining sodium and H_2O

Weak pulse
Cool, moist skin as peripheral vasoconstriction shunts blood to vital organs

Decreased cardiac output occurs when the heart fails as a pump and the circulation becomes backed up and congested. **Signs and symptoms** of heart failure come from two basic mechanisms: (1) the heart's inability to pump enough blood to meet the metabolic demands of the body; and (2) the kidney's compensatory mechanisms of abnormal retention of sodium and water to compensate for the decreased cardiac output. This increases blood volume and venous return, which causes further congestion.

Onset of heart failure may be: (1) *acute,* as following a myocardial infarction when the heart's contracting ability has been directly damaged; or (2) *chronic,* as with hypertension, when the ventricles must pump against chronically increased pressure. Heart failure may involve **systolic dysfunction,** in which the heart cannot contract properly, resulting in a low ejection fraction (the stroke volume divided by the end-diastolic volume, normally 60% to 80%). **Diastolic dysfunction** is a failure of the heart to relax fully between heartbeats; here the heart muscle wall is stiff and does not fill properly; there is low cardiac output but a normal ejection fraction. About 50% of patients with heart failure have a preserved ejection fraction.[20] The ejection fraction is normal at rest, but it may not increase appropriately with the stress of exercise, tachycardia, or hypertension.[20]

SOBOE, Shortness of breath on exertion.

ABNORMAL FINDINGS
FOR ADVANCED PRACTICE

TABLE 20.4 | Variations in S_1

The intensity of S_1 depends on three factors: (1) position of the atrioventricular (AV) valve at the start of systole, (2) structure of the valve leaflets, and (3) how quickly pressure rises in the ventricle.

	Factor	Examples
Loud (Accentuated) S_1 S_1 S_2	1. Position of AV valve at start of systole—Wide open and no time to drift together 2. Change in valve structure—Calcification of valve; needs increasing ventricular pressure to close the valve against increased atrial pressure	Hyperkinetic states in which blood velocity is increased: exercise, fever, anemia, hyperthyroidism Mitral stenosis with leaflets still mobile
Faint (Diminished) S_1 S_1 S_2	1. Position of AV valve—Delayed conduction from atria to ventricles. Mitral valve drifts shut before ventricular contraction closes it 2. Change in valve structure—Extreme calcification, which limits mobility 3. More forceful atrial contraction into noncompliant ventricle; delays or diminishes ventricular contraction	First-degree heart block (prolonged PR interval) Mitral insufficiency Severe hypertension—Systemic or pulmonary
Varying Intensity of S_1 S_1 S_2 S_1 S_2	1. Position of AV valve varies before closing from beat to beat 2. Atria and ventricles beat independently	Atrial fibrillation—Irregularly irregular rhythm Complete heart block with changing PR interval
Split S_1 S_1 S_2 T M	Mitral and tricuspid components are heard separately	Normal but uncommon

TABLE 20.5 | Variations in S_2

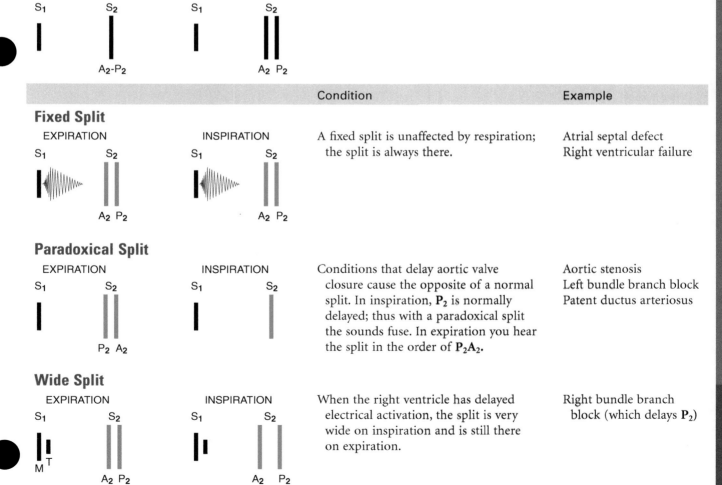

	Condition	Example
Accentuated S_2		
	1. Higher closing pressure	Systemic hypertension, ringing or booming S_2
	2. Exercise and excitement increase pressure in aorta	
	3. Pulmonary hypertension	Mitral stenosis, heart failure
	4. Semilunar valves calcified but still mobile	Aortic or pulmonic stenosis
Diminished S_2		
	1. A fall in systemic blood pressure causes a decrease in valve strength	Shock
	2. Semilunar valves thickened and calcified, with decreased mobility	Aortic or pulmonic stenosis

TABLE 20.6 | Variations in Split S_2

Normal Splitting

EXPIRATION   INSPIRATION

S_1 S_2 S_1 S_2

A_2-P_2 A_2 P_2

	Condition	Example
Fixed Split	A fixed split is unaffected by respiration; the split is always there.	Atrial septal defect Right ventricular failure
Paradoxical Split	Conditions that delay aortic valve closure cause the opposite of a normal split. In inspiration, P_2 is normally delayed; thus with a paradoxical split the sounds fuse. In expiration you hear the split in the order of P_2A_2.	Aortic stenosis Left bundle branch block Patent ductus arteriosus
Wide Split	When the right ventricle has delayed electrical activation, the split is very wide on inspiration and is still there on expiration.	Right bundle branch block (which delays P_2)

TABLE 20.7	Systolic Extra Sounds

Early systolic:	Mid/late systolic:
Ejection click	Midsystolic (mitral) click
Aortic prosthetic valve sounds	

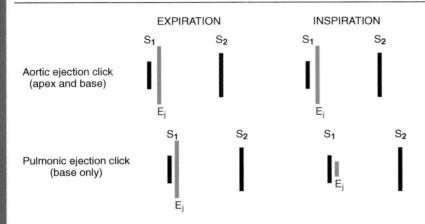

Ejection Click

The ejection click occurs early in systole at the start of ejection because it results from opening of the semilunar (SL) valves. Normally the SL valves open silently, but in the presence of stenosis (e.g., aortic stenosis, pulmonic stenosis) their opening makes a sound. It is short and high pitched, with a click quality and is heard better with the diaphragm.

The aortic ejection click is heard at the 2nd right interspace and apex and may be loudest at the apex. Its intensity does not change with respiration. The pulmonic ejection click is best heard in the 2nd left interspace and often grows softer with inspiration.

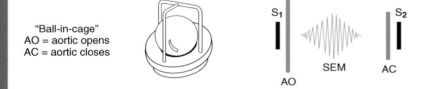

"Ball-in-cage"
AO = aortic opens
AC = aortic closes

Aortic Prosthetic Valve Sounds

As a sequela of modern technologic intervention for heart problems, some people now have *iatrogenically* induced heart sounds. The opening of a mechanical aortic ball-in-cage prosthesis produces an early systolic sound. This sound is less intense with a tilting disk prosthesis and is absent with a biologic tissue prosthesis (e.g., porcine).

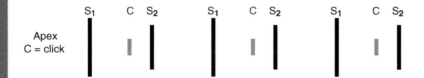

Apex
C = click

Midsystolic Click

Although it is systolic, this is not an ejection click. It is associated with **mitral valve prolapse,** in which the mitral valve leaflets not only close with contraction but balloon back up into the left atrium. During ballooning the sudden tensing of the valve leaflets and the chordae tendineae creates the click.

The sound occurs in mid-to-late systole and is short and high pitched with a click quality. It is best heard with the diaphragm, at the apex, but also may be heard at the left lower sternal border. The click usually is followed by a systolic murmur. The click and murmur move with postural change; when the person assumes a squatting position, the click may move closer to S_2, and the murmur may sound louder and delayed. The Valsalva maneuver also moves the click closer to S_2.

TABLE 20.8	Diastolic Extra Sounds

Early diastole:
  Opening snap
  Mitral prosthetic valve sound

Mid-diastole:
  Third heart sound
  Summation sound ($S_3 + S_4$)

Late diastole:
  Fourth heart sound
  Pacemaker-induced sound

Opening Snap

Normally the opening of the AV valves is silent. In the presence of stenosis, increasingly higher atrial pressure is required to open the valve. The deformed valve opens with a noise: the opening snap. It is sharp and high pitched with a snapping quality. It sounds after S_2 and is best heard with the diaphragm at the 3rd or 4th left interspace at the sternal border, less well at the apex.

    The opening snap usually is not an isolated sound. As a sign of mitral stenosis, the opening snap usually ushers in the low-pitched diastolic rumbling murmur of that condition.

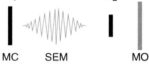

Mitral Prosthetic Valve Sound

An iatrogenic sound, the opening of a ball-in-cage mitral prosthesis gives an early diastolic sound: an opening click just after S_2. It is loud, heard over the whole precordium, and loudest at the apex and left lower sternal border.

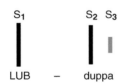 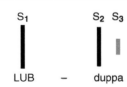

Third Heart Sound

The S_3 is a ventricular filling sound. It occurs in early diastole during the rapid filling phase. Your hearing quickly accommodates to the S_3; thus it is best heard when you listen initially. It sounds after S_2 but later than an opening snap would be. It is a dull, soft sound; and it is low pitched, like "distant thunder." It is heard best in a quiet room, at the apex, with the bell held lightly (just enough to form a seal), and with the person in the left lateral position.

    The S_3 can be confused with a split S_2. Use these guidelines to distinguish the S_3:

- *Location*—The S_3 is heard at the apex or left lower sternal border; the split S_2 at the base.
- *Respiratory variation*—The S_3 does not vary in timing with respirations; the split S_2 does.
- *Pitch*—The S_3 is lower pitched; the pitch of the split S_2 stays the same.

    The S_3 may be normal (physiologic) or abnormal (pathologic). The **physiologic S_3** is heard frequently in children and young adults; it occasionally may persist after 40 years, especially in women. The normal S_3 usually disappears when the person sits up.

    In adults the S_3 is usually abnormal. The **pathologic S_3** is also called a **ventricular gallop** or an S_3 gallop, and it persists when sitting up. The S_3 indicates decreased compliance of the ventricles, as in heart failure. It may be the earliest sign of heart failure. The S_3 may originate from either the left or the right ventricle; a left-sided S_3 is heard at the apex in the left lateral position, and a right-sided S_3 is heard at the left lower sternal border with the person supine and is louder in inspiration.

    The S_3 also occurs with conditions of volume overload such as mitral regurgitation and aortic or tricuspid regurgitation. The S_3 is also found in high cardiac output states in the absence of heart disease such as hyperthyroidism, anemia, and pregnancy. When the primary condition is corrected, the gallop disappears.

Continued

TABLE 20.8	**Diastolic Extra Sounds—cont'd**

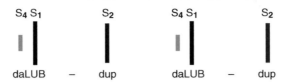

Fourth Heart Sound

The **S₄** is a ventricular filling sound. It occurs when the atria contract late in diastole. It is heard immediately before **S₁**. This is a very soft sound of very low pitch. You need a good bell, and you must be listening for it. It is heard best at the apex with the person in left lateral position.

A **physiologic S₄** may occur in adults older than 40 or 50 years with no evidence of cardiovascular disease, especially after exercise.

A **pathologic S₄** is termed an **atrial gallop** or an **S₄ gallop**. It occurs with decreased compliance of the ventricle (e.g., coronary artery disease, cardiomyopathy) and systolic overload (afterload), including outflow obstruction to the ventricle (aortic stenosis) and systemic hypertension. A left-sided **S₄** occurs with these conditions. It is heard best at the apex, in the left lateral position.

A right-sided **S₄** is less common. It is heard at the left lower sternal border and may increase with inspiration. It occurs with pulmonary stenosis or pulmonary hypertension.

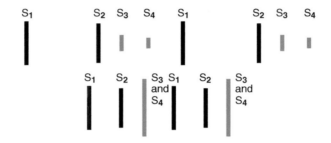

Summation Sound

When both the pathologic **S₃** and **S₄** are present, a quadruple rhythm is heard. Often in cases of cardiac stress, one response is tachycardia. During rapid rates the diastolic filling time shortens, and the **S₃** and **S₄** move closer together. They sound superimposed in mid-diastole, and you hear one loud, prolonged, summated sound, often louder than either **S₁** or **S₂**.

Extracardiac Sounds

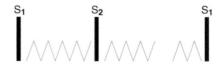

Pericardial Friction Rub

Inflammation of the pericardium gives rise to a friction rub. The sound is high pitched and scratchy, like sandpaper being rubbed. It is best heard with the diaphragm, with the person sitting up and leaning forward and the breath held in expiration.

A friction rub can be heard any place on the precordium but usually is best heard at the apex and left lower sternal border, places where the pericardium comes in close contact with the chest wall. Timing may be systolic and diastolic. The friction rub of pericarditis is common during the 1st week after a myocardial infarction and may last only a few hours.

TABLE 20.9 │ Abnormal Pulsations on the Precordium

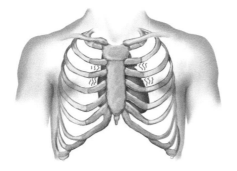

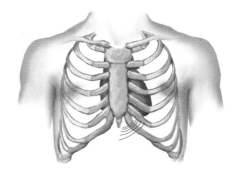

Base

A **thrill** in the 2nd and 3rd right interspaces occurs with severe aortic stenosis and systemic hypertension.

A **thrill** in the 2nd and 3rd left interspaces occurs with pulmonic stenosis and pulmonic hypertension.

Left Sternal Border

A **lift (heave)** occurs with right ventricular hypertrophy, as found in pulmonic valve disease, pulmonic hypertension, and chronic lung disease. You feel a diffuse lifting impulse during systole at the left lower sternal border. It may be associated with retraction at the apex because the left ventricle is rotated posteriorly by the enlarged right ventricle.

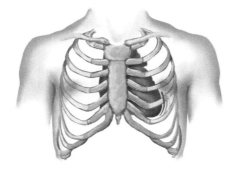

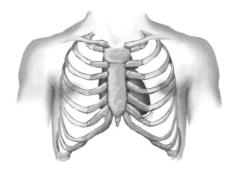

Apex

Cardiac enlargement displaces the apical impulse laterally and over a wider area when left ventricular hypertrophy and dilation are present. This is **volume overload,** as in heart failure, mitral regurgitation, aortic regurgitation, and left-to-right shunts.

Apex

The apical impulse is increased in force and duration but is not necessarily displaced to the left when left ventricular hypertrophy occurs alone without dilation. This is **pressure overload,** as found in aortic stenosis or systemic hypertension.

Images © Pat Thomas, 2006.

TABLE 20.10 | Congenital Heart Defects

	Description	Clinical Data

Patent Ductus Arteriosus (PDA)

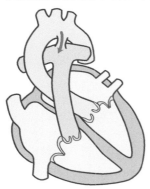

Persistence of the channel joining left pulmonary artery to aorta. This is normal in the fetus and usually closes spontaneously within hours of birth.

S: Usually no symptoms in early childhood; growth and development are normal.

O: Blood pressure has wide pulse pressure and bounding peripheral pulses from rapid runoff of blood into low-resistance pulmonary bed during diastole. Thrill is often palpable at left upper sternal border. The continuous murmur heard in systole and diastole is called a *machinery murmur.*

Atrial Septal Defect (ASD)

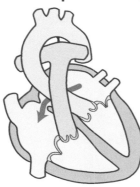

Abnormal opening in the atrial septum, resulting usually in left-to-right shunt and causing large increase in pulmonary blood flow.

S: Defect is remarkably well tolerated. Symptoms in infants are rare; growth and development normal. Children and young adults have mild fatigue and DOE.

O: Sternal lift is often present. S_2 has fixed split, with P_2 often louder than A_2. Murmur is systolic, ejection, medium pitch, best heard at base in 2nd left interspace. Murmur is caused not by shunt itself but by increased blood flow through pulmonic valve.

Ventricular Septal Defect (VSD)

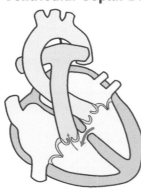

Abnormal opening in septum between the ventricles, usually subaortic area. The size and exact position vary considerably. If the VSD is large, the extra L→R blood volume can overload the right heart and lungs, causing right-sided heart failure.

S: Small defects are asymptomatic. Infants with large defects have poor growth, slow weight gain; later they look pale, thin, delicate. May have feeding problems; DOE; frequent respiratory infections; and, when the condition is severe, heart failure.

O: Loud, harsh holosystolic murmur, best heard at left lower sternal border, may be accompanied by thrill. Large defects also have soft diastolic murmur at apex (mitral flow murmur) caused by increased blood flow through mitral valve.

Continued

TABLE 20.10	Congenital Heart Defects—cont'd	
	Description	Clinical Data

Tetralogy of Fallot

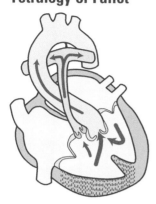

Four defects: (1) pulmonic (right ventricular outflow) stenosis, (2) VSD, (3) compensatory right ventricular hypertrophy, and (4) overriding aorta that receives blood from both R and L ventricles. *Result:* shunts a lot of venous blood directly into aorta away from pulmonary system; thus blood never gets oxygenated.

S: Severe cyanosis, not in first months of life but develops as infant grows and right ventricular outflow (i.e., pulmonic) stenosis gets worse. Cyanosis with crying and exertion at first, then at rest. Uses squatting posture after starts walking. DOE is common. Development is slowed.
O: Thrill palpable at left lower sternal border. S_1 normal; S_2 has A_2 loud and P_2 diminished or absent. Murmur is systolic, loud, crescendo-decrescendo.

Coarctation of the Aorta

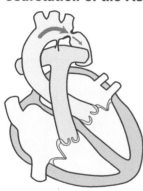

Severe narrowing of descending aorta, usually at the junction of the ductus arteriosus and the aortic arch, just distal to the origin of the left subclavian artery. Results in increased workload on left ventricle and obstruction of distal blood flow. Associated with defects of aortic valve in most cases, associated patent ductus arteriosus, and associated VSD.

S: In infants with associated lesions or symptoms, diagnosis occurs in the early months as heart failure develops. For asymptomatic children, growth and development are normal. Diagnosis follows abnormal BP findings. Adolescents may complain of vague lower-extremity cramping, worse with exercise.
O: Arm hypertension over 20 mm Hg higher than leg measures is a hallmark of coarctation. Another important sign is absent or greatly diminished femoral pulses. A systolic murmur is heard best at the left sternal border, radiating to the back.

S, Subjective data; *O,* objective data.

Images © Pat Thomas, 2006.

TABLE 20.11	Murmurs Caused by Valvular Defects

Midsystolic Ejection Murmurs

Caused by forward flow through semilunar valves. Examples below have the murmur pictured here:

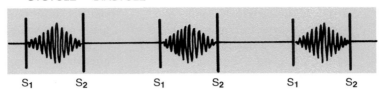

	Description	Clinical Data

Aortic Stenosis

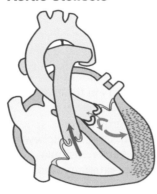

Calcification of aortic valve cusps restricts forward flow of blood during systole; LV hypertrophy develops.

S: Fatigue, DOE, palpitation, dizziness, fainting, anginal pain.

O: Pallor, slow diminished radial pulse, low BP, and auscultatory gap are common. Apical impulse sustained and displaced to left. Thrill in systole over 2nd and 3rd right interspaces and right side of neck. S_1 normal, often ejection click present, often paradoxical split S_2, S_4 present with LV hypertrophy.

Murmur: Loud, harsh, midsystolic, crescendo-decrescendo, loudest at second right interspace, radiates widely to side of neck, down left sternal border, or apex.

Pulmonic Stenosis

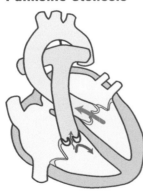

Calcification of pulmonic valve restricts forward flow of blood.

O: Thrill in systole at 2nd and 3rd left interspaces, ejection click often present after S_1, diminished S_2 and usually with wide split, S_4 common with RV hypertrophy.

Murmur: Systolic, medium pitch, coarse, crescendo-decrescendo (diamond shape), best heard at 2nd left interspace, radiates to the left and neck.

Continued

TABLE 20.11	Murmurs Caused by Valvular Defects—cont'd

Pansystolic Regurgitant Murmurs

Caused by backward flow of blood from area of higher pressure to one of lower pressure. Examples below have the murmur pictured here:

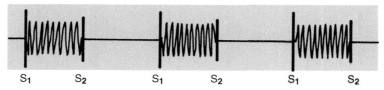

	Description	Clinical Data
Mitral Regurgitation 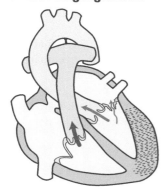	Stream of blood regurgitates back into LA during systole through incompetent mitral valve. In diastole, blood passes back into LV again along with new flow; results in LV dilation and hypertrophy.	S: Fatigue, palpitation, orthopnea, PND. O: Thrill in systole at apex. Lift at apex. Apical impulse displaced down and to left. S_1 diminished, S_2 accentuated, S_3 at apex often present. Murmur: Pansystolic, often loud, blowing; best heard at apex; radiates well to left axilla.
Tricuspid Regurgitation 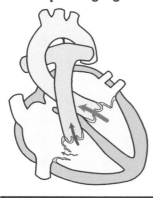	Backflow of blood through incompetent tricuspid valve into RA.	O: Engorged pulsating neck veins, liver enlarged. Lift at sternum if RV hypertrophy present; often thrill at left lower sternal border. Murmur: Soft, blowing, pansystolic; best heard at left lower sternal border; increases with inspiration.

Continued

TABLE 20.11 | Murmurs Caused by Valvular Defects—cont'd

Diastolic Rumbles of AV Valves

Filling murmurs at low pressures, best heard with bell lightly touching skin. Examples below have the murmur pictured here:

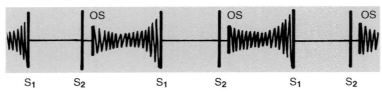

	Description	Clinical Data
Mitral Stenosis 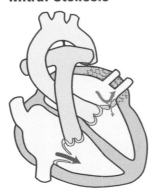	Calcified mitral valve does not open properly, impedes forward flow of blood into LV during diastole. Results in LA enlarged and LA pressure increased.	S: Fatigue, palpitations, DOE, orthopnea, occasional PND or pulmonary edema. O: Diminished, often irregular arterial pulse. Lift at apex, diastolic thrill common at apex. S_1 accentuated; opening snap after S_2 heard over wide area of precordium, followed by murmur. Murmur: Low-pitched diastolic rumble, best heard at apex, with person in left lateral position; does not radiate.
Tricuspid Stenosis 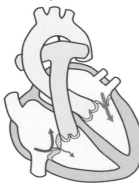	Calcification of tricuspid valve impedes forward flow into RV during diastole.	O: Diminished arterial pulse, jugular venous pulse prominent. Murmur: Diastolic rumble; best heard at left lower sternal border; louder in inspiration.

Continued

TABLE 20.11 | Murmurs Caused by Valvular Defects—cont'd

Early Diastolic Murmurs

Caused by emilunar valve incompetence. Examples below have the murmur pictured here:

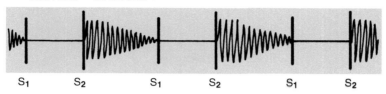

	Description	Clinical Data

Aortic Regurgitation

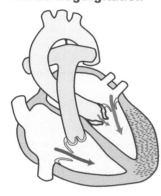

Stream of blood regurgitates back through incompetent aortic valve into LV during diastole. LV dilation and hypertrophy caused by increased LV stroke volume. Rapid ejection of large stroke volume into poorly filled aorta, then rapid runoff in diastole as part of blood pushed back into LV.

S: Only minor symptoms for many years, then rapid deterioration: DOE, PND, angina, dizziness.

O: Bounding "water-hammer" pulse in carotid, brachial, and femoral arteries. Blood pressure has wide pulse pressure. Pulsations in cervical and suprasternal area, apical impulse displaced to left and down, apical impulse feels brief.

Murmur starts almost simultaneously with **S₂**: soft, high pitched, blowing diastolic, decrescendo, best heard at 3rd left interspace at base as person sits up and leans forward, radiates down.

Pulmonic Regurgitation

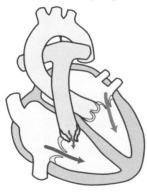

Backflow of blood through incompetent pulmonic valve from pulmonary artery to RV.

Murmur has same timing and characteristics as that of aortic regurgitation, and is hard to distinguish on physical examination.

O, Objective data; *S*, subjective data.

Images © Pat Thomas, 2006.

Summary Checklist: Heart and Neck Vessels Examination

Neck
1. Carotid pulse—Observe and palpate
2. Observe jugular venous pulse
3. Estimate jugular venous pressure

Precordium
Inspection and palpation
1. Describe location of apical impulse.
2. Note any heave (lift) or thrill.

Auscultation
1. Identify anatomic areas where you listen.
2. Note rate and rhythm of heartbeat.
3. Identify S_1 and S_2 and note any variation.
4. Listen in systole and diastole for any extra heart sounds.
5. Listen in systole and diastole for any murmurs.

6. Repeat sequence with bell.
7. Listen at the apex with person in left lateral position
8. Listen at the base with person in sitting position.

REFERENCES

1. Al Ghatrif, M., & Lakatta, E. G. (2015). The conundrum of arterial stiffness, elevated blood presssure, and aging. *Curr Hypertens Rep, 17*(2), 1.
2. Anderson, J. L., & Morrow, D. A. (2017). Acute myocardial infarction. *N Engl J Med, 376*(21), 2053–2064.
3. Benjamin, E. J., Blaha, M. J., Chiuve, S. E., et al. (2017). Heart Disease and Stroke Statistics—2017 Update: A report for the American Heart Association. *Circulation, 135*(10), e146–e603.
4. Blakeman, J. R., & Booker, K. J. (2016). Prodromal myocardial infarction symptoms experienced by women. *Heart Lung, 45,* 327–335.
5. Briggs, L. A. (2018). Deciphering chest pain in women. *Nurse Pract, 43*(4), 25–33.
6. Campo, D. L. (2016). Recognizing myocardial infarction in women. *Am J Nurs, 116*(9), 46–49.
7. Center for Disease Control (CDC). (2018). *American Heart Month 2018: You're in Control.* https://millionhearts.hhs.gov/news-media/events/heart-month.html.
8. DeVon, H. A., Burke, L. A., Vuckovic, K. M., et al. (2016). Symptoms suggestive of acute coronary syndrome. *J Cardiovasc Nurs, 32*(4), 383–392.
9. Grotta, J. C. (2013). Carotid stenosis. *N Engl J Med, 369*(12), 1143–1149.
10. Isaksson, R. M., Brulin, C., Eliasson, M., et al. (2013). Older women's prehospital experiences of their first myocardial infarction. *J Cardiovasc Nurs, 28,* 360–369.
11. Kaur, A., & Miller, M. (2017). General management principles of the pregnant woman. *Semin Respir Crit Care Med, 38,* 123–134. https://i1.ytimg.com/vi/nN6VR92V70M/mqdefault.jpgCare.
12. Khera, A. V., Emdin, C. A., Drake, I., et al. (2016). Genetic risk, adherence to a healthy lifestyle, and coronary disease. *N Engl J Med, 375*(24), 2349–2358.
13. Leveno, K. L., Corton, M. M., Dashe, J. S., et al. (2018). *Williams obstetrics* (25th ed.). New York: McGraw-Hill Education.
14. Mann, D. L., Zipes, D. P., Libby, P., et al. (2015). *Braunwald's heart disease: A textbook of cardiovascular medicine* (10th ed.). St. Louis: Elsevier.
15. McGee, S. (2018). *Evidence-based physical diagnosis* (4th ed.). St. Louis: Elsevier.
16. McSweeney, J. C., Rosenfeld, A. G., Abel, W. M., et al. (2016). Preventing and experiencing ischemic heart disease as a woman: State of the science. *Circulation, 133,* 1302–1331.
17. Melnyk, B. M., Orosilini, L., Gawlik, K., et al. (2016). The Million Hearts initiative: Guidelines and best practices. *Nurse Pract, 41*(2), 46–53.
18. O'Donovan, G., Lee, I.-M., & Hamer, M. (2017). Association of "Weekend Warrior" and other leisure time physical activity patterns with risks for all-cause, cardiovascular disease, and cancer mortality. *JAMA Intern Med, 177*(3), 335–342.
19. Pickett, C. A., Jackson, J. L., Hemann, B. A., et al. (2010). Carotid bruits and cerebrovascular disease risk: A meta-analysis. *Stroke, 41*(10), 2295–2302.
20. Redfield, M. (2016). Heart failure with preserved ejection fraction. *N Engl J Med, 375*(19), 1868–1877.
21. Richman, I. B., & Owens, D. K. (2017). Aspirin for primary prevention. *Med Clin North Am, 10,* 713–724.
22. Vaughan, A. S., Ritchey, M. D., Hannan, J., et al. (2017). Widespread recent increases in county-level heart disease mortality across age groups. *Ann Epidemiol, 27,* 796–800.
23. Wang, T. J. (2016). Vitamin D and cardiovascular disease. *Annu Rev Med, 67,* 261–272.
24. Wierwille, L. (2011). Pediatric heart murmurs: Evaluation and management in primary care. *Nurse Pract, 36*(3), 22–29.
25. Yeh, T. K., & Yeh, J. (2015). Chest pain in pediatrics. *Pediatr Ann, 44*(12), e274.

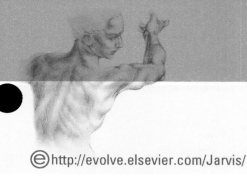

CHAPTER 21

Peripheral Vascular System and Lymphatic System

STRUCTURE AND FUNCTION

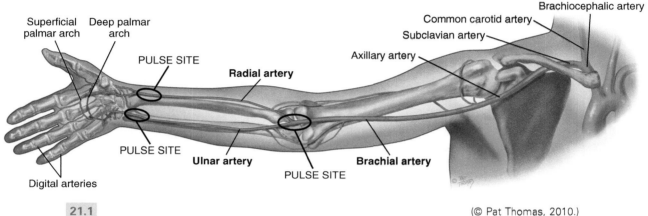

21.1

(© Pat Thomas, 2010.)

The vascular system consists of the vessels for transporting fluid such as the blood or lymph. Any disease in the vascular system impairs the delivery of oxygen and nutrients to the affected cells and retards the elimination of carbon dioxide and waste products from cellular metabolism.

ARTERIES

The heart pumps freshly oxygenated blood through the arteries to all body tissues (Fig. 21.1). The pumping heart makes this a high-pressure system. The artery walls are strong, tough, and tense to withstand pressure demands. Arteries contain elastic fibers, which allow their walls to stretch with systole and recoil with diastole. They also contain muscle fibers (vascular smooth muscle [VSM]), which control the amount of blood delivered to the tissues. The VSM contracts or dilates, which changes the diameter of the arteries to control the rate of blood flow.

Each heartbeat creates a pressure wave, which makes the arteries expand and then recoil. It is the recoil that propels blood through like a wave. All arteries have this pressure wave, or **pulse,** throughout their length, but you can feel it only at body sites where the artery lies close to the skin and over a bone. The following arteries are accessible to examination.

Temporal Artery. The temporal artery is palpated in front of the ear, as discussed in Chapter 14.

Carotid Artery. The carotid artery is palpated in the groove between the sternomastoid muscle and the trachea, as discussed in Chapter 20.

Arteries in the Arm. The major artery supplying the arm is the **brachial** artery, which runs in the biceps-triceps furrow of the upper arm and surfaces at the antecubital fossa in the elbow medial to the biceps tendon (see Fig. 21.1). Immediately below the elbow the brachial artery bifurcates into the ulnar and radial arteries. These run distally and form two arches supplying the hand; these are called the *superficial* and *deep palmar arches.* The radial pulse lies just medial to the radius at the wrist; the ulnar artery is in the same relation to the ulna, but it is deeper and often difficult to feel.

Arteries in the Leg. The major artery to the leg is the **femoral** artery, which passes under the inguinal ligament (Fig. 21.2). The femoral artery travels down the thigh. At the lower thigh it courses posteriorly; then it is termed the **popliteal** artery. Below the knee the popliteal artery divides. The anterior tibial artery travels down the front of the leg on to the dorsum of the foot, where it becomes the **dorsalis pedis.** In back of the leg the **posterior tibial** artery travels down behind the medial malleolus and forms the plantar arteries in the foot.

The function of the arteries is to supply oxygen and essential nutrients to the cells. **Ischemia** is a deficient supply of oxygenated arterial blood to a tissue caused by obstruction

501

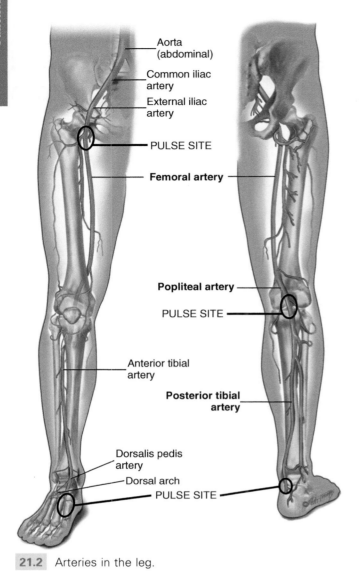

21.2   Arteries in the leg.

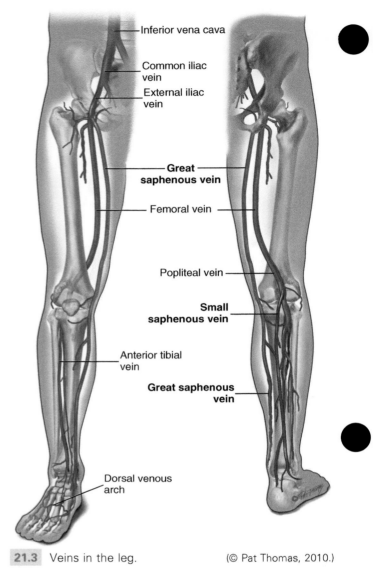

21.3   Veins in the leg.   (© Pat Thomas, 2010.)

of a blood vessel. A complete blockage leads to death of the distal tissue. A partial blockage creates an insufficient supply, and the ischemia may be apparent only at exercise when oxygen needs increase. **Peripheral artery disease (PAD)** affects noncoronary arteries and usually refers to arteries supplying the limbs. It usually is caused by atherosclerosis, and less commonly by embolism, hypercoagulable states, or arterial dissection.

VEINS

The course of the veins is parallel to the arteries, but the direction of flow is opposite; the veins absorb CO_2 and waste products from the periphery and carry them back to the heart. The body has more veins, and they lie closer to the skin surface. The following veins are accessible to examination.

Jugular Veins. Assessment of the jugular veins is presented in Chapter 20.

Veins in the Arm. Each arm has two sets of veins: superficial and deep. The superficial veins are in the subcutaneous tissue and are responsible for most of the venous return.

Veins in the Leg. The legs have three types of veins (Fig. 21.3):

1. The **deep veins** run alongside the deep arteries and conduct most of the venous return from the legs. These are the **femoral** and **popliteal** veins. As long as these veins remain intact, the superficial veins can be excised without harming the circulation.

2. The **superficial veins** are the **great** and **small saphenous** veins. The great saphenous vein, inside the leg, starts at the medial side of the dorsum of the foot. You can see it ascend in front of the medial malleolus; then it crosses the tibia obliquely and ascends along the medial side of the thigh. The small saphenous vein, outside the leg, starts on the lateral side of the dorsum of the foot and ascends behind the lateral malleolus, up the back of the leg, where it joins

the popliteal vein. Blood flows from the superficial veins into the deep leg veins.

3. **Perforators** (not illustrated) are connecting veins that join the two sets. They also have one-way valves that route blood from the superficial into the deep veins and prevent reflux to the superficial veins.

VENOUS FLOW

Veins drain the deoxygenated blood with its waste products from the tissues and return it to the heart. Unlike the arteries, veins are a low-pressure system. Because they do not have a pump to generate their blood flow, they need a mechanism to keep blood moving (Fig. 21.4). This is accomplished by (1) the contracting skeletal muscles that milk the blood proximally, back toward the heart; (2) the pressure gradient caused by breathing, in which inspiration makes the thoracic pressure decrease and the abdominal pressure increase; and (3) the intraluminal valves, which ensure unidirectional flow. Each valve is a paired semilunar pocket that opens toward the heart and closes tightly when filled to prevent backflow of blood.

In the legs this mechanism is called the *calf pump* or *peripheral heart*. When walking, the calf muscles alternately contract (systole) and relax (diastole). In the contraction phase the gastrocnemius and soleus muscles squeeze the veins and direct the blood flow proximally. Because of the valves, venous blood flows just one way—toward the heart.

Besides the presence of intraluminal valves, venous structure differs from arterial structure. Because venous pressure is lower, walls of the veins are thinner than those of the

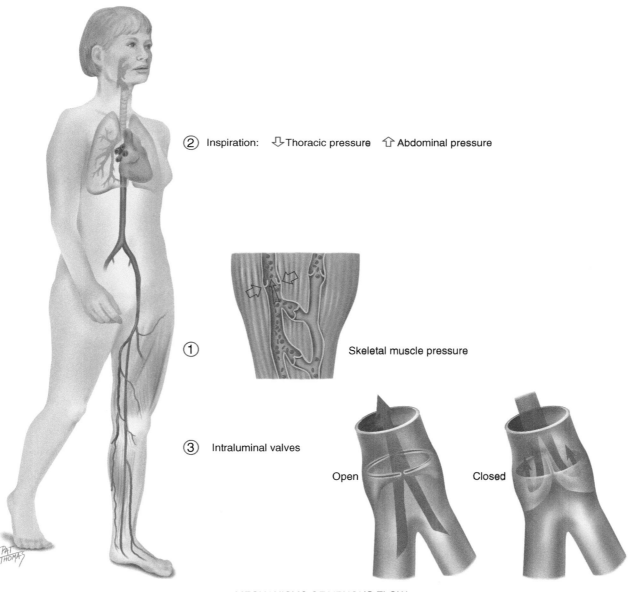

② Inspiration: ⬇Thoracic pressure ⬆Abdominal pressure

① Skeletal muscle pressure

③ Intraluminal valves

Open   Closed

MECHANISMS OF VENOUS FLOW

21.4

arteries. Veins have a larger diameter and are more distensible; they can expand and hold more blood when blood volume increases. This is a compensatory mechanism to reduce stress (preload) on the heart. Because of this ability to stretch, veins are called **capacitance vessels.**

Efficient venous return depends on contracting skeletal muscles, competent valves in the veins, and a patent lumen. Problems with any of these three elements lead to venous stasis. At risk for venous disease are people who undergo prolonged standing, sitting, or bed rest because they do not benefit from the milking action that walking accomplishes. Hypercoagulable states and vein wall trauma are other factors that increase risk for venous disease. Also, dilated and tortuous (varicose) veins create **incompetent valves,** wherein the lumen is so wide that the valve cusps cannot approximate. This condition increases venous pressure, which further dilates the vein. Some people have a genetic predisposition to varicose veins, but venous pooling also occurs in obese people and women following multiple pregnancies.

High hydrostatic pressure

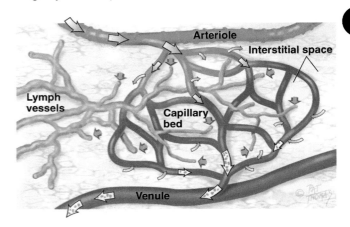

High oncotic pressure from plasma proteins

21.5 Microcirculation.   (© Pat Thomas, 2014.)

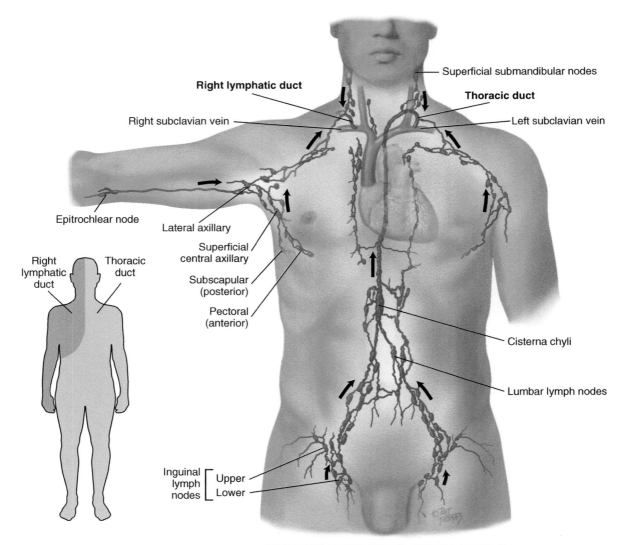

LYMPHATIC DUCTS AND DRAINAGE PATTERNS

21.6   (© Pat Thomas, 2010.)

LYMPHATICS

The lymphatics form a completely separate vessel system that retrieves excess fluid and plasma proteins from the interstitial spaces and returns them to the bloodstream. Fluid moves according to a pressure gradient (filtration). At the arterial end the *hydrostatic pressure* is caused by the pumping action of the heart and pushes somewhat more fluid out of the capillaries than the venules can absorb. This fluid is vacuumed out of the interstitial spaces by the lymph vessels (Fig. 21.5). Without lymphatic drainage, fluid would build up in the interstitial spaces and produce edema.

Substances pass around the microcirculation by a concentration gradient (diffusion). Most plasma proteins are too big to be pushed out of the arterioles; they remain and create the force for *colloid osmotic pressure* that pulls interstitial fluid back into the venules. A few smaller plasma proteins do escape the arterioles; they are captured by the lymph vessels and eventually returned to the bloodstream.

The vessels converge and drain into two main trunks, which empty into the venous system at the subclavian veins (Fig. 21.6):

1. The **right lymphatic duct** empties into the right sub-clavian vein. It drains the right side of the head and neck, right arm, right side of the thorax, right lung and pleura, right side of the heart, and right upper section of the liver.
2. The **thoracic duct** drains the rest of the body. It empties into the left subclavian vein.

The lymphatic system functions to (1) conserve fluid and plasma proteins that leak out of the capillaries, (2) form a major part of the immune system that defends the body against disease, and (3) absorb lipids from the small intestine.

The immune system is a complicated network of organs and cells that work together to protect the body. It detects and eliminates foreign pathogens, both those that come in from the environment and those arising from inside (abnormal or mutant cells). It accomplishes this by phagocytosis (digestion) of the substances by neutrophils and monocytes/macrophages and by production of specific antibodies or specific immune responses by the lymphocytes.

The lymphatic vessels have a unique structure. Lymphatic capillaries start as microscopic open-ended tubes, which siphon interstitial fluid. The capillaries converge to form vessels and drain into larger ones. The vessels have valves; therefore flow is one way from the tissue spaces into the bloodstream. The many valves make the vessels look beaded. The flow of lymph is slow compared with that of the blood. Lymph flow is propelled by contraction of the skeletal muscles, by pressure changes secondary to breathing, and by contraction of the vessel walls themselves.

Lymph nodes are small, oval clumps of lymphatic tissue located at intervals along the vessels. Most nodes are arranged in groups, both deep and superficial, in the body. Nodes filter the fluid before it is returned to the bloodstream and filter out microorganisms that could be harmful to the body. The pathogens are exposed to B and T lymphocytes in the lymph nodes, and these mount an antigen-specific response to eliminate the pathogens. With local inflammation the nodes in that area become swollen and tender.

The superficial groups of nodes are accessible to inspection and palpation and give clues to the status of the lymphatic system.

Cervical nodes drain the head and neck and are described in Chapter 14.

Axillary nodes drain the breast and upper arm. They are described in Chapter 18.

The **epitrochlear node** is in the antecubital fossa and drains the hand and lower arm.

The **inguinal nodes** in the groin drain most of the lymph of the lower extremity, the external genitalia, and the anterior abdominal wall.

Related Organs

The spleen, tonsils, and thymus aid the lymphatic system (Fig. 21.7). The **spleen** is located in the left upper quadrant of the abdomen. It has four functions: (1) to destroy old red blood cells; (2) to produce antibodies; (3) to store red blood cells; and (4) to filter microorganisms from the blood.

The **tonsils** (palatine, pharyngeal, and lingual) are located at the entrance to the respiratory and gastrointestinal tracts and respond to local inflammation.

The **thymus** is the flat, pink-gray gland located in the superior mediastinum behind the sternum and in front of the aorta. It is relatively large in the fetus and young child and atrophies after puberty. It is important in developing the T lymphocytes of the immune system in children. The B lymphocytes originate in the bone marrow and mature in the lymphoid tissue.

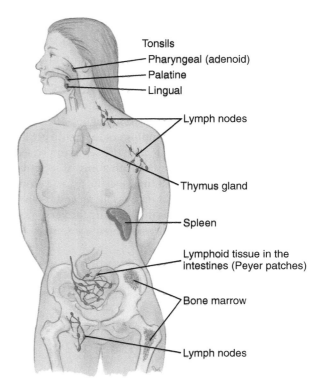

Tonsils
Pharyngeal (adenoid)
Palatine
Lingual

Lymph nodes

Thymus gland

Spleen

Lymphoid tissue in the intestines (Peyer patches)

Bone marrow

Lymph nodes

RELATED ORGANS IN IMMUNE SYSTEM

21.7

DEVELOPMENTAL COMPETENCE

Infants and Children

The lymphatic system has the same function in children as in adults. Lymphoid tissue is well developed at birth and grows rapidly until age 10 or 11 years. By 6 years of age the lymphoid tissue reaches adult size; it surpasses adult size by puberty, and then it slowly atrophies. It is possible that the excessive antigen stimulation in children causes the early rapid growth.

Lymph nodes are relatively large in children, and the superficial ones often are palpable even when the child is healthy. With infection, excessive swelling and hyperplasia occur. Enlarged tonsils are familiar signs in respiratory infections. The excessive lymphoid response also may account for the common childhood symptom of abdominal pain with seemingly unrelated problems such as upper respiratory infection (URI). Possibly the inflammation of mesenteric lymph nodes produces the abdominal pain.

The Pregnant Woman

Hormonal changes cause vasodilation and the resulting drop in blood pressure described in Chapter 20. The growing uterus obstructs drainage of the iliac veins and the inferior vena cava. This condition causes low blood flow and increases venous pressure. This in turn causes dependent edema, varicosities in the legs and vulva, and hemorrhoids.

The Aging Adult

Peripheral blood vessels grow more rigid with age, termed **arteriosclerosis.** This condition produces the rise in systolic blood pressure discussed in Chapter 10. Do not confuse this process with **atherosclerosis,** or the deposition of fatty plaques on the intima of the arteries. Both processes are present with PAD in aging adults. PAD is underdiagnosed and undertreated, yet it is a large cause of morbidity (painful walking, poor wound healing) and mortality in the United States. The prevalence of PAD increases dramatically with age; it is present in about 20% of people aged ≥70 years and 50% of those aged ≥85 years, and is likely to increase, given the growing aging population.[5] Only about 10% of people with PAD have the classic symptom of intermittent claudication (IC). About 40% do not state the symptom of leg pain, and the remaining 50% present with a mix of leg symptoms different from IC.[3] IC is pain in a specific muscle group (i.e., calf muscles) that is brought on by walking and is relieved by rest. IC impairs both walking distance and the person's quality of life.[21] Many older adults are disabled, suffer from arthritis or peripheral neuropathy, and cannot or will not walk. This delays PAD diagnosis and accounts for so many being undiagnosed by history alone.

Aging produces a progressive enlargement of the intramuscular calf veins. Prolonged bed rest, prolonged immobilization, and heart failure increase the risk for deep vein thrombosis (DVT) and subsequent pulmonary embolism. These conditions are common in aging and also with malignancy and myocardial infarction (MI). Low-dose anticoagulant medication reduces the risk for venous thromboembolism.

Loss of lymphatic tissue leads to fewer numbers of lymph nodes in older people and to a decrease in the size of remaining nodes.

 CULTURE AND GENETICS

Because family history of PAD is independently and strongly associated with PAD prevalence and severity,[7] it would follow that genetic factors have a role, but data here are limited. There is no ideal biomarker to screen for PAD, and genetic developments that would target therapeutic interventions are lagging.[11] For environmental factors, cigarette smoking is a particularly strong risk factor for all persons with PAD, as are diabetes and hypertension. Other risk factors are elevated levels of total cholesterol and obesity.[7] In the Heart and Soul Study examining risk factors by gender, data showed that depression was the strongest risk factor in women for PAD![10] Because PAD is underrecognized and undertreated in women, mental health screening may target more women in need of care. Across the age ranges, African Americans have twice the burden of PAD than do Caucasians.[4] Traditional risk factors for African Americans are high (cigarette smoking, diabetes, hypertension), but adjusting for these does not eliminate the higher prevalence. One study measured "Life's Simple 7" variables in a large African-American cohort.[6] These variables are smoking, blood pressure, total cholesterol, BMI, glucose, healthy diet, and physical activity. The researchers found the prevalence of PAD in African Americans increased with the frequency of poor health indicators in these 7 categories. A poor score in 3 or more of the health indicators increased the risk for PAD.[6] Thus the health care team must provide comprehensive screening for African Americans, women, and all aging persons, and tailor management of disease. The ankle-brachial index (ABI) is the first-line noninvasive test for PAD, and the technique is explained on p. 517.

SUBJECTIVE DATA

1. Leg pain or cramps
2. Skin changes on arms or legs
3. Swelling in arms or legs
4. Lymph node enlargement
5. Medications
6. Smoking history

Examiner Asks	Rationale

1. Leg pain or cramps. Any leg pain (cramps)? Where?

Examiner Asks	Rationale
• Describe the type of pain. Is it burning, aching, cramping, stabbing? Did this come on gradually or suddenly?	Peripheral vascular disease (PVD) includes PAD and venous disease—see pain profiles in Table 21.3, p. 524.
• Is it aggravated by activity, walking?	With PAD, blood flow cannot match muscle demand during exercise; therefore people feel muscle fatigue or pain when walking (claudication). But only 10% of those with PAD have this classic symptom.
• How many blocks (stairs) does it take to produce this pain?	**Claudication distance** is the number of blocks walked or stairs climbed to produce pain.
• Has this amount changed recently? • Is the pain worse with elevation? Worse with cool temperatures? • Does the pain wake you up at night?	Note sudden decrease in claudication distance or pain not relieved by rest. Night leg pain is common in aging adults. It may indicate the ischemic rest pain of PAD, severe night muscle cramping (usually the calf), or restless legs syndrome.
• Any recent change in exercise, a new exercise, or an increase in exercise?	Pain of musculoskeletal origin rather than vascular.
• What relieves this pain: dangling, walking, rubbing? Is the leg pain associated with any skin changes? • Is it associated with any change in sexual function (males)?	Aortoiliac occlusion is associated with erectile dysfunction (Leriche syndrome).
• Any history of vascular problems, heart problems, smoking, diabetes, obesity, pregnancy, hypertension, trauma, prolonged standing, or bed rest? [NOTE: Ask one at a time and pause for answer.]	Risk factors for PVD. Diabetes and smoking are stronger risk factors for PVD than they are even for heart disease.
2. Skin changes on arms or legs. Any **skin changes** on arms or legs? What color: redness, pallor, blueness, brown discolorations? • Any change in temperature—excess warmth or coolness? • Do your leg veins look bulging and crooked? How have you treated these? • Do you use support hose?	Coolness occurs with PAD. Varicose veins. Avoid compression stockings with PAD since they further impede blood flow. They are indicated to prevent leg swelling in standing workers or thrombus formation.
• Any leg sores or ulcers? Where on the leg? Any pain with the leg ulcer?	Leg ulcers occur with chronic arterial and venous disease (see Table 21.4, p. 525).
3. Swelling in arms or legs. Swelling in one or both legs? When did this swelling start? • What time of day is the swelling at its worst: morning or after being up most of the day? • Does the swelling come and go, or is it constant? • What seems to bring it on: trauma, standing all day, sitting? • What relieves swelling: elevation, support hose? • Is swelling associated with pain, heat, redness, ulceration, hardened skin?	**Edema** is bilateral when the cause is generalized (heart failure) or unilateral when it is the result of a local obstruction or inflammation.
4. Lymph node enlargement. Any "swollen glands" (lumps, kernels)? Where in body? How long have you had them? • Any recent change? • How do they feel to you: hard, soft? • Are the swollen glands associated with pain, local infection?	Enlarged lymph nodes occur with infection, malignancies, and immunologic diseases.
5. Medications. Which medications are you taking (e.g., oral contraceptives, hormone replacement)?	These may cause a hypercoagulable state. Also note that low-dose aspirin or clopidogrel is used to prevent blood clots in selected people.

Subjective Data

Examiner Asks	Rationale
6. **Smoking history.** Do you smoke cigarettes? How many packs per day would you say? At what age did you start? How many years have you smoked? Have you tried to quit? What helped for you? What did not help?	Tobacco constricts arteries, increases coagulability, injures endothelium, and promotes inflammation. Smoking is the strongest risk factor for PAD; starting smoking at ≤16 years more than doubles future PAD risk.

OBJECTIVE DATA

PREPARATION

During a complete physical examination, examine the arms at the very beginning when you are checking the vital signs and the person is sitting. Examine the legs directly after the abdominal examination while the person is still supine. Then have the person stand to evaluate the leg veins.

Examination of the arms and legs includes peripheral vascular characteristics (following here), the skin (see Chapter 13), musculoskeletal findings (see Chapter 23), and neurologic findings (see Chapter 24). A method of integrating these steps is discussed in Chapter 28.

Room temperature should be about 22° C (72° F) and draftless to prevent vasodilation or vasoconstriction. Use inspection and palpation. Compare your findings with the opposite extremity.

EQUIPMENT NEEDED

Occasionally need:
Paper tape measure
Tourniquet or blood pressure cuff
Stethoscope
Doppler ultrasonic probe

Normal Range of Findings	Abnormal Findings

Inspect and Palpate the Arms

Lift both the person's hands in your hands. Inspect and then turn the person's hands over, noting color of skin and nail beds; temperature, texture, and turgor of skin; and the presence of any lesions, edema, or clubbing. Use the **profile sign** (viewing the finger from the side) to detect early clubbing. The normal nail-bed angle is 160 degrees. (See Chapter 13 for a full discussion of skin color, lesions, and clubbing.)

Flattening of angle and clubbing (diffuse enlargement of terminal phalanges) occur with congenital cyanotic heart disease and cor pulmonale.

With the person's hands near the level of his or her heart, check **capillary refill.** This is an index of peripheral perfusion and cardiac output. Depress and blanch the nail beds; release and note the time for color return. Usually the vessels refill within a fraction of a second. Consider it normal if the color returns in less than 1 or 2 seconds. Note conditions that can skew your findings: a cool room, decreased body temperature, cigarette smoking, peripheral edema, and anemia.

The two arms should be symmetric in size.

Refill lasting more than 1 or 2 seconds signifies vasoconstriction or decreased cardiac output (hypovolemia, heart failure, shock). The hands are cold, clammy, and pale.

Edema of upper extremities occurs when lymphatic drainage is obstructed after breast surgery or radiation (see Table 21.2, p. 523).

Note the presence of any scars on hands and arms. Many occur normally with usual childhood abrasions or occupations involving hand tools.

Needle tracks in hands, arms, antecubital fossae occur with intravenous drug use; linear scars in wrists may signify past suicidal behavior.

Normal Range of Findings	Abnormal Findings

Palpate both radial pulses, noting rate, rhythm, elasticity of vessel wall, and equal force (Fig. 21.8). Grade the force (amplitude) on a 3-point scale:

3+, Increased, full, bounding

2+, **Normal**

1+, Weak

0, Absent

Full, bounding pulse (3+) occurs with hyperkinetic states (exercise, anxiety, fever), anemia, and hyperthyroidism.

Weak, "thready" pulse (1+) occurs with shock and PAD. See Table 21.1, p. 522, for illustrations of these and irregular pulse rhythms.

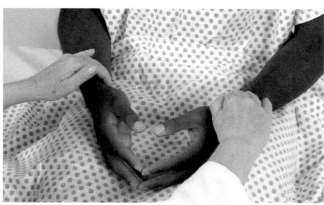

21.8

It usually is not necessary to palpate the ulnar pulses. If indicated, reach your hand under the person's arm and palpate along the medial side of the inner forearm (Fig. 21.9), although the ulnar pulses often are not palpable in the healthy person.

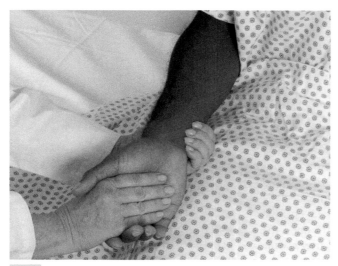

21.9   Palpate ulnar pulse.

Objective Data

Normal Range of Findings	Abnormal Findings

Palpate the brachial pulses if you suspect arterial insufficiency—their force should be equal bilaterally (Fig. 21.10).

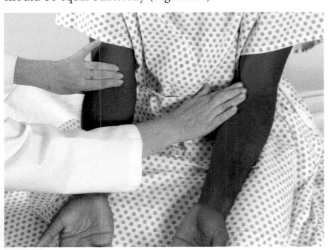

21.10 Palpate brachial pulse.

Check the epitrochlear lymph nodes in the depression 2 to 3 cm above and behind the medial condyle of the humerus. Do this by "shaking hands" with the person and reaching your other hand under the person's elbow to the groove between the biceps and triceps muscles, above the medial epicondyle (Fig. 21.11). These nodes normally are not palpable.

An enlarged epitrochlear node occurs with infection of the hand or forearm.

Epitrochlear nodes occur in conditions of generalized lymphadenopathy: lymphoma; chronic leukemia; infectious mononucleosis; HIV infection.

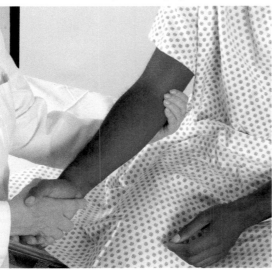

21.11 Search epitrochlear area.

The **modified Allen test** is used to evaluate the adequacy of collateral circulation before cannulating the radial artery (Fig. 21.12). **A,** Firmly occlude both the ulnar and radial arteries of one hand while the person makes a fist several times. This causes the hand to blanch. **B,** Ask the person to open the hand without hyperextending it; then release pressure on the ulnar artery while maintaining pressure on the radial artery. Adequate circulation is suggested by a palmar blush, a return to the normal color of the hand in less than 7 seconds. Although this test is simple and useful, it is relatively crude and subject to error (i.e., you must occlude both arteries uniformly with 11 pounds of pressure for the test to be accurate).

C, Pallor that persists or a sluggish return to color suggests occlusion of the collateral arterial flow. An equivocal result is 8 to 14 seconds; ≥15 seconds is a negative result. Avoid radial artery cannulation until adequate circulation is shown.

Normal Range of Findings	Abnormal Findings

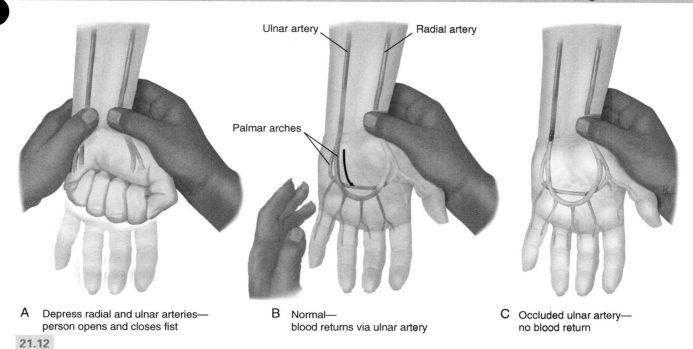

A   Depress radial and ulnar arteries—
    person opens and closes fist

B   Normal—
    blood returns via ulnar artery

C   Occluded ulnar artery—
    no blood return

21.12

Limitations of the modified Allen test are that it is subjective and requires patient cooperation that may not occur in emergency or critical care situations— just the times you need to cannulate the radial artery. Doppler flow studies can ensure collateral flow that is quantifiable. A small, flat probe is taped to the palm at the end of the patient's index finger. A baseline value for blood flow is recorded and then compared for change when the two arteries are occluded.

Inspect and Palpate the Legs

Uncover the legs while keeping the genitalia draped. Inspect both legs together, noting skin color, hair distribution, venous pattern, size (swelling or atrophy), and any skin lesions or ulcers.

Normally hair covers the legs. Even if leg hair is shaved, you will still note hair on the dorsa of the toes.

The venous pattern normally is flat and barely visible. Note obvious varicosities, although these are best assessed while standing.

Both legs should be symmetric in size without any swelling or atrophy. If the lower legs look asymmetric or if DVT is suspected, measure the calf circumference with a nonstretchable tape measure (Fig. 21.13). Measure at the widest point, taking care to measure the other leg in exactly the same place (i.e., the same number of centimeters down from the patella or other landmark). If lymphedema is suspected, measure also at the ankle, distal calf, knee, and thigh. Record your findings in centimeters.

Pallor with vasoconstriction; erythema with vasodilation; cyanosis.

Malnutrition: thin, shiny, atrophic skin; thick-ridged nails; loss of hair; ulcers; gangrene. Malnutrition, pallor, and coolness occur with arterial insufficiency.

Diffuse bilateral edema occurs with systemic illnesses.

Acute, unilateral, painful swelling and asymmetry of calves of 1 cm or more is abnormal; refer the person to determine whether DVT is present.

Objective Data

Normal Range of Findings	Abnormal Findings

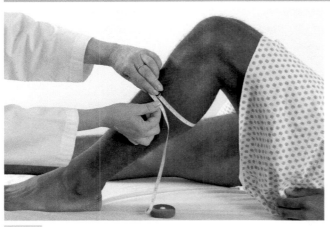

21.13 Measure calf circumference.

In the presence of skin discoloration, skin ulcers, or gangrene, note the size and the exact location.

Palpate for temperature along the legs down to the feet, comparing symmetric spots (Fig. 21.14). The skin should be warm and equal bilaterally. Bilateral cool feet may be caused by environmental factors such as cool room temperature, apprehension, and cigarette smoking. If any increase in temperature is present higher up the leg, note if it is gradual or abrupt.

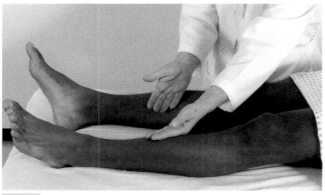

21.14

Flex the person's knee and then gently compress the length of gastrocnemius (calf) muscle anteriorly against the tibia; no tenderness should be present.

Palpate the inguinal lymph nodes. It is not unusual to find palpable nodes that are small (1 cm or less), movable, and nontender.

Abnormal Findings

Asymmetry of 1 to 3 cm occurs with mild lymphedema; 3 to 5 cm with moderate lymphedema; and more than 5 cm with severe lymphedema (see Table 21.2).

Asymmetric calf swelling of ≥2 cm occurs with DVT, but beware of diagnosing DVT with any one finding.[14] Use the Wells criteria instead on p. 518.

Brown discoloration occurs with chronic venous stasis caused by hemosiderin deposits from red blood cell degradation.

Venous ulcers occur usually at medial malleolus because of bacterial invasion of poorly drained tissues (see Table 21.4).

With arterial deficit, ulcers occur on tips of toes, metatarsal heads, and lateral malleoli.

A unilateral cool foot or leg or a sudden temperature drop as you move down the leg occurs with arterial ischemia.

Calf pain is not specific for DVT because it occurs also with superficial phlebitis, Achilles tendinitis, gastrocnemius and plantar muscle injury, and lumbosacral disorders.

Nodes that are enlarged, tender, or fixed in area.

Normal Range of Findings	Abnormal Findings

Palpate these peripheral arteries in both legs: femoral, popliteal, dorsalis pedis, and posterior tibial. Grade the force on the three-point scale. Locate the **femoral arteries** just below the inguinal ligament halfway between the pubis and anterior superior iliac spines (Fig. 21.15). To help expose the femoral area, particularly in obese people, ask the person to bend his or her knees to the side in a froglike position. Press firmly and then slowly release, noting the pulse tap under your fingertips. If this pulse is weak or diminished, auscultate the site for a bruit.

A bruit occurs with turbulent blood flow, indicating partial occlusion (see Table 21.6, p. 527).

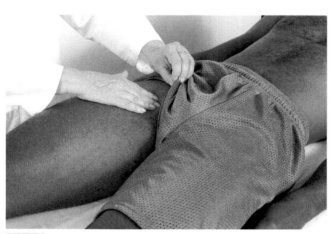

21.15 Femoral pulse.

The **popliteal pulse** is a more diffuse pulse and can be difficult to localize. With the leg extended but relaxed, anchor your thumbs on the knee and curl your fingers around into the popliteal fossa (Fig. 21.16). Press your fingers forward hard to compress the artery against the bone (the lower edge of the femur or the upper edge of the tibia). Often it is just lateral to the medial tendon.

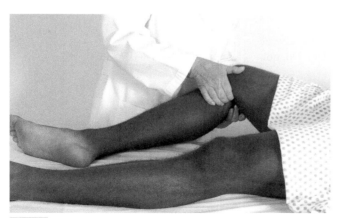

21.16 Popliteal pulse.

If you have difficulty, turn the person prone and lift up the lower leg (Fig. 21.17). Let the leg relax against your arm and press in deeply with your two thumbs. Often a normal popliteal pulse is impossible to palpate.

Objective Data

Normal Range of Findings	Abnormal Findings

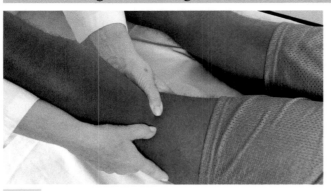

21.17 Popliteal pulse while prone.

For the **posterior tibial** pulse, curve your fingers around the medial malleolus (Fig. 21.18). Press softly. You will feel the tapping right behind it in the groove between the malleolus and the Achilles tendon. If you cannot, try passive dorsiflexion of the foot to make the pulse more accessible.

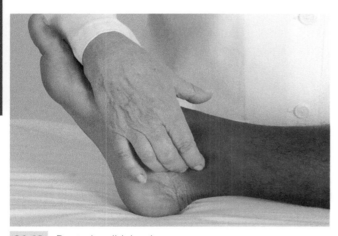

21.18 Posterior tibial pulse.

The **dorsalis pedis** pulse requires a very light touch. Normally it is just lateral to and parallel with the extensor tendon of the big toe (Fig. 21.19). Do not mistake the pulse in your own fingertips for that of the person.

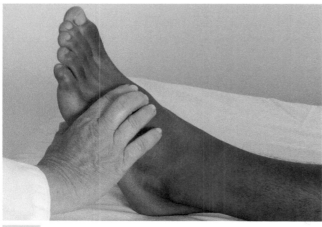

21.19 Dorsalis pedis pulse.

Normal Range of Findings	**Abnormal Findings**

In adults older than 45 years, occasionally either the dorsalis pedis or the posterior tibial pulse may be hard to find, but not both on the same foot.

Check for pretibial edema. Firmly depress the skin over the tibia or the medial malleolus for 5 seconds and release (Fig. 21.20, *A*). Normally your finger should leave no indentation, although a pit commonly is seen if the person has been standing all day or is pregnant.

Bilateral, dependent pitting edema occurs with heart failure, diabetic neuropathy, and hepatic cirrhosis (Fig. 21.20, *B*).

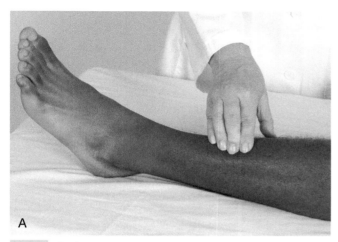

21.20   **A,** Check pretibial edema.

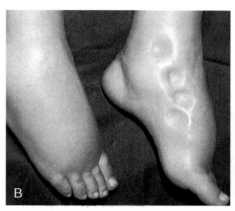

B, Pitting edema. (Bloom, Watkins, & Ireland, 1992.)

If pitting edema is present, grade it on the following scale:
1+, Mild pitting, slight indentation, no perceptible swelling of the leg
2+, Moderate pitting, indentation subsides rapidly
3+, Deep pitting, indentation remains for a short time, leg looks swollen
4+, Very deep pitting, indentation lasts a long time, leg is grossly swollen and distorted

This classic method of capturing pit depth and recovery time is commonly used. But it has not been proven to be an objective, reliable, or sensitive measurement for edema. The amount of pressure used is arbitrary, as is the judgment of the depth and rate of pitting. Ankle circumference is more reliable using a nonstretchable tape at a point 7 cm proximal to the midpoint of the medial malleolus. Because peripheral edema is a common clinical sign in a great number of conditions, it is important to detect true changes in the most accurate way available. Check with your own institution to conform to a consistently used scale.

Unilateral edema occurs with occlusion of a deep vein. Unilateral or bilateral edema occurs with lymphatic obstruction. With these factors it is "brawny" or nonpitting and feels hard to the touch.

Bilateral pitting edema calls for an examination of the neck veins (see Chapter 20). If the neck veins are abnormally distended, the peripheral edema may be related to heart disease or pulmonary hypertension).[14] If neck veins are normal, something else may cause the edema (e.g., liver disease, nephrosis, chronic venous insufficiency, antihypertensive or hormonal medications).

Ask the person to stand up so you can assess the venous system. Note any visible, dilated, and tortuous veins. If varicose veins are present, ask if they cause pain, swelling, fatigue, cramping.

Varicosities occur in the saphenous veins (see Table 21.5). Examination techniques to assess valve incompetency within varicose veins are not reliable because valve incompetence can be widely distributed throughout the leg.[12] Imaging by Doppler ultrasound is an objective, noninvasive measure of valvular incompetency.

Objective Data

Normal Range of Findings	Abnormal Findings

Color Changes

If you suspect an arterial deficit, raise the legs about 30 cm (12 inches) off the table and ask the person to wag the feet for about 30 seconds to drain off venous blood (Fig. 21.21). The skin color now reflects only the contribution of arterial blood. A light-skinned person's feet normally look a little pale but still should be pink. A dark-skinned person's feet are more difficult to evaluate, but the soles should reveal extreme color change.

Elevational pallor (marked) indicates arterial insufficiency.

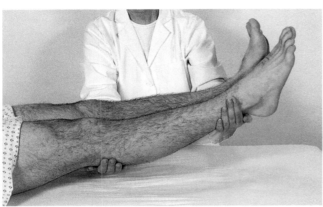

21.21

Now have the person sit up with the legs over the side of the table (Fig. 21.22, A). Compare the color of both feet. Note the time it takes for color to return to the feet—the normal time is 10 seconds or less. Note also the time it takes for the superficial veins around the feet to fill—the normal time is about 15 seconds. This test is unreliable if the person has concomitant venous disease with incompetent valves.

Dependent rubor (deep blue-red color) occurs with severe arterial insufficiency (Fig. 21.22, B). Chronic hypoxia produces loss of vasomotor tone and pooling of blood in the veins.

Delayed venous filling occurs with arterial insufficiency.

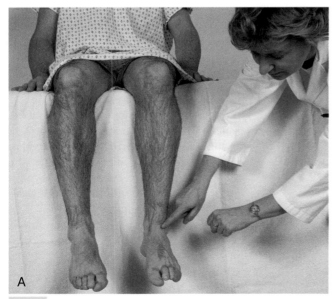

A

21.22

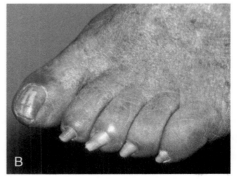

B

(**B,** Lemmi & Lemmi, 2011.)

Test the lower legs for strength (see Chapter 23) and sensation (see Chapter 24).

Motor loss occurs with severe arterial deficit.

Normal Range of Findings	Abnormal Findings

For those with a history of diabetes, PAD, or HIV, test for sensation on the sole of the foot using a monofilament, as described in Fig. 24.46 on p. 657.[15]

Sensory loss occurs with arterial deficit, especially diabetes.

The Doppler Ultrasonic Probe

Use this device to detect a weak peripheral pulse, to monitor blood pressure in infants or children, or to measure a low blood pressure or blood pressure in a lower extremity (Fig. 21.23). The Doppler probe magnifies pulsatile sounds from the heart and blood vessels. Position the person supine, with the legs externally rotated so you can reach the medial ankles easily. Place a drop of coupling gel on the end of the handheld transducer. Place the transducer over a pulse site at a 90-degree angle. Apply very light pressure; locate the pulse site by the swishing, whooshing sound.

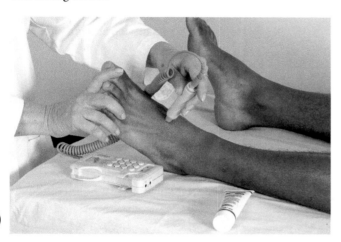

21.23

The Ankle-Brachial Index

Use of the Doppler stethoscope is a highly specific, noninvasive, and readily available way to determine the extent of peripheral arterial disease (PAD).

The patient is lying flat with the head and heels fully supported.[1] Confirm no smoking within 2 hours of the measurement and allow a 5- to 10-minute rest period supine before measurement. Choose the correct cuff width for the arm and the ankle; width should be 40% of limb circumference. Position the ankle cuff just above the malleoli with straight wrapping.

Use the Doppler probe for both brachial and ankle measurements. In all sites locate the pulse by Doppler and inflate the cuff 20 mm Hg above disappearance of flow signal; then deflate slowly to detect reappearance of flow signal.[1] Moving counterclockwise, measure: right arm, right posterior tibial (PT), right dorsalis pedis (DP), left PT, left DP, left arm. Calculate both ABI using this formula:

$$\text{Right ABI} = \frac{\text{Highest right ankle pressure (DP or PT)}}{\text{Highest arm pressure (right or left)}}$$

$$\text{Example:} \quad \frac{132 \text{ ankle systolic}}{124 \text{ arm systolic}} = \frac{1.06 \text{ or } 106\%, \text{ indicating}}{\text{no flow reduction}}$$

$$\text{Left ABI} = \frac{\text{Highest left ankle pressure (DP or PT)}}{\text{Highest arm pressure (right or left)}}$$

See Jarvis, *Lab Manual for Physical Examination and Health Assessment* (8th ed, Ch. 21), for a grid format to record your findings and for a link to an online calculator.

People with diabetes mellitus or chronic kidney disease may have calcified arteries that occasionally are noncompressible and give a falsely high (or negative) ankle pressure. Thus the presence or severity of PAD may be underestimated.[11]

An ABI between 0.91 and 1 is borderline cardiovascular risk.[1]

An ABI of 0.90 or less indicates PAD:
- 0.90 to 0.71—Mild PAD
- 0.70 to 0.41—Moderate PAD
- 0.40 to 0.30—Severe PAD, usually with rest pain except in the presence of diabetic neuropathy
- <0.30—Ischemia, with impending loss of tissue

Objective Data

Normal Range of Findings	Abnormal Findings

The Wells Score for Leg Deep Vein Thrombosis

Many of the assessment findings for DVT are unreliable and also occur with other conditions. Wells and others have combined findings into a simple scoring system. These criteria separate patients into groups of low, moderate, or high probability of DVT.[14]

Clinical Model for Predicting Pretest Probability of Deep-Vein Thrombosis[a]

Clinical Characteristic	Score
Active cancer (treatment ongoing, administered within previous 6 mo or palliative)	1
Paralysis, paresis, or recent plaster immobilization of the lower extremities	1
Recently bedridden >3 d or major surgery within previous 12 wk requiring general or regional anesthesia	1
Localized tenderness along the distribution of the deep venous system	1
Swelling of entire leg	1
Calf swelling >3 cm larger than asymptomatic side (measured 10 cm below tibial tuberosity)	1
Pitting edema confined to the symptomatic leg	1
Collateral superficial veins (nonvaricose)	1
Previously documented DVT	1
Alternative diagnosis at least as likely as DVT	-2

From Scarvelis, D., & Wells, P. S. (2006). Diagnosis and treatment of deep-vein thrombosis. *Can Med Assoc J, 175*(9), 1087-1092.
[a]A score of 0 or less = Low probability of DVT.

DVT presents with unilateral swelling of the affected leg, tenderness to severe pain, possibly warmth and redness from accompanying inflammation, and possibly superficial venous dilation. Evaluate these symptoms considering patient's current history and medical conditions.[17] For more accurate results, use the Wells criteria. Note that the Wells score has been validated in the outpatient and ED settings, but some evidence finds it insufficient to rule out DVT in the inpatient setting.[19] Doppler ultrasound imaging should be done.[23]

Score of 1 or 2 = moderate probability; score of 3 points or more = high probability of DVT.

❖ DEVELOPMENTAL COMPETENCE

Infants and Children

Transient acrocyanosis and skin mottling at birth are discussed in Chapter 13. Pulse force should be normal and symmetric. It also should be the same in the upper and lower extremities.

Weak pulses occur with vasoconstriction of diminished cardiac output.

Full, bounding pulses occur with patent ductus arteriosus from the large left-to-right shunt.

Diminished or absent femoral pulses but normal upper-extremity pulses suggest coarctation of aorta.

Palpable lymph nodes occur often in healthy infants and children. They are small, firm (shotty), mobile, and nontender. They may be the sequelae of past infection such as inguinal nodes from a diaper rash or cervical nodes from a respiratory infection. Vaccinations also can produce local lymphadenopathy. Note characteristics of any palpable nodes and whether they are local or generalized.

Enlarged, warm, tender nodes indicate current infection. Look for source of infection.

The Pregnant Woman

Expect diffuse bilateral pitting edema in the lower extremities, especially at the end of the day and into the third trimester. Nearly 80% of pregnant women have some peripheral edema because of increased water retention.[18] Varicose veins in the legs also are common in the third trimester.

Remain alert for generalized edema plus hypertension, which suggests preeclampsia, a dangerous obstetric condition.

Normal Range of Findings	Abnormal Findings

The Aging Adult

The DP and PT pulses may become more difficult to find. Trophic changes associated with arterial insufficiency (thin, shiny skin; thick-ridged nails; loss of hair on lower legs) also occur normally with aging.

HEALTH PROMOTION AND PATIENT TEACHING

Become familiar with the teaching points listed here, and adapt them for each patient's age and condition (e.g., heart failure, diabetes, obesity, PAD, arthritis). Present the relevant items.

We don't often think about our feet, but good foot care can prevent serious problems later on. First, check your feet often.

- Look for *red spots, sensitive areas, discoloration, cuts, blisters, and ingrown toenails. Use a mirror to check the bottoms of your feet. If you have diabetes, check your feet every day.*
- *Wash your feet regularly, especially between your toes. Dry feet carefully after a shower or bath; gently slide a towel between each toe.*
- *Keep toenails trimmed straight across, filed at the edges.*
- *Wear clean socks every day.*

Second, keep the blood flowing to your feet. Walking is a great way to do this. Or try these indoor exercises:

- *Sit down and rotate your ankles in one direction, then the other, or try writing the alphabet from A to Z!*
- *If you cannot walk far, put your feet up when sitting or lying down, stretching, wiggling toes. Having a gentle foot massage also helps.*

- *If sitting a long time, stand up and move around every half hour or hour.*
- *If you find yourself crossing your legs when sitting, uncross them often.*

Next, wear shoes that fit and are comfortable; wear them when you are outside, always.

- *Measure your feet toward the end of the day, when feet may be the largest.*
- *If you have one foot larger than the other, buy shoes that fit the larger one.*
- *Choose shoes so that the ball of the foot fits comfortably into the widest part of the shoe and toes are not crowded.*
- *Keep in mind that low-heeled shoes are safer and less damaging to the toes than are high-heeled shoes.*

Finally, keep the skin on your feet soft and smooth.

- *Use mild soap and mild skin lotion.*
- *Avoid adding oils or bubble bath to the bath; it makes the feet and tub very slippery.*

DOCUMENTATION AND CRITICAL THINKING

Sample Charting

SUBJECTIVE

No leg pain, no skin changes, no swelling or lymph node enlargement. No history of heart or vascular problems, diabetes, or obesity. Does not smoke. On no medications.

OBJECTIVE

Inspection: Extremities have pink-tan color without redness, cyanosis, or any skin lesions. Extremity size is symmetric without swelling or atrophy.

Palpation: Temperature is warm and = bilaterally. All pulses present, 2+ and = bilaterally. No lymphadenopathy.

ASSESSMENT

Healthy tissue
Effective tissue perfusion

Case Study 1

S.E. is a 30-year-old male office worker in general good health. Family history unremarkable. Recent basketball injury resulting in torn Achilles tendon.

SUBJECTIVE

3 weeks PTA—R ankle surgery to repair torn Achilles tendon. Lower leg placed in non–weight-bearing cast.

1 week PTA—Intermittent right calf pain. "Felt like cramping."

Present—Constant right calf pain. Rated at 7/10. Described as cramping, burning muscle pain. S.E. reports that "the cast feels tight."

Cast removed for assessment.

OBJECTIVE

Extremities inspection: Right calf red, toes pale. No cyanosis. Right calf 40 cm, left calf 36 cm in diameter. No varicosities. Left leg pink-tan. Right leg pink-tan with red area over posterior calf. Leg hair present.

Palpation: Right calf warm, toes cool. 2+ nonpitting edema. Painful to palpation.

Pulses: Femoral 2+, popliteal 0, DP 2+, PT 2+. All pulses equal bilaterally.

ASSESSMENT

Deep vein thrombosis R/T postoperative immobilization
Decreased tissue perfusion
Decreased mobility
Acute pain

Clinical Case Study 2

J.K. is a 43-year-old married male city sanitation worker, admitted to University Medical Center today for "bypass surgery tomorrow to fix my aorta and these black toes."

SUBJECTIVE

6 years PTA—Motorcycle accident with handlebars jammed into groin. Treated and released at local hospital. No apparent injury, although MD now thinks accident may have precipitated present stenosis of aorta.

1 year PTA—Radiating pain in right calf on walking 1 mile. Pain relieved by stopping walking.

3 months PTA—Problems with sex; unable to maintain erection during intercourse.

1 month PTA—Leg pain present after walking two blocks. Numbness and tingling in right foot and calf. Tips of three toes on right foot look black. Saw MD. Diagnostic studies showed stenosis of aorta "below vessels that go to my kidneys."

Present—Leg pain at rest, constant and severe, worse at night, partially relieved by dangling leg over side of bed.

Past history—No history of heart or vessel disease, hypertension, diabetes, obesity.

Personal habits—Smokes cigarettes, 3 packs per day (PPD) × 23 years. Now cut down to 1 PPD.

Walking is part of occupation, although has been driving city truck past 3 months because of leg pain. On no medications.

OBJECTIVE

Inspection: Lower extremity size = bilaterally with no swelling or atrophy. No varicosities. Color L leg pink-tan, R leg pink-tan when supine, but marked pallor to R foot on elevation. Black gangrene at tips of R 2nd, 3rd, 4th toes. Leg hair present but absent on involved toes.

Palpation: R foot cool and temperature gradually warms as proceed palpating up R leg.

Pulses: Femorals—both 1+; popliteals—both 0; PT—both 0 but present with Doppler; DP—0, but left DP is present with Doppler, and right is not present with Doppler.

ASSESSMENT

Ischemic rest pain R leg
Decreased tissue perfusion
Decreased mobility
Sexual dysfunction

Case Study 3

A.P. is a 17-year-old male who presents to the ED with pain and discoloration of his fingers. He is accompanied by his grandmother.

SUBJECTIVE

4 hours PTA—A.P. was waiting outside for the school bus "that took longer than usual 'cause of all the snow and ice." A.P. reports, "The tips of all my fingers are hard and feel like they're on fire. My grandma told me to run them under water to warm them up, but that made it hurt real bad."

OBJECTIVE

Vital signs: Temp 97.4° F (36.3° C) (oral). BP 118/78 mm Hg (sitting). Pulse 80 bpm (at rest). Resp 16/min.
General appearance: Grimacing with hands resting on thighs, palmar side up; not dressed appropriate for weather conditions (i.e., no gloves, hat, or winter coat).
Extremities: Skin brown with erythema, edema, waxy appearance, hard white plaques, and sensory deficit to phalanges (#1-5) bilat., distal portions of phalanges (#1-5) are cool to touch.

ASSESSMENT

Frostbite (stage I)
Acute pain
Decreased peripheral tissue perfusion

Documentation and Critical Thinking

TABLE 21.1 | Variations in Pulse Contour

Description	Associated With

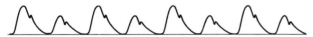

Weak, "Thready" Pulse—1+

Hard to palpate, need to search for it, may fade in and out, easily obliterated by pressure.

Decreased cardiac output, peripheral arterial disease, aortic valve stenosis

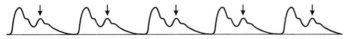

Full, Bounding Pulse—3+

Easily palpable, pounds under your fingertips.

Hyperkinetic states (exercise, anxiety, fever), anemia, hyperthyroidism

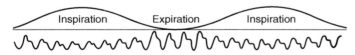

Water-Hammer (Corrigan) Pulse—3+

Greater than normal force, then collapses suddenly.

Aortic valve regurgitation, patent ductus arteriosus

Pulsus Bigeminus

Rhythm coupled, every other beat comes early, or normal beat followed by premature beat; force of premature beat decreased because of shortened cardiac filling time

Conduction disturbance (e.g., premature ventricular contraction, premature atrial contraction)

Pulsus Alternans

Rhythm regular, but force varies, with alternating beats of large and small amplitude

When heart rate (HR) is normal, pulsus alternans occurs with severe left ventricular failure, caused by ischemic heart disease, valvular heart disease, chronic hypertension, or cardiomyopathy

Pulsus Paradoxus

Beats have weaker amplitude with inspiration, stronger with expiration; best determined during blood pressure measurement; reading decreases (>10 mm Hg) during inspiration and increases with expiration

Common finding in cardiac tamponade (pericardial effusion in which high pressure compresses the heart and blocks cardiac output) and in severe bronchospasm of acute asthma

Pulsus Bisferiens

Each pulse has two strong systolic peaks with a dip in between; best assessed at the carotid artery

Aortic valve stenosis plus regurgitation

TABLE 21.2	Peripheral Vascular Disease in the Arms

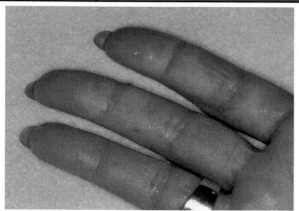

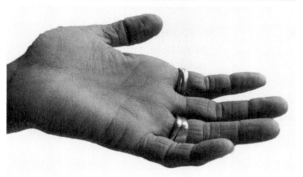

◀ Raynaud Phenomenon

Episodes of abrupt, progressive tricolor change of the fingers in response to cold, vibration, or stress: (1) white (pallor) in top figure from sympathetic-mediated vasoconstriction and resulting deficit in supply; (2) blue (cyanosis) in lower figure from slight relaxation of the spasm that allows a slow trickle of blood through the capillaries and increased oxygen extraction of hemoglobin; (3) finally red (rubor) in heel of hand caused by return of blood into the dilated capillary bed or reactive hyperemia.

May have cold, numbness, or pain along with pallor or cyanosis stage; then burning, throbbing pain, swelling along with rubor. Avoidance of cold is the most effective therapy; when episodes do occur, rewarm hands by donning gloves, rubbing in warm water, or using chemical rewarmers. After rewarming, a typical attack lasts 15 to 20 minutes. It is important to avoid smoking, sympathomimetic drugs, certain drugs for migraine headaches and for attention-deficit/hyperactivity disorder.[24]

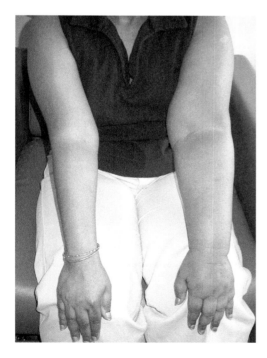

◀ Lymphedema

Lymphedema is the accumulation of protein-rich fluid in the interstitial spaces of the arm following breast surgery or treatment. It results from axillary lymph node removal, radiation therapy, fibrosis, or inflammation. Once protein-rich lymph builds up in the interstitial spaces, it further raises local colloid oncotic pressure, which promotes more fluid leakage. Acute lymphedema (within first 18 months) is reversible with treatment if no tissue damage has occurred. Chronic lymphedema is more difficult, and can lead to pain, disfigurement, mobility dysfunction, difficulty fitting into clothing, increased weight of arm making it hard to do daily activities, negative body image, and a constant emotional reminder of cancer. A cumulative incidence of 41% within 10 years is reported.[16] Risk factors of lymphedema include age, obesity, extent of axillary surgery, axillary radiation, infection, whether surgery occurred on dominant or nondominant side, and failure to use exercise and other activities to prevent lymphedema.[8] Objective data include unilateral swelling (compared to baseline presurgical measurement), measurement of arm volume, nonpitting brawny edema, overlying skin indurated. Early knowledge of lymphedema is important because there are treatments to prevent it: deep breathing and ball squeezing exercises, simple lymphatic drainage massage, elevation, compression garments, and strength training as long as no infection is present.[8,9]

See Illustration Credits for source information.

TABLE 21.3	Pain Profiles of Peripheral Vascular Disease	
Symptom Analysis	Chronic **Arterial** Symptoms (PAD)	Acute **Arterial** Symptoms
Arterial disease causes symptoms and signs of oxygen deficit.		
Location	Deep muscle pain, usually in calf, but may be lower leg or dorsum of foot	Varies, distal to occlusion, may involve entire leg
Character	Intermittent claudication, feels like "cramp," "numbness and tingling," "feeling of cold"	Throbbing
Onset and duration	Chronic pain, onset gradual after exertion	Sudden onset (within 1 hr)
Aggravating factors	Activity (walking, stairs); "claudication distance" is specific number of blocks, stairs it takes to produce pain Elevation (rest pain indicates severe involvement)	
Relieving factors	Rest (usually within 2 min [e.g., standing]) Dangling (severe involvement)	
Associated symptoms	Low ankle–brachial index; cool, pale skin; diminished pulses, pallor on elevation	Six Ps: *pain, pallor, pulselessness, paresthesia, poikilothermia* (coldness), *paralysis* (indicates severe)
Those at risk	Older and middle-age adults; African Americans have twice the incidence as other racial/ethnic groups; smoking is strongest risk, also hypertension, diabetes, hypercholesterolemia, obesity, vascular disease[13]	History of vascular surgery; arterial invasive procedure; abdominal aneurysm (emboli); trauma, including injured arteries; chronic atrial fibrillation
	Chronic Venous **Symptoms**	**Acute** Venous **Symptoms** (DVT)
Venous disease causes symptoms and signs of metabolic waste buildup.		
Location	Calf, lower leg	Calf
Character	Aching, tiredness, feeling of fullness	Moderate to intense, sharp; deep muscle tender to touch
Onset and duration	Chronic pain, increases at end of day	Sudden onset (within 1 hr)
Aggravating factors	Prolonged standing, sitting	Pain may increase with palpation
Relieving factors	Elevation, lying, walking	Pain medication
Associated symptoms	Edema, varicosities, weeping ulcers at ankles	Red, warm, swollen leg
Those at risk	Job with prolonged standing or sitting; obesity; multiple pregnancies; prolonged bed rest; history of heart failure, varicosities, or thrombophlebitis; veins crushed by trauma or surgery	

TABLE 21.4 | Leg Ulcers: Arterial, Venous, or Diabetic

Chronic **Arterial** Insufficiency	Chronic **Venous** Insufficiency

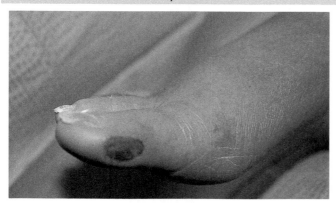

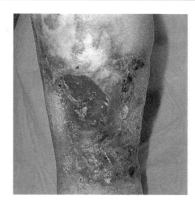

Arterial (Ischemic) Ulcer

Buildup of fatty plaques on intima (atherosclerosis) plus hardening, calcification of arterial wall (arteriosclerosis).

S: Deep muscle pain in calf or foot, claudication (pain with walking); pain worsens with leg elevation; pain at rest indicates worsening of condition.

O: Coolness in only one foot or leg, pallor, elevational pallor, and dependent rubor; diminished pulses; systolic bruits; signs of malnutrition (thin, shiny skin; thick-ridged nails; atrophy of muscles); distal gangrene.

Ulcers occur at toes, metatarsal heads, heels, and lateral ankle and are characterized by pale ischemic base, well-defined edges, and no bleeding; they look dry and punched out. Arterial ulcers are more common in those with smoking, diabetes, hyperlipidemia, and hypertension.[20]

Venous (Stasis) Ulcer

After acute DVT or chronic incompetent valves in deep veins. Venous ulcers account for 80% of lower leg ulcers.

S: Aching pain in calf or lower leg, worse at end of day, worse with prolonged standing or sitting; pain lessens with leg elevation. Itching with stasis dermatitis.

O: Lower leg edema that does not resolve with diuretic therapy. Firm, brawny edema; coarse, thickened skin; pulses normal; brown pigment discoloration; petechiae; dermatitis. Venous stasis causes increased venous pressure, which then causes red blood cells (RBCs) to leak out of veins and into skin. RBCs break down to hemosiderin (iron deposits), which are brown pigment deposits. Borders are irregular. Venous ulcers are shallow and may contain granulation tissue. A weepy, pruritic stasis dermatitis may be present.

Ulcers occur at medial malleolus and tibia; characterized by bleeding, uneven edges.

◄ Neuropathic Ulcer

Diabetes hastens changes described with arterial ischemic ulcer, with generalized dysfunction in all arterial areas: peripheral, coronary, cerebral, retinal, and renal. Peripheral diabetic ulcer has its pathogenesis in *sensory* neuropathy with loss of protective sensation, *autonomic* neuropathy with decreased sweating and dry skin, and *motor* neuropathy with foot deformity.[2] Ulcers then occur with repetitive stress over these at-risk areas. Over half of diabetic ulcers become infected, and about 20% of these infections lead to some level of amputation.[2] Symptoms include numbness and tingling, pain, weakness, loss of balance, falling, allodynia. Signs include decreased reflexes, loss of proprioception, loss of vibration sensation, small muscle wasting, loss of warm and cold sensation and pinprick, decreased reflexes, poor blood flow, and cold feet.[22] Without careful vigilance of pressure points on feet, ulcer may go unnoticed.

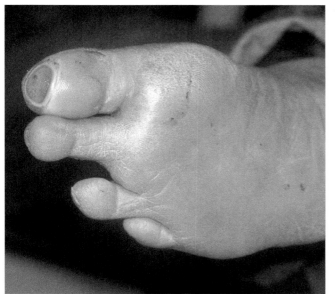

S, Subjective data; *O,* objective data.
See Illustration Credits for source information.

TABLE 21.5	Peripheral Vascular Disease in the Legs
Chronic Venous Disease	**Acute** Venous Disease

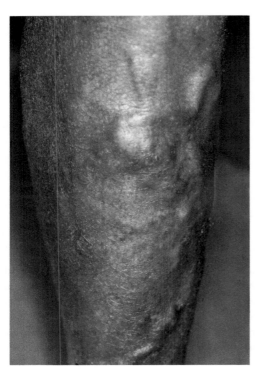

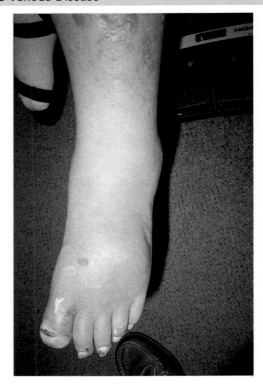

Superficial Varicose Veins

Normal leg veins have dilated as a result of chronic increased venous pressure (obesity, multiple pregnancies) and incompetent valves that permit reflux of blood back toward leg instead of forward toward heart. Varicose veins are 3 times more common in women than men. Older age increases risk as a result of thinning of elastic lamina of veins and degeneration of vascular smooth muscle. Size ranges from 1 mm to 1 cm in diameter; color ranges from red to blue or purple.

S: Aching, heaviness in calf, easy fatigability, restless legs, burning, throbbing, cramping.
O: Dilated, tortuous veins. New varicosities sit on surface of muscle or bone; older ones are deep and feel spongy.

Deep Vein Thrombophlebitis

A deep vein is occluded by a thrombus, causing inflammation, blocked venous return, cyanosis, and edema. Virchow triad is the classic 3 factors that promote thrombogenesis: stasis, hypercoagulability, and endothelial dysfunction.[17] Cause may be prolonged bed rest, history of varicose veins, trauma, infection, cancer, obesity, immobility, heart failure, or the use of estrogen hormones. Requires emergency referral because of risk for pulmonary embolism. Note that upper-extremity DVT is increasingly common as a result of frequent use of invasive lines such as central venous catheters.

S: Sudden onset of intense, sharp, deep muscle pain.
O: Increased warmth; swelling (to compare swelling, observe usual shoe size as in above photo); redness; dependent cyanosis is mild or may be absent; tender to palpation; apply Wells criteria as on p. 518.

See Illustration Credits for source information.

TABLE 21.6 | Peripheral Artery Disease

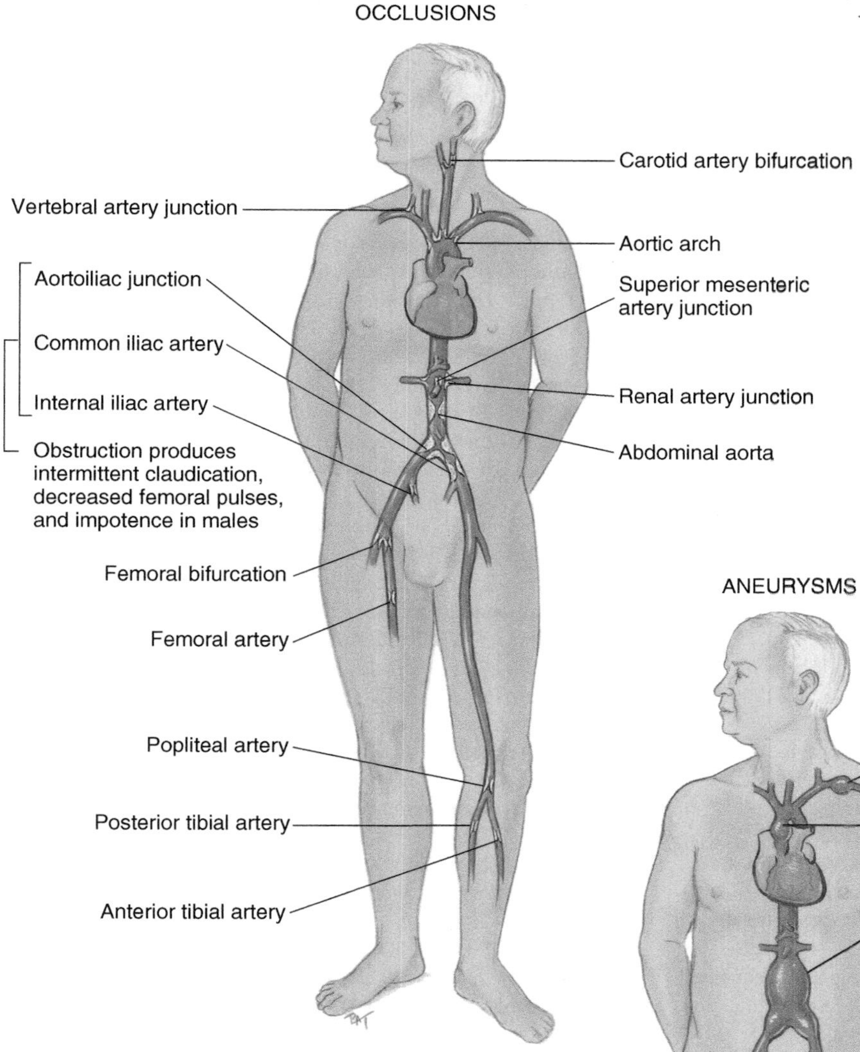

OCCLUSIONS

Vertebral artery junction

Aortoiliac junction

Common iliac artery

Internal iliac artery

Obstruction produces
intermittent claudication,
decreased femoral pulses,
and impotence in males

Femoral bifurcation

Femoral artery

Popliteal artery

Posterior tibial artery

Anterior tibial artery

Carotid artery bifurcation

Aortic arch

Superior mesenteric
artery junction

Renal artery junction

Abdominal aorta

◀ Occlusions

Occlusions in arteries are caused by atherosclerosis, which is the chronic gradual buildup of (in order) fatty streaks, fibroid plaque, calcification of the vessel wall, and thrombus formation. This reduces blood flow with vital oxygen and nutrients. Risk factors for atherosclerosis include obesity, cigarette smoking, hypertension, diabetes mellitus, elevated serum cholesterol, sedentary lifestyle, and family history of hyperlipidemia.

ANEURYSMS

Thoracic aneurysm

Aortic arch aneurysm

Abdominal aortic aneurysm (AAA)
Most common are fusiform in shape, extending from below the renal arteries to involve the entire infrarenal aorta and often involve the common iliac arteries.
Pressure causes lower abdominal pain and dull lower back pain.

Femoral aneurysm
(relatively uncommon)

Popliteal aneurysm
(relatively uncommon)–
occurs in 5%–20% of
people with AAA.

Aneurysms ▶

An aneurysm is a sac formed by dilation in the artery wall. Atherosclerosis weakens the middle layer (media) of the vessel wall. This stretches the inner and outer layers (intima and adventitia), and the effect of blood pressure creates the balloon enlargement. The most common site is the aorta, and the most common cause is atherosclerosis. The incidence increases rapidly in men older than 55 years and women older than 70 years; the overall occurrence is 4 to 5 times more frequent in men.

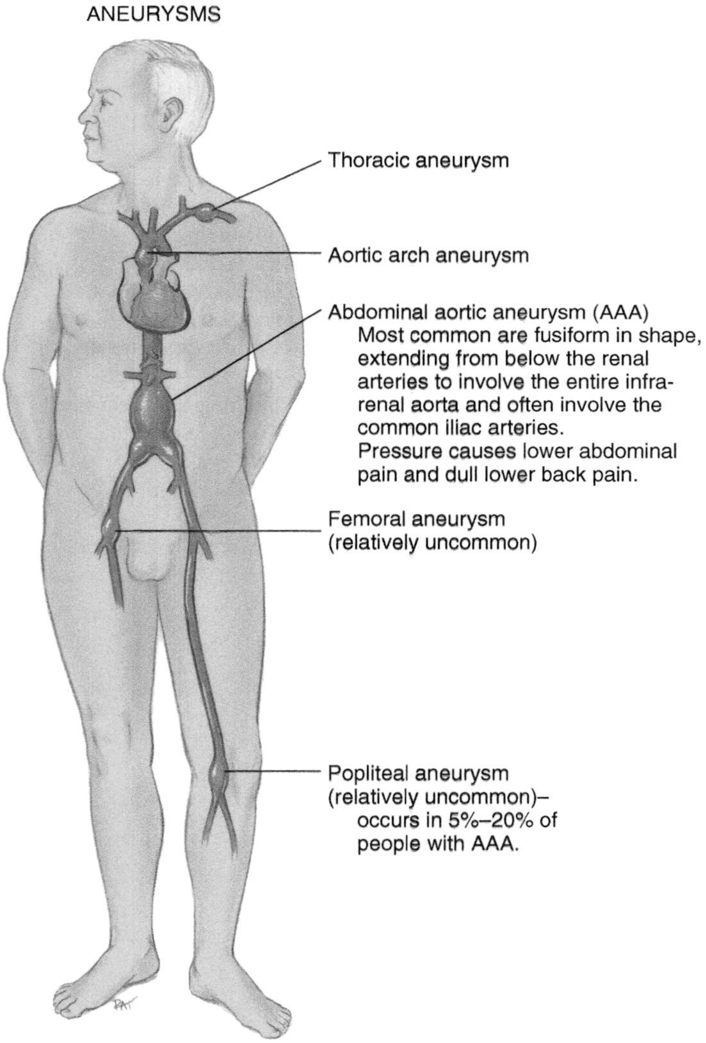

Summary Checklist: Peripheral Vascular Examination

1. Inspect arms for color, size, any lesions.
2. Palpate pulses: radial, brachial.
3. Check epitrochlear node.

4. Inspect legs for color, size, any lesions, trophic skin changes.
5. Palpate temperature of feet and legs.
6. Palpate inguinal nodes.

7. Palpate pulses: femoral, popliteal, posterior tibial, dorsalis pedis.
8. Touch sole of foot with microfilament.

REFERENCES

1. American Heart Association. (2012). Measurement and interpretation of the ankle-brachial index. *Circulation, 126*(24), 2890–2909.
2. Armstrong, D. G., Boulton, A., & Bus, S. A. (2017). Diabetic foot ulcers and their recurrence. *N Engl J Med, 376*(24), 2367–2375.
3. Benjamin, E. J., Blaha, M. J., Chiuve, S. E., et al. (2017). Heart disease and stroke statistics—2017 update: A report for the American Heart Association. *Circulation, 135*(10), e146–e603.
4. Carnethon, M. R., Jia, P., Howard, G., et al. (2017). Cardiovascular health in African Americans. *Circulation, 136*(21), e393–e423.
5. Chen, X., Stoner, J. A., Montgomery, R. S., et al. (2017). Prediction of 6-minute walk performance in patients with peripheral artery disease. *J Vasc Surg, 2017*(66), 1202–1209.
6. Collins, T. C., Slovut, D. P., Newton, R., et al. (2017). Ideal cardiovascular health and peripheral artery disease in African Americans. *Prevent Med Rep, 7*, 20–25.
7. Criqui, M. H., & Aboyans, V. (2015). Epidemiology of peripheral artery disease. *Circ Res, 116*, 1509–1526.
8. Donmez, A. A., & Kapuco, S. (2017). The effectiveness of a clinical and home-based activity program and simple lymphatic drainage in the prevention of breast cancer-related lymphedema. *Euro J Onc Nurs, 31*, 12–21.
9. Dunne, M., & Keenan, K. (2016). Late and long-term sequelae of breast cancer treatment. *Am J Nurs, 116*(6), 36–46.
10. Grenon, S. M., Cohen, B. E., Smolderen, K., et al. (2014). Peripheral arterial disease, gender, and depression in the Heart and Soul Study. *J Vasc Surg, 60*, 396–403.
11. Hazarika, S., & Annex, B. H. (2017). Biomarkers and genetics in peripheral artery disease. *Clin Chem, 63*(1), 236–244.
12. Jacobs, B. N., Andraska, E. A., Obi, A. T., et al. (2017). Pathophysiology of varicose veins. *J Vasc Surg: Venous Lymphat Disord, 5*, 460–467.
13. Kullo, I. J., & Rooke, T. W. (2016). Peripheral artery disease. *N Engl J Med, 374*(9), 861–870.
14. McGee, S. (2018). *Evidence-based physical diagnosis* (4th ed.). St. Louis: Elsevier.
15. National Institute on Aging. (2018). *Foot care.* https://go4life. nia.nih.gov/sites/default/files/Footcare.pdf.
16. Pereira, A., Koifman, R. J., & Bergmann, A. (2017). Incidence and risk factors of lymphedema after breast cancer treatment. *The Breast, 36*, 67–73.
17. Roberts, S. H., & Lawrence, S. M. (2017). Venous thromboembolism. *Am J Nurs, 117*(5), 38–48.
18. Sanghavi, M., & Rutherford, J. D. (2014). Cardiovascular physiology of pregnancy. *Circulation, 130*, 1003–1008.
19. Silveira, P. C., Ip, I. K., Goldhaber, S. Z., et al. (2015). Performance of Wells score for deep vein thrombosis in the inpatient setting. *JAMA Int Med, 175*(7), 1112–1117.
20. Singer, A. J., Tassiopoulos, A., & Kirsner, R. S. (2017). Evaluation and management of lower-extremity ulcers. *N Engl J Med, 377*(16), 1559–1566.
21. Skelly, C. L., & Cifu, A. S. (2016). Screening, evaluation, and treatment of peripheral arterial disease. *JAMA, 316*(14), 1486–1487.
22. Vinik, A. I. (2016). Diabetic sensory and motor neuropathy. *N Engl J Med, 374*(15), 1455–1462.
23. Wiegand, D. L. (Ed.), (2017). *AACN procedure manual for high acuity, progressive, and critical care* (7th ed.). St. Louis: Elsevier.
24. Wigley, F. M., & Flavahan, N. A. (2016). Raynaud's phenomenon. *N Engl J Med, 375*(6), 556–565.

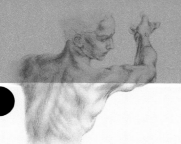

CHAPTER 22

Abdomen

STRUCTURE AND FUNCTION

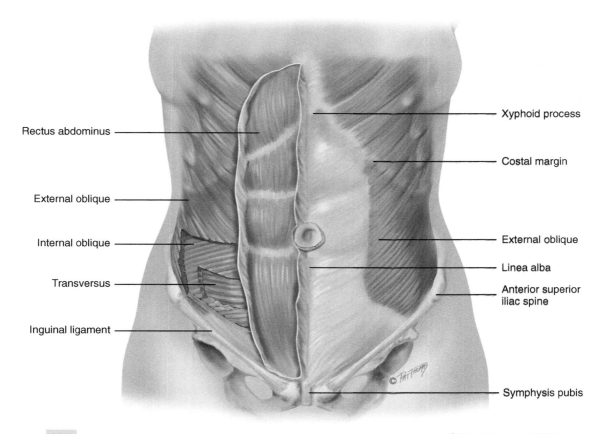

Rectus abdominus

External oblique

Internal oblique

Transversus

Inguinal ligament

Xyphoid process

Costal margin

External oblique

Linea alba

Anterior superior iliac spine

Symphysis pubis

22.1

(© Pat Thomas, 2006.)

SURFACE LANDMARKS

The **abdomen** is a large, oval cavity extending from the diaphragm down to the brim of the pelvis. It is bordered in back by the vertebral column and paravertebral muscles, and at the sides and front by the lower rib cage and abdominal muscles (Fig. 22.1). Four layers of large, flat muscles form the ventral abdominal wall. These are joined at the midline by a tendinous seam, the **linea alba.** One set, the **rectus abdominis,** forms a strip extending the length of the midline, and its edge is often palpable. The muscles protect and hold the organs in place, and they flex the vertebral column.

INTERNAL ANATOMY

Internal to the abdominal musculature lies the **peritoneum,** a double envelope of serous membrane that lines the abdominal wall (parietal peritoneum) and covers the surface of most abdominal organs (visceral peritoneum). **Mesenteries,** double layers of parietal peritoneum, extend from the abdominal wall as pathways for blood vessels, nerves, and lymphatics. Mesenteries also serve as supporting networks to suspend and stabilize the abdominal organs, called **viscera.** The **greater omentum** is a specialized fatty mesentery that overlies the ventral abdomen. It is important that you know

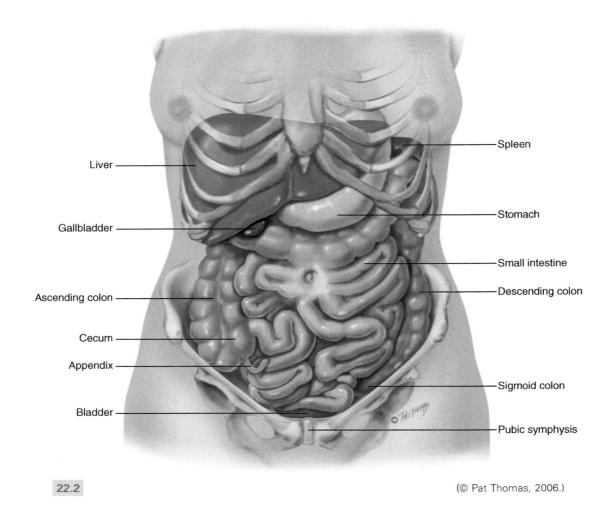

Liver

Gallbladder

Ascending colon

Cecum

Appendix

Bladder

Spleen

Stomach

Small intestine

Descending colon

Sigmoid colon

Pubic symphysis

22.2

(© Pat Thomas, 2006.)

the location of the abdominal organs so well that you could draw a map of them on the skin. Because of the overlying skin, subcutaneous layer, muscles, and omentum, you must be able to visualize each organ that you listen to or palpate through the abdominal wall.

The **solid viscera** are those that maintain a characteristic shape (liver, pancreas, spleen, adrenal glands, kidneys, ovaries, and uterus) (Fig. 22.2). The liver fills most of the right upper quadrant (RUQ) and extends over to the left midclavicular line (MCL). The lower edge of the liver and the right kidney normally may be palpable. The ovaries normally are palpable only on bimanual examination during the pelvic examination.

The shape of the **hollow viscera** (stomach, gallbladder, small intestine, colon, and bladder) depends on the contents. They usually are not palpable, although you may feel a colon distended with feces or a bladder distended with urine. The stomach is just below the diaphragm, between the liver and spleen. The gallbladder rests under the posterior surface of the liver, just lateral to the right MCL. Note that the small intestine is located in all four quadrants. It extends from the

pyloric valve of the stomach to the ileocecal valve in the right lower quadrant (RLQ), where it joins the colon.

The **spleen** is a soft mass of lymphatic tissue on the left posterolateral wall of the abdominal cavity, immediately under the diaphragm (Fig. 22.3). It lies obliquely with its long axis behind and parallel to the 10th rib, lateral to the midaxillary line. Its width extends from the 9th to the 11th rib, about 7 cm. It is not palpable normally. If it becomes enlarged, its lower pole moves downward and toward the midline.

The **aorta** is just to the left of midline in the upper part of the abdomen (Fig. 22.4). It descends behind the peritoneum, and at 2 cm below the umbilicus it bifurcates into the right and left common iliac arteries opposite the 4th lumbar vertebra. You can palpate the aortic pulsations easily in the upper anterior abdominal wall. The right and left iliac arteries become the femoral arteries in the groin area. Their pulsations are easily palpated at a point halfway between the anterior superior iliac spine and the symphysis pubis.

The **pancreas** is a soft, lobulated gland located behind the stomach. It stretches obliquely across the posterior abdominal wall to the left upper quadrant.

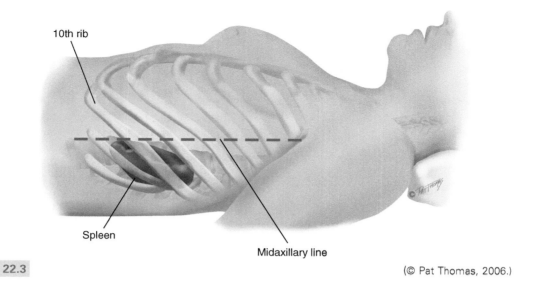

10th rib

Spleen

Midaxillary line

22.3

(© Pat Thomas, 2006.)

The bean-shaped **kidneys** are retroperitoneal, or behind the peritoneal cavity along the posterior abdominal wall (Fig. 22.5). They are well protected by the posterior ribs and musculature. The 12th rib forms an angle with the vertebral column, the **costovertebral angle.** The left kidney lies here at the 11th and 12th ribs. Because of the placement of the liver, the right kidney rests 1 to 2 cm lower than the left kidney and sometimes may be palpable.

For convenience in description, the abdominal wall is divided into **four quadrants** by a vertical and a horizontal

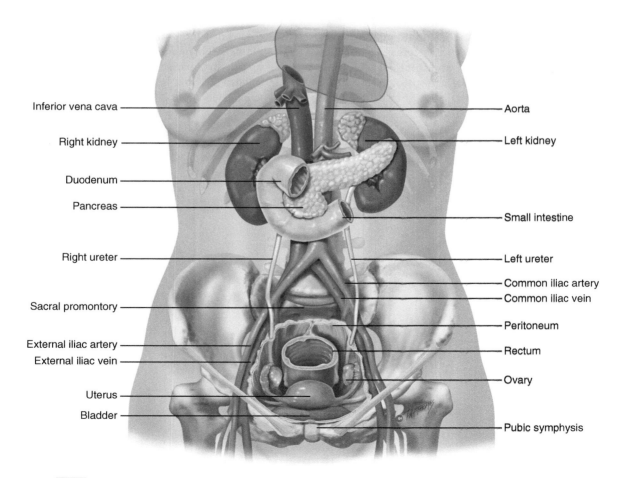

Inferior vena cava

Right kidney

Duodenum

Pancreas

Right ureter

Sacral promontory

External iliac artery

External iliac vein

Uterus

Bladder

Aorta

Left kidney

Small intestine

Left ureter

Common iliac artery

Common iliac vein

Peritoneum

Rectum

Ovary

Pubic symphysis

22.4

(© Pat Thomas, 2006.)

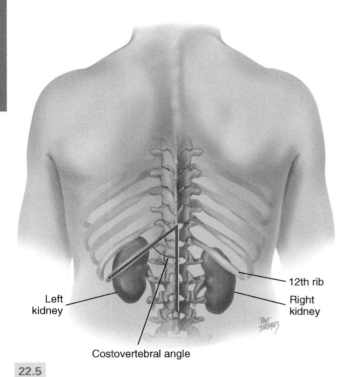

22.5

The anatomic location of the organs by quadrants is:

Right Upper Quadrant (RUQ)	**Left Upper Quadrant (LUQ)**
Liver	Stomach
Gallbladder	Spleen
Duodenum	Left lobe of liver
Head of pancreas	Body of pancreas
Right kidney and adrenal	Left kidney and adrenal
Hepatic flexure of colon	Splenic flexure of colon
Part of ascending and transverse colon	Part of transverse and descending colon

Right Lower Quadrant (RLQ)	**Left Lower Quadrant (LLQ)**
Cecum	Part of descending colon
Appendix	Sigmoid colon
Right ovary and tube	Left ovary and tube
Right ureter	Left ureter
Right spermatic cord	Left spermatic cord

Midline

Aorta
Uterus (if enlarged)
Bladder (if distended)

line bisecting the umbilicus (Fig. 22.6). (An older, more complicated scheme divided the abdomen into nine regions; and some regional names persist, such as **epigastric** for the area between the costal margins, **umbilical** for the area around the umbilicus, and **hypogastric** or **suprapubic** for the area above the pubic bone.)

❖ DEVELOPMENTAL COMPETENCE

Infants and Children

In the newborn the umbilical cord shows prominently on the abdomen. It contains two arteries and one vein. The liver takes up proportionately more space in the abdomen at birth than in later life. In a healthy term neonate the lower edge may be palpated 0.5 to 2.5 cm below the right costal margin.

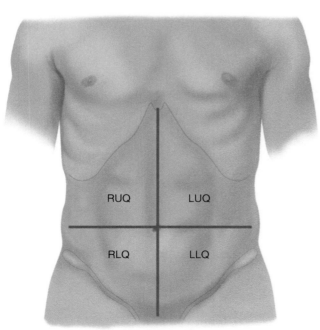

Four quadrants

22.6

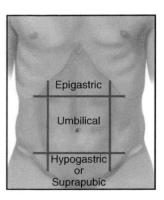

The urinary bladder is located higher in the abdomen than in the adult. It lies between the symphysis and the umbilicus. In addition, during early childhood the abdominal wall is less muscular; therefore the organs may be easier to palpate.

The Pregnant Woman

Nausea and vomiting, or "morning sickness," is an early sign of pregnancy for most pregnant women, starting between the 1st and 2nd missed periods. The cause may be the result of hormonal changes such as the production of human chorionic gonadotropin (hCG). Another symptom is "acid indigestion" or heartburn (pyrosis) caused by esophageal reflux. Gastrointestinal (GI) motility decreases, which prolongs gastric emptying time. The decreased motility causes more water to be resorbed from the colon, which leads to constipation. The constipation, in addition to increased venous pressure in the lower pelvis, may lead to hemorrhoids.

The enlarging uterus displaces the intestines upward and posteriorly. Bowel sounds are diminished. The appendix may be displaced upward and to the right, but any appendicitis-related pain during pregnancy would still be felt in the RLQ.[19] Finally, skin changes on the abdomen such as striae and linea nigra are discussed later in this chapter on p. 539 and in Chapter 31, respectively.

The Aging Adult

Aging alters the appearance of the abdominal wall. After middle age, some fat accumulates in the suprapubic area in females as a result of decreased estrogen levels. Males also show some fat deposits in the abdominal area, which accentuates with a more sedentary lifestyle. With further aging adipose tissue is redistributed away from the face and extremities and to the abdomen and hips. The abdominal musculature relaxes.

Age-related changes occur in the GI system but do not significantly affect function as long as no disease is present.

- Salivation decreases, causing a dry mouth and a decreased sense of taste (discussed in Chapter 17).
- Esophageal emptying is delayed. If an aging person is fed in the supine position, it increases risk for aspiration.
- Gastric acid secretion decreases with aging. This may cause pernicious anemia (because it interferes with vitamin B_{12} absorption), iron-deficiency anemia, and malabsorption of calcium.
- The incidence of gallstones increases with age, occurring in 10% to 20% of middle-age and older adults, being more common in females.
- Liver size decreases by 25% between the ages of 20 and 70 years, although most liver function remains normal. Drug metabolism by the liver is impaired, in part because blood flow through the liver and liver size are decreased.[18] Therefore the liver metabolism that is responsible for the enzymatic oxidation, reduction, and hydrolysis of drugs is substantially decreased with age. Prolonged liver metabolism causes increased side effects (e.g., older people

taking benzodiazepines have an increased risk of falling and thus of hip fracture).

- Aging people frequently report constipation. Chronic constipation occurs more frequently in the aging than in the general population, and aging women are affected 2 to 3 times more than their male counterparts. A higher incidence of constipation in the aging results in greater use of laxatives, with up to 74% of aging patients in nursing homes using laxatives every day.[16] Because many adults are confused as to what defines constipation, the Rome III standardizes symptom criteria for functional constipation. These symptoms include reduced stool frequency (less than 3 bowel movements per week) and other common and troubling associated symptoms (i.e., straining, lumpy or hard stool, feeling of incomplete evacuation, feeling of anorectal blockage, use of manual maneuvers).

Constipation is not a physiologic consequence of aging. Common causes of constipation include decreased physical activity, inadequate intake of water, a low-fiber diet, side effects of medications (opioids, tricyclic antidepressants), irritable bowel syndrome, bowel obstruction, hypothyroidism, and inadequate toilet facilities (i.e., difficulty ambulating to the toilet may cause the person to deliberately retain the stool until it becomes hard and difficult to pass).

CULTURE AND GENETICS

Lactase is the digestive enzyme necessary for absorption of the carbohydrate *lactose* (milk sugar). In some racial groups lactase activity is high at birth but declines to low levels by adulthood. These people are **lactose intolerant** and have abdominal pain, bloating, and flatulence when milk products are consumed. Millions of American adults have the potential for lactose-intolerance symptoms; although 70% to 80% of white Americans produce lactase adequately into adulthood, only 30% of Mexican Americans, 20% of African Americans, and no American Indians will maintain adequate ability to digest lactose without adverse symptoms.[1] This is clinically significant because dairy foods meet crucial nutritional requirements, including calcium, magnesium, potassium, proteins, and vitamins A, D, B_{12}, and riboflavin. If people perceive themselves to be lactose intolerant based on racial heritage, the lowered calcium intake may affect bone health. Health care providers should encourage low-fat or fat-free dairy foods and monitor any symptoms. In addition, even in lactose-intolerant individuals, regular lactose consumption may be tolerated when the colonic flora adapt to aid digestion of lactose.[1]

NOTE: Content on obesity has been moved to Chapter 12.

Celiac disease is an autoimmune disorder that affects less than 1% of the population, although the incidence has been increasing in recent years.[4] Affected persons are permanently intolerant of gluten, a protein found in wheat, barley, rye, and some commercially produced oats. When gluten is ingested, immune-mediated inflammation results in damage to the small intestine and in malabsorption.[20] Onset can occur in childhood or adulthood with common symptoms of diarrhea, abdominal pain, and abdominal distention. Other symptoms include anemia, osteoporosis, neuropathy, abnormal liver function, and skin lesions.[15,17] Persons with evidence of malabsorption or at increased risk for celiac disease (family history, other autoimmune diseases) should undergo testing for celiac disease through serology and small bowel biopsy.[15,20]

Celiac disease is treated through a gluten-free diet. Persons with wheat allergy and non-celiac gluten sensitivity should also follow a gluten-free diet. There is currently a trend for persons without these disease-specific indications to follow a gluten-free diet because of the perception that a gluten-free diet is healthier or for the treatment of other symptoms or disorders, such as irritable bowel syndrome, autism, and chronic fatigue syndrome. Due to inadequate and/or inconclusive research, there is controversy regarding the benefits of a gluten-free diet in persons without celiac disease, gluten sensitivity, or wheat allergy. In addition, gluten-free diets are not without risks.[8] Gluten-free diets may result in deficiencies in fiber, vitamin D, vitamin B_{12}, folate, iron, zinc, magnesium, and calcium. Persons following a gluten-free diet also may have increased intake of saturated and hydrogenated fatty acids.[21] Regardless of the reason for adhering to a gluten-free diet, it is essential to refer patients who adopt this diet to registered dietitians to prevent micronutrient deficiency and optimize quality of nutritional choices.

SUBJECTIVE DATA

1. Appetite	4. Abdominal pain	7. Past abdominal history
2. Dysphagia	5. Nausea/vomiting	8. Medications
3. Food intolerance	6. Bowel habits	9. Nutritional assessment

Examiner Asks	Rationale
1. Appetite • Any change in **appetite?** Is it a loss of appetite? • Any change in weight? How much weight gained or lost? Over what time period? Is the weight loss caused by diet?	**Anorexia** is a loss of appetite from GI disease as a side effect to some medications, with pregnancy, or with mental health disorders.
2. Dysphagia • Any difficulty in swallowing? When did you first notice it? Is there any associated pain? Any coughing or choking when swallowing? Any worse with liquids versus solids?	**Dysphagia** occurs with disorders of the throat or esophagus, such as thrush (candida infection), neurologic changes (e.g., stroke), or obstruction (e.g., solid mass or tumor).
3. Food intolerance • Are there any foods you cannot eat? What happens if you do eat them: allergic reaction, heartburn, belching, bloating, indigestion? • Do you use antacids? How often?	**Food intolerance** (e.g., lactase deficiency resulting in bloating or excessive gas after taking milk products). **Pyrosis** (heartburn), a burning sensation in esophagus and stomach from reflux of gastric acid. Eructation (belching).
4. Abdominal pain • Any **abdominal pain?** Please point to it. • Is the pain in one spot, or does it move around? • How did it start? How long have you had it? • Constant, or does it come and go? Occur before or after meals? Does it peak? When? • How would you describe the character: cramping (colic type), burning in pit of stomach, dull, stabbing, aching? • Is the pain relieved by food or worse after eating?	Abdominal pain may be *visceral* from an internal organ (dull, general, poorly localized); *parietal* from inflammation of overlying peritoneum (sharp, precisely localized, aggravated by movement); or *referred* from a disorder in another site (see Table 22.3, p. 562). Acute pain requiring urgent diagnosis occurs with appendicitis, cholecystitis, bowel obstruction, or a perforated organ. Chronic pain of gastric ulcers occurs usually on an empty stomach; pain of duodenal ulcers occurs 2 to 3 hours after a meal and is relieved by more food.

Examiner Asks	Rationale

- Is the pain associated with menstrual period or irregularities, stress, dietary indiscretion, fatigue, nausea and vomiting, gas, fever, rectal bleeding, frequent urination, vaginal or penile discharge?
- What makes the pain worse: food, position, stress, medication, activity?
- What have you tried to relieve pain: rest, heating pad, change in position, medication?

5. Nausea/vomiting

- Any **nausea** or **vomiting?** How often? How much comes up? What is the color? Is there an odor?
- Is it bloody?

Nausea/vomiting is common with GI disease, many medications, pregnancy.
Hematemesis occurs with stomach or duodenal ulcers and esophageal varices.

- Is the nausea or vomiting associated with colicky pain, diarrhea, fever, chills?
- What foods did you eat in the past 24 hours? Where? At home, school, restaurant? Is there anyone else in the family with same symptoms in past 24 hours?

Consider food poisoning or other types of bacterial or viral gastroenteritis.

- Any recent travel? Where to? Drink the local water or eat fruit? Swimming in public beaches or pools?

Nausea, vomiting, and diarrhea can occur when exposed to new local pathogens in developing countries. Water supply may be contaminated.

6. Bowel habits

- How often do you have a **bowel movement?**
- What is the color? Consistency?
- Any diarrhea or constipation? How long?
- Any recent change in bowel habits?
- Use laxatives? Which ones? How often do you use them?

Assess usual **bowel habits.**
Black stools may be tarry due to occult blood (melena) from GI bleeding or nontarry from iron medications. Gray stools occur with hepatitis.
Red blood in stools occurs with GI bleeding or localized bleeding around the anus (e.g., hemorrhoids).

7. Past abdominal history

- Any **history** of GI problems: ulcer, gallbladder disease, hepatitis/jaundice, appendicitis, colitis, hernia?
- Ever had any abdominal operations? Please describe.
- Any problems after surgery?
- Any abdominal x-ray studies? How were the results?

8. Medications

- Which **medications** are you taking currently?
- How about alcohol—how much would you say you drink each day? Each week? When was your last alcoholic drink?
- How about cigarettes—do you smoke? How many packs per day? For how long?

Peptic ulcer disease occurs with frequent use of nonsteroidal antiinflammatory drugs (NSAIDs), alcohol, smoking, and *Helicobacter pylori* infection.

9. Nutritional assessment

- Now I would like to ask you about your diet. Please tell me all the food you ate yesterday, starting with breakfast.
- Which fresh food markets are located in your neighborhood?

Nutritional assessment via 24-hour recall (see Chapter 12 for full discussion).
Many inner-city neighborhoods are fresh food "deserts," lacking produce markets but full of fast-food restaurants.

Examiner Asks	Rationale

Additional History for Infants and Children

1. Are you breastfeeding or bottle-feeding the baby? If bottle-feeding, how does baby tolerate the formula?

2. Which table foods have you introduced? How does the infant tolerate the food?

Consider a new food as a possible allergen. Adding only one new food at a time to the infant's diet helps identify allergies.

3. How often does your toddler/child eat? Does he or she eat regular meals? How do you feel about your child's eating problems?
- Please describe all that your child had to eat yesterday, starting with breakfast. Which foods does the child eat for snacks?

- Does toddler/child ever eat nonfoods: grass, dirt, paint chips?

Irregular eating patterns are common and a source of parental anxiety. As long as the child shows normal growth and development and only nutritious foods are offered, parents may be reassured.

Pica: Although a toddler may attempt nonfoods at some time, he or she should recognize edibles by age 2 years.

4. Does your child have constipation? How long?

Constipation may affect from 0.7% to almost 30% of children. This is almost always functional constipation, meaning the bowel is otherwise healthy, but there may be inadequate fiber and fluids, inactivity, stress, medications, or other contributing diseases. Children may also ignore the urge to defecate or withhold or delay defecation, especially during toilet training.[6]

- What is the number of stools/day? Stools/week?
- How much water, juice is in the diet?
- Does the constipation seem to be associated with toilet training?
- What have you tried to treat the constipation?

5. Does the child have abdominal pain? Please describe what you have noticed and when it started.

Pain is hard to assess with children. Many conditions of unrelated organ systems have vague abdominal pain (e.g., otitis media). They cannot articulate specific symptoms and often focus on "the tummy." Abdominal pain accompanies inflammation of the bowel, constipation, urinary tract infection, and anxiety.

6. For the overweight child: How long has weight been a problem?
- At what age did the child first seem overweight? Did any change in diet pattern occur then?
- Describe the diet pattern now.
- Do any others in family have a similar problem?
- How does child feel about his or her own weight?

Reduced physical activity and food marketing practices contribute to current obesity epidemic.

Family history of obesity.

Assess body image and social adjustment.

Additional History for Adolescents

1. What do you eat at regular meals? Do you eat breakfast? What do you eat for snacks?

Adolescent takes control of eating and may reject family values (e.g., skipping breakfast, consuming junk foods and soda

Examiner Asks	Rationale

• How many calories do you figure you consume?

pop). The only control parents have is what food is in the house.

You probably cannot change adolescent eating patterns, but you can supply nutritional facts.

2. What is your exercise pattern?

Boys need an average 4000 cal/day to maintain weight; more calories if exercise is pursued. Girls need 20% fewer calories and the same nutrients as boys. Fast food is high in fat, calories, and salt and has low fiber.

3. If weight is less than body requirements: How much have you lost? By diet, exercise, or how?

Screen any extremely thin teenager for **anorexia nervosa,** a serious psychosocial disorder that includes loss of appetite, voluntary starvation, and grave weight loss. This person may augment weight loss by purging (self-induced vomiting) and use of laxatives.

• How do you feel? Tired, hungry? How do you think your body looks?

Denial of these feelings is common. Although thin, teen insists that she looks fat, "disgusting." Distorted body image.

• What is your activity pattern?

The adolescent with anorexia may have healthy activity and exercise but often is hyperactive.

• Is the weight loss associated with any other body change, such as menstrual irregularity?
• What do your parents say about your eating? What do your friends say?

Amenorrhea is common with anorexia nervosa.

This is a family problem involving control issues. Anyone at risk warrants immediate referral to a physician and mental health professional.

Additional History for the Aging Adult

1. How do you acquire your groceries and prepare your meals?

Assess risk for nutritional deficit: limited access to grocery store, income, or cooking facilities; physical disability (impaired vision, decreased mobility, decreased strength, neurologic deficit).

2. Do you eat alone or share meals with others?

Assess risk for nutritional deficit if living alone; may not bother to prepare all meals; social isolation; depression.

3. Please tell me all that you had to eat yesterday, starting with breakfast.

NOTE: 24-hour recall may not be sufficient because daily pattern may vary. Attempt week-long diary of intake. Food pattern may differ during the month if monthly income (e.g., Social Security check) runs out.

• Do you have any trouble swallowing these foods?
• What do you do right after eating: walk, take a nap?

4. How often do your bowels move?
• If the person reports constipation: What do you mean by constipation? How much liquid is in your diet? How much bulk or fiber?

Examiner Asks	Rationale
• Do you take anything for constipation, such as laxatives? Which ones? How often? • Which medications do you take?	Consider GI side effects (e.g., nausea, upset stomach, anorexia, dry mouth).

OBJECTIVE DATA

PREPARATION

The lighting should include a strong overhead light and a secondary stand light. Expose the abdomen so that it is fully visible. Drape the genitalia and female breasts.

The following measures enhance abdominal wall relaxation:

- The person should have emptied the bladder, saving a urine specimen if needed.
- Keep the room warm to avoid chilling and tensing of muscles.
- Position the person supine, with the head on a pillow, the knees bent or on pillow, and the arms at the sides or across the chest. (NOTE: Discourage the person from placing his or her arms over the head because this tenses abdominal musculature.)
- To avoid abdominal tensing, the stethoscope endpiece must be warm, your hands must be warm, and your fingernails must be very short.
- Inquire about any painful areas. Examine such an area last to avoid any muscle guarding.
- Finally, learn to use distraction: Enhance muscle relaxation through breathing exercises; emotive imagery; your low, soothing voice; by engaging in conversation; or by having the person relate his or her abdominal history while you palpate.

EQUIPMENT NEEDED
Stethoscope
Alcohol wipe (to clean endpiece)

Normal Range of Findings	Abnormal Findings

Inspect the Abdomen

Contour

Stand on the person's right side and look down on the abdomen. Then stoop or sit to gaze across the abdomen. Your head should be slightly higher than the abdomen. Determine the profile from the rib margin to the pubic bone. The contour describes the nutritional state and normally ranges from flat to rounded (Fig. 22.7).

Scaphoid abdomen caves in. Protuberant abdomen indicates abdominal distention (see Table 22.1, p. 559).

Flat

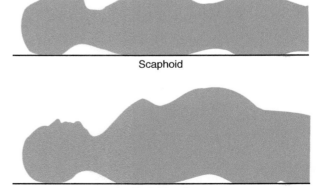
Scaphoid

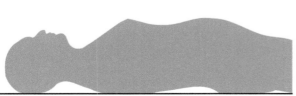
Rounded

Protuberant

22.7

Normal Range of Findings	Abnormal Findings

Symmetry

Shine a light across the abdomen toward you or lengthwise across the person. The abdomen should be symmetric bilaterally (Fig. 22.8). Note any localized bulging, visible mass, or asymmetric shape. Even small bulges are highlighted by shadow. Step to the foot of the examination table to recheck symmetry.

Bulges, masses.

Hernia—Protrusion of abdominal viscera through abnormal opening in muscle wall (see Table 22.4, Abnormalities on Inspection, p. 563).

Sister Mary Joseph nodule is a hard nodule in umbilicus that occurs with metastatic cancer of stomach, large intestine, ovary, or pancreas.[10]

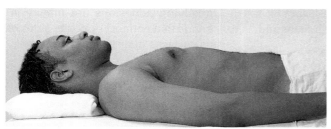

22.8

Ask the person to take a deep breath to further highlight any change. The abdomen should stay smooth and symmetric. Or ask the person to perform a sit-up without pushing up with his or her hands.

Note any localized bulging.

Hernia or enlarged liver or spleen may show.

Umbilicus

Normally it is midline and inverted, with no sign of discoloration, inflammation, or hernia. It becomes everted and pushed upward with pregnancy.

The umbilicus is a common site for piercings. The site should not be red or crusted.

Everted with ascites or underlying mass (Table 22.1).

Deeply sunken with obesity.

Enlarged, everted with umbilical hernia.

Bluish periumbilical color occurs (though rarely) with intraperitoneal bleeding (Cullen sign).[10]

Skin

The surface is smooth and even, with homogeneous color. This is a good area to judge pigment because it is often protected from sun.

Redness with localized inflammation.

Jaundice (shows best in natural daylight).

Skin glistening and taut with ascites.

Striae also occur with ascites.

One common pigment change is **striae** (lineae albicantes)—silvery white, linear, jagged marks about 1 to 6 cm long (Fig. 22.9). They occur when elastic fibers in the reticular layer of the skin are broken after rapid or prolonged stretching as in pregnancy or excessive weight gain. Recent striae are pink or blue; then they turn silvery white.

Striae look purple-blue with Cushing syndrome (excess adrenocortical hormone causes the skin to be fragile and easily broken from normal stretching).

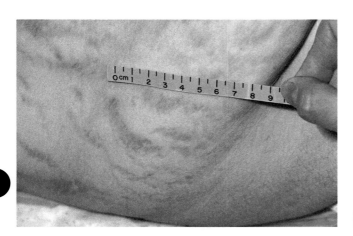

22.9 Striae.

Normal Range of Findings	Abnormal Findings

Pigmented nevi (moles)—circumscribed brown macular or papular areas—are common on the abdomen.

Normally no lesions are present, although you may note well-healed surgical scars. If a scar is present, draw its location in the person's record, indicating the length in centimeters (Fig. 22.10). (NOTE: Infrequently a person may forget a past operation when providing the history. If you note a scar now, ask about it.) A surgical scar alerts you to the possible presence of underlying adhesions and excess fibrous tissue.

Unusual color or change in shape of mole (see Chapter 13).

Petechiae.

Spider angiomas occur with portal hypertension or liver disease.

Lesions, rashes (see Chapter 13).

Underlying adhesions are inflammatory bands that connect opposite sides of serous surfaces after trauma or surgery.

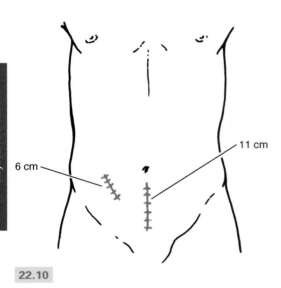

6 cm

11 cm

22.10

Veins usually are not seen, but a fine venous network may be visible in thin persons.

Prominent, dilated veins (caput medusae) occur with portal hypertension, cirrhosis, ascites, or vena caval obstruction.

Veins are more visible with malnutrition as a result of thinned adipose tissue.

Poor turgor occurs with dehydration, which often accompanies GI disease.

Good skin turgor reflects adequate hydration. Gently pinch up a fold of skin; then release to note the immediate return of the skin to original position.

Pulsation or Movement

Normally you may see the pulsations from the aorta beneath the skin in the epigastric area, particularly in thin people with good muscle wall relaxation. Respiratory movement also shows in the abdomen, particularly in males. Finally, waves of peristalsis sometimes are visible in very thin people. They ripple slowly and obliquely across the abdomen.

Marked pulsation of aorta occurs with widened pulse pressure (e.g., hypertension, aortic insufficiency, thyrotoxicosis) and aortic aneurysm.

Marked visible peristalsis, together with a distended abdomen, indicates intestinal obstruction.

Hair Distribution

The pattern of pubic hair growth normally has a diamond shape in adult males and an inverted triangle shape in adult females (see Chapters 25 and 27).

Patterns alter with endocrine or hormone abnormalities, chronic liver disease.

Normal Range of Findings	Abnormal Findings

Demeanor

A comfortable person is relaxed quietly on the examining table and has a benign facial expression and slow, even respirations.

Restlessness and constant turning to find comfort occur with the colicky pain of gastroenteritis or bowel obstruction (see Table 22.2, p. 561, and Table 22.3, p. 562).

Absolute stillness, resisting any movement, occurs with the pain of peritonitis.

Knees flexed up, facial grimacing, and rapid, uneven respirations also indicate pain.

Auscultate Bowel Sounds and Vascular Sounds

Depart from the usual examination sequence and auscultate the abdomen next. This is done because percussion and palpation can increase peristalsis, which would give a false interpretation of bowel sounds. Use the diaphragm endpiece because bowel sounds are relatively high-pitched. Hold the stethoscope lightly against the skin; pushing too hard may stimulate more bowel sounds (Fig. 22.11). Begin in the RLQ at the ileocecal valve area because bowel sounds normally are always present here.

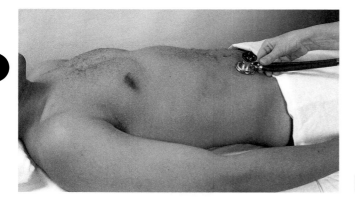

22.11

Bowel Sounds

Note the character and frequency of bowel sounds. Although the origin of bowel sounds is not fully understood, they may originate from the movement of air and fluid within the stomach and large and small intestine. A wide range of normal sounds can occur. Normal bowel sounds are high-pitched, gurgling, cascading sounds, occurring irregularly anywhere from 5 to 30 times per minute. Do not bother to count them. In addition, because the sounds radiate widely over the abdomen, the gurgle you hear in the RLQ may originate in the stomach. Therefore listening in all four quadrants is not necessary.[10] Just judge if they are present or are hypoactive or hyperactive.

One type of hyperactive bowel sounds is fairly common: hyperperistalsis, when you feel your "stomach growling," termed **borborygmus.**

Bowel sound interpretation is highly subjective and can vary widely among clinicians, and bowel sounds are likely not a reliable indicator of bowel function in many circumstances.[5,19a] For example, when assessing for the return of GI function after abdominal surgery, bowel sounds are less reliable than the passage of flatus and stool, as well as tolerance of oral intake.[13] A perfectly "silent abdomen" is uncommon; you must listen for 5 minutes by your watch before deciding whether bowel sounds are completely absent.

Two distinct patterns of abnormal bowel sounds may occur:
1. **Hyperactive sounds** are loud, high-pitched, rushing, tinkling sounds that signal increased motility.
2. **Hypoactive or absent sounds** follow abdominal surgery or with inflammation of the peritoneum (see Table 22.5, Abnormal Bowel Sounds, p. 564, and Table 22.2, p. 561).

Objective Data

Normal Range of Findings	Abnormal Findings

Vascular Sounds

As you listen to the abdomen, note the presence of any vascular sounds or **bruits.** Using firmer pressure, check over the aorta, renal arteries, iliac, and femoral arteries, especially in people with hypertension (Fig. 22.12). Usually no such sound is present. However, about 4% to 20% of healthy people (usually younger than 40 years) may have a normal bruit originating from the celiac artery.[10] It is systolic, medium to low in pitch, and heard between the xiphoid process and the umbilicus.

Note location, pitch, and timing of a vascular sound.

A systolic bruit is a pulsatile blowing sound and occurs with stenosis, partial occlusion, or aneurysm of an artery.

Venous hum and peritoneal friction rub are rare (see Table 22.6, Friction Rubs and Vascular Sounds, p. 565).

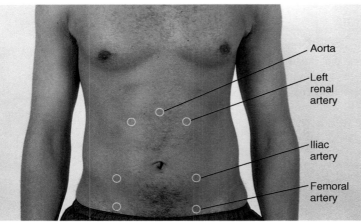

Aorta

Left renal artery

Iliac artery

Femoral artery

22.12

For safe practice, do *NOT* use auscultation of the abdomen for the correct placement of nasogastric tubes. Despite evidence showing that auscultation of an air bolus is not adequate to determine placement in the stomach or lung, you may see some nurses still practicing this method. Current evidence mandates confirming initial placement by chest x-ray and supports continuing assessment by measuring the external portion of the tube and testing the pH of stomach aspirates (pH less than 5.5 is acceptable). Ongoing visualization of gastric aspirates is also important to ensure that the tube has not migrated; fasting gastric secretions range from clear to green or brown.[2]

The auscultation method can wrongly suggest that the feeding tube is correctly placed in the stomach; serious harm or even fatality can result from administering tube-feeding material or medications into the lung.

Percussion

Percuss to assess the relative density of abdominal contents and to screen for abnormal fluid or masses.

General Tympany

First percuss lightly in all four quadrants to determine the prevailing amount of tympany and dullness (Fig. 22.13). Move clockwise. Tympany should predominate because air in the intestines rises to the surface when the person is supine.

Dullness occurs over a distended bladder, adipose tissue, fluid, or a mass.

Hyperresonance is present with gaseous distention.

Normal Range of Findings	Abnormal Findings

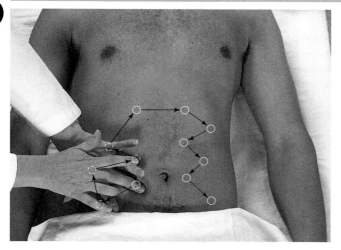

22.13

Liver Span, Splenic Dullness, and Bladder Percussion

Traditionally, the upper and lower borders of the liver were identified by percussion to estimate liver span. This technique of measuring liver span underestimates the true liver size because clinicians place the upper border too low and/or the lower border too high.[10] Percussion also yields highly variable results between examiners and frequently does not identify hepatomegaly even when present. Therefore, this examination technique is not recommended. Please see information on palpation of the liver on p. 546 for further assessment.

Screening for splenomegaly through percussion of splenic dullness is omitted because detection through palpation is more reliable.[10]

Detection of a distended bladder through percussion is also omitted due to unreliability.[10] Bedside bladder scanning with ultrasound is commonly used to estimate bladder volume.

The upper liver border is overestimated if chronic obstructive lung disease is present, and both upper and lower edges are obscured if obesity or ascites is present.

Costovertebral Angle Tenderness

Indirect fist percussion causes the tissues to vibrate instead of producing a sound. To assess the kidney, place one hand over the 12th rib at the costovertebral angle on the back (Fig. 22.14). Thump that hand with the ulnar edge of your other fist. The person normally feels a thud but no pain. (Although this step is explained here with percussion techniques, its usual sequence in a complete examination is with thoracic assessment, when the person is sitting up and you are standing behind.)

Sharp pain occurs with inflammation of the kidney or paranephric area, as in pyelonephritis.

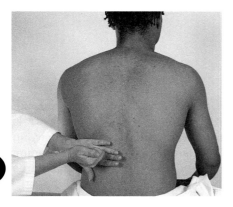

22.14

Objective Data

| **Normal Range of Findings** | **Abnormal Findings** |

Palpate Surface and Deep Areas

Perform palpation to judge the size, location, and consistency of certain organs and to screen for an abnormal mass or tenderness. Review comfort measures on p. 538. Because most people are naturally inclined to protect the abdomen, you need to use additional measures to enhance complete muscle relaxation.

1. Bend the person's knees.
2. Keep your palpating hand low and parallel to the abdomen. Holding the hand high and pointing down would make anyone tense up.
3. Teach the person to breathe slowly (in through the nose and out through the mouth).
4. Keep your own voice low and soothing. Conversation may relax the person.
5. Try "emotive imagery." For example, you might say, "Now I want you to imagine that you are dozing on the beach, with the sun warming your muscles and the sound of the waves lulling you to sleep. Let yourself relax."
6. With a very ticklish person, keep the person's hand under your own with your fingers curled over his or her fingers. Move both hands around as you palpate; people are not ticklish to themselves.
7. Alternatively perform palpation just after auscultation. Keep the stethoscope in place and curl your fingers around it, palpating as you pretend to auscultate. People do not perceive a stethoscope as a ticklish object. You can slide the stethoscope out when the person is used to being touched.

Light and Deep Palpation

Begin with **light palpation.** With the first four fingers close together, depress the skin about 1 cm (Fig. 22.15). Make a gentle rotary motion, sliding the fingers and skin together. Then lift the fingers (do not drag them) and move clockwise to the next location around the abdomen. The objective here is not to search for organs but to form an overall impression of the skin surface and superficial musculature. Save the examination of any identified tender areas until last. This method avoids pain and the resulting muscle rigidity that would obscure deep palpation later in the examination.

Muscle guarding.
Rigidity.
Large masses.
Tenderness.

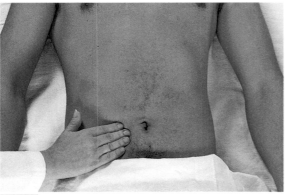

22.15

As you circle the abdomen, discriminate between voluntary muscle guarding and involuntary rigidity. **Voluntary guarding** occurs when the person is cold, tense, or ticklish. It is bilateral, and you will feel the muscles relax slightly during exhalation. Use the relaxation measures to try to eliminate this type of guarding, or it will interfere with deep palpation. If the rigidity persists, it is probably involuntary.

Involuntary rigidity is a constant, boardlike hardness of the muscles. It is a protective mechanism accompanying acute inflammation of the peritoneum. It may be unilateral, and the same area

Normal Range of Findings	Abnormal Findings

Now perform **deep palpation** using the technique described earlier but push down about 5 to 8 cm (2 to 3 inches) (Fig. 22.16). Moving clockwise, explore the entire abdomen.

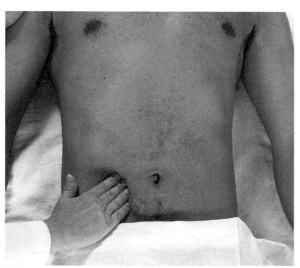

22.16

To overcome the resistance of a very large or obese abdomen, use a bimanual technique. Place your two hands on top of one another (Fig. 22.17). The top hand does the pushing; the bottom hand is relaxed and can concentrate on the sense of palpation. With either technique note the location, size, consistency, and mobility of any palpable organs and the presence of any abnormal enlargement, tenderness, or masses.

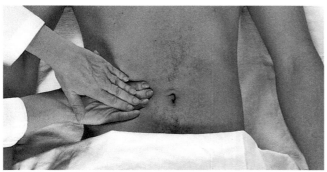

22.17

Making sense of what you are feeling is more difficult than it looks. Inexperienced examiners complain that the abdomen "all feels the same," as if they are pushing their hand into a soft sofa cushion. It helps to memorize the anatomy and visualize what is under each quadrant as you palpate. Also remember that some structures are normally palpable, as illustrated in Fig. 22.18.

Objective Data

Normal Range of Findings   **Abnormal Findings**

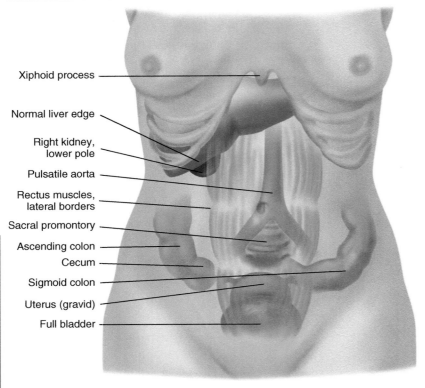

Xiphoid process

Normal liver edge

Right kidney, lower pole

Pulsatile aorta

Rectus muscles, lateral borders

Sacral promontory

Ascending colon

Cecum

Sigmoid colon

Uterus (gravid)

Full bladder

NORMALLY PALPABLE STRUCTURES

22.18

Mild tenderness normally is present when palpating the sigmoid colon in the left lower quadrant. Any other tenderness should be investigated.

Tenderness occurs with local inflammation, inflammation of the peritoneum or underlying organ, and with an enlarged organ whose capsule is stretched.

If you identify a mass, first distinguish it from a normally palpable structure or an enlarged organ. Then note the following:
1. Location
2. Size
3. Shape
4. Consistency (soft, firm, hard)
5. Surface (smooth, nodular)
6. Mobility (including movement with respirations)
7. Pulsatility
8. Tenderness

Liver

Next palpate for specific organs, beginning with the liver in the RUQ (Fig. 22.19). Place your left hand under the person's back parallel to the 11th and 12th ribs and lift up to support the abdominal contents. Place your right hand on the RUQ, with fingers parallel to the midline. Push deeply down and under the right costal margin. Ask the person to breathe slowly. With every exhalation, move your palpating hand up 1 or 2 cm. It is normal to feel the edge of the liver bump your fingertips as the diaphragm pushes it down during inhalation. It feels like a firm, regular ridge. Often the liver is not palpable and you feel nothing firm.

Objective Data

Normal Range of Findings	Abnormal Findings

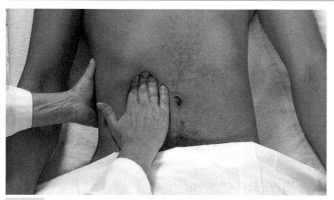

22.19

One variation occurs in people with chronic emphysema, in which the liver is displaced downward by the hyperinflated lungs. Although you palpate the lower edge well below the right costal margin, the overall size is still within normal limits.

Hooking Technique. An alternative method of palpating the liver is to stand up at the person's shoulder and swivel your body to the right so that you face the person's feet (Fig. 22.20). Hook your fingers over the costal margin from above. Ask the person to take a deep breath. Try to feel the liver edge bump your fingertips.

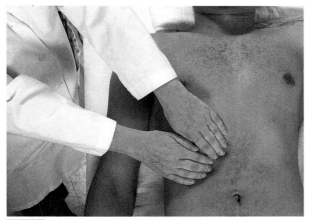

22.20

Scratch Test. This traditional technique uses auscultation to detect the lower border of the liver. Place the stethoscope over the xiphoid process while lightly stroking the skin with one finger up the MCL from the RLQ and parallel to the liver border. When you reach the liver edge, the sound is magnified in the stethoscope. However, there are many variations in the technique, and evidence is mixed as to its value.[10] One study found moderate agreement between the results by scratch test and ultrasound.[7] The researchers recommend the scratch test if the abdomen is distended, obese, or too tender for palpation or if muscles are rigid or guarded.[7]

Abnormal Findings

Except with a depressed diaphragm, a liver palpated more than 1 to 2 cm below the right costal margin is enlarged. Record the number of centimeters it descends and note its consistency (hard, nodular) and tenderness (see Table 22.7, Palpation of Enlarged Organs, p. 566). For example, an abnormally firm liver may indicate cirrhosis.[10]

Objective Data

Normal Range of Findings	Abnormal Findings

Spleen

Normally the spleen is not palpable and must be enlarged 3 times its normal size to be felt. To search for it, reach your left hand over the abdomen and behind the left side at the 11th and 12th ribs (Fig. 22.21A). Lift up for support. Place your right hand obliquely on the LUQ with the fingers pointing toward the left axilla and just inferior to the rib margin. Push your hand deeply down and under the left costal margin and ask the person to take a deep breath. You should feel nothing firm. Imaging by ultrasound is more precise.

The spleen enlarges with mononucleosis, trauma, leukemia and lymphomas, portal hypertension, and HIV infection (see Table 22.7). Consider malaria in persons with fever and splenomegaly returning from travel to areas where malaria is endemic. If you feel an enlarged spleen, refer the person but do not continue to palpate it. An enlarged spleen is friable and can rupture easily with overpalpation.

Describe the number of centimeters that it extends below the left costal margin.

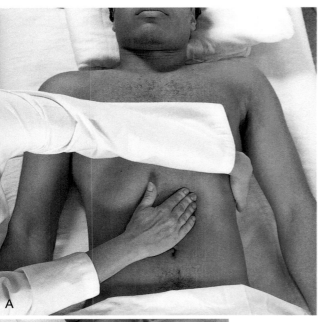

A

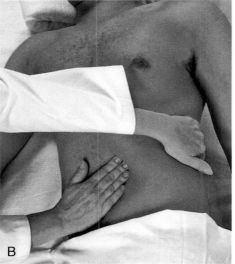

B

22.21

When enlarged, the spleen slides out and bumps your fingertips. It can grow so large that it extends into the lower quadrants. When this condition is suspected, start low so that you will not miss it. An alternative position is to roll the person onto his or her right side to displace the spleen more forward and downward (Fig. 22.21B). Then palpate as described earlier.

Normal Range of Findings	Abnormal Findings

Kidneys

Search for the right kidney by placing your hands together in a "duck-bill" position at the person's right flank (Fig. 22.22A). Press your two hands together firmly (you need deeper palpation than that used with the liver or spleen), and ask the person to take a deep breath. In most people you will feel no change. Occasionally you may feel the lower pole of the right kidney as a round, smooth mass that slides between your fingers. Either condition is normal.

Enlarged kidney.
Kidney mass.

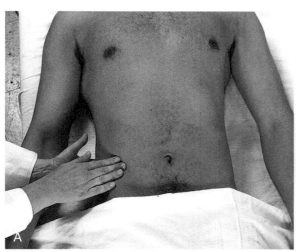
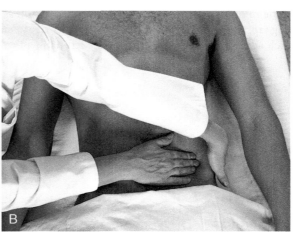

22.22

The left kidney sits 1 cm higher than the right kidney and is not palpable normally. Search for it by reaching your left hand across the abdomen and behind the left flank for support (Fig. 22.22B). Push your right hand deep into the abdomen and ask the person to breathe deeply. You should feel no change with the inhalation.

Aorta

Using your opposing thumb and fingers, palpate the aortic pulsation in the upper abdomen slightly to the left of midline (Fig. 22.23). Normally it is 2.5 to 4 cm wide in the adult and pulsates in an anterior direction.

Widened with abdominal aortic aneurysm (see Table 22.6, p. 565, and Table 22.7, p. 567).

Prominent lateral pulsation with aortic aneurysm pushes the examiner's two fingers apart. Palpation may have poor accuracy detecting aneurysm due to interference of the skin and adipose tissue, as well as the retroperitoneal location of the aorta.[10]

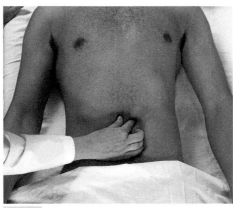

22.23

Normal Range of Findings	Abnormal Findings

Procedures for Advanced Practice

Percussion

At times you may suspect that a person has **ascites** (free fluid in the peritoneal cavity) because of a distended abdomen, bulging flanks, and an umbilicus that is protruding and displaced downward. You can differentiate ascites from gaseous distention by performing two percussion tests.

Fluid Wave. First test for a **fluid wave** by standing on the person's right side. Place the ulnar edge of another examiner's hand or the patient's own hand firmly on the abdomen in the midline (Fig. 22.24). (This stops transmission across the skin of the upcoming tap.) Place your left hand on the person's right flank. With your right hand reach across the abdomen and give the left flank a firm strike.

Ascites occurs with heart failure, portal hypertension, cirrhosis, hepatitis, pancreatitis, and cancer.

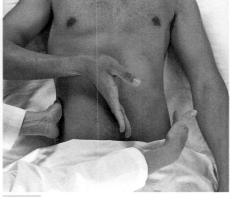

22.24   Fluid wave.

If ascites is present, the blow will generate a fluid wave through the abdomen, and you will feel a distinct tap on your left hand. If the abdomen is distended from gas or adipose tissue, you will feel no change.

Shifting Dullness. The second test for ascites is percussing for **shifting dullness.** In a supine person ascitic fluid settles by gravity into the flanks, displacing the air-filled bowel to the periumbilical space. You will hear a tympanitic note as you percuss over the top of the abdomen because gas-filled intestines float over the fluid (Fig. 22.25). Then percuss down the side of the abdomen. If fluid is present, the note will change from tympany to dull as you reach its level. Mark this spot.

A positive fluid wave test occurs with large amounts of ascitic fluid. Also note edema in the legs.

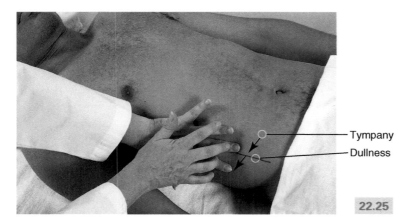

Tympany
Dullness

22.25

Normal Range of Findings	Abnormal Findings

Now turn the person onto the right side (roll him or her toward you) (Fig. 22.26). The fluid will gravitate to the dependent (in this case, right) side, displacing the lighter bowel upward. Begin percussing the upper side of the abdomen and move downward. The sound changes from tympany to a dull sound as you reach the fluid level; but this time the level of dullness is higher, upward toward the umbilicus. This **shifting level of dullness** indicates the presence of fluid.

This test has less diagnostic value than the fluid wave test. Shifting dullness is positive with a large volume of ascitic fluid; it will not detect less than 500 to 1100 mL of fluid.[10]

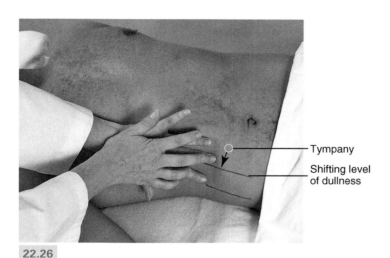

Tympany

Shifting level of dullness

22.26

Both tests, fluid wave and shifting dullness, are not completely reliable. Ultrasound study is the definitive tool.

Palpation

Rebound Tenderness. Assess rebound tenderness when the person reports abdominal pain or when you elicit tenderness during palpation. Choose a site remote from the painful area. Hold your hand 90 degrees, or perpendicular, to the abdomen. Push down slowly and deeply (Fig. 22.27A); then lift up *quickly* (Fig. 22.27B). This makes structures that are indented by palpation rebound suddenly. A normal, or negative, response is no pain on release of pressure. Perform this test at the end of the examination because it can cause severe pain and muscle rigidity.

Pain on release of pressure confirms rebound tenderness, which is a reliable sign of peritoneal inflammation. Peritoneal inflammation accompanies appendicitis.

Cough tenderness that is localized to a specific spot also signals peritoneal irritation.

Rebound tenderness occurring in the right lower quadrant when pressure is applied to the left lower quadrant (**Blumberg sign**) may indicate appendicitis. Refer the person with suspected appendicitis for computed tomography (CT) scanning.

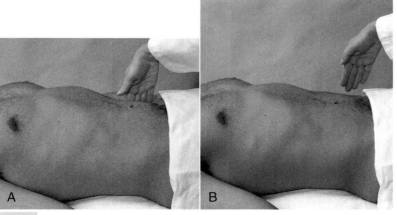

A   B

22.27

Objective Data

Normal Range of Findings

Inspiratory Arrest (Murphy Sign). Normally, palpating the liver causes no pain. In a person with inflammation of the gallbladder (cholecystitis), pain occurs. Hold your fingers under the liver border. Ask the person to take a deep breath. A normal response is to complete the deep breath without pain. (NOTE: This sign is less accurate in patients older than 60 years; evidence shows that 25% of them do not have any abdominal tenderness).[10]

Other Special Tests for Appendicitis

McBurney Point Tenderness. Draw a straight line from the anterior superior spinous process of the ileum to the umbilicus. McBurney point is located 1.5 to 2 inches from the ileum along this line. (McBurney point is at the hand placement in Fig. 22.16, p. 545.)

Iliopsoas Muscle Test. Perform the iliopsoas muscle test when the acute abdominal pain of appendicitis is suspected. With the person supine, lift the right leg straight up, flexing at the hip (Fig. 22.28); then push down over the lower part of the right thigh as the person tries to hold the leg up. When the test is negative, the person feels no change.

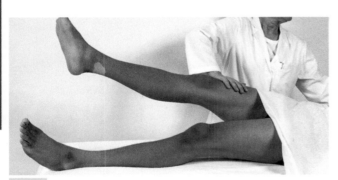

22.28 Iliopsoas muscle test.

Obturator Test. For the obturator test, lift the person's right leg, flexing at the hip, and 90 degrees at the knee. Hold his or her ankle, and rotate the leg internally and externally. There should be no pain. This test is less specific.[10]

The Alvarado Score. This scoring system combines findings to assist evaluation in patients with RLQ pain. Also called the **MANTRELS score**, from the mnemonic in the following list, a score of 4 or less significantly decreases the probability of appendicitis.[10]

Finding	Points
Symptoms	
Migration to right iliac fossa	1
Anorexia[a]	1
Nausea and vomiting	1
Signs	
Tenderness, RLQ	2
Rebound tenderness	1
Elevation of temperature (oral ≥37.3° C)	1
Laboratory Findings	
Leukocytosis (white blood cell count >10,000/μL)	2
Shift to the left (>75% neutrophils)	1
Total Possible Points	10

[a]For *anorexia*, may substitute acetone in urine.[10]

Abnormal Findings

When the test is positive, as the descending liver pushes the inflamed gallbladder onto the examining hand, the person feels sharp pain and abruptly stops inspiration midway.

Inflammation of the appendix usually produces RLQ pain to palpation, with maximal tenderness sometimes occurring over McBurney point.[10]

When the iliopsoas muscle is inflamed (which occurs with an inflamed or perforated appendix), pain is felt in the RLQ, and the test is positive.

An inflamed appendix irritates the obturator muscle, and this leg movement produces pain in a positive finding.

An Alvarado score of ≥7 increases the probability of appendicitis.

Normal Range of Findings	Abnormal Findings

❖ DEVELOPMENTAL COMPETENCE

The Infant

Inspection. The contour of the abdomen is protuberant because of the immature abdominal musculature. The skin contains a fine, superficial venous pattern. This may be visible in lightly pigmented children up to the age of puberty.

Inspect the umbilical cord throughout the neonatal period. At birth it is white and contains two umbilical arteries and one vein surrounded by mucoid connective tissue, called *Wharton's jelly.* The umbilical stump dries within a week, hardens, and falls off by 10 to 14 days. Skin covers the area by 3 to 4 weeks.

The abdomen should be symmetric, although two bulges are common. You may note an **umbilical hernia.** It appears at 2 to 3 weeks and is especially prominent when the infant cries. The hernia reaches maximum size at 1 month (up to 2.5 cm or 1 inch) and usually disappears by 1 year. Another common variation is **diastasis recti,** a separation of the rectus muscles with a visible bulge along the midline (see Table 22.4). The condition is more common with black infants, and it usually disappears by early childhood.

The abdomen shows respiratory movement. The only other abdominal movement you should note is occasional peristalsis, which may be visible because of the thin musculature.

Auscultation. Auscultation yields only bowel sounds, the metallic tinkling of peristalsis. No vascular sounds should be heard.

Percussion. Percussion finds tympany over the stomach (the infant swallows some air with feeding) and dullness over the liver. The abdomen sounds tympanitic, although it is normal to percuss dullness over the bladder. This dullness may extend up to the umbilicus.

Palpation. Aid palpation by flexing the baby's knees with one hand while palpating with the other (Fig. 22.29). Alternatively you may hold the upper back and flex the neck slightly with one hand. Offer a pacifier to a crying baby. The abdomen feels soft and supple.

Scaphoid shape occurs with dehydration.
Dilated veins.

The presence of only one artery signals the risk for congenital defects.
Inflammation.
Drainage after cord falls off.
Refer any umbilical hernia larger than 2.5 cm (see Table 22.4); continuing to grow after 1 month; or lasting for more than 2 years in a white child or for more than 7 years in a black child.
Refer diastasis recti lasting more than 6 years.
Marked peristalsis with pyloric stenosis (see Table 22.5, p. 564).

Bruit.
Venous hum.

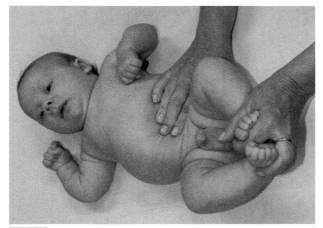

22.29

The liver fills the RUQ. It is normal to feel the liver edge at the right costal margin or 1 to 2 cm below. Normally you may palpate the spleen tip and both kidneys and the bladder. Also easily palpated are the cecum in the RLQ and the sigmoid colon, which feels like a sausage in the left inguinal area.

Objective Data

Normal Range of Findings	Abnormal Findings

Make note of the newborn's first stool, a sticky, greenish-black meconium stool within 24 hours of birth. By the 4th day, stools of breastfed babies are golden yellow, pasty, and smell like sour milk, whereas those of formula-fed babies are brown-yellow, firmer, and more fecal smelling.

The Child

Younger than 4 years, the abdomen looks protuberant when the child is both supine and standing. After age 4 years the potbelly remains when standing because of lumbar lordosis, but the abdomen looks flat when supine. Normal movement on the abdomen includes respirations, which remain abdominal until 7 years of age.

To palpate the abdomen, position the young child on the parent's lap as you sit knee-to-knee with the parent. Flex the knees up and elevate the head slightly. The child can "pant like a dog" to further relax abdominal muscles. Hold your entire palm flat on the abdominal surface for a moment before starting palpation. This accustoms the child to being touched (Fig. 22.30). If the child is very ticklish, hold his or her hand under your own as you palpate or apply the stethoscope and palpate around it.

A scaphoid abdomen is associated with dehydration or malnutrition.

Younger than 7 years, the absence of abdominal respirations occurs with inflammation of the peritoneum.

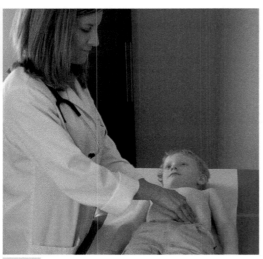

22.30

The liver remains easily palpable 1 to 2 cm below the right costal margin. The edge is well-defined and moves easily. On the left the spleen also is easily palpable with a well-defined movable edge. Usually you can feel 1 to 2 cm of the right kidney and the tip of the left kidney.

In assessing abdominal tenderness, remember that the young child often answers this question affirmatively no matter how the abdomen actually feels. Use objective signs to aid assessment, such as a cry changing in pitch as you palpate, facial grimacing, moving away from you, and guarding.

The school-age child has a slim abdominal shape as he or she loses the potbelly. This slimming trend continues into adolescence. Variation in body image means that some adolescents are comfortable with exposure to the abdomen and others may be embarrassed. Be sensitive to this and use adequate draping or keep her or him in personal clothing (Fig. 22.31). The physical findings are the same as those listed for the adult.

Normal Range of Findings	Abnormal Findings

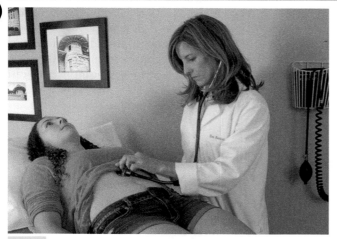

22.31 Aim to keep adolescent in own clothing.

The Aging Adult

On inspection you may note increased deposits of subcutaneous fat on the abdomen and hips because it is redistributed away from the extremities. The abdominal musculature is thinner and has less tone than that of the younger adult; thus in the absence of obesity, you may note peristalsis.

Because of the thinner, softer abdominal wall, the organs may be easier to palpate (in the absence of obesity). The liver is easier to palpate. Normally you will feel the liver edge at or just below the costal margin. With distended lungs and a depressed diaphragm, the liver is palpated lower, descending 1 to 2 cm below the costal margin with inhalation. The kidneys are easier to palpate.

Abdominal rigidity with acute abdominal conditions is less common in aging.

With an acute abdomen the aging person often complains of less pain than a younger person would.

HEALTH PROMOTION AND PATIENT TEACHING

HEPATITIS B AND HEPATITIS C

Let's talk about your potential risks for viral hepatitis, which is a liver infection. There are three major types of hepatitis: A, B, and C. Hepatitis B and C are spread through blood and body fluids, for example by sharing contaminated needles or by sexual contact. Both hepatitis B and C can cause a brief period of illness, then either be cleared from the body entirely or go on to cause a long-term, or chronic, infection. Chronic infection is especially common with hepatitis C. Chronic hepatitis can eventually cause the liver to fail by causing liver scarring (fibrosis and cirrhosis). Chronic hepatitis also increases your risk for liver cancer.[3,9,12]

For high-risk individuals, the U.S. Preventive Services Task Force recommends screening for hepatitis B and C through blood testing. Risk for hepatitis B virus (HBV) is highest among people born in countries with high HBV infection prevalence, people born in the United States but not vaccinated in infancy with parents who were born in high-risk countries, people with HIV-positive status, users of injection drugs, men who have sex with men, and people with sexual partners with HBV or who have household contacts with HBV.[9] Those at highest risk for HCV include people with a current or past history of injection drug use and people with additional risk factors: blood transfusion before 1992, birth year between 1945 and 1965, unregulated tattoos, birth to an HCV-infected mother, and long-term hemodialysis.[11] High-risk individuals should be screened at least once and at periodic intervals if the risk persists (e.g., if the person continues to use injection drugs).

Health promotion and disease prevention teaching are essential components of the disease screening process. Providers should be aware of the sensitive nature of risk assessment and should use open-ended and direct questioning to explore patients' risks for viral hepatitis to determine whether screening is warranted. Primary prevention involves risk-factor modification, which includes the provision of resources to make the necessary lifestyle modifications to reduce risk of exposure. For example, be prepared to provide referrals to drug treatment programs, information about condom use, and recommendations for vaccines. Although there is no vaccination for HCV, there is a safe, effective vaccine against HBV. All infants should receive the hepatitis B vaccine, as well as people in high-risk groups and all health care workers. For a complete list of who should be vaccinated against HBV, along with recommended vaccines and vaccination schedule, visit https://www.cdc.gov/hepatitis/hbv/hbvfaq.htm#vaccFAQ. For both HBV- and HCV-infected people, secondary prevention includes antiviral treatment regimens to prevent the long-term complications that can lead to significant liver disease and death.

DOCUMENTATION AND CRITICAL THINKING

Sample Charting

SUBJECTIVE

States appetite is good with no recent change, no dysphagia, no food intolerance, no pain, no nausea/vomiting. Has one formed BM/day. Takes OTC multivitamins, no other prescribed or over-the-counter medication. No history of abdominal disease, injury, or surgery. Diet recall of past 24 hours listed at end of history.

OBJECTIVE

Inspection: Abdomen flat, symmetric, with no apparent masses. Skin smooth with no striae, scars, or lesions.
Auscultation: Bowel sounds present, no bruits.
Percussion: Tympany predominates in all 4 quadrants.
Palpation: Abdomen soft, no organomegaly, no masses, no tenderness.

ASSESSMENT

Healthy abdomen; bowel sounds present

Clinical Case Study 1

O.W. is a 33-year-old male who underwent gastric bypass surgery 1 week PTA. Preoperative BMI 62.8 (height 180 cm; weight 204 kg). Past medical history of type 2 diabetes mellitus, morbid obesity, hypertension, obstructive sleep apnea, and venous stasis ulcers on bilateral lower extremities.

SUBJECTIVE

1 week PTA—Endoscopic gastric bypass surgery performed without complication.
5 days PTA—Patient discharged home in stable condition on a pureed diet. No postoperative complications.
1 day PTA—O.W. noticed increased nausea and nonspecific shoulder pain.
Present—"I feel terrible." Reports fever with chills, nausea, constant pain in back and shoulders, abdominal pain, and palpitations. O.W. denies changes in diet or deviation from prescribed diet.

OBJECTIVE

Vital signs: Temp 102° F (39° C). Pulse 130 bpm. Resp 20/min. BP 90/56 mm Hg, right arm, supine.
Inspection: Lying on side with knees tucked. Abdomen uniformly round. Grimacing with movement.
Auscultation: Hypoactive bowel sounds. No vascular sounds.
Percussion: Tympany predominates. Scattered dullness caused by adipose tissue. Percussion elicits tenderness.
Palpation: Extreme tenderness. Rebound tenderness present RLQ and LLQ. Unable to palpate organs because of tenderness and obesity.

ASSESSMENT

Acute abdomen
Possible anastomotic leaking at gastric bypass site
Acute abdominal pain due to peritoneal inflammation
Potential for intra-abdominal infection

Clinical Case Study 2

E.J. is a 63-year-old retired homemaker with a history of lung cancer with metastasis to the liver.

SUBJECTIVE

Feeling "puffy and bloated" for the past week. States unable to get comfortable. Also short of breath "all the time now." Difficulty sleeping. "I feel like crying all the time now."

OBJECTIVE

Inspection: Weight increase of 8 lb in 1 week. Abdomen is distended with everted umbilicus and bulging flanks. Girth at umbilicus is 85 cm. Prominent dilated venous pattern present over abdomen.
Auscultation: Bowel sounds present. No vascular sounds.
Percussion: When supine, tympany present at dome of abdomen, dullness over flanks. Shifting dullness present. Positive fluid wave present.
Palpation: Abdominal wall firm, able to feel liver with deep palpation at 6 cm below right costal margin. Liver feels firm, nodular, nontender. 4+ pitting edema in both ankles.

ASSESSMENT

Ascites
Grieving
Shortness of breath due to increased intra-abdominal pressure
Pain due to distended abdomen
Potential for skin breakdown due to ascites, edema, and faulty metabolism
Insomnia

Clinical Case Study 3

D.G. is a 17-year-old male high school student who enters the emergency department with abdominal pain for 2 days.

SUBJECTIVE

2 days PTA, D.G. noted abdominal pain in umbilical region. Now pain is sharp and severe, and he points to location in RLQ. No BM for 2 days. No appetite. Nausea and vomiting off and on 1 day; no blood in vomitus.

OBJECTIVE

Inspection: Temp 100.4° F (38° C). Pulse 116 bpm. Resp 18/min. BP 112/70 mm Hg.
Lying on side with knees drawn up under chin. Resists any movement. Face tight and occasionally grimacing. Cries out with any sudden movement.
Auscultation: No bowel sounds present. No vascular sounds.
Percussion: Tympany. Percussion over RLQ leads to tenderness.
Palpation: Abdominal wall is rigid and boardlike. Extreme tenderness to palpation in RLQ. Rebound tenderness is present in RLQ. Positive iliopsoas muscle test. Alvarado score 7 with no laboratory results available yet.

ASSESSMENT

Acute abdomen, possible appendicitis
Acute abdominal pain in RLQ
Nausea and vomiting

Clinical Case Study 4

G.C. is a 5-week-old male who was brought to the clinic today by his parents for vomiting.

SUBJECTIVE

Since birth G.C. has been a "great eater who nursed all the time without problems."

10 days PTA—G.C. continues to want to nurse all the time but now "projectile vomits" soon after he feeds and "never appears comfortable."

4 days PTA—Vomiting continued post-feeds; last reported stool at that time; 7 wet diapers/day.

1 day PTA—Vomiting continued; "only had 3 wet diapers today."

Birth weight—9 lb 9 oz (4.3 kg)

OBJECTIVE

Vital signs: Temp 98.6° F (37° C) (axillary). Pulse 128 bpm. Resp 42/min. Weight 11 lb 3 oz (5.1 kg). BP 76/40 mm Hg (sleeping).

General appearance: Infant resting comfortably in mom's arms.

HEENT: Anterior and posterior fontanels slightly sunken; eyes clear and moist; TM pearly gray bilat; nares patent bilat; oral mucosa slightly moist

Cardiovascular: Sinus arrhythmia; no abnormal heart sounds.

Respiratory: Breath sounds clear and equal bilat; unlabored.

Abdomen: Visible gastric peristalsis and olive-shaped mass palpated in the epigastrium just right of umbilicus.

ASSESSMENT

Pyloric stenosis
Potential for protein calorie malnutrition due to vomiting secondary to pyloric sphincter obstruction
Acute abdominal pain due to abdominal fullness
Dehydration due to vomiting

ABNORMAL FINDINGS

| TABLE 22.1 | Abdominal Distention |

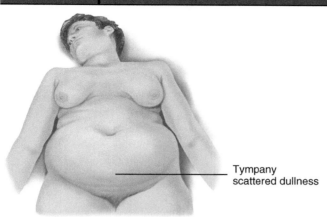

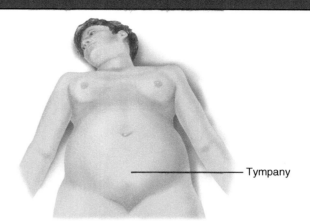

Obesity

Inspection. Uniformly rounded. Umbilicus sunken (it adheres to peritoneum, layers of fat are superficial to it).
Auscultation. Normal bowel sounds.
Percussion. Tympany. Scattered dullness over adipose tissue.
Palpation. Normal. May be hard to feel through thick abdominal wall.

Air or Gas

Inspection. Single round curve.
Auscultation. Depends on cause of gas (e.g., decreased or absent bowel sounds with ileus); hyperactive with early intestinal obstruction.
Percussion. Tympany over large area.
Palpation. May have muscle spasm of abdominal wall.

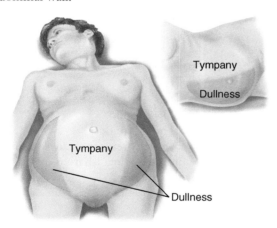

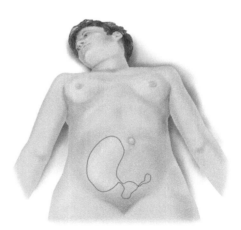

Ascites

Inspection. Single curve. Everted umbilicus. Bulging flanks when supine. Taut, glistening skin due to recent weight gain; increase in abdominal girth.
Auscultation. Normal bowel sounds over intestines. Diminished over ascitic fluid.
Percussion. Tympany at top where intestines float. Dull over fluid. Produces fluid wave and shifting dullness.
Palpation. Taut skin and increased intra-abdominal pressure limit palpation.

Ovarian Cyst (Large)

Inspection. Curve in lower half of abdomen, toward midline. Everted umbilicus.
Auscultation. Normal bowel sounds over upper abdomen where intestines pushed superiorly.
Percussion. Top dull over fluid. Intestines pushed superiorly. Large cyst produces fluid wave and shifting dullness.
Palpation. Transmits aortic pulsation, whereas ascites does not.

Continued

TABLE 22.1	Abdominal Distention—cont'd

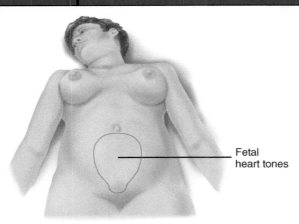

Fetal
heart tones

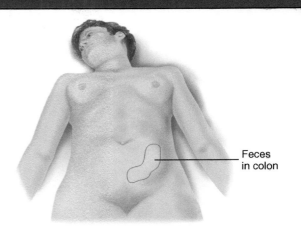

Feces
in colon

Pregnancy[a]

Inspection. Single curve. Umbilicus protruding. Breasts engorged.

Auscultation. Fetal heart tones. Bowel sounds diminished.

Percussion. Tympany over intestines. Dull over enlarging uterus.

Palpation. Uterine fundus. Fetal parts. Fetal movements.

Feces

Inspection. Localized distention.

Auscultation. Normal bowel sounds.

Percussion. Tympany predominates. Scattered dullness over fecal mass.

Palpation. Plastic-like or ropelike mass with feces in intestines.

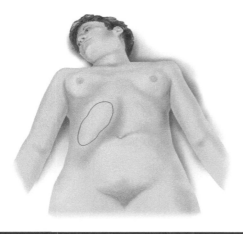

◀ Tumor

Inspection. Localized distention.

Auscultation. Normal bowel sounds.

Percussion. Dull over mass if reaches up to skin surface.

Palpation. Define borders. Distinguish from enlarged organ or normally palpable structure.

[a]Obviously a normal finding, pregnancy is included for comparison of conditions causing abdominal distention.

TABLE 22.2 | Clinical Portrait of Intestinal Obstruction

Patient History and Symptoms

- History of previous abdominal surgery with adhesions
- Vomiting
- Fever
- Absence of stool or gas passage
- Colicky pain from strong peristalsis above the obstrucion

Physical Examination Findings

- Restless, ill-appearing patient
- Distended abdomen
- Hyperactive bowel sounds in early obstruction, hypoactive or silent in late obstruction
- Tenderness to palpation
- Hypovolemic shock due to dehydration and sepsis may occur (increased pulse, decrease BP, cool skin, dry mucous membranes)

Diagnostic Tests

- Laboratory: Evidence of dehydration, loss of electrolytes, and possibly sepsis
- Radiology: Accumulation of fluid and gas in bowel proximal to (above) obstruction[14]

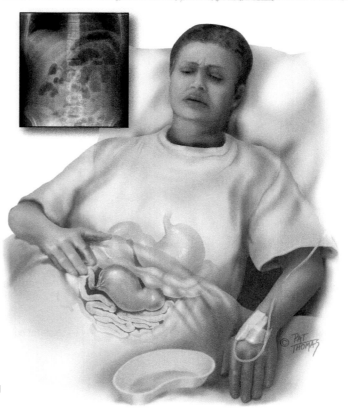

© Pat Thomas, 2014.

TABLE 22.3	Common Sites of Referred Abdominal Pain

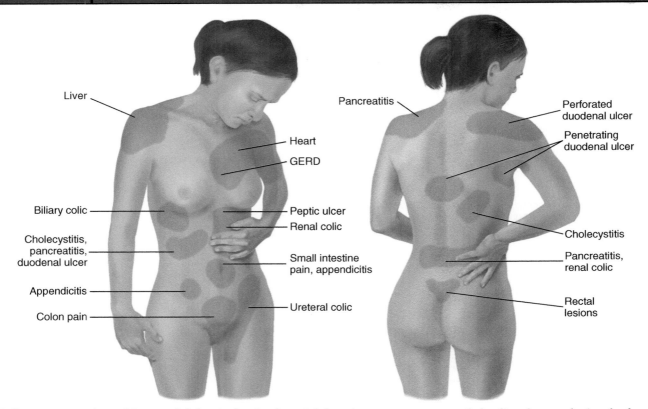

Liver

Heart

GERD

Biliary colic

Peptic ulcer

Renal colic

Cholecystitis, pancreatitis, duodenal ulcer

Appendicitis

Small intestine pain, appendicitis

Colon pain

Ureteral colic

Pancreatitis

Perforated duodenal ulcer

Penetrating duodenal ulcer

Cholecystitis

Pancreatitis, renal colic

Rectal lesions

When a person gives a history of abdominal pain, the pain's location may not necessarily be directly over the involved organ because the human brain has no felt image for internal organs. Rather, pain is referred to a site where the organ was located in fetal development. Although the organ migrates during fetal development, its nerves persist in referring sensations from the former location. The following are examples, not a complete list.

Liver. Hepatitis may have mild-to-moderate dull pain in right upper quadrant (RUQ) or epigastrium, along with anorexia, nausea, malaise, low-grade fever.

Esophagus. Gastroesophageal reflux disease (GERD) is a complex of symptoms of esophagitis, including burning pain in midepigastrium or behind lower sternum that radiates upward, or "heartburn." Occurs 30 to 60 minutes after eating; aggravated by lying down or bending over.

Gallbladder. Cholecystitis is biliary colic, sudden pain in RUQ that may radiate to right or left scapula and that builds over time, lasting 2 to 4 hours, after ingestion of fatty foods, alcohol, or caffeine. Associated with nausea and vomiting and with positive Murphy sign or sudden stop in inspiration with RUQ palpation.

Pancreas. Pancreatitis has acute, boring midepigastric pain radiating to the back and sometimes to the left scapula or flank, severe nausea, and vomiting.

Duodenum. Duodenal ulcer typically has dull, aching, gnawing pain; does not radiate; may be relieved by food; and may awaken the person from sleep.

Stomach. Gastric ulcer pain is dull, aching, gnawing epigastric pain, usually brought on by food and radiates to back or substernal area. Pain of perforated ulcer is burning epigastric pain of sudden onset that refers to one or both shoulders.

Appendix. Appendicitis typically starts as dull, diffuse pain in periumbilical region that later shifts to severe, sharp, persistent pain and tenderness localized in RLQ (McBurney point). Pain is aggravated by movement, coughing, deep breathing; associated with anorexia, then nausea and vomiting, fever.

Kidney. Kidney stones prompt a sudden onset of severe, colicky flank or lower abdominal pain.

Small intestine. Gastroenteritis has diffuse, generalized abdominal pain with nausea, diarrhea.

Colon. Large bowel obstruction has moderate, colicky pain of gradual onset in lower abdomen and bloating. Irritable bowel syndrome (IBS) has sharp or burning cramping pain over a wide area; does not radiate. Brought on by meals; relieved by bowel movement.

TABLE 22.4 | Abnormalities on Inspection

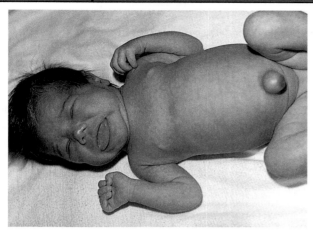

Umbilical Hernia

This is a soft, skin-covered mass, the protrusion of the omentum or intestine through a weakness or incomplete closure in the umbilical ring. It is accentuated by increased intra-abdominal pressure as with crying, coughing, vomiting, or straining; but the bowel rarely incarcerates or strangulates. More common in premature infants. Most resolve spontaneously by 1 year; parents should avoid affixing a belt or coin at the hernia because this will not help closure and may cause contact dermatitis. In an adult it occurs with pregnancy, chronic ascites, or chronic increased intrathoracic pressure (e.g., asthma, chronic bronchitis).

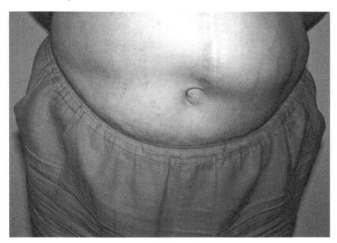

Incisional Hernia

A bulge near an old operative scar that may not show when person is supine but is apparent when the person increases intra-abdominal pressure by a sit-up, by standing, or by the Valsalva maneuver.

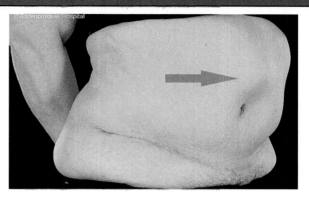

Epigastric Hernia

Protrusion of abdominal structures presents as a small, fatty nodule at epigastrium in midline, through the linea alba. Usually one can feel it rather than observe it. May be palpable only when standing.

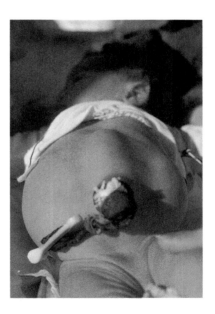

Diastasis Recti

A midline longitudinal ridge that is a separation of the abdominal rectus muscles. Ridge is revealed when intra-abdominal pressure is increased by raising head while supine. Occurs congenitally (here) and as a result of pregnancy or marked obesity in which prolonged distention or a decrease in muscle tone has occurred. Usually it is not clinically significant.

See Illustration Credits for source information.

TABLE 22.5 | Abnormal Bowel Sounds

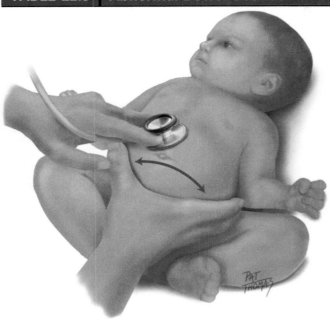

◀ Succussion Splash

Unrelated to peristalsis, this is a very loud splash auscultated over the upper abdomen when the infant is rocked side to side. It indicates increased air and fluid in the stomach, as seen with pyloric obstruction or large hiatus hernia.

Marked peristalsis together with projectile vomiting in the newborn suggests pyloric stenosis, an obstruction of the pyloric valve of the stomach. Pyloric stenosis is a congenital defect and appears in the 2nd or 3rd week. After feeding, pronounced peristaltic waves cross from left to right, leading to projectile vomiting. Then one can palpate an olive-size mass in the RUQ midway between the right costal margin and umbilicus. Refer promptly because of risk for weight loss.

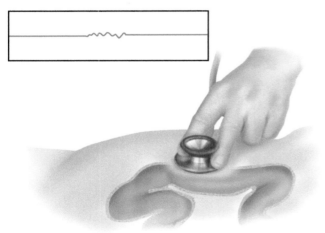

Hypoactive Bowel Sounds

Diminished or absent bowel sounds signal decreased motility as a result of inflammation as seen with peritonitis; from paralytic ileus as following abdominal surgery; or from late bowel obstruction. Occurs also with pneumonia.

Hyperactive Bowel Sounds

Loud, gurgling sounds, **"borborygmi,"** signal increased motility. They occur with early mechanical bowel obstruction (high-pitched), gastroenteritis, brisk diarrhea, laxative use, and subsiding paralytic ileus.

TABLE 22.6	Friction Rubs and Vascular Sounds

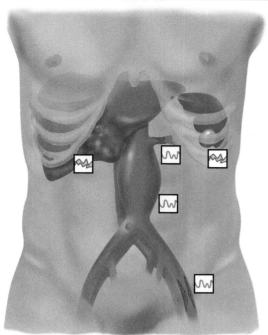

Peritoneal friction rub

Vascular sounds

◀ **Peritoneal Friction Rub**

A rough, grating sound, like two pieces of leather rubbed together, indicates peritoneal inflammation. Occurs rarely. Usually occurs over organs with a large surface area in contact with the peritoneum.

Liver—Friction rub over lower right rib cage from abscess or metastatic tumor.

Spleen—Friction rub over lower left rib cage in left anterior axillary line from abscess, infection, or tumor.

◀ **Vascular Sounds**

Arterial—A **bruit** indicates turbulent blood flow, as found in constricted, abnormally dilated, or tortuous vessels. Listen with the bell. Occurs with the following:

- *Aortic aneurysm*—Murmur is harsh, systolic, or continuous and accentuated with systole. Note in person with hypertension.
- *Renal artery stenosis*—Murmur is midline or toward flank, soft, low-to-medium pitch.
- *Partial occlusion of femoral arteries.*

Venous hum—Occurs rarely. Heard in periumbilical region. Originates from inferior vena cava. Medium pitch, continuous sound, pressure on bell may obliterate it. May have palpable thrill. Occurs with portal hypertension and cirrhotic liver.

TABLE 22.7 | Palpation of Enlarged Organs

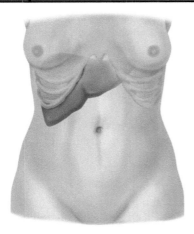

Enlarged Liver

An enlarged, smooth, nontender liver occurs with fatty infiltration, portal obstruction or cirrhosis, high obstruction of inferior vena cava, and lymphocytic leukemia.

The liver feels enlarged and smooth but is tender to palpation with early heart failure, acute hepatitis, or hepatic abscess.

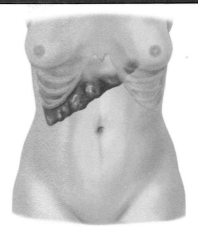

Enlarged Nodular Liver

An enlarged and nodular liver occurs with late portal cirrhosis, metastatic cancer, or tertiary syphilis. Often with cirrhosis the liver is smaller, but the edge is firmer than normal, and the edge is easily palpable.

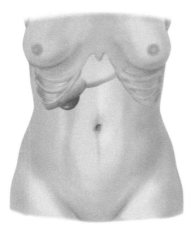

Enlarged Gallbladder

An enlarged, tender gallbladder suggests acute cholecystitis. Feel it behind the liver border as a smooth and firm mass like a sausage, although it may be difficult to palpate because of involuntary rigidity of abdominal muscles. The area is exquisitely painful to fist percussion, and inspiratory arrest (Murphy sign) is present.

An enlarged, nontender gallbladder also feels like a smooth, sausagelike mass. It occurs when the gallbladder is filled with stones, as with common bile duct obstruction.

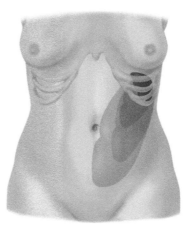

Enlarged Spleen

Because any enlargement superiorly is stopped by the diaphragm, the spleen enlarges down and to the midline. When extreme, it can extend down to the left pelvis. It retains the splenic notch on the medial edge. When splenomegaly occurs with acute infections (mononucleosis), it is moderately enlarged and soft, with rounded edges. When the result of a chronic cause, the enlargement is firm or hard, with sharp edges. An enlarged spleen is usually not tender to palpation; it is tender only if the peritoneum is also inflamed.

Continued

TABLE 22.7 | **Palpation of Enlarged Organs—cont'd**

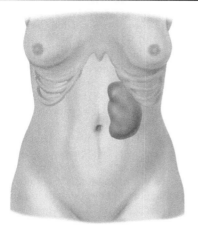

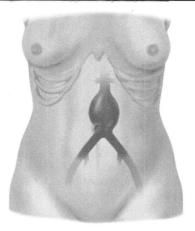

Enlarged Kidney

Enlarged with hydronephrosis, cyst, or neoplasm. May be difficult to distinguish an enlarged kidney from an enlarged spleen because they have a similar shape. Both extend forward and down. However, the spleen may have a sharp edge, whereas the kidney never does. The spleen retains the splenic notch, whereas the kidney has no palpable notch. Percussion over the spleen is dull, whereas over the kidney it is tympanitic because of the overriding bowel.

Aortic Aneurysm

Most aortic aneurysms (>95%) are located below the renal arteries and extend to the umbilicus. A focal bulging >5 cm is palpable in about 80% of cases during routine physical examination and feels like a pulsating mass in the upper abdomen just to the left of midline. You will hear a bruit. Femoral pulses are present but decreased. Additional information on abdominal aneurysm is illustrated in Table 22.6.

Summary Checklist: Abdomen Examination

1. **Inspection**
   Contour
   Symmetry
   Umbilicus
   Skin
   Pulsation or movement
   Hair distribution
   Demeanor

2. **Auscultation**
   Bowel sounds
   Note any vascular sounds

3. **Percussion**
   Percuss all four quadrants

4. **Palpation**
   Light palpation in all four quadrants
   Deeper palpation in all four quadrants
   Palpate for liver, spleen, kidneys

REFERENCES

1. Bayless, T. M., Brown, E., & Paige, D. M. (2017). Lactase non-persistence and lactose intolerance. *Curr Gastroenterol Rep, 19*, 23.
2. Boullata, J. I., et al. (2017). ASPEN safe practices for enteral nutrition therapy. *JPEN J Parenter Enteral Nutr, 41*(1), 15–103.
3. Centers for Disease Control. (2016). *Hepatitis B FAQs for health professionals.* https://www.cdc.gov/hepatitis/hbv/hbvfaq.htm#overview.
4. Choung, R. S., et al. (2015). Trends and racial/ethnic disparities in gluten-sensitive problems in the United States: Findings from the National Health and Nutrition Examination Surveys from 1988-2012. *Am J Gastroenterol, 110*, 455–461.
5. Felder, S., Margel, D., Murrell, Z., et al. (2014). Usefulness of bowel sound auscultation: A prospective evaluation. *J Surg Educ, 71*, 768–773.
6. Ferrara, L. R., & Saccomano, S. J. (2017). Constipation in children: Diagnosis, treatment, and prevention. *Nurse Pract, 42*(7), 30–34.

Abnormal Findings

7. Gupta, K., Dhawan, A., Abel, C., et al. (2013). A re-evaluation of the scratch test for locating the liver edge. *BMC Gastroenterol, 13*(1), 35.

8. Johanson, L. (2015). The gluten-free frenzy: Fad or fitting? *Medsurg Nurs, 24*, 213–217.

9. LeFevre, M. L. (2014). Screening for hepatitis B infection in nonpregnant adolescents and adults: U.S. Preventive Services Task Force Recommendation Statement. *Ann Intern Med, 161*, 58–67.

10. McGee, S. R. (2018). *Evidence-based physical diagnosis* (4th ed.). St. Louis: Elsevier.

11. Moyer, V. A. (2013). Screening for hepatitis C infection in adults: U.S. Preventive Services Task Force recommendation statement. *Ann Intern Med, 159*, 349–358.

12. Pozza, R., Hill, C., Hefner, A. M., et al. (2017). Hepatitis C infection: Updates on treatment guidelines. *Nurse Pract, 42*(5), 15–24.

13. Read, T. E., Brozovich, M., Andujar, J. E., et al. (2017). Bowel sounds are not associated with flatus, bowel movement, or tolerance of oral intake in patients after major abdominal surgery. *Dis Colon Rectum, 60*, 608–613.

14. Reddy, S. R., & Cappell, M. S. (2017). A systematic review of the clinical presentation, diagnosis, and treatment of small bowel obstruction. *Curr Gastroenterol Rep, 19*, 28.

15. Robinson, B. L., Davis, S. C., & Vess, J. (2015). Primary care management of celiac. *Nurse Pract, 40*(2), 28–34.

16. Roque, M. V., & Bouras, E. P. (2015). Epidemiology and management of chronic constipation in elderly patients. *Clin Interv Aging, 10*, 919–930.

17. Rubio-Tapia, A., Hill, I. D., Kelly, C. P., et al. (2013). ACG Clinical Guidelines: Diagnosis and management of celiac disease. *Am J Gastroenterol, 108*, 656–676.

18. Ryan, D. J., O'Sullivan, F., & Jackson, S. H. D. (2016). Prescribing medicines for older patients. *Medicine (Baltimore), 44*, 433–437.

19. Theilen, L. H., et al. (2016). Acute appendicitis in pregnancy: Predictive clinical factors and pregnancy outcomes. *Am J Perinatol, 34*, 523–528.

19a. Van Bree, S. H. W., Prins, M. M. C., & Juffermans, N. P. (2018). Auscultation for bowel sounds in patients with ileus: An outdated practice in the ICU? *Neth J Crit Care, 26*, 142–146.

20. U.S. Preventive Services Task Force. (2017). Screening for celiac disease: US Preventive Services Task Force recommendation statement. *JAMA, 317*, 1252–1257.

21. Vici, G., Belli, L., Biondi, M., et al. (2016). Gluten free diet and nutrient deficiencies: A review. *Clin Nutr, 35*, 1236–1241.

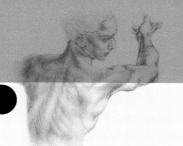

CHAPTER 23

Musculoskeletal System

STRUCTURE AND FUNCTION

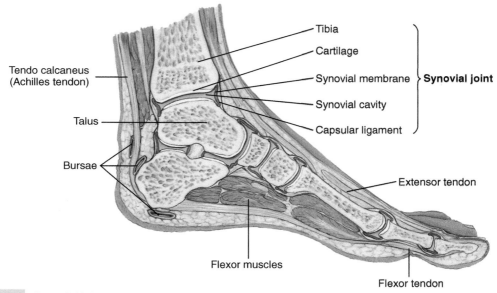

Tibia

Cartilage

Tendo calcaneus
(Achilles tendon)

Synovial membrane } **Synovial joint**

Synovial cavity

Talus

Capsular ligament

Bursae

Extensor tendon

Flexor muscles

Flexor tendon

23.1 Synovial joints.

The musculoskeletal system consists of the body's **bones, joints,** and **muscles.** Humans need this system (1) for *support* to stand erect, and (2) for *movement*. The musculoskeletal system also functions (3) to encase and *protect* the inner vital organs (e.g., brain, spinal cord, heart); (4) to *produce* the red blood cells, white blood cells, and platelets in the bone marrow (hematopoiesis); and (5) as a *reservoir* for *storage* of essential minerals such as calcium and phosphorus in the bones.

MUSCULOSKELETAL COMPONENTS

The skeleton is the bony framework of the body. It has 206 bones, which support the body like the posts and beams of a building. **Bone** and cartilage are specialized forms of connective tissue. Bone is hard, rigid, and very dense. Its cells are continually turning over and remodeling. The **joint** (or articulation) is the place of union of two or more bones. Joints are the functional units of the musculoskeletal system because they permit the mobility needed for activities of daily living (ADLs).

Fibrous, Cartilaginous, and Synovial Joints

In **fibrous** joints the bones are united by interjacent fibrous tissue or cartilage and are immovable (e.g., the sutures in the skull). **Cartilaginous** joints are separated by fibrocartilaginous discs and are only slightly movable (e.g., the vertebrae). **Synovial** joints are freely movable because their bones are separated from one another and enclosed in a joint cavity (Fig. 23.1). This cavity is lined with a synovial membrane that secretes a lubricant, or synovial fluid. Just like grease on gears, synovial fluid allows sliding of opposing surfaces, and this sliding permits movement.

In synovial joints a layer of resilient **cartilage** covers the surface of opposing bones. Cartilage is avascular; it receives nourishment from synovial fluid that circulates during joint movement. It is a very stable connective tissue with a slow cell turnover. It has a tough, firm consistency yet is flexible. This cartilage cushions the bones and gives a smooth surface to facilitate movement.

The joint is surrounded by a fibrous capsule and supported by ligaments. **Ligaments** are fibrous bands running directly from one bone to another bone that strengthen the joint and

569

help prevent movement in undesirable directions. A **bursa** is an enclosed sac filled with viscous synovial fluid, much like a joint. Bursae are located in areas of potential friction (e.g., subacromial bursa of the shoulder, prepatellar bursa of the knee) and help muscles and tendons glide smoothly over bone.

Muscles

Muscles account for 40% to 50% of body weight. When they contract they produce movement. Muscles are of three types: skeletal, smooth, and cardiac. This chapter is concerned with **skeletal,** or voluntary, muscles—those under conscious control.

Each **skeletal muscle** is composed of bundles of muscle fibers or **fasciculi.** The skeletal muscle is attached to bone by a **tendon**—a strong fibrous cord. Skeletal muscles produce the following movements (Fig. 23.2):

1. Flexion—Bending a limb at a joint
2. Extension—Straightening a limb at a joint
3. Abduction—Moving a limb away from the midline of the body

4. Adduction—Moving a limb toward the midline of the body
5. Pronation—Turning the forearm so the palm is down
6. Supination—Turning the forearm so the palm is up
7. Circumduction—Moving the arm in a circle around the shoulder
8. Inversion—Moving the sole of the foot inward at the ankle
9. Eversion—Moving the sole of the foot outward at the ankle
10. Rotation—Moving the head around a central axis
11. Protraction—Moving a body part forward and parallel to the ground
12. Retraction—Moving a body part backward and parallel to the ground
13. Elevation—Raising a body part
14. Depression—Lowering a body part

Temporomandibular Joint

The temporomandibular joint (TMJ) is the articulation of the mandible and the temporal bone (Fig. 23.3). You can feel

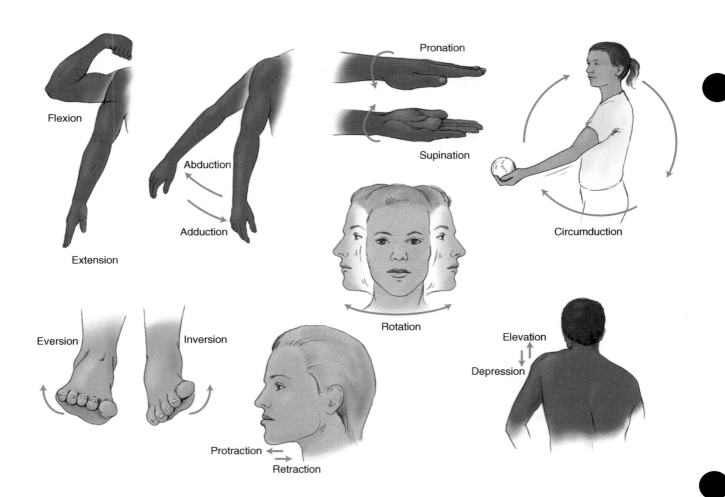

SKELETAL MUSCLE MOVEMENTS

23.2

© Pat Thomas, 2006.

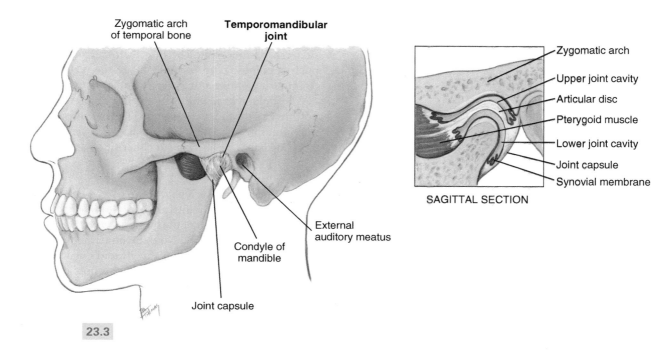

Zygomatic arch of temporal bone

Temporomandibular joint

External auditory meatus

Condyle of mandible

Joint capsule

Zygomatic arch

Upper joint cavity

Articular disc

Pterygoid muscle

Lower joint cavity

Joint capsule

Synovial membrane

SAGITTAL SECTION

23.3

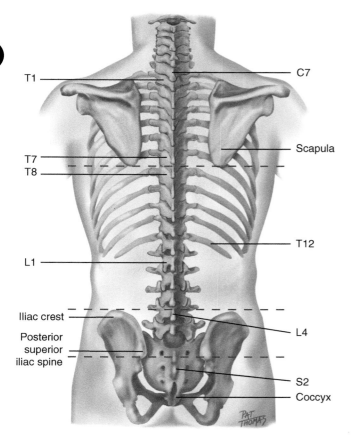

T1

T7

T8

L1

Iliac crest

Posterior superior iliac spine

C7

Scapula

T12

L4

S2

Coccyx

LANDMARKS OF THE SPINE

23.4

it in the depression anterior to the tragus of the ear. The TMJ permits jaw function for speaking and chewing. The joint allows three motions: (1) hinge action to open and close the jaws; (2) gliding action for protrusion and retraction; and (3) gliding for side-to-side movement of the lower jaw.

Spine

The **vertebrae** are 33 connecting bones stacked in a vertical column (Fig. 23.4). You can feel their spinous processes in a furrow down the midline of the back. The furrow has para-vertebral muscles mounded on either side down to the sacrum, where it flattens. Humans have 7 cervical, 12 thoracic, 5 lumbar, 5 sacral, and 3 or 4 coccygeal vertebrae. The following surface landmarks will orient you to their levels:

- The spinous processes of C7 and T1 are prominent at the base of the neck (see Fig. 23.4).
- The inferior angle of the scapula normally is at the level of the interspace between T7 and T8.
- An imaginary line connecting the highest point on each iliac crest crosses L4.
- An imaginary line joining the two symmetric dimples that overlie the posterior superior iliac spines crosses the sacrum.

A lateral view shows that the vertebral column has four curves (a double-**S**–shape) (Fig. 23.5). The cervical and lumbar curves are concave (inward or anterior), and the thoracic and sacrococcygeal curves are convex. The balanced or compensatory nature of these curves, together with the resilient intervertebral discs, allows the spine to absorb a great deal of shock.

The **intervertebral discs** are elastic fibrocartilaginous plates that constitute one-fourth of the length of the column

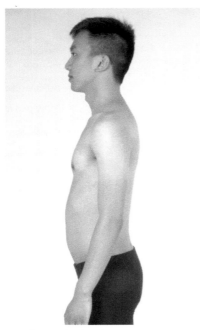

23.5 Curves of vertebral column.

(Fig. 23.6). Each disc center has a **nucleus pulposus** made of soft, semifluid, mucoid material that has the consistency of toothpaste in the young adult. The discs cushion the spine like a shock absorber and help it move. As the spine moves,

the elasticity of the discs allows compression on one side, with compensatory expansion on the other. Sometimes compression can be too great. The disc then can rupture; and the nucleus pulposus can herniate out of the vertebral column, compressing on the spinal nerves and causing pain.

The unique structure of the spine enables both upright posture and flexibility for motion. The motions of the vertebral column are flexion (bending forward), extension (bending back), abduction (to either side), and rotation.

Shoulder

The **shoulder girdle** is a belt of three large bones (humerus, scapula and clavicle), joints, and muscles. The **glenohumeral joint** is the articulation of the humerus with the glenoid fossa of the scapula (Fig. 23.7). Note the humeral head's articular surface is much greater than the glenoid's articular surface. This ball-and-socket action allows great mobility of the arm on many axes, more than any other joint. The joint is enclosed by a group of four powerful muscles and tendons that support and stabilize it. Together these are called the **rotator cuff.** The four muscles are the SITS muscles (supraspinatus, infraspinatus, teres minor, and subscapularis). These form a cover around the head of the humerus. They rotate the arm laterally and stabilize the head of the humerus against the shallow glenoid fossa of the scapula. The large **subacromial bursa** helps during abduction of the arm so that the greater tubercle of the humerus moves easily under the acromion process of the scapula.

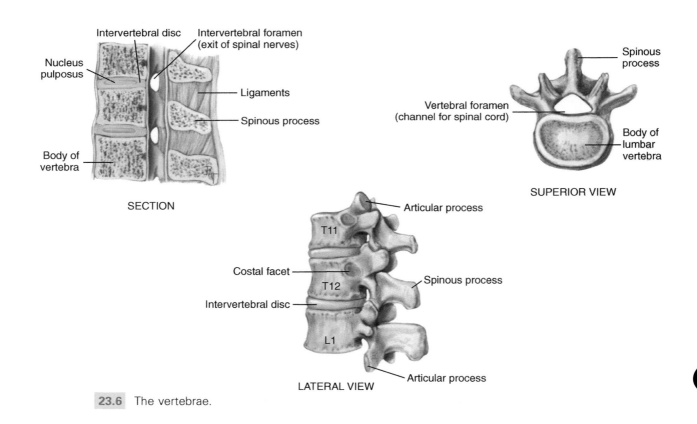

23.6 The vertebrae.

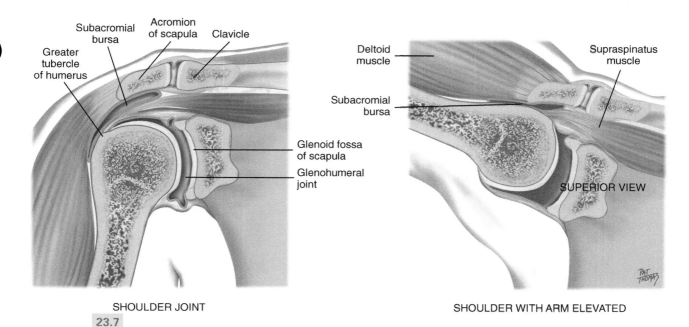

SHOULDER JOINT

23.7

SHOULDER WITH ARM ELEVATED

The bones of the shoulder have palpable landmarks to guide your examination (Fig. 23.8). You can feel the bump of the scapula's **acromion process** at the very top of the shoulder. Move your fingers in a small circle outward, down, and around. The next bump is the **greater tubercle** of the humerus a few centimeters down and laterally, and from that the **coracoid process** of the scapula is a few centimeters medially. The coracoid process projects anteriorly and laterally from the neck of the scapula. These surround the deeply situated joint.

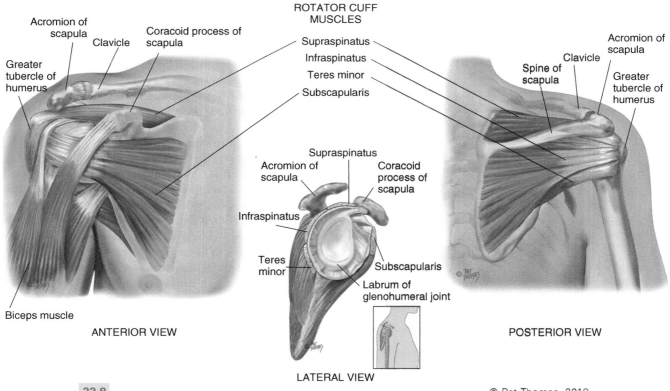

ANTERIOR VIEW

LATERAL VIEW

POSTERIOR VIEW

23.8

© Pat Thomas, 2018.

Wrist and Carpals

Of the body's 206 bones, over half are in the hands and feet. The wrist, or **radiocarpal joint,** is the articulation of the distal radius (on the thumb side) and a row of 8 carpal bones (Fig. 23.9). Its condyloid action permits movement in two planes at right angles: flexion and extension, and side-to-side deviation. You can feel the groove of this joint on the dorsum of the wrist.

The **midcarpal** joint is the articulation between the two parallel rows of carpal bones. It allows flexion, extension, and some rotation. The **metacarpophalangeal** (MCP) and the **interphalangeal** joints (DIP and PIP) permit finger flexion and extension. The flexor tendons of the wrist and hand are enclosed in synovial sheaths.

Elbow

The elbow joint contains the three bony articulations of the humerus, radius, and ulna of the forearm (Fig. 23.10). Its hinge action moves the forearm (radius and ulna) on one plane, allowing flexion and extension. The muscles are the biceps and brachioradialis for flexion, and the triceps and brachialis for extension. The olecranon bursa lies between the olecranon process and the skin.

Palpable landmarks are the **medial** and **lateral epicondyles** of the humerus and the large **olecranon process** of the ulna between them. The sensitive ulnar nerve runs between the olecranon process and the medial epicondyle.

The radius and ulna articulate with one another at two radioulnar joints, one at the elbow and one at the wrist. These move together to permit pronation and supination of the hand and forearm.

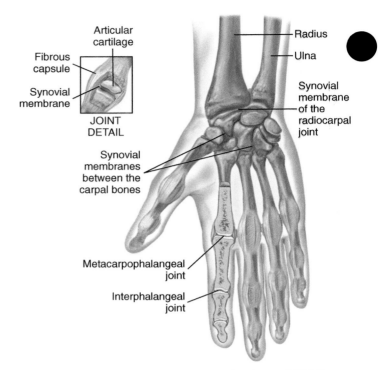

BONES OF THE HAND – PALMAR VIEW

23.9

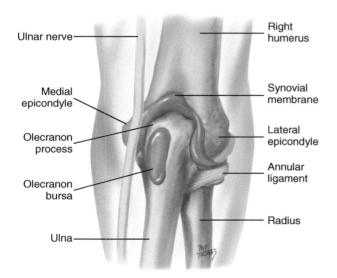

RIGHT ELBOW – POSTERIOR VIEW

23.10

Hip

The hip joint is the articulation between the cup-shaped acetabulum and the head of the femur (Fig. 23.11). As in the shoulder, ball-and-socket action permits a wide range of motion (ROM) on many axes. The hip has somewhat less ROM than the shoulder, but it has more stability as befits its weight-bearing function. Hip stability is the result of powerful muscles that spread over the joint, a strong fibrous articular capsule, and the very deep insertion of the head of the femur. The muscles include the anterior flexor (iliopsoas), the posterior extensor (gluteus maximus), adductor muscles that swing the thigh toward the midline, and abductor muscles that swing it away. Three bursae facilitate movement.

Palpation of these bony landmarks will guide your examination. You can feel the entire iliac crest, from the **anterior superior iliac spine** to the posterior. The **ischial tuberosity** lies under the gluteus maximus muscle and is palpable when the hip is flexed. The **greater trochanter** of the femur is normally the width of the person's palm below the iliac crest and halfway between the anterior superior iliac spine and the ischial tuberosity. Feel it when the person is standing, in a flat depression on the upper lateral side of the thigh.

Knee

The knee joint is the articulation of three bones—the femur, the tibia, and the patella (kneecap)—in one common articular cavity (Fig. 23.12). It is the largest joint in the body and

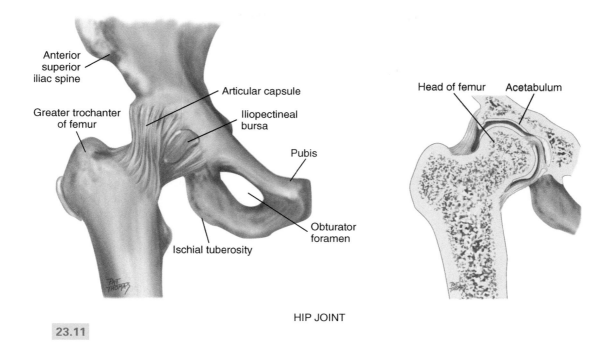

HIP JOINT

23.11

is complex. It is a hinge joint, permitting flexion and extension of the lower leg on a single plane. There is no overlying fat or muscle; only the ligaments hold the tibia and femur in place, making the knee vulnerable to injury.

The knee's synovial membrane is the largest in the body. It forms a sac at the superior border of the patella, called the **suprapatellar pouch** (or bursa), which extends up as much as 6 cm behind the quadriceps muscle. Two wedge-shaped cartilages, called the **medial** and **lateral menisci,** cushion the

tibia and femur. The joint is stabilized by two sets of ligaments. The **cruciate ligaments** (not shown) crisscross within the knee; they give anterior and posterior stability and help control rotation. The **collateral ligaments** connect the joint at both sides; they give medial and lateral stability and prevent dislocation. Numerous bursae prevent friction. One, the **prepatellar bursa,** lies between the patella and the skin. The **infrapatellar fat pad** is a small, triangular fat pad below the patella behind the patellar ligament.

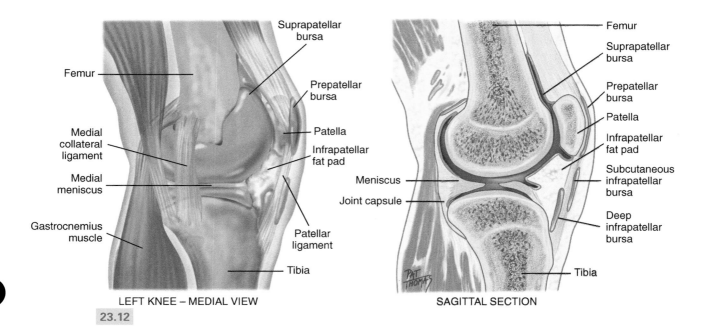

LEFT KNEE – MEDIAL VIEW

SAGITTAL SECTION

23.12

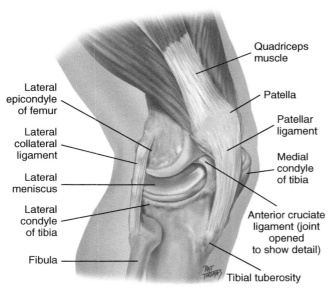

LANDMARKS OF THE RIGHT KNEE JOINT

23.13

Landmarks of the knee joint start with the large **quadriceps** muscle, which you can feel on your anterior and lateral thigh (Fig. 23.13). The quadriceps extends the knee, and its four heads merge into a common tendon that continues down to enclose the round bony patella. Then the tendon inserts down on the **tibial tuberosity,** which you can feel as a bony prominence in the midline. Move to the sides and a bit superiorly and note the lateral and medial condyles of the tibia. Superior to these on either side of the patella are the medial and lateral epicondyles of the femur. Posteriorly, the hamstring muscles flex the knee.

Ankle and Foot

The ankle, or **tibiotalar joint,** is the articulation of the tibia, fibula, and talus (Fig. 23.14). It is a hinge joint, limited to flexion (dorsiflexion) and extension (plantar flexion) on one plane. Landmarks are two bony prominences on either side: the **medial malleolus** and the **lateral malleolus.** Strong, tight medial and lateral ligaments extend from each malleolus onto the foot. These help the lateral stability of the ankle joint, although they may be torn in eversion or inversion sprains of the ankle. The **calcaneus** (heel) is under the talus and points posteriorly.

Joints distal to the ankle give additional mobility to the foot. The subtalar joint permits inversion and eversion of the foot. The foot has a longitudinal arch, with weight-bearing distributed between the parts that touch the ground—the heads of the metatarsals and the calcaneus (heel). Muscles include the gastrocnemius and toe flexors for plantar flexion and the anterior tibialis and toe extensors for dorsiflexion.

❖ DEVELOPMENTAL COMPETENCE

Infants and Children

By 3 months' gestation, the fetus has formed a "scale model" of the skeleton that is made up of cartilage. During succeeding months in utero, the cartilage ossifies into true bone and starts to grow. Bone growth continues after birth—rapidly during infancy and then steadily during childhood—until adolescence, when both boys and girls undergo a rapid growth spurt.

Long bones grow in two dimensions. They increase in width or diameter by deposition of new bony tissue around the shafts. Lengthening occurs at the **epiphyses,** or growth plates. These specialized growth centers are transverse discs located at the ends of long bone. Any trauma or infection at this location puts the growing child at risk for bone deformity. This longitudinal growth continues until closure of the epiphyses; the last closure occurs at about age 20 years.

Skeletal contour changes are apparent at the vertebral column. At birth the spine has a single C-shaped curve. At 3 to 4 months, raising the baby's head from prone position develops the anterior curve in the cervical neck region. From 1 year to 18 months, standing erect develops the anterior curve in the lumbar region.

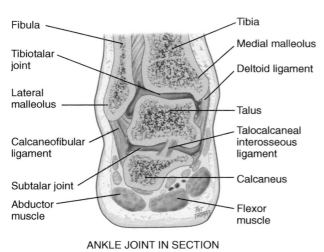

ANKLE JOINT IN SECTION

23.14

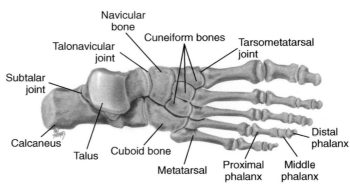

DORSAL VIEW (TOP OF FOOT)

Although the skeleton contributes to linear growth, muscles and fat are significant for weight increase. Individual muscle fibers grow throughout childhood, but growth is marked during the adolescent growth spurt. Then muscles respond to increased secretion of growth hormone to adrenal androgens and in boys to further stimulation by testosterone. Muscles vary in size and strength in different people. This is because of genetic programming, nutrition, and exercise. All through life muscles increase with use and atrophy with disuse.

The Pregnant Woman

Increased levels of circulating hormones (estrogen, relaxin from the corpus luteum, and corticosteroids) cause increased mobility in the joints. Increased mobility in the sacroiliac, sacrococcygeal, and symphysis pubis joints in the pelvis contributes to the noticeable changes in maternal posture. The most characteristic change is progressive **lordosis,** which compensates for the enlarging fetus; otherwise the center of balance would shift forward. Lordosis compensates by shifting the weight farther back on the lower extremities. This shift in balance in turn creates strain on the low back muscles, which in some women is felt as low back pain during late pregnancy.

Anterior flexion of the neck and slumping of the shoulder girdle are other postural changes that compensate for the lordosis. These upper-back changes may put pressure on the ulnar and median nerves during the third trimester. Nerve pressure creates aching, numbness, and weakness in the upper extremities in some women.

The Aging Adult

Peak bone mass or bone mineral density (BMD) is reached in the early to late 20s for Caucasians, with females reaching their peaks significantly earlier than males.[18] After that bone **remodeling** occurs, which is the cyclic process of bone resorption and deposition responsible for skeletal maintenance at sites that need repair or replacement. The standard pattern is for bone resorption to equal bone replacement. When bone resorption (loss of bone matrix) occurs more rapidly, the net effect is a gradual loss of bone density or **osteoporosis.** Osteoporosis is a disease involving the loss of mineralized bone mass and leading to porous bone and thus the risk of fractures. Although aging women have a greater amount of bone loss compared with aging men, decreased levels of estrogen in both sexes are partly responsible because osteoblasts that form new bone have estrogen receptors. Resistance and weight-bearing exercise may increase bone density at the hip and lumbar spine, but exercise needs to be regular and high intensity.[2] Further, its effects may be lost once exercise is stopped. (See Health Teaching on p. 608 for more lifestyle changes to retard osteoporosis.)

Postural changes are evident with aging. Long bones do not shorten with age. Decreased height of 3 to 5 cm occurs with shortening of the vertebral column, caused by loss of water content and thinning of the intervertebral discs and by

a decrease in the height of individual vertebrae from osteoporosis. A progressive decrease in height is not significant until 60 years. A greater decrease occurs in the 70s and 80s as a result of osteoporotic collapse of the vertebrae. Other postural changes are an increase in the thoracic curve (kyphosis), a backward head tilt to compensate for the kyphosis, and a slight flexion of hips and knees.

The distribution of subcutaneous fat changes through life. Usually men and women gain weight in their 40s and 50s. They begin to lose fat in the face and deposit it in the abdomen and hips. In the 80s and 90s, fat further decreases in the periphery, especially noticeable in the forearms, and increases over the abdomen and hips.

Loss of subcutaneous fat leaves bony prominences more marked (e.g., tips of vertebrae, ribs, iliac crests) and body hollows deeper (e.g., cheeks, axillae). An absolute loss in muscle mass occurs; some muscles decrease in size, and some atrophy, producing weakness.

Lifestyle affects musculoskeletal changes; a sedentary lifestyle hastens musculoskeletal changes of aging. However, physical exercise increases skeletal mass and helps prevent or delay osteoporosis. Physical activity delays or prevents bone loss in postmenopausal women in a dose-dependent manner[23] (see Patient Teaching on p. 608).

CULTURE AND GENETICS

Substantial racial/ethnic differences exist in bone mineral density (BMD) among women in the United States and globally. A higher BMD value means a denser bone; a low BMD value is a strong and consistent predictor of hip and vertebral fracture among postmenopausal women. Evidence comparing BMD in older women in four countries showed, in comparison with U.S. Caucasian women, that the BMD hip site measurements were 21% to 31% higher in Afro-Caribbean women and 13% to 23% higher in African-American women, similar in Hong Kong Chinese women, and higher in South Korean women.[24] The higher BMD values confer a lower fracture risk among women of African heritage. Why such high hip BMD values for Afro-Caribbean women? Perhaps it was that they reported all their parents and grandparents to be of African ancestry with little European mixture, higher weight-bearing activity, and more sun exposure in Caribbean countries.[24]

Women have been studied regarding age at attaining peak BMD. In the spine, women of all races gained BMD up to 30 to 33 years of age.[1] But at the femoral neck in the hip joint, BMD peaked earlier among white women (≤16 years) than among African Americans (21 years) and Hispanics (20 years). An earlier peak BMD and a more rapid decline following is a trend that may explain the increased fracture risk for white women later in life. These data plus physical activity data discussed earlier suggest that weight-bearing physical activity (e.g., fast walking) is imperative during the reproductive and middle adult years to slow the process of decline in BMD.

SUBJECTIVE DATA

1. Joints
   Pain
   Stiffness
   Swelling, heat, redness
   Limitation of movement
2. Knee joint (if injured)

3. Muscles
   Pain (cramps)
   Weakness
4. Bones
   Pain
   Deformity
   Trauma (fractures, sprains, dislocations)

5. Functional assessment (ADLs)
6. Patient-centered care

Examiner Asks	Rationale
1. Joints • Any problems with your joints? Any **pain?** • Location: Which joints? On one side or both sides? • Quality: What does the pain feel like: aching, stiff, sharp or dull, shooting? Severity: How strong is it? • Onset: When did it start? • Timing: What time of day does the pain occur? How long does it last? How often does it occur? • Is the pain aggravated by movement, rest, position, weather? Is it relieved by rest, medications, application of heat or ice? • Is the pain associated with chills, fever, recent sore throat, trauma, repetitive activity? • Any **stiffness** in your joints? • Any **swelling, heat, redness** in the joints? • Any tick bite? • Any **limitation of movement** in any joint? Which joint? • Which activities give you problems? (See Functional Assessment on p. 579 and on p. 607.)	**Joint pain** and loss of function are the most common musculoskeletal concerns that prompt a person to seek care. Rheumatoid arthritis (RA) involves symmetric joints; other musculoskeletal illnesses involve isolated or unilateral joints. Exquisitely tender with acute inflammation. RA pain is worse in the morning when arising; osteoarthritis is worse later in the day; tendinitis is worse in the morning, improves during the day. Movement increases most joint pain except in RA, in which movement decreases pain. Joint pain 10 to 14 days after an untreated strep throat suggests rheumatic fever. Joint injury occurs from trauma or repetitive motion. RA stiffness occurs in the morning and after rest periods. Suggests acute inflammation. Assess risk of Lyme disease. Decreased ROM may be caused by joint injury to cartilage or capsule or to muscle contracture.
2. Knee joint (if injury reported) • How did you injure your knee? Hit inside of knee? Outside? Twisting or pivoting? Overuse such as jumping or kneeling? • Hear a "pop" at injury? Can you stand on that leg? Can you flex the knee? Point to where it hurts the most.	Inside knee injury can strain or rupture medial ligament; outside injury can strain or rupture lateral ligament; abrupt twisting can injure anterior cruciate ligament.[28] Pop may mean tear in ligament or fracture. With direct knee trauma, obtain x-ray if the patient is unable to flex knee to 90 degrees or unable to bear weight for 4 steps, if pain is experienced at fibula head or patella, or if patient is over age 55 years (Ottawa knee rules).[28]

Examiner Asks	Rationale

3. Muscles

- Any problems in the muscles such as any **pain** or **cramping?** Which muscles?
- If in calf muscles: Is the pain with walking? Does it go away with rest?

- Are your muscle aches associated with fever, chills, the "flu"?
- Any **weakness** in muscles?
- Location: Where is the weakness? How long have you noticed it?
- Do the muscles look smaller there?

Myalgia is usually felt as cramping or aching.

Suggests intermittent claudication (see Chapter 21).

Viral illness often includes myalgia.

Weakness may involve musculoskeletal or neurologic systems (see Chapter 24).

Atrophy.

4. Bones

- Any **bone pain?** Is the pain affected by movement?
- Any **deformity** of any bone or joint? Is the deformity caused by injury or trauma? Does it affect ROM?
- Any **accidents** or **trauma** ever affect the bones or joints: fractures; joint strain, sprain, dislocation? Which ones?
- When did this occur? What treatment was given? Any problems or limitations now as a result?
- Any back pain? In which part of your back? Is pain felt anywhere else, such as shooting down leg?

- Any numbness and tingling? Any limping?
- Have you been feeling worried or anxious?

Fracture causes sharp pain that increases with movement. Other bone pain usually feels "dull" and "deep" and is unrelated to movement.

Low back pain occurs with degenerative discs, osteoporosis, lumbar stenosis, or is nonspecific.[21]

Chronic pain can increase anxiety symptoms.[13]

5. Functional assessment (ADLs).

Do your joint (muscle, bone) problems create any limits on your usual ADLs? Which ones? (NOTE: Ask about each category; if the person answers "yes," ask specifically about each activity in category.)
- Bathing—Getting in and out of the tub, turning faucets?
- Toileting—Urinating, moving bowels, able to get self on/off toilet, wipe self?
- Dressing—Buttoning or zipping clothes, fastening opening behind neck, pulling dress or sweater over head, pulling up pants, tying shoes, getting shoes that fit?
- Grooming—Shaving, brushing teeth, brushing or fixing hair, applying makeup?
- Eating—Preparing meals, pouring liquids, cutting up foods, bringing food to mouth, drinking?
- Mobility—Walking, walking up or down stairs, getting in/out of bed, getting out of house?
- Communicating—Talking, using phone, writing?

Functional assessment screens the safety of independent living, the need for home health services, and quality of life (see Chapter 32).

Assess any self-care deficit.

Impaired physical mobility.

Impaired verbal communication.

6. Patient-centered care.

Any occupational hazards that could affect the muscles and joints? Does your work involve heavy lifting? Or any repetitive motion or chronic stress to joints? Any efforts to alleviate these?
- Tell me about your exercise program. Describe the type of exercise, frequency, the warm-up program.

- Any pain during exercise? How do you treat it?
- Have you had any recent weight gain? Please describe your usual daily diet. (Note the person's usual caloric intake, all four food groups, daily amount of protein, calcium.)

Assess risk for back pain or carpal tunnel syndrome.

A strict program of regular high-dose exercises increases bone strength and reduces fracture risk.[23]

Examiner Asks	Rationale
• Are you taking any medications for musculoskeletal system: bisphosphonates, aspirin, antiinflammatory, muscle relaxant, pain reliever? Hormone therapy?	Review daily aspirin and NSAID schedule; screen for adverse effects such as GI pain, bleeding. Bisphosphonates are first-line therapy for osteoporosis for specific guidelines; hormone therapy is not recommended due to risk factors.[16]
• How about supplemental medications, calcium, or vitamin D? How many dairy products eaten per day? How many over-the-counter (OTC) medications taken daily?	Dietary calcium is better absorbed than supplements. Serum levels of vitamin D can be checked, and supplements recommended.
• If person has chronic disability or crippling illness: How has your illness affected: Your interaction with family? Your interaction with friends? The way you view yourself?	Assess for: • Self-esteem disturbance. • Loss of independence. • Body image disturbance. • Role performance disturbance. • Social isolation.
• How about cigarettes—How much do you smoke per day? And alcohol use—How many drinks per day? Per week?	Smoking increases bone loss and risk of fracture in older women; moderate-to-heavy alcohol drinking increases falls risk.

Additional History for Infants and Children

1. Were you told about any trauma to infant during labor and delivery? Did the baby's head come first? Was there a need for forceps? Did the baby need resuscitation?

   Traumatic delivery increases risk for fractures, (e.g., humerus, clavicle).
   Period of anoxia may result in hypotonia of muscles.

2. Were the baby's motor milestones achieved at about the same time as siblings or age-mates?

3. Has your child ever broken any bones? Any dislocations? How were these treated?

4. Have you ever noticed any bone deformity? Spinal curvature? Unusual shape of toes or feet? At what age? Have you ever sought treatment for any of these?

Additional History for Adolescents

1. Involved in any sports at school or after school? How frequently (times per week)? How does your sport fit in with other school demands and other activities?

   Assess safety of sport for child. Note if child's height and weight are adequate for the particular sport (e.g., football).

2. Do you use any special equipment? Does any training program exist for your sport?

   Use of safety equipment and presence of adult supervision decrease risk for sports injuries.

3. What do you do if you get hurt?

   Students may not report injury or pain for fear of limiting participation in sport.

Additional History for the Aging Adult

Use functional assessment history questions to elicit any loss of function, self-care deficit, or safety risk that may occur as a process of aging or musculoskeletal illness. (Review the complete functional assessment in Chapter 32.)

1. Any change in weakness over the past months or years? Any increase in falls or stumbling over the past months or years?

   Encourage exercise to the best of person's ability and safety.
   A history of falls increases risk of future falling.

Examiner Asks	Rationale
2. Do you use any mobility aids to help you get around: cane, walker?	
3. The U.S. government recommends screening women ages 65 years or older for osteoporosis with a low-dose x-ray called DXA. Have you had that image? Know the results? Do you have access to that test?	Screening interval of 2 years is suggested to measure any change in BMD.[33] Recent evidence shows if baseline BMD is normal or osteopenia is mild, rescreening intervals of 15 years may suffice, and intervals of 5 years for women with moderate osteopenia.[8]

OBJECTIVE DATA

PREPARATION

The purposes of the musculoskeletal examination are to assess function for ADLs and to screen for any abnormalities. You already will have considerable data regarding ADLs through the history. Note additional ADL data as the person goes through the motions necessary for an examination: gait; posture; how the person sits in a chair, rises from chair, takes off jacket, manipulates small object such as a pen, raises from supine.

A **screening** musculoskeletal examination suffices for most people:
- Inspection and palpation of joints integrated with each body region
- Observation of ROM as person proceeds through motions described earlier
- Age-specific screening measures such as Ortolani sign for infants or scoliosis screening for adolescents

A **complete** musculoskeletal examination as described in this chapter is appropriate for people with articular disease, a history of musculoskeletal symptoms, or any problems with ADLs.

Make the person comfortable before and throughout the examination. Drape for full visualization of the body part you are examining without needlessly exposing the person. Take an orderly approach—head to toe, proximal to distal (from the midline outward).

Support each joint at rest. Muscles must be soft and relaxed to assess the joints under them accurately. Take care when examining any inflamed area where rough manipulation could cause pain and muscle spasm. To avoid this, use firm support, gentle movement, and gentle return to a relaxed state.

Compare corresponding paired joints. Expect symmetry of structure and function and normal parameters for that joint.

EQUIPMENT NEEDED
Tape measure
Skin marking pen
Goniometer (occasional)

Normal Range of Findings	Abnormal Findings
Order of the Examination	
Inspection	
Note the **size** and **contour** of every joint. Inspect the skin and tissues over the joints for **color, swelling,** and any **masses** or **deformity.** Presence of swelling is significant and signals joint irritation. Use the contralateral side for comparison.	Swelling may be excess joint fluid (effusion), thickening of the synovial lining, inflammation of surrounding soft tissue (bursae, tendons), or bony enlargement.

Normal Range of Findings	Abnormal Findings

Deformities include **fracture** (a break in a bone), **dislocation** (complete loss of contact between the two bones in a joint), **subluxation** (two bones in a joint stay in contact, but their alignment is off), **contracture** (shortening of a muscle leading to limited ROM of joint), or **ankylosis** (stiffness or fixation of a joint).

Palpation

Palpate each joint, including its skin for temperature, its muscles, bony articulations, and area of joint capsule. Notice any heat, tenderness, swelling, or masses. Joints normally are not tender to palpation. If any tenderness does occur, try to localize it to specific anatomic structures (e.g., skin, muscles, bursae, ligaments, tendons, fat pads, or joint capsule).

Warmth and tenderness signal inflammation.

The synovial membrane normally is not palpable. When thickened, it feels "doughy" or "boggy." A small amount of fluid is present in the normal joint, but it is not palpable.

Palpable fluid is abnormal. Because fluid is contained in an enclosed sac, if you push on one side of the sac, the fluid will shift and cause a visible bulging on another side.

Range of Motion

Ask for **active (voluntary) ROM** while modeling the movements yourself as appropriate; thus you can use your own movements as a control. You may stabilize the body area proximal to that being moved. Familiarize yourself with the type of each joint and its normal ROM so you can recognize limitations. If you see a limitation, gently attempt **passive motion** with the person's muscles relaxed while you move the body part. Anchor the joint with one hand while your other hand slowly moves it to its limit. The normal ranges of active and passive motion should be the same.

Limitation in ROM is the most sensitive sign of joint disease.[19] The amount of limitation may alert you to the cause of disease. **Articular** disease (inside the joint capsule [e.g., arthritis]) produces swelling and tenderness around the whole joint, and it limits all planes of ROM in both active and passive motion. **Extra-articular** disease (injury to a specific tendon, ligament, nerve) produces swelling and tenderness to that one spot in the joint and affects only certain planes of ROM, especially during active (voluntary) motion.

Joint motion normally causes no tenderness, pain, or crepitation. Do not confuse crepitation with the normal discrete "crack" heard as a tendon or ligament slips over bone during motion, such as when you do a knee bend.

Crepitation is an audible and palpable crunching or grating that accompanies movement. It occurs when the articular surfaces in the joints are roughened, as with RA (see Table 23.1, Abnormalities Affecting Multiple Joints, p. 611).

Muscle Testing

Test the strength of the prime-mover muscle groups for each joint. Repeat the motions that you elicited for active ROM. Now ask the person to flex and hold as you apply opposing force. Muscle strength should be equal bilaterally and fully resist your opposing force. (NOTE: Muscle status and joint status are interdependent and should be interpreted together. Chapter 24 discusses the examination of muscles for size and development, tone, and presence of tenderness.)

A wide variability of strength exists among people. Use a grading system from no voluntary movement to full strength, as shown.

Normal Range of Findings				Abnormal Findings

Grade	Description	% Normal	Assessment
5	Full ROM against gravity, full resistance	100	Normal
4	Full ROM against gravity, some resistance	75	Good
3	Full ROM with gravity	50	Fair
2	Full ROM with gravity eliminated (passive motion)	25	Poor
1	Slight contraction	10	Trace
0	No contraction	0	Zero

Temporomandibular Joint

With the person seated, **inspect** the area just anterior to the ear. Place the tips of your first two fingers in front of each ear and ask the person to open and close the mouth. Drop your fingers into the depressed area over the joint and note smooth motion of the mandible. An audible and palpable snap or click occurs in many healthy people as the mouth opens (Fig. 23.15). Then ask the person to:

Instructions to Person

- Open mouth maximally.

- Partially open mouth, protrude lower jaw, and move it side to side.
- Stick out lower jaw.

Motion and Expected Range

Vertical motion. You can measure the space between the upper and lower incisors. Normal is 3 to 6 cm or three fingers inserted sideways.
Lateral motion. Normal extent is 1 to 2 cm (Fig. 23.16).

Protrude without deviation.

Swelling looks like a round bulge over the joint, although it must be moderate or marked to be visible.
Crepitus and pain occur with TMJ dysfunction during movement or chewing. Malocclusion of teeth also causes palpable crepitus or audible dick.

Decreased ROM occurs with TMJ inflammation and arthritis.

Lateral motion may be lost earlier and more significantly than vertical motion.

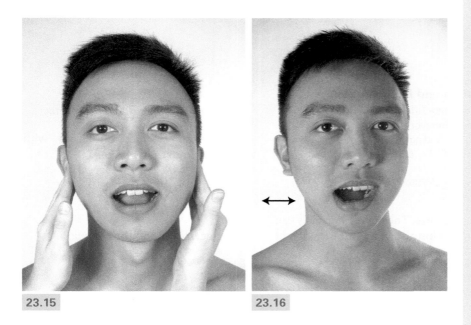

23.15   23.16

Palpate the contracted temporalis and masseter muscles as the person clenches the teeth. Compare right and left sides for size, firmness, and strength. Ask the person to move the jaw forward and laterally against your resistance and open mouth against resistance. This also tests the integrity of cranial nerve V (trigeminal).

TMJ dysfunction causes tenderness with palpation.

Objective Data

Normal Range of Findings	**Abnormal Findings**

Cervical Spine

Inspect the alignment of head and neck. The spine should be straight, and the head erect. **Palpate** the spinous processes and the sternomastoid, trapezius, and paravertebral muscles. They should feel firm, with no muscle spasm or tenderness.

Head tilted to one side.
Asymmetry of muscles.
Tenderness and hard muscles with muscle spasm. Tenderness with arthritis or postural disorders with desk or office work.[3]

Ask the person to follow these motions (Fig. 23.17)[a]:

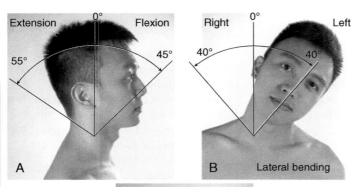

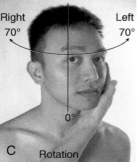

23.17

Instructions to Person	**Motion and Expected Range**
• Touch chin to chest.	Flexion of 45 degrees (Fig. 23.17, *A*).
• Lift the chin toward the ceiling.	Hyperextension of 55 degrees.
• Touch each ear toward the corresponding shoulder. Do not lift the shoulder.	Lateral bending of 40 degrees (Fig. 23.17, *B*).
• Turn the chin toward each shoulder.	Rotation of 70 degrees (Fig. 23.17, *C*).

Limited ROM occurs with arthritis.

Pain with movement occurs with arthritis or muscle overuse.

Repeat the motions while applying opposing force. The person normally can maintain flexion against your full resistance. This also tests the integrity of cranial nerve XI (spinal).

The person cannot hold flexion.

Upper Extremity

Shoulder

Inspect and compare both shoulders posteriorly and anteriorly. Check the size and contour of the joint and compare shoulders for equality of bony landmarks.

Redness. Inequality of bony landmarks occurs with scoliosis. Atrophy, shows as

---

[a]Do not attempt if you suspect neck trauma.

Normal Range of Findings

Normally no redness, muscular atrophy, deformity, or swelling is present. Check the anterior aspect of the joint capsule and the subacromial bursa for abnormal swelling.

If the person reports any shoulder pain, ask that he or she point to the spot with the hand of the unaffected side. Be aware that shoulder pain may be from local causes or it may be referred pain from a hiatal hernia or a cardiac or pleural condition, which could be potentially serious. Pain from a local cause is reproducible during the examination by palpation or motion.

While standing in front of the person, **palpate** both shoulders, noting any muscular spasm or atrophy, swelling, heat, or tenderness. Start at the clavicle and methodically explore the acromioclavicular joint, scapula, greater tubercle of the humerus, area of the subacromial bursa, the biceps groove, and anterior aspect of the glenohumeral joint. Palpate the pyramid-shaped axilla; no adenopathy or masses should be present.

Test ROM by asking the person to perform four motions (Fig. 23.18). Cup one hand over the shoulder during ROM to note any crepitation; normally none is present.

Abnormal Findings

lack of fullness, can signal rotator cuff problem or disuse.

Dislocated shoulder loses normal rounded shape and looks flattened laterally.

Swelling from excess fluid is best seen anteriorly. Considerable fluid must be present to cause a visible distention because the capsule normally is so loose (see Table 23.2, Shoulder Abnormalities, p. 613).

Swelling of subacromial bursa is localized under deltoid muscle and may be accentuated when the person tries to abduct the arm.

Swelling.
Hard muscles with muscle spasm.
Tenderness or pain.

Objective Data

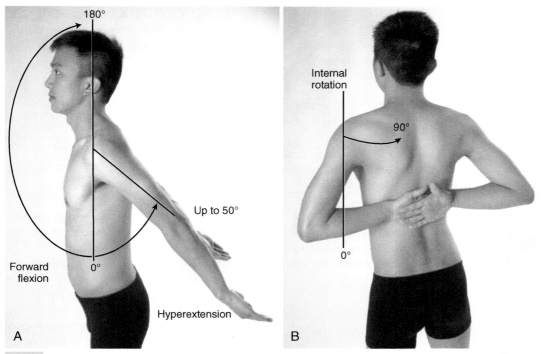

180°

Internal
rotation

90°

Up to 50°

Forward
flexion

0°

Hyperextension

0°

A

B

23.18

Continued

Normal Range of Findings	Abnormal Findings

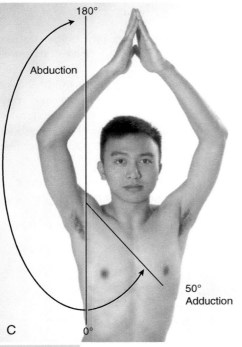

C

D

23.18, cont'd

Instructions to Person	**Motion and Expected Range**	Limited ROM.

Instructions to Person

- With arms at sides and elbows extended, move both arms forward and up in wide vertical arcs and then move them back.
- Rotate arms internally behind back; place back of hands as high as possible toward scapulae.
- With arms at sides and elbows extended, raise both arms in wide arcs in the coronal plane. Touch palms together above head.
- Touch both hands behind the head with elbows flexed and rotated posteriorly.

Motion and Expected Range

Forward flexion of 180 degrees. Hyperextension up to 50 degrees (Fig. 23.18, *A*).

Internal rotation of 90 degrees (Fig. 23.18, *B*).

Abduction of 180 degrees. Adduction of 50 degrees (Fig. 23.18, *C*).

External rotation of 90 degrees (Fig. 23.18, *D*).

Limited ROM.
Asymmetry.
Pain with motion.

Crepitus with motion.
Rotator cuff lesions may cause limited ROM, pain, and muscle spasm during abduction, whereas forward flexion stays fairly normal.

Test the strength of the shoulder muscles by asking the person to shrug the shoulders, flex forward and up, and abduct against your resistance. The shoulder shrug also tests the integrity of cranial nerve XI, the spinal accessory.

Elbow

Inspect the size and contour of the elbow in both flexed and extended positions. Look for any deformity, redness, or swelling. Check the olecranon bursa and the normally present hollows on either side of the olecranon process for abnormal swelling.

Subluxation of the elbow shows the forearm dislocated posteriorly.

Swelling and redness of olecranon bursa are localized and easy to observe because of the close proximity of the bursa to skin.

Effusion or synovial thickening shows first as a bulge or fullness in groove on either side of the olecranon process, and it occurs with gouty arthritis and bursitis.

Normal Range of Findings	Abnormal Findings

Palpate with the elbow flexed about 70 degrees and as relaxed as possible (Fig. 23.19). Use your left hand to support the person's left forearm and palpate the extensor surface of the elbow—the olecranon process and the medial and lateral epicondyles of the humerus—with your right thumb and fingers.

With your thumb in the lateral groove and your index and middle fingers in the medial groove, palpate either side of the olecranon process using varying pressure. Normally present tissues and fat pads feel fairly solid. Check for any synovial thickening, swelling, nodules, or tenderness.

Epicondyles, head of radius, and tendons are common sites of inflammation and local tenderness, or "tennis elbow."

Soft, boggy, or fluctuant swelling in both grooves occurs with synovial thickening or effusion.

Local heat or redness (signs of inflammation) can extend beyond synovial membrane.

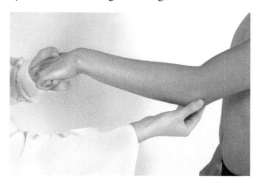

23.19

Palpate the area of the olecranon bursa for heat, swelling, tenderness, consistency, or nodules.

Subcutaneous nodules are raised, firm, and nontender, and overlying skin moves freely. Common sites are in the olecranon bursa and along the extensor surface of the ulna. These nodules occur with RA (see Table 23.3, Elbow Abnormalities, p. 614).

Test ROM by asking the person to:

Instructions to Person	Motion and Expected Range
• Bend and straighten the elbow (Fig. 23.20).	Flexion of 150 to 160 degrees; extension at 0. Some healthy people lack 5 to 10 degrees of full extension, and others have 5 to 10 degrees of hyperextension.
• Movement of 90 degrees in pronation and supination (Fig. 23.21).	Hold the hand midway; then touch front and back sides of hand to table.

After a fall or trauma, full extension of the elbow can usually rule out fracture.

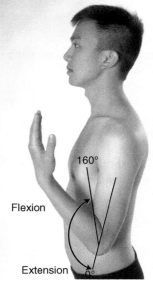

160°

Flexion

Extension

23.20

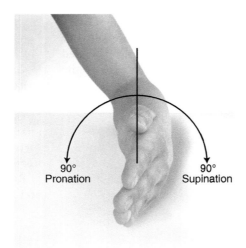

90°
Pronation

90°
Supination

23.21

Normal Range of Findings	Abnormal Findings

While testing **muscle strength,** stabilize the person's arm with one hand (Fig. 23.22). Have him or her flex the elbow against your resistance applied just proximal to the wrist. Then ask the person to extend the elbow against your resistance.

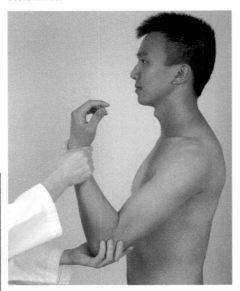

23.22

Wrist and Hand

Inspect the hands and wrists on the dorsal and palmar sides, noting position, contour, and shape. The normal functional position of the hand shows the wrist in slight extension. This way the fingers can flex efficiently, and the thumb can oppose them for grip and manipulation. The fingers lie straight in the same axis as the forearm. Normally no swelling or redness, deformity, or nodules are present.

The skin looks smooth with knuckle wrinkles present and no swelling or lesions. Muscles are full, with the palm showing a rounded mound proximal to the thumb (the **thenar eminence**) and a smaller rounded mound proximal to the little finger.

Palpate each joint in the wrist and hands. Facing the person, support the hand with your fingers under it and palpate the wrist firmly with both of your thumbs on its dorsum (Fig. 23.23). Make sure that the person's wrist is relaxed and in straight alignment. Move your palpating thumbs side to side to identify the normal depressed areas that overlie the joint space. Use gentle but firm pressure. Normally the joint surfaces feel smooth, with no swelling, bogginess, nodules, or tenderness.

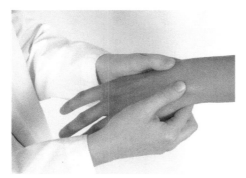

23.23

Subluxation (partial dislocation) of wrist.

Ulnar deviation; fingers list to ulnar side.

Ankylosis; wrist in extreme flexion.

Dupuytren contracture; flexion contracture of finger(s).

Swan-neck or boutonnière deformity in fingers.

Atrophy of the thenar eminence with carpal tunnel syndrome (see Table 23.4, Wrist and Hand Abnormalities, p. 615).

Ganglion cyst is a localized swelling in wrist (see Table 23.4).

Synovial swelling on dorsum.

Generalized swelling with arthritis and infection.

Tenderness after a fall—check for fracture.

Rheumatoid arthritis (RA) shows bilateral swelling and tenderness.

Normal Range of Findings	Abnormal Findings

Palpate the metacarpophalangeal joints with your thumbs, just distal to and on either side of the knuckle (Fig. 23.24).

RA shows boggy or tender MCPs; this does not occur in osteoarthritis (OA).

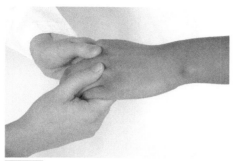

23.24

Use your thumb and index finger in a pinching motion to palpate the sides of the interphalangeal joints (Fig. 23.25). Normally no synovial thickening, tenderness, warmth, or nodules are present.

Heberden and Bouchard nodules are hard and nontender and occur with osteoarthritis (see Table 23.4).

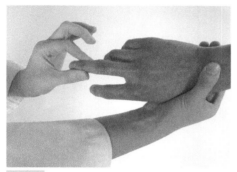

23.25

Test ROM (Fig. 23.26) by asking the person to:

Instructions to Person	Motion and Expected Range
• Bend hand up at wrist.	Hyperextension of 70 degrees (Fig. 23.26, *A*).
• Bend hand down at wrist.	Palmar flexion of 90 degrees.
• Bend fingers up and down at metacarpophalangeal joints.	Flexion of 90 degrees. Hyperextension of 30 degrees (Fig. 23.26, *B*).
• With palms flat on table, turn them outward and in.	Ulnar deviation of 50 to 60 degrees and radial deviation of 20 degrees (Fig. 23.26, *C*).
• Spread fingers apart; make a fist.	Abduction of 20 degrees; fist tight. The responses should be equal bilaterally (Fig. 23.26, *D, E*).
• Touch thumb to each finger and to base of little finger.	The person is able to perform, and the responses are equal bilaterally (Fig. 23.26, *F*).

Loss of ROM here is the most common and most significant functional loss of the wrist.
Limited motion.
Pain on movement.

Normal Range of Findings	Abnormal Findings

Objective Data

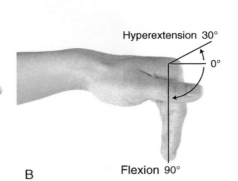

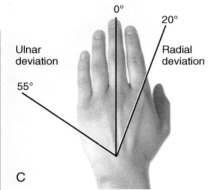

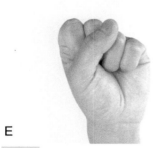

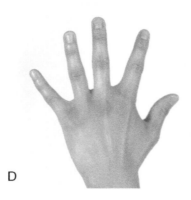

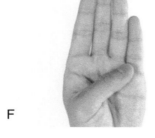

23.26

For **muscle testing,** position the person's forearm supinated (palm up) and resting on a table (Fig. 23.27). Stabilize by holding your hand at the person's midforearm. Ask the person to flex the wrist against your resistance at the palm.

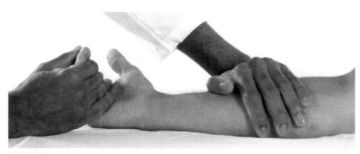

23.27

Normal Range of Findings	Abnormal Findings

Phalen Test

Ask the person to hold both hands back to back while flexing the wrists 90 degrees. Acute flexion of the wrist for 60 seconds produces no symptoms in the normal hand (Fig. 23.28).

Phalen test reproduces numbness and burning in a person with carpal tunnel syndrome (see Table 23.4).

Tinel Sign

Direct percussion of the location of the median nerve at the wrist produces no symptoms in the normal hand (Fig. 23.29).

In carpal tunnel syndrome percussion of the median nerve produces burning and tingling along its distribution, which is a positive Tinel sign.

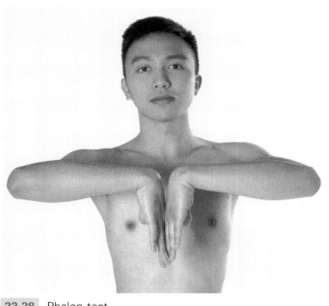

23.28 Phalen test.

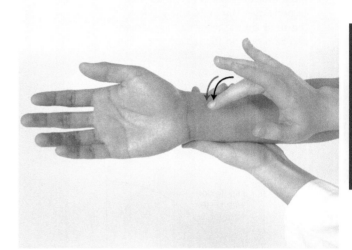

23.29 Tinel sign.

Lower Extremity

Hip

Wait to **inspect** the hip joint together with the spine a bit later in the examination as the person stands. At that time note symmetric levels of iliac crests, gluteal folds, and equally sized buttocks. A smooth, even gait reflects equal leg lengths and functional hip motion.

Help the person into a supine position and **palpate** the hip joints. The joints should feel stable and symmetric, with no tenderness or crepitus.

Pain with palpation.
Crepitation.

Assess **ROM** (Fig. 23.30) by asking the person to:

Instructions to Person	Motion and Expected Range
• Raise each leg with knee extended.	Hip flexion of 90 degrees (Fig. 23.30, *A*).
• Bend each knee up to the chest while keeping the other leg straight.	Hip flexion of 120 degrees. The opposite thigh should remain on the table (Fig. 23.30, *B*).

Limited motion.
Pain with motion.
Flexion flattens the lumbar spine; if this reveals a flexion deformity in the opposite hip, it is a positive *Thomas test.*

Normal Range of Findings

- Flex knee and hip to 90 degrees. Stabilize by holding the thigh with one hand and the ankle with the other hand. Swing the foot outward. Swing the foot inward. (Foot and thigh move in opposite directions.)
- Swing leg laterally, then medially, with knee straight. Stabilize pelvis by pushing down on the opposite anterior superior iliac spine.
- When standing (later in examination), swing straight leg back behind body. Stabilize pelvis to eliminate exaggerated lumbar lordosis. The most efficient way is to ask person to bend over the table and support the trunk on the table. Or the person can lie prone on the table.

Internal rotation of 40 degrees. External rotation of 45 degrees (Fig. 23.30, C).

Abduction of 40 to 45 degrees. Adduction of 20 to 30 degrees (Fig. 23.30, D).

Hyperextension of 15 degrees when stabilized.

Abnormal Findings

Limited internal rotation of hip is an early and reliable sign of hip disease.

Limitation of abduction of the hip while supine is the most common motion dysfunction found in hip disease.

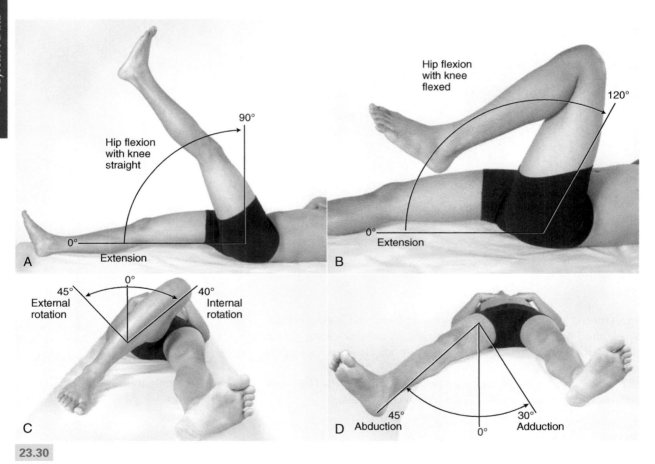

23.30

Knee

The person should remain supine with legs extended, although some examiners prefer the knees to be flexed and dangling for **inspection.** The skin normally looks smooth, with even coloring and no lesions.

Shiny and atrophic skin.
Swelling or inflammation (see Table 23.5, Knee Abnormalities, p. 618).
Lesions (e.g., psoriasis).

Normal Range of Findings	Abnormal Findings

Inspect lower leg alignment. The lower leg should extend in the same axis as the thigh.

Angulation deformity:
- Genu varum (bowlegs) (see p. 604)
- Genu valgum (knock-knees)
- Flexion contracture

Inspect the knee's shape and contour. Normally distinct concavities, or hollows, are present on either side of the patella, the "peripatellar grooves." Check them for any sign of fullness or swelling. Note other locations such as the prepatellar bursa and the suprapatellar pouch for any abnormal swelling.

Hollows disappear; then they may bulge with synovial thickening or effusion.

Check the quadriceps muscle in the anterior thigh for any atrophy. Because it is the prime mover of knee extension, this muscle is important for joint stability during weight bearing.

Atrophy occurs with disuse or chronic disorders. It first appears in the medial part of the muscle, although it is difficult to note because the vastus medialis is relatively small.

Enhance **palpation** with the knee in the supine position with complete relaxation of the quadriceps muscle. Start high on the anterior thigh, about 10 cm above the patella. Palpate with your left thumb and fingers in a grasping fashion (Fig. 23.31). Proceed down toward the knee, exploring the region of the suprapatellar pouch. Note the consistency of the tissues. The muscles and soft tissues should feel solid, and the joint should feel smooth, with no warmth, tenderness, thickening, or nodularity.

Feels fluctuant or boggy with synovitis of suprapatellar pouch.

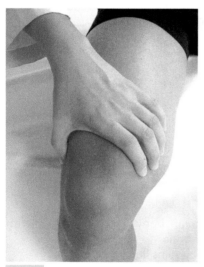

23.31

When swelling occurs, you need to distinguish whether it is caused by soft tissue swelling or increased fluid in the joint. Comparison with the unaffected knee is important. The tests for the **bulge sign** and **ballottement** of the patella aid this assessment.

Bulge Sign

For swelling in the suprapatellar pouch, the bulge sign confirms the presence of small amounts of fluid as you try to move the fluid from one side of the joint to the other. Firmly stroke up on the medial aspect of the knee 2 or 3 times to displace any fluid (Fig. 23.32, *A*). Tap the lateral aspect (Fig. 23.32, *B*). Watch the medial side in the hollow for a distinct bulge from a fluid wave. Normally none is present.

The bulge sign occurs with very small amounts of effusion, 4 to 8 mL, from fluid flowing across the joint (Fig. 23.32, *C*).

Normal Range of Findings	Abnormal Findings

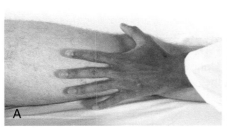 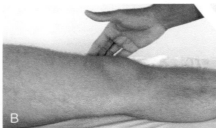 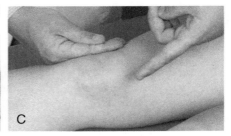

23.32 *A*, Stroke medial aspect.   *B*, Elicit bulge sign.   *C*, Note bulge sign.   (Dieppe, 1991.)

Ballottement of the Patella

This test is reliable when larger amounts of fluid are present. Use your left hand to compress the suprapatellar pouch to move any fluid into the knee joint. With your right hand push the patella sharply against the femur. If no fluid is present, the patella is already snug against the femur (Fig. 23.33, *A*).

If fluid has collected, your tap on the patella moves it through the fluid, and you will hear a tap as the patella bumps up on the femoral condyles (Fig. 23.33, *B*).

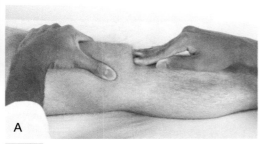

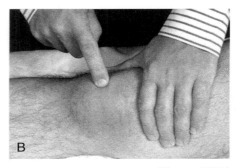

23.33 Ballottement.

(Dieppe, 1991.)

Continue palpation and explore the tibiofemoral joint (Fig. 23.34). Note smooth joint margins and absence of pain. Palpate the infrapatellar fat pad and the patella. Check for crepitus by holding your hand on the patella as the knee is flexed and extended. Some crepitus in an otherwise asymptomatic knee may occur.

Irregular bony margins occur with osteoarthritis.

Pain at joint line.

Pronounced crepitus is significant, and it occurs with degenerative diseases of the knee.

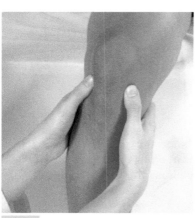

23.34

Normal Range of Findings	Abnormal Findings

Check ROM (Fig. 23.35) by asking the person to:

Instructions to Person	Motion and Expected Range
• Bend each knee. • Extend each knee.	Flexion of 130 to 150 degrees. A straight line of 0 degrees in some people; a hyperextension of 15 degrees in others.
• Check knee ROM during ambulation. • (optional) If able, squat and try a duck walk.	Duck walk shows intact ligaments and no effusion or arthritis.

Limited ROM.
Contracture.
Pain with motion.
Limp.
Sudden locking—The person is unable to extend the knee fully. This usually occurs with a painful and audible "pop" or "click." Sudden buckling, or "giving way," occurs with ligament injury, which causes weakness and instability.

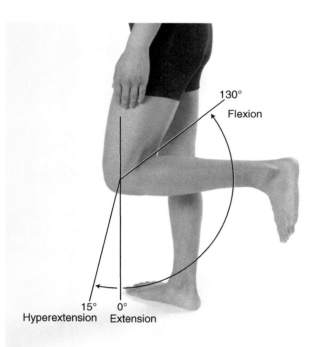

130°
Flexion

15°   0°
Hyperextension   Extension

23.35

Check **muscle strength** by asking the person to maintain knee flexion while you oppose by trying to pull the leg forward. Muscle extension is demonstrated by the person's success in rising from a seated position in a low chair or by rising from a squat without using the hands for support.

Special Test for Meniscal Tears

Mcmurray Test. Perform this test when the person has reported a history of trauma followed by locking, giving way, or local pain in the knee. Position the person supine as you stand on the affected side. Hold the heel and flex the knee and hip. Place your other hand on the knee with fingers on the medial side. Rotate the leg in and out to loosen the joint. Externally rotate the leg, and push a valgus (inward) stress on the knee. Slowly extend the knee. Normally the leg extends smoothly with no pain (Fig. 23.36).

If you hear or feel a "click," McMurray test is positive for a torn meniscus. This must be referred to orthopedics for imaging and possible surgical repair.

Objective Data

Objective Data

Normal Range of Findings

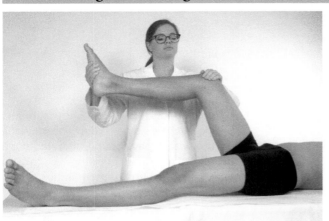

23.36   McMurray test.

Ankle and Foot

Inspect while the person is in a sitting, non–weight-bearing position and when standing and walking. Compare both feet, noting position of feet and toes, contour of joints, and skin characteristics. The foot should align with the long axis of the lower leg; an imaginary line would fall from midpatella to between the first and second toes.

Weight bearing should fall on the middle of the foot, from the heel, along the midfoot, to between the 2nd and 3rd toes. Most feet have a longitudinal arch, although that can vary normally from "flat feet" to a high instep.

The toes point straight forward and lie flat. The ankles (malleoli) are smooth bony prominences. Normally the skin is smooth, with even coloring and no lesions. Note the locations of any calluses or bursal reactions because they reveal areas of abnormal friction. Examining well-worn shoes helps assess areas of wear and accommodation.

Support the ankle by grasping the heel with your fingers while palpating with your thumbs (Fig. 23.38). Explore the joint spaces. They should feel smooth and depressed, with no fullness, swelling, or tenderness.

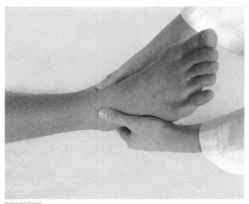

23.38

Palpate the metatarsophalangeal joints between your thumb on the dorsum and your fingers on the plantar surface (Fig. 23.39).

Using a pinching motion of your thumb and forefinger, palpate the interphalangeal joints on the medial and lateral sides of the toes.

Abnormal Findings

Use the Ottawa knee rules for any knee pain with injury for referral for imaging: (1) isolated pain of patella or head of fibula; (2) age ≥55 years; (3) cannot flex knee to 90 degrees; (4) cannot bear weight for 4 steps.[15]

In **hallux valgus** the distal part of the great toe is directed *away* from the body midline (Fig. 23.37).

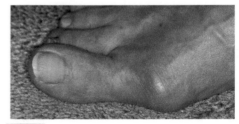

23.37   Hallux valgus with bunion.
(Lemmi & Lemmi, 2011.)

Hammertoes.
Calluses.
Ulcers.
Swelling or inflammation.
Tenderness, occurs with arthritis, trauma to ligaments.
Plantar fasciitis shows localized tenderness under heel where fascia is torn (see Table 23.6, Ankle and Foot Abnormalities, p. 620).

Swelling or inflammation, tenderness, occur with arthritis or trauma.

Normal Range of Findings	Abnormal Findings

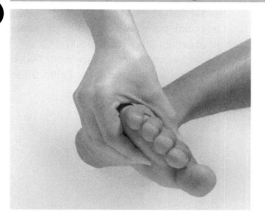

23.39

Test ROM (Fig. 23.40) by asking the person to:

Instructions to Person

- Point toes toward the floor.
- Point toes toward the nose.

- Turn soles of feet out, then in. (Stabilize ankle with one hand and hold heel with the other to test the subtalar joint.)
- Flex and straighten toes.

Motion and Expected Range

Plantar flexion of 45 degrees.
Dorsiflexion of 20 degrees (Fig. 23.40, *A*).
Eversion of 20 degrees.
Inversion of 30 degrees (Fig. 23.40, *B*).

Limited ROM.
Pain with motion.

Assess **muscle strength** by asking the person to maintain dorsiflexion and plantar flexion against your resistance.

Unable to hold flexion.

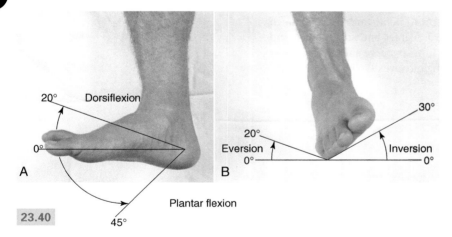

23.40

Spine

The person should be standing, draped in a gown open at the back. Place yourself far enough back so you can see the entire back. **Inspect** and note whether the spine is straight (1) by following an imaginary vertical line from the head through the spinous processes and down through the gluteal cleft; and (2) by noting equal horizontal positions for the shoulders, scapulae, iliac crests, and gluteal folds and equal spaces between the arm and lateral thorax on the two sides (Fig. 23.41, *A*). The person's knees and feet should be aligned with the trunk and pointing forward.

From the side note the normal convex thoracic curve and concave lumbar curve (Fig. 23.41, *B*). An enhanced thoracic curve, or kyphosis, is common in aging people. A pronounced lumbar curve, or lordosis, is common in obese people.

A difference in shoulder elevation and in level of scapulae and iliac crests occurs with scoliosis (see Table 23.7, Spine Abnormalities, p. 621).

Lateral tilting and forward bending occur with a herniated nucleus pulposus (see Table 23.7).

Objective Data

Normal Range of Findings

Palpate the spinous processes. Normally they are straight and not tender. Palpate the paravertebral muscles; they should feel firm with no tenderness or spasm.

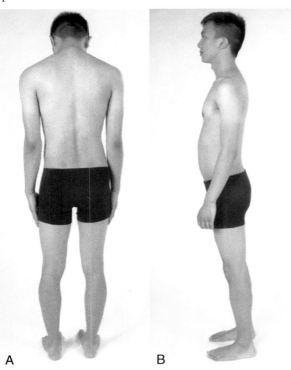

A　　　　　B

23.41

Check **ROM** of the spine by asking the person to bend forward and touch the toes (Fig. 23.42). Look for flexion of 75 to 90 degrees and smoothness and symmetry of movement. Note that the concave lumbar curve should disappear with this motion and the back should have a single convex C-shaped curve.

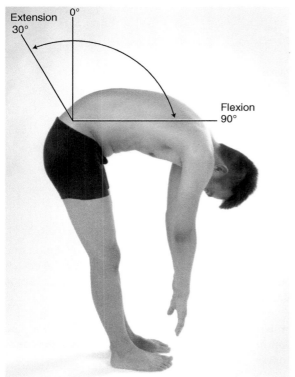

23.42

Abnormal Findings

Spinal curvature. Tenderness.

Low back pain and spasm of paravertebral muscles (see Table 23.1).

Chronic axial skeletal pain occurs with fibromyalgia syndrome (see Table 23.9, p. 623).

Normal Range of Findings	Abnormal Findings

If you suspect a spinal curvature during inspection, this may be seen more clearly when the person touches the toes. While the person is bending over, mark a dot on each spinous process. When the person resumes standing, the dots should form a straight vertical line.

If the dots form a slight S-shape when the person stands, a spinal curve is present.

Stabilize the pelvis with your hands. Check ROM (Fig. 23.43) by asking the person to:

Instructions to Person	Motion and Expected Range
• Bend sideways.	Lateral bending of 35 degrees (Fig. 23.43, *A*).
• Bend backward.	Hyperextension of 30 degrees.
• Twist shoulders to one side, then the other.	Rotation of 30 degrees, bilaterally (Fig. 23.43, *B*).

Limited ROM occurs with osteoarthritis and ankylosing spondylitis (Table 23.1).
Pain with motion.

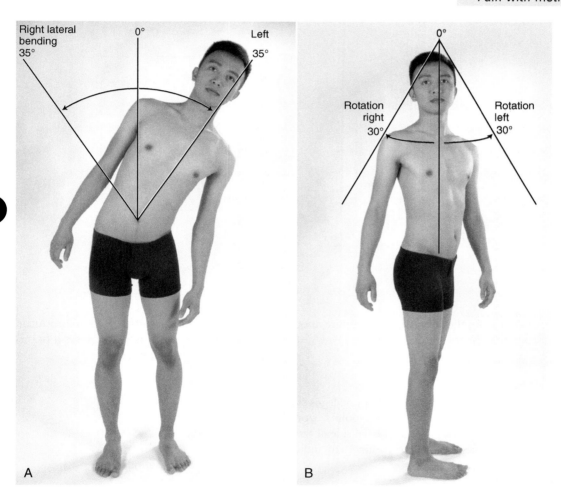

A

B

23.43

These maneuvers reveal only gross restriction. Movement is still possible even if some spinal fusion has occurred.

Finally ask the person to walk on his or her toes for a few steps and return walking on the heels.

Special Procedures for Advanced Practice

With a history of **recent ankle trauma** or a fall, palpate the length of the lateral and medial ankle ligaments in the position of Fig. 23.38. If no sprain, there will be no tenderness, swelling, or bruising. Follow the Ottawa rule for possible ankle or midfoot fracture listed at right.[19]

An x-ray image is needed only if there is pain near the malleoli/midfoot and inability to bear weight (4 steps) or bone tenderness.

Normal Range of Findings	Abnormal Findings

Straight Leg Raising or Lasègue Test

These maneuvers reproduce back and leg pain and help confirm the presence of sciatica and a herniated nucleus pulposus. Straight leg raising while keeping the knee extended normally produces no pain. Raise the affected leg just short of the point where it produces pain. Then dorsiflex the foot (Fig. 23.44).

Lasègue's test stretches the nerve route over the disc protrusion and gives a painful response of muscle contraction.[26] Test is positive if it reproduces or worsens sciatic pain and if person resists further leg elevation. This strongly suggests herniated disc and more so if person has increased pain on dorsiflexion of the foot.

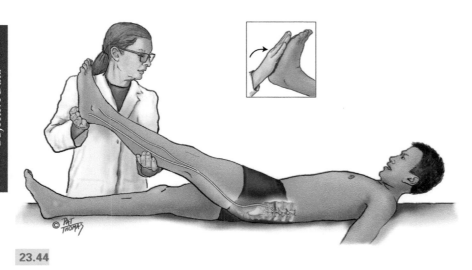

23.44

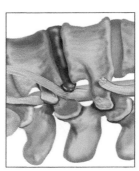

(© Pat Thomas, 2018.)

Raise the unaffected leg while leaving the other leg flat. Inquire about the involved side.

If lifting the unaffected leg reproduces sciatic pain, it strongly suggests a herniated nucleus pulposus.

Measure Leg Length Discrepancy

Perform this measurement if you need to determine whether one leg is shorter than the other. For *true leg length,* measure between *fixed* points, from the anterior iliac spine to the medial malleolus, crossing the medial side of the knee (Fig. 23.45). Normally these measurements are equal or within 1 cm, indicating no true bone discrepancy.

Unequal leg lengths.

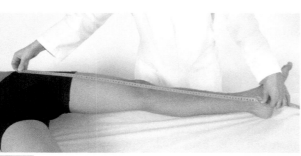

23.45

Objective Data

Normal Range of Findings	Abnormal Findings
Sometimes the true leg length is equal, but the legs still look unequal. For *apparent leg length,* measure from a nonfixed point (the umbilicus) to a fixed point (medial malleolus) on each leg.	True leg lengths are equal, but apparent leg lengths unequal—this condition occurs with pelvic obliquity or adduction or flexion deformity in the hip.

❖ DEVELOPMENTAL COMPETENCE

Be familiar with the developmental milestones. Keep handy a concise chart of the usual sequence of motor development so you can refer to expected findings for the age of each child you are examining. Use the Denver II test to screen the fine and gross motor skills for the child's age.

Because some overlap exists between the musculoskeletal and neurologic examinations, the assessments of muscle tone, resting posture, and motor activity are discussed in Chapter 24.

Infants

Examine the infant fully undressed and lying on the back. Take care to place the newborn on a warming table to maintain body temperature.

Feet and Legs. Start with the feet and work your way up the extremities. Note any *positional deformities,* a residual of fetal positioning. Often the newborn's feet are not held straight but instead in a varus (apart) or valgus (together) position. It is important to distinguish whether this position is flexible (and thus usually self-correctable) or fixed. Scratch the outside of the bottom of the foot. If the deformity is self-correctable, the foot assumes a normal right angle to the lower leg. Or immobilize the heel with one hand and gently push the forefoot to the neutral position with the other hand. If you can move it to neutral position, it is flexible.

> A true deformity is fixed and assumes a right angle only with forced manipulation or not at all.

Note the relationship of the forefoot to the hindfoot. Commonly the hindfoot is in alignment with the lower leg, and just the forefoot angles inward. This forefoot adduction is *metatarsus adductus.* It is usually present at birth and usually resolves spontaneously by age 3 years.

> Metatarsus varus—adduction and inversion of forefoot.
>
> Talipes equinovarus (see Table 23.8, Congenital or Pediatric Abnormalities, p. 622).

Check for *tibial torsion,* a twisting of the tibia. Place both feet flat on the table and push to flex up the knees. With the patella and the tibial tubercle in a straight line, place your fingers on the malleoli. In an infant note that a line connecting the four malleoli is parallel to the table.

> More than 20 degrees of deviation; or if lateral malleolus is anterior to medial malleolus, it indicates tibial torsion.

Tibial torsion may originate from intrauterine positioning and then be exacerbated at a later age by continuous sitting in a reverse tailor position, the "TV squat" (i.e., sitting with the buttocks on the floor and the lower legs splayed back and out on either side).

Hips. Check the hips for *developmental dysplasia of the hip* (DDH). The most reliable method is **Ortolani maneuver,** which should be done at every professional visit until the infant is 1 year old. With the infant supine, flex the knees holding your thumbs on the inner midthighs and your fingers outside on the hips touching the greater trochanters. Adduct the legs until your thumbs touch (Fig. 23.46, *A).* Then gently lift and *abduct,* moving the knees apart and down so their lateral aspects touch the table (Fig. 23.46, *B).* This normally feels smooth and has no sound.

> With a dislocated hip the head of the femur is not cupped in the acetabulum but rests posterior to it.
>
> Hip instability feels like a clunk as the head of the femur pops back into place. This is a *positive Ortolani sign* and warrants referral.

Objective Data

Normal Range of Findings	Abnormal Findings

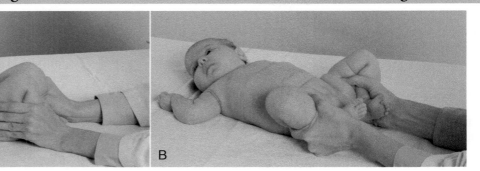

23.46   Ortolani maneuver.

The **Allis test** also is used to check for hip dislocation by comparing leg lengths (Fig. 23.47). Place the baby's feet flat on the table and flex the knees up. Scan the tops of the knees; normally they are at the same elevation.

Finding one knee significantly lower than the other is a positive indication of Allis sign and suggests hip dislocation (see Table 23.8, p. 622).

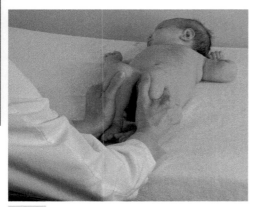

23.47   Allis test.

Note the gluteal folds. Normally they are equal on both sides. However, some asymmetry may occur in healthy children.

Hands and Arms. Inspect the hands, noting shape, number, and position of fingers and palmar creases.

Unequal gluteal folds may accompany hip dislocation after 2 to 3 months of age.

Polydactyly is the presence of extra fingers or toes. Syndactyly is webbing between adjacent fingers or toes (see Table 23.4).

A single transverse crease is a palmar crease that occurs with Down syndrome, accompanied by short broad fingers, incurving of little fingers, and low-set thumbs.

Palpate the length of the clavicles because the clavicle is the bone most frequently fractured during birth. The clavicles should feel smooth, regular, and without crepitus. Also note equal ROM of arms during Moro reflex.

Fractured clavicle: Note irregularity at the fracture site, crepitus, and angulation. The site has rapid callus formation with a palpable lump within a few weeks. Observe limited arm ROM and unilateral response to Moro reflex.

Normal Range of Findings	Abnormal Findings

Back. Lift the infant and examine the back. Note the normal single C-curve of the newborn's spine (Fig. 23.48). By 2 months the infant can lift the head while prone on a flat surface. This builds the concave cervical spinal curve and indicates normal forearm strength. Inspect the length of the spine for any tuft of hair, dimple in midline, cyst, or mass. Normally none are present.

A tuft of hair over a dimple in the midline may indicate spina bifida.

A small dimple in the midline—anywhere from the head to the coccyx—suggests dermoid sinus.

Mass, such as meningocele.

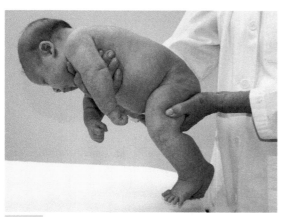

23.48

Observe ROM through spontaneous movement of extremities.

Test muscle strength by lifting the infant with your hands under the axillae (Fig. 23.49). A baby with normal muscle strength wedges securely between your hands.

A baby who starts to "slip" between your hands shows weakness of the shoulder muscles.

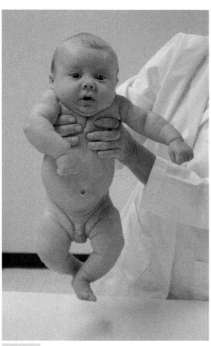

23.49

Normal Range of Findings	Abnormal Findings

Preschool-Age and School-Age Children

Once the infant learns to crawl and then walk, the waking hours show perpetual motion. This is convenient for your musculoskeletal assessment; you can observe the muscles and joints during spontaneous play before a table-top examination. Most young children enjoy showing off their physical accomplishments. For specific motions coax the toddler: "Show me how you can walk to Mom" or "Climb the step stool." Ask the preschooler to hop on one foot or jump.

Back. While the child is standing, note the posture. From behind you should note a "plumb line" from the back of the head, along the spine, to the middle of the sacrum. Shoulders are level within 1 cm, and scapulae are symmetric. From the side lordosis is common throughout childhood, appearing more pronounced in children with a protuberant abdomen.

Legs and Feet. Anteriorly note the leg position. A "bowlegged" stance *(genu varum)* is a lateral bowing of the legs (Fig. 23.50, *A*). It is present when you measure a persistent space of more than 2.5 cm between the knees when the medial malleoli are together. Genu varum is normal for 1 year after the child begins walking. The child may walk with a waddling gait. This resolves with growth; no treatment is indicated.

Lordosis is marked with muscular dystrophy and rickets.

Severe bowing or unilateral bowing also occurs with rickets.

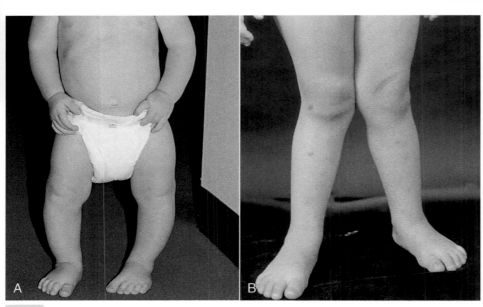

23.50 *A,* Genu varum. *B,* Genu valgum. (Zitelli, 2007.)

"Knock-knees" *(genu valgum)* are present when there is more than 2.5 cm between the medial malleoli when the knees are together (Fig. 23.50, *B*). It occurs normally between 2 and 3½ years. Treatment is not indicated. (NOTE: To remember the two conditions, link the r's and g's: genu va<u>r</u>um—knees apa<u>r</u>t; genu val<u>g</u>um—knees to<u>g</u>ether.)

Often parents tell you that they are concerned about the child's foot development. The most common questions are about "flatfeet" and "pigeon toes." Flatfoot *(pes planus)* is pronation, or turning in, of the medial side of the foot. The young child may look flatfooted because the normal longitudinal arch is concealed by a fat pad until age 3 years. When standing begins, the child takes a broad-based stance, which causes pronation. Thus pronation is common between 12 and 30 months. You can see it best from behind the child, where the medial side of the foot drops down and in.

Genu valgum also occurs with rickets, poliomyelitis, and syphilis.

Pronation beyond 30 months.

Normal Range of Findings	Abnormal Findings

Pigeon toes (i.e., toeing in) are demonstrated when the child tends to walk on the lateral side of the foot and the longitudinal arch looks higher than normal. It often starts as a forefoot adduction, which usually corrects spontaneously by 3 years of age as long as the foot is flexible.

Check the child's gait while walking away from and returning to you. Let him or her wear socks because a cold tile floor distorts the usual gait. From 1 to 2 years expect a broad-based gait, with arms out for balance. Weight-bearing falls on the inside of the foot. From 3 years the base narrows, and the arms are closer to the sides. Inspect the shoes for spots of greatest wear to aid your judgment of the gait. Normally the shoes wear more on the outside of the heel and the inside of the toe.

The child may sit for the remainder of the examination. Start with the feet and hands of the child from 2 to 6 years because he or she is happy to show these off and proceed through the examination described earlier (Fig. 23.51).

Toeing in from forefoot adduction that is fixed or lasts beyond age 3 years.
Toeing in from tibial torsion.

Limp, usually caused by trauma, fatigue, or hip disease.
Abnormal gait patterns (see Chapter 24).

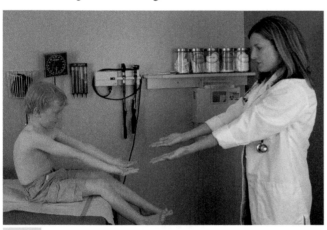

23.51

Particularly check the arm for full ROM and presence of pain. Look for subluxation of the elbow (head of the radius). This occurs most often between 2 and 4 years as a result of forceful removal of clothing or dangling while adults suspend the child by the hands.

Palpate the bones, joints, and muscles of the extremities as described in the adult examination.

Inability to supinate the hand while the arm is flexed, together with pain in the elbow, indicates subluxation of the head of the radius.

Pain or tenderness in extremities is usually caused by trauma or infection.

Fractures caused by trauma show as an inability to use the area, a deformity, or an excess motion in the involved bone with pain and crepitation.

Enlargement of the tibial tubercles with tenderness suggests Osgood-Schlatter disease (see Table 23.5, p. 617).

Adolescents

Proceed with the musculoskeletal examination that you provide for the adult, except pay special note to spinal posture. Kyphosis is common during adolescence because of chronic poor posture. Be aware of the risk for sports-related injuries with the adolescent because sports participation and competition often peak with this age-group.

The U.S. Preventive Services Task Force[32] does not support the routine screening of asymptomatic adolescents for idiopathic scoliosis. They found that most cases detected through screening did not progress to clinically significant

Objective Data

Normal Range of Findings	Abnormal Findings

scoliosis. In addition, the harm of unnecessary imaging, follow-up visits, and psychological adverse effects of brace wear did not offset any potential benefits of screening. However, when idiopathic scoliosis is discovered incidentally or when the teen or parent expresses concern, clinicians should be prepared to evaluate.

Screen for scoliosis with the *forward bend test*. Seat yourself behind the standing child and ask him or her to stand with the feet shoulder-width apart and bend forward slowly to touch the toes. Expect a straight vertical spine while standing and also while bending forward. Posterior ribs should be symmetric, with equal elevation of shoulders, scapulae, and iliac crests.

Scoliosis is most apparent during the preadolescent growth spurt; marked asymmetry suggests scoliosis—ribs hump up on one side as child bends forward, with unequal landmark elevation (see Table 23.7).

The Pregnant Woman

Proceed through the examination described in the adult section. Expected postural changes in pregnancy include progressive lordosis and, toward the third trimester, anterior cervical flexion, kyphosis, and slumped shoulders (Fig. 23.52, *A*). When the pregnancy is at term, the protuberant abdomen and relaxed mobility in the joints create the characteristic "waddling" gait (Fig. 23.52, *B*).

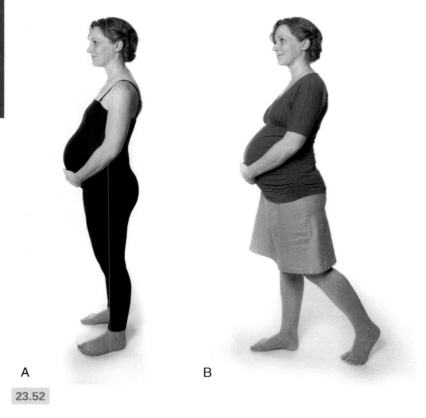

A   B

23.52

The Aging Adult

Postural changes include a decrease in height, more apparent in the 70s and 80s (Fig. 23.53). The expression "lengthening of the arm-trunk axis" describes this shortening of the trunk with comparatively long extremities. Kyphosis is common, with a backward head tilt to compensate. This creates the outline of a figure 3 when you view this older adult from the left side. Slight flexion of hips and knees is also common.

Objective Data

| **Normal Range of Findings** | **Abnormal Findings** |

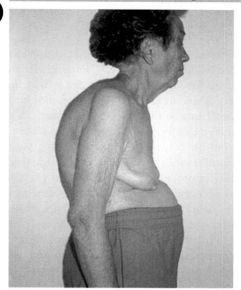

23.53

Contour changes include a decrease of fat in the body periphery and fat deposition over the abdomen and hips. The bony prominences become more marked.

For most older adults ROM testing proceeds as described earlier. ROM and muscle strength are much the same as with the younger adult, provided no musculoskeletal illnesses or arthritic changes are present.

Get Up and Go Test. Evidence shows that this timed test helps to identify older adults at increased risk of falling. Watch the time it takes the person to rise from an armchair, walk 10 feet, turn, walk back, and sit down again. A healthy adult over 60 years can manage this test in fewer than 10 seconds.[22]

Performance >10 seconds together with history of falls and mobility problems increases risk for future falling.

Functional Assessment. For those with advanced aging changes, arthritic changes, or musculoskeletal disability, perform a **functional assessment for ADLs.** This applies the ROM and muscle strength assessments to the accomplishment of specific activities. You need to determine adequate and safe performance of functions essential for independent home life. See Chapter 32 for further assessments.

Instructions	**Common Adaptation for Aging Changes**
1. Walk (with shoes on).	Shuffling pattern; swaying; arms out to help balance; broader base of support; person may watch feet.
2. Climb up stairs.	Person holds handrail; may haul body up with it; may lead with favored (stronger) leg.
3. Walk down stairs.	Holds handrail, sometimes with both hands. If person is weak, he or she may descend sideways, lowering weaker leg first. If person is unsteady, he or she may watch feet.
4. Pick up object from floor.	Person often bends at waist instead of bending knees; holds furniture to support while bending and straightening.
5. Rise up from sitting in chair.	Person uses arms to push off chair arms, upper trunk leans forward before body straightens, feet planted wide in broad base of support.
6. Rise up from lying in bed.	May roll to one side, push with arms to lift up torso, grab bedside table to increase leverage.

Objective Data

HEALTH PROMOTION AND PATIENT TEACHING

DIET

Peak bone mass is a major determinant for osteoporosis in later life,[34] and you can teach your patients many ways to decrease their risk of osteoporosis. Say, "*Eat the rainbow. Choose colorful plates with green, red, orange, yellow, and purple foods.*" Starting in childhood, a diet rich in dark green and deep yellow vegetables (spinach, romaine lettuce, broccoli, carrots, sweet potatoes) and low in fried foods helps lower fat mass and promotes bone mass accrual. This evidence comes from a study of children ages 4 to 8 that periodically measured bone mass by dual-energy x-ray absorptiometry (DEXA).[36] Also for pregnant women and parents, "*Try to keep visits to fast-food outlets as an occasional treat only.*" Another DEXA study of 1107 infants and young children showed that neighborhood exposure to fast-food restaurants was associated with lower bone mineral density in infancy.[34] Increasing exposure to healthy food markets and butchers was associated with higher BMD at 4 and 6 years of age. Of course fast food often is less expensive, but diet patterns encouraged in childhood will continue in adolescence and adulthood.[34]

"*Protect your bones by getting enough calcium and vitamin D.*" About 99% of calcium in the body is in bones and teeth, and calcium is lost every day though skin, nails, hair, sweat, urine, and feces. The body does not produce new calcium; we must get it through food, or the body takes it from our bones. "*The amount of calcium you need every day depends on your age and sex. Women ages 50 years or younger need 1000 mg daily, and those over 50 need 1200 mg daily. Men ages 70 years and younger need 1000 mg daily, increasing to 1200 mg daily for men over 70.*" Sources include dairy products (milk, cheese, yogurt), juices, breakfast foods, soy milk. Check the nutrition facts panel on food packaging for the percentage of daily value provided in 1 serving. "*Your body needs vitamin D to absorb the calcium. Women and men under age 50 need 400 to 800 IU daily; those over age 50 need 800 to 1000 IU daily.*" The skin makes vitamin D from the ultraviolet rays in sunlight, but because of skin cancer concerns, people now stay out of the sun, cover up, or use sunscreen. Vitamin D has been added to foods, so check the nutrition facts panel. One 8-oz glass of milk usually has 25% of daily value of vitamin D. A blood test can measure the body's level of vitamin D; if the level is low, a vitamin D supplement can be prescribed.

Finally, tobacco smoking and excessive alcohol drinking are harmful to bone health.[16] Smoking is linked to reduced BMD, and excess drinking increases the risk of falls.[2] "*We recommend no more than 1 standard drink of alcohol daily for women and no more than 2 standard drinks per day for men.*" "*If you smoke, let's find a method to help you quit.*"

EXERCISE

Obesity and osteoporosis have their origins in childhood, and both are affected by diet and exercise.[36] "*Physical activity delays or prevents bone loss; the more you do, the greater the benefit to your bones. If you are just getting started, aim for 2 or 3 days a week. Start easy so that you don't get hurt. Then work up to 30 minutes a day for 5 days a week.*" Fast walking is the best prevention for osteoporosis; the faster the pace, the higher the preventive effect on the risk for hip fracture. Physical activity also improves muscle strength to prevent falls and increase balance and posture control, decreases back pain, and increases quality of life.[29] Further evidence shows that older adults who had a physical training program with resistance, balance, and functional training showed significant increases in strength, flexibility, heart rate after exercise, and balance.[29] "*Have a little fun—try dancing!*" A review of 18 studies of all types of dancing showed an improvement of physical health among older adults—in flexibility, muscular strength and endurance, balance, cardiovascular endurance, and cognitive function.[12] "*Have you tried yoga or tai chi?*" These increase balance and muscle tone and may help reduce falls.[2]

OSTEOPOROSIS SCREENING

"*All women should get a bone mineral density scan by DEXA by age 65 years; men by age 70 years.*" A BMD measurement by DEXA is the best predictor of future hip fracture risk.[16] The test is noninvasive, takes very little time, and has a low level of radiation exposure. Another assessment tool is the FRAX, a computerized fracture risk algorithm developed by the World Health Organization (available at www.shef.ac.uk/FRAX—click on the Calculation Tool tab). It has been validated for men and women ages 40 to 90 years in most countries of the world and is most useful for people with low hip BMD.[16]

The FRAX algorithm helps in the decision for treatment; if the absolute risk of hip fracture in the next 10 years is 3% or more, or the risk of major osteoporotic fracture is 20% or more, treatment can decrease the rate of possible fractures.[30,35]

FALL PREVENTION

"*Falls put you at risk of serious injury. Build your strength with an exercise program. Review your medicines with your provider to check which ones hurt your balance. Check your vision and hearing every year—eyes and ears keep you on your feet. Safety-proof your home: increase lighting, make stairs safe, remove trip hazards such as throw rugs, and install grab bars wherever needed.*"[25]

DOCUMENTATION AND CRITICAL THINKING

Sample Charting

SUBJECTIVE

States no joint pain, stiffness, swelling, or limitation. No muscle pain or weakness. No history of bone trauma or deformity. Able to manage all usual daily activities with no physical limitations. Occupation involves no musculoskeletal risk factors. Exercise pattern is brisk walk 1 mile 5×/week.

OBJECTIVE

Joints and muscles symmetric; no swelling, masses, deformity; normal spinal curvature. No tenderness to palpation of joints; no heat, swelling, or masses. Full ROM; movement smooth, no crepitus, no tenderness. Muscle strength—able to maintain flexion against resistance and without tenderness.

ASSESSMENT

Muscles and joints—healthy and functional

Clinical Case Study 1

M.T. is a 45-year-old female salesperson with a diagnosis of rheumatoid arthritis 3 years PTA, who seeks care now for "swelling and burning pain in my hands" for 1 day.

SUBJECTIVE

M.T. was diagnosed as having rheumatoid arthritis at age 41 years by staff at this agency. Since that time her "flare-ups" seem to come every 6 to 8 months. Acute episodes involve hand joints and are treated with aspirin, which gives relief. Typically experiences morning stiffness, lasting ½ to 1 hour. Joints feel warm, swollen, tender. Has had weight loss of 15 lbs over past 4 years and feels fatigued much of the time. States should rest more, but "I can't take the time." Daily exercises have been prescribed but doesn't do them regularly. Takes aspirin for acute flare-ups, feels better in a few days, and decreases dose by herself.

OBJECTIVE

Body joints within normal limits with exception of joints of wrist and hands. Radiocarpal, metacarpophalangeal, and proximal interphalangeal joints are red, swollen, tender to palpation. Spindle-shaped swelling of proximal interphalangeal joints of 3rd digit right hand and 2nd digit left hand; ulnar deviation of metacarpophalangeal joints.

ASSESSMENT

Acute pain
Decreased physical mobility
Needs health teaching on aspirin treatment
Needs exercise teaching
Needs health teaching on rest periods

Clinical Case Study 2

L.M. is a 58-year-old woman employed in housekeeping in a local hotel for 10 years who presents now with "much pain in right knee for 1 day."

SUBJECTIVE

L.M. reports being overweight since having children in her 20s and having bilateral knee pain for the past 2 years. No morning stiffness, but pain increases during working day. For last 6 months takes 6 extra-strength acetaminophen (500 mg each) in 3 divided doses daily, but pain persists. One day PTA, walking downstairs at work carrying load of sheets, reports right knee gave way and almost fell. Continued working, but today pain is increased. Able to bear weight and walk to car but unable to work. No history of stomach pain or stomach bleeding. No smoking, no alcohol.

OBJECTIVE

Vital signs: Pulse 76 bpm. Resp 12/min. BP 146/86 mm Hg. No fever. Height 64 in, weight 180 lbs. BMI 31.
Right knee has no swelling or increased pain on palpation. ROM both hips full on external and internal rotation, abduction and adduction. Unable to flex hip with knee straight (says has not done that in years); hip flexion with knee flexed is 90 degrees and painful on right. ROM knees: unable to hyperextend; flexion when standing with support is 90 degrees and painful on right. Gait is slow but no limp.

ASSESSMENT

Chronic knee pain with activity; increased knee pain with injury
Weakened quadriceps muscles
Obesity
Stage 1 hypertension

Clinical Case Study 3

A.S. is a 2-year-old boy who presents to the ED with his parents with refusal to use right upper extremity.

SUBJECTIVE

2 hours PTA—Each of A.S.'s parents were on one side of him and were "swinging him" as they walked. On the last "swing" A.S. started crying and since that time has refused to use his right arm.

OBJECTIVE

Vital signs: Temp 37.2° C (oral). Pulse 122 bpm (resting). Resp 30/min. BP (unable to obtain due to movement).
General appearance: Quiet child who is holding his right arm against his body in the extended, pronated, and adducted position.
Extremities: No visible swelling, masses, and/or deformities; winces when right arm palpated and clunk heard on supination and flexion of right forearm.

ASSESSMENT

Radial head subluxation (nursemaid's elbow)
Acute pain
Potential for injury R/T unstable joint

ABNORMAL FINDINGS
FOR ADVANCED PRACTICE

TABLE 23.1 | Abnormalities Affecting Multiple Joints

Inflammatory Conditions

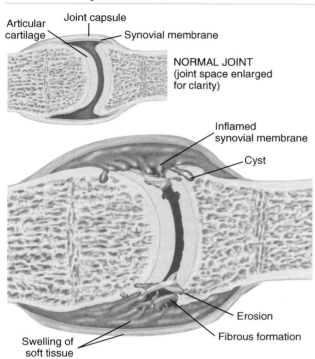

Articular cartilage — Joint capsule — Synovial membrane

NORMAL JOINT (joint space enlarged for clarity)

Inflamed synovial membrane

Cyst

Erosion

Fibrous formation

Swelling of soft tissue

◀ Rheumatoid Arthritis (RA)

RA is a chronic inflammatory pain condition that is possibly started by an autoimmune response, inflammatory event, or infection.[7] It occurs 2.5 times more in women than in men; its peak is ages 30 to 60 years although it can occur at any age. The inflammation of synovial tissues, hyperplasia, and swelling lead to fibrosis, cartilage and bone destruction, which limit motion and show as deformity. Joint involvement is symmetric and bilateral, with heat, redness, swelling, and painful motion of affected joints. Rheumatoid arthritis (RA) symptoms include fatigue, weakness, anorexia, weight loss, low-grade fever, and lymphadenopathy. RA carries increased cardiovascular risk of heart attack and stroke. Associated signs are described in the following tables, especially Table 23.4.

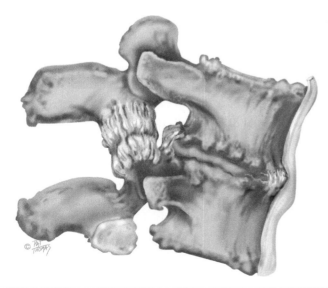

◀ Ankylosing Spondylitis (AS)

AS is chronic inflamed vertebrae (spondylitis) that in extreme form leads to bony fusion of vertebral joints (ankyloses). It affects the spine, pelvis, and thoracic cage, and is characterized by inflammatory back pain that is dull and deep in lower back or buttocks.[31] It also has morning back stiffness that lasts ≥30 minutes and decreases with activity, nighttime awakening with pain, age at onset ≤45 years. It affects males by a 2:1 ratio, beginning in late adolescence or early 20s. Spasm of paraspinal muscles pulls spine into forward flexion, obliterating cervical and lumbar curves. Thoracic curve exaggerated into single kyphotic rounding. Also includes flexion deformities of hips and knees as they compensate for spinal flexion.

Continued

TABLE 23.1 | **Abnormalities Affecting Multiple Joints—cont'd**

Degenerative Conditions

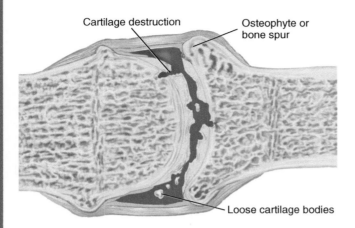

Cartilage destruction

Osteophyte or bone spur

Loose cartilage bodies

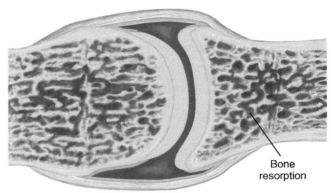

Bone resorption

Osteoarthritis (OA) (Degenerative Joint Disease)

Noninflammatory, localized, progressive disorder involving deterioration of articular cartilages (cushion between the ends of bones) and subchondral bone remodeling, synovial inflammation, and formation of new bone (osteophytes) at joint surfaces. Increased risk occurs with older age, females, and Caucasians. Obesity increases risk and progression of OA, especially in the knee.[11] Asymmetric joint involvement commonly affects hands, knees, hips, and lumbar and cervical segments of the spine. Affected joints have stiffness; swelling with hard, bony protuberances; pain with motion; and limitation of motion (see Table 22.4).

Osteoporosis

Decrease in skeletal bone mass leading to low bone mineral density (BMD) and impaired bone density. The weakened bone state increases risk for fractures, especially at wrist, hip, and vertebrae. Occurs primarily in postmenopausal white women. Osteoporosis risk also is associated with smaller height and weight, younger age at menopause, lack of physical activity, and lack of estrogen in women.

TABLE 23.2 | **Shoulder Abnormalities**

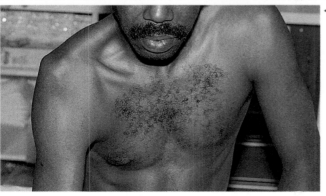

◀ Dislocated Shoulder

Glenohumeral dislocation is the most frequent type of joint dislocation.[15] Anterior dislocation (95%) shows when hunching the shoulder forward and the tip of the clavicle dislocates. It occurs with trauma involving abduction, extension, and rotation (e.g., falling on an outstretched arm or diving into a pool), showing obvious deformity and severe pain. Needs radiography. At risk for further dislocations due to injury to ligaments.

Continued

| TABLE 23.2 | Shoulder Abnormalities—cont'd |

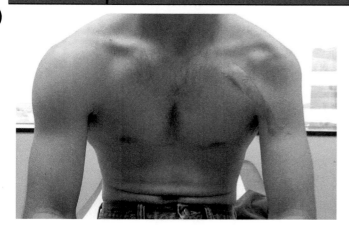

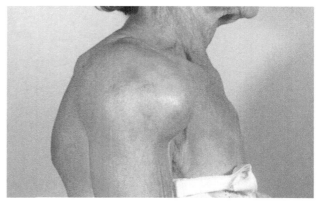

Atrophy

Loss of muscle mass is exhibited as a lack of fullness surrounding the deltoid muscle, here in left shoulder from brachial plexus injury. Atrophy also occurs from disuse, muscle tissue damage, or motor nerve damage.

Joint Effusion

Swelling from excess fluid in the joint capsule, here from rheumatoid arthritis. Best observed anteriorly. Fluctuant to palpation. Considerable fluid must be present to cause a visible distention because the capsule normally is so loose.

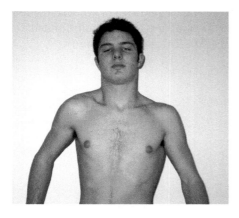

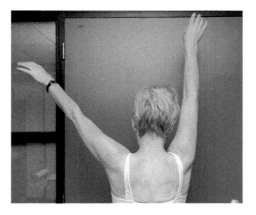

Tear of Rotator Cuff

Characteristic "hunched" position and limited abduction of arm. Occurs from traumatic adduction while arm is held in abduction or from fall on shoulder, throwing, or heavy lifting. Positive drop arm test: if the arm is passively abducted at the shoulder, the person is unable to sustain the position and shrugs or hitches the shoulder forward to compensate with remaining intact muscles. Needs ultrasound imaging, possibly MRI.[15]

Frozen Shoulder—Adhesive Capsulitis

Fibrous tissues form in the joint capsule, causing stiffness, progressive limitation of motion, and pain, especially unilateral nocturnal pain. Motion limited in abduction and external rotation; unable to reach overhead. It may lead to atrophy of shoulder girdle muscles. Gradual onset; prevalence in 20% of diabetics. Also associated with prolonged bed rest or shoulder immobility.

See Illustration Credits for source information.

| TABLE 23.3 | Elbow Abnormalities |

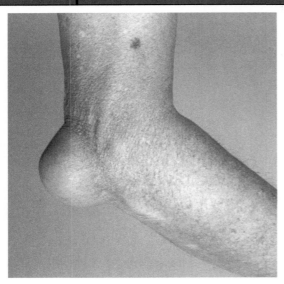

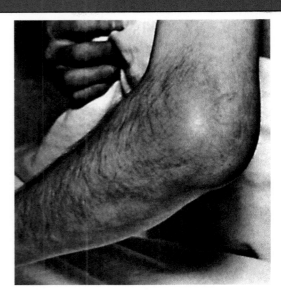

Olecranon Bursitis

Large, soft knob, or "goose egg," and redness from swelling and inflammation of olecranon bursa. Localized and easy to see because bursa lies just under skin. Occurs with trauma, gout, or RA.

Arthritis

Joint effusion or synovial thickening, seen first as bulge or fullness in grooves on either side of olecranon process. Redness and heat can extend beyond area of synovial membrane. Soft, boggy, or fluctuant fullness to palpation. Limited extension of elbow. Occurs with RA, gout, OA, trauma.

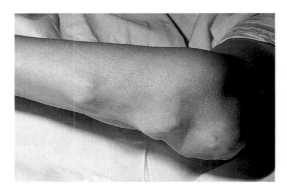

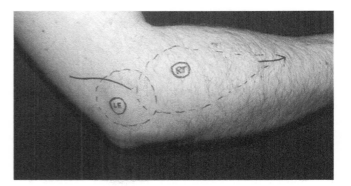

Rheumatoid Nodules

These raised firm nodules are granulomatous lesions that grow along small blood vessels in people with RA. Can be tender or nontender, movable or fixed; skin slides freely over nodules. Develop over pressure points such as extensor surface of arm (ulna) and olecranon.

Epicondylitis—Tennis Elbow

Chronic disabling pain at lateral epicondyle (LE) of humerus; radiates down extensor surface of forearm. Pain can be located with one finger. Resisting extension of the hand increases the pain. Inflammation along flexor and extensor tendons of elbow joint with overuse.[15] Occurs with excessive pronation and supination of forearm with an extended wrist (e.g., racquet sports or using a screwdriver).

See Illustration Credits for source information.

TABLE 23.4 | Wrist and Hand Abnormalities

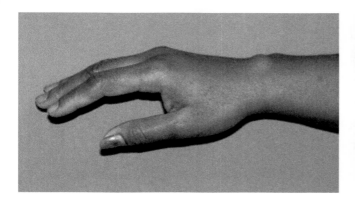

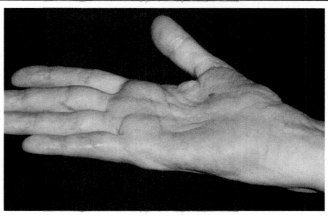

Ganglion Cyst

Round, cystic, nontender nodule overlying a tendon sheath or joint capsule, usually on dorsum of wrist. Flexion makes it more prominent. The fluid-filled mass is more common in women ages 30 to 60 years.[37] Nonpainful ganglion cysts are a cosmetic concern; painful ones may compress the median or ulnar nerve, causing numbness and tingling or weakness.

Colles Fracture (not illustrated)

Nonarticular fracture of distal radius, with or without fracture of ulna at styloid process. Usually from a fall on an outstretched hand; occurs more often in older women. Wrist looks puffy with "silver fork" deformity, a characteristic hump when viewed from the side.

Carpal Tunnel Syndrome With Atrophy of Thenar Eminence

Pain along thumb and index and middle fingers and atrophy occur from interference with motor function from compression of the median nerve inside the carpal tunnel. Caused by chronic repetitive motion; occurs between 40 and 60 years and is more common in women. Symptoms of carpal tunnel syndrome include pain, nighttime pain, burning and numbness, positive findings on Phalen test, positive Tinel sign, and often atrophy of thenar muscles.

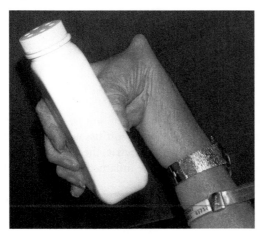

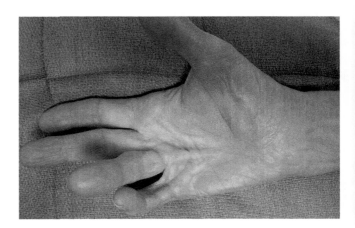

Ankylosis

Wrist in extreme flexion with ruptures of wrist and finger extensors, caused by severe rheumatoid arthritis (RA). This is a functionally compromised hand because, when the wrist is palmar flexed, a good deal of power is lost from the fingers, and often the thumb cannot oppose the fingers.

Dupuytren Contracture

Chronic hyperplasia of the palmar fascia causes flexion contractures of the digits, first in the 4th digit, then the 5th digit, and then the 3rd digit. Note the bands that extend from the midpalm to the digits and the puckering of palmar skin. Common in men older than 40 years and is usually bilateral. It occurs with diabetes, epilepsy, and alcoholic liver disease and as an inherited trait. The contracture is painless but impairs hand function.

Continued

TABLE 23.4 **Wrist and Hand Abnormalities—cont'd**

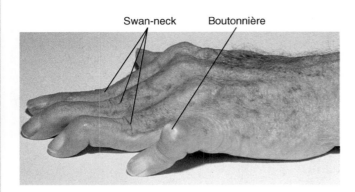

Swan-neck   Boutonnière

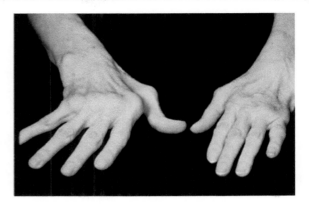

Swan-Neck and Boutonnière Deformity

Flexion contracture resembles curve of a **swan's neck**, as in metacarpophalangeal joint. Then hyperextension of the PIP joint, and flexion of the DIP joint. It occurs with chronic RA, often accompanied by ulnar drift of the fingers. In **boutonnière deformity** the knuckle looks as if being pushed through a buttonhole. It is a common deformity.

Ulnar Deviation or Drift

Fingers drift to the ulnar side because of stretching of the articular capsule and muscle imbalance. Also note subluxation and swelling in the joints and muscle atrophy on the dorsa of the hands. This is caused by chronic RA.

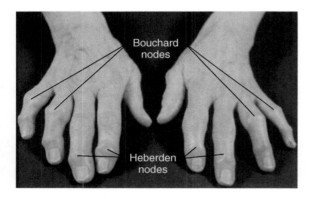

Bouchard nodes

Heberden nodes

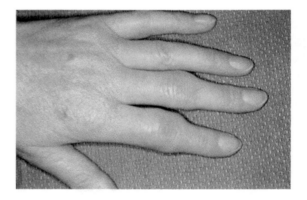

Osteoarthritis (OA)

Different from RA, OA is characterized by hard, nontender, noninflammatory nodules, 2 to 3 mm or more. These osteophytes (bony overgrowths) of the DIP joints are called *Heberden nodes*. Those of the PIP joints are called *Bouchard nodes* and are less common.

Acute Rheumatoid Arthritis

Painful swelling and stiffness of joints, with fusiform or spindle-shaped swelling of the soft tissue of PIP joints. Fusiform swelling is usually symmetric, the hands are warm, and the veins are engorged. The inflamed joints have a limited range of motion.

Continued

TABLE 23.4	Wrist and Hand Abnormalities—cont'd

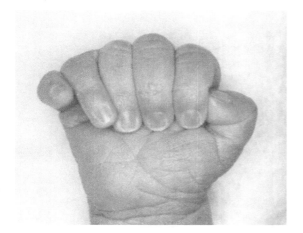

Polydactyly

Extra digits are a congenital deformity, usually occurring at the 5th finger or the thumb. Surgical removal is considered for cosmetic appearance. The 6th finger shown here was not removed because it had full ROM and sensation and a normal appearance.

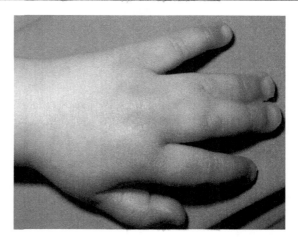

Syndactyly

Webbed fingers are a congenital deformity requiring surgical separation. The metacarpals and phalanges of the webbed fingers are different lengths and the joints do not line up. To leave the fingers fused would thus limit their flexion and extension.

See Illustration Credits for source information.

TABLE 23.5	Knee Abnormalities

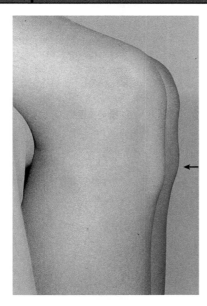

Osgood-Schlatter Disease

Painful swelling of the tibial tubercle just below the knee, from overuse injury that places traction and microtrauma on the bone.[17] Occurs most in puberty during rapid growth and before closure of the growth plate. Pain increases with kicking, running, bike riding, volleyball, basketball, soccer. It is usually self-limited, and symptoms resolve with rest.

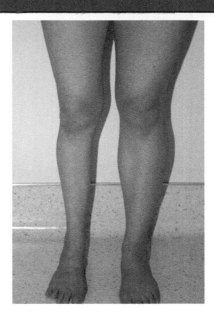

Post-Polio Muscle Atrophy

Right leg and foot muscle atrophy as a result of childhood polio. Poliomyelitis epidemics peaked in the United States in the 1940s and 1950s. The development of the oral polio vaccine (1962) has almost eradicated the disease. However, thousands of polio survivors have this muscle atrophy.

Continued

Abnormal Findings

TABLE 23.5 | **Knee Abnormalities—cont'd**

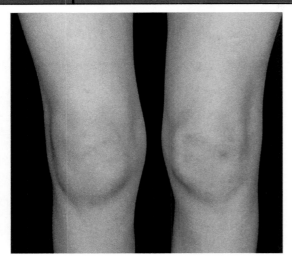

Mild Synovitis

Loss of normal hollows on either side of the patella, which are replaced by mild distention. Occurs with synovial thickening or effusion (excess fluid) as in RA. Also note mild distention of the suprapatellar pouch.

Prepatellar Bursitis

Localized swelling on anterior knee between patella and skin. A tender, fluctuant mass indicates swelling; infection may spread to surrounding soft tissue. The condition is limited to the bursa, and the knee joint itself is not involved. Overlying skin may be red, shiny, atrophic, or coarse and thickened.

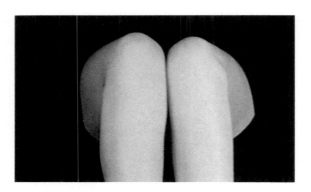

◄ Swelling of Menisci

Localized soft swelling from cyst in lateral meniscus shows at the midpoint of the anterolateral joint line. Semiflexion of the knee makes swelling more prominent. Other meniscal injuries present as a sharp acute pain at lateral or medial joint line together with catching, locking, or popping.[17] Tears in the menisci occur with severe ligament injury and present with joint instability, swelling, and pain. Suspected tears are referred to orthopedics due to future increased risk of osteoarthritis.

See Illustration Credits for source information.

TABLE 23.6 | **Ankle and Foot Abnormalities**

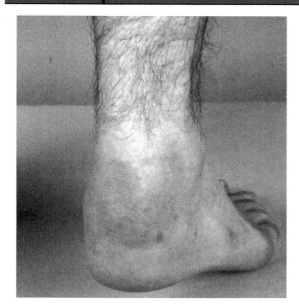

Achilles Tenosynovitis

Inflammation of a tendon sheath near the ankle (here the Achilles tendon) produces a superficial linear swelling and a localized tenderness along the route of the sheath. Movement of the involved tendon usually causes pain.

Tophi With Chronic Gout

Hard nodules (tophi) most often in the metatarsophalangeal joint of first toe. Tophi are collections of sodium urate crystals caused by chronic gout in and around the joint. Crystals are stong inflammation triggers that cause extreme painful swelling and joint deformity. They may erode through skin with a chalky discharge.[9]

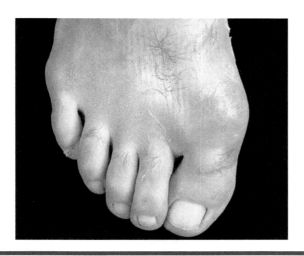

◀ Acute Gout

Gout is a painful inflammatory arthritis characterized by excess uric acid in the blood and deposits of urate crystals in the joint space.[27] Acute episodes are triggered by surgery, trauma, diuretics, alcohol intake. Episodes are characterized by redness, swelling, heat, and extreme pain such as a continuous throbbing. Increased prevalence in obesity, metabolic syndrome, hypertension, hyperlipidemia.

Continued

Abnormal Findings

TABLE 23.6 | Ankle and Foot Abnormalities—cont'd

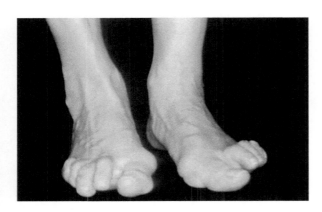

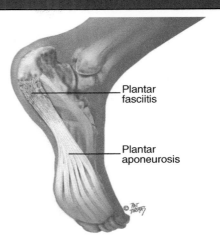

Hallux Valgus With Bunion and Hammertoes

Hallux valgus, a common deformity from RA, is a lateral or outward deviation of the great toe with medial prominence of the head of the 1st metatarsal. The **bunion** is the inflamed bursa that forms at the pressure point. The great toe loses power to push off while walking; this stresses the 2nd and 3rd metatarsal heads, and they develop calluses and pain. Chronic sequelae include corns, calluses, hammertoes, and joint subluxation. Note the **hammertoe** deformities in the 2nd, 3rd, 4th, and 5th toes that include hyperextension of the metatarsophalangeal joint and flexion of the proximal interphalangeal joint. **Corns** (thickening of soft tissue) develop on the dorsum over the bony prominence from prolonged pressure from shoes.

Plantar Fasciitis

The plantar fascia is a band of connective tissue that extends lengthwise from the medial tubercle of the heel to the metatarsal heads and the five proximal phalanges of the toes.[14] An inflammatory response to repetitive microtrauma to this fascia is the most frequent cause of heel pain. Risk factors include obesity, high-arched foot, running, standing long periods on hard flooring, or recent activity changes. Pain is unilateral, "throbbing, searing, or piercing," and is localized to the plantar medial part of the heel; it is worse in the morning or after periods of long rest. Ultrasound imaging often aids in diagnosis. It is self-limiting; treatments include rest and oral pain medications or steroids, a 2- to 4-month stretching program, orthotics for shoes, or night splints.[14]

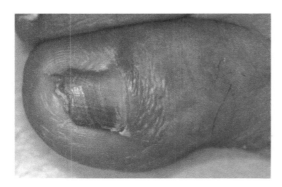

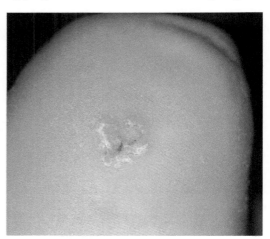

Ingrown Toenail

A misnomer; the nail does not grow in, but the soft tissue grows over the nail and obliterates the groove. It occurs almost always on the great toe on the medial or lateral side. It is caused by trimming the nail too short or toe crowding in tight shoes. The area becomes infected when the nail grows and its corner penetrates the soft tissue.

Plantar Wart

Vascular papillomatous growth is caused by *human papillomavirus* and occurs on the sole of the foot, commonly at the ball and has small dark spots. Although it looks like a callus, it is extremely painful. The wart is tender if you pinch it side to side, whereas a callus is tender to direct pressure.

See Illustration Credits for source information.

TABLE 23.7	Spine Abnormalities

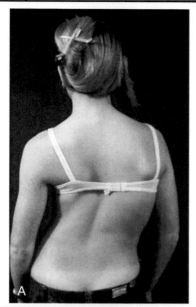

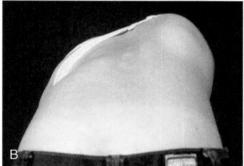

◀ **Scoliosis**

Lateral curvature of thoracic and lumbar segments of the spine, usually with some rotation of involved vertebral bodies. *Functional* scoliosis is flexible; appears with standing and disappears with forward bending. It may compensate for other abnormalities (leg length discrepancy).

Structural scoliosis is fixed; the curvature shows both on standing and on bending forward. Note rib hump with forward flexion. When the person is standing, note unequal shoulder elevation, unequal scapulae, obvious curvature, and unequal hip level. *Idiopathic* scoliosis shows at 10 years of age through adolescence during the peak of the growth spurt; usually not progressive and more common in girls.[10]

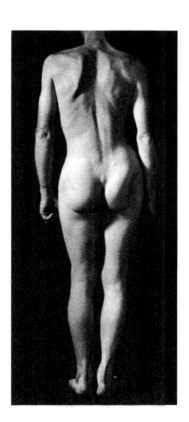

Herniated Intervertebral Disc ▶

The nucleus pulposus (the center of the disc) ruptures into the spinal canal and puts pressure on the local spinal nerve root, causing pain and inflammation. Usually occurs from strenuous activities (lifting, twisting, continuous flexion with lifting, fall on buttocks), mostly in men 20 to 45 years of age, more in smokers.[6] Lumbar herniations occur mainly in interspaces L4 to L5 and L5 to S1. NOTE: Sciatic pain, numbness, and paresthesia of involved dermatome; listing away from affected side; decreased mobility; low back tenderness; and decreased motor and sensory function in leg. Straight leg raising tests reproduce sciatic pain (see p. 600).

See Illustration Credits for source information.

TABLE 23.8	Congenital or Pediatric Abnormalities

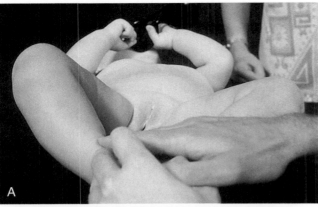

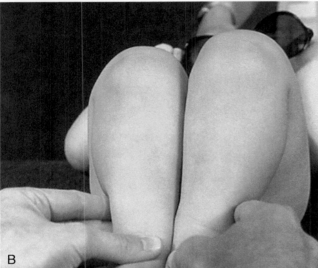

◄ **Developmental Dysplasia of the Hip**

With a dislocated hip the head of the femur is displaced out of the cup-shaped acetabulum. The degree varies; subluxation may occur as stretched ligaments allow partial displacement of femoral head, and acetabular dysplasia may develop because of excessive laxity of hip joint capsule.

Occurrence is 1:500 to 1:1000 births; common in girls by 7:1 ratio. Signs include limited abduction of flexed thigh (illustration A), positive indications of Ortolani sign, asymmetric skin creases or gluteal folds, unequal knee elevation (illustration B), limb length discrepancy, and positive indication of Trendelenburg sign in older children.

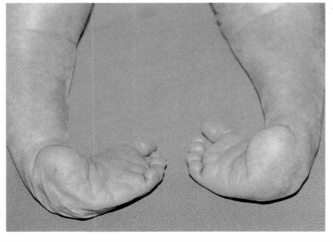

◄ **Talipes Equinovarus (Clubfoot)**

Congenital, rigid, and fixed malposition of foot, including (1) inversion, (2) forefoot adduction, and (3) foot pointing downward (equinus). A common birth defect, with an incidence of 1:1000 to 3:1000 live births. Males are affected twice as frequently as females.

Continued

TABLE 23.8	Congenital or Pediatric Abnormalities—cont'd

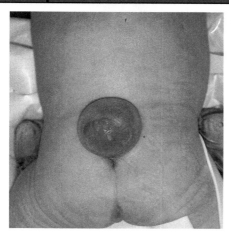

◄ **Spina Bifida**

Incomplete closure of posterior part of vertebrae results in a neural tube defect. Seriousness varies from skin defect along the spine to protrusion of the sac containing meninges, spinal fluid, or malformed spinal cord. The most serious type is myelomeningocele (shown here), in which the meninges and neural tissue protrude. In these cases the child is usually paralyzed below the level of the lesion.

Coxa Plana (Legg-Calvé-Perthes Syndrome) (not illustrated)

Avascular necrosis of the femoral head, occurring primarily in males between 3 and 12 years of age, with peak at age 6 years. In initial inflammatory stage interruption of blood supply to femoral epiphysis occurs, halting growth. Revascularization and healing occur later, but significant residual deformity and dysfunction may be present.

See Illustration Credits for source information.

TABLE 23.9	Fibromyalgia Syndrome

Chronic widespread musculoskeletal pain lasting >3 months, associated with fatigue, insomnia, and psychosocial distress. Most (90%) are adult women. The pain is amplified centrally in the brain. Because it is not a peripheral pain condition, medications for peripheral pain (NSAIDs) will not help.[4]

The 2010 revised criteria stopped the tender point on the body count and substituted interview criteria.[20] These include a widespread pain index or a 0-19 count of the person's report of the number of painful body regions. The 2010 criteria also assess characteristic symptoms (fatigue, nonrefreshed sleep, cognitive problems, somatic symptoms) on a 0-3 severity scale.

Summary Checklist: Musculoskeletal Examination

For each joint to be examined:
1. **Inspection**
   Size and contour of joint
   Skin color and characteristics
2. **Palpation of joint area**
   Skin
   Muscles

Bony articulations
Joint capsule
3. **ROM**
   Active
   Passive (if limitation in active ROM
   is present)

Measure with goniometer (if
   abnormality in ROM is present)
4. **Muscle testing**

REFERENCES

1. Berenson, A. B., Rahman, M., & Wilkinson, G. (2009). Racial difference in the correlates of bone mineral content/density and age at peak among reproductive-aged women. *Osteopor Int, 20*(8), 1439–1449.
2. Black, D. M., & Rosen, C. J. (2016). Postmenopausal osteoporosis. *N Engl J Med, 374*(3), 254–262.
3. Browne, K. L., & Merrill, E. (2015). Musculoskeletal management matters: Principles of assessment and triage for the nurse practitioner. *J Nurse Pract, 11*(10), 929–939.
4. D'Arcy, Y., Kraus, S., Clair, A., et al. (2016). Fibromyalgia: Timely diagnosis and treatment options. *Nurse Pract, 41*(9), 37–43.
5. Reference deleted in proofs.
6. Deyo, R. A., & Mirza, S. K. (2016). Herniated lumbar intervertebral disk. *N Engl J Med, 374*(18), 1763–1772.
7. Durham, C. O., Fowler, T., Donato, A., et al. (2015). Pain management in patients with rheumatoid arthritis. *Nurse Pract, 40*(5), 38–45.
8. Gourlay, M. L., Fine, J. P., Preisser, J. S., et al. (2012). Bone-density testing interval and transition to osteoporosis in older women. *N Engl J Med, 366*(3), 225–233.
9. Harding, M. (2016). An update on gout for primary care providers. *Nurse Pract, 41*(4), 14–22.
10. Hresko, M. T. (2013). Idiopathic scoliosis in adolescents. *N Engl J Med, 368*(9), 834–841.
11. Hunter, D. J. (2015). Viscosupplementation for osteoarthritis of the knee. *N Engl J Med, 372*, 1040–1047.
12. Hwang, P. W., & Braun, K. L. (2015). The effectiveness of dance interventions to improve older adults' health. *Alt Thera, 21*(5), 64–70.
13. Janzen, K., & Peters-Watral, B. (2016). Treating co-occurring chronic low back pain & generalized anxiety disorder. *Nurse Pract, 41*(1), 12–19.
14. Johnson, R. E., Haas, K., Lindow, K., et al. (2014). Plantar fasciitis: What is the diagnosis and treatment? *Orthop Nurs, 33*(4), 198–204.
15. Khan, M. S., Shuaib, W., Evans, D. D., et al. (2014). Evidence-based practice: Best imaging practice in musculoskeletal disorders. *J Trauma Nurs, 21*(4), 170–181.
16. Kling, J. M., Clarke, B. L., & Sandhu, N. P. (2014). Osteoporosis prevention, screening, and treatment. *J Womens Health, 23*(7), 563–572.
17. Lipman, R., & John, R. M. (2015). A review of knee pain in adolescent females. *Nurse Pract, 40*(7), 28–36.
18. Lu, J., Shin, Y., Yen, M., et al. (2016). Peak bone mass and patterns of change in total bone mineral density and bone mineral contents from childhood into young adulthood. *J Clin Densitom, 19*(2), 180–191.
19. McGee, S. (2018). *Evidence-based physical diagnosis* (4th ed.). St. Louis: Saunders.
20. Menzies, V. (2016). Fibromyalgia syndrome: Current considerations in symptom management. *Am J Nurs, 116*(1), 24.
21. Metzger, R. L. (2016). Evidence-based practice guidelines for the diagnosis and treatment of lumbar spinal conditions. *Nurse Pract, 41*(12), 30–37.
22. Moyer, V. A. (2012). Prevention of falls in community-dwelling older adults. *Ann Intern Med, 157*(3), 197–204.
23. Muir, J. M., Ye, C., Bhandari, M., et al. (2013). The effect of regular physical activity on bone mineral density in post-menopausal women aged 75 and over. *BMC Musculoskelet Disord, 14*, 253–261.
24. Nam, H. S., Kweon, S. S., Choi, J. S., et al. (2013). Racial/ethnic differences in bone mineral density among older women. *J Bone Mineral Metabol, 31*(2), 190–198.
25. National Council on Aging (NCOA). *Take control of your health: 6 steps to prevent a fall.* https://www.ncoa.org/healthy-aging?falls-prevention.
26. Ropper, A. H., & Zafonte, R. D. (2015). Sciatica. *N Engl J Med, 372*(13), 1240–1248.
27. Saccomano, S. J., & Ferrara, L. R. (2015). Treatment and prevention of gout. *Nurse Pract, 40*(8), 24–30.
28. Schraeder, T. L., Terek, R. M., & Smith, C. C. (2010). Clinical evaluation of the knee. *N Engl J Med, 363*(4).
29. Seco, J., Abecia, L. C., Echevarria, E., et al. (2013). A long-term physical activity training program increases strength and flexibility, and improves balance in older adults. *Rehabil Nurs, 38*(1), 37–47.
30. Shuler, F. D., Conjeski, J. M., & Hamilton, R. L. (2011). Incorporating the WHO FRAX assessment tool into nursing practice. *Am J Nurs, 111*(8), 59–62.
31. Taurog, J. D., Chhabra, A., & Colbert, A. A. (2016). Ankylosing spondylitis and axial spondyloarthritis. *N Engl J Med, 374*(26), 2563–2574.
32. U.S. Preventive Services Task Force. (2005). Screening for idiopathic scoliosis for adolescents. *Am Fam Physician, 71*, 1975–1976.
33. U.S. Preventive Services Task Force. (2011). Screening for osteoporosis. *Ann Intern Med, 154*(5), 356–364.
34. Vogel, D., Parsons, C., Godfrey, K., et al. (2016). Greater access to fast-food outlets is associated with poorer bone health in young children. *Osteoporos Int, 27*, 1011–1019.
35. World Health Organization (WHO). *FRAX calculation tool.* http://shef.ac.uk/FRAX/tool.aspx?country=9.
36. Wosje, K. S., Khoury, P. R., Claytor, R. P., et al. (2010). Dietary patterns associated with fat and bone mass in young children. *Am J Clin Nutr, 92*(2), 294–303.
37. Zychowicz, M. E. (2013). A closer look at hand and wrist complaints. *Nurse Pract, 38*(3), 46–53.

Neurologic System

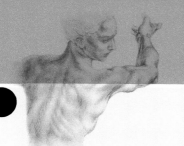

STRUCTURE AND FUNCTION

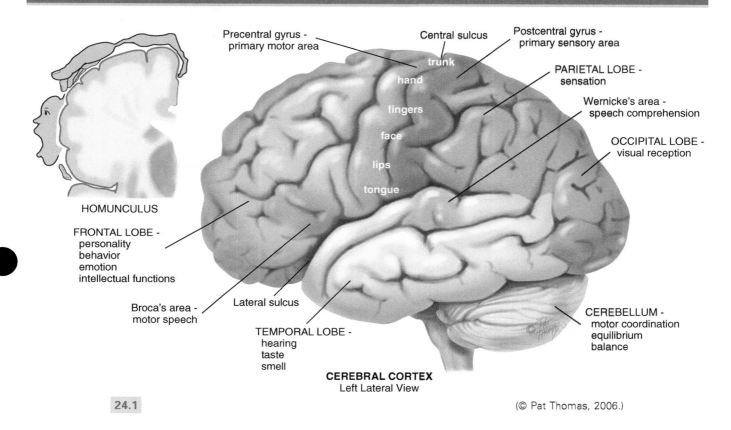

Precentral gyrus - primary motor area

Central sulcus

Postcentral gyrus - primary sensory area

trunk

hand

fingers

face

lips

tongue

PARIETAL LOBE - sensation

Wernicke's area - speech comprehension

OCCIPITAL LOBE - visual reception

HOMUNCULUS

FRONTAL LOBE - personality behavior emotion intellectual functions

Broca's area - motor speech

Lateral sulcus

TEMPORAL LOBE - hearing taste smell

CEREBELLUM - motor coordination equilibrium balance

CEREBRAL CORTEX
Left Lateral View

24.1

(© Pat Thomas, 2006.)

The nervous system can be divided into two parts: central and peripheral. The **central nervous system** (CNS) includes the brain and spinal cord. The **peripheral nervous system** includes all the nerve fibers *outside* the brain and spinal cord: the 12 pairs of cranial nerves, the 31 pairs of spinal nerves, and all their branches. The peripheral nervous system carries sensory (**a**fferent) messages *to* the CNS from sensory receptors, motor (**e**fferent) messages *from* the CNS out to muscles and glands, and autonomic messages that govern the internal organs and blood vessels.

THE CENTRAL NERVOUS SYSTEM

Cerebral Cortex. The cerebral cortex is the outer layer of nerve cell bodies; it looks like "gray matter" because it lacks myelin. Myelin is the white insulation on the axon that increases the conduction velocity of nerve impulses.

The cerebral cortex is the center for a human's highest functions, governing thought, memory, reasoning, sensation, and voluntary movement (Fig. 24.1). Each half of the cerebrum is a **hemisphere;** the left hemisphere is dominant in most (95%) people, including those who are left-handed.

Each hemisphere is divided into four **lobes:** frontal, parietal, temporal, and occipital. The lobes have certain areas that mediate specific functions.

- The **frontal** lobe has areas concerned with personality, behavior, emotions, and intellectual function.
- The precentral gyrus of the frontal lobe initiates voluntary movement.
- The **parietal** lobe's postcentral gyrus is the primary center for sensation.
- The **occipital** lobe is the primary visual receptor center.
- The **temporal** lobe behind the ear has the primary

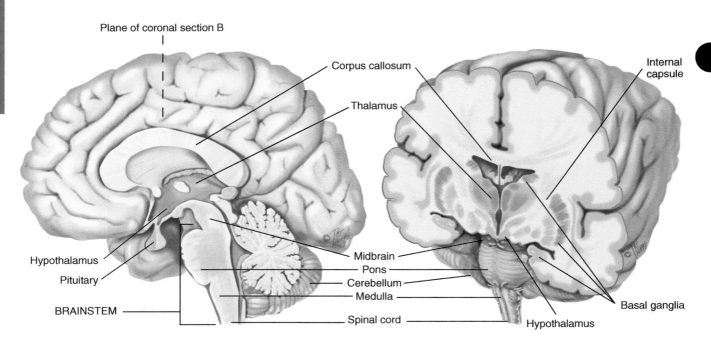

Plane of coronal section B

Corpus callosum

Thalamus

Internal capsule

Hypothalamus

Pituitary

BRAINSTEM

Midbrain
Pons
Cerebellum
Medulla
Spinal cord

Basal ganglia

Hypothalamus

A. Medial view of right hemisphere

B. Coronal section

COMPONENTS OF THE CENTRAL NERVOUS SYSTEM

24.2

(© Pat Thomas, 2006.)

auditory reception center, with functions of hearing, taste, and smell.

- **Wernicke's area** in the temporal lobe is associated with language comprehension. When damaged in the person's dominant hemisphere, *receptive aphasia* results. The person hears sound, but it has no meaning, like hearing a foreign language.
- **Broca's area** in the frontal lobe mediates motor speech. When injured in the dominant hemisphere, *expressive aphasia* results; the person cannot talk. The person can understand language and knows what he or she wants to say but can produce only a garbled sound.

Damage to any of these specific cortical areas produces a corresponding loss of function: motor weakness, paralysis, loss of sensation, or impaired ability to understand and process language. Damage occurs when the highly specialized neurologic cells are deprived of their blood supply such as when a cerebral artery becomes occluded (ischemic stroke) or when vascular bleeding (hemorrhagic stroke) occurs.

Basal Ganglia. The basal ganglia are large bands of gray matter buried deep within the two cerebral hemispheres that form the subcortical-associated motor system (the extrapyramidal system) (Fig. 24.2). They help to initiate and coordinate movement and control automatic associated movements of the body (e.g., the arm swing alternating with the legs during walking).

Thalamus. The thalamus is the main relay station where the sensory pathways of the spinal cord, cerebellum, basal

ganglia, and brainstem form **synapses** (sites of contact between two neurons) on their way to the cerebral cortex. It is an integrating center with connections that are crucial to human emotion and creativity.

Hypothalamus. The hypothalamus is a major respiratory center with basic vital functions: temperature, appetite, sex drive, heart rate, and blood pressure (BP) control; sleep center; anterior and posterior pituitary gland regulator; and coordinator of autonomic nervous system activity and stress response.

Cerebellum. The cerebellum is a coiled structure located under the occipital lobe that is concerned with motor coordination of voluntary movements, equilibrium (i.e., the postural balance of the body), and muscle tone. It does not initiate movement but coordinates and smooths it (e.g., the complex and quick coordination of many different muscles needed in playing the piano, swimming, or juggling). It is like the "automatic pilot" on an airplane in that it adjusts and corrects the voluntary movements but operates entirely below the conscious level.

Brainstem. The brainstem is the central core of the brain consisting of mostly nerve fibers. Cranial nerves III through XII originate from nuclei in the brainstem. It has three areas:

1. **Midbrain**—The most anterior part of the brainstem that still has the basic tubular structure of the spinal cord. It merges into the thalamus and hypothalamus. It contains many motor neurons and tracts.
2. **Pons**—The enlarged area containing ascending sensory and descending motor tracts. It has two respiratory

centers (pneumotaxic and apneustic) that coordinate with the main respiratory center in the medulla.

3. **Medulla**—The continuation of the spinal cord in the brain that contains all ascending and descending fiber tracts. It has vital autonomic centers (respiration, heart, gastrointestinal function) and nuclei for cranial nerves VIII through XII. Pyramidal decussation (crossing of the motor fibers) occurs here (see p. 629).

Spinal Cord. The spinal cord is the long, cylindric structure of nervous tissue about as big around as your little finger. It occupies the upper 2/3 of the vertebral canal from the medulla to lumbar vertebrae L_1-L_2. Its white matter is bundles of myelinated axons that form the main highway for ascending and descending fiber tracts that connect the brain to the spinal nerves. It mediates reflexes of posture control, urination, and pain response. Its nerve cell bodies, or gray matter, are arranged in a butterfly shape with anterior and posterior "horns."

The vertebral canal continues down beyond the spinal cord for several inches. The lumbar cistern is inside this space and is the favored spot to withdraw samples of cerebrospinal fluid (CSF).

Pathways of the CNS

Crossed representation is a notable feature of the nerve tracts; the *left* cerebral cortex receives sensory information from and controls motor function to the *right* side of the body, whereas *the right* cerebral cortex likewise interacts with the *left* side of the body. Knowledge of where the fibers cross the midline helps you interpret clinical findings.

Sensory Pathways

Millions of sensory receptors are embroidered into the skin, mucous membranes, muscles, tendons, and viscera. They monitor conscious sensation, internal organ functions, body position, and reflexes. Sensation travels in the afferent fibers in the peripheral nerve, through the posterior (dorsal) root, and into the spinal cord. There it may take one of two routes: the anterolateral (or spinothalamic) tract or the posterior (or dorsal) columns (Fig. 24.3).

Anterolateral Tract. The anterolateral tract (formerly spinothalamic) contains sensory fibers that transmit the sensations of pain, temperature, itch, and crude touch (i.e.,

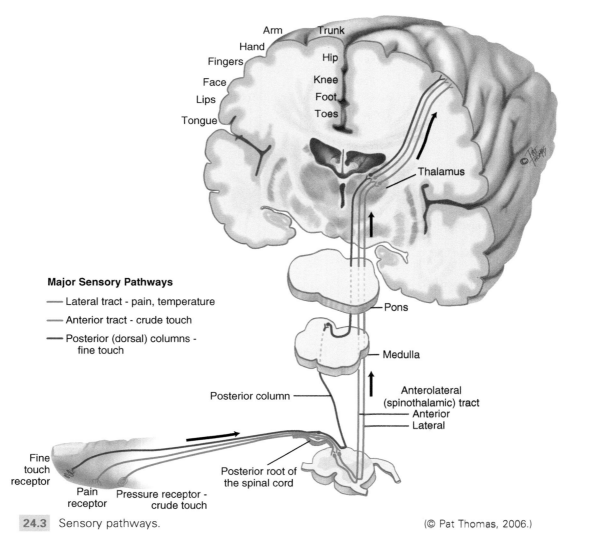

Arm   Trunk
Hand
Fingers   Hip
Face   Knee
Lips   Foot
Tongue   Toes

Thalamus

Major Sensory Pathways

—— Lateral tract - pain, temperature

—— Anterior tract - crude touch

—— Posterior (dorsal) columns -
    fine touch

Pons

Medulla

Posterior column

Anterolateral
(spinothalamic) tract
Anterior
Lateral

Fine
touch
receptor

Pain
receptor

Pressure receptor -
crude touch

Posterior root of
the spinal cord

24.3   Sensory pathways.   (© Pat Thomas, 2006.)

not precisely localized). The fibers enter the dorsal root of the spinal cord and synapse with a second sensory neuron. The second-order neuron fibers cross directly to the opposite side and ascend up the anterolateral tract to the thalamus. Fibers carrying pain and temperature sensations ascend the more lateral tract, whereas those of crude touch form the more anterior tract. At the thalamus the fibers synapse with a third sensory neuron, which carries the message to the sensory cortex for full interpretation.

Posterior (Dorsal) Columns. These fibers conduct the sensations of position, vibration, and finely localized touch.

- **Position** (proprioception)—Without looking you know where your body parts are in space and in relation to one another.
- **Vibration**—You can feel vibrating objects.
- **Finely localized touch** (stereognosis)—Without looking you can identify familiar objects by touch.

These fibers enter the dorsal root and proceed immediately up the same side of the spinal cord to the brainstem. At the medulla they synapse with a second sensory neuron and then cross. They travel to the **thalamus,** synapse again, and proceed to the sensory cortex, which localizes the sensation and makes full discrimination.

The sensory cortex is arranged in a specific pattern forming a corresponding "map" of the body (see the homunculus in Fig. 24.1). Pain in the right hand is perceived at its specific spot on the left cortex map. Some organs are absent from the brain map such as the heart, liver, or spleen. You know you have one but you have no "felt image" of it. Pain originating in these organs is referred because no felt image exists in which to have pain. Pain is felt "by proxy" by another body part that does have a felt image. For example, pain in the heart is referred to the chest, shoulder, and left arm, which were its neighbors in fetal development. Pain originating in the spleen is felt on the top of the left shoulder.

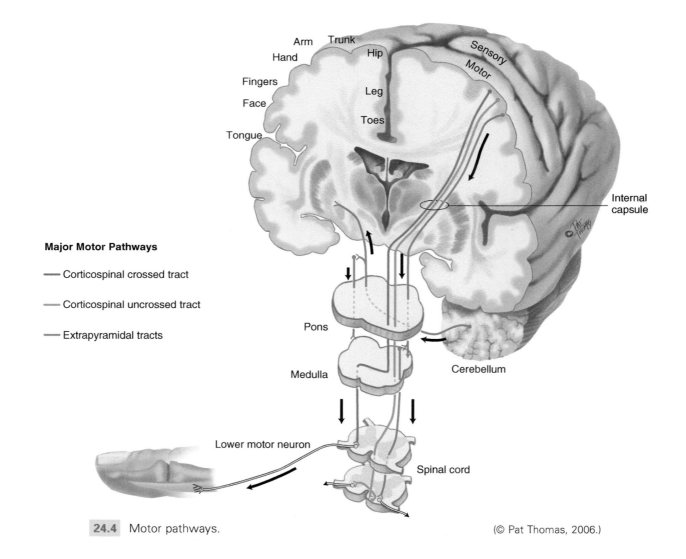

Major Motor Pathways

—— Corticospinal crossed tract

—— Corticospinal uncrossed tract

—— Extrapyramidal tracts

24.4   Motor pathways.   (© Pat Thomas, 2006.)

Motor Pathways

Corticospinal or Pyramidal Tract (Fig. 24.4). The area has been named *pyramidal* because it originates in pyramidal-shaped cells in the motor cortex. Motor nerve fibers originate in the motor cortex and travel to the brainstem, where they cross to the opposite or contralateral side *(pyramidal decussation)* and then pass down in the lateral column of the spinal cord. At each cord level they synapse with a lower motor neuron contained in the anterior horn of the spinal cord. Ten percent of corticospinal fibers do not cross, and these descend in the anterior column of the spinal cord. Corticospinal fibers mediate voluntary movement, particularly very skilled, discrete, purposeful movements such as writing.

The corticospinal tract is a newer, "higher" motor system that permits humans to have very skilled and purposeful movements. The origin of the tract in the motor cortex is arranged in a specific pattern called *somatotopic organization.* It is another body map, this one of a person, or *homunculus,* hanging "upside down" (see Fig. 24.1). Body parts are not equally represented on the map, and the homunculus looks distorted. To use political terms, it is more like an electoral map than a geographic map. That is, body parts with movements that are relatively more important to humans (e.g., the hand) occupy proportionally more space on the brain map.

Extrapyramidal Tracts. The extrapyramidal tracts include all the motor nerve fibers originating in the motor cortex, basal ganglia, brainstem, and spinal cord that are *outside* the pyramidal tract. This is a phylogenetically older, "lower," more primitive motor system. These subcortical motor fibers maintain muscle tone and control body movements, especially gross automatic movements such as walking.

Cerebellar System. This complex motor system coordinates movement, maintains equilibrium, and helps maintain posture. The cerebellum receives information about the position of muscles and joints, the equilibrium of the body, and what kind of motor messages are being sent from the cortex to the muscles. The information is integrated, and the cerebellum uses feedback pathways to exert its control back on the cortex or down to lower motor neurons in the spinal cord. This entire process occurs on a subconscious level.

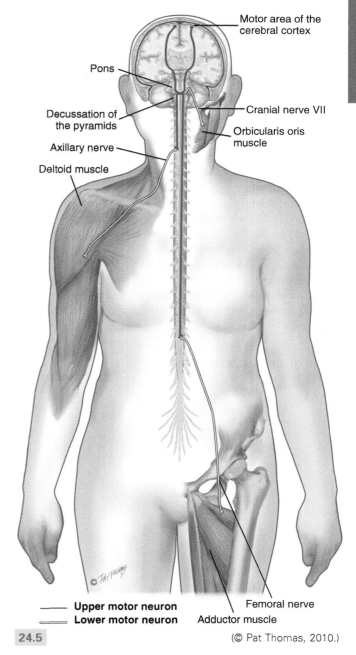

Upper motor neuron
Lower motor neuron

Motor area of the cerebral cortex
Pons
Decussation of the pyramids
Axillary nerve
Deltoid muscle
Cranial nerve VII
Orbicularis oris muscle
Femoral nerve
Adductor muscle

24.5
(© Pat Thomas, 2010.)

Upper and Lower Motor Neurons

Upper motor neurons (UMNs) are a complex of all the descending motor fibers that can influence or modify the lower motor neurons. They are located completely within the CNS. The UMNs convey impulses from motor areas of the cerebral cortex to the lower motor neurons in the anterior horn cells of the spinal cord (Fig. 24.5). Examples of UMNs are corticospinal, corticobulbar, and extrapyramidal tracts. Examples of UMN diseases are stroke, cerebral palsy, and multiple sclerosis.

Lower motor neurons (LMNs) are located mostly in the peripheral nervous system. The cell body of the LMN is located in the anterior gray column of the spinal cord, but the nerve fiber extends from here to the muscle. The LMN is the "final common pathway" because it funnels many neural signals here and provides the final direct contact with the muscles. Any movement must be translated into action by LMN fibers. Examples of LMNs are cranial nerves and spinal nerves of the peripheral nervous system. Examples of LMN diseases are Bell palsy in the face (cranial nerve VII), spinal cord lesions, and poliomyelitis.

Structure and Function

THE PERIPHERAL NERVOUS SYSTEM

A **nerve** is a bundle of fibers *outside* the CNS. The peripheral nerves carry input to the CNS via their sensory afferent fibers and deliver output from the CNS via the efferent fibers.

Reflex Arc

Reflexes are basic defense mechanisms of the nervous system. They are involuntary, operating below the level of conscious control and permitting a quick reaction to potentially painful or damaging situations. Reflexes also help the body maintain balance and appropriate muscle tone. There are 3 types of reflexes: (1) **Stretch or/deep tendon reflexes** (myotatic), e.g., patellar (or knee jerk) (Fig. 24.6); (2) **superficial (cutaneous)**, e.g., plantar reflex; (3) **visceral** (organic), e.g., pupillary response to light and accommodation.

The fibers that mediate the reflex are carried by a specific spinal nerve. In the simplest reflex tapping the tendon stretches the muscle spindles in the muscle, which activates

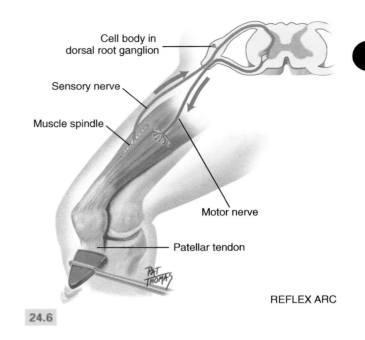

24.6 REFLEX ARC

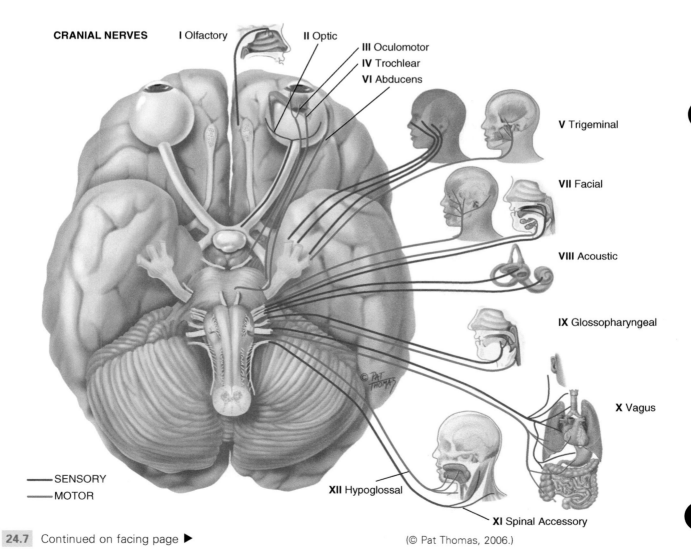

24.7 Continued on facing page ▶

(© Pat Thomas, 2006.)

the sensory afferent nerve. The sensory afferent fibers carry the message from the receptor and travel through the dorsal root into the spinal cord (see Fig. 24.6). They synapse directly in the cord with the motor neuron in the anterior horn. Motor efferent fibers leave via the ventral root and travel to the muscle, stimulating a sudden contraction.

The deep tendon (myotatic, or stretch) reflex has 5 components: (1) an intact sensory nerve (afferent), (2) a functional synapse in the cord, (3) an intact motor nerve fiber (efferent), (4) the neuromuscular junction, and (5) a competent muscle.

Cranial Nerves

Cranial nerves are LMNs that enter and exit the brain rather than the spinal cord (Fig. 24.7). Cranial nerves I and II extend from the cerebrum; cranial nerves III through XII extend from the midbrain and brainstem. The 12 pairs of cranial nerves supply primarily the head and neck, except the vagus nerve (Lat. *vagus,* or wanderer, as in "vagabond"), which travels to the heart, respiratory muscles, stomach, and gallbladder.

Spinal Nerves

The 31 pairs of **spinal nerves** arise from the length of the spinal cord and supply the rest of the body (Fig. 24.8). They are named for the region of the spine from which they exit:

8 cervical, 12 thoracic, 5 lumbar, 5 sacral, and 1 coccygeal. They are "mixed" nerves because they contain both sensory and motor fibers. The nerves enter and exit the cord through roots—sensory afferent fibers through the posterior or dorsal roots and motor efferent fibers through the anterior or ventral roots.

The nerves exit the spinal cord in an orderly ladder. Each nerve innervates a particular segment of the body. **Dermal segmentation** is the cutaneous distribution of the various spinal nerves.

A **dermatome** is a circumscribed skin area that is supplied mainly from one spinal cord segment through a particular spinal nerve (see Fig. 24.8). The dermatomes overlap, which is a form of biologic insurance, i.e., if one nerve is severed, most of the sensations can be transmitted by the one above and the one below. Do not attempt to memorize all dermatome segments; just focus on the following as useful landmarks:

- The **thumb, middle finger,** and **fifth finger** are each in the dermatomes of C_6, C_7, and C_8.
- The **axilla** is at the level of T_1.
- The **nipple** is at the level of T_4.
- The **umbilicus** is at the level of T_{10}.
- The **groin** is in the region of L_1.
- The **knee** is at the level of L_4.

Cranial Nerve	Type	Function
I: Olfactory	Sensory	Smell
II: Optic	Sensory	Vision
III: Oculomotor	Mixed*	Motor—most extraocular muscle movement, opening of eyelids
		Parasympathetic—pupil constriction, lens shape
IV: Trochlear	Motor	Down and inward movement of eye
V: Trigeminal	Mixed	Motor—muscles of mastication
		Sensory—sensation of face and scalp, cornea, mucous membranes of mouth and nose
VI: Abducens	Motor	Lateral movement of eye
VII: Facial	Mixed	Motor—facial muscles, close eye, labial speech, close mouth
		Sensory—taste (sweet, salty, sour, bitter) on anterior two thirds of tongue
		Parasympathetic—saliva and tear secretion
VIII: Acoustic	Sensory	Hearing and equilibrium
IX: Glossopharyngeal	Mixed	Motor—pharynx (phonation and swallowing)
		Sensory—taste on posterior one third of tongue, pharynx (gag reflex)
		Parasympathetic—parotid gland, carotid reflex
X: Vagus	Mixed	Motor—pharynx and larynx (talking and swallowing)
		Sensory—general sensation from carotid body, carotid sinus, pharynx, viscera
		Parasympathetic—carotid reflex
XI: Spinal accessory	Motor	Movement of trapezius and sternomastoid muscles
XII: Hypoglossal	Motor	Movement of tongue

Mixed refers to a nerve carrying a combination of fibers: motor + sensory; motor + parasympathetic; or motor + sensory + parasympathetic.

24.7, cont'd

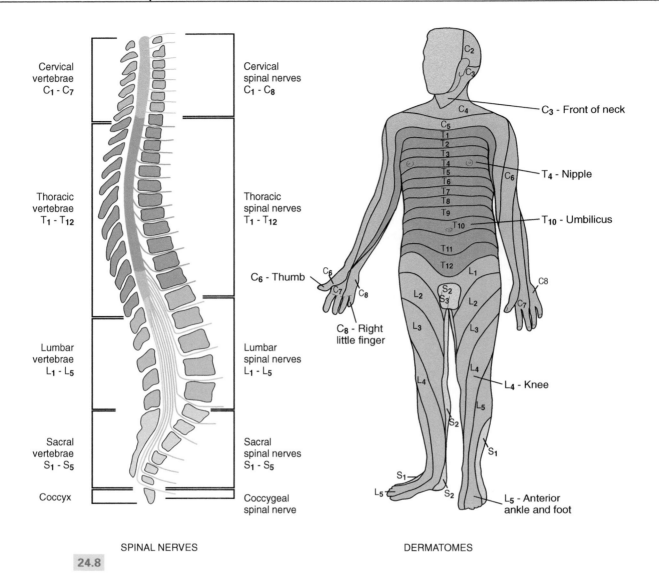

SPINAL NERVES

DERMATOMES

24.8

Autonomic Nervous System

The peripheral nervous system is composed of cranial nerves and spinal nerves. These nerves carry fibers that can be divided functionally into two parts: somatic and autonomic. The somatic fibers innervate the skeletal (voluntary) muscles; the autonomic fibers innervate smooth (involuntary) muscles, cardiac muscle, and glands. The autonomic system mediates unconscious activity. Although a description of the autonomic system is beyond the scope of this book, its overall function is to maintain homeostasis of the body.

❖ DEVELOPMENTAL COMPETENCE

Infants

The neurologic system is not completely developed at birth. Motor activity in the newborn is under the control of the spinal cord and medulla. Very little cortical control exists, and the neurons are not yet myelinated. Movements are directed primarily by primitive reflexes. As the cerebral cortex develops during the first year, it inhibits these reflexes, and they disappear at predictable times. Persistence of the primitive reflexes is an indication of CNS dysfunction.

The infant's sensory and motor development proceeds along with the gradual acquisition of myelin because myelin is needed to conduct most impulses. The process of myelinization follows a cephalocaudal and proximodistal order (head, then neck, trunk, and out to extremities). This is just the order in which we observe the infant gaining motor control (lifts head, lifts head and shoulders, rolls over, moves whole arm, uses hands, walks). As the milestones are achieved, each is more complex and coordinated. Milestones occur in an orderly sequence, although the exact age of occurrence may vary.

Sensation also is rudimentary at birth. The newborn needs a strong stimulus and then responds by crying and with whole body movements. As myelinization develops, the infant is able to localize the stimulus more precisely and make a more accurate motor response.

The Aging Adult

The aging process causes a general atrophy with a steady loss of neuron structure in the brain and spinal cord. This causes a decrease in weight and volume with a thinning of the cerebral cortex, reduced subcortical brain structures, and expansion of the ventricles.[9] Neuron loss leads many people older than 65 years to show signs that in the younger adult would be considered abnormal, such as general loss of muscle bulk; loss of muscle tone in the face, in the neck, and around the spine; decreased muscle strength; impaired fine coordination and agility; loss of vibratory sense at the ankle; decreased or absent Achilles reflex; loss of position sense at the big toe; pupillary miosis; irregular pupil shape; and decreased pupillary reflexes.

Alzheimer Disease (AD) is a slow-onset dementia affecting millions of people in the United States. Because AD is characterized as brain atrophy that may progress for years before symptoms of dementia become apparent, it has been difficult to distinguish age-related memory loss (e.g., lost car keys) from AD memory loss (e.g., forgetting recently learned information). Reductions in brain volume are normal in healthy aging, but more increased atrophy occurs with AD.[9] See Chapter 5, *Mental Status Assessment,* for more content on AD; also see Table 24.1, p. 670, to compare the warning signs of AD with changes present in normal aging.

The velocity of nerve conduction decreases between 5% and 10% with aging, making the reaction time slower in some older people. An increased delay at the synapse also occurs, so the impulse takes longer to travel. As a result, touch and pain sensation, taste, and smell may be diminished.

The motor system may show a general slowing of movement. Muscle strength and agility decrease. A generalized decrease occurs in muscle bulk, which is most apparent in the dorsal hand muscles. Muscle tremors may occur in the hands, head, and jaw, along with possible repetitive facial grimacing (dyskinesias).

Aging is accompanied by a progressive decrease in cerebral blood flow and oxygen consumption. In some people this causes dizziness and a loss of balance with position change. These people need to be taught to get up slowly. Otherwise they have an increased risk for falls and resulting injuries.[23] In addition, older people may forget they fell, which makes it hard to diagnose the cause of the injury.

When they are in good health, aging people walk about as well as they did during their middle and younger years, except more slowly and deliberately. Some survey the ground for obstacles or uneven terrain. Some show a hesitation and a slightly wayward path.

CULTURE AND GENETICS

Stroke is an interruption of blood supply to the brain and is the 5th most common cause of death in the United States.[18] There is racial/ethnic disparity here because 4.6% of American Indian/Alaska natives have had a stroke, 4.6% of other races as multiracial people, 4% of African Americans, 2.3% of Hispanics, 2.5% of whites, and only 1.3% of Asian/Pacific Islanders. Further, African Americans, American Indian/Alaska natives (AI/AN), and Asian/Pacific Islanders die from stroke at younger ages than do whites.[18]

Evidence shows that rates of ischemic stroke have declined in the past 2 decades in whites and in Medicare beneficiaries aged >65 years. This decline in stroke rates coincides with a significant increase in the use of medications that lower stroke risk; the use of statin drugs and antihypertensive drugs has greatly increased in the general population since 1992.[18] More work must be done to screen for hyperlipidemia and high BP and to make evidence-proven medications available to all racial and ethnic groups.

There is geographic disparity too; 8 states with high stroke mortality are concentrated in the U.S. southeast region, called the *stroke belt.* Within the stroke belt even higher stroke mortality occurs in the coastal plain of North Carolina, South Carolina, and Georgia, now called the *buckle* region.[18] Stroke mortality is approximately 20% higher in the stroke belt and approximately 40% higher in the stroke buckle than in the rest of the United States. This disparity is due partly to an increased incidence of traditional risk factors (high BP, diabetes, atrial fibrillation, hyperlipidemia, smoking, physical inactivity) in these states and partly to a greater knowledge deficit of the stroke warning signs.[18] However, another factor is geographic access to a Primary Stroke Center (PSC) within 60 minutes of calling 911 by ground transport. Time is crucial for stroke intervention, with an estimated 1.9 million neurons dying every minute during an acute stroke.[19] Access to PSCs is worse in the stroke belt and in rural areas. In major cities 87% of people had ≤60-minute access, 59% in minor cities, 9% in suburbs, and only 1% in rural regions.[19]

In the age group of 45 to 64 years, African Americans have 2 to 3 times the risk of stroke as whites. About 40% of this risk is due to traditional stroke risk factors, especially high systolic BP.[18] African Americans have a triple threat here: 1) more likely to have high BP; 2) less likely to have their high BP controlled; and 3) suboptimal control; this combination yields a stroke risk 3 times higher in African Americans than in whites.[10] Metabolic syndrome (high blood glucose, dyslipidemia, obesity, hypertension) is 40% to 46% more prevalent among Mexican Americans than among non–Mexican-American whites and blacks; this is more evident in men than in women.[18] These symptoms increase the risk for stroke. There also are disparities in access to care regarding stroke symptoms. Hispanic and Asian men and women are much less likely to use emergency medical services (EMS) transport to a hospital than are their white counterparts, and black women are less likely to use EMS than are white women.[17] Thus these groups experience longer delays before brain imaging and thrombolysis therapy.

Evidence from 188 countries across the globe over 23 years of data collection shows that 90% of the stroke burden was due to modifiable risk factors, including behavioral risk factors (smoking, poor diet, low physical activity), metabolic factors (high systolic BP, high BMI, high fasting glucose, high total cholesterol), and environmental factors (air pollution, lead exposure).[8] Study authors post that controlling behavioral and metabolic risk factors could stop over three-quarters of global stroke burden. Air pollution (especially in low- and middle-income countries) has emerged as a significant risk factor and should be a main priority.[8]

SUBJECTIVE DATA

1. Headache	6. Weakness	11. Patient-centered care
2. Head injury	7. Incoordination	12. Environmental/occupational
3. Dizziness/vertigo	8. Numbness or tingling	hazards
4. Seizures	9. Difficulty swallowing	
5. Tremors	10. Difficulty speaking	

Examiner Asks	Rationale
1. **Headache.** Any unusually frequent or severe headaches? • When did they start? How often do they occur? • Where in your head do you feel the headaches? Do they seem to be associated with anything? (Headache history is discussed in Chapter 14.)	A patient who says, "This is the worst headache of my life," needs emergency referral to screen possible stroke.
2. **Head injury.** Ever had any **head injury?** Please describe. • What part of your head was hit? • Did you have a loss of consciousness? For how long? • Do you remember details of the event?	**Concussion** comes from a direct blow that causes rotation of the brain inside the skull and shear injury.[5]
3. **Dizziness/vertigo.** Ever feel light-headed, a swimming sensation, like feeling faint? • When have you noticed this? How often does it occur? Does it occur with activity, change in position? • Do you ever feel a sensation called **vertigo,** a rotational spinning sensation? (NOTE: Distinguish vertigo from dizziness.) Do you feel as if the room spins (objective vertigo)? Or do you feel that you are spinning (subjective vertigo)? Did this come on suddenly or gradually?	**Syncope** is a sudden loss of strength, a temporary loss of consciousness (a faint) caused by lack of cerebral blood flow, e.g., low BP. True **vertigo** is rotational spinning caused by neurologic disease in the vestibular apparatus in the ear or the vestibular nuclei in the brainstem.
4. **Seizures.** Ever had convulsions? When did they start? How often do they occur? • Course and duration—When a seizure starts, do you have any warning sign? What type of sign? • Motor activity—Where in your body do the seizures begin? Do they travel through your body? On one side or both? Does your muscle tone seem tense or limp? • Any associated signs—Color change in face or lips, loss of consciousness (for how long), automatisms (eyelid fluttering, eye rolling, lip smacking), incontinence? • Postictal phase—After the seizure, are you told that you spent time sleeping or had any confusion? Do you have weakness, headache, or muscle ache?	**Seizures** occur with epilepsy, a paroxysmal disease characterized by altered or loss of consciousness, involuntary muscle movements, and sensory disturbances. *Aura* is a subjective sensation that precedes a seizure; it could be auditory, visual, or motor.

Examiner Asks	Rationale

- Precipitating factors—Does anything seem to bring on the seizures: activity, discontinuing medication, fatigue, stress?
- Do you take any medication?
- Coping strategies—How have the seizures affected daily life, occupation?

5. **Tremors.** Any shakes or **tremors** in the hands or face? When did they start?
   - Do they seem to grow worse with anxiety, intention, or rest?
   - Are they relieved with rest, activity, alcohol? Do they affect daily activities?

Tremor is an involuntary shaking, vibrating, or trembling (see Table 24.4, Abnormalities in Muscle Movement, p. 673).

6. **Weakness.** Any **weakness** or problem moving any body part? Is it generalized or local? Does weakness occur with any particular movement (e.g., with proximal or large muscle weakness, it is hard to get up out of a chair or reach for an object; with distal or small muscle weakness, it is hard to open a jar, write, use scissors, or walk without tripping)?

Paresis is a partial or incomplete paralysis. *Paralysis* is a total loss of motor function caused by a lesion in the neurologic or muscular system or loss of sensory innervation.

7. **Incoordination.** Any problem with **coordination?** Any problem with balance when walking? Do you list to one side? Any falling? Which way? Do your legs seem to give way? Any clumsy movement?

Dysmetria is the inability to control the distance, power, and speed of a muscular action.

8. **Numbness or tingling.** Any **numbness or tingling** in any body part? Does it feel like pins and needles? When did it start? Where do you feel it? Does it occur with activity?

Paresthesia is an abnormal sensation (e.g., burning, tingling).

9. **Difficulty swallowing.** Any problem **swallowing?** Occur with solids or liquids? Have you experienced excessive saliva, drooling?

10. **Difficulty speaking.** Any problem **speaking:** with forming words or with saying what you intended to say? When did you first notice this? How long did it last?

Dysarthria is difficulty forming words; *dysphasia* is difficulty with language comprehension or expression (see Table 5.2, p. 76).

11. **Patient-centered care. Past history** of stroke, spinal cord injury, meningitis or encephalitis, congenital defect, or alcohol use problem?

12. **Environmental/occupational hazards.** Are you exposed to any environmental/occupational hazards: insecticides, organic solvents, lead?
    - Are you taking any medications now?
    - How much alcohol do you drink? Each week? Each day?
    - How about other mood-altering drugs: marijuana, cocaine, barbiturates, tranquilizers?

Review anticonvulsants and antitremor, antivertigo, and pain medication. Review moderate to heavy alcohol use.

Additional History for Infants and Children

1. Did the baby's mother have any health problems during the pregnancy: any infections or illnesses, medications taken, toxemia, hypertension, alcohol or drug use, diabetes?

Prenatal history may affect infant's neurologic development.

2. Please tell me about this baby's birth. Was the baby at term or premature? Birth weight?
   - Any birth trauma? Did the baby breathe immediately?
   - Were you told the baby's Apgar scores?
   - Any congenital defects?

Examiner Asks	Rationale

3. Reflexes—What have you noticed about the baby's behavior? Do sucking and swallowing seem coordinated? When you touch the cheek, does the baby turn his or her head toward touch? Does the baby startle with a loud noise or shaking of crib? Does the baby grasp your finger?

4. Does the child seem to have any problem with balance? Have you noted any unexplained falling, clumsy or unsteady gait, progressive muscular weakness, problem with going up or down stairs, problem with getting up from lying position?

If it occurs, may not be noticed until starts to walk in late infancy.
Screens for muscular dystrophy.

5. Has this child had any seizures? Please describe. Did the seizure occur with a high fever? Did any loss of consciousness occur—how long? How many seizures occurred with this same illness (if occurred with high fever)?

Seizures may occur with high fever in infants and toddlers. Or they may be a sign of neurologic disease.

6. Did this child's motor or developmental milestones seem to come at about the right age? Seem to be growing and maturing normally to you? How does his or her development compare with siblings or age-mates?

7. Do you know if your child has had any environmental exposure to lead? When was he or she tested for lead levels?

Tested at 1 year. Chronically elevated lead levels cause developmental delay or loss of a newly acquired skill or may be asymptomatic.

8. Have you been told about any learning problems in school: problems with attention span, inability to concentrate, hyperactivity?

9. Any family history of seizure disorder, cerebral palsy, muscular dystrophy?

10. Does your teen play sports? Which ones? Collision sports such as football, ice hockey, soccer, lacrosse?
   • Ever had injury to head? What symptoms did he or she have—headache, nausea and vomiting, poor balance, blurred vision, loss of consciousness, memory loss, mental fogginess?

Teens are more susceptible to concussion because of thinner cranial bones, larger head-to-body ratio, immature central nervous system, and larger subarachnoid space in which brain can rattle.[12] Detailed history with evidence of direct impact helps diagnosis.

   • Screened for concussion? What did they tell you about when to return to play?

If asymptomatic, gradual return to play every 24 hours in stepwise fashion: physical and cognitive rest, light aerobics, sport-specific exercise, noncontact drills, full-contact practice, return to game play.[5]

Additional History for the Aging Adult

1. Any problem with dizziness? Does it occur when you first sit or stand up, when you move your head, when you get up and walk just after eating? Does it occur with any of your medications? Any recent falls?

Decreased blood to brain (orthostatic hypotension) increases the risk for falls. Major risks for falls: balance and gait disorder, polypharmacy, history of recent falls. Other risks: older age, female, poor vision, cognitive decline, environmental clutter, and alcohol use.
Micturition syncope.

   • (For men) Do you ever get up at night and then feel faint while standing to urinate?
   • How does dizziness affect your daily activities? Are you able to drive safely and maneuver within your house safely?
   • Which safety modifications have you applied at home?

Examiner Asks	Rationale
2. Have you noticed any decrease in memory, change in mental function? Have you felt any confusion? Did it seem to come on suddenly or gradually?	Memory loss and cognitive decline occur early with AD and are confused with normal cognitive decline of aging (see Table 24.1, 10 Warning Signs of Alzheimer Disease, p. 670).
3. Have you ever noticed any tremor? Is it in your hands or face? Is it worse with anxiety, activity, rest? Does it seem to be relieved with alcohol, activity, rest? Does it interfere with daily or social activities?	Alcohol relieves senile tremor but this is not recommended. Assess any alcohol use or abuse in an effort to relieve tremor.
4. Have you ever had any sudden vision change, fleeting blindness? Did it occur along with weakness? Did you have any loss of consciousness?	Screen symptoms of stroke.

OBJECTIVE DATA

PREPARATION

Perform a **screening neurologic examination** on seemingly well people who have no significant subjective findings from the history.

1. Mental status (level of alertness, appropriateness of responses, orientation to date and place)
2. Cranial nerves (II–visual acuity, pupillary light reflex; III, IV, VI–eye movements; VII–facial strength (smile, eye closure); VIII–hearing
3. Motor function: Strength (shoulder abduction, elbow extension, wrist extension, finger abduction, hip flexion, knee flexion, ankle dorsiflexion); coordination (fine finger movements, finger to nose); gait (casual, tandem)
4. Sensation (one modality at toes can be light touch, pain/temperature, or proprioception)
5. Reflexes: Deep tendon reflexes (biceps, patellar, Achilles); plantar responses

Perform a **complete neurologic examination** on people who have neurologic concerns (e.g., headache, weakness, loss of coordination) or who have shown signs of neurologic dysfunction.

Perform a **neurologic recheck** examination on people who have neurologic deficits and require periodic assessments (e.g., hospitalized people or those in extended care), using the examination sequence beginning on p. 653.

Integrate the steps of the neurologic examination with the examination of each particular part of the body as much as you are able. For example, test cranial nerves while assessing the head and neck (recall Chapters 14 through 17). However, when recording your findings, consider all neurologic data as a functional unit and record them all together.

Position the person sitting up with the head at your eye level.

EQUIPMENT NEEDED

Penlight
Tongue blade
Cotton swab
Cotton ball
Tuning fork (128 Hz or 256 Hz)
Percussion hammer

Sequence for complete neurologic examination:

1. Mental status (see Chapter 5)
2. Cranial nerves
3. Motor system
4. Sensory system
5. Reflexes

Normal Range of Findings	Abnormal Findings
Test Cranial Nerves	
Cranial Nerve I—Olfactory Nerve	
Do not test routinely. With the person's eyes closed, occlude one nostril and present an aromatic substance. Use familiar, obtainable, and nonnoxious smells such as coffee, toothpaste, orange, vanilla, soap, or peppermint. Alcohol wipes smell familiar and are easy to find.	Air passages are occluded with upper respiratory infection or sinusitis. Anosmia—Decrease or loss of smell occurs bilaterally with tobacco smoking, allergic rhinitis, and cocaine use.

Normal Range of Findings	Abnormal Findings

Normally a person can identify an odor on each side of the nose. Smell normally is decreased bilaterally with aging. Any asymmetry in the sense of smell is important.

Unilateral loss of smell in the absence of nasal disease is *neurogenic anosmia* (e.g., head trauma, brain lesion; see Table 24.2, Abnormalities in Cranial Nerves, p. 671).

Cranial Nerve II—Optic Nerve

Test visual acuity and visual fields by confrontation (see Chapter 15).

Using the ophthalmoscope, examine the ocular fundus to determine the color, size, and shape of the optic disc (see Chapter 15).

Visual field loss (see Table 15.5, p. 310).

Papilledema with increased intracranial pressure; optic atrophy (see Table 15.9, p. 314).

Cranial Nerves III, IV, and VI—Oculomotor, Trochlear, and Abducens Nerves

Palpebral fissures are usually equal in width or nearly so.

Ptosis (drooping) occurs with myasthenia gravis, dysfunction of cranial nerve III, or Horner syndrome (see Table 15.2, p. 306).

Check pupils for size, regularity, equality, direct and consensual light reaction, and accommodation (see Chapter 15).

Increasing intracranial pressure causes a sudden, unilateral, dilated, and nonreactive pupil.

Assess extraocular movements by the cardinal positions of gaze (see Chapter 15).

Nystagmus is a back-and-forth oscillation of the eyes. End-point nystagmus, a few beats of horizontal nystagmus at extreme lateral gaze, occurs normally.

Assess any other nystagmus carefully, noting:

Pendular movement (oscillations move equally left to right) or *jerk* (a quick phase in one direction, then a slow phase in the other); classify the jerk nystagmus in the direction of the quick phase;

Amplitude (degree of movement is fine, medium, or coarse);

Frequency (constant or fade after a few beats);

Plane of movement (horizontal, vertical, rotary, or a combination).

Strabismus (deviated gaze) or limited movement (see Table 15.1, p. 305).

Nystagmus occurs with disease of the vestibular system, cerebellum, or brainstem.

Cranial Nerve V—Trigeminal Nerve

Motor Function. Assess the muscles of mastication by palpating the temporal and masseter muscles as the person clenches the teeth (Fig. 24.9). Muscles should feel equally strong on both sides. Next try to separate the jaws by pushing down on the chin; normally you cannot.

Decreased strength on one or both sides.

Asymmetry in jaw movement.

Pain with clenching of teeth.

Unilateral weakness occurs with lesion of the pons (same side) and cancer metastases to skull.

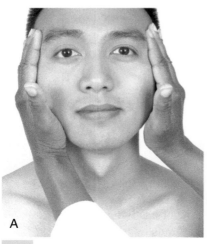
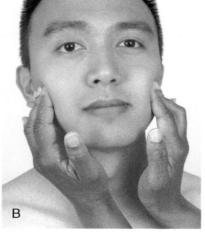

A   B

24.9

Normal Range of Findings	Abnormal Findings

Sensory Function. With the person's eyes closed, test light touch sensation by touching a cotton wisp to these designated areas on person's face: forehead, cheeks, and chin (Fig. 24.10). Ask the person to say "Now" whenever the touch is felt. This tests all three divisions of the nerve: (1) ophthalmic, (2) maxillary, and (3) mandibular.

Decreased or unequal sensation. With a stroke, sensation of face and body is lost on the opposite side of the lesion. Hemiparesis and aphasia often are associated.

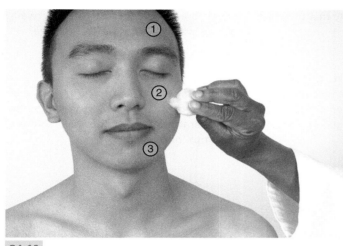

24.10

Cranial Nerve VII—Facial Nerve

Motor Function. Note mobility and facial symmetry as the person responds to these requests: smile, frown, close eyes tightly (against your attempt to open them), lift eyebrows (Fig. 24.11), show teeth, and puff cheeks (Fig. 24.12). Press the person's puffed cheeks in and note that the air should escape equally from both sides.

Muscle weakness is shown by flattening of the nasolabial fold, drooping of one side of the face, lower eyelid sagging, and escape of air from only one cheek that is pressed in.

Loss of movement and asymmetry of movement occur with both CNS lesions (e.g., stroke that affects lower face on one side) and peripheral nervous system lesions (e.g., Bell palsy that affects the upper *and* lower face on one side).

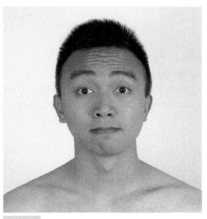

24.11

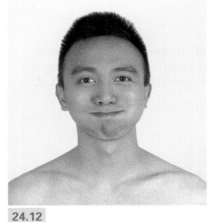

24.12

Cranial Nerve VIII—Acoustic (Vestibulocochlear) Nerve

Test hearing acuity by the ability to hear normal conversation and by the whispered voice test (see Chapter 16).

Objective Data

Normal Range of Findings	Abnormal Findings

Cranial Nerves IX and X—Glossopharyngeal and Vagus Nerves

Motor Function. Depress the tongue with a tongue blade and note pharyngeal movement as the person says "ahhh" or yawns; the uvula and soft palate should rise in the midline, and the tonsillar pillars should move medially.

Touch the posterior pharyngeal wall with a cotton applicator stick and note presence of pharyngeal sensation. Avoid the gag reflex. Also note that the voice sounds smooth and not strained.

Absence or asymmetry of soft palate movement or tonsillar pillar movement. Following a stroke, dysfunction in swallowing increases risk for aspiration.

Hoarse or brassy voice occurs with vocal cord dysfunction; nasal twang occurs with weakness of soft palate.

Cranial Nerve XI—Spinal Accessory Nerve

Examine the sternomastoid and trapezius muscles for equal size. Check equal strength by asking the person to rotate the head forcibly against resistance applied to the side of the chin (Fig. 24.13). Then ask the person to shrug the shoulders against resistance (Fig. 24.14). These movements should feel equally strong on both sides.

Atrophy.

Muscle weakness or paralysis occurs with a stroke or following injury to the peripheral nerve (e.g., surgical removal of lymph nodes).

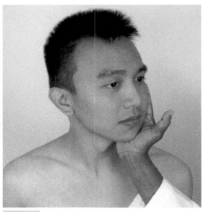

24.13

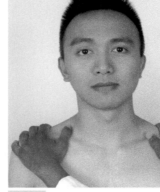

24.14

Cranial Nerve XII—Hypoglossal Nerve

Inspect the tongue. No wasting or tremors should be present. Note the forward thrust in the midline as the person protrudes the tongue. Also ask the person to say "light, tight, dynamite" and note that lingual speech (sounds of letters l, t, d, n) is clear and distinct.

Atrophy. Fasciculations.

Tongue deviates to side when stroke affects the hypoglossal nerve (when this occurs, deviation is toward the paralyzed side).

Inspect and Palpate the Motor System

Muscles

Size. As you proceed through the examination, inspect all muscle groups for size. Compare the right side with the left. Muscle groups should be within the normal size limits for age and symmetric bilaterally. When muscles in the extremities look asymmetric, measure each in centimeters and record the difference. A difference of 1 cm or less is not significant. Note that it is difficult to assess muscle mass in very obese people.

Strength. (See Chapter 23.) Test the power of homologous muscles simultaneously. Test muscle groups of the extremities, neck, and trunk.

Atrophy—Abnormally small muscle with a wasted appearance; occurs with disuse, injury, LMN disease such as polio, diabetic neuropathy.

Hypertrophy—Increased size and strength; occurs with isometric exercise.

Paresis or weakness is diminished strength; paralysis or plegia is absence of strength.

Normal Range of Findings	Abnormal Findings

Tone. Tone is the normal degree of tension (contraction) in voluntarily relaxed muscles. It shows as a mild resistance to passive stretch. To test muscle tone, move the extremities through a passive range of motion. First persuade the person to relax completely, to "go loose like a rag doll." Move each extremity smoothly through a full range of motion. Support the arm at the elbow (Fig. 24.15) and the leg at the knee. Normally you will note a mild, even resistance to movement.

Limited range of motion.
Pain with motion.
Flaccidity—Decreased resistance, hypotonia occur with peripheral weakness.

Spasticity and rigidity—Types of increased resistance that occur with central weakness (see Table 24.3, Abnormalities in Muscle Tone, p. 672).

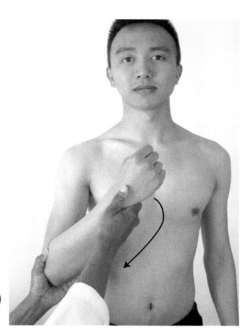

24.15

Involuntary Movements. Normally no involuntary movements occur. If they are present, note their location, frequency, rate, and amplitude. Note if the movements can be controlled at will.

Tic, tremor, fasciculation, myoclonus, chorea, and athetosis (see Table 24.4, p. 672).

Cerebellar Function

Coordination and Skilled Movements Tests of Ataxia

Rapid Alternating Movements (RAM). Ask the person to pat the knees with both hands, lift up, turn hands over, and pat the knees with the backs of the hands (Fig. 24.16). Then ask the person to do this faster. Normally this is done with equal turning and a quick, rhythmic pace.

Lack of coordination.
Slow, clumsy, and sloppy response is termed *dysdiadochokinesia* and occurs with cerebellar disease.

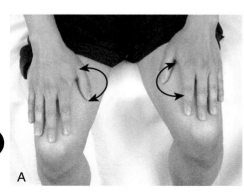
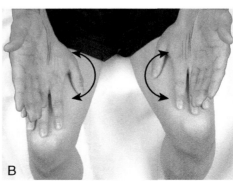

A   B   24.16

Normal Range of Findings	Abnormal Findings

Alternatively ask the person to touch the thumb to each finger on the same hand, starting with the index finger; then reverse direction (Fig. 24.17). Normally this can be done quickly and accurately.

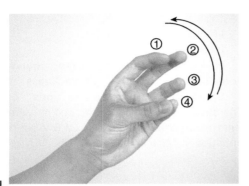

24.17

Finger-Nose-Finger Test. With the person's eyes open, ask that he or she use the index finger to touch your finger and then his or her own nose (Fig. 24.18). After a few times, move your finger to a different spot. The person's movement should be smooth and accurate.

Lack of coordination.

Dysmetria is clumsy movement with overshooting the mark and occurs with cerebellar disorders, alcohol intoxication.

Past-pointing is a constant deviation to one side.

Intention tremor when reaching to a visually directed object.

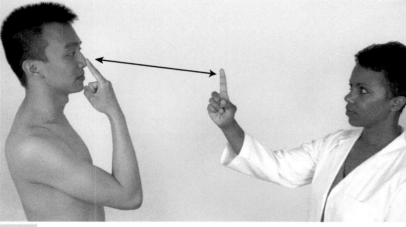

24.18

Heel-to-Shin Test. Test lower-extremity coordination by asking the person, who is in a supine position, to place the heel on the opposite knee and run it down the shin from the knee to the ankle (Fig. 24.19). Normally the person moves the heel in a straight line down the shin.

Lack of coordination, heel falls off shin; occurs with cerebellar disease.

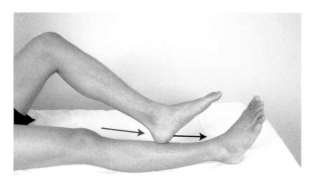

24.19

Normal Range of Findings	Abnormal Findings

Balance Tests

Gait. Observe as the person walks 10 to 20 feet, turns, and returns to the starting point. Normally the person moves with a sense of freedom. The gait is smooth, rhythmic, and effortless; the opposing arm swing is coordinated; the turns are smooth. The step length is about 15 inches from heel to heel.

(NOTE: To minimize position changes, observe these balance tests at the end of the examination.)

Stiff, immobile posture. Staggering or reeling. Wide base of support.

Lack of arm swing or rigid arms.

Unequal rhythm of steps. Slapping of foot. Scraping of toe of shoe.

Ataxia—Uncoordinated or unsteady gait (see Table 24.6, Abnormal Gaits, p. 675).

Ask the person to walk a straight line in a heel-to-toe fashion (tandem walking) (Fig. 24.20). This decreases the base of support and will accentuate any problem with coordination. Normally the person can walk straight and stay balanced.

Crooked line of walk.

Widens base to maintain balance.

Staggering, reeling, loss of balance.

An ataxia that did not appear with regular gait may appear now. Inability to tandem walk is sensitive for an upper motor neuron lesion such as multiple sclerosis and for acute cerebellar dysfunction such as alcohol intoxication.

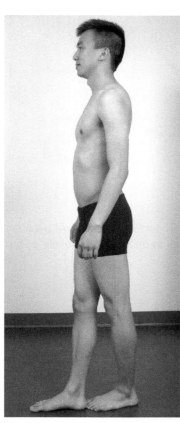

24.20   Tandem walking.

You may also test for balance by asking the person to walk on his or her toes and then on the heels for a few steps. Normally plantar flexion and dorsiflexion are strong enough to permit this.

The Romberg Test. Ask the person to stand up with feet together and arms at the sides. Once in a stable position, ask him or her to close the eyes and to hold the position (Fig. 24.21A). Wait about 20 seconds. Normally a person can maintain posture and balance even with the visual orienting information blocked, although slight swaying may occur. (Stand close to catch the person in case he or she falls.)

Muscle weakness in the legs prevents this.

Sways, falls, widens base of feet to avoid falling (see Fig. 24.21B).

Positive Romberg sign is loss of balance that occurs when closing the eyes. You eliminate the advantage of orientation with the eyes, which had compensated for sensory loss. A positive Romberg sign occurs with cerebellar ataxia (multiple sclerosis, alcohol intoxication), loss of proprioception, and loss of vestibular function.

Objective Data

Normal Range of Findings

Abnormal Findings

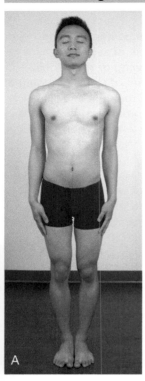

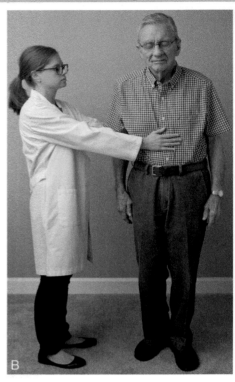

24.21 Romberg test.

Ask the person to perform a shallow knee bend, first on one leg and then the other, either standing alone or with hand supported on table (Fig. 24.22). This demonstrates normal position sense, muscle strength, and cerebellar function. Note that some individuals cannot hop because of aging or obesity. Alternatively you can ask them to rise from a chair without using the arm rests for support.

Unable to perform knee bend because of weakness in quadriceps muscle or hip extensors.

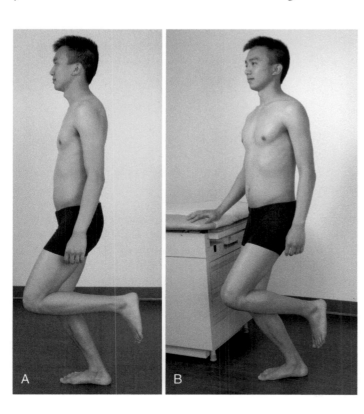

24.22

Normal Range of Findings	Abnormal Findings

Assess the Sensory System

Ask the person to identify various sensory stimuli to test the intactness of the peripheral nerve fibers, the sensory tracts, and higher cortical discrimination.

Ensure validity of sensory system testing by making sure that the person is alert, cooperative, and comfortable and has an adequate attention span. Otherwise you may get misleading and invalid results. Testing the sensory system can be fatiguing. You may need to repeat the examination later or to break it into parts when the person is tired.

You do not need to test the entire skin surface for every sensation. Screening procedures are sufficient—testing superficial pain or light touch and vibration in a few distal locations and testing stereognosis. Complete testing of the sensory system is warranted only in those with neurologic symptoms (e.g., localized pain, numbness, and tingling) or when you discover abnormalities (e.g., motor deficit). Then test all sensory modalities and cover most dermatomes of the body.

Compare sensations on symmetric parts of the body. When you find a definite decrease in sensation, map it out by systematic testing in that area. Proceed from the point of decreased sensation toward the sensitive area. By asking the person to tell you where the sensation changes, you can map the exact borders of the deficient area. Draw your results on a diagram.

Avoid asking leading questions, "Can you feel this pinprick?" This creates an expectation of how the person should feel the sensation, which is called *suggestion.* Instead, use unbiased directions, "Tell me what you feel."

The person's eyes should be closed during each of the tests. Take time to explain what will be happening and how you expect the person to respond.

Note if the topographic pattern of sensory loss is distal (i.e., over the hands and feet in a "glove and stocking" distribution) or if it is over a specific dermatome.

Anterolateral (Spinothalamic) Tract

Pain. Pain is tested by the person's ability to perceive a pinprick. Break a tongue blade lengthwise, forming a sharp point at the fractured end and a dull spot at the rounded end. Lightly apply the sharp point or the dull end to the person's body in a random, unpredictable order (Fig. 24.23). Ask the person to say "sharp" or "dull," depending on the sensation felt. (Note that the sharp edge is used to test for pain; the dull edge is used as a general test of the person's responses.)

Hypoalgesia—Decreased pain sensation.
Analgesia—Absent pain sensation.
Hyperalgesia—Increased pain sensation.

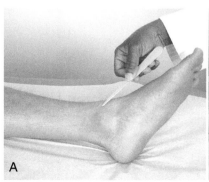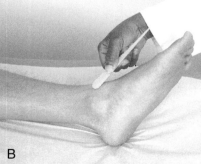

A   B

24.23

Let at least 2 seconds elapse between each stimulus to avoid *summation.* With summation, frequent consecutive stimuli are perceived as one strong stimulus. Discard tongue blade to prevent transmitting any possible infection.

Normal Range of Findings	Abnormal Findings

Light Touch. Apply a wisp of cotton to the skin. Stretch a cotton ball to make a long end and brush it over the skin in a random order of sites and at irregular intervals (Fig. 24.24). This prevents the person from responding just from repetition. Include the arms, forearms, hands, chest, thighs, and legs. Ask the person to say "now" or "yes" when touch is felt. Compare symmetric points.

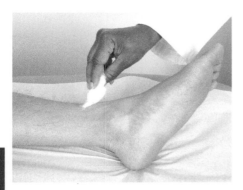

24.24

Posterior (Dorsal) Column Tract

Vibration. Test the person's ability to feel vibrations of a tuning fork over bony prominences. Use a low-pitch tuning fork (128 Hz or 256 Hz) because its vibration has a slower decay. Strike the tuning fork on the heel of your hand and hold the base on a bony surface of the fingers and great toe (Fig. 24.25). Ask the person to indicate when the vibration starts and stops. If he or she feels a normal vibration or buzzing sensation on these distal areas, you may assume that proximal spots are normal and proceed no further. If no vibrations are felt, move proximally and test ulnar processes and ankles, patellae, and iliac crests. Compare the right side with the left side. If you find a deficit, note whether it is gradual or abrupt.

Unable to feel vibration. Loss of vibration sense occurs with peripheral neuropathy (e.g., diabetes and alcoholism). Often this is the first sensation lost.

Peripheral neuropathy is worse at the feet and gradually improves as you move up the leg, as opposed to a specific nerve lesion, which has a clear zone of deficit for its dermatome (see Table 24.9, Patterns of Sensory Loss, p. 678).

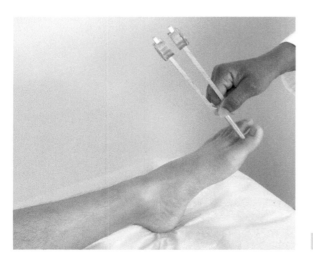

24.25

Position (Kinesthesia). Test the person's ability to perceive passive movements of the extremities. Move a finger or the big toe up and down and ask the person to tell you which way it is moved (Fig. 24.26). The test is done with the eyes closed; but, to be sure that it is understood, have the person watch a few trials first. Vary the order of movement up or down. Hold the digit by the sides since upward or downward pressure on the skin may provide a clue as to how it has been moved. Normally a person can detect movement of a few millimeters.

Objective Data

Normal Range of Findings	**Abnormal Findings**

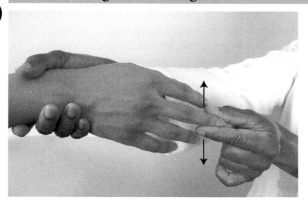

24.26

Loss of position sense occurs with peripheral neuropathy (diabetes mellitus), multiple sclerosis, spinal cord lesions.

Tactile Discrimination (Fine Touch). The following tests also measure the discrimination ability of the sensory cortex. As a prerequisite the person needs a normal or near-normal sense of touch and position sense.

Stereognosis. With his or her eyes closed, place a familiar object (paper clip, key, coin, cotton ball, or pencil) in the person's hand and ask him or her to identify it (Fig. 24.27). Normally a person will explore it with the fingers and correctly name it. Test a different object in each hand; testing the left hand assesses right parietal lobe functioning.

Problems with tactile discrimination occur with lesions of the sensory cortex or posterior column.

Astereognosis—Inability to identify object correctly. Occurs in sensory cortex lesions (e.g., stroke).

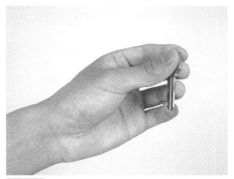

24.27   Stereognosis.

Graphesthesia. Graphesthesia is the ability to "read" a number by having it traced on the skin. With the person's eyes closed, use a blunt instrument to trace a single digit number or a letter on the palm (Fig. 24.28). Ask the person to tell you what it is. Graphesthesia is a good measure of sensory loss if the person cannot make the hand movements needed for stereognosis, as occurs in arthritis.

Inability to distinguish number occurs with lesions of the sensory cortex.

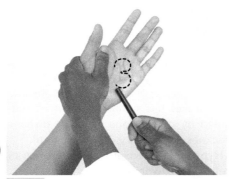

24.28   Graphesthesia.

Objective Data

Normal Range of Findings	Abnormal Findings

Extinction. Simultaneously touch both sides of the body at the same point. Ask the person to state how many sensations are felt and where they are. Normally both sensations are felt.

Point Location. Touch the skin and withdraw the stimulus promptly. Tell the person, "Put your finger where I touched you." You can perform this test simultaneously with light touch sensation.

The ability to recognize only one of the stimuli occurs with sensory cortex lesion; the stimulus is extinguished on the side *opposite* the cortex lesion.

With a sensory cortex lesion, the person cannot localize the sensation accurately, even though light touch sensation may be retained.

Test the Reflexes

Stretch Reflexes or Deep Tendon Reflexes (DTRs)

Measurement of the stretch reflexes reveals an involuntary muscle contraction, the intactness of the reflex arc at specific spinal levels, and the normal override on the reflex of the higher cortical levels.

For an adequate response, the limb should be relaxed and the muscle partially stretched. Stimulate the reflex by directing a short, snappy blow of the reflex hammer onto the insertion tendon of the muscle. Use a relaxed hold on the hammer (Fig. 24.29).

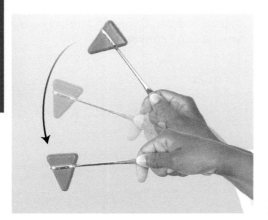

24.29

As with the percussion technique, the action takes place at your wrist. Strike a brief, well-aimed blow and bounce up promptly; do not let the hammer rest on the tendon. It is the swing of the hammer, not the strength of the strike, that gets the best result. Use the pointed end of the reflex hammer when aiming at a smaller target such as your thumb on the tendon site; use the flat end when the target is wider or to diffuse the impact and prevent pain.

Use just enough force to get a response. Compare right and left sides—the responses should be equal. The reflex response is graded on a 4-point scale:

4+ Very brisk, hyperactive with clonus, indicative of disease
3+ Brisker than average, may indicate disease, probably normal
2+ Average, normal
1+ Diminished, low normal, or occurs only with reinforcement
0   No response

This is a subjective scale and requires some clinical practice. Even then, the scale is not completely reliable because no standard exists to say *how* brisk a reflex should be to warrant a grade of 3+. Also, a wide range of normal exists in reflex responses. Healthy people may have diminished reflexes, or they may have brisk ones. Your best plan is to interpret DTRs *only* within the context of the rest of the neurologic examination.

Clonus is a set of rapid, rhythmic contractions of the same muscle.

Hyperreflexia is the exaggerated reflex seen when the monosynaptic reflex arc is released from the usually inhibiting influence of higher cortical levels. This occurs with upper motor neuron lesions (e.g., stroke). It is significant when accompanied by other signs of UMN disease (weakness, spasticity, Babinski sign).[16]

Hyporeflexia, which is the absence of a reflex, is a lower motor neuron problem.

Normal Range of Findings	Abnormal Findings

Objective Data

Sometimes the reflex response fails to appear. Try further encouragement of relaxation, varying the person's position or increasing the strength of the blow. **Reinforcement** is another technique to relax the muscles and enhance the response (Fig. 24.30). Ask the person to perform an isometric exercise in a muscle group somewhat away from the one being tested. For example, to enhance a patellar reflex, ask the person to lock the fingers together and "pull as hard as you can." Then strike the tendon. To enhance a biceps response, ask the person to clench the teeth or to grasp the thigh with the opposite hand.

Abnormal Findings: It occurs with interruption of sensory afferents or destruction of motor efferents and anterior horn cells (e.g., spinal cord injury). It is significant only when other findings of LMN disense occur also (weakness, atrophy, fasciculations).

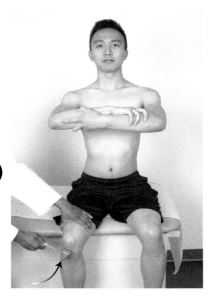

24.30   Reinforcement.

Biceps Reflex (C5 to C6). Support the person's forearm on yours; this position relaxes and partially flexes the person's arm. Place your thumb on the biceps tendon and strike a blow on your thumb. You can feel as well as see the normal response, which is contraction of the biceps muscle and flexion of the forearm (Fig. 24.31).

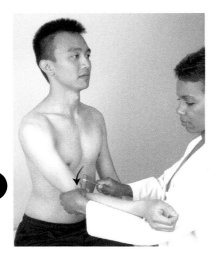

24.31   Biceps reflex.

Normal Range of Findings	Abnormal Findings

Triceps Reflex (C7 to C8). Tell the person to let the arm "just go dead" as you suspend it by holding the upper arm. Strike the triceps tendon directly just above the elbow (Fig. 24.32). The normal response is extension of the forearm. Alternatively hold the person's wrist across the chest to flex the arm at the elbow and tap the tendon.

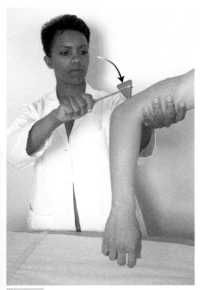

24.32 Triceps reflex.

Brachioradialis Reflex (C5 to C6). Hold the person's thumbs to suspend the forearms in relaxation. Strike the forearm directly, about 2 to 3 cm above the radial styloid process (Fig. 24.33). The normal response is flexion and supination of the forearm.

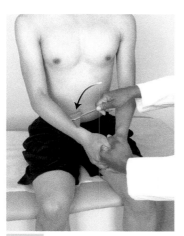

24.33 Brachioradialis reflex.

Quadriceps Reflex ("Knee Jerk") (L2 to L4). Let the lower legs dangle freely to flex the knee and stretch the tendons. Strike the tendon directly just below the patella (Fig. 24.34). Extension of the lower leg is the expected response. You also will palpate contraction of the quadriceps.

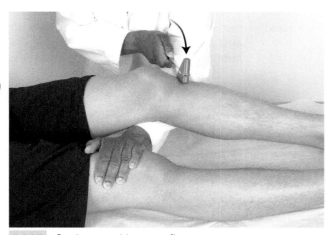

24.34 Quadriceps reflex.

For the person in the supine position, use your own arm as a lever to support the weight of one leg against the other (Fig. 24.35). This maneuver also flexes the knee.

24.35 Supine quadriceps reflex.

Achilles Reflex ("Ankle Jerk") (L_5 to S_2). Position the person with the knee flexed and the hip externally rotated. Hold the foot in dorsiflexion and strike the Achilles tendon directly (Fig. 24.36). Feel the normal response as the foot plantar flexes against your hand.

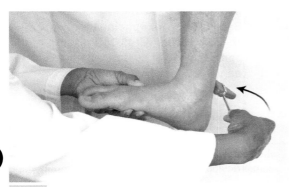

24.36 Achilles reflex.

| **Normal Range of Findings** | **Abnormal Findings** |

For the person in the supine position, flex one knee and support that lower leg against the other leg so it falls "open." Dorsiflex the foot and tap the tendon (Fig. 24.37).

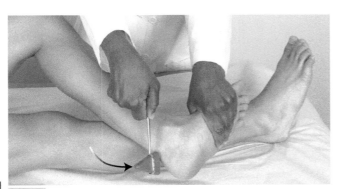

24.37 Supine Achilles reflex.

Clonus. Test for clonus, particularly when the reflexes are hyperactive. Support the lower leg in one hand. With your other hand move the foot up and down a few times to relax the muscle. Then stretch the muscle by briskly dorsiflexing the foot. Hold the stretch (Fig. 24.38). With a normal response you feel no further movement. When clonus is present, you feel and see rapid, rhythmic contractions of the calf muscle and movement of the foot.

Clonus is repeated reflex muscular movements. A hyperactive reflex with sustained clonus (lasting as long as the stretch is held) occurs with UMN disease.

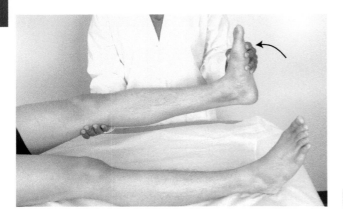

24.38

Superficial (Cutaneous) Reflexes[a]

Plantar Reflex (L₄ to S₂). Position the thigh in slight external rotation. With the reflex hammer draw a slow (5- to 6-second) stroke up the lateral side of the sole of the foot and inward across the ball of the foot, like an upside-down J (Fig. 24.39, *A*). The normal response is plantar flexion of the toes and inversion and flexion of the forefoot.

Except in infancy, the abnormal response is dorsiflexion of the big toe and fanning of all toes, which is a positive Babinski sign, or upgoing toes (Fig. 24.39, *B*). This occurs with UMN disease of the corticospinal (or pyramidal) tract. Accompanied by foot weakness.

---

[a]A traditional superficial cutaneous reflex, the abdominal reflex, is omitted in this edition because evidence shows that its clinical value is slight.[16] It is absent in many healthy people, especially in aging people. Even the asymmetric abdominal reflexes or reflexes in only upper quadrants are common in healthy people.

Normal Range of Findings	Abnormal Findings

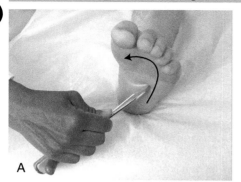

A

24.39   Plantar reflex.

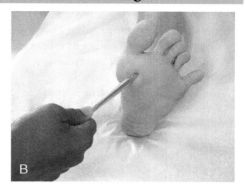

B

Neurologic Recheck

Some hospitalized people have head trauma or a neurologic deficit caused by a systemic disease. Monitor these people closely for any improvement or deterioration in neurologic status and for any indication of increasing intracranial pressure. Signs of increasing intracranial pressure signal impending cerebral disaster and death and require early and prompt intervention.

Use an abbreviation of the neurologic examination in the following sequence:
1. Level of consciousness
2. Motor function
3. Pupillary response
4. Vital signs

Level of Consciousness. A *change* in the level of consciousness is the single most important factor in this examination. It is the earliest and most sensitive index of change in neurologic status. Note the ease of *arousal* and the state of awareness, or *orientation.* Assess orientation by asking questions about:
- Person—Own name, occupation, names of workers around person, their occupations
- Place—Where person is, nature of building, city, state
- Time—Day of week, month, year

Vary the questions during repeat assessments so the person is not merely memorizing answers. Note the quality and content of the verbal response; articulation, fluency, manner of thinking; and any deficit in language comprehension or production (see Chapter 5).

When the person is intubated and cannot speak, you have to ask questions that require a nod or shake of the head (e.g., "Is this a hospital?" "Are you at home?" "Are we in Texas?")

A person is fully alert when his or her eyes open at your approach or spontaneously; when he or she is oriented to person, place, and time; and when he or she is able to follow verbal commands appropriately.

If the person is not fully alert, increase the amount of stimulus used in this order:
1. Name called
2. Light touch on person's arm
3. Vigorous shake of shoulder
4. Pain applied (pinch nail bed, pinch trapezius muscle, rub your knuckles on the person's sternum)

Record the stimulus used and the person's response to it.

A change in consciousness may be subtle. Note any decreasing level of consciousness, disorientation, memory loss, uncooperative behavior, or even complacency in a previously combative person.

Review Table 5.1, Levels of Consciousness, p. 75.

Objective Data

Normal Range of Findings	Abnormal Findings

Motor Function. Check the voluntary movement of each extremity by giving the person specific commands. (This procedure also tests level of consciousness by noting the person's ability to follow commands.)

Ask the person to lift the eyebrows, frown, bare teeth. Note symmetric facial movements and bilateral nasolabial folds (cranial nerve VII).

You can check upper arm strength by checking hand grasps. Ask the person to squeeze your fingers. Offer your two fingers, one on top of the other, so a strong hand grasp does not hurt your knuckles (Fig. 24.40). Be judicious about asking the person to squeeze your hands; some people with diffuse brain damage, especially frontal lobe injury, have a grasp that is a reflex only.

A weak grip occurs with upper and lower motor neuron disease and with local hand problems (arthritis, carpal tunnel syndrome).

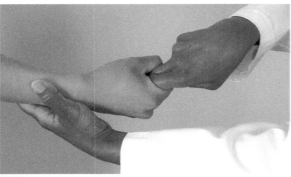

24.40

Alternatively ask the person to lift each hand or to hold up one finger. You also can check upper-extremity strength by palmar drift. Ask the person to extend both arms forward or halfway up, palms up, eyes closed, and hold for 10 to 20 seconds (Fig. 24.41, *A*). Normally the arms stay steady with no downward drift.

Pronator drift is a downward unilateral drift and turning in of the forearm that occurs with mild hemiparesis (Fig. 24.41, *B*).

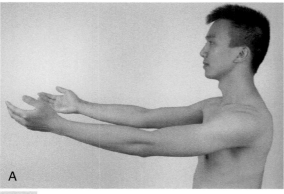

A

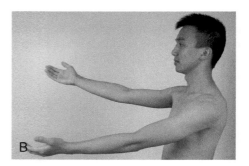

B

24.41

Check lower extremities by asking the person to do straight leg raises. Ask the person to lift one leg at a time straight up off the bed (Fig. 24.42). Full strength allows the leg to be lifted 90 degrees. If multiple trauma, pain, or equipment precludes this motion, ask the person to push one foot at a time against the resistance in your hand, "like putting your foot on the gas pedal of your car" (Fig. 24.43).

Normal Range of Findings	Abnormal Findings

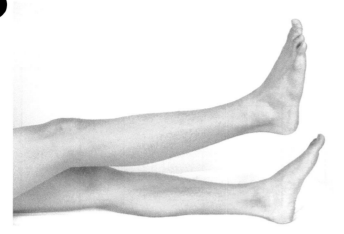

24.42

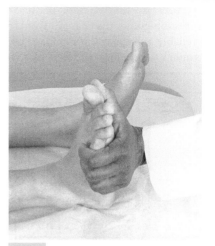

24.43

For the person with decreased level of consciousness, note if movement occurs spontaneously and as a result of noxious stimuli such as pain or suctioning. An attempt to push away your hand after such stimuli is called *localizing* and is characterized as purposeful movement.

Pupillary Response. Note the size, shape, and symmetry of both pupils. Shine a light into each pupil, and note the direct and consensual light reflex. Both pupils should constrict briskly. (Allow for the effects of any medication that could affect pupil size and reactivity.) When recording, pupil size is expressed in millimeters. Use a millimeter scale and hold it next to the person's eyes for the most accurate measurement (Fig. 24.44). Note that subjective assessments of pupil diameter are prone to inconsistencies. Early evidence shows that pupil diameters are underestimated as pupil size increases and that pupil reactivity (sluggishness) often is misidentified.[14] Standardization may be improved by a new tool, the pupilometer, a noninvasive handheld device that measures pupil diameter and reactivity.

Any abnormal posturing, decorticate rigidity, or decerebrate rigidity indicates diffuse brain injury (see Table 24.10).

In a brain-injured person a sudden unilateral dilated and nonreactive pupil is ominous. Cranial nerve III runs parallel to the brainstem. When increasing intracranial pressure pushes the brainstem down (uncal herniation), it puts pressure on cranial nerve III, causing pupil dilation.

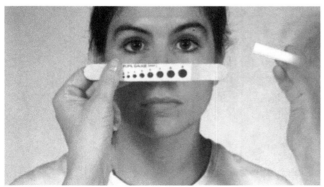

24.44

Vital Signs. Measure the temperature, pulse, respiration, and BP as often as the person's condition warrants. Although they are vital to the overall assessment of the critically ill person, pulse and BP are notoriously unreliable parameters of CNS deficit. Any changes are late consequences of rising intracranial pressure.

The Cushing reflex shows signs of increasing intracranial pressure: BP—sudden elevation with widening pulse pressure; pulse—decreased rate, slow and bounding.

Objective Data

Normal Range of Findings	Abnormal Findings

The Glasgow Coma Scale. Because the terms describing levels of consciousness are ambiguous, the Glasgow Coma Scale (GCS) was developed as an accurate and reliable *quantitative* tool (Fig. 24.45). The GCS is a standardized, objective assessment that defines the level of consciousness by giving it a numeric value.

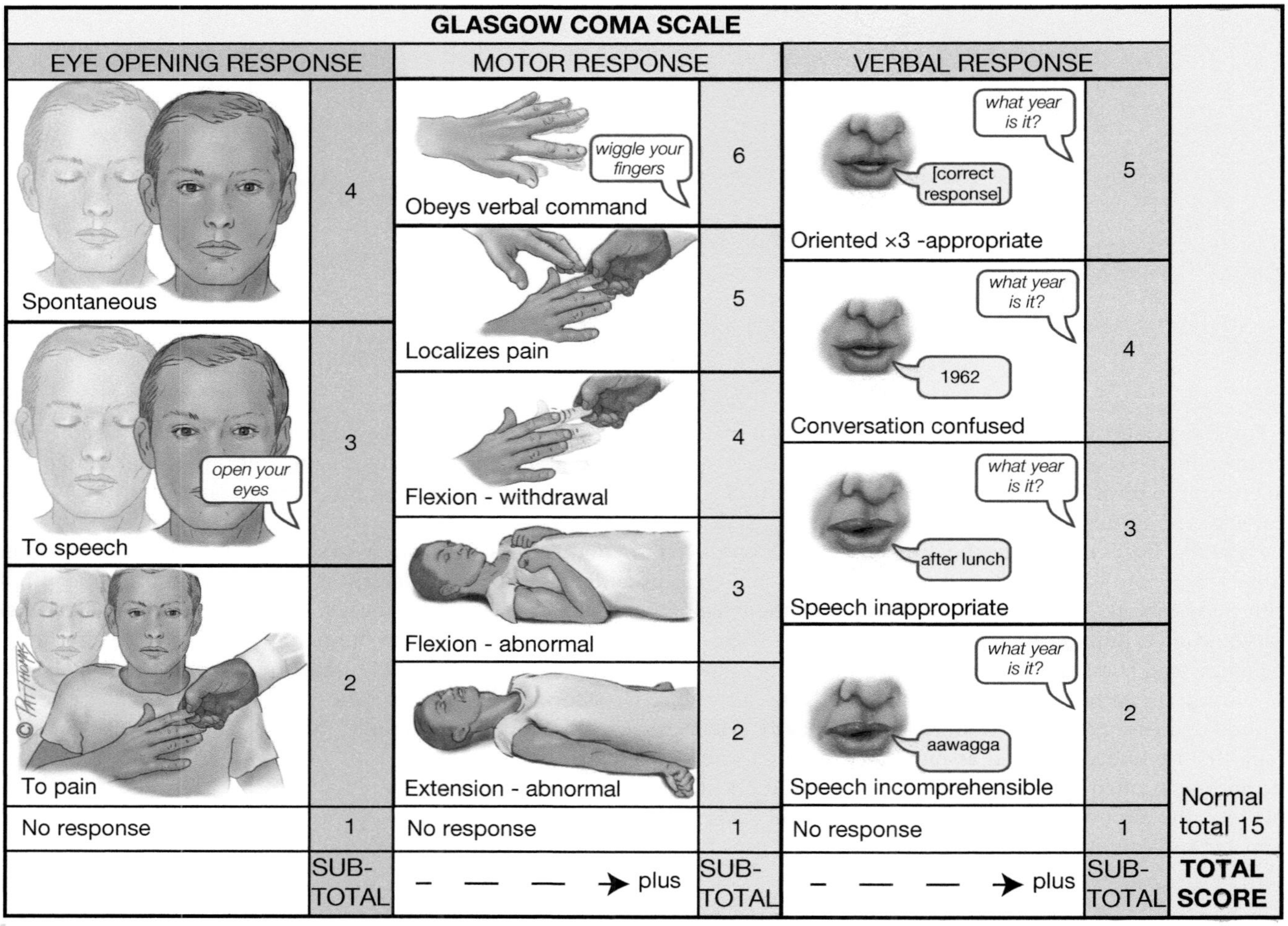

GLASGOW COMA SCALE

EYE OPENING RESPONSE		MOTOR RESPONSE		VERBAL RESPONSE		
Spontaneous	4	Obeys verbal command — *wiggle your fingers*	6	Oriented ×3 -appropriate — *what year is it?* [correct response]	5	
To speech — *open your eyes*	3	Localizes pain	5	Conversation confused — *what year is it?* 1962	4	
To pain	2	Flexion - withdrawal	4	Speech inappropriate — *what year is it?* after lunch	3	
		Flexion - abnormal	3	Speech incomprehensible — *what year is it?* aawagga	2	
		Extension - abnormal	2			Normal total 15
No response	1	No response	1	No response	1	
	SUB-TOTAL	— — — → plus	SUB-TOTAL	— — — → plus	SUB-TOTAL	**TOTAL SCORE**

24.45

(Images © Pat Thomas, 2014.)

The scale is divided into three areas: eye opening, verbal response, and motor response. Each area is rated separately, and a number is given for the person's best response. The three numbers are added; the total score reflects the functional level of the brain. A fully alert, normal person has a score of 15, whereas a score of 7 or less reflects coma. Serial assessments can be plotted on a graph to illustrate visually whether the person is stable, improving, or deteriorating.

The GCS assesses the functional state of the brain as a whole, not of any particular site in the brain. The scale is easy to learn and master, has good interrater reliability, and enhances interprofessional communication by providing a common language.

Diabetic Neuropathy Screening

For peoples with type 1 and type 2 diabetes, test skin sensation on the soles of the feet. Hold the filament by the paper handle and touch the filament to the skin at each numbered site for only 1 to 2 seconds (Fig. 24.46, *A*). Push the filament to make it bend, and ask the person to say "now" or "yes" at each site. Use all 10 sites indicated.

Normal Range of Findings	Abnormal Findings

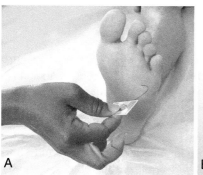 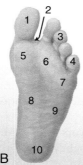

24.46

Diabetes increases the risk of peripheral neuropathy. If the patient cannot feel any one of the 10 sites, referral is necessary (Fig. 24.46, *B*).

✧ DEVELOPMENTAL COMPETENCE

Infants (Birth to 12 Months)

The neurologic system shows dramatic growth and development during the first year of life. Assessment includes noting that milestones you normally would expect for each month have indeed been achieved and that the early, more primitive reflexes are eliminated from the baby's repertory when they are supposed to be.

At birth the newborn is very alert, with the eyes open, and demonstrates strong, urgent sucking. The normal cry is loud, lusty, and even angry. The next 2 or 3 days may be spent mostly sleeping as the baby recovers from the birth process. After that the pattern of sleep and waking activity is highly variable; it depends on the baby's individual body rhythm and external stimuli.

The behavioral assessment should include your observations of the infant's spontaneous waking activity, responses to environmental stimuli, and social interaction with the parents and others.

By 2 months, the baby smiles responsively and recognizes the parent's face. Babbling occurs at 4 months, and one or two words (mama, dada) are used nonspecifically after 9 months.

The cranial nerves cannot be tested directly, but you can infer their proper functioning by the following maneuvers:

II, III, IV, VI
- Optical blink reflex—Shine light in open eyes, note rapid closure
- Size, shape, equality of pupils
- Regards face or close object
- Eyes follow movement

V
- Rooting reflex, sucking reflex

VII
- Facial movements (e.g., wrinkling forehead and nasolabial folds) symmetric when crying or smiling

VIII
- Loud noise yields Moro reflex (until age 4 months)
- Acoustic blink reflex—Infant blinks in response to loud hand clap 30 cm (12 inches) from head (avoid making air current)
- Eyes follow direction of sound

IX, X
- Swallowing, gag reflex
- Coordinate sucking and swallowing

XII
- Pinch nose and infant's mouth opens and tongue rises in midline

Failure to attain a skill by expected time.
Persistence of reflex behavior beyond the normal time.

A high-pitched, shrill cry or cat-sounding screech occurs with CNS damage.
A weak, groaning cry or expiratory grunt occurs with respiratory distress.
Lethargy, hyporeactivity, hyperirritability, and parent's report of significant change in behavior all warrant referral.

| Normal Range of Findings | Abnormal Findings |

The Motor System

Observe spontaneous motor activity for smoothness and symmetry. Smoothness of movement suggests proper cerebellar function, as does the coordination involved in sucking and swallowing. To screen gross- and fine-motor coordination, use the Denver II test with its age-specific developmental milestones. You also can assess movement by testing the reflexes listed in the following section. Note their smoothness of response and symmetry. Also note whether their presence or absence is appropriate for the infant's age.

Assess muscle tone by first observing resting posture. The newborn favors a flexed position; extremities are symmetrically folded inward, the hips are slightly abducted, and the fists are tightly flexed (Fig. 24.47). However, infants born by breech delivery do not have flexion in the lower extremities.

Delay in motor activity occurs with brain damage, mental disability, peripheral neuromuscular damage, prolonged illness, and parental neglect.

Abnormal postures:
Frog position—Hips abducted and almost flat against the table, externally rotated (normal only after breech delivery).
Opisthotonos—Head arched back, stiffness of neck, and extension of arms and legs; occurs with meningeal or brainstem irritation and kernicterus (see Table 24.10, Abnormal Postures, p. 680).
Extension of limbs may occur with intracranial hemorrhage.
Any type of continual asymmetry (e.g., asymmetry of upper limbs) occurs with brachial plexus palsy.

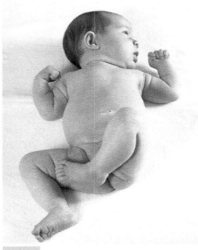

24.47

After 2 months, flexion gives way to gradual extension, beginning with the head and continuing in a cephalocaudal direction. Now is the time to check for spasticity; none should be present. Test for spasticity by flexing the infant's knees onto the abdomen and then quickly releasing them. They will unfold but not too quickly. Also gently push the head forward—the baby should comply.

Spasticity is an early sign of cerebral palsy. After releasing flexed knees, legs will quickly extend and adduct, even to a "scissoring" motion when spasticity is present. The baby also often resists head flexion and extends back against your hand when spasticity is present.

The fists normally are held in tight flexion for the first 3 months. Then they open for part of the time.

A purposeful reach for an object with both hands occurs around 4 months, a transfer of an object from hand to hand at 7 months, a grasp using fingers and opposing thumb at 9 months, and a purposeful release at 10 months. Babies are normally ambidextrous for the first 18 months.

Note persistent one-hand preference in baby younger than 18 months of age, which may indicate a motor deficit on the opposite side.

Head control is an important milestone in motor development. You can incorporate the following two movements into every infant assessment to check the muscle tone necessary for head control.

First, with the baby supine, pull to a sit holding the wrists and note head control (Fig. 24.48). The newborn will hold the head almost in the same plane as the body, and it will balance briefly when the baby reaches a sitting position and then flop forward. (Even a premature infant shows some head flexion.) At 4 months, the head stays in line with the body and does not flop.

Because development progresses in a cephalocaudal direction, head lag is an early sign of brain damage.
After 6 months refer any baby with failure to hold head in midline when sitting.

Normal Range of Findings	Abnormal Findings

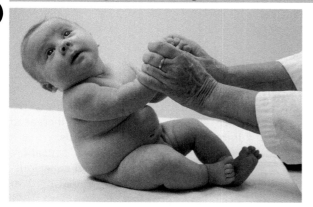

24.48

Second, lift up the baby in a prone position, with one hand supporting the chest (Fig. 24.49). The term newborn holds the head at an angle of 45 degrees or less from horizontal, the back is straight or slightly arched, and the elbows and knees are partly flexed.

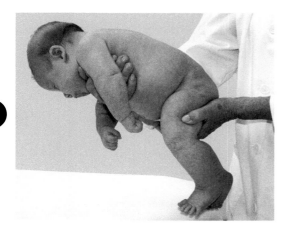

24.49

At 3 months the baby raises the head and arches the back, as in a swan dive. This is the *Landau reflex*, which persists until 1½ years of age (Fig. 24.50).

Head lag; a limp, floppy trunk; and dangling arms and legs.

Absence of the reflex indicates motor weakness, upper motor neuron disease, or mental disability.

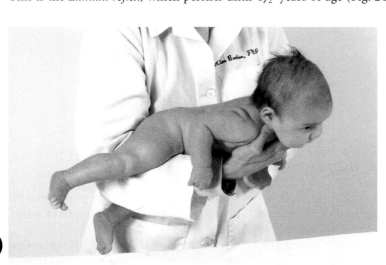

24.50

Normal Range of Findings	Abnormal Findings

Assess muscle strength by noting the strength of sucking and of spontaneous motor activity. Normally no tremors are present, and no continual overshooting of the mark occurs when reaching.

The Sensory System

You will perform very little sensory testing with infants and toddlers. The newborn normally has hypoesthesia and requires a strong stimulus to elicit a response. The baby responds to pain by crying and a general reflex withdrawal of all limbs. By 7 to 9 months, the infant can localize the stimulus and shows more specific signs of withdrawal. Other sensory modalities are not tested.

Unusually rapid withdrawal is *hyperesthesia*, which occurs with spinal cord lesions, CNS infections, increased intracranial pressure, peritonitis.

No withdrawal is decreased sensation, which occurs with decreased consciousness, mental deficiency, spinal cord or peripheral nerve lesions.

Reflexes

Infantile automatisms are reflexes that have a predictable timetable of appearance and departure. The reflexes most commonly tested are listed in the following section. For the screening examination you can just check the rooting, grasp, tonic neck, and Moro reflexes.

Rooting Reflex. Brush the infant's cheek near the mouth. Note whether he or she turns the head toward that side and opens the mouth (Fig. 24.51). Appears at birth and disappears at 3 to 4 months.

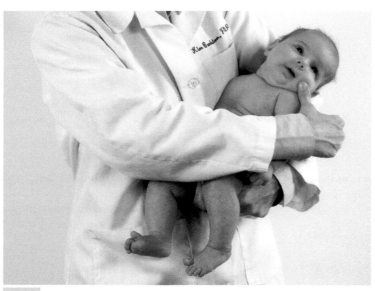

24.51

Sucking Reflex. Touch the lips and offer your gloved little finger to suck. Note strong sucking reflex. The reflex is present at birth and disappears at 10 to 12 months.

Palmar Grasp. Place the baby's head midline to ensure symmetric response. Offer your finger from the baby's ulnar side, away from the thumb. Note tight grasp of all the baby's fingers (Fig. 24.52). Sucking enhances grasp. Often you can pull baby to a sit from grasp. The reflex is present at birth, is strongest at 1 to 2 months, and disappears at 3 to 4 months.

The palmar grasp reflex is absent with brain damage and local muscle or nerve injury.

Persistence of palmar grasp reflex after 4 months of age occurs with frontal lobe lesion.

Normal Range of Findings	Abnormal Findings

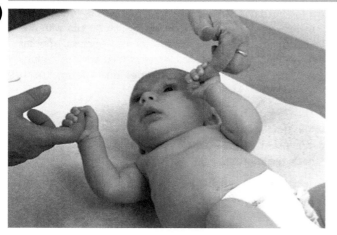

24.52 Palmar grasp.

Plantar Grasp. Touch your thumb at the ball of the baby's foot. Note that the toes curl down tightly (Fig. 24.53). The reflex is present at birth and disappears at 8 to 10 months.

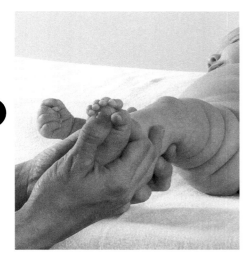

24.53 Plantar grasp.

Babinski Reflex. Stroke your finger up the lateral edge and across the ball of the infant's foot. Note fanning of toes (positive Babinski reflex) (Fig. 24.54). The reflex is present at birth and disappears (changes to the adult response) by 24 months of age (variable).

Positive Babinski reflex after 2 or $2\frac{1}{2}$ years occurs with pyramidal tract disease.

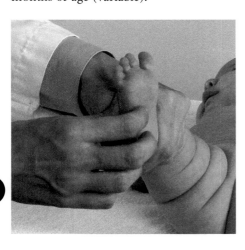

24.54 Babinski reflex.

Objective Data

Normal Range of Findings	Abnormal Findings

Tonic Neck Reflex. With the baby supine, relaxed, or sleeping, turn the head to one side with the chin over shoulder. Note ipsilateral extension of the arm and leg and flexion of the opposite arm and leg; this is the "fencing" position. If you turn the infant's head to the opposite side, positions will reverse (Fig. 24.55). The reflex appears by 2 to 3 months, decreases at 3 to 4 months, and disappears by 4 to 6 months.

Persistence later in infancy occurs with brain damage.

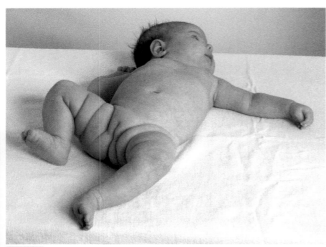

24.55 Tonic neck reflex.

Moro Reflex. Startle the infant by jarring the crib, making a loud noise, or supporting the head and back in a semi-sitting position and quickly lowering the infant to 30 degrees. The baby looks as if he or she is hugging a tree: symmetric abduction and extension of the arms and legs, fanning fingers, and curling of the index finger and thumb to C-position occur. The infant then brings in both arms and legs (Fig. 24.56). The reflex is present at birth and disappears at 1 to 4 months.

Absence of the Moro reflex in the newborn or persistence after 5 months indicates severe CNS injury.

Absence of movement in just one arm occurs with fracture of the humerus or clavicle and with brachial nerve palsy.

Absence in one leg occurs with a lower spinal cord problem or a dislocated hip.

A hyperactive Moro reflex occurs with tetany or CNS infection.

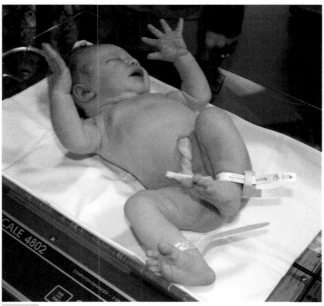

24.56 Moro reflex.

Normal Range of Findings	Abnormal Findings

Placing Reflex. Hold the infant upright under the arms, close to a table. Let the dorsal "top" of foot touch the underside of the table. Note flexing of hip and knee, followed by extension at the hip, to place foot on table (Fig. 24.57). Reflex appears at 4 days after birth.

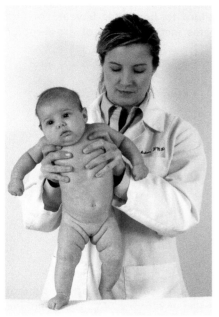

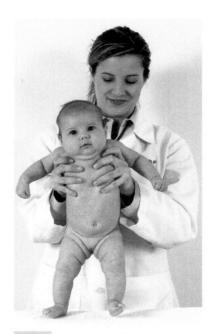

24.57   Placing reflex.   **24.58**   Stepping reflex.

Stepping Reflex. Hold the infant upright under the arms, with the feet on a flat surface. Note regular alternating steps (Fig. 24.58). The reflex disappears before voluntary walking.

Extensor thrust, or "scissoring"; crossing of lower extremities.

Preschool- and School-Age Children

Assess the child's general behavior during play activities, reaction to parent, and cooperation with parent and with you. Complete details are described in Chapter 5, Mental Status Assessment.

When testing visual fields (cranial nerve II) and cardinal positions of gaze (cranial nerves III, IV, VI), you often need to gently immobilize the head, or the child will track with the whole head. Make a game out of asking the child to imitate your funny "faces" (cranial nerve VII); thus the child has fun and you win a friend.

Much of the motor assessment can be derived from watching the child undress and dress and manipulate buttons. This indicates muscle strength, symmetry, joint range of motion, and fine-motor skills. Use the Denver II to screen gross- and fine-motor skills that are appropriate for the child's specific age. Be familiar with developmental milestones for each age.

Muscle hypertrophy or atrophy occurs with muscular dystrophy.
Muscle weakness.
Incoordination.

Normal Range of Findings

Abnormal Findings

Note the child's gait during both walking and running. Allow for the normal wide-based gait of the toddler and the normal knock-kneed walk of the preschooler. Normally the child can balance on one foot for about 5 seconds by 4 years, can balance for 8 to 10 seconds at 5 years, and can hop at 4 years. Children enjoy performing these tests (Fig. 24.59).

Causes of motor delay are listed earlier in the infant section.

Staggering, falling.

Weakness climbing up or down stairs occurs with muscular dystrophy.

Broad-based gait beyond toddlerhood, scissor gait (see Table 24.6).

Failure to hop after 5 years of age indicates incoordination of gross-motor skill.

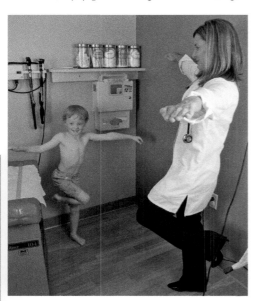

24.59

Observe the child as he or she rises from a supine position on the floor to a sitting position and then to a stand. Note the muscles of the neck, abdomen, arms, and legs. Normally the child curls up in the midline to sit up and pushes off with both hands against the floor to stand (Fig. 24.60, *A*).

Weak pelvic muscles are a sign of muscular dystrophy; from the supine position the child will roll to one side, bend forward to all four extremities, plant hands on legs, and literally "climb" up himself or herself. This is the *Gower sign* (Fig. 24.60, *B*).

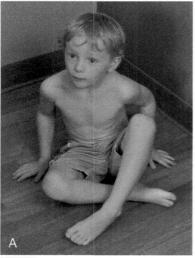

A

24.60

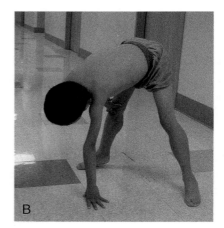

B

(Braddom, 2011.)

Assess fine coordination by using the finger-to-nose test if you can be sure that the young child understands your directions. Demonstrate the procedure first; then ask the child to do the test with the eyes open and then with the eyes closed. Fine coordination is not fully developed until the child has reached 4 to 6 years. Consider it normal if a younger child can bring the finger to within 2 to 5 cm (1 to 2 inches) of the nose.

Failure of the finger-to-nose test with the eyes open indicates gross incoordination; failure of the test with the eyes closed indicates minor incoordination or lack of position sense.

Normal Range of Findings

Testing sensation is very unreliable in toddlers and preschoolers. You may test light touch by asking the child to close the eyes and then to point to the spot where you touch or tickle. A child younger than 6 years is not usually tested for vibration, position, stereognosis, graphesthesia, or two-point discrimination. In addition, do not test for perception of superficial pain. In children older than 6 years, you may perform sensory testing as with adults. Use a fractured tongue blade if you need to test superficial pain.

The DTRs usually are not tested in children younger than 5 years because of lack of cooperation in relaxation. When you need to test DTRs in a young child, use your finger to percuss the tendon (Fig. 24.61). Use a reflex hammer only with an older child. Coax the child to relax or distract and percuss discreetly when the child is not paying attention. The knee jerk is present at birth, then the ankle jerk and brachial reflex appear, and the triceps reflex is present at 6 months.

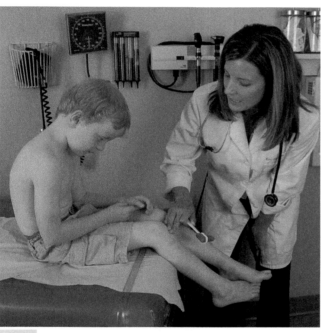

24.61

When a child is feverish or acts very sick and irritable, test for nuchal rigidity as an indicator of meningeal irritation. With the child sitting upright, ask the child to touch his or her chin to the chest (see Fig. 24.61). This can be done easily when the brain meninges are healthy and not inflamed.

The Aging Adult

Use the same examination as used with the younger adult. Be aware that some aging adults show a slower response to your requests, especially to those calling for coordination of movements.

Any decrease in muscle bulk is most apparent in the hand, as seen by guttering between the metacarpals. These dorsal hand muscles often look wasted, even with no apparent arthropathy. The grip strength remains relatively good.

Senile tremors occasionally occur. These benign tremors include an intention tremor of the hands, head nodding (as if saying "yes" or "no"), and tongue protrusion. *Dyskinesias* are the repetitive stereotyped movements in the jaw, lips, or tongue that may accompany senile tremors. No associated rigidity is present.

Abnormal Findings

Sensory loss occurs with decreased consciousness, mental deficiency, or spinal cord or peripheral nerve dysfunction.

Hyperactivity of DTRs occurs with UMN lesion, hypocalcemia, and hyperthyroidism and with muscle spasm associated with early poliomyelitis.

Decreased or absent reflexes occur with a LMN lesion, muscular dystrophy, and flaccidity or flaccid paralysis.

Clonus may occur with fatigue, but it usually indicates hyperreflexia.

Nuchal rigidity is an extreme resistance to any direction of head movement and occurs with inflammation of the meninges due to meningitis, bleeding, or tumor.

Hand muscle atrophy is worsened with disuse and degenerative arthropathy.

Distinguish senile tremors from tremors of parkinsonism. The latter includes rigidity and slowness and weakness of voluntary movement.

Objective Data

Normal Range of Findings	Abnormal Findings
The gait may be slower and more deliberate than that in the younger person, and it may deviate slightly from a midline path.	Absence of a rhythmic reciprocal gait pattern is seen in parkinsonism and hemiparesis (see Table 24.6).
The aging adult may have more difficulty performing rapid alternating movements (e.g., pronating and supinating the hands on the thigh).	
After 65 years, loss of the sensation of vibration at the ankle malleolus is common and is usually accompanied by loss of the ankle jerk. Position sense in the big toe may be lost, although this is less common than vibration loss. Tactile sensation may be impaired. The aging person may need stronger stimuli for light touch and especially for pain.	Note any difference in sensation between right and left sides, which may indicate a neurologic deficit.
The DTRs are less brisk. Those in the upper extremities are usually present, but the ankle jerks commonly are lost. Knee jerks may be lost, but this occurs less often. Because aging people find it difficult to relax their limbs, always use reinforcement when eliciting the DTRs.	
The plantar reflex may be absent or difficult to interpret. Often you will not see a definite normal flexor response.	Still consider a definite extensor response to be abnormal.

HEALTH PROMOTION AND PATIENT TEACHING

"Know about Stroke. Know the Signs so you can Act in Time." A stroke or brain attack occurs when blood flow is interrupted to a part of the brain. Stroke is the most common cause of adult disability and is the 4th leading killer in the United States.[20,25] Because stroke symptoms usually do not hurt, many people ignore them or delay seeking medical attention. Sometimes people can have a "ministroke," or transient ischemic attack (TIA). In these cases, the stroke symptoms last only temporarily and disappear, often within an hour. Because the symptoms "go away," people often do not report them or seek medical attention. However, a TIA is a warning sign that should not be ignored. Anyone who suffers a TIA should seek help to rule out the possibility of a future brain attack. Know stroke's warning signs and stroke's risk factors. Paying attention to these can save lives.

Common symptoms of stroke include *sudden* onset of:
- Weakness or numbness in the face, arms, or legs, especially when it is on one side of the body
- Confusion, trouble speaking or understanding
- Changes in vision, such as blurry vision or partial or complete loss of vision in one or both eyes
- Trouble with walking, dizziness, loss of balance, or coordination
- Severe headache with no reason or explanation[20]

The F.A.S.T. plan, promoted by the American Stroke Association, is an easy way to remember the sudden signs of stroke:
- F = Face drooping
- A = Arm weakness
- S = Speech difficulty
- T = Time to call 9-1-1

"Let's review the risk factors for stroke and talk about the ones that are treatable." The risk of stroke does increase with age, but there are other important factors you can help control: (1) **High blood pressure.** High BP increases the risk of stroke by 2 to 4 times.[20] Keeping your weight in healthy limits and regular exercise help, but if your BP remains high, medications can be used to bring it down. (2) **Cigarette smoking.** Smoking increases stroke risk by 2 to 4 times. The main artery carrying blood to your brain is the carotid artery. Smoking is linked to the buildup of fatty plaque in that artery (atherosclerosis). And that's not all. The nicotine in cigarettes raises BP; the carbon monoxide in cigarettes decreases the oxygen in the blood; and smoking makes the blood more likely to clot.[20] We can find a program or medication to help a person quit smoking. (3) **Heart disorders.** Atrial fibrillation, a rapid irregular heartbeat, is a risk factor for stroke, as is coronary heart disease. There are medications to control these heart conditions, and we can help each person decide when blood thinners or anticholesterol drugs are the right choices.

"Vaccination can decrease the risk of herpes zoster (HZ), or shingles, in older adults." Infection with herpes zoster results from the reactivation of latent varicella virus (chickenpox).[6] HZ shows as a painful red blistered rash along a nerve route on one side of the body. It often is followed by a chronic lingering pain along the nerve (postherpetic neuralgia) that decreases physical functioning, interrupts sleep,[2] and causes fatigue and anxiety or depression. However, HZ does not need to happen. The herpes zoster vaccine is approved for use in people over 50 years and recommended for those over 60 years. This vaccine reduces the risk of developing shingles in those over 70 years by 91.3%.[6] The vaccine comes in one dose as a shot and can be given in a provider's office or pharmacy. If you are over 60 years, you should get the vaccine even if you do not remember having had chickenpox. Evidence shows that over 99% of Americans aged 40 and older have had chickenpox, even if they don't remember getting the disease. There is no maximum age for getting shingles vaccine.[4]

DOCUMENTATION AND CRITICAL THINKING

SUBJECTIVE

No unusually frequent or severe headaches; no head injury, dizziness or vertigo, seizures, or tremors. No weakness, numbness or tingling, or difficulty swallowing or speaking. Has no past history of stroke, spinal cord injury, meningitis, or alcohol disorder.

OBJECTIVE

Mental status: Appearance, behavior, and speech appropriate; alert and oriented to person, place, and time; recent and remote memory intact.

Cranial nerves:

II: Vision 20/20 left eye, 20/20 right eye; peripheral fields intact by confrontation; fundi normal.

III, IV, VI: EOMs intact, no ptosis or nystagmus; pupils equal, round, react to light and accommodation (PERRLA).

V: Sensation intact and equal bilaterally; jaw strength equal bilaterally.

VII: Facial muscles intact and symmetric.

VIII: Hearing—whispered words heard bilaterally.

IX, X: Swallowing intact, uvula rises in midline on phonation.

XI: Shoulder shrug, head movement intact and equal bilaterally.

XII: Tongue protrudes midline, no tremors.

Motor: No atrophy, weakness, or tremors. Rapid alternating movements—finger-to-nose smoothly intact. Gait smooth and coordinated, able to tandem walk, negative Romberg.

Sensory: Sharp and dull, light touch, vibration intact. Stereognosis—able to identify key.

Reflexes: No Babinski sign, DTRs 2+ and = bilaterally with downgoing toes; see following drawing:

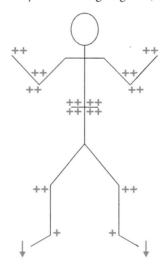

ASSESSMENT

Neurologic system intact; healthy function

J.T. is a 61-year-old male carpenter with a large building firm who is admitted to the Rehabilitation Institute with a diagnosis of right hemiplegia and aphasia following a stroke (CVA) 4 weeks PTA.

SUBJECTIVE

Because of J.T.'s speech dysfunction, history provided by wife.

4 weeks PTA—Complaint of severe headache; then sudden onset of collapse and loss of consciousness while at work. Did not strike head as he fell. Transported by ambulance to Memorial Hospital where admitting physician said J.T. "probably had a stroke." Right arm and leg were limp, and he remained unconscious. Admitted to critical care unit. Regained consciousness day 3 after admission, unable to move right side, unable to speak clearly or write. Remained in ICU 4 more days until "doctors were sure heart and breathing were steady."

3 weeks PTA—Transferred to medical floor where care included physical therapy 2 ×/day and passive ROM 4 ×/day.

Now—Some improvement in right motor function. Bowel control achieved with use of commode same time each day (after breakfast). Bladder control improved. Some occasional incontinence, usually when he cannot tell people he needs to urinate.

OBJECTIVE

Mental status: Dressed in jogging suit, sitting in wheelchair, appears alert with appropriate eye contact, listening intently to history. Speech is slow, requires great effort, able to give one-word answers that are appropriate but lack normal tone. Seems to understand all language spoken to him. Follows requests appropriately, within limits of motor weakness.

Cranial nerves:

II: Acuity normal; fields by confrontation—right homonymous hemianopsia; fundi normal.

III, IV, VI: EOMs intact, no ptosis or nystagmus, PERRLA.

V: Sensation intact to pinprick and light touch. Jaw strength weak on right.

VII: Flat nasolabial fold on right, motor weakness on right lower face. Able to wrinkle forehead bilaterally but unable to smile or bare teeth on right.

VIII: Hearing intact.

IX, X: Swallowing intact, uvula rises midline on phonation.

XI: Shoulder shrug, head movement weaker on right.

XII: Tongue protrudes midline; no tremors.

Sensory: Sharp and dull, light touch present but diminished on right arm and leg. Vibration intact. Position sense impaired on right side. Stereognosis intact.

Motor: Right hand grip weak, right arm drifts, right leg weak, unable to support weight. Spasticity in right arm and leg muscles, limited range of motion on passive motion. Unable to stand up and walk unassisted. Unable to perform finger-to-nose or heel-to-shin on right side; left side smoothly intact.

Reflexes: Hyperactive 4+ with clonus, and upgoing toes in right leg.

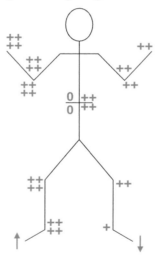

ASSESSMENT

Decreased verbal communication

Decreased physical mobility

Disturbed body image

Self-care deficits: feeding, bathing, toileting, dressing/grooming

Disturbed sensory perception (absent right visual fields)

Potential for injury

Clinical Case Study 2

L.B. is a 38-year-old premenopausal female who recently underwent treatment for breast cancer. Her treatment included a right radical mastectomy followed by chemotherapy. Her cancer is in remission, and she is in the clinic for her annual follow-up. During her course of chemotherapy L.B. described symptoms of peripheral neuropathy in her hands and feet.

SUBJECTIVE

L.B. reports difficulty walking, including balance problems for the past 6 months. "It feels like my feet and hands are burning all the time." L.B. describes episodes of sharp, shooting pain—"like an electric shock"—that occur approximately 2 to 3 times per week. No precipitating factors identified. "I kept thinking it'd get better now that I'm off chemo." Reports pain with computer use and difficulty using her cell phone because of inability to "hit the right key."

OBJECTIVE

Mental status: Dressed appropriately for weather, age, and sex. Appears alert. Crying as she relays current symptoms. Avoids eye contact.
Cranial nerves: Grossly intact.
Motor: No atrophy or tremors. Bilateral lower extremity strength 3+. Grips weak but equal. Gait smooth and coordinated. Unable to tandem walk without losing balance. Rapid alternating movement smoothly intact.
Sensory: Sharp and dull, light touch, and vibration intact on arms. Unable to identify sharp or dull, light touch, or vibration on hands to the wrists and feet to the ankles. Stereognosis—unable to identify key or coin bilaterally.
Reflexes: No Babinski sign, DTRs 2+ and equal bilaterally with downgoing toes.

ASSESSMENT

Severe chemotherapy-induced peripheral neuropathy
Potential for impaired skin integrity
Potential for depression
Decreased physical mobility
Decreased sensory perception: tactile

Clinical Case Study 3

S.S., an 11-month-old male, is brought to the ED via ambulance after parents called 911.

SUBJECTIVE

45 minutes PTA—S.S. was crawling when he "just stiffened, collapsed on his tummy, and then his arms and legs started shaking for about 2 minutes. We tried to talk to him, but he acted 'out of it.'" Parents report that S.S. had been experiencing a "cold since yesterday but no fever until today." They deny S.S. experiencing any vomiting or diarrhea and state that he has been eating, drinking, and voiding "as usual."

OBJECTIVE

Vital signs: Temp 102.9° F (39.4° C) (rectal). Pulse 146 bpm. Resp 42/min. BP 94/56 mm Hg (resting).
General appearance: Quiet and appears drowsy but quickly awakens when touched or spoken to.
HEENT: Fontanels closed; conjunctivae clear, sclera white; bilat TMs dull red and bulging, no light reflex, no mobility on pneumatic otoscopy; no lymphadenopathy.
Neuro: All CNs intact without deficit; no atrophy, weakness, or tremors; sensory intact w/light and deep touch and vibration; DTRs 2+, Babinski +.
Cardiovascular: Regular rate and rhythm w/o abnormal heart sounds.
Respiratory: Breath sounds clear and equal bilat; unlabored

ASSESSMENT

Simple febrile seizure
Need for health teaching regarding fever reduction
Potential for ineffective airway clearance
Potential for injury

Documentation and Critical Thinking

ABNORMAL FINDINGS

TABLE 24.1	10 Warning Signs of Alzheimer Disease (Alzheimer's Association, 2009)	
	Alzheimer Disease (AD)	**Normal Aging**
1 MEMORY LOSS	Memory loss: Forgetting recently learned information is one of the most common early signs of dementia. A person begins to forget more often and is unable to recall the information later.	Forgetting names or appointments occasionally but later remembering
2 LOSING TRACK	Difficulty performing familiar tasks: People with dementia often find it hard to plan or complete everyday tasks. Individuals may lose track of the steps involved in preparing a meal, placing a telephone call, or playing a game.	Occasionally forgetting why you came into a room or what you planned to say
3 FORGETTING WORDS	Problems with language: People with AD often forget simple words or substitute unusual words, making their speech or writing hard to understand. For example, they may be unable to find the toothbrush and instead ask for "that thing for my mouth."	Sometimes having trouble finding the right word
4 GETTING LOST	Disorientation to time and place: People with AD can become lost in their own neighborhood, forget where they are and how they got there, and not know how to get back home.	Forgetting the day of the week or where you were going
5 POOR JUDGMENT	Poor or decreased judgment: Those with AD may dress inappropriately, wearing several layers on a warm day or little clothing in the cold. They may show poor judgment such as giving away large sums of money to telemarketers.	Making a questionable or debatable decision from time to time
6 ABSTRACT FAILING	Problems with abstract thinking: Someone with AD may have unusual difficulty performing complex mental tasks such as forgetting what numbers are for and how they should be used.	Finding it challenging to balance a checkbook
7 LOSING THINGS	Misplacing things: A person with AD may put things in unusual places (e.g., an iron in the freezer or a wristwatch in the sugar bowl).	Misplacing keys or a wallet temporarily
8 MOOD SWINGS	Changes in mood or behavior: Someone with AD may show rapid mood swings—from calm to tears to anger—for no apparent reason.	Occasionally feeling sad or moody
9 PERSONALITY CHANGE	Changes in personality: The personalities of people with dementia can change dramatically. They may become extremely confused, suspicious, fearful, or dependent on a family member.	People's personalities do change somewhat with age
10 GROWING PASSIVE	Loss of initiative: A person with AD may become very passive, sitting in front of the television for hours, sleeping more than usual, or not wanting to do usual activities.	Sometimes feeling weary of work or social obligations

Adapted from Leifer, B.P. (2009). Alzheimer's disease: seeing the signs early. *J Acad Nurse Pract, 21*(11), 588-595.

TABLE 24.2 | Abnormalities in Cranial Nerves

Nerve	Test	Abnormal Findings	Possible Causes
I: Olfactory	Identify familiar odors	Anosmia	Tobacco or cocaine use; fracture of cribriform plate or ethmoid area; frontal lobe lesion; tumor in olfactory bulb or tract; Parkinson disease
II: Optic	Visual acuity	Defect in or absent central vision	Congenital blindness; refractive error; acquired vision loss from numerous diseases (e.g., stroke, diabetes); trauma to globe or orbit (see discussion of CN III)
	Visual fields	Defect in peripheral vision, hemianopsia	
	Shine light in eye	Absent light reflex	
	Direct inspection	Papilledema	Increased intracranial pressure; glaucoma; diabetes
		Optic atrophy	
		Retinal lesions	
III: Oculomotor	Inspection	Dilated pupil, ptosis, eye turns out and slightly down	Paralysis in CN III from internal carotid aneurysm; tumor; inflammatory lesions; uncal herniation with increased intracranial pressure
	Extraocular muscle movement	Failure to move eye up, in, down	Ptosis from myasthenia gravis; oculomotor nerve palsy; Horner syndrome
	Shine light in eye	Absent light reflex	Blindness; drug influence; increased intracranial pressure; CNS injury; circulatory arrest; CNS syphilis
IV: Trochlear	Extraocular muscle movement	Failure to turn eye down or out	Fracture of orbit; brainstem tumor
V: Trigeminal	Superficial touch—three divisions	Absent touch and pain, paresthesias	Trauma; tumor; pressure from aneurysm; inflammation; sequelae of alcohol injection for trigeminal neuralgia
	Corneal reflex	No blink	
	Clench teeth	Weakness of masseter or temporalis muscles	Unilateral weakness with CN V lesion; bilateral weakness with UMN or LMN disorder
VI: Abducens	Extraocular muscle movement to right and left sides	Failure to move laterally, diplopia on lateral gaze	Brainstem tumor or trauma; fracture of orbit
VII: Facial	Wrinkle forehead, close eyes tightly	Absent or asymmetric facial movement	Bell palsy (LMN lesion) causes paralysis of entire half of face
	Smile, puff cheeks	Loss of taste	UMN lesions (stroke, tumor, inflammatory) cause paralysis of lower half of face, leaving forehead intact; other LMN causes of paralysis: swelling from ear or meningeal infections
	Identify tastes		
VIII: Acoustic	Hearing acuity	Decrease or loss of hearing	Inflammation; occluded ear canal; otosclerosis; presbycusis; drug toxicity; tumor
IX: Glossopharyngeal	Gag reflex	See CN X	
X: Vagus	Phonates "ahh"	Uvula deviates to side	Brainstem tumor; neck injury; CN X lesion
	Gag reflex	No gag reflex	Vocal cord weakness
	Note voice quality	Hoarse or brassy	Soft palate weakness
		Nasal twang	Unilateral CN X lesion
		Husky	
	Note swallowing	Dysphagia, fluids regurgitate through nose	Bilateral CN X lesion
XI: Spinal accessory	Turn head, shrug shoulders against resistance	Absent movement of sternomastoid or trapezius muscles	Neck injury, torticollis
XII: Hypoglossal	Protrude tongue	Deviates to side	LMN lesion
	Wiggle tongue from side to side	Slowed rate of movement	Bilateral UMN lesion

TABLE 24.3 — Abnormalities in Muscle Tone

Condition	Description	Associated With
Flaccidity	Decreased muscle tone or *hypotonia;* muscle feels limp, soft, and flabby; muscle is weak and easily fatigued; limb feels like a rag doll	**Lower motor neuron** injury anywhere from the anterior horn cell in the spinal cord to the peripheral nerve (peripheral neuritis, poliomyelitis, Guillain-Barré syndrome); early stroke and spinal cord injury are flaccid at first
Spasticity	Increased tone or *hypertonia;* increased resistance to passive lengthening; then may suddenly give way (clasp-knife phenomenon) like a pocket knife sprung open	**Upper motor neuron** injury to corticospinal motor tract (e.g., paralysis with stroke develops spasticity days or weeks after incident)
Rigidity	Constant state of resistance (lead-pipe rigidity); resists passive movement in any direction; dystonia	Injury to extrapyramidal motor tracts (e.g., basal ganglia with parkinsonism)
Cogwheel rigidity	Type of rigidity in which the increased tone is released by degrees during passive range of motion so it feels like small, regular jerks	Parkinsonism

TABLE 24.4 — Abnormalities in Muscle Movement

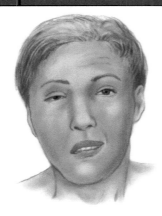

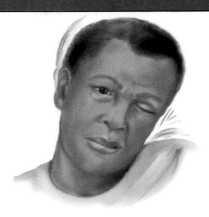

Paralysis

Decreased or loss of motor power caused by problem with motor nerve or muscle fibers. Causes: acute—trauma, spinal cord injury, stroke, poliomyelitis, polyneuritis, Bell palsy; chronic—muscular dystrophy, diabetic neuropathy, multiple sclerosis; episodic—myasthenia gravis.

Patterns of paralysis: *hemiplegia*—spastic or flaccid paralysis of one side (right or left) of body and extremities; *paraplegia*—symmetric paralysis of both lower extremities; *quadriplegia*—paralysis in all four extremities. *Paresis*—weakness of muscles rather than paralysis.

Tic

Involuntary, compulsive, repetitive twitching of a muscle group (e.g., wink, grimace, head movement, shoulder shrug); due to a neurologic cause (e.g., tardive dyskinesias, Tourette syndrome) or a psychogenic cause (habit tic).

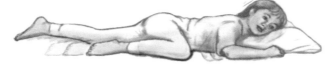

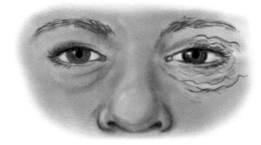

Myoclonus

Rapid, sudden jerk or a short series of jerks at fairly regular intervals. A hiccup is a myoclonus of diaphragm. Single myoclonic arm or leg jerk is normal when the person is falling asleep; myoclonic jerks are severe with grand mal seizures.

Fasciculation

Rapid, continuous twitching of resting muscle or part of muscle without movement of limb, which can be seen by clinicians or felt by patients. Types: fine—occurs with LMN disease, associated with atrophy and weakness; coarse—occurs with cold exposure or fatigue and is not significant.

Continued

| TABLE 24.4 | **Abnormalities in Muscle Movement—cont'd** |

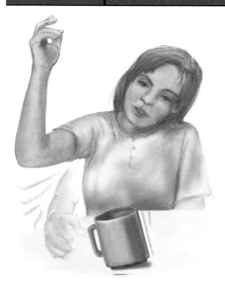

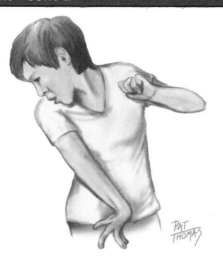

Chorea

Sudden, rapid, jerky, purposeless movement involving limbs, trunk, or face. Occurs at irregular intervals, not rhythmic or repetitive, more convulsive than a tic. Some are spontaneous, and some are initiated; all are accentuated by voluntary acts. Disappears with sleep. Common with Sydenham chorea and Huntington disease.

Athetosis

Slow, twisting, writhing, continuous movement, resembling a snake or worm. Involves the distal more than the proximal part of the limb. Occurs with cerebral palsy. Disappears with sleep. "Athetoid" hand—Some fingers are flexed, and some are extended.

Tremor

Involuntary contraction of opposing muscle groups. Results in rhythmic, back-and-forth movement of one or more joints. May occur at rest or with voluntary movement. All tremors disappear while sleeping. Tremors may be slow (3 to 6 per second) or rapid (10 to 20 per second).

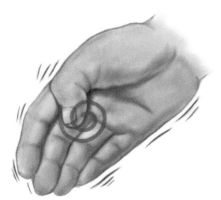

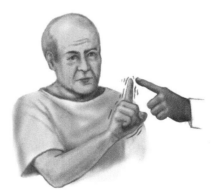

Rest Tremor

It occurs when muscles are quiet and supported against gravity (hand in lap). Coarse and slow (3 to 6 per second); partly or completely disappears with voluntary movement (e.g., "pill rolling" tremor of parkinsonism, with thumb and opposing fingers).[28]

Intention Tremor

Rate varies; worse with voluntary movement as in reaching toward a visually guided target. Occurs with cerebellar disease and multiple sclerosis.

Essential tremor (familial)—A type of intention tremor; most common tremor with older people. Benign (no associated disease) but causes emotional stress in business or social situations. Improves with sedatives, propranolol; discourage alcohol because of risk for addiction.

Continued

Abnormal Findings

TABLE 24.4	Abnormalities in Muscle Movement—cont'd

Seizure Disorder (not illustrated)

A seizure is a time-limited event caused by excessive, hypersynchronous discharge of neurons in the brain. It may be from a clear provocation such as cerebral trauma, structural lesions (tumor, blood clot, infection), hyponatremia, acute alcohol withdrawal, or medication overdose. Also, epilepsy has unprovoked recurrent seizures due to cerebrovascular disease or in 70% of patients of unknown cause. Generalized seizures involve the entire brain such as the tonic-clonic or grand mal seizure. This type of seizure has distinct phases: (1) loss of consciousness; (2) tonic phase with muscular rigidity, opening of mouth and eyes, tongue biting, and high-pitched cry; (3) clonic phase with violent muscular contractions, facial grimacing, and increased heart rate; and (4) postictal phase with deep sleeping, disorientation, and confusion.

TABLE 24.5	Ischemic and Hemorrhagic Stroke

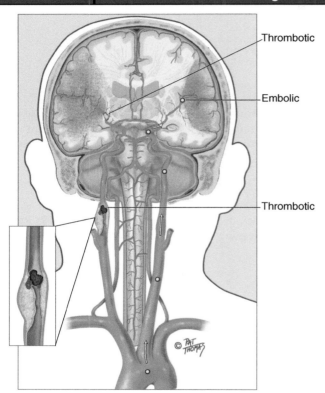

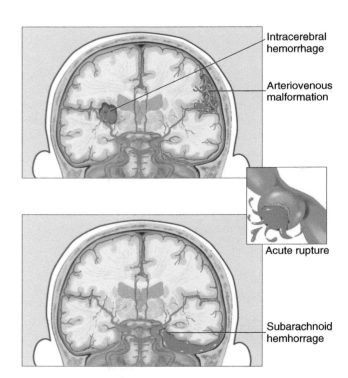

Ischemic stroke is a sudden interruption of blood flow to the brain and accounts for 87% of all strokes. These are of two types. **Thrombotic** strokes result from atherosclerotic plaque formation. A vulnerable plaque ruptures, and a local thrombus forms that deprives the brain tissue in the region of crucial oxygen and glucose. **Embolic** strokes result from a traveling clot caused by atrial fibrillation or flutter, recent heart attack, growth around prosthetic heart valves, and endocarditis. Acute ischemic stroke symptoms include unilateral facial droop, arm drift, weakness or paralysis on one half of the body, difficulty speaking or understanding speech, confusion, sudden onset of dizziness, loss of balance, clouding of vision.[1,13,24,25]

Hemorrhagic stroke results from acute rupture and bleeding from a weakened artery in the brain and accounts for only 13% of all strokes. Most are intracerebral hemorrhages caused by ruptured aneurysm, arteriovenous malformation, disturbed coagulation cascade, tumor, or cocaine abuse. Arteriovenous malformations are congenital networks of arteries and veins that do not have capillaries in between and are at risk for rupture. Think of a snarl of tendrils. A subarachnoid hemorrhage is less common and is due to an aneurysm between the base of the cerebral cortex and the arachnoid layer of the meninges. Symptoms include sudden severe headache, nausea and vomiting, sudden loss of consciousness, and focal seizures.[3,15,26,27]

ABNORMAL FINDINGS
FOR ADVANCED PRACTICE

TABLE 24.6	Abnormal Gaits	
Type	**Characteristic Appearance**	**Possible Causes**
Spastic Hemiparesis	Arm is immobile against the body, with flexion of the shoulder, elbow, wrist, and fingers and adduction of shoulder; does not swing freely. Leg is stiff and extended and circumducts with each step (drags toe in a semicircle).	UMN lesion of the corticospinal tract (e.g., stroke, trauma)
Cerebellar Ataxia	Staggering, wide-based gait; difficulty with turns; uncoordinated movement with positive Romberg sign.	Alcohol or barbiturate effect on cerebellum; cerebellar tumor; multiple sclerosis
Parkinsonian (Festinating)	Posture is stooped; trunk is pitched forward; elbows, hips, and knees are flexed. Steps are short and shuffling. Hesitation to begin walking, and difficult to stop suddenly. The person holds the body rigid. Walks and turns body as one fixed unit. Difficulty with any change in direction.	Parkinsonism
Scissors	Knees cross or are in contact, like holding an orange between the thighs. The person uses short steps, and walking requires effort.	Paraparesis of legs, multiple sclerosis
Steppage or Footdrop	Slapping quality—Looks as if walking up stairs and finding no stair there. Lifts knee and foot high and slaps it down hard and flat to compensate for footdrop.	Weakness of peroneal and anterior tibial muscles; caused by LMN lesion at spinal cord (e.g., poliomyelitis)

Continued

TABLE 24.6	Abnormal Gaits—cont'd	
Type	Characteristic Appearance	Possible Causes
Waddling	Weak hip muscles—When the person takes a step, the opposite hip drops, which allows compensatory lateral movement of pelvis. Often the person also has marked lumbar lordosis and a protruding abdomen.	Hip girdle muscle weakness caused by muscular dystrophy, dislocation of hips
Short Leg	Leg length discrepancy >2.5 cm (1 inch). Vertical telescoping of affected side, which dips as person walks. Appearance of gait varies, depending on amount of accompanying muscle dysfunction.	Congenital dislocated hip; acquired shortening from disease, trauma

TABLE 24.7	Characteristics of Upper and Lower Motor Neuron Lesions	
	Upper Motor Neuron Lesion	Lower Motor Neuron Lesion
Weakness/paralysis	In muscles corresponding to distribution of damage in pyramidal tract lesion; usually in hand grip, arm extensors, leg flexors	In specific muscles served by damaged spinal segment, ventral root, or peripheral nerve
Location	Descending motor pathways that originate in motor areas of cerebral cortex and carry impulses to anterior horn cells of spinal cord	Nerve cells that originate in anterior horn of spinal cord or brainstem and carry impulses by spinal or cranial nerves to muscles, the "final common pathway"
Example	Stroke (brain attack)	Poliomyelitis, herniated intervertebral disk
Muscle tone	Increased tone; spasticity	Loss of tone; flaccidity
Bulk	May have some atrophy from disuse; otherwise normal	Atrophy (wasting), may be marked
Abnormal movements	None	Fasciculations
Reflexes	Hyperreflexia, ankle clonus; diminished or absent superficial abdominal reflexes; positive Babinski sign	Hyporeflexia or areflexia; no Babinski sign, no pathologic reflexes
Possible nursing diagnoses	Risk for contractures; impaired physical mobility	Impaired physical mobility

TABLE 24.8	Patterns of Motor System Dysfunction

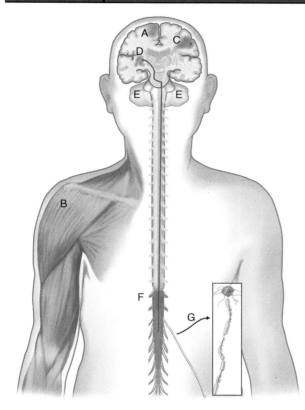

A—Cerebral palsy. Mixed group of paralytic neuromotor disorders of infancy and childhood; due to damage to cerebral cortex from a developmental defect, intrauterine meningitis or encephalitis, birth trauma, anoxia, or kernicterus.

B—Muscular dystrophy. Chronic, progressive wasting of skeletal musculature, which produces weakness, contractures, and in severe cases respiratory dysfunction and death. Onset of symptoms occurs in childhood. Many types exist; the most severe is Duchenne dystrophy, characterized by the waddling gait described in Table 24.6.

C—Hemiplegia. Damage to corticospinal tract (stroke). UMN damage occurs above the pyramidal decussation crossover; thus motor impairment is on contralateral (opposite) side. Initially flaccid when lesion is acute; later the muscles become spastic, and abnormal reflexes appear. Characteristic posture: arm—shoulder adducted, elbow flexed, wrist pronated, leg extended; face—weakness only in lower muscles. Hyperreflexia and possible clonus occur on the involved side; loss of corneal, abdominal, and cremasteric reflexes; positive Babinski and Hoffman reflexes.

D—Parkinsonism. Loss of dopamine-producing neurons in the substantia nigra and through the basal ganglia, causing motor tract disorder. Cardinal symptoms are resting tremor, bradykinesia, cogwheel rigidity, loss of balance; also anxiety, depression, and urinary incontinence. Cognitive impairment is widespread, including loss of executive function, visual-spatial impairment, and memory loss.[7] Body tends to stay immobile; facial expression is flat, staring, expressionless; excessive salivation occurs; eye blinking is reduced. Posture is stooped; equilibrium is impaired; balance is easily lost; gait is described in Table 24.6.

E—Cerebellar. A lesion in one hemisphere produces motor abnormalities on the ipsilateral side. Characterized by ataxia, lurching forward of affected side while walking; rapid alternating movements are slow and arrhythmic; finger-to-nose test reveals ataxia and tremor with overshoot or undershoot; and eyes display coarse nystagmus.

F—Paraplegia. LMN damage caused by spinal cord injury. A severe injury or complete transection initially produces "spinal shock," which is defined as no movement or reflex activity below level of lesion. Gradually deep tendon reflexes reappear and become increased; flexor spasms of legs occur; and finally extensor spasms of legs occur; these spasms lead to prevailing extensor tone.

G—Multiple sclerosis (MS). Chronic, progressive, immune-mediated disease in which axons experience inflammation, demyelination, degeneration and, finally, sclerosis. Structures most frequently involved are the optic nerve, oculomotor nerve, corticospinal tract, posterior column tract, and cerebellum. Thus symptoms include nystagmus, diplopia, extreme fatigue, weakness, spasticity, loss of balance, hyperreflexia, Babinski sign (upgoing toes). MS affects young adults in their productive years, with onset between 20 and 40 years.[11,21]

Image © Pat Thomas, 2010.

TABLE 24.9 | Patterns of Sensory Loss

Type	Characteristics	Possible Causes
Peripheral Neuropathy 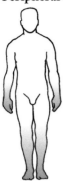	Loss of all sensation that affects nerves of the same length but spares the face.[16] Polyneuropathy affects longest nerves first (feet, then fingertips) and is termed a stocking-and-glove sensory loss. May also see atrophy of the small muscles of feet and hands and absent ankle reflexes.[16] As sensory testing moves more proximally, anesthesia zone at toes and fingertips merges into a hypoesthesia zone and gradually becomes healthy.	The long-term complications of diabetes that cause neuropathy may be due to abnormal thickening of the basement membrane of the capillaries. Chronic alcoholism also leads to polyneuropathy.
Individual Nerves or Roots 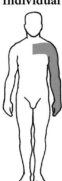	Radiculopathy causes a decrease or loss of all sensory modalities in a dermatome pattern. Area of sensory loss corresponds to distribution of involved nerve.	Cervical radiculopathy, carpal tunnel syndrome, trauma, vascular occlusion
Spinal Cord Hemisection (Brown-Séquard Syndrome) 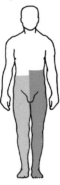	Injury to one-half of the cord, causing *contralateral* loss of pain and temperature, starting one to two segments below level of lesion. The *ipsilateral* side of the lesion has paralysis and loss of vibration and touch sensation. A pure Brown-Séquard syndrome is rare; most people with unilateral cord lesions have bilateral weakness and loss of sensation, with ipsilateral weakness greatest on the side of the lesion and sensory loss greatest contralaterally.[16]	Meningioma, neurofibroma, cervical spondylosis, multiple sclerosis

Continued

TABLE 24.9 | Patterns of Sensory Loss—cont'd

Type	Characteristics	Possible Causes
Acute Compression of the Spinal Cord 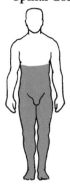	Acute spinal cord compression yields symmetric loss of sensation under a circumferential boundary (the "sensory level").[22] Accompanied by symmetric paralysis of the limbs and torso below the level of the lesion, urinary retention, or incontinence. Limbs may be flaccid and have loss of reflexes and systemic hypotension during initial phase of spinal shock.	Acute traumatic spinal compression is caused by fractured vertebrae or movement of bone fragments, disk herniation, and movement of vertebral bodies.[22] The cervical spine is vulnerable to trauma because it lacks protection from the rib cage, its joints are smaller, and the large cranium pivots on the fulcrum of the neck.[22] Cord damage also occurs with degenerative spondylosis that narrows the spinal canal, tumor growth, epidural hematoma, or abscess.
Thalamus 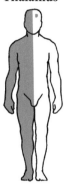	Loss of *all* sensory modalities on the face, arm, and leg on side contralateral to lesion. Also, pupil miosis and aphasia.	Vascular occlusion (stroke)
Cortex Lesion 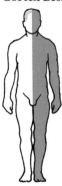	Because pain, vibration, and crude touch are mediated by the thalamus, little loss of these sensory functions occurs with a cortex lesion. Loss of discrimination occurs on contralateral side. Loss of graphesthesia, loss of stereognosis (recognition of shapes and weights), loss of finger finding.	Cerebral cortex, parietal lobe lesion (e.g., stroke)

| TABLE 24.10 | Abnormal Postures |

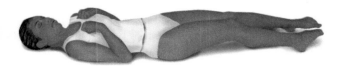

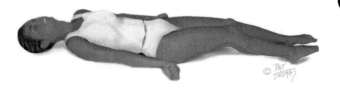

Decorticate Rigidity

Upper extremities—flexion of arm, wrist, and fingers; adduction of arm (i.e., tight against thorax). Lower extremities—extension, internal rotation, plantar flexion. This indicates hemispheric lesion of cerebral cortex.

Decerebrate Rigidity

Upper extremities stiffly extended, adducted; internal rotation, palms pronated. Lower extremities stiffly extended; plantar flexion; teeth clenched; hyperextended back. More ominous than decorticate rigidity; indicates lesion in brainstem at midbrain or upper pons.

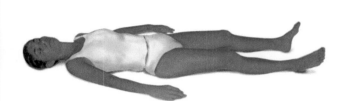

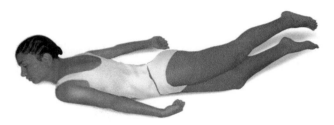

Flaccid Quadriplegia

Complete loss of muscle tone and paralysis of all four extremities, indicating completely nonfunctional brainstem.

Opisthotonos

Prolonged arching of back, with head and heels bent backward. This indicates meningeal irritation.

Images © Pat Thomas, 2006.

| TABLE 24.11 | Pathologic Reflexes |

Reflex	Method of Testing	Abnormal Response (Reflex is Present)	Indications
Babinski	Stroke lateral aspect and across ball of foot.	Extension of great toe, fanning of toes	Corticospinal (pyramidal) tract disease (e.g., stroke, trauma)
Oppenheim	Using heavy pressure with your thumb and index finger, stroke anterior medial tibial muscle.	Same as above	Same
Gordon	Firmly squeeze calf muscles.	Same as above	Same
Hoffmann	With patient's hand relaxed, wrist dorsiflexed, and fingers slightly flexed, sharply flick nail of distal phalanx of middle or index finger.	Clawing of fingers and thumb	Same
Kernig	In flat-lying supine position raise leg straight or flex thigh on abdomen and extend knee.	Resistance to straightening (because of hamstring spasm), pain down posterior thigh	Meningeal irritation (e.g., meningitis, infections)
Brudzinski	With one hand under neck and other hand on person's chest, sharply flex chin on chest and watch hips and knees.	Resistance and pain in neck, with flexion of hips and knees	Meningeal irritation (e.g., meningitis, infections)

TABLE 24.12	Frontal Release Signs

Reflex

Snout reflex

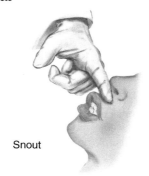

Snout

Method of testing
Gently percuss oral region
Abnormal response (reflex is present)
Puckers lips
Indications
Frontal lobe disease, cerebral degenerative disease (Alzheimer), amyotrophic
sclerosis, corticobulbar lesions

Sucking reflex

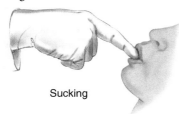

Sucking

Method of testing
Touch oral region
Abnormal response (reflex is present)
Sucking movement of lips, tongue, jaw, swallowing
Indications
Same as for snout reflex

Grasp reflex

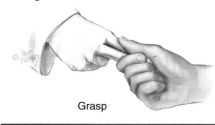

Grasp

Method of testing
Touch palm with your finger
Abnormal response (reflex is present)
Uncontrolled, forced grasping (grasp is usually last of these signs to appear;
thus its presence indicates severe disease)
Indications
When unilateral, frontal lobe lesion on contralateral side; when bilateral,
diffuse bifrontal lobe disease

Images © Pat Thomas, 2006.

Abnormal Findings

Summary Checklist: Neurologic Examination

Neurologic Screening Examination
1. **Mental status**
2. **Cranial nerves**
   II: Optic
   III, IV, VI: Extraocular muscles
   V: Trigeminal
   VII: Facial mobility
3. **Motor function**
   Gait and balance
   Knee flexion—hop or shallow knee
   bend

4. **Sensory function**
   Superficial pain and light touch—
   arms and legs
   Vibration—arms and legs
5. **Reflexes**
   Biceps
   Triceps
   Patellar
   Achilles

Neurologic Complete Examination
1. **Mental status**
2. **Cranial nerves II through XII**

3. **Motor system**
   Muscle size, strength, tone
   Rapid alternating movements
   Gait and balance
4. **Sensory function**
   Superficial pain and light touch
   Vibration, position sense
   Stereognosis, graphesthesia,
   two-point discrimination
5. **Reflexes**
   DTRs: Biceps, triceps,
   brachioradialis, patellar, Achilles
   Superficial: Plantar

REFERENCES

1. Anderson, J. A. (2014). The golden hour: Performing an acute ischemic stroke workup. *Nurse Pract, 39*(9), 22–30.
2. Beuscher, L., Reeves, G., & Harrell, D. (2017). Managing herpes zoster in older adults: Prescribing considerations. *Nurse Pract, 42*(6), 24–30.
3. Bushnell, C., McCullough, L. D., Awad, I. A., et al. (2014). Guidelines for the prevention of stroke in women. *Stroke, 45*(5), 1545–1588.
4. Centers for Disease Control (CDC). (2017). *What everyone should know about shingles vaccine.* https://www.cdc.gov/vaccines/vpd/shingles/public.
5. Chadehumbe, M. A. (2016). Neurologic care in concussion and post-concussive encephalopathy. *Curr Probl Pediatr Adolesc Health Care, 46*, 52–57.
6. Cunningham, A. L., Lal, H., Kovac, M., et al. (2016). Efficacy of the herpes zoster subunit vaccine in adults 70 years of age or older. *N Engl J Med, 375*(11), 1019–1032.
7. Dancis, A., & Cotter, V. T. (2015). Diagnosis and management of cognitive impairment in Parkinson's disease. *J Nurse Pract, 11*(3), 307–313.
8. Feigin, V. L., Roth, G. A., Naghavi, M., et al. (2016). Global burden of stroke and risk factors in 188 countries during 1990-2013. *Lancet Neurol, 15*(9), 913–924.
9. Fjell, A. M., McEvoy, L., Holland, D., et al. (2013). Brain changes in older adults at very low risk for Alzheimer's disease. *J Neurosci, 33*(19), 8237–8242.
10. Gutierrez, J., & Williams, O. A. (2014). A decade of racial and ethnic stroke disparities in the United States. *Neurology, 82*(12), 1080–1082.
11. Hunter, S. F. (2016). Overview and diagnosis of multiple sclerosis. *Am J Manag Care, 226*(6 Suppl.), S141–S150.
12. Jamault, V., & Duff, E. (2013). Adolescent concussions: When to return to play. *Nurse Pract, 38*(2), 16–22.
13. Jovin, T. G., Chamorro, A., Cobo, E., et al. (2015). Original article: Thrombectomy within 8 hours after symptom onset in ischemic stroke. *N Engl J Med, 372*, 2296–2306.
14. Kerr, R. G., Bacon, A. M., Baker, L. L., et al. (2016). Underestimation of pupil size by critical care and neurosurgical nurses. *Am J Crit Care, 25*(3), 213–219.
15. Lawton, M. T., & Vates, E. (2017). Subarachnoid hemorrhage. *N Engl J Med, 377*(3), 257–266.
16. McGee, S. (2018). *Evidence-based physical diagnosis* (4th ed.). St Louis: Elsevier.
17. Mochari-Greenberger, H., Xian, Y., Hellkamp, A. S., et al. (2015). Racial/ethnic and sex differences in emergency medical services transport among hospitalized US stroke patients. *J Am Heart Assoc, 4*(8), e002099.
18. Mozaffarian, D., Benjamin, E. J., Go, A. S., et al. (2016). Heart disease and stroke statistics—2016 update. *Circulation, 133*, e38–e360.
19. Mullen, M. T., Wiebe, D. J., Bowman, A., et al. (2014). Disparities in accessibility of certified primary stroke centers. *Stroke, 45*(11), 3381–3388.
20. National Institute of Neurological Disorders and Stroke (NINDS). (2017). *Brain basics: Preventing stroke.* https://www.ninds.nih.gov/Disorders/Patient-Caregiver-Education/Preventing-Stroke.
21. Reich, D. S., Lucchinetti, C. F., & Calabrese, P. A. (2018). Multiple sclerosis. *N Engl J Med, 378*(2), 169–179.
22. Ropper, A. E., & Ropper, A. H. (2017). Acute spinal cord compression. *N Engl J Med, 376*(14), 1358–1368.
23. Saccomano, S. J., & Ferrara, L. R. (2015). Fall prevention in older adults. *Nurse Pract, 40*(6), 40–47.
24. Schweickert, P. A., Gaughen, J. R., Kreitel, E. M., et al. (2016). An overview of antithrombotics in ischemic stroke. *Nurse Pract, 41*(6), 48–55.
25. Sofer, D. (2016). Study assesses the global stroke burden. *Am J Nurs, 116*(9), 16.
26. Solomon, R. A., & Connolly, E. S. (2017). Arteriovenous malformations of the brain. *N Engl J Med, 376*(19), 1859–1866.
27. Thompson, B. G., Brown, R. J., Amin-Hanjani, S., et al. (2015). Guidelines for the management of patients with unruptured intracranial aneurysms. *Stroke, 46*(8), 2368–2400.
28. Vernon, G. M., Leiningen, C., Thomas, C. A., et al. (2017). Essential tremor & Parkinson disease: Recognizing the differences. *Nurse Pract, 42*(10), 35–40.

Male Genitourinary System

STRUCTURE AND FUNCTION

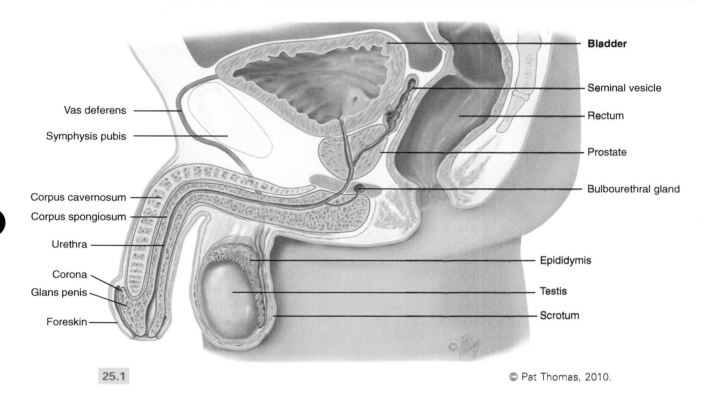

Vas deferens

Symphysis pubis

Corpus cavernosum

Corpus spongiosum

Urethra

Corona

Glans penis

Foreskin

Bladder

Seminal vesicle

Rectum

Prostate

Bulbourethral gland

Epididymis

Testis

Scrotum

25.1

© Pat Thomas, 2010.

THE MALE GENITALIA

The male genital structures include the penis and scrotum externally and the testis, epididymis, and vas deferens internally. Glandular structures accessory to the genital organs (the prostate, seminal vesicles, and bulbourethral glands) are discussed in Chapter 26.

Penis

The **penis** is composed of three cylindric columns of erectile tissue: the two corpora cavernosa on the dorsal side and the corpus spongiosum ventrally (Fig. 25.1). At the distal end of the shaft the corpus spongiosum expands into a cone of erectile tissue, the **glans.** The shoulder where the glans joins the shaft is the **corona.** The **urethra** is a conduit for both the genital and the urinary systems. It transverses the corpus spongiosum, and its meatus forms a slit at the glans tip. Over

the glans, the skin folds in and back on itself, forming a hood or flap. This is the **foreskin** or **prepuce.** Often it is surgically removed shortly after birth by circumcision. The **frenulum** is a fold of the foreskin extending from the urethral meatus ventrally.

Scrotum

The **scrotum** is a loose protective sac, which is a continuation of the abdominal wall. After adolescence the scrotal skin is deeply pigmented and has large sebaceous follicles. The scrotal wall consists of thin skin lying in folds, or **rugae,** and the underlying cremaster muscle. The **cremaster muscle** controls the size of the scrotum by responding to ambient temperature. This is to keep the testes at 3° C below abdominal temperature, the best temperature for producing sperm. When it is cold, the muscle contracts, raising the sac and bringing the testes closer to the body to absorb heat necessary

683

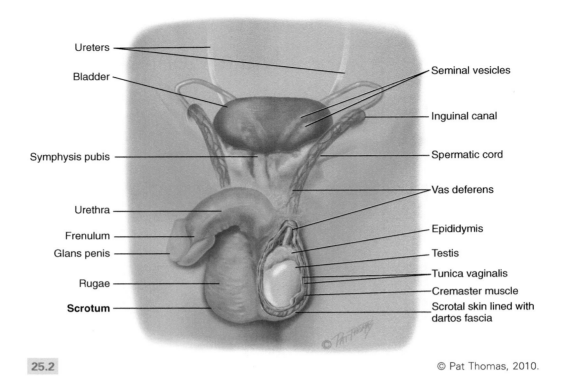

25.2

© Pat Thomas, 2010.

for sperm viability. As a result the scrotal skin looks corrugated. When it is warmer, the muscle relaxes, the scrotum lowers, and the skin looks smoother.

Inside a septum separates the sac into two halves. In each scrotal half is a **testis,** which produces sperm. The testis has a solid oval shape, which is compressed laterally and measures 4 to 5 cm long by 3 cm wide in the adult. It is suspended vertically by the spermatic cord (Fig. 25.2). The left testis is lower than the right because the left spermatic cord is longer. Each testis is covered by a double-layered membrane, the tunica vaginalis, which separates it from the scrotal wall. The two layers are lubricated by fluid so the testis can slide a little within the scrotum; this helps prevent injury.

Sperm are transported along a series of ducts. First the testis is capped by the **epididymis,** which is a markedly coiled duct system and the main storage site of sperm. It is a comma-shaped structure, curved over the top and the posterior surface of the testis. Occasionally (in 6% to 7% of males), the epididymis is anterior to the testis.

The lower part of the epididymis is continuous with a muscular duct, the **vas deferens.** This duct approximates with other vessels (arteries and veins, lymphatics, nerves) to form the **spermatic cord.** The spermatic cord ascends along the posterior border of the testis and runs through the tunnel of the inguinal canal into the abdomen. Here the vas deferens continues back and down behind the bladder, where it joins the duct of the seminal vesicle to form the **ejaculatory duct.** This duct empties into the urethra.

The **lymphatics** of the penis and scrotal surface drain into the inguinal lymph nodes, whereas those of the testes drain into the abdomen. Abdominal lymph nodes are not accessible to clinical examination.

Inguinal Area

The **inguinal area,** or groin, is the juncture of the lower abdominal wall and the thigh (Fig. 25.3). Its diagonal borders are the anterior superior iliac spine and the symphysis pubis. Between these landmarks lies the **inguinal ligament** (Poupart ligament). Superior to the ligament lies the **inguinal canal,** a narrow tunnel passing obliquely between layers of abdominal muscle. It is 4 to 6 cm long in the adult. Its openings are an internal ring, located 1 to 2 cm above the midpoint of the inguinal ligament, and an external ring, located just above and lateral to the pubis.

Inferior to the inguinal ligament is the **femoral canal.** It is a potential space located 3 cm medial to and parallel with the femoral artery. You can use the artery as a landmark to find this space.

Knowledge of these anatomic areas in the groin is useful because they are potential sites for a hernia, which is a loop of bowel protruding through a weak spot in the musculature.

❖ DEVELOPMENTAL COMPETENCE

Infants

Prenatally the testes develop in the abdominal cavity near the kidneys. During the later months of gestation the testes migrate, pushing the abdominal wall in front of them and dragging the vas deferens, blood vessels, and nerves behind. The testes descend along the inguinal canal into the scrotum before birth. At birth each testis measures 1.5 to 2 cm long and 1 cm wide. Only a slight increase in size occurs during the prepubertal years.

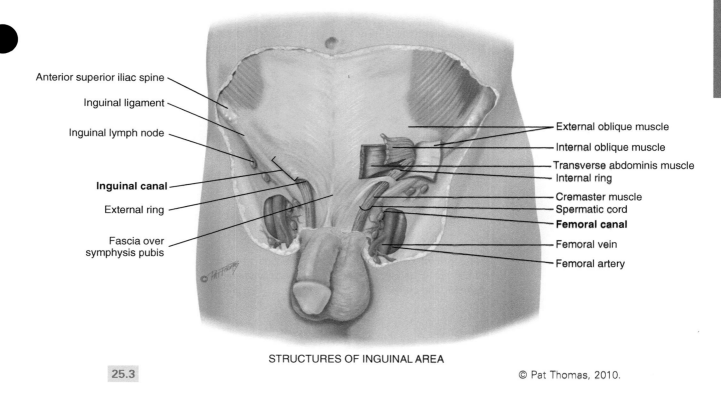

Anterior superior iliac spine

Inguinal ligament

Inguinal lymph node

Inguinal canal

External ring

Fascia over
symphysis pubis

External oblique muscle

Internal oblique muscle

Transverse abdominis muscle

Internal ring

Cremaster muscle

Spermatic cord

Femoral canal

Femoral vein

Femoral artery

STRUCTURES OF INGUINAL AREA

25.3

© Pat Thomas, 2010.

Adolescents

The most current evidence shows that signs of puberty in the United States begin now at an average of age 9 for African-American boys and age 10 for Caucasians and Hispanics.[10] The first sign is enlargement of the testes. Next pubic hair appears, and then penis size increases. The stages of development are documented in Tanner's sexual maturity ratings (SMRs) (Table 25.1).

Compared with earlier studies, the onset of Tanner stage 2 (testes enlargement and pubic hair growth) is now about 2 years earlier for African-American boys and about 1½ years earlier for Caucasians.[10] This earlier onset of puberty has also been noted in other countries. In the United States it may relate to environmental factors such as chemical exposure, diet changes, and less physical activity. Just because physical maturity occurs earlier does not mean that boys have the psychological or emotional maturity to go with the physical changes. It is important for clinicians and parents to be aware of physical changes so they can help boys negotiate the emotions and behaviors associated with puberty.

Gender Identity

Do not assume sexual orientation by feminine or masculine clothing, hairstyle, physical appearance, or sports preference. Adolescence is a time of sexual expression and experimentation and identity formation. "Sexual minority" includes those who self-identify as gay if male; lesbian if female; bisexual when sexually attracted to both males and females; transgender when having an innate, deep-seated knowledge that their own orientation differs from their birth assignment[4];

and questioning if struggling with sexual attractions and identity formation.[12] Transgender youth may be struggling with transition to the desired gender; MTF is males transitioning to females. Sexual minority also includes men having settled themselves into same-sex relationships, MSM or men having sex with men. It is crucial that clinicians have an open, accepting attitude in order to provide health care that is factual and confidential.[12] Many youth and young adults have experienced discrimination, bullying, and homophobia. Most young people are resilient, and given family support, school support, and acceptance by friends, they will emerge and lead happy, meaningful lives. Those who lack this support experience high-risk sexual behaviors, drug behaviors, and mental health concerns.

Adults and Aging Adults

The older man does not experience a definite end to fertility as the woman does. The production of sperm begins to decrease around 40 years, although it continues into the 80s and 90s. Testosterone production declines after age 30 but very gradually, so resulting physical changes are not evident until later in life.

In the aging male the amount of pubic hair decreases and turns gray. Penis size decreases. Because of decreased tone of the dartos muscle, the scrotal contents hang lower, the rugae decrease, and the scrotum looks pendulous. The testes decrease in size and are less firm to palpation. The prostate gland surrounding the upper urethra undergoes an expected tissue hyperplasia in about 80% of men over 60 years. While this is NOT cancer, benign prostatic hyperplasia (BPH)

TABLE 25.1 Sexual Maturity Rating (SMR) in Boys

DEVELOPMENTAL STAGE	PUBIC HAIR	PENIS	SCROTUM
1	No pubic hair; fine body hair on abdomen (vellus hair) continues over pubic area	Preadolescent, size and proportion the same as during childhood	Preadolescent, size and proportion the same as during childhood
2	Few straight, slightly darker hairs at base of penis; hair is long and downy	Little or no enlargement	Testes and scrotum begin to enlarge; scrotal skin reddens and changes in texture
3	Sparse growth over entire pubis; hair is darker, coarser, and curly	Penis begins to enlarge, especially in length	Further enlarged
4	Thick growth over pubic area but not on thighs; hair coarse and curly as in adult	Penis grows in length and diameter, with development of glans	Testes almost fully grown; scrotum darker
5	Growth spread over medial thighs, although not yet up toward umbilicus; after puberty, pubic hair growth continues until the mid-20s, extending up the abdomen toward the umbilicus	Adult size and shape	Adult size and shape

Adapted from Tanner, J. M. (1962). *Growth at adolescence.* Oxford, England: Blackwell Scientific Publications.

causes an obstructed urine stream and risk for urinary tract infection (UTI). (See Chapter 26 for a full discussion of BPH.)

In general, declining testosterone production leaves the older male with a slower and less intense sexual response, and an erection takes longer to develop and is less full or firm. Ejaculation is shorter and less forceful, and the volume of seminal fluid is less than when the man was younger. After ejaculation, rapid detumescence (return to the flaccid state) occurs, especially after 60 years.

Sexual Expression in Later Life. Chronologic age by itself should not mean a halt in sexual activity. The just-mentioned physical changes need not interfere with the libido and pleasure from sexual intercourse. The older male is capable of sexual function as long as he is in reasonably good health and has an interested, willing partner. In the absence of disease, a withdrawal from sexual activity may be caused by loss of spouse; depression; preoccupation with work; marital or family conflict; side effects of medications such as antihypertensives, psychotropics, antidepressants, antispasmodics, sedatives, tranquilizers or narcotics, and estrogens; heavy use of alcohol; lack of privacy (living with adult children or in a nursing home); economic or emotional stress; poor nutrition; or fatigue.

🌐 CULTURE AND GENETICS

Circumcision. Early in pregnancy expectant parents make the decision about whether to circumcise their newborn son. Circumcision is an elective surgical procedure to remove all or part of the foreskin (prepuce) from the penis. Parents need an unbiased presentation of the risks and benefits of this procedure.

Medical benefits of male circumcision include a reduced risk of acquiring HIV infection through heterosexual contact. Studies showing this reduced risk emerged from sub-Saharan Africa, where HIV is endemic; results may not generalize to other countries where HIV prevalence is lower and routes of acquiring HIV are different.[9] Most HIV transmission in the United States is by drug needle sharing and by men having sex with men. However, HIV is a global infection, and the World Health Organization has proposed reaching 80% male circumcision in HIV-endemic countries to decrease heterosexual transmission.[19]

In addition to the benefit of reduced heterosexual HIV risk, the American Academy of Pediatrics (AAP) proposes that the health benefits of newborn male circumcision outweigh the risks and that all families should have access to male circumcision if they choose it.[2] The procedure should be covered by insurance and Medicaid. Further benefits listed are reduced risk of urinary tract infections in infancy and in adults a reduced risk of STIs such as human papillomavirus (HPV) infection, herpes simplex virus, and genital ulcer disease in men, and a decreased risk of bacterial vaginosis and trichomoniasis in female partners.[2,19] These data are supported by a Mayo Clinic review claiming circumcision benefits exceed risks by 100 to 1 and that circumcision of newborn boys should be public health policy.[13]

However, other reports refute the claimed health benefits of infant male circumcision and state that the only benefit may be protection against urinary tract infections in infant boys and that this can be treated with antibiotics.[9] The other benefits are questionable and are not compelling reasons for surgery before boys are old enough to decide for themselves.[9] While the current findings are mixed, nurses and other health providers must discuss circumcision early in pregnancy so

that families have time to ask questions, discuss current information, and make their best decision.[15]

Circumcision is a nontherapeutic surgical procedure with a small but possible risk for complications. Most are minor and treatable: pain, bleeding, swelling, or inadequate skin removal. A review of adverse events of male circumcision in U.S. medical settings found the incidence at less than 0.5% during infancy, but adverse events increased when performed at older ages.[7] Neonates certainly are capable of perceiving pain; therefore parents need to be apprised of pain-relief measures for the circumcision procedure. These include dorsal penile nerve block and a lidocaine-prilocaine cream (EMLA).[2]

Kidney Disease. Chronic kidney disease (CKD) is determined by blood tests, urinalysis, and imaging studies that show decreased kidney function or kidney damage lasting 3 months or longer. This can lead progressively and irreversibly to end-stage renal disease (ESRD), when the person survives only by kidney transplant or dialysis. CKD is a global health problem. It has two main causes, hypertension and diabetes, which comprise 70% or more of patients who progress to ESRD and are undergoing dialysis.

The prevalence of diabetes and hypertension is higher in some racial groups, which reflects the higher ESRD. Compared with Caucasians, ESRD is 3.7 times greater in African Americans, 1.4 times greater in American Indians, and 1.5 times greater in Asian Americans. Hispanics are 1.5 times more likely to develop ESRD than non-Hispanics.[14] An analysis of a nationally representative sample of the U.S. population identified the association between low socioeconomic status (SES) and CKD.[22] The lower SES groups were younger, less likely to be male, and comprised of more non-Hispanic blacks and Mexican Americans than were the high-SES groups. In the low-SES groups, there was a higher proportion of adverse health-related behaviors (current smoking, high alcohol intake, high sedentary time, unhealthy diet), a higher proportion of comorbid conditions (diabetes, hypertension, obesity, hypercholesterolemia), as well as more people having no health insurance and no routine health care visits in the past year.[22] All these are seen as mediators by which low SES contributes substantially to the development of CKD, and the association was highest in non-Hispanic blacks. Because these mediators are potentially modifiable, our health care system could design interventions targeting them, and these interventions may be most helpful for non-Hispanic blacks.

Bladder Cancer. This is the fourth most common cause of cancer in men, with a higher incidence in white Americans than in African Americans. Smoking is the most common risk factor, responsible for about two-thirds of cancers. Other risk factors include occupational exposure to aniline dyes and other chemicals used in the textile, paint, plastic, printing, and rubber industries.[8] The initial sign is painless hematuria. This can be present in other conditions, but bladder cancer should always be tested, especially with a history of smoking.

Subjective Data

SUBJECTIVE DATA

1. Frequency, urgency, and nocturia
2. Dysuria
3. Hesitancy and straining
4. Urine color

5. Past genitourinary history
6. Penis—pain, lesion, discharge
7. Scrotum, self-care behaviors, lump

8. Sexual activity and contraceptive use
9. Sexually transmitted infection (STI) contact

Examiner Asks	Rationale
1. Frequency, urgency, and nocturia. Urinating more often than usual? • Feel as if you cannot wait to urinate? • Awaken during the night because you need to urinate? How often? Is this a recent change?	**Frequency.** Average adult voids 5-6 times/day, varying with fluid intake, individual habits. Polyuria—Excessive quantity. Oliguria—Diminished, <400 mL/24 hours. **Urgency.** **Nocturia** occurs together with frequency and urgency in urinary tract disorders. Other origins: cardiovascular, habitual, diuretic medication.
2. Dysuria. Any pain or burning with urinating?	**Dysuria.** Burning is common with acute cystitis, prostatitis, urethritis.
3. Hesitancy and straining. Any trouble starting the urine stream? • Need to strain to start or maintain stream? • Any change in force of stream: narrowing, becoming weaker? • Dribbling such that you must stand closer to the toilet? • Afterward do you still feel you need to urinate? • Ever had any urinary tract infections?	**Hesitancy.** Straining. Loss of force and decreased caliber. Terminal dribbling. Sense of residual urine. Recurrent episodes of acute cystitis. Symptoms suggest bladder outlet obstruction from chronic BPH.
4. Urine color. Is the usual **urine** clear or discolored, cloudy, foul-smelling, bloody (Fig. 25.4)?	Cloudy in urinary tract infection. Hematuria—A danger sign that warrants further workup. Some color changes are temporary or harmless. However, for blood in urine or for a color change lasting longer than a day, seek health care. It may be a UTI with dysuria symptoms. Or hematuria may signal glomerulonephritis or cancers of prostate or bladder. A history of smoking is the most common risk factor for bladder cancer, with 4 times the risk of nonsmokers.[8] For a complete description, see Table 25.2, Urine Color and Discolorations, p. 703.

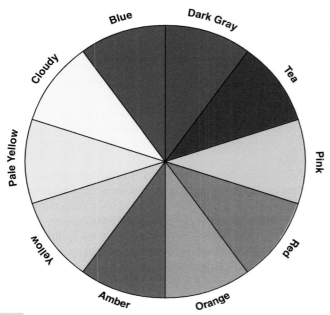

25.4

Courtesy Connie Cooper.

Examiner Asks	Rationale

5. Past genitourinary history. Any difficulty controlling your urine?

Urge incontinence—Involuntary urine loss from overactive detrusor muscle in bladder.
Stress incontinence—Involuntary urine loss with physical strain, sneezing, or coughing caused by weakness of pelvic floor.

- Accidentally urinate when you sneeze, laugh, cough, or bear down?

- Any **history** of kidney disease, kidney stones, flank pain, urinary tract infections, prostate trouble?

6. Penis. Any problem with penis—**pain, lesions?**
- Any **discharge?** How much? Has it increased or decreased since start?
- The color? Any odor? Discharge associated with pain or urination?

Urethral discharge occurs with infection (see Table 25.3, Urinary Problems, p. 704).

7. Scrotum, self-care behaviors. Any problem with the scrotum or testicles?
- Any **lump** or **swelling** on testes?
- Any change in size of the scrotum? Any history of undescended testicle as infant?
- Noted any bulge or swelling in the scrotum? For how long? Ever been told you have a hernia? Any dragging, heavy feeling in scrotum?

Concern about any self-discovered mass (spermatocele, hydrocele, varicocele, rarely testicular cancer) alerts you to careful exploration during examination.
Possible hernia.

8. Sexual activity and contraceptive use. Are you in a relationship involving sexual intercourse now? [NOTE: Use gender-neutral terms.]
- Are aspects of sex satisfactory to you and your partner?
- Are you satisfied with the way you and your partner communicate about sex?
- Occasionally a man notices a change in ability to have an erection when aroused. Have you noticed any changes?[a]

Questions about **sexual activity** should be routine in review of body systems for these reasons:
- Communicates that you accept individual's sexual activity and believe that it is important.
- Your comfort with discussion prompts person's interest and possibly relief that topic has been introduced.
- Establishes a database for comparisons with any future sexual activities.
- Provides opportunity to screen sexual problems.
Your questions should be objective and matter-of-fact.
Gay and bisexual men need to feel acceptance to discuss their health concerns. Young MSM who report unprotected anal intercourse in the previous 6 months are at increased risk for gonorrhea, chlamydia, syphilis, and HIV.[12]

- Do you and your partner use a condom or a contraceptive? Which method? Is it satisfactory? Any questions about this method?
- How many sexual partners have you had in the past 6 months?

- What is your sexual preference—relationship with a woman, a man, both?

9. STI contact. Any sexual contact with a partner having an STI such as gonorrhea, herpes, HIV, chlamydia, human papilloma virus (HPV), venereal warts, syphilis?
- When was this contact? Did you get the disease?
- How was it treated? Any complications?
- Do you use condoms to help prevent STIs?
- Any questions or concerns about any of these diseases?

Additional History for Infants and Children

1. Does your child have any problem urinating? Urine stream look straight?
- Any pain with urinating, crying, or holding the genitals?
- Any urinary tract infection?

[a]At times, phrase your questions so that all is right for the person to acknowledge a problem.

Examiner Asks	Rationale

2. If your boy is uncircumcised, do not retract the foreskin forcibly. It will retract on its own when the child has spontaneous erections (no liquid comes out) or when your boy can retract it himself easily. Then have him clean the glans gently.

Forced retractions can hurt and tear adhesions normal at birth. Adhesions resolve spontaneously in early months or years and then foreskin slides easily.

3. (If child older than 2 to 2½ years.) Has toilet training started? How is it progressing?
   • (If child 5 years or older.) Wet the bed at night? Is this a problem for child or for you (parents)? What have you done? How does the child feel about it?

Nocturnal enuresis—Involuntarily urinating at night after age 5 to 6 years.

4. Any problem with child's penis or scrotum: sores, swelling, discoloration?
   • Told if his testes are descended or undescended?
   • Ever had a hernia or hydrocele?
   • Swelling in his scrotum during crying or coughing?

5. (Ask directly to preschooler or young school-age child.) Has anyone ever touched your penis or in between your legs, and you did not want them to? Sometimes that happens to children, and it's not okay. They should remember that they have not been bad. They should try to tell a big person about it. Can you tell me 3 different big people whom you trust to whom you could talk?

Screen for sexual abuse. For prevention, teach the child that it is NOT okay for someone to look at or touch his private parts while telling him it is a secret. Naming 3 trusted adults will include someone outside the family—important, since most molestation is by a parent.

Additional History for Preadolescents and Adolescents

Ask questions that seem appropriate for boy's age, but be aware that norms vary widely. When you are in doubt, it is better to ask too many questions than to omit something. Children obtain information, often misinformation, from the media, Internet, and peers at very early ages. You may be sure that your information will be more thoughtful and accurate.

Ask direct, matter-of-fact questions. Avoid sounding judgmental.

Start with a *permission statement*. "Often boys your age experience. ..." This conveys that it is normal and all right to think or feel a certain way.

Try the *ubiquity approach*. "When did you ...?" rather than "Do you ...?" This method is less threatening because it implies that the topic is normal and unexceptional.

Do not be concerned if a boy will not discuss sexuality with you or respond to offers for information. He may not wish to let on that he needs or wants more information. You do well to "open the door." The adolescent may come back at a future time.

1. Around age 10 to 12 years, boys start to change and grow around the penis and scrotum. What changes have you noticed?

   Who can you talk to about your body changes and for sex information? How do these talks go? Do you think you get enough information? What about sex education classes at school? How about your parents? Is there a favorite teacher, nurse, doctor, minister, or counselor to whom you can talk?

2. Boys around age 12 years have a normal experience of fluid coming out of the penis at night, called nocturnal emissions, or "wet dreams." Have you had this?

An occasional boy confuses this with a sign of STI or feels guilty.

Examiner Asks	Rationale

3. Teenage boys have other normal experiences and wonder if they are the only ones who ever had them, such as having an erection at embarrassing times, having sexual fantasies, or masturbating. Also, a boy might have a thought about touching another boy's genitals and wonder if this means he might be homosexual. Would you like to talk about any of these things?

A boy may feel guilty about experiencing these things if not informed that they are normal.

4. Often boys your age have questions about sexual activity. What questions do you have? How about things such as birth control or STIs such as gonorrhea or herpes? Any questions about these?
- Are you dating? Someone steady? Have you had intercourse? Are you using condoms?

- (If relationship is heterosexual) Which kind of birth control did you use the *last* time you had intercourse?

Assess level of knowledge. Many boys will not admit that they need more knowledge.

Avoid the term "having sex." It is ambiguous, and teens can take it to mean anything from foreplay to intercourse. Use behavior-specific words.

This particular question often reveals that the teen is not using any method of birth control.

5. Has a nurse or doctor ever taught you how to examine your own testicles to make sure they are healthy?

Assess knowledge of testicular self-examination.

6. Has anyone ever touched your genitals when you did not want them to? Another boy, or an adult, even a relative? Sometimes that happens to teenagers. They should remember it is not their fault. They should tell another adult about it.

Screen for sexual abuse.

7. Routine vaccinations include the vaccine Gardasil. Have you had these?

First approved in 2009 for boys and men ages 9 to 26 years for prevention of STI genital warts in men and for reducing HPV-related cervical cancer in women.

Additional History for the Aging Adult

1. Any difficulty urinating? Any hesitancy and straining? A weakened force of stream? Any dribbling? Any incomplete emptying?

Early symptoms of enlarging prostate may be tolerated or ignored. Later symptoms are more dramatic: hematuria, urinary tract infection.[20,23]

2. Do you ever leak water/urine when you don't want to? Do you use pads/tissue to catch urine in your underwear?

Incontinence is any involuntary leaking of urine.

3. Do you need to get up at night to urinate? Which medications are you taking? What fluids do you drink in the evening?

Nocturia may be caused by diuretic medication, habit, or fluid ingestion 3 hours before bedtime; coffee and alcohol especially have a diuretic effect.

Fluid retention from mild heart failure or varicose veins produces nocturia because recumbency at night mobilizes fluid.

4. Is it all right to ask you about your sexual function? This is something I ask all the men. For example, it is normal for an erection to develop slowly at this age. This is not a sign of impotence, but a man might wonder if it is.

Excluding physical illness, an older man is fully capable of sexual function. But some assume that normal changes mean they are "old men," and they withdraw from sexual

Subjective Data

Examiner Asks	Rationale
• Any change in your ability to have an erection? • Wanting to have an erection is normal, and it is treatable with medication.	activity. The older person is not reluctant to discuss sexual activity, and most welcome the opportunity. Depressants to sexual desire and function include antihypertensives, sedatives, tranquilizers, estrogens, and alcohol. Alcohol decreases the sexual response even more dramatically in the older person.

OBJECTIVE DATA

PREPARATION

Entering the Room

Knock and wait for permission to enter. Before the exam, say, "If at any time you want me to stop the exam, just say 'stop.'" Ask the male to stand and lower undershorts down to knees. You the examiner should be sitting, or the male can be supine on the table for the initial exam and then stand to check for hernia.

It is normal for a male to feel apprehensive about having his genitalia examined, especially by a female examiner. Younger adolescents usually have more anxiety than older adolescents. But any male may have difficulty dissociating a necessary, matter-of-fact step in the physical examination from the feeling that this is an invasion of his privacy. His concerns are modesty, fear of pain, cold hands, negative judgment, or fear of having an erection during the examination and that this would be misinterpreted by the examiner.

Take time to consider these feelings and to explore your own. It is normal for you to feel embarrassed and apprehensive too. You may worry about your age, lack of clinical experience, causing pain, or even that your movements might "cause" an erection. Accept these feelings and work through them so you can examine the male in a professional way. Discuss concerns with an experienced examiner. Your demeanor is important. Your unresolved discomfort magnifies any discomfort the man may have.

Your demeanor should be *confident* and relaxed, unhurried yet businesslike. Do not discuss genitourinary history or sexual practices while you are performing the examination. This may be perceived as judgmental. Instead say, "I'm just checking for changes" and "You are normal and healthy."

Use a firm, deliberate touch, not a soft, stroking one. Start your touch by leading with the back of your hand. If an erection does occur, say, "This is only a normal physiologic response to touch." Proceed with the rest of the examination.

EQUIPMENT NEEDED

Collect a urine screen for gonorrhea and chlamydia

Gloves: wear gloves during every male genitalia examination

Occasional: Materials for cytology

Flashlight

Normal Range of Findings	Abnormal Findings
Inspect and Palpate the Penis The skin normally looks wrinkled, hairless, and without lesions. The dorsal vein may be apparent (Fig. 25.5).	Inflammation. Lesions: nodules, solitary ulcer (chancre), grouped vesicles or superficial ulcers, wartlike papules (see Table 25.4, Male Genital Lesions, p. 705).

Normal Range of Findings	**Abnormal Findings**

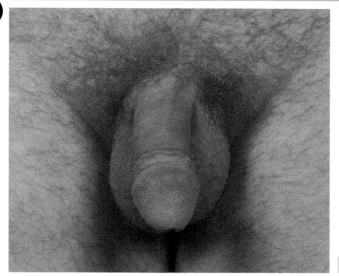

25.5

The glans looks smooth and without lesions. Ask the uncircumcised male to retract the foreskin, or you retract it. It should move easily. Some cheesy smegma may have collected under the foreskin. After inspection slide the foreskin back to the original position.

The urethral meatus is positioned just about centrally.

At the base of the penis, pubic hair distribution is consistent with age. Hair is without pest inhabitants.

Compress the glans anteroposteriorly between your thumb and forefinger (Fig. 25.6). The meatus edge should appear pink, smooth, and without discharge.

Inflammation. Lesions on glans or corona.

Phimosis—Narrowed opening of prepuce so cannot retract the foreskin. **Paraphimosis**—Painful constriction of glans by retracted foreskin.

Hypospadias—Ventral location of meatus. **Epispadias**—Dorsal location of meatus (see Table 25.5, Penis Abnormalities, p. 706).

Pubic lice or nits can be seen with the unaided eye. Excoriated skin usually accompanies.

Stricture—Narrowed opening.

Edges that are red, everted, edematous, along with purulent discharge, suggest urethritis (see Table 25.3, p. 704). Urethritis occurs with gonorrhea and/or chlamydia infection.

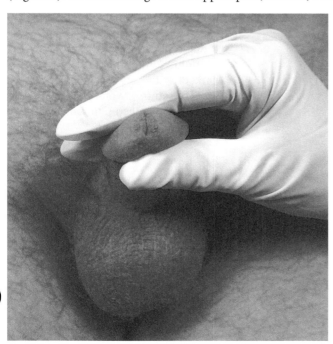

25.6

Objective Data

Normal Range of Findings	Abnormal Findings

Palpate the shaft of the penis between your thumb and first two fingers. Normally it feels smooth, semifirm, and nontender.

Nodule or induration.
Tenderness.

Inspect and Palpate the Scrotum

Inspect the scrotum as the male holds the penis out of the way. Alternatively you hold the penis out of the way with the back of your hand (Fig. 25.7). Scrotal size varies with ambient room temperature. Asymmetry is normal, with the left scrotal half usually lower than the right.

Scrotal swelling (edema) may be taut and pitting. This occurs with heart failure, renal failure, or local inflammation.
Lesions.

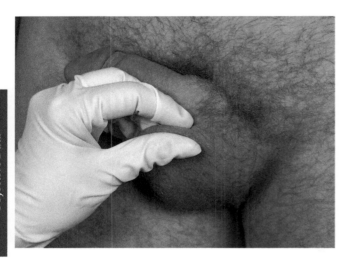

25.7

Spread rugae out between your fingers. Lift the sac to inspect the posterior surface. Normally no scrotal lesions are present, except for the commonly found sebaceous cysts. These are yellowish, 1-cm nodules and are firm, nontender, and often multiple.

Palpate gently each scrotal half between your thumb and first two fingers (Fig. 25.8). The scrotal contents should slide easily. Testes normally feel oval, firm and rubbery, smooth, and equal bilaterally and are freely movable and slightly tender to moderate pressure. Each epididymis normally feels discrete, softer than the testis, smooth, and nontender.

Inflammation.

Absent testis—May be a temporary migration or true cryptorchidism (see Table 25.6, Scrotum Abnormalities, p. 708).
Atrophied testes—Small and soft.
Fixed testes.
Nodules on testes or epididymides warrant ultrasound imaging.
Marked tenderness.
An indurated, swollen, and tender epididymis indicates epididymitis.

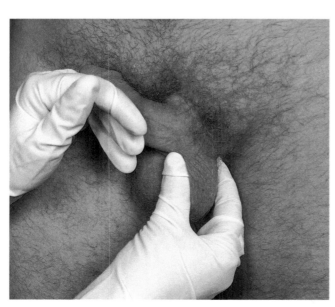

25.8

Objective Data

Normal Range of Findings	Abnormal Findings

Palpate each spermatic cord between your thumb and forefinger along its length from the epididymis up to the external inguinal ring (Fig. 25-9, *A*). You should feel a smooth, nontender cord.

Thickened cord.
Soft, swollen, and tortuous cord—left-sided varicocele (see Table 25.6, p. 709, and Fig. 25.9, *B*).

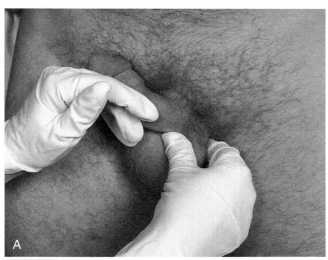

25.9, A

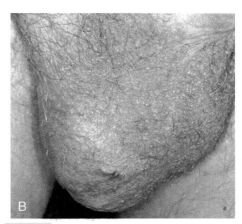

25.9, B   Varicocele. (Lemmi & Lemmi, 2011.)

Normally no other scrotal contents are present. If you do find a mass, note:
- Any tenderness?
- Is the mass distal or proximal to testis?
- Can you place your fingers over it?
- Does it reduce when the person lies down?
- Can you auscultate bowel sounds over it?

Abnormalities in the scrotum: hernia, tumor, orchitis, epididymitis, hydrocele, spermatocele, varicocele (see Table 25.6, Scrotum Abnormalities, p. 709).

Transillumination. Perform this maneuver only if you note a swelling or mass. Darken the room. Shine a strong flashlight from behind the scrotal contents. Solid scrotal contents do not transilluminate.

Serous fluid does transilluminate and shows as a red glow (e.g., hydrocele or spermatocele). Solid tissue and blood do not transilluminate (e.g., hernia, epididymitis, or tumor) (see Table 25.6).

Inspect and Palpate for Hernia

Inspect the inguinal region for a bulge as the person stands and as he strains down. Normally none is present.

Bulge at external inguinal ring or femoral canal. (A hernia may be present but easily reduced and appear only with an increase in intra-abdominal pressure.)

Palpate the inguinal canal (Fig. 25.10). For the right side, ask the male to shift his weight onto the left (unexamined) leg. Place your right index finger low on the right scrotal half so you carry as much skin as possible as you proceed. Palpate up the length of the spermatic cord, invaginating the scrotal skin as you go, to the external inguinal ring. It feels like a triangular slitlike opening. If positioned properly, it will admit your finger; gently insert it into the canal and ask the man to "bear down." Normally you feel no change. Repeat the procedure on the left side.

Palpable herniating mass bumps your fingertip or pushes against the side of your finger (see Table 25.7, Inguinal and Femoral Hernias, p. 711).

Normal Range of Findings	Abnormal Findings

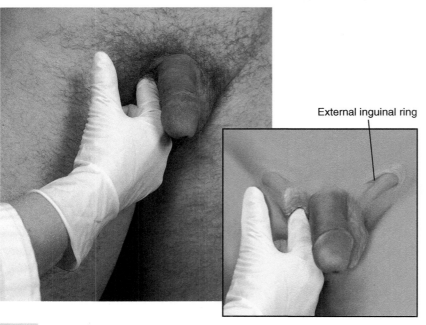

External inguinal ring

25.10

Place your right hand upright on the man's right upper thigh, remembering the acronym NAVEL (*N*erve, *A*rtery, *V*ein, *E*mpty space, *L*ymphatics). Locate the femoral artery pulse with your index finger; the empty space will be under your 4th finger. Ask the man to bear down and palpate the femoral area for a bulge. Normally you feel none. Change sides, using your left hand for the man's left side.

Palpate Inguinal Lymph Nodes

Palpate the horizontal chain along the groin inferior to the inguinal ligament and the vertical chain along the upper inner thigh.

It is normal to palpate an isolated node on occasion; it then feels small (<1 cm), soft, discrete, and movable (Fig. 25.11).

Enlarged, hard, matted, fixed nodes. Painful nodes.

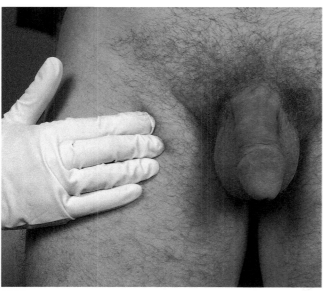

25.11

Normal Range of Findings	Abnormal Findings

Self-Care—Testicular Self-Examination (TSE)

Encourage self-care by teaching every male (from 13 to 14 years old through adulthood) how to examine his own testicles.

Testicular cancer is not common, but it has no early symptoms. When detected early and treated before metastasis, the cure rate is almost 100%. Therefore include the teaching but adjust your message to emphasize familiarity with the young man's own body rather than only cancer detection as the goal.

Early detection is enhanced if the male is familiar with his normal consistency. Points to include during health teaching are:

- **T** = timing, once a month
- **S** = shower, warm water relaxes scrotal sac
- **E** = examine, check for changes, report changes immediately

Phrase your teaching something like this (Fig. 25.12):

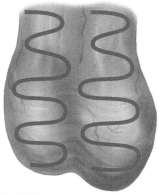

25.12

A good time to examine the testicles is during the shower or bath, when your hands are warm and soapy and the scrotum is warm. Cold hands stimulate a muscle (cremasteric) reflex, retracting the scrotal contents. The procedure is simple. Hold the scrotum in the palm of your hand and gently feel each testicle using your thumb and first two fingers. If it hurts, you are using too much pressure. The testicle is egg shaped and movable. It feels rubbery with a smooth surface, like a peeled hard-boiled egg. The epididymis is on top and behind the testicle; it feels a bit softer. The spermatic cord feels like thick, straight strands of string. Abnormal lumps are rare and usually not worrisome. But, if you ever notice a firm, painless lump; a hard area; or an overall enlarged testicle, call your provider for a further check.

Assess Urinary Function

A urinalysis shows a color of pale yellow to amber caused by the presence of urochrome pigments. Normal urine is clear and slightly acidic with a pH range of 4.5 to 8.0. Specific gravity measures the concentration of urine, from very dilute at 1.003 to concentrated at 1.030. There is little or no protein, no glucose, and fewer than 5 red blood cells (RBCs) or white blood cells (WBCs) per high-powered field in the microscope.

Abnormal Findings

The overall incidence of testicular cancer is rare, accounting for about 8000 new cases annually. It occurs most often between 15 and 35 years. It is associated with a history of cryptorchidism and other factors (see p. 709).

Cloudiness suggests presence of WBCs, bacteria, casts. Certain drugs or foods can change urine color (see Table 25.2). Proteinuria indicates glomerular disease in the nephron. Glycosuria suggests hyperglycemia occurring with diabetes. Increased WBCs occur with UTI; increased RBCs occur with UTI, glomerulonephritis, renal calculi, trauma, and cancer.

Objective Data

Objective Data

Normal Range of Findings	Abnormal Findings

Serum analysis of kidney function is measured with creatinine, an end-product of muscle metabolism. Normal levels range from 0.7 to 1.5 mg/dL and are fairly constant from day to day. Blood urea nitrogen (BUN) measures urea, an end-product of protein metabolism. It measures 10 to 20 mg/dL and rises with dehydration or an increase in protein intake.

Creatinine measures glomerular filtration rate (GFR). The GFR is the product of filtration pressure in the glomeruli, normally 125 mL/min. When the GFR decreases by half, the serum creatinine level doubles, indicating decreased kidney function. The BUN rises with decreased kidney function but is less specific.

❖ DEVELOPMENTAL COMPETENCE

Infants and Children

For an infant or a toddler, perform this procedure right after the abdominal examination. In a preschool-age to young school-age child (3 to 8 years), leave underpants on until just before the examination. In an older school-age child or adolescent, offer an extra drape, as with the adult. Reassure child and parents of normal findings.

Inspect the penis and scrotum. Penis size is usually small in infants (2 to 3 cm) (Fig. 25.13) and in young boys until puberty. In the obese boy the penis looks even smaller because of folds of skin covering the base.

Rarely a very small penis may be an enlarged clitoris in a genetically female infant. Families with newborns with ambiguous genitalia need reassurance that they will be active in the evaluation and in recommendations to determine sex assignment.[24]

Redness, swelling, lesions.

Discharge.

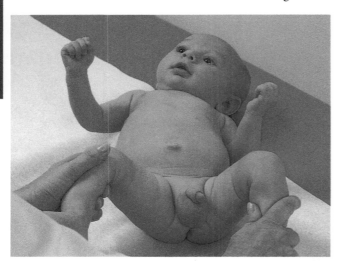

25.13

In the circumcised infant the glans looks smooth, with the meatus centered at the tip. While the child wears diapers, the meatus may become ulcerated from ammonia irritation. This is more common in circumcised infants.

Hypospadias, epispadias (see Table 25.5). Stricture—Narrowed opening.

Occasionally ulceration may produce a stricture, shown by a pinpoint meatus and a narrow stream. This increases the risk for urine obstruction.

If possible, observe the newborn's first voiding to assess strength and direction of stream.

Poor stream is significant because it may indicate a stricture or neurogenic bladder.

If uncircumcised, leave the foreskin alone and do not retract it because this can hurt and cause tearing of the adhesions attaching the foreskin to the shaft. Forced retraction leads to scarring; most adhesions resolve spontaneously in the early months or even by 2 to 4 years. Leave it alone until the parent says it retracts itself (with early erections) or until it is easily retracted by the child. The area is very sensitive, so just inspect glans and meatus. Foreskin should return to its original position easily.

The scrotum looks pink in light-skinned infants and dark brown in dark-skinned infants. Rugae are well formed in the full-term infant. Size varies

Phimosis—Unable to retract the foreskin.

Paraphimosis—The foreskin cannot be slipped forward once it is retracted.

Dirt and smegma collecting under foreskin.

Normal Range of Findings	Abnormal Findings

with ambient temperature, but overall the infant's scrotum looks large in relation to the penis. No bulges, either constant or intermittent, are present.

Palpate the scrotum and testes. The cremasteric reflex is strong in the infant, pulling the testes up into the inguinal canal and abdomen from exposure to cold, touch, exercise, or emotion. Take care not to elicit the reflex: (1) keep your hands warm and palpate from the external inguinal ring down, and (2) block the inguinal canals with the thumb and forefinger of your other hand to prevent the testes from retracting (Fig. 25.14).

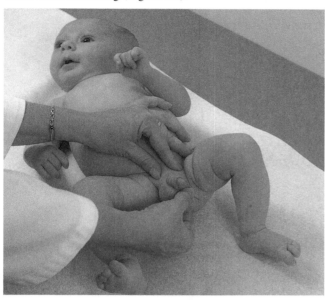

25.14

Normally the testes are descended and equal in size bilaterally (1.5 to 2 cm until puberty). It is important to document that you have palpated the testes. Once palpated, they are considered descended, even if they have retracted momentarily at the next visit.

If the scrotal halves feel empty, search for the testes along the inguinal canal and try to milk them down. Ask the toddler or child to squat with the knees flexed up; this pressure may force the testes down. Or have the young child sit cross-legged to relax the reflex (Fig. 25.15).

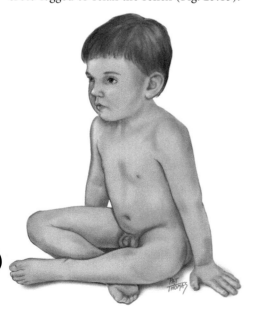

25.15

Cryptorchidism—Undescended testes (those that have never descended). Undescended testes are common in premature infants. They occur in 3% to 4% of term infants, although most have descended by 3 months of age. Age at which child should be referred differs among clinicians (see Table 25.6).

Objective Data

Normal Range of Findings	Abnormal Findings
Migratory testes (physiologic cryptorchidism) are common because of the strength of the cremasteric reflex and the small mass of the prepubertal testes. Note that the affected side has a normally developed scrotum (with true cryptorchidism, the scrotum is atrophic) and that the testis can be milked down. These testes descend at puberty and are normal.	
Palpate the epididymis and spermatic cord as described in the adult section. A common scrotal finding in the boy younger than 2 years is a **hydrocele,** or fluid in the scrotum. It appears as a large scrotum and transilluminates as a faint pink glow. It usually disappears spontaneously.	A hydrocele is a cystic collection of serous fluid in the tunica vaginalis, surrounding the testis. (See Table 25.6.)
Inspect the inguinal area for a bulge. If you do not see a bulge but the parent gives a positive history of one, try to elicit it by increasing intra-abdominal pressure. Ask the boy to hold his breath and strain down, or have him blow up a balloon.	
If a hernia is suspected, palpate the inguinal area. Use your little finger to reach the external inguinal ring.	

The Adolescent

The adolescent shows a wide variation in normal development of the genitals. Using the SMR charts, note: (1) enlargement of the testes and scrotum, (2) pubic hair growth, (3) darkening of scrotal color, (4) roughening of scrotal skin, (5) increase in penis length and width, and (6) axillary hair growth.

Be familiar with the normal sequence of growth.

The Aging Adult

In the older male you may note thinner, graying pubic hair and the decreased size of the penis. The size of the testes may be decreased and may feel less firm. The scrotal sac is pendulous with less rugae. The scrotal skin may become excoriated if the man continually sits on it.

Male hypogonadism (testosterone deficiency) occurs in 40% of men after age 45 years and may present as depression, fatigue, loss of muscle mass or strength, or decreased libido, although these symptoms occur also with obesity, diabetes, metabolic syndrome.[11] Serum testosterone levels do not yet have a clearly defined normal range nor a level when treatment is indicated.[11]

HEALTH PROMOTION AND PATIENT TEACHING

"We have described the technique of testicular self-examination during your exam. Now let's discuss the benefits and risks, and how often you may want to perform the exam yourself." Having a risk factor does not mean that you will get testicular cancer, just as having no risk factors does not mean you are free of getting the disease, but some risk factors do increase the likelihood. These are: (1) an undescended testicle, one that fails to move from the belly into the scrotum before birth; (2) family history of testicular cancer in a father or brother; (3) HIV infection, especially AIDS, though no other infections increase the risk; (4) cancer in your other testicle; (5) race and ethnicity—Caucasian men are 4 to 5 times more likely to develop testicular cancer than are African-American or Asian-American men.[3]

The benefits of TSE are in becoming comfortable with your own body and if you do find a lump or thickening, checking it with your provider. Most lumps are not cancerous, but when a lump is cancerous, early detection and treatment result in the highest rates of survival, almost 100%. This drops to a 5-year survival rate of 73% (still high) for most other stages of the disease.[18] The risks of TSE are additional office visits, testing and radiologic imaging, and possible anxiety while the tests are conducted. The American Cancer Society has no official recommendation on regular performance of TSE, but that is because the condition is rare and to have a clinical study showing the usefulness of TSE would take a sample size of millions of men.[18] One interesting study was done, however—a cost-utility study.[1] They compared the cost of a great number of clinical exams based on the TSE when it turns out to be heathy to the cost of missing 1 advanced-stage tumor and all the treatment that resulted. This study found a 2.4-to-1 cost benefit ratio for early detection of testicular cancer versus finding and treating cancer at advanced stages.[1] So we have this information to discuss and your personal decision.

DOCUMENTATION AND CRITICAL THINKING

Sample Charting

SUBJECTIVE

Urinates 4 or 5 times/day, clear, straw-colored. No nocturia, dysuria, or hesitancy. No pain, lesions, or discharge from penis. Does not do testicular self-examination. No history of genitourinary disease. Sexually active in a monogamous relationship. Sexual life satisfactory to self and partner. Uses birth control via barrier method (partner uses diaphragm). No known STI contact.

OBJECTIVE

No lesions, inflammation, or discharge from penis. Scrotum—testes descended, symmetric, no masses. No inguinal hernia.

ASSESSMENT

Genital structures normal and healthy.

Case Study 1

H.P. is a 75-year-old retired college professor. Past medical history includes prostatectomy 2 weeks PTA due to severe benign prostatic hypertrophy; also hypertension, type 2 diabetes, and COPD.

SUBJECTIVE

H.P. presents to the emergency department in severe pain, rated at 10/10. "My balls hurt so bad I can't walk straight." Reports urinary frequency and "pink" urine. Low-grade fever for 24 hours.

OBJECTIVE

Vital signs: Temp 100.4° F (38° C). Pulse 118 bpm, regular. Resp 18/min. BP 146/88 mm Hg, right arm, sitting.
Inspection: Scrotum appears reddened and enlarged.
Palpation: Extreme tenderness with palpation. Epididymis enlarged bilaterally. Difficult to identify testicles. Scrotal skin edematous. No discharge.
Laboratory data: White blood cell count 15,000/mcL with a shift to the left; *E. coli* in urine

ASSESSMENT

Epididymitis
Acute pain

Clinical Case Study 2

R.C. is a 19-year-old male student who 2 days PTA noted acute onset of painful urination, frequency, and urgency. Noted some thick penile discharge.

SUBJECTIVE

States has no side pain, no abdominal pain, no fever, and no genital skin rash. R.C. is concerned that he has an STI because of an episode of unprotected intercourse with a new partner 6 days PTA. Has no known allergies.

OBJECTIVE

Vital signs: Temp 98.6° F (37° C). Pulse 72 bpm. Resp 16/min. No lesions or inflammation around penis or scrotum. Urethral meatus has mild edema with purulent urethral discharge. No pain on palpation of genitalia. Testes symmetric with no masses. No lymphadenopathy.

ASSESSMENT

Urethral discharge
Need for health teaching about STI prevention

Case Study 3

J.T. is a 13-year-old male who presents to the ED with abdominal pain, nausea, and testicular pain.

SUBJECTIVE

4 hours PTA: J.T. was in summer camp playing basketball when pain to groin "came on all of a sudden." Reports pain began in left testicle but now radiates to entire scrotum (10 on 1-10 pain scale). Rest and scrotal support do not provide relief.

OBJECTIVE

Vital signs: Temp 97.9° F (36.6° C) (oral). Pulse 72 bpm. Resp 16/min. BP 119/70 mm Hg (standing).
General appearance: Bent over, anxious, grimacing, and guarding stomach and genital area.
Abdomen: BS active in all 4 quadrants; nausea; denies vomiting and/or pain on palpation.
Genitourinary: Red, warm, edematous scrotum w/pain on palpation. L testicle especially painful, elevated and lying transversely; cremasteric reflex absent on L side; no pelvic lymphadenopathy; denies sexual activity

ASSESSMENT

Testicular (left) torsion
Acute pain
Decreased tissue perfusion

ABNORMAL FINDINGS

TABLE 25.2	Urine Color and Discolorations

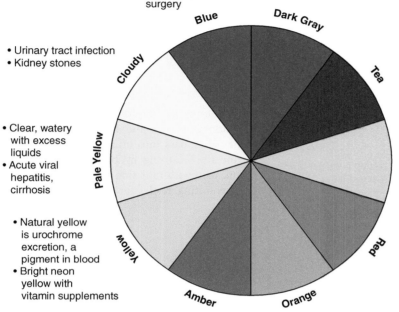

- Medication side effect: amitriptyline, Indocin
- Foods: asparagus
- Dye after prostate surgery

- Urine contains melanin, melanuria

- Liver disease, especially with pale stools, jaundice
- Myoglobinuria
- Some medications or food dyes
- Blood in urine

- Urinary tract infection
- Kidney stones

- With menses
- Some foods: beets, berries, food dyes
- Some laxatives
- Kidney stones
- Urinary tract infection

- Clear, watery with excess liquids
- Acute viral hepatitis, cirrhosis

- Natural yellow is urochrome excretion, a pigment in blood
- Bright neon yellow with vitamin supplements

- Blood in urine
- Nephritis, cystitis
- Cancer (prostate, bladder)
- Following prostate surgery

- Gold or concentrated with dehydration
- Some laxatives
- Food or supplements with B-complex vitamins

- Medication side effect: rifampin for meningitis, Pyridium, warfarin (Coumadin)
- Some foods, food dyes, laxatives
- Dehydration
- Jaundice (bilirubinemia)

Wheel labels: Blue, Dark Gray, Tea, Pink, Red, Orange, Amber, Yellow, Pale Yellow, Cloudy

See Illustration Credits for source information.

TABLE 25.3	Urinary Problems

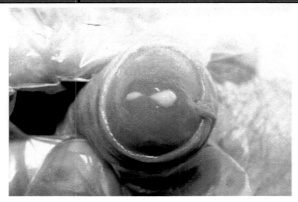

◀ **Urethritis (Urethral Discharge and Dysuria)**

Infection of urethra causes painful, burning urination or pruritus. Meatus edges are reddened, everted, and swollen with purulent discharge. Urine is cloudy with discharge and mucus shreds. Cause determined by urine screen: (1) gonococcal urethritis has thick, profuse, yellow or gray-brown discharge; (2) nongonococcal urethritis (NGU) may have similar discharge but often has scanty, mucoid discharge. Of these, about 40% are caused by chlamydia infection. Guidelines are to treat for both infections if either are found.[5]

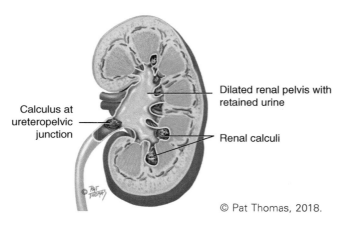

Calculus at ureteropelvic junction

Dilated renal pelvis with retained urine

Renal calculi

© Pat Thomas, 2018.

◀ **Renal Calculi**

Renal stones (crystals of calcium oxalate or uric acid) form in kidney tubules and then migrate and become urgent when they pass into ureter, become lodged, and obstruct urine flow, causing hydronephrosis. Cause abrupt severe flank pain with radiation to the groin or abdomen, nausea and vomiting, restlessness, gross or microscopic hematuria.

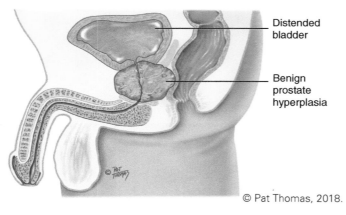

Distended bladder

Benign prostate hyperplasia

© Pat Thomas, 2018.

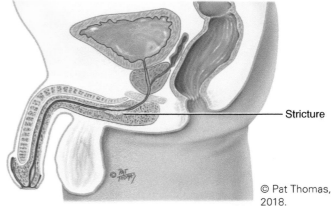

Stricture

© Pat Thomas, 2018.

Acute Urinary Retention and Urinary Tract Infection

Inability to pass urine with bladder distention and lower abdominal pain. Common in older men due to bladder outlet obstruction of BPH (see Chapter 26). This can cause UTI, owing to stasis and turbulent flow. UTI incidence increases among men ages ≥60 years and presents with dysuria, frequency, urgency, nocturia, suprapubic pain, occasionally gross hematuria, possibly fever.[16] Treat with antibiotics and address underlying problem.

Urethral Stricture

Pinpoint, constricted opening at meatus or inside along urethra. Occurs congenitally or secondary to urethral injury. Gradual decrease in force and caliber of urine stream is most common symptom. Shaft feels indurated along ventral aspect at site of stricture.

See Illustration Credits for source information.

ABNORMAL FINDINGS
FOR ADVANCED PRACTICE

TABLE 25.4 | **Male Genital Lesions**

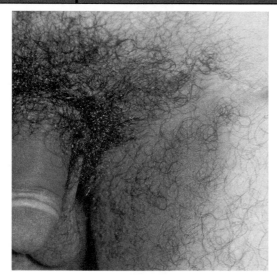

Tinea Cruris

A fungal infection in the crural fold, not extending to scrotum, occurring in postpubertal males ("jock itch") after sweating or wearing layers of occlusive clothing. It forms a red-brown half-moon shape with well-defined borders.

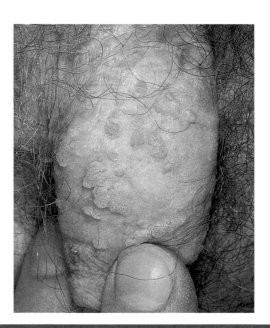

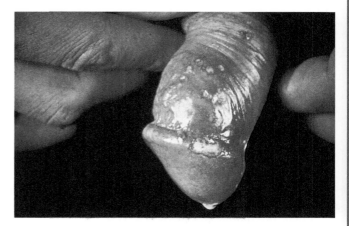

Genital Herpes—HSV-2 Infection

Clusters of small vesicles with surrounding erythema, which are often painful and erupt on the glans, foreskin, or anus. These rupture to form superficial ulcers. May have mild tingling before outbreak or shooting pain in buttock or leg. An STI, the initial infection lasts 7 to 10 days and is treated with oral antivirals. The virus remains dormant indefinitely; recurrent infections last 3 to 10 days with milder symptoms.

◀ **Genital Warts**

Soft, pointed, moist, fleshy, painless papules may be single or multiple in a cauliflower-like patch. Color may be gray, pale yellow, or pink in white males and black or translucent gray-black in black males. They occur on shaft of penis, behind corona, or around the anus where they may grow into large, grapelike clusters.

These are caused by the human papillomavirus (HPV) and are one of the most common STIs. The HPV infection is correlated with early onset of sexual activity, infrequent use of contraception, and multiple sexual partners.

The vaccine Gardasil is indicated for prevention of genital warts; approval was re-confirmed in 2014 for boys and men ages 9 to 26 years. It also reduces HPV-related disease in women, such as cervical cancer.[21]

Continued

TABLE 25.4	Male Genital Lesions—cont'd

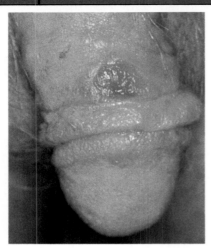

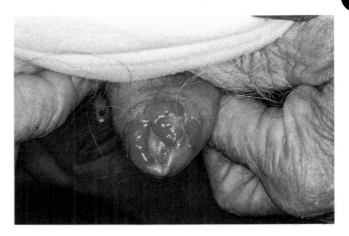

Syphilitic Chancre

Begins within 2 to 4 weeks of infection as a small, solitary, silvery papule that erodes to a red, round or oval, superficial ulcer with a yellowish serous discharge. Palpation reveals a nontender indurated base that can be lifted like a button between the thumb and the finger. Lymph nodes enlarge early but are nontender. This is an STI easily treated with penicillin G; but untreated it leads to cardiac and neurologic problems and blindness. Almost eradicated in the United States in 1957; epidemics recur cyclically every 7 to 10 years.

Carcinoma

Begins as red, raised, warty growth or as an ulcer with watery discharge. As it grows, may necrose and slough. Usually painless. Almost always on glans or inner lip of foreskin and following chronic inflammation. Enlarged lymph nodes are common.

See Illustration Credits for source information.

TABLE 25.5	Penis Abnormalities

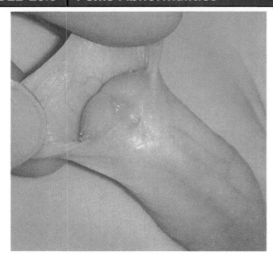

◄ Hypospadias

A congenital disorder of the urethra (1 in 300 baby boys)[17] in which the urethral meatus opens on the ventral (under) side of the glans or shaft. About 90% of openings are on or near the head of the penis with a groove extending from the meatus to the expected location at the tip. Shiny tissue extends from the meatus to the tip and the foreskin is not fully developed, leaving the ventral side of the glans uncovered. Circumcision can proceed if parents desire this; surgical correction of hypospadias can be at age 3 months or older.[17]

Priapism (not illustrated)

Prolonged painful erection of penis without sexual stimulation and unrelieved by intercourse or masturbation. When lasting 4 hours or longer can cause ischemia of penis, fibrosis of tissue, erectile dysfunction. Can occur as a rare side effect of drugs for erectile dysfunction and street drugs; with sickle-cell trait or disease; with leukemia in which excess white blood cells produce engorgement; with malignancy; from local trauma; or as a result of spinal cord injuries with autonomic nervous system dysfunction.

Continued

TABLE 25.5 | **Penis Abnormalities—cont'd**

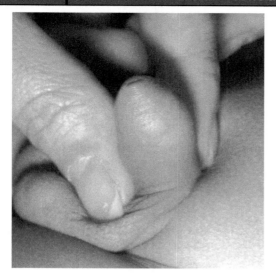

Phimosis

Nonretractable foreskin forming a pointy tip with a tiny orifice. Foreskin is advanced and so tight that it is impossible to retract over glans. May be congenital or acquired from adhesions secondary to infection. Poor hygiene leads to retained dirt and smegma, which increases risk for inflammation, calculus formation, obstructive uropathy.

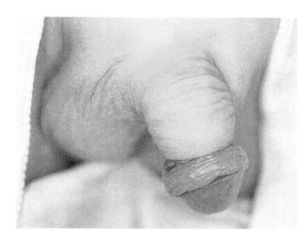

Paraphimosis

Foreskin is retracted and fixed. Once retracted behind glans, a tight or inflamed foreskin cannot return to its original position. Constriction impedes circulation, so glans swells. A medical emergency; the constricting band prevents venous and lymphatic return from the glans and compromises arterial circulation.

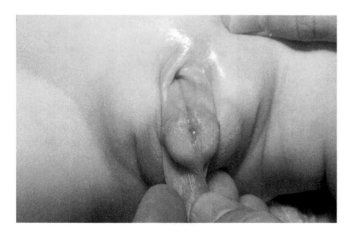

Epispadias

Meatus opens on the dorsal (upper) side of glans or shaft above a broad, spadelike penis. Rare; less common than hypospadias but more disabling because of associated urinary incontinence and separation of pubic bones.

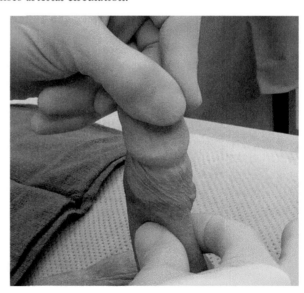

Peyronie Disease

Hard, nontender, subcutaneous plaques on dorsal or lateral surface palpated by stretching the penis. May be single or multiple and asymmetric. They are associated with painful bending of the penis during erection. Usually occurs after age 45 years. Its cause is trauma to the penis with resulting scar, deformity, and often erectile dysfunction. More common in men with diabetes, gout, and Dupuytren contracture of the palm.

See Illustration Credits for source information.

TABLE 25.6 | Scrotum Abnormalities

Disorder	Clinical Findings	Discussion
Absent Testis, Cryptorchidism 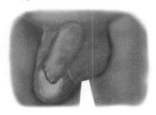	S: Empty scrotal half O: Inspection—In true maldescent, atrophic scrotum on affected side Palpation—No testis A: Absent testis	True cryptorchidism—Testes that have never descended. Incidence at birth is 3% to 4%; one-half of these descend in first month. Incidence with premature infants is 30%; in the adult, 0.7% to 0.8%. True undescended testes have a histologic change by 6 years, causing decreased spermatogenesis and infertility. Also increases risk for testicular cancer.
Small Testis 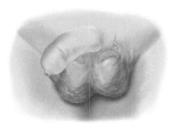	S: (None) O: Palpation—Small and soft (rarely may be firm) A: Small testis	Small and soft (<3.5 cm) indicates atrophy as with cirrhosis or hypopituitarism, following estrogen therapy, or as a sequelae of orchitis. Small and firm (<2 cm) occurs with Klinefelter syndrome (hypogonadism).
Testicular Torsion 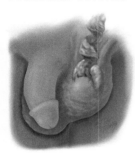	S: Excruciating unilateral pain in testicle of sudden onset, often during sleep or following trauma; may also have lower abdominal pain, nausea and vomiting, no fever O: Inspection—Red, swollen scrotum, one testis (usually left) higher owing to rotation and shortening Palpation—Cord feels thick, swollen, tender; epididymis may be anterior; cremasteric reflex absent on side of torsion	Sudden twisting of spermatic cord. Occurs in late childhood, early adolescence; rare after age 20 years. Torsion usually on left side; faulty anchoring of testis on wall of scrotum allows testis to rotate. The anterior testis rotates medially toward the other testis. Blood supply is cut off, resulting in ischemia and engorgement. An emergency requiring surgery; testis can become gangrenous in a few hours.
Epididymitis 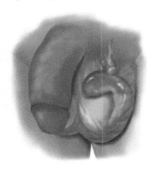	S: Severe pain of sudden onset in scrotum, relieved by elevation (positive Prehn sign); also rapid swelling, fever O: Inspection—Enlarged scrotum; reddened Palpation—Exquisitely tender; epididymis enlarged, indurated; hard to distinguish from testis. Overlying scrotal skin may be thick and edematous Laboratory—White blood cells and bacteria in urine A: Tender swelling of epididymis	Acute infection of epididymis commonly caused by prostatitis; after prostatectomy because of trauma of urethral instrumentation; or from chlamydia, gonorrhea, or other bacterial infection. Often difficult to distinguish between epididymitis and testicular torsion.

Continued

TABLE 25.6	Scrotum Abnormalities—cont'd	
Disorder	**Clinical Findings**	**Discussion**
Varicocele 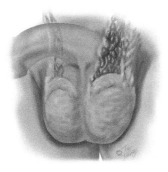	S: Dull pain; constant pulling or dragging feeling; or may be asymptomatic O: Inspection—Usually no sign; or bluish color through light scrotal skin Palpation—When standing, feel soft, irregular mass posterior to and above testis; collapses when supine, refills when upright; feels distinctive, like a "bag of worms" Testis on side of varicocele may be smaller due to impaired circulation A: Soft mass on spermatic cord	A varicocele is dilated, tortuous internal spermatic varicose veins caused by incompetent valves, which permit reflux of blood; 90% left-sided because left spermatic vein inserts at a right angle into left renal vein.[6] Occurs in 15% by age 15 years. Screen at early adolescence; obtain scrotal ultrasound; early treatment important to prevent potential infertility when an adult.
Spermatocele 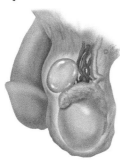	S: Painless, usually found on examination O: Inspection—Does transilluminate higher in the scrotum than a hydrocele, and the sperm may fluoresce Palpation—Round, freely movable mass lying above and behind testis; if large, feels like a third testis A: Free cystic mass on epididymis	Retention cyst in epididymis; cause unclear but may be obstruction of tubules. Filled with thin, milky fluid that contains sperm. Most spermatoceles are small (<1 cm); occasionally they may be larger and mistaken for hydrocele.
Early Testicular Tumor 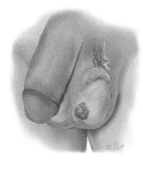	S: Painless, found on examination; may have history of undescended testicle or familial testicular cancer. O: Palpation—Firm nodule or harder-than-normal section of testicle; testicular swelling occurs in most A: Solitary nodule	Most testicular tumors occur between ages 18 and 35; practically all are malignant. More common in whites; must biopsy to confirm. Most important risk factor is undescended testis, even those surgically corrected. Early detection important in prognosis, but practice of testicular self-examination is low.
Diffuse Tumor 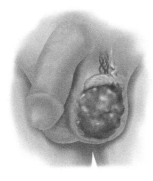	S: Enlarging testis (most common symptom). When enlarges, has feel of increased weight O: Inspection—Enlarged, does not transilluminate Palpation—Enlarged, smooth, ovoid, firm Important—Firm palpation does *not* cause usual sickening discomfort as with normal testis A: Nontender swelling of testis	Diffuse tumor maintains shape of testis.

TABLE 25.6	Scrotum Abnormalities—cont'd	
Disorder	Clinical Findings	Discussion
Hydrocele 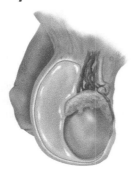	S: Painless swelling, although person may complain of weight and bulk in scrotum O: Inspection—Enlarged mass does transilluminate with a pink or red glow (in contrast to a hernia) Palpation—Nontender mass; able to get fingers above mass (in contrast to scrotal hernia) A: Nontender swelling of testis	Cystic. Circumscribed collection of serous fluid in tunica vaginalis surrounding testis. May occur following epididymitis, trauma, hernia, tumor of testis, or spontaneously in the newborn. Usually resolves during first year; if large or enlarging, may need surgical decompression.
Scrotal Hernia 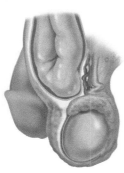	S: Swelling, may have pain with straining O: Inspection—Enlarged, may reduce when supine, does not transilluminate Palpation—Soft, mushy mass; palpating fingers cannot get above mass. Mass is distinct from testicle that is normal A: Nontender swelling of scrotum	Scrotal hernia usually caused by indirect inguinal hernia (see Table 25.7). Requires surgery. Teach patient or boy's parents signs of incarcerated hernia; proceed to ED if these occur before planned surgery.
Orchitis 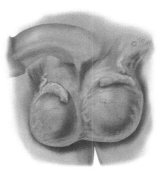	S: Acute or moderate pain of sudden onset, swollen testis, feeling of weight, fever O: Inspection—Enlarged, edematous, reddened; does not transilluminate Palpation—Swollen, congested, tense, and tender; hard to distinguish testis from epididymis A: Tender swelling of testis	Acute inflammation of testis. Most common cause is mumps; can occur with any infectious disease. May have associated hydrocele that does transilluminate.
Scrotal Edema 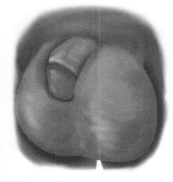	S: Tenderness O: Inspection—Enlarged, may be reddened (with local irritation) Palpation—Taut with pitting. Probably unable to feel scrotal contents A: Scrotal edema	Accompanies marked edema in lower half of body (e.g., congestive heart failure, renal failure, and portal vein obstruction). Occurs with local inflammation: epididymitis, torsion of spermatic cord. Also, obstruction of inguinal lymphatics produces lymphedema of scrotum.

S, Subjective data; *O,* objective data; *A,* assessment.

Images © Pat Thomas, 2006.

TABLE 25.7	Inguinal and Femoral Hernias

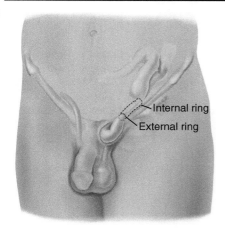 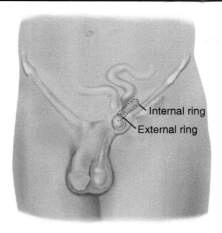 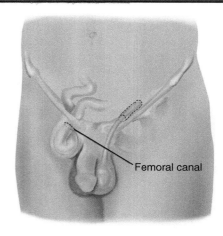

	Indirect Inguinal	**Direct Inguinal**	**Femoral**
Course	Sac herniates through internal inguinal ring; can remain in canal or pass into scrotum	Directly behind and through external inguinal ring, above inguinal ligament; rarely enters scrotum	Through femoral ring and canal, below inguinal ligament, more often on right side
Clinical Symptoms and Signs	Pain with straining; soft swelling that increases with increased intra-abdominal pressure; may decrease when lying down	Usually painless; round swelling close to the pubis in area of internal inguinal ring; easily reduced when supine[b]	Pain may be severe; may become strangulated
Frequency	Most common; 60% of all hernias. More common in infants <1 year and males 16 to 20 years of age	Less common; occurs most often in men older than 40 years, rare in women	Least common, 4% of all hernias; more common in women
Cause	Congenital or acquired	Acquired weakness; brought on by heavy lifting, muscle atrophy, obesity, chronic cough, or ascites	Acquired; due to increased abdominal pressure, muscle weakness, or frequent stooping

Images © Pat Thomas, 2006.

[b]**Reducible**—Contents will return to abdominal cavity by lying down or gentle pressure. **Incarcerated**—Herniated bowel cannot be returned to abdominal cavity. **Strangulated**—Blood supply to hernia is shut off. Accompanied by nausea, vomiting, and tenderness.

Summary Checklist: Male Genitalia Examination

1. Inspect and palpate the penis.
2. Inspect and palpate the scrotum.
3. If a mass exists, transilluminate it.
4. Palpate for an inguinal hernia.
5. Palpate the inguinal lymph nodes.

REFERENCES

1. Aberger, M., Wilson, B., Holzbeierlein, J. M., et al. (2014). Testicular self-examination and testicular cancer: A cost-utility analysis. *Cancer Med, 3*(6), 1629–1634.
2. American Academy of Pediatrics. (2012). Male circumcision. *Pediatrics, 130*(3), e756–e3785.
3. American Cancer Society (ACS). (2016). *About testicular cancer*. Atlanta: ACS. http://www/camcer/prg/cancer/testicular-cancer.html.
4. Baker, K. E. (2017). The future of transgender coverage. *N Engl J Med, 376*(19), 1801–1804.
5. Centers for Disease Control and Prevention. (CDC) (2015). *Diseases characterized by urethritis and cervicitis.* Atlanta:

CDC. https://www/cdc/gpv/std/tg2015/urethritis-and-cervicitis.htm.

6. El Abiad, Y., & Qarro, A. (2016). Acute varicocele revealing renal cancer. *N Engl J Med, 374*(21), 2075.

7. El Bcheraoui, C., Zhang, X., Cooper, C. S., et al. (2014). Rates of adverse events associated with male circumcision in U.S. medical settings, 2001 to 2010. *JAMA Pediatr, 168*(7), 625–634.

8. Farling, K. B. (2017). Bladder cancer risk factors, diagnosis, and management. *Nurse Pract, 42*(3), 26–34.

9. Frisch, M., Aigrain, Y., Barauskas, V., et al. (2013). Cultural bias in the AAP's 2012 Technical Report and Policy Statement on male circumcision. *Pediatrics, 131*(4), 796–800.

10. Herman-Giddens, M. E., Steffes, J., Harris, D., et al. (2012). Secondary sexual characteristics in boys. *Pediatrics, 130*(5), e1058–e1068.

11. Lawrence, K. L., Stewart, F., & Larson, B. M. (2017). Approaches to male hypogonadism in primary care. *Nurse Pract, 42*(2), 32–37.

12. Levine, D. A. (2013). Office-based care for lesbian, gay, bisexual, transgender, and questioning youth. *Pediatrics, 132*(1), 198–203.

13. Morris, B. J., Bailis, S. A., & Wiswell, T. E. (2014). Circumcision rates in the United States: Rising or falling? *Mayo Clin Proc, 89*, 677–686.

14. National Institutes of Health (NIH) (2016). *Kidney disease statistics for the United States.* Washington: NIH. https://niddk.nih.gov/health-information/health-statistics/kidney-disease.

15. Sardi, L., & Livingston, K. (2015). Parental decision making in male circumcision. *MCN Am J Matern Child Nurs, 40*(2), 110.

16. Schaeffer, A. J., & Nicolle, L. E. (2016). Urinary tract infections in older men. *N Engl J Med, 374*(6), 562.

17. Snodgrass, W. T., & Bush, N. C. (2016). Hypospadias. In A. J. Wein, et al. (Eds.), *Campbell-Walsh Urology* (11th ed.). Philadelphia: Elsevier.

18. Thornton, C. P. (2016). Best practice in teaching male adolescents and young men to perform testicular self-examinations. *J Ped Healthcare, 30*(6), 518–527.

19. Tobian, A. A., Kacker, S., & Quinn, T. C. (2014). Male circumcision: A globally relevant but under-utilized method for the prevention of HIV and other sexually transmitted infections. *Ann Rev Med, 65*(1), 293–306.

20. Tsodilov, A., Gulati, R., Heijnsdijk, A. M., et al. (2017). Reconciling the effects of screening on prostate cancer mortality in the ERSPC and PLCO trials. *Ann Intern Med, 167*(7), 449–455.

21. Valentino, K., & Poronsky, C. B. (2016). Human Papillomavirus infection and vaccination. *J Ped Nurs, 31*, e155–e166.

22. Vart, P., Gansevoort, R. T., Crews, D. C., et al. (2015). Mediators of the association between low socioeconomic status and chronic kidney disease in the United States. *Am J Epidemiol, 181*(6), 385–396.

23. Vickers, A. J. (2017). Prostate cancer screening. *Ann Intern Med, 167*, 509–510.

24. Yatsenko, S. A., & Witchel, S. F. (2017). Genetic approach to ambiguous genitalia and disorders of sex development: What clinicians need to know. *Semin Perinatol, 41*(4), 232–243.

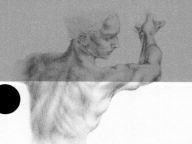

CHAPTER 26

Anus, Rectum, and Prostate

http://evolve.elsevier.com/Jarvis/

STRUCTURE AND FUNCTION

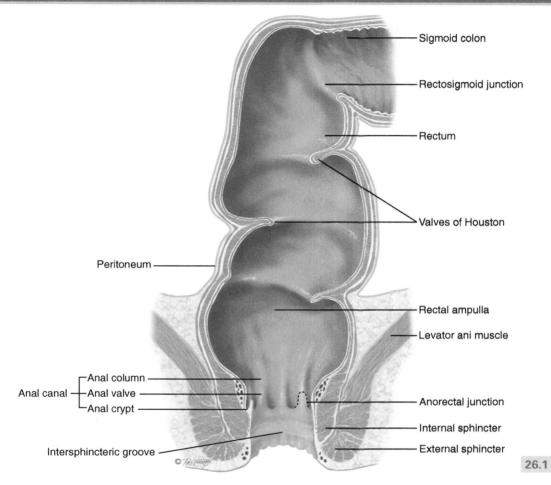

- Sigmoid colon
- Rectosigmoid junction
- Rectum
- Valves of Houston
- Peritoneum
- Rectal ampulla
- Levator ani muscle
- Anal column
- Anal canal
- Anal valve
- Anal crypt
- Anorectal junction
- Internal sphincter
- External sphincter
- Intersphincteric groove

26.1

ANUS AND RECTUM

The **anal canal** is the outlet of the gastrointestinal (GI) tract; it is about 3.8 cm long in the adult. It is lined with modified skin (having no hair or sebaceous glands) that merges with rectal mucosa at the anorectal junction.

The anal canal is surrounded by two concentric layers of muscle, the **sphincters** (Fig. 26.1). The internal sphincter is under involuntary control by the autonomic nervous system. The external sphincter surrounds the internal sphincter but also has a small section overriding the tip of the internal sphincter at the opening. It is under voluntary control. Except for the passing of feces and gas, the sphincters keep the anal canal tightly closed. The **intersphincteric groove** separates the internal and external sphincters and is palpable.

The **anal columns** (or columns of Morgagni) are folds of mucosa. These extend vertically down from the rectum and end in the **anorectal junction** (also called the **dentate** line). This junction is not palpable, but it is visible on proctoscopy. Each anal column contains an artery and a vein. Under conditions of chronic increased venous pressure, the vein may enlarge, forming a hemorrhoid. At the lower end of each column is a small crescent fold of mucous membrane, the **anal valve.** The space above the anal valve (between the columns) is a small recess, the **anal crypt.**

The anal canal slants forward toward the umbilicus, forming a distinct right angle with the rectum, which rests back in the hollow of the sacrum (Fig. 26.2). Although the rectum contains only autonomic nerves, numerous somatic sensory nerves are present in the anal canal and external skin;

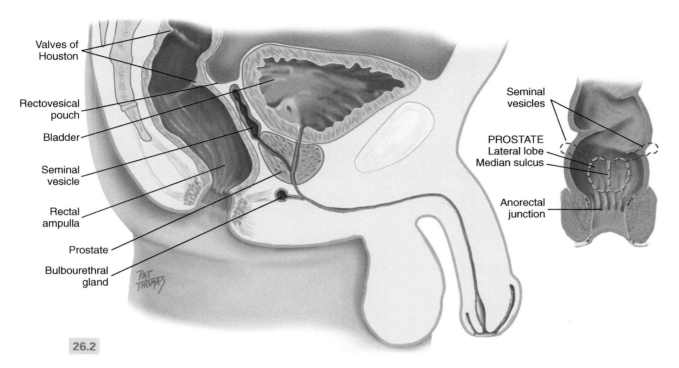

26.2

therefore a person feels sharp pain from any trauma to the anal area.

The **rectum,** which is 12 cm long, is the distal portion of the large intestine. It extends from the sigmoid colon, at the level of the 3rd sacral vertebra, and ends at the anal canal. Just above the anal canal the rectum dilates and turns posteriorly, forming the rectal ampulla. The rectal interior has 3 semilunar transverse folds called the **valves of Houston.** These cross one-half the circumference of the rectal lumen. Their function is unclear, but they may serve to hold feces as the flatus passes. The lowest is within reach of palpation, usually on the person's left side—do not mistake for an intrarectal mass.

Peritoneal Reflection. The peritoneum covers only the upper two-thirds of the rectum. In the male the anterior part of the peritoneum reflects down to within 7.5 cm of the anal opening, forming the **rectovesical pouch** (see Fig. 26.2) and then covers the bladder. In the female this is termed the **recto-uterine pouch** and extends down to within 5.5 cm of the anal opening.

PROSTATE

In the male the **prostate gland** lies in front of the anterior wall of the rectum and 2 cm behind the symphysis pubis. It surrounds the bladder neck and urethra and has 15 to 30 ducts that open into the urethra. The prostate secretes a thin, milky, alkaline fluid that supports sperm. It is a bilobed structure with a round or heart shape. It measures 2.5 cm long and 4 cm in diameter. The two lateral lobes are separated by a shallow groove called the **median sulcus.**

The two **seminal vesicles** project like rabbit ears above the prostate. They secrete a fluid that is rich in fructose, which nourishes the sperm and contains prostaglandins. The two **bulbourethral** (Cowper) glands are each the size of a pea and

are located inferior to the prostate on either side of the urethra (also see Fig. 26.5). They secrete a clear, viscid mucus.

Regional Structures

In the female the uterine cervix lies in front of the anterior rectal wall and may be palpated through it.

The combined length of the anal canal and the rectum is about 16 cm in the adult. The average length of the examining finger is from 6 cm to 10 cm, bringing many rectal structures within reach.

The sigmoid colon is named from its S-shaped course in the pelvic cavity. It extends from the iliac flexure of the descending colon and ends at the rectum. It is 40 cm long and is accessible to examination only through the colonoscope. The flexible fiberoptic scope provides a view of the entire mucosal surface of the sigmoid and the colon.

❖ DEVELOPMENTAL COMPETENCE

The first stool passed by the newborn is dark green meconium and occurs within 24 to 48 hours of birth, indicating anal patency. From that time on the infant usually has a stool after each feeding. This response to eating is a wave of peristalsis called the *gastrocolic reflex.* It continues throughout life, although children and adults usually produce no more than one or two stools per day.

The infant passes stools by reflex. Voluntary control of the external anal sphincter cannot occur until the nerves supplying the area have become fully myelinated, usually around $1\frac{1}{2}$ to 2 years of age. Toilet training usually starts after age 2 years.

At male puberty the prostate gland undergoes a very rapid increase to more than twice its prepubertal size. During young adulthood its size remains fairly constant.

The prostate gland commonly starts to enlarge during the middle adult years, but this is NOT cancer. This **benign** prostatic hyperplasia (BPH) is present in 80% of men over 60 years. The **hyperplasia** is an imbalance between cell proliferation and programmed cell death (apoptosis). The prostatic growth creates bladder outlet obstruction because it constricts the urethra. This impedes urine output like putting a clamp on a garden hose.

CULTURE AND GENETICS

Prostate cancer (PC) is the most frequently diagnosed cancer in men. These cancers are heterogeneous; many are indolent, nonlethal and slow growing; some are aggressive. Known risk factors include increasing age, African ancestry, a family history of PC (brother or father), and inherited mutations of *BRCA1* and *BRCA2* genes. The risk of PC is 74% higher in African-American and African-Caribbean men.[2] Reasons are not known but may be related to inherited genetic factors. Other risk factors affect prostate cancer progression once it occurs and is treated.[18] Not smoking, keeping a healthy body weight, and maintaining regular vigorous exercise seem to delay prostate cancer progression. Early evidence suggests that some foods (tomatoes rich in the antioxidant lycopene, broccoli, cauliflower, and other cruciferous vegetables) and healthy sources of vegetable fats (olive oil and nuts) may reduce the risk of cancer progression, although data are sparse.[18] Obesity is strongly associated with an increased risk of aggressive PC and is associated with PC progression and mortality. Mechanisms here may be insulin and insulin-like growth factors, change in levels of sex hormones, or fat cell (adipokine) signaling.[18]

Men with metastatic PC are more likely to have a lower socioeconomic status (SES), to lack insurance or have Medicaid, and to be of black or Hispanic race/ethnicity.[28] This is associated with lack of access to preventive PSA screening, lack of high-quality insurance coverage, and barriers to full evaluation. Evidence shows that nonwhite men with high-risk PC were less likely to have full treatment but that high-quality insurance coverage decreased the racial disparity in PC treatment; and access to high-technology cancer centers decreased the disparity of treatment based on race and insurance status.[9]

Because it is known that men of color have an increased risk of PC, screening guidelines should be tailored to individual risk. The American Urological Association recommends that men of African ancestry and men with a family history of prostate cancer should be offered the blood test of PSA screening. Further, they recommend that men between ages 55 to 69 years of average risk and with a life expectancy of >10 years should have counseling with their provider on the risks and benefits of PSA screening; then they may have the test if they so choose.[13] PSA risks and benefits are described under Health Promotion on p. 722.

Colorectal cancer (CRC) incidence rates are higher in Alaska Natives and African Americans when compared to whites, and lower in Asian/Pacific Islanders. Also, rates are 30% to 40% higher in men than in women.[22] These rates actually have worsened since the 1970s, when more effective screening, early detection, and treatment helped to increase 5-year survival rates.[21] Reasons appear to relate to screening and treatment differences that occur along racial/ethnic lines and to insurance status. Therefore, racial differences are not inevitable if counties in the United States work to equalize their health care workforce and health screening for all.[21]

By age an interesting paradox has occurred. CRC incidence in those over 50 years has declined by about 5% but increased in those under 50 years by 22%. Similarly, death rates decreased by 34% in those over 50 years but increased by 13% in those under 50 years. Recommendations include beginning screening at age 50 for those at average risk but earlier with a family history of CRC.[22] We need more research as to causes for increasing CRC in younger adults.[5] Hereditary factors that increase CRC risk include family history, as mentioned, inherited genetic Lynch syndrome (hereditary nonpolyposis colorectal cancer [HNPCC]), and familial adenomatous polyposis (FAP), as well as a personal history of chronic inflammatory bowel disease (ulcerative colitis or Crohn disease) or type 2 diabetes.[2] For patient teaching on when to have CRC screening, see the Health Promotion section on p. 722.

SUBJECTIVE DATA

1. Usual bowel routine
2. Change in bowel habits
3. Rectal bleeding, blood in the stool
4. Medications (laxatives, stool softeners, iron)
5. Rectal conditions (pruritus, hemorrhoids, fissure, fistula)
6. Family history
7. Patient-centered care (diet of high-fiber foods, most recent examinations)

Examiner Asks	Rationale
1. **Usual bowel routine.** Bowels move regularly? How often? Usual color? Hard or soft? • Any straining at stool, incomplete evacuation, urge to have bowel movement but nothing comes?	Rome III criteria for constipation: ≤3 stools/wk, straining, lumpy or hard stools, incomplete evacuation, sensation of blockage.[23,27] Risks: older age, women, inactivity.

Subjective Data

Examiner Asks	Rationale
• Eat breakfast? (This increases colon motility and prompts a bowel movement in many.) • Pain while passing a bowel movement?	**Dyschezia.** Pain due to local condition (hemorrhoid, fissure) or constipation.
2. Change in bowel habits. Any loose stools or diarrhea? When did it start? How long has it lasted? How severe? Number of stools per day? Character: watery, bloody, mucus-filled, purulent? Also have nausea and vomiting, abdominal pain?	Diarrhea occurs with gastroenteritis, colitis, irritable colon syndrome. Risks include: child-care center, eating raw shellfish, undercooked meat or eggs, contaminated water. Noninflammatory diarrhea is milder and usually viral; inflammatory is more severe and bacterial; associated with travel, foodborne illness, fever, abdominal pain. Check for dehydration (decreased urine, thirst, dizziness, change in mental status).[6]
• Eaten at a restaurant recently? Anyone else in your group or family have the same symptoms? Traveled to a developing country during the past 6 months?	Consider foodborne illness, unclear water. Consider parasitic or bacterial infection. *E. coli* is most frequent cause of traveler's diarrhea.
• Been hospitalized recently? On antibiotics?	Diarrhea is a side effect of antibiotics, also *Clostridium difficile* has explosive diarrhea.
3. Rectal bleeding, blood in the stool. Ever had black or bloody stools? When did you first notice blood in the stools? What is the color—bright red or dark red–black? How much blood: spotting on the toilet paper or outright passing of blood with the stool? Do the bloody stools have a particular smell?	**Melena.** Black stools may be tarry due to occult blood (melena) from GI bleeding or non-tarry from ingestion of iron medications. Red blood occurs with GI bleeding, local bleeding around the anus, with colon and rectal cancer.
• Ever had clay-colored stools? • Ever had mucus or pus in stool? • Frothy stool? • Need to pass gas frequently?	Clay color indicates absent bile pigment: biliary cirrhosis, gallstones, alcoholic or viral hepatitis. **Steatorrhea** is excessive fat in stool: malabsorption as in celiac disease, cystic fibrosis, chronic pancreatitis, Crohn disease. Flatulence occurs with some medications, nutritional supplements, Crohn disease, certain foods.
4. Medications. Which **medications** do you take—prescription and over-the-counter? Laxatives or stool softeners? Which ones? How often? Iron pills? Do you ever use enemas to move your bowels? How often?	Over $800 million annually is spent in the United States on OTC laxatives![23]
5. Rectal conditions. Any problems in rectal area: itching, pain or burning, hemorrhoids? How do you treat these? Any hemorrhoid preparations? Ever had a fissure or fistula? How was it treated? • Ever had a problem controlling your bowels?	Symptomatic hemorrhoids: pruritus, painless rectal bleeding, red blood on tissue or in bowl. Fissure has painful bowel movements like "shards of glass." Fecal incontinence is leaking of solid or liquid stool involuntarily. Mucoid discharge and soiled underwear occur with prolapsed hemorrhoids.
6. Family history. Any **family history:** polyps or cancer in colon or rectum, inflammatory bowel disease, prostate cancer?	Risk factors for CRC, PC.

Examiner Asks	Rationale
7. Patient-centered care. What is the usual amount of **high-fiber foods** in your daily diet: cereals, apples or other fruits, vegetables, whole-grain breads? How many glasses of water do you drink each day?	High-fiber foods of the soluble type (beans, prunes, barley, carrots, broccoli, cabbage) lower cholesterol levels, whereas insoluble fiber foods (cereals, wheat germ) reduce risk for colon cancer. Also, fiber foods fight obesity, stabilize blood sugar, and help some GI disorders.
• Date of last: digital rectal examination, stool blood test, colonoscopy, prostate-specific antigen blood test (for men).	Early detection for cancer: colonoscopy after age 50 years then every 10 years; fecal occult blood test annually after age 50 years; age 45 years for African Americans[2]; information about PSA blood test annually for men older than 50 years or African-American men beginning at age 45 years.[3]

Additional History for Infants and Children

1. Have you ever noticed any irritation in your child's anal area: redness, raised skin, frequent itching?	Pinworms are a common cause of intense itching and irritated anal skin.
2. How are your child's bowel movements (BMs)? Frequency? Any problems? Any pain or straining with BM?	Assess usual stooling pattern. Constipation is decrease in BM frequency, with difficult passing of very hard, dry stools. **Encopresis** is persistent passing of stools into clothing in a child older than 4 years, at which age continence would be expected.

OBJECTIVE DATA

PREPARATION

Perform a rectal examination on all adults and particularly those in middle and late years. Help the person assume one of the following positions (Fig. 26.3):

Place the male in left lateral decubitus, standing, or lithotomy position. Instruct the standing male to rest elbows on exam table and point toes together; this relaxes the regional muscles, making it easier to spread the buttocks.

Place the female in the lithotomy position if examining genitalia as well; use the left lateral decubitus position for the rectal area alone.

EQUIPMENT NEEDED

Penlight
Lubricating jelly
Gloves
Fecal occult blood test container

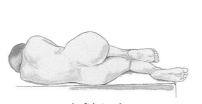
Left lateral

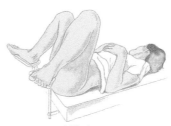
Lithotomy

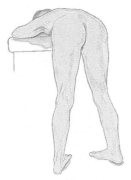
Standing

26.3 Positions for rectal examination.

Normal Range of Findings

Abnormal Findings

Inspect the Perianal Area

Spread the buttocks wide apart with both gloved hands and observe the perianal region. The anus normally looks moist and hairless, with coarse, folded skin that is more pigmented than the perianal skin. The anal opening is tightly closed. No lesions are present.

Inflammation. Lesions or scars.
Linear split—Fissure.
Flabby skin sac—Hemorrhoid. Shiny blue skin sac—Thrombosed hemorrhoid.
Small round opening in anal area—Fistula (see Table 26.1, Anal Region Abnormalities, p. 724).

Inspect the sacrococcygeal area. Normally it appears smooth and even.

Inflammation or tenderness, swelling, tuft of hair, or dimple at tip of coccyx may indicate pilonidal cyst (see Table 26.1).

Instruct the person to hold the breath and bear down by performing a Valsalva maneuver. No break in skin integrity or protrusion through the anal opening should be present. Describe any abnormality in clock-face terms, with the 12 o'clock position as the anterior point toward the symphysis pubis and the 6 o'clock position toward the coccyx.

Appearance of fissure or hemorrhoids.
Circular red doughnut of tissue—Rectal prolapse.

Procedures for Advanced Practice

Palpate the Anus and Rectum

Drop lubricating jelly onto your gloved index finger. Instruct the person that palpation is not painful but may feel like needing to move the bowels. Ask the man to take a deep breath and hold it. Place the pad of your index finger gently against the anal verge (Fig. 26.4). You will feel the sphincter tighten and then relax. As it relaxes ask the man to exhale and flex the tip of your finger and slowly insert it into the anal canal in a direction toward the umbilicus. *Never* approach the anus at right angles with your index finger extended. Such a jabbing motion causes sphincter tightening and is painful.

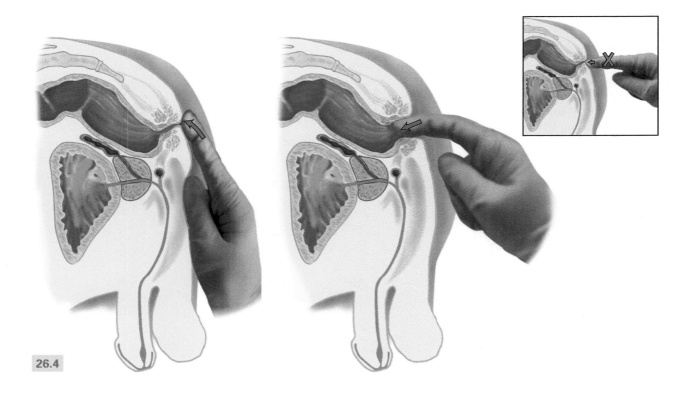

26.4

Normal Range of Findings

Rotate your examining finger to palpate the entire muscular ring. The canal should feel smooth and even. Note the intersphincteric groove circling the canal wall. To assess tone, ask the person to tighten the muscle. The sphincter should tighten evenly around your finger with no pain to the person.

Use a bidigital palpation with your thumb against the perianal tissue (Fig. 26.5). Press your examining finger toward it. This maneuver highlights any swelling or tenderness and helps assess the bulbourethral glands.

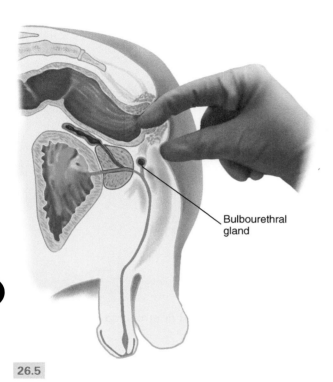

Bulbourethral gland

26.5

Above the anal canal the rectum turns posteriorly, following the curve of the coccyx and sacrum. Insert your finger farther and explore all around the rectal wall. It normally feels smooth with no nodularity. Promptly report any mass you discover for further examination.

Prostate Gland. On the anterior wall in the male, note the elastic, bulging prostate gland (Fig. 26.6). Find the median sulcus and palpate the entire prostate in a systematic manner, but note that only the superior and part of the lateral surfaces are accessible to examination. Press *into* the gland at each location because when a nodule occurs, it will not project into the rectal lumen. The surface should feel smooth and muscular; search for any distinct nodule or diffuse firmness. Note these characteristics:

Abnormal Findings

Decreased tone.
Increased tone occurs with inflammation and anxiety.
Tenderness.

Internal hemorrhoid above anorectal junction is not palpable unless thrombosed.
A soft, slightly movable mass may be a polyp.
A firm or hard mass with irregular shape or rolled edges may be CRC (see Table 26.2, Rectum Abnormalities, p. 726).

Normal Range of Findings	Abnormal Findings

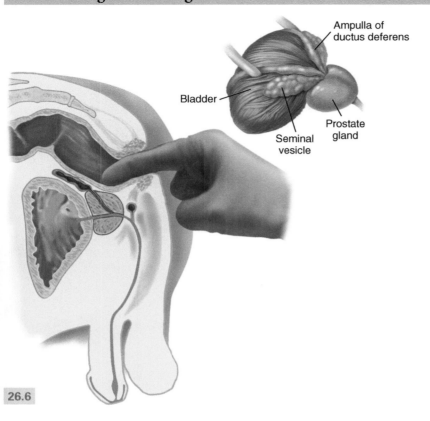

Ampulla of ductus deferens

Bladder

Seminal vesicle

Prostate gland

26.6

Size—2.5 cm long by 4 cm wide; should not protrude more than 1 cm into the rectum

Enlarged or atrophied gland.

Shape—Heart shape, with palpable central groove

Flat with no groove.

Surface—Smooth

Nodular.

Consistency—Elastic, rubbery

Hard; or boggy, soft, fluctuant.

Mobility—Slightly movable

Fixed.

Sensitivity—Nontender to palpation

Tender. Swollen, exquisitely tender gland accompanies prostatitis.

Enlarged, firm, smooth gland with central groove obliterated suggests BPH.

Any stone-hard, irregular, fixed nodule indicates PC (see Table 26.3, Prostate Gland Abnormalities, p. 727).

In the female palpate the cervix through the anterior rectal wall. It normally feels like a small, round mass. You also may palpate a retroverted uterus or a tampon in the vagina. Do not mistake the cervix or a tampon for a tumor.

Withdraw your examining finger; normally no bright red blood or mucus is on the glove. To complete the examination, offer the person tissues to remove the lubricant and help him or her to a more comfortable position.

Examination of Stool. Inspect any feces remaining on the glove. Normally the color is brown, and the consistency is soft.

Jellylike mucus shreds mixed in stool indicate inflammation.

Bright red blood on stool surface indicates rectal bleeding. Bright red blood mixed with feces indicates possible colonic bleeding.

Normal Range of Findings	Abnormal Findings

Test any stool on the glove for **occult blood**. A negative response is normal. If the stool is *Hematest* positive, it indicates occult blood. The fecal immunochemical test (FIT) is newer and can be used without the diet or medication restrictions of the older guaiac-based tests. There are two types of FITs: liquid-based tests that store the stool sample in a hemoglobin stabilizing buffer, and dry-slide cards that are analyzed manually.

Enhance self-care by providing the average-risk patient an at-home collection kit to screen for asymptomatic colorectal cancer and precancerous lesions (high-risk adenomas). A patient collects the stool specimen at home and mails it to the laboratory. Evidence shows that the newer fecal immunochemical test is easier and requires only one stool sample. It detects antibodies specific for human hemoglobin and is sensitive to invasive cancers and precancerous lesions.

Black tarry stool with distinct malodor indicates upper GI bleeding with blood partially digested. (Must lose more than 50 mL from upper GI tract to be considered melena.)

Black stool—Also occurs with ingesting iron or bismuth preparations.

Gray, tan stool—Absent bile pigment (e.g., obstructive jaundice).

Pale yellow, greasy stool—Increased fat content (steatorrhea), as occurs with malabsorption syndrome.

Occult bleeding usually indicates cancer of the colon.

❖ DEVELOPMENTAL COMPETENCE

Infants and Children

For the newborn, hold the feet with one hand and flex the knees up onto the abdomen. Note the presence of the anus. Confirm a patent rectum and anus by noting the first meconium stool passed within 24 to 48 hours of birth. To assess sphincter tone, check the *anal reflex*. Gently stroke the anal area and note a quick contraction of the sphincter.

For each infant and child, note that the buttocks are firm and rounded with no masses or lesions. Recall that the *mongolian spot* is a common variation of hyperpigmentation in black, American Indian, Mediterranean, and Asian newborns (see Chapter 13).

The perianal skin is free of lesions. However, diaper rash is common in children younger than 1 year and is exhibited as a generalized reddened area with papules or vesicles.

Omit palpation unless the history or symptoms warrant. When internal palpation is needed, position the infant or child on the back with the legs flexed and gently insert a gloved, well-lubricated finger into the rectum. Use your gloved and lubricated pinky finger; its smaller size is more comfortable for the infant or child.

Inspect the perianal region of the school-age child and adolescent during examination of the genitalia. Internal palpation is not performed routinely.

Imperforate anus.

Flattened buttocks in cystic fibrosis or celiac syndrome.

Coccygeal mass. Meningocele (sac containing meninges that protrude through a defect in the bony spine).

Tuft of hair or pilonidal dimple.

Pustules indicate secondary infection of diaper rash.

Signs of physical or sexual abuse (e.g., anal abrasions, perianal tears).

Fissure—Common cause of constipation or rectal bleeding in child. (Painful, so the child does not defecate.)

Anal impatency. Fecal impaction may warrant rectal palpation by an experienced clinician.

The Aging Adult

As an aging person performs the Valsalva maneuver, you may note relaxation of the perianal musculature and decreased sphincter control. Otherwise the full examination proceeds as that described earlier for the younger adult.

Objective Data

HEALTH PROMOTION AND PATIENT TEACHING

"You have asked about the PSA blood test as a warning for prostate cancer. Let's talk about the pros and possible cons of this test. Then you can decide whether you want to have your PSA followed." We have this discussion at age 50 years for men who are at average risk of prostate cancer; at age 45 years for African-American men and for men who have a father, brother, or son diagnosed with prostate cancer at an early age (younger than 65 years); and at age 40 years for men at even higher risk, that is, men with more than one first-degree relative with prostate cancer at an early age.[3]

PSA stands for prostate-specific antigen, a small protein made only by the prostate gland when it is metabolically active. We follow the test once a year and watch for a sustained rise in the PSA level. A rising PSA does not mean that a person has cancer for sure; it means that the gland is active, which occurs also with noncancerous growth, infection such as prostatitis, and ejaculation. Screening the PSA is effective in detecting early prostate cancer, but it cannot tell whether a possible cancer is slow-growing (latent) or aggressive. A rising PSA can lead to further testing, such as radiologic imaging and a biopsy. A biopsy involves a needle insertion into the gland to harvest some cells for the microscope to tell whether they are cancerous and what type. These tests can be expensive, depending on insurance; slightly painful; and can lead to worry while you wait for results. With PSA screening, 5-, 10-, and 15-year survival rates are close to 100%, 98%, and 94%, respectively.[18,19] It is not yet clear whether early detection and treatment lead to any change in the outcome of the slow-growing cancers. Please discuss these points with your loved ones, and let us know whether to follow your PSA blood test.

"Screening for colorectal cancer starts at age 50 years, and a colonoscopy is recommended for men and women." Colorectal cancer is a commonly diagnosed cancer in the United States, but it can be detected at a curable stage in people who have no warning symptoms. We have many good clinical trials showing lower death rates among people who have screening than among those who do not.[11,15,26] The colonoscopy also can show precancerous polyps, and these are removed during the test, which further decreases the risk of colorectal cancer. If the first colonoscopy shows no cancer and no polyps, the next test can be 10 years later. Screening starts at younger ages for patients with symptoms (blood around stool, anemia, change in bowel habits).[1] Or if a patient's history has 2 or more first-degree relatives with colorectal cancer, we can test the patient for genetic syndromes showing increased risk; if present, the screening can begin at age 20 or 25 years.

"Another test is one you can do at home, the fecal immunochemical test (FIT), which is done on your stool sample. This starts at age 40 years."[7,20] The FIT detects blood from any ulcer in the colon, which can come from cancer or from large polyps. With a manual liquid-based FIT, you apply a test strip inside the sampling tube to the stool sample. The change in color shows a positive or negative result. The stool sample can be mailed to our office and testing done here. This is done every year; if it ever turns positive, a colonoscopy is the next step.

(For men under 26 years): *"Routine immunizations now include the HPV vaccine. The Gardasil and Gardasil-9 became available in 2009 and 2015, respectively, to prevent HPV infection in adolescents and men. Vaccines are approved for ages 9 to 26 years, and younger boys ages 11 to 12 years need only 2 doses of the vaccine."*[17] HPV stands for human papillomavirus and is the most common sexually transmitted infection. It can cause genital or anal cancers. The vaccine prevents this. Men ages 17 to 25 years are at greater risk of contracting HPV if they have high-risk sexual activity: intercourse with multiple partners, unprotected sexual intercourse, or anal receptive intercourse with men. But even if these behaviors do not apply to you, protecting yourself against HPV also keeps you from spreading an HPV infection to your female partner; HPV can cause cervical cancer in women. The vaccine has been used for many years and is safe.

DOCUMENTATION AND CRITICAL THINKING

Sample Charting

SUBJECTIVE

Has one BM daily, soft, brown, no pain, no change in bowel routine. On no medications. Has no history of pruritus, hemorrhoids, fissure, or fistula. Diet includes 1 to 2 servings daily each of fresh fruits and vegetables but no whole-grain cereals or breads.

OBJECTIVE

No fissure, hemorrhoids, fistula, or skin lesions in perianal area. Sphincter tone good; no prolapse. Rectal walls smooth; no masses or tenderness. Prostate not enlarged; no masses or tenderness. Stool brown; Hematest negative.

Health Promotion and Patient Teaching

Documentation and Critical Thinking

ASSESSMENT

Rectal structures intact; no palpable lesions

Clinical Case Study 1

D.R. is a 55-year-old male. Employed as a database analyst. No personal or family history of GI disease or colon cancer. Personal history of obesity (BMI 42.5); low-fiber, high-fat diet; hypertension; recent knee replacement. Medications include antihypertensive agent and hydrocodone prn for knee pain.

SUBJECTIVE

D.R. presents with inability to sit without pain, constipation, and "bleeding when I wipe." Last bowel movement 1 day PTA. D.R. reports stool was difficult to expel.

OBJECTIVE

Abdomen: Rounded appearance. Bowel sounds present. Tympany predominates. Dull over LLQ. Firm, nontender LLQ. No organomegaly.

Rectal: Skin sac indicative of hemorrhoid located at 6 o'clock. Grade IV thrombosed hemorrhoids located at 12 o'clock and 2 o'clock. Sphincter tone good. Rectal walls smooth; no masses. Reports tenderness with rectal exam. No stool present.

ASSESSMENT

Thrombosed hemorrhoids
Acute pain
Constipation from opioid use and low-fiber diet

Clinical Case Study 2

C.M. is a 62-year-old male with COPD for 15 years who today has had "diarrhea for 3 days."

SUBJECTIVE

7 days PTA—C.M. seen at this agency for acute respiratory infection that was diagnosed as acute bronchitis and treated with oral ampicillin. No hospitalization. Took medication as directed.

3 days PTA—Symptoms of respiratory infection improved. Ingesting usual diet. Onset of 4-5 loose, unformed brown stools a day. No abdominal pain or cramping. No nausea.

Now—Diarrhea continues. No blood or mucus noticed in stool. No new foods or restaurant food in past 3 days. Wife not ill.

OBJECTIVE

Vital signs: Temp 98.6° F (37° C). Pulse 88 bpm. Resp 18/min. BP 142/82 mm Hg.

Respiratory: Respirations unlabored. Barrel chest. Hyperresonant to percussion. Lung sounds clear but diminished. No crackles or rhonchi today.

Abdomen: Flat. Bowel sounds present. No organomegaly or tenderness to palpation.

Rectal: No lesions in perianal area. Sphincter tone good. Rectal walls smooth; no masses or tenderness. Prostate smooth and firm, no median sulcus palpable, no masses or tenderness. Stool brown; Hematest negative.

ASSESSMENT

Diarrhea from effects of antibiotic medication

Documentation and Critical Thinking

ABNORMAL FINDINGS

TABLE 26.1   Anal Region Abnormalities

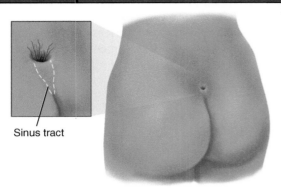

Sinus tract

◄ Pilonidal Cyst or Sinus

A hair-containing cyst or sinus located in the midline over the coccyx or lower sacrum. Often opens as a dimple with visible tuft of hair and possibly an erythematous halo. Or may appear as a palpable cyst. When advanced, has a palpable sinus tract. Although a congenital disorder, it is first diagnosed between 15 and 30 years.

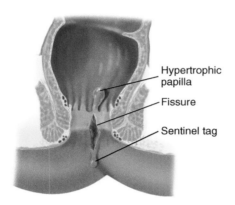

Hypertrophic papilla

Fissure

Sentinel tag

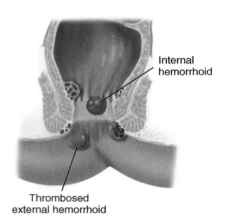

Internal hemorrhoid

Thrombosed external hemorrhoid

Fissure

An exquisitely painful longitudinal tear in the superficial mucosa at the anal margin. Most (>90%) occur in the posterior midline area. Pain with passing stool is described as passing "shards of glass"; may have bright red blood in the stool. Inspection shows an acute fissure as having sharp edges and a chronic fissure as indurated and accompanied by a papule of skin, *sentinel tag,* on the anal margin below or a polyp above. Fissures are caused by trauma, ischemia, and elevated anal pressure. Occurs with constipation, obesity, and hypothyroidism.[16] Medical treatments are stool softeners, nitroglycerin ointment, topical nifedipine or diltiazem cream, but injection of botulinum toxin into internal anal sphincter is slightly more effective.[8]

Hemorrhoids

These common, flabby papules are a varicosed vein. An *external hemorrhoid* starts below the anorectal junction covered by anal skin. When *thrombosed,* it contains clotted blood and becomes a painful, swollen, shiny blue mass that itches and bleeds with defecation. When resolved, it leaves a painless, flabby skin sac around the anal orifice. An *internal hemorrhoid* starts above the anorectal junction covered by mucous membrane. Hemorrhoids result from increased pressure: with straining at stool, chronic constipation, pregnancy, obesity, or a low-fiber diet. Accompanied by painless rectal bleeding, red blood on tissue or toilet bowl, pruritus, anal swelling and pain, fecal soilage, mucus discharge. Treat with fiber supplement, laxative, decreased time on toilet, rubber band ligation.[8,12]

Continued

TABLE 26.1	Anal Region Abnormalities—cont'd

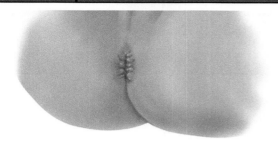

◀ Pruritus Ani

Intense itching and burning in the perineum has myriad causes: soaps, restrictive clothing, fecal soiling or hemorrhoids, eczema or psoriasis, STIs (herpes, condylomata), candida infection from moist or sweaty folds of skin in obese or aging persons, systemic causes (such as diabetes, liver disease), and pinworm infestation in children. Persistent scratching makes an inflammatory response and shows as red, raised, thickened, excoriated skin; may be swollen and moist. Careful history leads to treatment of underlying cause. Urge not to scratch, to avoid scented soap, prepared wipes, tight underclothing.[4,25]

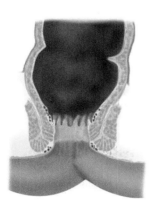

◀ Fecal Impaction (FI)

A complete colon blockage by hard, desiccated immovable stool, which presents as constipation or overflow incontinence. FI is common, potentially serious, and not routinely discussed.[10] At highest risk are children, incapacitated patients (spinal cord injuries, stroke), aging adults, and those in institutions. Causes of constipation and FI are many, including immobility, low fiber, dehydration, neurologic diseases, opioids and other medications. Exams of some aging people may lead to confusion, agitation. Inspect abdominal distention with tympany, palpable cord in left lower quadrant; may not palpate stool on rectal exam if higher impaction. Warrants radiologic imaging. Complications are bowel obstruction, perforation, peritonitis. Treatment is disimpaction with endoscopy (manual can cause perforation, rectal bleeding, and vagal stimulation), then distal colon cleansing with enemas, and a bowel regimen to prevent recurrence.[10] Usually treated in outpatient setting, but between 2006 and 2011, the frequency of constipation visits in Emergency Departments increased by 41.5%.[23]

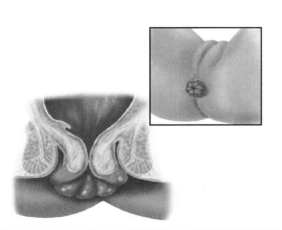

◀ Rectal Prolapse

The complete rectal mucous membrane protrudes through the anus, appearing as a moist red doughnut with radiating lines. When prolapse is incomplete, only the mucosa bulges. When complete, it includes the anal sphincters. Occurs following a Valsalva maneuver such as straining at stool or with exercise. Caused by weakened pelvic support muscles and requires surgery.

ABNORMAL FINDINGS
FOR ADVANCED PRACTICE

TABLE 26.2 | **Rectum Abnormalities**

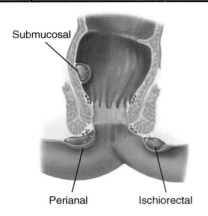

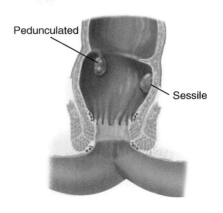

Abscess

A localized cavity of pus from infected anorectal gland. Characterized by persistent throbbing rectal pain, and appears red, hot, swollen, indurated, and tender. In internal abscess may be palpated as boggy area on rectal exam. Must be incised and drained to prevent spread, recurrence, and formation of fistula.

Rectal Polyp

A protruding growth from the rectal mucous membrane is fairly common. The polyp may be *pedunculated* (on a stalk) or *sessile* (a mound on the surface, close to the mucosal wall). The soft nodule is difficult to palpate. Colonoscopy, removal, and biopsy screen for a malignant growth. Removal of adenomatous polyps has been shown to prevent deaths from colorectal cancer. Particularly larger sizes of polyps increase risk of cancer.[24]

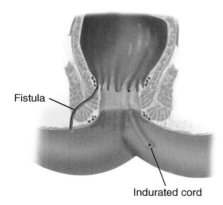

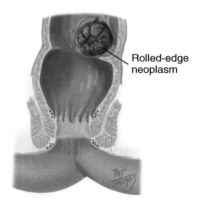

Anorectal Fistula

Anorectal abscess (see Table 26.2) starts from an infected anorectal gland; the infection channels through the perianal tissues to form a fistula, a connection between the infected gland and the outside perineum.[8] Fistulae also occur with Crohn disease or radiation therapy. Persistent pain and swelling occur with abscess; fistulae are sometimes painful and itch. The fistula track feels like an indurated cord on bidigital palpation; may drain purulent or serosanguineous matter.

Carcinoma

A malignant neoplasm in the colon or rectum is asymptomatic; thus the importance of routine imaging by colonoscopy and DRE. An early lesion may be a single firm nodule, may have an ulcerated center with rolled edges. As the lesion grows it has an irregular cauliflower shape and is fixed and stone-hard. Refer a person with any rectal lesion for cancer screening. Suggest screening guidelines: careful family history, fecal occult blood tests annually, and colonoscopy every 10 years, starting at age 50 years for those at average risk, earlier for those at high risk.[1]

TABLE 26.3	Prostate Gland Abnormalities

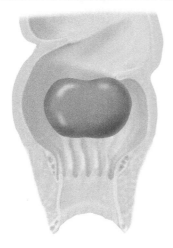

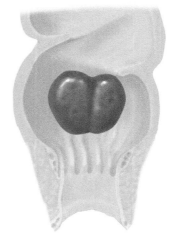

Benign Prostatic Hypertrophy (BPH)

S: Urinary frequency, urgency, hesitancy, straining to urinate, weak stream, intermittent stream, sensation of incomplete emptying, nocturia.

O: A symmetric nontender enlargement; commonly occurs in males beginning in the middle years. The prostate surface feels smooth, rubbery, or firm (like the consistency of the nose), with the median sulcus obliterated.

Prostatitis

S: Fever, chills, malaise, urinary frequency and urgency, dysuria, urethral discharge; dull, aching pain in perineal and rectal area.

O: An exquisitely tender enlargement is *acute* inflammation, yielding a swollen, slightly asymmetric gland.

With a chronic inflammation the signs can vary from tender enlargement with a boggy feel to isolated firm areas caused by fibrosis. Or the gland may feel normal.

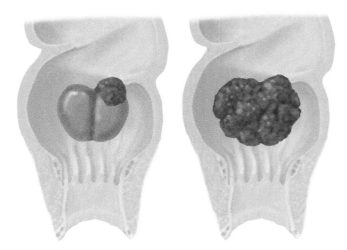

◄ Carcinoma

S: Frequency, nocturia, hematuria, weak stream, hesitancy, pain or burning on urination; continuous pain in lower back, pelvis, thighs.

O: A malignant neoplasm often starts as a single hard nodule on the posterior surface, producing asymmetry and a change in consistency. As it invades normal tissue, multiple hard nodules appear, or the entire gland feels stone-hard and fixed. The median sulcus is obliterated.

S, Subjective data; *O,* objective data.

Abnormal Findings

| Summary Checklist: Anus, Rectum, and Prostate Examination |

1. **Inspect anus** and perianal area.
2. Inspect during Valsalva maneuver.
3. **Palpate anal canal** and rectum on all adults.
4. **Test stool** for occult blood.

REFERENCES

1. Abdelsattar, Z. M., Wong, S. L., Regenbogen, S. E., et al. (2016). Colorectal cancer outcomes and treatment patterns in patients too young for average-risk screening. *Cancer, 122*(6), 929–934.
2. American Cancer Society (ACS). (2017). *Cancer Facts & figures 2017.* ACS. https://www.cancer.org/cancer-facts-and-figures-2017.pdf.
3. American Cancer Society (ACS). (2017). *ACS recommendations for prostate cancer early detection.* https://www.cancer.org/cancer/prostate-cancer/early-detection/acs-recommendations.html.
4. Ansari, P. (2016). Pruritus ani. *Clin Colon Rectal Surg, 29*(1), 38–42.
5. Baron, J. A., Barry, E. L., Mott, L. A., et al. (2015). A Trial of calcium and vitamin D for the prevention of colorectal adenomas. *N Engl J Med, 373*(16), 1519.
6. Barr, W., & Smith, A. (2014). Acute diarrhea. *Am Fam Physician, 89*(3), 180–189.
7. Chen, C. H., Tsai, M. K., & Wen, C. P. (2016). Extending colorectal cancer screening to persons aged 40 to 49 years with immunochemical fecal occult blood test. *J Clin Gastroenterol, 50*(9), 761–768.
8. Foxx-Orenstein, A. E., Umar, S. B., & Crowell, M. D. (2014). Common anorectal disorders. *Gastroenterol Hepatol, 10*(5), 294–301.
9. Gerhard, R. S., Patil, D., Liu, Y., et al. (2017). Treatment of men with high-risk prostate cancer based on race, insurance coverage, and access to advanced technology. *Urol Oncol, 35*, 250–256.
10. Hussain, Z., Whitehead, D., & Lacy, B. (2014). Fecal impaction. *Curr Gastroenterol Rep, 16*(404), 1–7.
11. Inadomi, J. M. (2017). Screening for colorectal neoplasia. *N Engl J Med, 376*(2), 149–156.
12. Jacobs, D. (2014). Hemorrhoids. *N Engl J Med, 371*(10), 944–951.
13. Katz, A. (2015). Early localized prostate cancer. *Am J Nurs, 115*(3), 34–46.
14. Reference deleted in proofs.
15. Mahon, S. M. (2017). Colorectal cancer screening: Using evidence-based guidelines. *Nurse Pract, 42*(10), 18–26.
16. Mapel, D. W., Schum, M., & Von Worley, A. (2014). The epidemiology and treatment of anal fissures in a population-based cohort. *BMC Gastroenterol, 14*(1), 129–135.
17. McCutcheon, T., & Schaar, G. (2017). HPV knowledge and vaccination rates in college-aged males: Implications for practice. *Nurse Pract, 42*(1), 49–53.
18. Peisch, S. F., Van Blarigan, E. L., Chan, J. M., et al. (2017). Prostate cancer progression and mortality. *World J Urol, 35*(6), 867–874.
19. Pinsky, P. F., Prorok, P. C., & Kramer, B. S. (2017). Prostate cancer screening. *N Engl J Med, 376*(13), 1285–1289.
20. Robertson, D. J., Lee, J. K., Boland, C. R., et al. (2017). Recommendations on fecal immunochemical testing to screen for colorectal neoplasia. *Gastrointest Endosc, 85*(1), 2–21.
21. Rust, G., Zhang, S., Yu, Z., et al. (2016). Counties eliminating racial disparities in colorectal cancer mortality. *Cancer, 22*(11), 1735–1748.
22. Siegel, R. L., Miller, K. D., Fedewa, S. A., et al. (2017). Colorectal cancer statistics, 2017. *CA Cancer J Clin, 67*(2), 177–193.
23. Sommers, T., Corban, C., Sengupta, N., et al. (2015). Emergency department burden of constipation in the United States from 2006 to 2011. *Am J Gastroenterol, 110*(4), 572–579.
24. Strum, W. B. (2016). Colorectal adenomas. *N Engl J Med, 374*(11), 1065–1075.
25. Swamiappan, M. (2016). Anogenital pruritus. *J Clin Diagn Res, 10*(4), 1–3.
26. U.S. Preventive Services Task Force (USPSTF). (2016). Screening for colorectal cancer. *JAMA, 315*(23), 2564–2575.
27. Vazquez Roque, M., & Bouras, E. (2015). Epidemiology and management of chronic constipation in elderly patients. *Clin Interv Aging, 10*, 919–930.
28. Weiner, A., Matulewicz, R., Tosoian, J., et al. (2017). PD03-07 The impact of socioeconomic status, race, and insurance type on the risk of newly diagnosed metastatic prostate cancer in the United States. *J Urology, 197*(4S), e59.

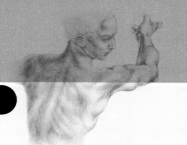

CHAPTER 27

Female Genitourinary System

Ⓔhttp://evolve.elsevier.com/Jarvis/

STRUCTURE AND FUNCTION

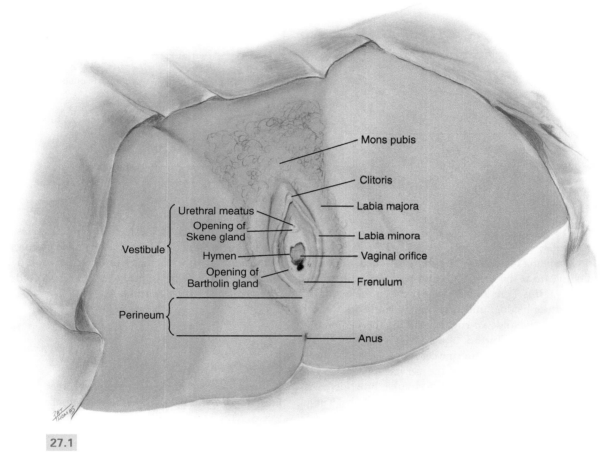

Mons pubis

Clitoris

Urethral meatus

Opening of
Skene gland

Labia majora

Labia minora

Vestibule

Hymen

Vaginal orifice

Opening of
Bartholin gland

Frenulum

Perineum

Anus

27.1

EXTERNAL GENITALIA

The external genitalia are called the **vulva,** or pudendum (Fig. 27.1). The **mons pubis** is a round, firm pad of adipose tissue covering the symphysis pubis. After puberty it is covered with hair in the pattern of an inverted triangle. The **labia majora** are two rounded folds of adipose tissue extending from the mons pubis down and around to the perineum. After puberty hair covers the outer surfaces of the labia, whereas the inner folds are smooth and moist and contain sebaceous follicles.

Inside the labia majora are two smaller, darker folds of skin, the **labia minora.** These are joined anteriorly at the clitoris where they form a hood, or prepuce. The labia minora are joined posteriorly by a transverse fold, the **frenulum,** or fourchette. The **clitoris** is a small, pea-shaped erectile body, homologous with the male penis and highly sensitive to tactile stimulation.

The labial structures encircle a boat-shaped space, or cleft, termed the **vestibule.** Within it are numerous openings. The **urethral meatus** appears as a dimple 2.5 cm posterior to the clitoris. Surrounding the urethral meatus are the tiny, multiple **paraurethral (Skene) glands.** Their ducts are not visible but open posterior to the urethra at the 5 and 7 o'clock positions.

The **vaginal orifice** is posterior to the urethral meatus. It appears either as a thin median slit or a large opening with irregular edges, depending on the presentation of the membranous **hymen.** The hymen is a thin, circular or crescent-shaped fold that may cover part of the vaginal orifice or may be absent completely. On either side and posterior to the vaginal orifice are two **vestibular (Bartholin) glands,** which secrete a clear lubricating mucus during intercourse. Their ducts are not visible but open in the groove between the labia minora and the hymen.

729

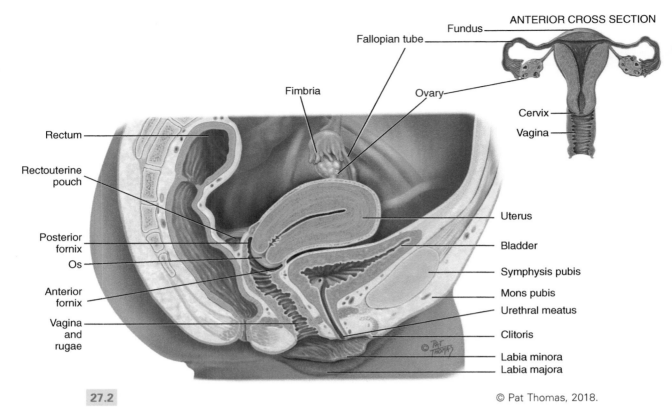

ANTERIOR CROSS SECTION

Fundus

Fallopian tube

Fimbria

Ovary

Cervix

Vagina

Rectum

Rectouterine pouch

Uterus

Posterior fornix

Bladder

Os

Symphysis pubis

Anterior fornix

Mons pubis

Urethral meatus

Vagina and rugae

Clitoris

Labia minora

Labia majora

27.2

© Pat Thomas, 2018.

INTERNAL GENITALIA

The internal genitalia include the **vagina,** a flattened, tubular canal extending from the orifice up and backward into the pelvis (Fig. 27.2). It is 9 cm long and sits between the rectum posteriorly and the bladder and urethra anteriorly. Its walls are in thick transverse folds, or **rugae,** enabling the vagina to dilate widely during childbirth.

At the end of the canal, the uterine **cervix** projects into the vagina. In the nulliparous female the cervix appears as a smooth doughnut shape with a small circular hole, or **os.** After childbirth the os is slightly enlarged and irregular. The cervical epithelium is of two distinct types. The vagina and cervix are covered with smooth, pink, stratified squamous epithelium. Inside the os the endocervical canal is lined with columnar epithelium that looks red and rough. The point where these two tissues meet is the **squamocolumnar junction** and is not visible.

A continuous recess is present around the cervix, termed the **anterior fornix** in front and the **posterior fornix** in back. Behind the posterior fornix another deep recess is formed by the peritoneum. It dips down between the rectum and cervix to form the **rectouterine pouch,** or **cul-de-sac of Douglas.**

The **uterus** is a pear-shaped, thick-walled, muscular organ. It is flattened anteroposteriorly, measuring 5.5 to 8 cm long by 3.5 to 4 cm wide and 2 to 2.5 cm thick. It is freely movable, not fixed, and usually tilts forward and superior to the bladder (a position labeled as *anteverted* and *anteflexed,* see p. 748).

The **fallopian tubes** are two pliable, trumpet-shaped tubes, 10 cm in length, extending from the uterine fundus laterally to the brim of the pelvis. There they curve posteriorly, their fimbriated ends located near the **ovaries.** The two ovaries are located one on each side of the uterus at the level of the anterior superior iliac spine. Each is oval shaped, 3 cm long by 2 cm wide by 1 cm thick, and serves to develop ova (eggs) and the female hormones.

❖ DEVELOPMENTAL COMPETENCE

Infants and Adolescents

At birth the external genitalia are engorged because of the presence of maternal estrogen. The structures recede in a few weeks, remaining small until puberty. The ovaries are located in the abdomen during childhood. The uterus is small with a straight axis and no anteflexion.

At puberty estrogens stimulate the growth of cells in the reproductive tract and the development of secondary sex characteristics. The first signs of puberty are breast development (thelarche) and pubic hair development, beginning between the ages of 8 to 10 years (mean = 11.6 years).[24] Puberty culminates with the first menstrual cycle (menarche) just after the peak of growth velocity. Irregularity of the menstrual cycle is common during adolescence because of the occasional failure to ovulate. With menarche the uterine body flexes on the cervix. The ovaries now are in the pelvic cavity.

Tanner's table on the 5 stages of pubic hair development (sexual maturity rating [SMR]) is helpful in teaching girls the expected sequence of sexual development (Table 27.1). These data were developed on Caucasian girls and may not generalize to all racial groups, i.e., mature Asian women normally have fine, sparse pubic hair.

The National Health and Nutrition Examination Survey (NHANES) gives a cross-sectional snapshot of U.S. health characteristics. Data from NHANES on reproductive milestones shows a trend in achieving menarche at younger ages over the last hundred years. In the first half of the 20th century, this was attributed to better nutrition and treatment of infectious disease, but by the turn into the 21st century, obesity and physical inactivity were factors. By race/ethnicity, the mean age at onset of pubic hair and menarche was 9.5 and 12.06 years for African-American girls; 10.3 and 12.09 years for Mexican-American girls; and 10.5 and 12.52 years for white girls. Thus African-American and Mexican-American girls are entering puberty about one-half year earlier than white girls.[2]

Does this matter? Well, yes. The concerns are that girls enter physical puberty before they are emotionally mature, that increased exposure to environmental estrogens may be a contributing factor, and that earlier menarche may increase risk for some reproductive cancers.[2] The biggest concern is that the epidemic of childhood and adolescent overweight and obesity is a major contributor to early menarche.

During the past 4 decades the prevalence of overweight and obesity in U.S. children has more than tripled,[22] with African-American, Hispanic, and American Indian girls at especially high risk. Evidence shows that increased weight and body mass index (BMI) contribute to earlier pubertal development, with a median age of menarche occurring 5.4 months earlier in obese preteen girls than in girls with normal BMI.[24] African-American girls enter puberty before Caucasian and Hispanic girls, but it is not clear if obesity alone contributes to this earlier onset or if socioeconomic or environmental factors contribute as well.[22]

The Pregnant Woman

A complete discussion of the pregnant woman follows in Chapter 31. Shortly after the first missed menstrual period the genitalia show signs of the growing fetus. See p. 758 for the changes in the cervix on internal examination.

The greatest change is in the uterus itself. The nonpregnant uterus has a flattened pear shape. Its early growth encroaches on the space occupied by the bladder, producing the symptom of urinary frequency. By 10 to 12 weeks' gestation, the uterus becomes globular in shape and is too large to stay in the pelvis. At 20 to 24 weeks, the uterus has an oval shape. It rises almost to the liver, displacing the intestines superiorly and laterally.

Cervical and vaginal secretions increase during pregnancy and are thick, white, and more acidic because of *Lactobacillus acidophilus*, which changes glycogen into lactic acid. The acidic pH keeps pathogenic bacteria from multiplying in the vagina, but the increase in glycogen increases the risk for candidiasis (commonly called a *yeast infection*) during pregnancy.

Sexual Identity

Women who have sex with women (WSW) include lesbian and bisexual women. The first consideration for these women is simply access to health care. Evidence is mixed as to whether lesbians report being negatively affected by their health care providers if they disclose their status.[23] Trust is crucial so that women and providers are comfortable in discussing sexual behaviors, risks, and health maintenance. The placement of pamphlets, stickers, and posters that are inclusive of WSW signals that this provider (office, clinic) is inclusive and approachable. Some lesbian women may lack insurance coverage if same-sex partners are not eligible for

TABLE 27.1 Sexual Maturity Rating (SMR) in Girls	
Stage 1 Preadolescent. No pubic hair. Mons and labia covered with fine vellus hair as on abdomen.	

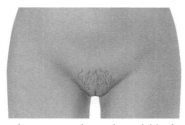 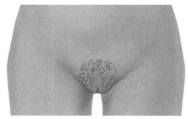

Stage 2 Growth sparse and mostly on labia. Long, downy hair, slightly pigmented, straight or only slightly curly.	**Stage 3** Growth sparse and spreading over mons pubis. Hair is darker, coarser, curlier.

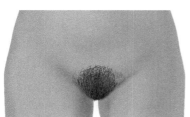 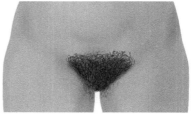

Stage 4 Hair is adult in type but over smaller area; none on medial thigh.	**Stage 5** Adult in type and pattern; inverse triangle. Also on medial thigh surface.

Adapted from Tanner, J.M. (1962). *Growth at adolescence*. Oxford, England: Blackwell Scientific.

Structure and Function

shared insurance benefits. Next are myths and misconceptions to break down. The risk of cervical cancer among lesbians is underestimated because of perceived and real lack of sexual contact with men, and lesbian women may not present themselves for screening. Almost all cervical cancers result as a long-term consequence of human papillomavirus (HPV). HPV is transmitted by skin-to-skin contact, so the virus can be spread through women's genital-to-genital, oral-genital, or digital-genital contact.[33] Further, many lesbian women have had earlier male sex partners. Therefore, all women who have a cervix (heterosexual, homosexual, bisexual) need cervical cancer screening by a Papanicolaou test every 3 years from ages 21 to 65 years.[31]

Transgender girls/women are those who had sex assignment as males at birth but who continually identify and live as female. Be aware that transgender women are not cross-dressers or drag queens. Transgender girls may be going through transition to alter birth sex to their confirming gender. This includes family transition, legal steps, hormone therapy, and sometimes gender confirmation surgery.

The Aging Woman

In contrast to the slowly declining hormones in the aging male, the female's hormonal milieu decreases rapidly. *Menopause* is cessation of the menses. Usually this occurs around 48 to 51 years, although a wide variation of age from 35 to 60 years exists. The preceding 1 to 2 years of decline in ovarian function shows irregular menses that gradually become farther apart and produce a lighter flow. Ovaries stop producing progesterone and estrogen. Because cells in the reproductive tract are estrogen dependent, decreased estrogen levels during menopause bring dramatic physical changes.

The uterus shrinks in size because of decreased myometrium. The ovaries atrophy to 1 to 2 cm and are not palpable after menopause. Ovulation still may occur sporadically after menopause. The sacral ligaments relax, and the pelvic musculature weakens; thus the uterus droops. The cervix shrinks and looks paler with a thick, glistening epithelium.

The vagina becomes shorter, narrower, and less elastic. Without sexual activity the vagina atrophies to one-half its former length and width. The vaginal epithelium atrophies, becoming thinner, drier, and itchy. This results in a fragile mucosal surface that is at risk for bleeding and vaginitis. Decreased vaginal secretions leave the vagina dry and at risk for irritation and pain with intercourse (dyspareunia). The vaginal pH becomes more alkaline, and glycogen content decreases from the decreased estrogen. These factors also increase the risk for vaginitis because they create a suitable medium for pathogens.

However, these physical changes need not affect sexual pleasure and function. As with the male, the older female is capable of sexual expression and function given reasonably good health and an interested partner. Aging women greatly outnumber their male counterparts, and aging women are more likely to be single, whereas males their same age are more likely to be married.

 ## CULTURE AND GENETICS

In the United States, rates of cervical cancer have decreased substantially since the introduction of Pap test screening in the 1950s and HPV testing since. There has been a decrease in racial disparity in cervical cancer in recent years, with Pap test use slightly higher among black women (84.7%) than among non-Hispanic whites (83.1%). Further, there was no difference among racial groups in adherence to follow-up after an abnormal Pap test.[37] However, black women still have higher cervical cancer incidence rates and lower relative survival rates than whites. Factors related to these statistics are (1) presenting with cancer at later stages and being less likely to receive the best treatment due to patient refusal, (2) inappropriate physician recommendation, (3) poorer health, and (4) comorbid conditions.[37] There is also a geographic disparity—incidence rates were highest among non-Hispanic blacks in the South. Also in the South, incidence rates among whites decreased after age 40 years and rates for black women increased with greater age. Thus one population to target to decrease cervical cancer rates and mortality would be older black women living in the Southern United States.[37]

The HPV vaccine has been linked to steep declines in the presence of the virus in teenage girls and young women, just 6 years after its introduction—a 64% decrease in quadrivalent HPV types in teens ages 14 to 19 years and a 34% decrease in those ages 20 to 24 years.[14] The American Cancer Society (ACS) recommends the vaccine for all boys and girls at 11 and 12 years, with late vaccination as soon as possible for those not vaccinated.[26] HPV causes almost all cervical cancers, as well as vulvar, vaginal, anal, and oropharyngeal cancers in females and most oropharyngeal, anal, and penile cancers in males. The ACS predicts 28,500 cancers could be prevented annually by HPV vaccination in the United States.[26]

While cervical cancer does not even appear on the list of the 10 most common new cancers in the United States, cervical cancer is the 4th most common cancer among women globally. In less developed countries, it is the 2nd most commonly diagnosed cancer and the 3rd leading cause of death in women.[21] No woman should die of cervical cancer in this day and age,[30] yet look at how many do. There is development of better screening technologies for low- and middle-income countries, particularly visual inspection with acetic acid (VIA) with follow-up point-of-care cryotherapy.[21,30]

Female *genital mutilation,* or "cutting," is an invasive, coercive surgical procedure performed on girls before puberty. It is practiced within Aboriginal, Christian, and Muslim families who have immigrated to the United States from western and southern Asia, the Middle East, and large areas of Africa. It is a social custom, not a religious practice, and is illegal in the United States. This procedure involves removal, partial or total, of the clitoris and is believed to inhibit sexual pleasure. However the procedure can cause severe bleeding, death, sterility, infection, psychological trauma, and have severe consequences during childbirth. As such, genital mutilation violates the human and reproductive rights of women.[3]

SUBJECTIVE DATA

1. Menstrual history	5. Acute pelvic pain	9. Sexual activity
2. Obstetric history	6. Urinary symptoms	10. Contraceptive use
3. Menopause	7. Vaginal discharge	11. Sexually transmitted infection
4. Patient-centered care	8. Past history	(STI) contact

Examiner Asks	Rationale
1. Menstrual history. Tell me about your menstrual periods: • Date of your last menstrual period? • Age at first period? • How often are your periods? • How many days does your period last? • Usual amount of flow: light, medium, heavy? How many pads or tampons do you use each day or hour? • Any clotting? • Any pain or cramps before or during period? How do you treat it? Interfere with daily activities? Any other associated symptoms: bloating, breast tenderness, moodiness? Any spotting between periods?	**Menstrual history** is usually nonthreatening; thus it is a good place to start. LMP—Last menstrual period. Menarche—Mean age at onset at 12 to 13 years; delayed onset suggests endocrine or underweight problem. Cycle—Normally every 28 days; varies from 18 to 45 days. Amenorrhea—Absent menses.[19] Duration—Average 3 to 7 days. Menorrhagia—Heavy menses. Clotting indicates heavy flow or vaginal pooling. **Dysmenorrhea** responds to ibuprofen because it works on uterine smooth muscle.
2. Obstetric history. Have you ever been pregnant? • How many times? • How many babies have you had? • Any miscarriage or abortion? • For each pregnancy describe: duration, any complication, labor and delivery, baby's sex, birth weight, condition. • Do you think you may be pregnant now? What symptoms have you noticed?	Gravida—Number of pregnancies. Para—Number of births. Abortions—Interrupted pregnancies, including elective abortions and spontaneous miscarriages.
3. Menopause. Have your periods slowed down or stopped? • Any associated symptoms of menopause (e.g., hot flashes, night sweats, numbness and tingling, headache, palpitations, drenching sweats, mood swings, vaginal dryness, itching)? Any treatment? • If hormone replacement therapy (HRT), how much? How is it working? Any side effects? • How do you feel about going through menopause?	**Menopause,** cessation of menstruation. Perimenopausal period from ages 40 to 55 years has hormone shifts, resulting in vasomotor instability. Side effects of HRT include fluid retention, breast pain, vaginal bleeding, and cardiovascular and breast cancer risk. Some women with severe vasomotor symptoms may choose HRT but at the lowest effective dose for the shortest time. Although a normal life stage, reaction varies from acceptance to feelings of loss.

Subjective Data

4. Patient-centered care. How often do you have a gynecologic checkup? The recommended screening for cervical cancer prevention by age: (1) no Pap tests if you are under 21 years, regardless of sexual activity; (2) Pap test once every 3 years for women ages 21-30 years; (3) HPV and Pap "co-testing" every 3 years for women ages 30-65 years.[10] Your last Pap test? Results?

We do recommend yearly screening for chlamydial infection in all sexually active women under 25 years and in older women with a new sex partner, more than one sex partner, or a sex partner with other partners. We do this by testing first-catch urine.[5]

5. Acute pelvic pain. Any pain in the lower abdomen or pelvis? When did it start? Constant or come and go? Associated with periods? On a scale of 1 to 10, with 10 being the strongest, how would you rate your pain?

6. Urinary symptoms. Any problems with urinating? Frequently and small amounts?

- Sudden urge; cannot wait to urinate?
- Any burning or pain on urinating?
- Awaken during night to urinate?
- Blood in the urine?

- Urine dark, cloudy, foul smelling?
- Any difficulty controlling urine or wetting yourself? Full bladder, "must go *now*"?

- Urinate with a sneeze, laugh, cough, bearing down?

7. Vaginal discharge. Any unusual **vaginal discharge?** Increased amount?

- Character or color: white, yellow-green, gray, curdlike, foul smelling?

- When did it begin?
- Is the discharge associated with vaginal itching, rash, pain with intercourse?

- Taking any medications?

- Family history of diabetes?
- In which part of your menstrual cycle are you now?

Although Pap tests save lives, adolescents and young women have high rates of HPV infection that their own immune systems can clear. Delaying Pap testing until age 21 allows the HPV infections to regress spontaneously in adolescents, avoiding overtreatment.[10]

Chlamydia is the most frequent STI in the United States and has serious sequelae from lack of treatment: PID, ectopic pregnancy, infertility.[5]

Acute pain lasts <3 months. Consider urgent conditions: pelvic inflammatory disease (PID), appendicitis, ruptured ovarian cysts, ovarian torsion, which need transvaginal ultrasound imaging.[11]

Urinary incontinence (UI) is important to ask about because UI can decrease quality of life, limit activities, and increase falls and fracture risk.

Urgency.

Dysuria.

Nocturia.

Hematuria occurs with urinary tract infection (UTI) and kidney disease.

Bile in urine or UTI.

Urge incontinence—overactive detrusor muscle in bladder. Overactive bladder occurs in 55% of women ages 66-75 years and in 64% of women ages 76-85 years.[18]

Stress incontinence—Involuntary urine loss with physical strain, sneezing, or coughing.

Normal discharge is small, clear or cloudy, and always nonirritating.

Suggests vaginal infection; character of discharge often suggests causative organism (see Table 27.5, p. 760).

Acute versus chronic problem.

Rash is result of irritation from discharge. Dyspareunia occurs with vaginitis of any cause.

Oral contraceptives increase glycogen content of vaginal epithelium, providing fertile medium for some organisms. Broad-spectrum antibiotics alter balance of normal flora.

Diabetes increases glycogen content.

Menses, postpartum, menopause have a more alkaline vaginal pH.

Examiner Asks	Rationale

- Use a vaginal douche? How often?
- Use feminine hygiene spray?
- Wear nonventilating underpants, pantyhose?
- Treated the discharge with anything? Result?

Frequent douching alters pH.
Spray has risk for contact dermatitis.
Local irritation.

8. **Past history.** Any other problems in the genital area? Sores or lesions—now or in the past? How were they treated? Any abdominal pain?
   - Any past surgery on uterus, ovaries, vagina?

Assess feelings. Some fear loss of sexual response after hysterectomy, which may affect intimate relationships.

9. **Sexual activity.** Often women have a question about their **sexual relationship** and how it affects their health. Do you?
   - Are you in a relationship involving sex now?
   - Are aspects of sex satisfactory to you and your partner?
   - Satisfied with the way you and partner communicate about sex?
   - Satisfied with your ability to respond sexually?
   - Do you have more than one sexual partner?

   - What is your sexual preference: relationship with a man, with a woman, both?

Begin with open-ended question to assess individual needs. Include appropriate questions as a routine. Communicates that you accept individual's sexual activity and believe that it is important.

Your comfort with discussion prompts person's interest and possibly relief that the topic has been introduced. Provides opportunity to screen sexual problems.

The practice environment must be welcoming and respectful of lesbians and bisexual women to discuss their health concerns.

10. **Contraceptive use.** Currently planning a pregnancy or avoiding pregnancy?
    - Do you and your partner use a **contraceptive?** Which method? Is it satisfactory? Do you have any questions about method?
    - Which methods have you used in the past? Have you and partner discussed having children?
    - Have you ever had any problems becoming pregnant?

Assess smoking history. Oral contraceptives, together with cigarette smoking, increase the risk for vascular problems.

Infertility is considered after 1 year of unprotected sexual intercourse without conceiving.

11. **STI contact.** Any sexual contact with partner having an STI such as gonorrhea, herpes, HIV/AIDS, chlamydial infection, venereal warts, syphilis? When? How was it treated? Were there any complications?

    - Any precautions to reduce risk for STIs? Use condoms at each episode of sexual intercourse?

A STI can be transmitted during vaginal, oral, and anal sexual contact with an infected partner. Treating patient and the sex partner(s) prevents reinfection and infection of others.

Additional History for Infants and Children

1. Does your child have any problem urinating? Pain with urinating, crying, holding genitals? UTI?
   - (If the child is older than 2 to 2½ years) Has toilet training started? How is it progressing?
   - Does the child wet bed at night? Is this a problem for child or you (parents)? What have you (parents) done?

Reassure that nocturnal enuresis is common with sound sleepers and may persist until 7 years.

Examiner Asks	Rationale
2. Problem with genital area: itching, rash, vaginal discharge?	Occurs with poor perineal hygiene or insertion of foreign body into vagina.
3. (To child) Has anyone ever touched you in between your legs when you did not want them to? Sometimes that happens to children. They should remember that they have not been bad. They should try to tell a big person about it. Can you tell me three different big people you trust whom you could talk to?	Screen for sexual abuse (see Chapter 7). For prevention, teach the child that it is not okay for someone to look at or touch her private parts while telling her it is a secret. Naming three trusted adults will include someone outside the family—important because most molestation is by a parent.

Additional History for Preadolescents and Adolescents

Assess sexual growth and development and sexual behavior. First, ask questions that seem appropriate for girl's age, but norms vary widely. Children obtain information, often misinformation, from the media and from peers at surprisingly early ages. You can be sure your information will be more thoughtful and accurate.

- Ask direct, matter-of-fact questions. Avoid sounding judgmental.
- Start with a **permission statement:** "Often girls your age experience …." This conveys that it is normal to think or feel a certain way.
- Try the open-ended question: "When did you …?" rather than "Do you …?" This is less threatening because it implies that the topic is normal and unexceptional.

Examiner Asks	Rationale
1. Around age 9 or 10 years, girls start to develop breasts and pubic hair. Have you ever seen charts and pictures of normal growth patterns for girls? Let us go over these now.	
2. Have your periods started? How did you feel? Were you ready or surprised?	Assess attitude of girl and parents. Note inadequate preparation or distaste.
3. To whom in your family do you talk about your body changes and sex information? How do these talks go? Do you think you get enough information? What about sex education classes at school? Is there a teacher, a nurse or doctor, a minister, a counselor to whom you can talk? 　　Often girls your age have questions about sexual intercourse. Do you have questions? Are you dating? Someone steady? 　　Do you and your boyfriend have intercourse? Are you using condoms? What kind of protection did you use the last time you had sex?	Avoid the term "sexually active," which is ambiguous. Also, a Pap test is not needed to safely prescribe oral contraceptives; just weight, BP, and health history. Requiring a pelvic exam for asymptomatic teens is a barrier to access for some teens.
4. Has anyone ever talked to you about sexually transmitted infections such as chlamydia, herpes, gonorrhea, or HIV/AIDS?	Teach STI risk reduction.
5. Routine vaccinations include the human papillomavirus (HPV) vaccine (Gardasil, Cervarix). It is given before girls have sexual intercourse.	HPV is the most common STI in the United States. The 2-dose series of Gardasil 9 is recommended for girls and boys 9–14 years, doses separated by 6–12 months.[9]
6. Sometimes a person touches a girl in a way that she does not want them to. Has that ever happened to you? If that happens, the girl should remember that it is not her fault. She should tell another adult about it.	Screen for sexual abuse.

Subjective Data

Examiner Asks	Rationale

Additional History for the Aging Adult

1. After menopause, noted any vaginal bleeding?

Postmenopausal bleeding warrants pelvic exam, transvaginal ultrasonography, and referral.

2. Any vaginal itching, discharge, pain with intercourse? Tried any products? Lubricants? Estrogen cream or vaginal tablet?

Vaginal dryness, decreased lubrication are common with decreased estrogen. Many treatments are available.[17]

3. Any pressure in genital area, loss of urine with cough or sneeze, back pain, or constipation?

Occurs with weakened pelvic musculature and uterine prolapse.

4. Are you in a relationship involving sex now? Are aspects of sex satisfactory to you and your partner? Is there adequate privacy for a sexual relationship?

OBJECTIVE DATA

PREPARATION

Assemble the equipment and arrange within easy reach. Familiarize yourself with the vaginal speculum before the examination. Practice opening and closing the blades, locking them into position, and releasing them. Note that the plastic speculum locks and unlocks with a resounding click that can be alarming to the uninformed woman.

EQUIPMENT NEEDED

Urine specimen for STI screening
Gloves
Gooseneck lamp with a strong light
Vaginal speculum of appropriate size (Fig. 27.3):
    Graves speculum for most adult women, available in varying lengths and widths
    Pederson speculum, narrow blades for young or postmenopausal women with narrowed introitus
Large cotton-tipped applicators (rectal swabs)
Materials for cytologic study:
    Cytobrush and liquid-based cytology vial for Pap test
    Specimen container for gonorrhea culture (GC)/chlamydia
    Small bottles of normal saline, potassium hydroxide (KOH), and acetic acid (white vinegar)
Water-based lubricant
Roll of pH test tape

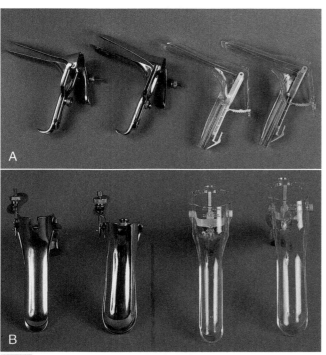

27.3

Objective Data

POSITION

Initially the woman should be sitting to establish trust and rapport before the vaginal examination.

For the examination, place the woman in the lithotomy position with the examiner sitting on a stool. Help the woman into supine position with feet in stirrups and knees apart, and buttocks at edge of examining table (Fig. 27.4). Ask the woman to lift her hips as you guide them to the edge of the table. Leave on shoes or socks. Or you can place an examination glove over each of the stirrups to warm the stirrups and keep her feet from slipping.

Elevate her head to a 45-degree angle so you can see her face. The 45-degree table angle also helps locate internal structures. Place her arms at her sides or across the chest, not over the head, because this position only tightens the abdominal muscles. Be sure to push down the drape between the woman's legs.

The lithotomy position leaves many women feeling helpless and vulnerable. Indeed, many women tolerate the pelvic examination because they consider it basic for health care, yet they find it embarrassing and uncomfortable. Previous examinations may have been painful, or the previous examiner's attitude may have been hurried and patronizing. The examination need not be this way. You can help the woman relax, decrease her anxiety, and retain a sense of control by using these measures:

- Have her empty the bladder before the examination.
- Position the examination table so her perineum is not exposed to an inadvertent open door.
- Ask if she would like a friend, family member, or chaperone to be present. Position this person by the woman's head to maintain privacy.
- Elevate her head and shoulders to a semisitting position to maintain eye contact.
- Place the stirrups so the legs are not abducted too far.
- Explain each step in the examination before you do it.
- Assure the woman she can say "stop" at any point should she feel any discomfort.
- Use a gentle, firm touch and gradual movements.
- Communicate throughout the examination. Maintain a dialogue to share information.
- Use the techniques of the *educational* or *mirror pelvic examination* (Fig. 27.5). This has some modifications in attitude, position, and communication. First the woman is an active participant, one who is learning and sharing decisions about her own health care. She holds a mirror between her legs, above the examiner's hands. She can see all you are doing and has a full view of her genitalia.

The mirror works well for teaching normal anatomy and its relationship to sexual behavior. Even women who are in a sexual relationship or who have had children may be surprisingly uninformed about their own anatomy. You will find that the woman's enthusiasm on seeing her own cervix is rewarding too. The mirror pelvic examination also works well when abnormalities arise because the woman can see the rationale for treatment and monitor progress at the next appointment. She is more willing to comply with treatment when she shares in the decision.

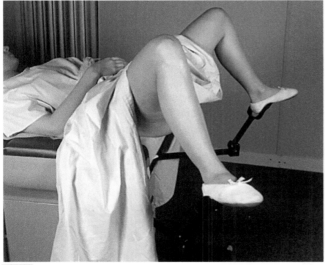

27.4

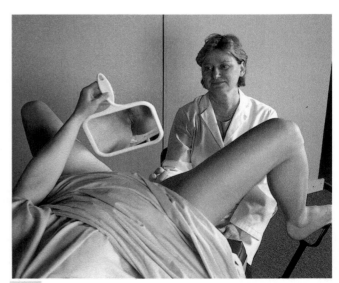

27.5

Normal Range of Findings	Abnormal Findings

External Genitalia

Inspection

NOTE:
- Skin color is even; labia minora are a darker pink (Fig. 27.6).

Normal Range of Findings	Abnormal Findings

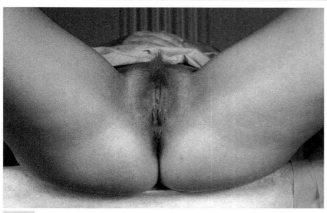

27.6

Note any pigmented nevus or lesion that the woman cannot see. Refer any suspicious lesion for biopsy.

- Hair distribution is in the usual female pattern of inverted triangle, although it normally may trail up the abdomen toward the umbilicus.

Consider delayed puberty if no pubic hair or breast development has occurred by age 13 years.
Nits or lice at the base of pubic hair.
Swelling.

- Labia majora normally are symmetric, plump, and well formed. In the nulliparous woman labia meet in the midline; after a vaginal delivery the labia are gaping and slightly shriveled.
- No lesions should be present, except for occasional sebaceous cysts. These are yellowish, 1-cm nodules that are firm, nontender, and often multiple.

With your gloved hand separate the labia majora to inspect:
- Labia minora are dark pink and moist, usually symmetric (Fig. 27.7).

Excoriation, nodules, rash, or lesions (see Table 27.2, External Genitalia Abnormalities, p. 756).

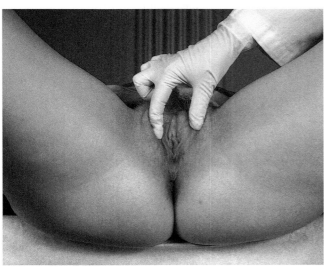

27.7

- Clitoris.
- Urethral opening appears stellate or slitlike and is midline.
- Vaginal opening, or introitus, may appear as a narrow vertical slit or as a larger opening.
- Perineum is smooth. A well-healed episiotomy scar, midline or mediolateral, may be present after a vaginal birth.
- Anus has coarse skin of increased pigmentation (see Chapter 26 for assessment).

Inflammation or lesions.
Polyp. Discharge.
Foul-smelling, irritating discharge.

Objective Data

Normal Range of Findings	Abnormal Findings

Palpation

Assess Bartholin glands. Palpate the posterior parts of the labia majora with your gloved index finger in the vagina and your thumb outside at 5 and 7 o'clock positions (Fig. 27.8). Normally the labia feel soft and homogeneous.

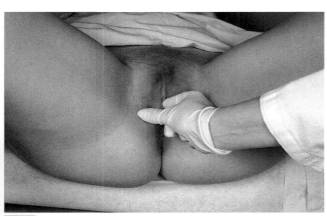

27.8

Palpate the perineum. Normally it feels thick, smooth, and muscular in the nulliparous woman and thin and rigid in the multiparous woman.

Using your index and middle fingers, separate the vaginal orifice and ask the woman to strain down. Normally no bulging of vaginal walls or urinary incontinence occurs.

Internal Genitalia

Speculum Examination

Select the proper-size speculum. Warm and lubricate it under warm running water. Regarding Pap test cytology, evidence shows that applying a small amount (dime size) of water-soluble gel lubricant (with no carbomer thickeners) on the outer blades increases patient comfort and does not obscure interpretation of conventional or liquid-based cytology).[13] Further, use of lubricant decreases pain and may increase compliance in older women with vaginal atrophy or postradiation therapy.[13]

A good technique is to dedicate one hand to the patient and the other hand to picking up equipment in the room. For example, hold the speculum in your left hand (the equipment hand), with the index and middle fingers surrounding the blades and your thumb under the thumbscrew. This prevents the blades from opening painfully during insertion. With your right index and middle fingers (the patient hand), push the introitus down and open to relax the pubococcygeal muscle (Fig. 27.9). Tilt the width of the blades obliquely and insert the speculum past your right fingers, applying any pressure *downward*. This avoids pressure on the sensitive urethra above it.

Abnormal Findings column:

Swelling (see Table 27.2).
Induration.
Pain with palpation.
Erythema around or discharge from duct opening.

Tenderness.
Paper-thin perineum.
Bulging of the vaginal wall indicates cystocele, rectocele, or uterine prolapse (see Table 27.3, Pelvic Musculature Abnormalities, p. 758).
Urinary incontinence.

Normal Range of Findings	Abnormal Findings

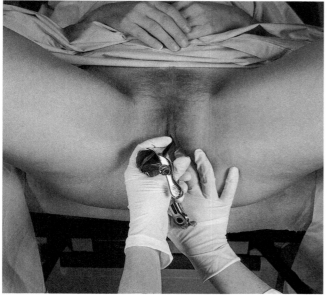

27.9

Ease insertion by asking the woman to bear down. This method relaxes the perineal muscles and opens the introitus. (With experience you can combine speculum insertion with assessing the support of the vaginal muscles.) As the blades pass your right fingers, withdraw your fingers. Now move the speculum to your right hand and turn the width of the blades horizontally. Continue to insert in a 45-degree angle *downward* toward the small of the woman's back (Fig. 27.10). This matches the natural slope of the vagina.

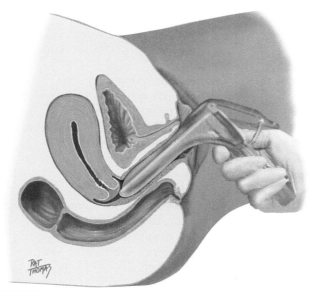

27.10

Normal Range of Findings	Abnormal Findings

After the blades are fully inserted, open them by squeezing the handles together (Fig. 27.11). The cervix should be in full view. Sometimes this does not occur (especially with beginning examiners) because the blades are angled above the location of the cervix. Try closing the blades, withdrawing about halfway, and reinserting in a more *downward* plane. Then slowly sweep upward. Once you have the cervix in full view, lock the blades open by tightening the thumbscrew.

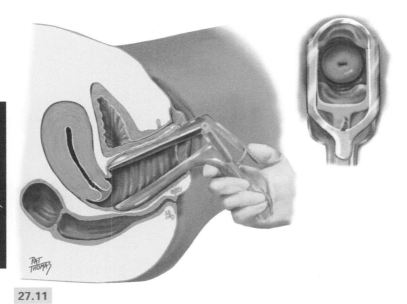

27.11

Inspect the Cervix and Its Os

NOTE:

- **Color.** Normally the cervical mucosa is pink and even (Fig. 27.12, *A*). During the 2nd month of pregnancy it looks blue (Chadwick sign), and after menopause it is pale.

- **Position.** Midline, either anterior or posterior. Projects 1 to 3 cm into the vagina.

- **Size.** Diameter is 2.5 cm (1 inch).

- **Os.** This is small and round in the nulliparous woman. In the parous woman it is a horizontal, irregular slit and also may show healed lacerations on the sides (see Fig. 27.12, *A* and *B*).

- **Surface.** This is normally smooth, but **cervical eversion,** or ectropion, may occur normally after vaginal deliveries (Fig. 27.12, *B*). The endocervical canal is everted or "rolled out." It looks like a red, beefy halo inside the pink cervix surrounding the os. It is difficult to distinguish this normal variation from an abnormal condition (e.g., erosion or carcinoma), and biopsy may be needed.

Redness, inflammation.

Pallor with anemia.

Cyanotic other than with pregnancy (see Table 27.4, Cervix Abnormalities, p. 758).

Lateral position may be due to adhesion or tumor. Projection of more than 3 cm may be a prolapse.

Hypertrophy of more than 4 cm occurs with inflammation or tumor.

Surface reddened, granular, and asymmetric, particularly around os.

Friable, bleeds easily.

Any lesions: white patch on cervix; strawberry spot.

Objective Data

Normal Range of Findings	Abnormal Findings

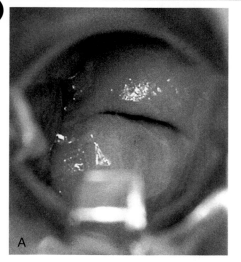

A

NORMAL VARIATIONS OF THE CERVIX

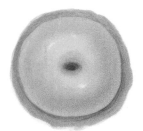
Nulliparous

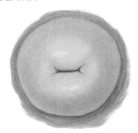
Parous (after childbirth)

LACERATIONS

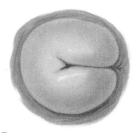
B Unilateral transverse

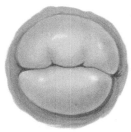
Bilateral transverse

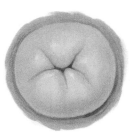
Stellate

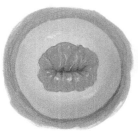
Cervical eversion

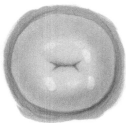
Nabothian cysts

27.12

Nabothian cysts are benign growths that commonly appear on the cervix after childbirth. They are small, smooth, yellow nodules that may be single or multiple. Less than 1 cm, they are retention cysts caused by obstruction of cervical glands.

- **Note the cervical secretions.** Depending on the day of the menstrual cycle, secretions may be clear and thin, or thick, opaque, and stringy. Always they are odorless and nonirritating.

Swab the area with a thick-tipped rectal swab. This method sponges away secretions, and you have a better view of the structures.

Refer any suspicious red, white, or pigmented lesion for biopsy (see Erosion and Cervical Cancer sections in Table 27.4).

Cervical polyp—Bright red growth protruding from the os (see Table 27.4).

Foul-smelling, irritating, with yellow, green, white, or gray discharge (see Table 27.5, Vulvovaginal Inflammations, p. 760).

Objective Data

Normal Range of Findings	Abnormal Findings

Obtain Cervical Tests and Cultures

The Pap test screens for cervical cancer and not for endometrial or ovarian cancer. Do not obtain during the woman's menses or if a heavy infectious discharge is present. Instruct the woman not to douche, have intercourse, or put anything into the vagina within 24 hours before collecting the specimens.

Obtain the Pap test before other specimens so you will not disrupt or remove cells. The vast majority of U.S. cervical cancer screening now uses liquid-based cytology vials. Using liquid-based cytology, the cervical specimens are dipped into a vial with a semipermeable membrane that filters out debris, blood, and lubricants that interfere with specimen accuracy.[13] Conventional glass slides can be "unsatisfactory" because of obscuring by blood, inflammation, or clumped distribution of cells. After liquid-based cytology examination, pathologists can further study the liquid remnant, such as testing for high-risk HPV types. Whichever collection method you are using, collect the cellular specimens from the following three locations.

Vaginal Pool. Gently rub the cytobrush or the blunt end of an Ayre spatula over the vaginal wall under and lateral to the cervix (Fig. 27.13). Dip the cytobrush into a liquid vial or wipe the spatula on a glass slide. If the mucosa is very dry (as in a postmenopausal woman), moisten a sterile swab with normal saline solution to collect this specimen.

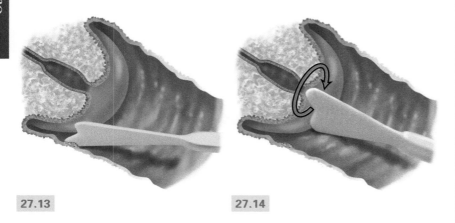

27.13   27.14

Cervical Scrape (Fig. 27.14). Use a cytobrush or insert the bifid end of the Ayre spatula into the vagina with the more pointed bump into the cervical os. Rotate it 360 to 720 degrees, using firm pressure. The rounded cervix fits snugly into the spatula's groove. The spatula scrapes the surface of the squamocolumnar junction (SCJ) and cervix as you turn the instrument. Dip into a liquid vial or spread the specimen from both sides of the spatula onto a glass slide. Use a single stroke to thin out the specimen, not a back-and-forth motion. This specimen is important for the adolescent whose endocervical cells have not yet migrated into the endocervical canal.

Endocervical Specimen (Fig. 27.15). Insert a cytobrush into the os. A cytobrush gives a higher yield of endocervical cells at the SCJ and is safe for use during pregnancy. The woman may feel a slight pinch with the brush, and scant bleeding may occur. For this reason collect the endocervical specimen last so bleeding will not obscure cytologic evaluation.

Normal Range of Findings

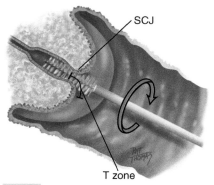

SCJ

T zone

27.15

Rotate the brush 720 degrees in ONE direction in the endocervical canal, either clockwise or counterclockwise. Then stir the cytobrush gently into the liquid vial. Or rotate it gently on a slide to deposit all the cells. Rotate in the opposite direction from the one in which you obtained the specimen. Avoid leaving a thick specimen that would be hard to read under the microscope. Immediately (within 2 seconds) spray the slide with fixative to avoid drying.

For the woman after hysterectomy whose cervix has been removed, collect a scrape from the end of the vagina and a vaginal pool.

Label the frosted ends of the slides or the vial with the woman's name. Send specimens to the laboratory with the following necessary data:

- Date of specimen
- Woman's date of birth
- Date of last menstrual period
- Any hormone medication
- If pregnant, estimated date of delivery

- Known infections
- Prior surgery or radiation
- Prior abnormal cytology
- Abnormal findings on physical examination

To screen for STIs and if you note any abnormal vaginal discharge, obtain the GC/chlamydia culture. Female vaginal swab specimens are the best specimen type.[1] Insert a sterile cotton applicator into the os, rotate it 360 degrees, and leave it in place 10 to 20 seconds for complete saturation. Insert into labeled container. NOTE: Self-collected vaginal swab specimens are equal in quality, and women are highly accepting of this screening.[5]

Occasionally you will need the following samples:

Saline Mount, or "Wet Prep." Spread a sample of the discharge onto a glass slide and add one drop of normal saline solution and a coverslip.

KOH Prep. To a sample of the discharge on a glass slide, add one drop of potassium hydroxide and a coverslip.

Anal Culture. Insert a sterile cotton swab into the anal canal about 1 cm. Rotate it and move it side to side. Leave in place 10 to 20 seconds. If the swab collects feces, discard it and begin again. Insert into specimen container.

Abnormal Findings

These data are important for accurate interpretation (e.g., a specimen may be interpreted as positive unless the laboratory technicians know that the woman has had prior radiation treatment).

Trichomonads show on slide with protozoal infection *Trichomonas vaginalis.* Clue cells show as epithelial cells with stippled edges with bacterial vaginosis. Fishy odor exudes after KOH on slide "whiff test."

Branching hyphae of *Candida* vaginitis show on slide.

Screens for GC/chlamydia in those with anal receptive intercourse. Self-collected specimens are highly acceptable too.

Objective Data

Normal Range of Findings	**Abnormal Findings**

Acetic Acid Wash. Acetic acid (white vinegar) screens for asymptomatic HPV, which causes genital warts and cervical cancer. After all other specimens are gathered, soak a thick-tipped cotton rectal swab with acetic acid and "paint" the cervix. Acetic acid dissolves mucus and temporarily causes intracellular dehydration and coagulation of protein. A normal response (indicating no HPV infection) is no change in the cervical epithelium.

Rapid acetowhitening or blanching, especially with irregular borders, suggests HPV infection (see Table 27.2).

Inspect the Vaginal Wall

Loosen the thumbscrew but continue to hold the speculum blades open. Slowly withdraw the speculum, rotating it as you go, to fully inspect the vaginal wall. Normally the wall looks pink, deeply rugated, moist and smooth, and free of inflammation or lesions. Normal discharge is thin and clear or opaque and stringy but always odorless.

Inflammation or lesions.

Leukoplakia appears as spot of dried white paint.

Vaginal discharge: thick, white, and curdlike with candidiasis; profuse, watery, gray-green, and frothy with trichomoniasis; or any gray, green-yellow, white, or foul-smelling discharge (see Table 27.5).

When the blade ends are near the vaginal opening, let them close, but be careful not to pinch the mucosa or catch any hairs. Turn the blades obliquely to avoid stretching the opening. Place the metal speculum in a basin to be cleaned later and soaked in a sterilizing and disinfecting solution; discard the plastic variety. Discard your gloves and wash hands.

Bimanual Examination

Rise to a stand and have the woman remain in lithotomy position. Drop lubricant onto the first two fingers of your regloved intravaginal hand (Fig. 27.16).

Assume the "obstetric" position with the first two fingers extended, the last two flexed onto the palm, and the thumb abducted. Insert your fingers into the vagina, with any pressure directed posteriorly. Wait until the vaginal walls relax and then insert your fingers fully.

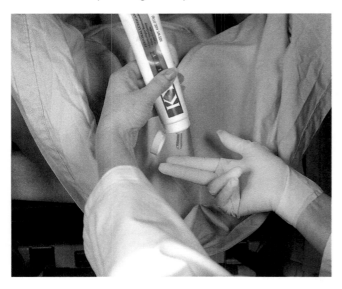

27.16

You will use both hands to palpate the internal genitalia to assess their location, size, and mobility and to screen for any tenderness or mass. One hand is on the abdomen while the other hand (often the dominant, more sensitive hand) inserts two fingers into the vagina (Fig. 27.17). It does not matter which you choose as the intravaginal hand; try each way and settle on the most comfortable method for you.

Normal Range of Findings	Abnormal Findings

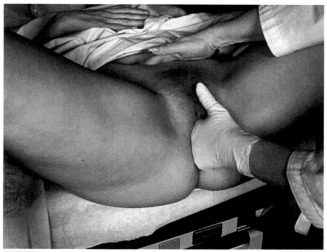

27.17 Bimanual examination.

Palpate the vaginal wall. Normally it feels smooth and has no area of induration or tenderness.

Cervix. Locate the cervix in the midline, often near the anterior vaginal wall. The cervix points in the opposite direction of the fundus of the uterus. Palpate with the palmar surface of the fingers. Note these characteristics of a normal cervix:

- **Consistency**—Feels smooth and firm, as the consistency of the tip of the nose. It softens and feels velvety at 5 to 6 weeks of pregnancy (Goodell sign).
- **Contour**—Evenly rounded.
- **Mobility**—With a finger on either side, move the cervix gently from side to side. Normally this produces no pain (Fig. 27.18).

Palpate all around the fornices; the wall should feel smooth.

Nodule.
Tenderness.

Hard with malignancy.
Nodular.
Irregular.
Immobile with malignancy.
Painful with inflammation, pelvic inflammatory disease (PID), ectopic pregnancy.

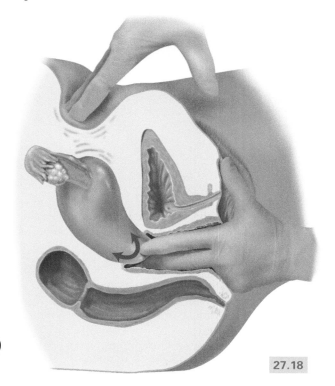

27.18

Normal Range of Findings	Abnormal Findings

Next use your abdominal hand to push the pelvic organs closer for your intravaginal fingers to palpate. Place your hand midway between the umbilicus and the symphysis; push down in a slow, firm manner, fingers together and slightly flexed. Brace the elbow of your pelvic arm against your hip and keep it horizontal. The woman must be relaxed.

Uterus. With your intravaginal fingers in the anterior fornix, assess the uterus. Determine the position, or *version*, of the uterus (Fig. 27.19). This compares the long axis of the uterus with the long axis of the body. In many women the uterus is anteverted; you palpate it at the level of the pubis with the cervix pointing posteriorly. Two other positions occur normally (midposition and retroverted); two aspects of flexion also occur, in which the long axis of the uterus is not straight but is flexed.

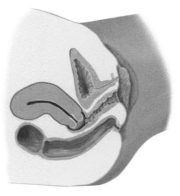

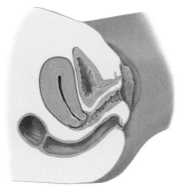

Anteverted

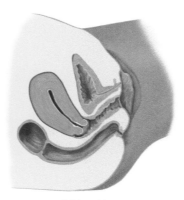

Midposition

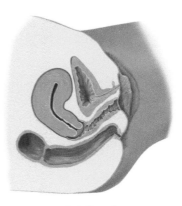

Anteflexed

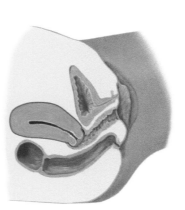

Retroverted

Retroflexed

27.19

Palpate the uterine wall with your fingers in the fornices. Normally it feels firm and smooth, with the contour of the fundus rounded. It softens during pregnancy. Bounce the uterus gently between your abdominal and intravaginal hand. It should be freely movable and nontender.

If the retroverted uterus is fixed and immobile, there may be endometriosis or PID adhering it.

Enlarged uterus (see Table 27.6, Uterine Enlargement, p. 762).
Lateral displacement.
Nodular mass. Irregular, asymmetric uterus.
Fixed and immobile.
Tenderness.

Normal Range of Findings	Abnormal Findings

Adnexa. Move both hands to the right to explore the adnexa. Place your abdominal hand on the lower quadrant just inside the anterior iliac spine and your intravaginal fingers in the lateral fornix (Fig. 27.20). Push the abdominal hand in and try to capture the ovary. Often you cannot feel it. When you can, it normally feels smooth, firm, and almond-shaped and is highly movable, sliding through the fingers. It is slightly sensitive but not painful. The fallopian tube is not palpable normally. No other mass or pulsation should be felt.

Enlarged adnexa. Nodules or mass in adnexa.

Immobile.
Markedly tender (see Table 27.7, Adnexal Enlargement, p. 763).
Pulsation or palpable fallopian tube suggests ectopic pregnancy; this warrants immediate referral.

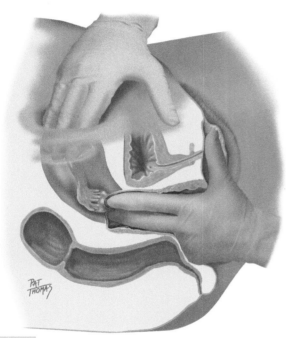

27.20

A note of caution—normal adnexal structures often are not palpable. Be careful not to mistake an abnormality for a normal structure. To be safe, consider abnormal any mass that you cannot *positively* identify and refer the woman for further study.

Move to the left to palpate the other side. Then, withdraw your hand and check secretions on the fingers before discarding the glove. Normal secretions are clear or cloudy and odorless.

Rectovaginal Examination

Use this technique to assess the rectovaginal septum, posterior uterine wall, cul-de-sac, and rectum. Change gloves to avoid spreading any possible infection. Lubricate the first two fingers. Instruct the woman that this may feel uncomfortable and will mimic the feeling of moving her bowels. Ask her to bear down as you insert your index finger into the vagina and your middle finger gently into the rectum (Fig. 27.21).

Objective Data

Normal Range of Findings	Abnormal Findings

Objective Data

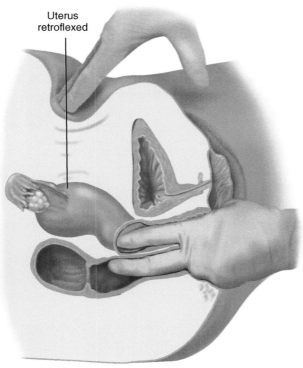

Uterus
retroflexed

RECTOVAGINAL PALPATION

27.21

While pushing with the abdominal hand, repeat the steps of the bimanual examination. Try to keep the intravaginal finger on the cervix so the intrarectal finger does not mistake the cervix for a mass. Note:
- Rectovaginal septum should feel smooth, thin, firm, and pliable.
- Rectovaginal pouch, or cul-de-sac, is a potential space and usually not palpated.
- Uterine wall and fundus feel firm and smooth.

Nodular or thickened.

Rotate the intrarectal finger to check the rectal wall and anal sphincter tone. (See Chapter 26 for assessment of anus and rectum.) Check your gloved finger as you withdraw; test any adherent stool for occult blood.

Use tissues to wipe the area and help her up. Remind her to slide her hips back from the edge before sitting up so she will not fall.

❖ DEVELOPMENTAL COMPETENCE

Infants and Children

Preparation
- **Infant**—Place on examination table.
- **Toddler/preschooler**—Place on parent's lap.
  - Frog-leg position—Hips flexed, soles of feet together and up to bottom.
  - Preschool child may want to separate her own labia.
  - No drapes—The young girl wants to see what you are doing.
- **School-age child**—Place on examination table, frog-leg position, no drapes.

During childhood a routine screening is limited to inspection of the external genitalia to determine that (1) the structures are intact, (2) the vagina is present, and (3) the hymen is patent (open).

Normal Range of Findings

The newborn's genitalia are somewhat engorged. The labia majora are swollen, the labia minora are prominent and protrude beyond the labia majora, the clitoris looks relatively large, and the hymen appears thick. Because of transient engorgement, the vaginal opening is more difficult to see now than it will be later. Place your thumbs on the labia majora. Push laterally while pushing the perineum down and try to note the vaginal opening above the hymenal ring. Do not palpate the clitoris because it is very sensitive.

A sanguineous vaginal discharge or leukorrhea (mucoid discharge) is normal during the first few weeks because of the maternal estrogen effect. (This also may cause transient breast engorgement and secretion.) During the early weeks the genital engorgement resolves, and the labia minora atrophy and remain small until puberty (Fig. 27.22).

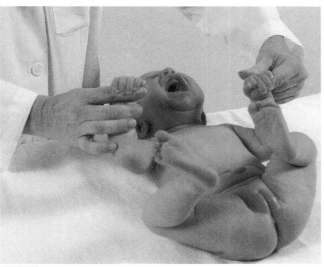

27.22

Between the ages of 2 months and 7 years, the labia majora are flat, the labia minora are thin, the clitoris is relatively small, and the hymen is tissue-paper thin. Normally no irritation or foul-smelling discharge is present.

In the young school-age girl (7 to 10 years), the mons pubis thickens, the labia majora thicken, and the labia minora become slightly rounded. Pubic hair appears beginning around age 11 years, although sparse pubic hair may occur as early as age 8 years. Normally the hymen is perforate. Menarche closely follows the adolescent growth spurt, accompanied by normal body odor and acne.

Almost always in these age-groups an external examination will suffice. If needed, an internal pelvic examination is best performed by a pediatric gynecologist using specialized instruments.

The Adolescent

The adolescent girl has special needs during the genitalia examination. Examine her alone, without the mother present. Assure her of privacy and confidentiality. Allow plenty of time for health education and discussion of pubertal progress. Assess her growth velocity and menstrual history, and use the SMR charts to teach breast and pubic hair development. Assure her that increased vaginal fluid (physiologic *leukorrhea*) is normal because of the estrogen effect.

Abnormal Findings

Ambiguous genitalia are rare but are suggested by a markedly enlarged clitoris, fusion of the labia (resembling scrotum), and palpable mass in fused labia (resembling testes) (see Table 27.8, Pediatric Genitalia Abnormalities, p. 765).

Imperforate hymen warrants referral.

Lesions, rash.

Poor perineal hygiene.

Pest inhabitants. Excoriations.

During and after toddler age, foul-smelling discharge occurs with lodging of foreign body, pinworms, or infection.

Absence of pubic hair by 13 years indicates delayed puberty.

Amenorrhea in adolescent, together with bluish and bulging hymen, indicates imperforate hymen and warrants referral.

Objective Data

Normal Range of Findings

Perform a pelvic examination when the history suggests abnormal vaginal discharge, missed periods, and a positive pregnancy test, or at 21 years of age. Start Pap tests at age 21 years. Although the techniques of the examination are listed in the adult section, you will need to provide additional time and psychological support for the adolescent having her first pelvic examination.

The experience of the first pelvic examination determines how the adolescent will approach future care. Your accepting attitude and gentle, unhurried approach are important. You have a unique teaching opportunity here. Take the time to teach, using the girl's own body as illustration. Your frank discussion of anatomy and sexual behavior communicates that these topics are acceptable to discuss and not taboo with health care providers. This affirms the girl's self-concept.

During the bimanual examination note that the adnexa are not palpable in the adolescent.

The Pregnant Woman

Depending on the week of gestation of the pregnancy, inspection shows the enlarging abdomen and other signs (see Fig. 31.2 on p. 802). The height of the fundus ascends gradually as the fetus grows.

The external genitalia show hyperemia of the perineum and vulva because of increased vascularity. Internally the walls of the vagina appear violet or blue (Chadwick sign) because of hyperemia. The vaginal walls are deeply rugated, and the vaginal mucosa thickens. The cervix looks blue, feels velvety, and feels softer than in the nonpregnant state, making it a bit more difficult to differentiate from the vaginal walls.

During bimanual examination the isthmus of the uterus feels softer and is more easily compressed between your two hands (Hegar sign). The fundus balloons between your two hands; it feels connected to, but distinct from, the cervix because the isthmus is so soft.

Search the adnexal area carefully during early pregnancy. Normally the adnexal structures are not palpable.

The Aging Adult

Natural lubrication is decreased; to avoid a painful examination, take care to lubricate instruments and the examining hand adequately. Use the Pedersen speculum (rather than the Graves) because its narrower, flatter blades are more comfortable in women with vaginal stenosis or dryness.

Menopause and the resulting decrease in estrogen production cause numerous physical changes. Pubic hair gradually decreases, becoming thin and sparse in later years. The skin is thinner, and fat deposits decrease, leaving the mons pubis smaller and the labia flatter with a hanging appearance. Clitoris size also decreases after age 60 years.

Internally the rugae of the vaginal walls decrease, and the walls look pale pink because of the thinned epithelium. The cervix shrinks and looks pale and glistening. It may retract, appearing to be flush with the vaginal wall. In some it is hard to distinguish the cervix from the surrounding vaginal mucosa. Or the cervix may protrude into the vagina if the uterus has prolapsed.

With the bimanual examination you may need to insert only one gloved finger if vaginal stenosis exists. The uterus feels smaller and firmer, and the ovaries are not palpable normally.

Abnormal Findings

Because the STI rates are higher among adolescents than other age-groups, screen for STIs (1) with history of multiple sexual partners; (2) with previous STI treatment; (3) chlamydia and gonorrhea screening annually for sexually active adolescents; and (4) syphilis screening for teens who are commercial sex workers, use IV drugs, or have contacts with syphilis.[1]

Pelvic or adnexal mass.

An ectopic pregnancy has serious consequences (see Table 27.7).

Refer any suspicious red, white, or pigmented lesion for biopsy.

Vaginal atrophy increases the risk for infection and trauma.

Refer any mass for prompt evaluation.

Normal Range of Findings	Abnormal Findings

Be aware that older women may have special needs and will appreciate the following plans of care: for those with arthritis, taking a mild analgesic or antiinflammatory before the appointment may ease joint pain in positioning; schedule appointment times when joint pain or stiffness is at its least; allow extra time for positioning and "unpositioning" after the examination; and be careful to maintain dignity and privacy.

Women ages 65+ years may choose to stop cervical cancer screening if they have ≥3 consecutive negative Pap tests or ≥2 consecutive negative HPV and Pap tests within the last 10 years. Also, women with a total hysterectomy for benign findings may stop cervical cancer screening.[36] However, the woman and clinician should consider also her individual health states, comorbidities, and life expectancy.

HEALTH PROMOTION AND PATIENT TEACHING

THE ADOLESCENT

Clinicians can open discussions with teens about potentially risky behavior and preventive sexual health before their first sexual encounter. Your goal is to remove barriers to health care, to promote youth-friendly services, and to assure private confidential discussions. Here are some talking points you can adapt to your setting.[25]

Talking Points	Conversation Openers
Routine HPV vaccination with completion of series	*Have you started the HPV vaccine series? Finished the 2 doses? 3 doses? This protects you against cervical cancer and other cancers caused by the human papillomavirus.*
Preparation for possible sexual activity	*Are you dating anyone? Someone special? Is he (she) urging you to have sex? How do you feel about having sex at this time? Let's talk about how you can stop sex at this time. Or, if you are ready, let's talk about using a condom every time. Do you have access to condoms?*
Providing information on how to prevent unintended pregnancy and STIs for adolescents in a committed heterosexual relationship	*Would you like to become pregnant? How would this affect your health? Your education? (If not) What kinds of contraception have you thought of to prevent pregnancy? Use of condoms? Use of long-acting reversible methods such as IUDs and hormonal implants?[26] Let me explain the advantages of these, but they do not protect against sexually transmitted infections such as chlamydia or gonorrhea. You need to use condoms to help protect against infections.*
Providing information about STI prevention for adolescents who are having intercourse	*Have you had a new sex partner this year? Do you think your boyfriend (girlfriend) may be having sex with another person? These are ways to spread chlamydia, a vaginal infection that is easily treated but that could cause serious problems if it is not treated. Your best protection is to use a condom every time you have sex. We also test for chlamydia every year by a urine sample or with a special swab you can put into the vagina yourself and bring in for testing.*
Sexual identity	*Are you attracted to boys or to girls? Or maybe to both? Or maybe to neither!? Let's talk about this. Anyone at home you can talk to about this? How about at school?*
Use of alcohol and drugs	*Some teens your age experiment with drugs or alcohol. They need to know the dangers of using drugs at this age, especially in sexual situations. How would you feel if you were out with your best friend and she (he) wanted to start drinking? Have you thought about being with your boyfriend (girlfriend) and he (she) urges you to start drinking? Let's talk about what you could say.*
Physical safety in family and sexual relationships	*I always ask all teens this: Do you feel safe at home? With your boyfriend (girlfriend)? Have you ever been hit, punched, slapped, or pushed into wall, thrown onto floor?*
Cyberbullying, bullying behaviors at school	*I always ask all teens this: Has anyone sent you text messages that feel harmful or dangerous? As if you are being pressured to do something you do not want to? Anyone you can talk to about this? Let's talk about this now.*

DOCUMENTATION AND CRITICAL THINKING

Sample Charting

SUBJECTIVE

Menarche age 12 years, cycle usually q 28 days, duration 5 days, flow moderate, no dysmenorrhea, LMP April 3. Grav 0/Para 0/ Ab 0. Gyne checkup and last Pap test 1 year PTA, negative.

No urinary problems, no irritating or foul-smelling vaginal discharge, no sores or lesions, no history pelvic surgery. Satisfied with sexual relationship with husband, uses vaginal diaphragm for birth control, no plans for pregnancy at this time. Not aware of any STI contact to herself or husband.

OBJECTIVE

External genitalia: No swelling, lesions, or discharge. No urethral swelling or discharge.
Internal: Vaginal walls have no bulging or lesions; cervix pink with no lesions. Scant clear mucoid discharge.
Bimanual: No pain on moving cervix; uterus anteflexed and anteverted, no enlargement or irregularity.
Adnexa: Ovaries not enlarged.
Rectal: No hemorrhoids, fissures, or lesions; no masses or tenderness; stool brown with FIT test negative.

ASSESSMENT

Genital structures intact and appear healthy

Clinical Case Study 1

J.K., 27-year-old married woman with type 1 diabetes, Grav 0/Para 0/Ab 0. Presents at clinic with "urinary burning, vaginal itching, and curdy discharge × 4 days."

SUBJECTIVE

4 to 5 days PTA—Noted burning on urination; intense vaginal itching; thick, white, "smelly" discharge. Warm water douche—no relief. Intercourse is painful.

No previous history of vaginal infection, urinary tract infection, or pelvic surgery. Type 1 diabetes since age 12, well managed with insulin and diet, HbA1c is <6.5%. Monogamous heterosexual relationship, has used low-estrogen birth control pills for 3 years with no side effects.

OBJECTIVE

Vulva and vagina erythematous and edematous. Thick, white, curdlike discharge clinging to vaginal walls. Cervix pink, no lesions.
Bimanual examination: No pain on palpating cervix, uterus not enlarged, ovaries not enlarged.
Specimens: Pap test, GC/chlamydia to lab. Vaginal pH <4.5. KOH prep shows mycelia and spores of *Candida albicans*.

ASSESSMENT

Candida albicans vaginitis
Pain from vaginal infection

Clinical Case Study 2

B.L., 17-year-old female high school student, comes to clinic for oral contraceptives.

SUBJECTIVE

Menarche 12 years, cycle q 30 days, duration 6 days, mild cramps relieved by naproxen. LMP March 10. No dysuria, vaginal discharge, vaginal itching. Relationship involving vaginal intercourse with one boyfriend for 8 months PTA. Thinks he has other heterosexual contacts. For birth control boyfriend uses condoms "sometimes." Wants to start birth control pills. Never had pelvic examination. Never had teaching about breast self-examination or STIs except AIDS. Smokes cigarettes, ½ PPD; started age 11 years. Has not had HPV vaccines.

OBJECTIVE

Breasts: Symmetric, no lesions or discharge. Palpation reveals no mass or tenderness.
External genitalia: No redness, lesions, or discharge.
Internal genitalia: Vaginal walls and cervix pink with no lesions or discharge. GC/chlamydia specimens obtained.
Bimanual: No tenderness to palpation. Uterus anteverted with no enlargement; ovaries not enlarged.
Specimens: GC/chlamydia, to lab.

ASSESSMENT

Breast and pelvic structures appear healthy
Needs teaching on breast self-examination, birth control measures, STI prevention, cigarette smoking
Needs routine HPV vaccines

Clinical Case Study 3

K.B. is a 65-year-old female, retired elementary school teacher. Takes multivitamins daily. No prescription medications. No significant past medical history.

SUBJECTIVE

Menarche age 14 years, cycle q30 days. Menopause at age 60. Gyne checkups yearly. Last Pap test negative. Grav 2/ Para 2/ Ab 0. No urinary problems. No history of STIs. Monogamous relationship for 45 years. No sexual intercourse × 2 years due to fatigue of self and husband. Husband recently cleared for sexual activity post myocardial infarction. After resumption of sexual activity, K.B. noticed bloody vaginal discharge. Dyspareunia. Vaginal itching. Not aware of any STI contact in self or husband.

OBJECTIVE

External genitalia: Thin, gray pubic hair. Labia appear flat and hanging. No lesions, swelling, or discharge. Introitus constricted.
Internal: Vaginal walls pale pink. Cervix pale pink, retracted, flush with vaginal wall. Abraded areas on posterior vaginal wall. Bloody, mucoid discharge. Tenderness reported during exam.
Bimanual: No pain with cervical movement. Unable to palpate ovaries. Uterus small, firm.
Rectal: No hemorrhoids, fissures, or tenderness. Stool brown, FIT test negative.

ASSESSMENT

Atrophic vaginitis
Sexual dysfunction and dyspareunia
Potential for vaginal infection

Clinical Case Study 4

C.P. is a 9-year-old female who is being seen at the clinic today for vulva pain.

SUBJECTIVE

1 day PTA—States, "My foot slipped off the pedal while I was riding my brother's bike, and I fell." Reports pain localized to vulva. Denies menarche and/or urinary problems.

OBJECTIVE

External genitalia: Swelling and ecchymosis noted to labia majora; no lacerations, no rash, no lesions, and no vaginal discharge; no urethral swelling or discharge; internal and bimanual exam deferred at this time.

ASSESSMENT

Genital structures intact
Acute pain from trauma of falling off bike

Documentation and Critical Thinking

ABNORMAL FINDINGS
FOR ADVANCED PRACTICE

TABLE 27.2	External Genitalia Abnormalities

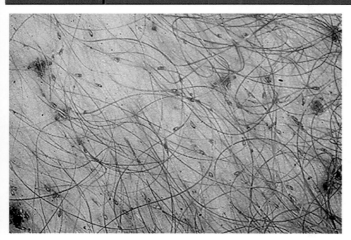

Pediculosis Pubis (Crab Lice)

S: Severe perineal itching.

O: Excoriations and erythematous areas. May see little dark spots (lice are small), nits (eggs) or lice adherent to pubic hair near roots. Usually localized in pubic hair, occasionally in eyebrows or eyelashes. Transmission usually sexual contact though may be contaminated clothing, bedding.

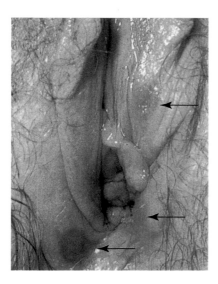

Syphilitic Chancre

O: This STI begins as a small, solitary silvery papule that erodes to a red, round or oval, superficial ulcer with a yellowish serous discharge. Palpation—Nontender indurated base; can be lifted like a button between thumb and finger. Nontender inguinal lymphadenopathy. May go unnoticed; resolves spontaneously. But secondary syphilis follows: fever, lymphadenopathy, mucocutaneous red rash, sore throat.

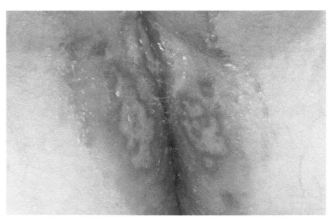

Herpes Simplex Virus—Type 2 (Herpes Genitalis)

S: Episodes of local pain, dysuria, fever, headache, malaise, or asymptomatic.[8]

O: HSV2 presents as clusters of small, shallow vesicles with surrounding erythema; erupts on genital areas and inner thigh, usually bilaterally. Also inguinal adenopathy, edema. Progresses through short-lived vesicles (1–3 days), painful ulcers, crusts (2–3 weeks). Virus remains dormant; symptomatic recurrence in 1st year about 70% to 90%, then less frequent.

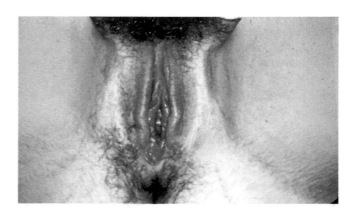

Red Rash—Contact Dermatitis

S: History of skin contact with allergenic substance in environment, intense pruritus.

O: Primary lesion—Red, swollen vesicles. Then may have weeping of lesions, crusts, scales, thickening of skin, excoriations from scratching. May result from reaction to feminine hygiene spray or synthetic underclothing.

Continued

TABLE 27.2 | External Genitalia Abnormalities—cont'd

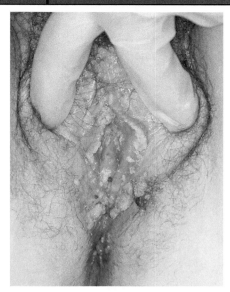

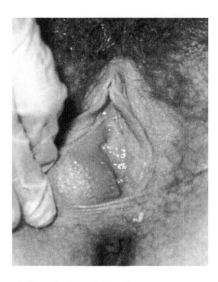

Human Papillomavirus Genital Warts

S: Painless warty growths; may be unnoticed by woman.

O: Pink or flesh-colored, soft, pointed, moist, warty papules. Single or multiple in a cauliflower-like patch. Occur around vulva, introitus, anus, vagina, cervix. (NOTE: Advanced case shown here.) HPV infection is the most common STI, especially in adolescents. Risk factors: early age at menarche and multiple sexual partners. Genital warts are less common than cervical lesions but must be treated with topical medication or surgical removal. Abstain from sex while warts are present.

Abscess of Bartholin Gland

S: Local pain; can be severe.

O: Overlying skin red, shiny, and hot. Posterior part of labia swollen; palpable fluctuant mass and tenderness. (Compare with wrinkled skin on the other, normal side.) Mucosa shows red spot at site of duct opening. Requires incision and drainage, antibiotic therapy.

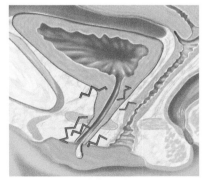

Urethritis

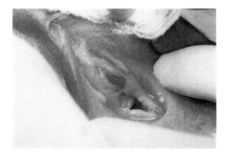

Urethritis and UTI

S: Inflamed urethra and UTI present with dysuria, frequency, urgency, flank or suprapubic pain. Older adults may only have communication problems, confusion, and lethargy.

O: Anterior vaginal wall shows erythema, pain along urethra, maybe purulent discharge. *Escherichia coli* is the most frequent cause and should receive antibiotics though there is a growing emergence of resistant organisms. Urine culture, not urinalysis, is used to diagnose UTI because asymptomatic bacteria are common in older people, and the latter should not be treated by antibiotics.[16]

Urethral Caruncle

S: Tender, pain with urination, urinary frequency, hematuria, dyspareunia, or asymptomatic.

O: Small, deep red, benign mass protruding from meatus; usually secondary to urethritis or skenitis; lesion may bleed on contact. More common in postmenopausal women.

S, Subjective data; *O,* objective data.
See Illustration Credits for source information.

Abnormal Findings

TABLE 27.3 Pelvic Musculature Abnormalities

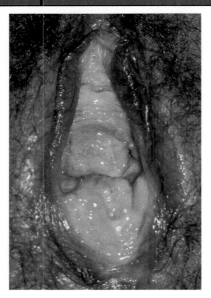

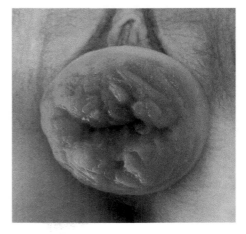

Cystocele

S: Feeling of pressure in vagina, stress incontinence.
O: With straining, note introitus widening and the presence of a soft, round *anterior* bulge. The bladder, covered by vaginal mucosa, prolapses into the vagina.

Rectocele

S: Feeling of pressure in vagina, possibly constipation.
O: With straining, note introitus widening and the presence of a soft, round bulge from *posterior*. Here, part of the rectum, covered by vaginal mucosa, prolapses into the vagina.

Uterine Prolapse

O: With straining or standing, uterus protrudes into vagina. Nontender, nonfluctuant, smooth hemisphere; may cause a broad-based gait. Prolapse is graded: 1st degree, cervix appears at introitus with straining; 2nd degree, cervix bulges outside introitus with straining; 3rd degree (in this case), cervix is enlarged, edematous, protrudes markedly and without straining.

S, Subjective data; *O,* objective data.
See Illustration Credits for source information.

TABLE 27.4 Cervix Abnormalities

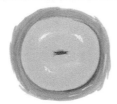

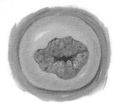

Bluish Cervix—Cyanosis

O: Bluish discoloration of the mucosa occurs normally in pregnancy (Chadwick sign at 6 to 8 weeks' gestation) and with any other condition causing hypoxia or venous congestion (e.g., heart failure, pelvic tumor).

Erosion

O: Cervical lips inflamed and eroded. Reddened granular surface is superficial inflammation, with no ulceration (loss of tissue). Usually secondary to purulent or mucopurulent cervical discharge. Biopsy needed to distinguish erosion from carcinoma; cannot rely on inspection.

Continued

TABLE 27.4   Cervix Abnormalities—cont'd

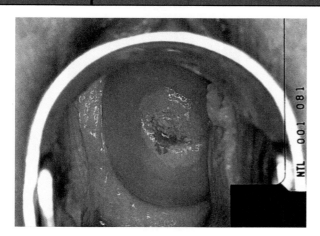

Human Papillomavirus (HPV, Condylomata)

O: Virus can appear in various forms when affecting cervical epithelium. Here warty growth appears as abnormal thickened white epithelium. Visibility of lesion is enhanced by acetic acid (vinegar) wash, which dissolves mucus and temporarily causes intracellular dehydration and coagulation of protein. Must be treated or will progress to cervical cancer (see Cervical Cancer).

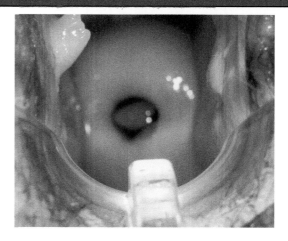

Polyp

S: May have mucoid discharge or bleeding.
O: Bright red, soft, pedunculated growth emerges from os. It is benign, but this must be determined by biopsy. May be lined with squamous or columnar epithelium.

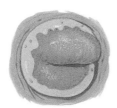

Diethylstilbestrol (DES) Syndrome

S: Prenatal exposure to DES causes rare tumor and cervical and vaginal abnormalities not apparent until adolescence. DES was given to some pregnant women from 1940 to 1970.
O: Red, granular patches of columnar epithelium extend beyond normal squamocolumnar junction onto cervix and into fornices (a wide transformation zone). Cervical abnormalities: circular groove, transverse ridge, protuberant anterior lip, "cockscomb" formation. The DES exposure causes infertility, ectopic pregnancy, spontaneous abortion, and preterm labor. Women exposed to DES in utero have 2× risk of high-grade squamous neoplasia and should continue annual cytology screening up to mid-40s.[29]

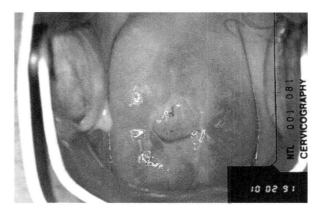

Cervical Cancer

S: Bleeding between menstrual periods, after sex, after menopause; unusual vaginal discharge.
O: Chronic ulcer and induration are early signs of carcinoma, although the lesion may or may not show on the exocervix. (Here lesion is around the external os.)
Diagnosed by Pap test and biopsy. Caused by persistent HPV infection. Risk factors are early age at first intercourse, multiple sex partners, cigarette smoking, undetected HPV. Prevention lies in HPV vaccines and early detection.

S, Subjective data; *O*, objective data.
See Illustration Credits for source information.

Abnormal Findings

TABLE 27.5	Vulvovaginal Inflammations

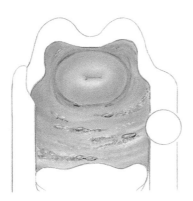

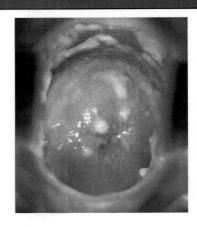

Atrophic Vaginitis

S: Postmenopausal vaginal itching, dryness, burning sensation, dyspareunia, mucoid discharge (may be flecked with blood), postcoital bleeding. Symptoms occur gradually due to thinning of epithelial layers.

O: Pale, dry mucosa with abraded areas that bleed easily, decreased rugae; may have bloody discharge. Decrease in usual shiny vaginal secretions. Vagina may be shortened and narrowed; cervix may be less protuberant.[32] Estrogen normally keeps tissues thick, moist, rugated, and glycogen rich; so loss of estrogen creates signs and increases risk for trauma and infection.

Candidiasis (Moniliasis)

S: Intense pruritus; thick, whitish, clumpy discharge.

O: Vulva and vagina are erythematous and edematous. Discharge is usually thick, white, curdy, "like cottage cheese," not malodorous. Microscopic examination of discharge on KOH wet mount shows branched hyphae.

Causes: Recent use of antibiotics, some oral contraceptives, uncontrolled or undiagnosed diabetes, douching that disrupts normal flora balance, wearing tight or nylon underwear, pregnancy with increased glycogen, more alkaline vaginal pH as in menses, postpartum, or menopause.

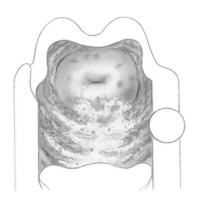

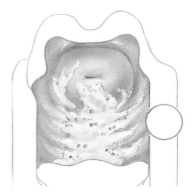

Trichomoniasis

S: Pruritus, watery and often malodorous vaginal discharge, urinary frequency, terminal dysuria, itching. Symptoms are worse during menstruation when the pH is optimal for organism's growth.

O: Vulva may be erythematous. Vagina diffusely red; granular; occasionally with red, raised papules and petechiae ("strawberry" appearance). Frothy, yellow-green, foul-smelling discharge. Vaginal pH >4.5. Microscopic examination of saline wet mount specimen shows characteristic flagellated cells.

Bacterial Vaginosis (*Gardnerella vaginalis, Haemophilus vaginalis,* or Nonspecific Vaginitis)

S: Profuse discharge, "constant wetness" with "foul, fishy, rotten" odor.

O: Thin, creamy, gray-white, malodorous discharge. No inflammation on vaginal wall or cervix because this is a surface parasite. Vaginal pH >4.5. Microscopic view of saline wet mount specimen shows typical "clue cells" (epithelial cells with stippled borders). Sniff for fishy odor after adding KOH to slide ("whiff test"). These signs are termed *Amsel criteria.*

Continued

TABLE 27.5   Vulvovaginal Inflammations—cont'd

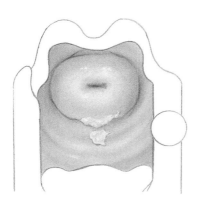

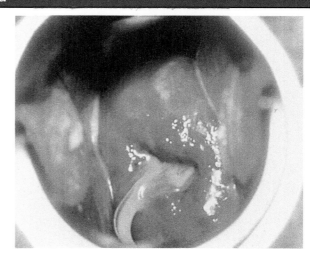

Chlamydia

S: Minimal or no symptoms. May have urinary frequency, dysuria, vaginal discharge, postcoital bleeding.

O: May have yellow or green mucopurulent discharge, friable cervix, cervical motion tenderness. Signs are subtle, easily mistaken for gonorrhea. If untreated, chlamydia can ascend to cause PID and result in infertility. The most common STI; the highest prevalence is among sexually active adolescents. Urine chlamydia testing using nucleic acid amplification tests (NAAT) is a noninvasive method to screen.[34] Use a single urine specimen to detect both pregnancy and chlamydia.

Gonorrhea

S: Variable: Vaginal discharge, dysuria, abnormal uterine bleeding, abscess in Bartholin or Skene glands; 95% of cases are asymptomatic.

O: Often no signs are apparent. May have purulent vaginal discharge. Diagnose by positive culture of organism. If the condition is untreated, it may progress to acute salpingitis, PID. Treat with antibiotics and retest in 3 to 6 months.

S, Subjective data; *O,* objective data.
See Illustration Credits for source information.

TABLE 27.6   Uterine Enlargement

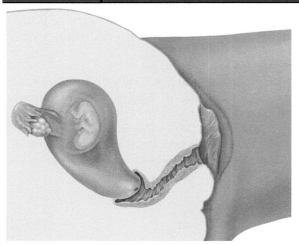

◀ Pregnancy

Obviously a normal condition, pregnancy is included here for comparison.

S: Amenorrhea, fatigue, breast engorgement, nausea, change in food tolerance, weight gain.

O: Early signs—Cyanosis of vaginal mucosa and cervix (Chadwick sign). Palpation—Soft consistency of cervix, enlarging uterus with compressible fundus and isthmus (Hegar sign at 10 to 12 weeks).

Continued

TABLE 27.6	Uterine Enlargement—cont'd

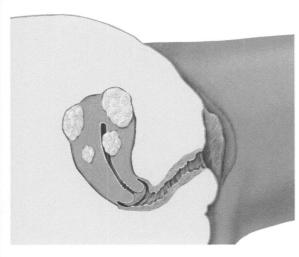

◄ Myomas (Leiomyomas, Uterine Fibroids)

S: Varies, depending on size and location. Often no symptoms. Symptoms that occur include vague discomfort, bloating, heaviness, pelvic pressure, dyspareunia, urinary frequency, backache, or excessive uterine bleeding and resulting anemia.

O: Uterus irregularly enlarged; firm; mobile; and nodular with hard, painless nodules in the uterine wall. Heavy bleeding produces anemia. Confirmed by ultrasound imaging.

These benign tumors are common; by age 50 years 70% of white women and >80% of black women will have at least one.[28] Myomas are estrogen dependent; after menopause the lesions regress but do not disappear. Surgery may be indicated.

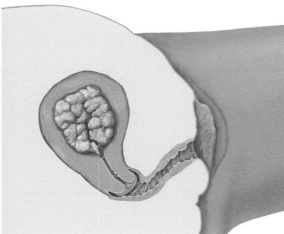

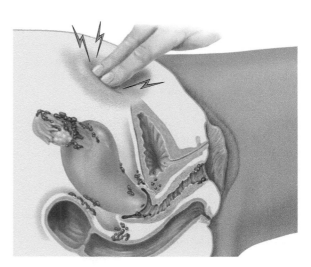

Carcinoma of the Endometrium

S: Abnormal and intermenstrual bleeding before menopause; postmenopausal bleeding or mucosanguineous discharge. Pain and weight loss occur late in the disease.

O: Uterus may be enlarged.

The Pap test is rarely effective in detecting endometrial cancer. Women with abnormal vaginal bleeding or at high risk should have an endometrial tissue sample. Risk factors are early menarche, late menopause, history of infertility, failure to ovulate, tamoxifen, unopposed estrogen therapy (which continually stimulates the endometrium, causing hyperplasia), and obesity (which increases endogenous estrogen).

Endometriosis

S: Cyclic or chronic pelvic pain, occurring as dysmenorrhea or dyspareunia, low backache. May have irregular uterine bleeding, hypermenorrhea, or be asymptomatic.

O: Uterus fixed, tender to movement. Small, firm nodular masses tender to palpation on posterior aspect of fundus, uterosacral ligaments, ovaries, sigmoid colon. Ovaries often enlarged.

Masses are aberrant growths of endometrial tissue scattered throughout pelvis, probably transplanted tissue by retrograde menstruation. Ectopic tissue responds to hormone stimulation; builds up between periods, sloughs during menstruation. May cause infertility from pelvic adhesions, tubal obstruction, decreased ovarian function.

S, Subjective data; *O,* objective data.

TABLE 27.7 | Adnexal Enlargement

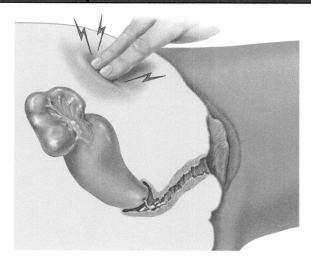

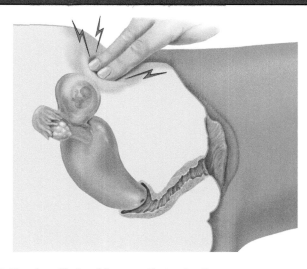

Fallopian Tube Mass—Acute Salpingitis (PID)

S: Sudden fever >38° C or 100.4° F, suprapubic pain and tenderness.

O: Acute—Rigid, boardlike lower abdominal musculature. May have purulent discharge from cervix. Movement of uterus and cervix causes intense pain. Pain in lateral fornices and adnexa. Bilateral adnexal masses difficult to palpate because of pain and muscle spasm. Chronic—Bilateral, tender, fixed adnexal masses.

Complications include ectopic pregnancy, infertility, and reinfection. PID usually caused by *Chlamydia trachomatis* and *Neisseria gonorrhoeae*.[4]

Fallopian Tube Mass—Ectopic Pregnancy

S: Sharp, stabbing abdominal or pelvic pain, vaginal spotting or new-onset bleeding, although < half of women have these classic symptoms; positive urine pregnancy test.

O: Softening of cervix and fundus; movement of cervix and uterus cause pain; palpable tender, round, mobile swelling, lateral to uterus. Late signs may indicate rupture: decreased BP, tachycardia, diaphoresis, shock; regard as emergency. Transvaginal ultrasonography crucial for all suspected ectopic pregnancies. This is an implanted fertilized ovum in the fallopian tube; incidence is 1% to 2% of pregnancies; up to 4% of those using assisted reproductive technology.[7] Crucial to identify before fallopian tube ruptures and fatal hemorrhage ensues. This is leading cause of first-trimester pregnancy-related death.

Continued

TABLE 27.7 | **Adnexal Enlargement—cont'd**

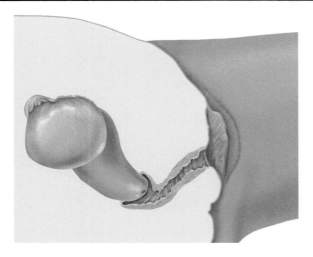

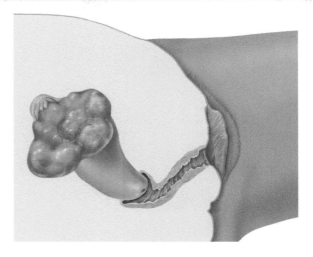

Fluctuant Ovarian Mass—Ovarian Cyst

S: Usually asymptomatic; when cyst is large, can be painful; may have dyspareunia.

O: Bimanual palpation shows smooth, round, fluctuant, mobile, nontender mass on ovary. Ultrasound image shows location of cyst. Follicular cysts are most common; follicle around ovum does not burst as usual to release egg but grows into cyst. Most resolve on their own, with follow-up at 2 to 3 months.

Solid Ovarian Mass—Ovarian Cancer

S: Vague symptoms; may have abdominal pain, pelvic pain, increased abdominal size, bloating, difficulty eating, red spotting, or may be asymptomatic.

O: May or may not palpate solid tumor on ovary. Heavy, solid, fixed, poorly defined mass suggests malignancy; benign mass may feel mobile and solid.

Biopsy necessary to distinguish. The Pap test does not detect ovarian cancer. Screening with serum CA 125 test, transvaginal ultrasound, and a new biomarker HE4 are done but still tests are not specific.[27]

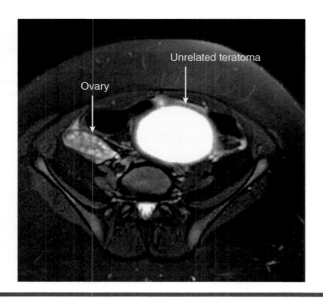

Ovary

Unrelated teratoma

◄ Polycystic Ovary Syndrome (PCOS)

S: Amenorrhea for 3 months or infrequent menses, infertility, hyperandrogenism (acne, hirsutism, hair loss), weight gain.

O: Bimanual palpation may reveal enlarged ovary with multiple fluctuant balloonlike masses. MRI image shows patient's right ovary with multiple cysts, also unrelated benign teratoma in left ovary. PCOS affects 6% to 15% of reproductive-age women, with infertility, weight gain, and hirsutism, causing significant distress. May also have insulin resistance and diabetes. May be treated with metformin, hormonal regulation of menses, and infertility specialists.[15,20]

S, Subjective data; *O,* objective data.

TABLE 27.8	Pediatric Genitalia Abnormalities

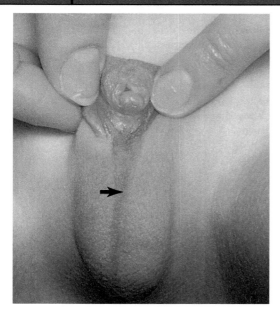

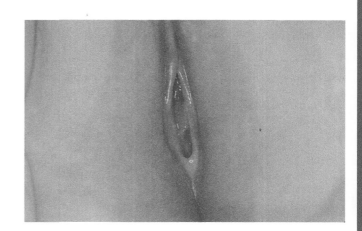

Ambiguous Genitalia

Female pseudohermaphroditism is a congenital anomaly resulting from hyperplasia of the adrenal glands, which exposes the female fetus to excess amounts of androgens. This causes masculinized external genitalia, here shown as enlargement of the clitoris and fusion of the labia. *Ambiguous* means that the enlarged clitoris here may look like a small penis with hypospadias and the fused labia look like an incompletely formed scrotum with absent testes. Other forms of intersexual conditions occur, and the family must be referred for diagnostic evaluation.

Vulvovaginitis in Child

This is acute, nonspecific vulvovaginitis.
Causes in the prepubertal child include infection from a respiratory or bowel pathogen, STI, presence of a foreign body, or *Candida albicans* in a child with diabetes.

See Illustration Credits for source information.

Summary Checklist: Female Genitalia Examination

1. **Inspect external genitalia.**
2. **Palpate labia,** Skene and Bartholin glands.
3. Using **vaginal speculum,** inspect cervix and vagina.
4. Obtain **specimens** for cytologic study.
5. Perform **bimanual examination:** cervix, uterus, adnexa.
6. Perform **rectovaginal** examination.
7. **Test stool** for occult blood.

REFERENCES

1. American Academy of Pediatrics (AAP). (2014). Screening for nonviral sexually transmitted infections in adolescents and young adults. *Pediatrics, 134*(1), 1–26.
2. Anderson, S., & Must, A. (2005). Interpreting the continued decline in the average age at menarche: Results from two nationally representative surveys of U.S. girls studied 10 years apart. *J Pediatr, 147*(6), 753–760.
3. Banayya Jungari, S. (2016). Female genital mutilation is a violation of reproductive rights of women. *Health Soc Work, 41*(1), 25–31.
4. Brunham, R. C., Gottlieb, S. L., & Paavonen, J. (2015). Pelvic inflammatory disease. *N Engl J Med, 372*(21), 2039.
5. Centers for Disease Control and Prevention (CDC). (2015). *Chlamydial infections.* https://cdc.gov/std/tg2015/chlamydia. htm.

6. Curtis, K. M., & Peipert, J. F. (2017). Long-acting reversible contraception. *N Engl J Med, 376*(5), 461–468.

7. Gatzke, N., & Johnson, L. (2014). Ectopic pregnancy: A red flag diagnosis. *Nurse Pract, 39*(12), 42–47.

8. Gnann, J. W., Jr., & Whitley, R. J. (2016). Genital herpes. *N Engl J Med, 375*(7), 666–674.

9. Jones, A. N., Bartlett, J. W., Bates, R. A., et al. (2017). Primary immunization of human papillomavirus vaccine in the pediatric population. *Clin Pediatr, 56*(7), 605.

10. Karjane, N., & Chelmow, D. (2013). New cervical cancer screening guidelines, again. *Obstet Gynecol Clin North Am, 40*(2), 211–223.

11. Kessenich, C. R., & Coyne, J. P. (2017). Using transvaginal ultrasound to determine the cause of chronic pelvic pain. *Nurse Pract, 42*(5), 10–12.

12. Reference deleted in proofs.

13. Lin, S. N., Taylor, J., Alperstein, S., et al. (2014). Does speculum lubricant affect liquid-based Papanicolaou test adequacy? *Cancer Cytopathol, 122*(3), 221.

14. Markowitz, L. E., Hariri, S., Steinav, M., et al. (2016). Prevalence of HPV after introduction of the vaccination program in the United States. *Pediatrics, 137*(3), 1–9.

15. McCartney, C. R., & Marshall, J. C. (2016). Polycystic ovary syndrome. *N Engl J Med, 375*(1), 54–64.

16. Nelson, J., & Good, E. (2015). Urinary tract infections and asymptomatic bacteriuria in older adults. *Nurse Pract, 40*(8), 43–48.

17. Pace, D. T. (2017). The menopausal woman. *Nurse Pract, 42*(12), 43–49.

18. Palmer, M. H., & Willis-Gray, M. G. (2017). Overactive bladder in women. *Am J Nurs, 117*(4), 34–43.

19. Pereira, K., & Brown, J. A. (2017). Secondary amenorrhea. *Nurse Pract, 42*(9), 34–41.

20. Pereira, K., & Kreider, K. E. (2017). Caring for women with polycystic ovary syndrome. *Nurse Pract, 42*(2), 39–47.

21. Pimple, S., Mishra, G., & Shastri, S. (2016). Global strategies for cervical cancer prevention. *Curr Opin Obstet Gynecol, 28*(1), 4–10.

22. Ramnitz, M. S., & Lodish, M. B. (2013). Racial disparities in pubertal development. *Semin Reprod Med, 31*(5), 333–339.

23. Roberts, S. J. (2015). Primary care of women who have sex with women. *Nurse Pract, 40*(12), 24–32.

24. Rosenfield, R. L., Lipton, R. B., & Drum, M. L. (2009). Thelarche, pubarche, and menarche attainment in children with normal and elevated body mass index. *Pediatrics, 123*(1), 84–88.

25. Santa Maria, D., Guilamo-Ramos, V., Jemmott, L. S., et al. (2017). Nurses on the front lines: Improving adolescent sexual and reproductive health. *Am J Nurs, 117*(1), 42–51.

26. Saslow, D., Andrews, K. S., Manassaram-Baptiste, D., et al. (2016). Human papillomavirus vaccination guideline update: American Cancer Society guideline endorsement. *CA Cancer J Clin, 66*(5), 375–385.

27. Slatnik, C. P., & Duff, E. (2015). Ovarian cancer. *Nurse Pract, 40*(9), 47–54.

28. Stewart, E. A. (2015). Uterine fibroids. *N Engl J Med, 372*(17), 1646–1655.

29. Troisi, R., Hatch, E. E., Palmer, J. R., et al. (2016). Prenatal diethylstilbestrol exposure and high-grade squamous cell neoplasia of the lower genital tract. *Am J Obstet Gynecol, 215*(3), 322.e1–322.e8.

30. Tsu, V., & Jerónimo, J. (2016). Saving the world's women from cervical cancer. *N Engl J Med, 374*(26), 2509–2511.

31. United States Preventive Services Task Force (USPSTF) (2012). *The guide to clinical preventative services: screening for cervical cancer.* AHRQ Publication no. 11-05156-EF-3). Baltimore, MD: Lippincott Williams & Wilkins.

32. Ward, K., & Deneris, A. (2016). Genitourinary syndrome of menopause. *Nurs Pract, 41*(7), 28–33.

33. Waterman, L., & Voss, J. (2015). HPV, cervical cancer risks, and barriers to care for lesbian women. *Nurse Pract, 40*(1), 46–54.

34. Wiesenfeld, H. C. (2017). Screening for *Chlamydia trachomatis* infections in women. *N Engl J Med, 376*(8), 765.

35. Reference deleted in proofs.

36. Wuerthner, B. A., & Avila-Wallace, M. (2016). Cervical cancer screening, management, and prevention. *Nurse Pract, 41*(9), 18–23.

37. Yoo, W., Kim, S., Huh, W. K., et al. (2017). Recent trends in racial and regional disparities in cervical cancer incidence and mortality in United States. *PLoS ONE, 12*(2), 1–13.

CHAPTER 28

The Complete Health Assessment: Adult

The choreography of the complete history and physical examination is the art of arranging all the separate steps you have learned into a fluid whole. Your first examination may seem awkward and contrived; you may have to pause and think of what comes next rather than moving smoothly between assessments. Repeated rehearsals will make the choreography smoother. You will come to the point at which the procedure flows naturally; and even if you forget a step, you will be able to insert it gracefully into the next logical place.

The following examination sequence is one suggested route. It is intended to minimize the number of position changes for the patient and for you. With experience you may wish to adapt this and arrange a sequence that feels natural for you. As you identify an order that works for you, make sure to be consistent and always perform the assessment in the same order. This will minimize the risk of forgetting an assessment.

A complete examination is performed at a patient's first entry into an outpatient setting or initial admission to the hospital. Perform all the steps listed here for a complete examination. With experience you will learn to strike a balance between which steps you must retain to be thorough and which corners you may safely cut when time is pressing. The steps for the follow-up in-hospital assessment are described in Chapter 30.

Have all equipment prepared and accessible before the examination. Review Chapter 8 for the list of necessary equipment, the setting, the patient's emotional state, your demeanor, and the preparation of the patient considering his or her age.

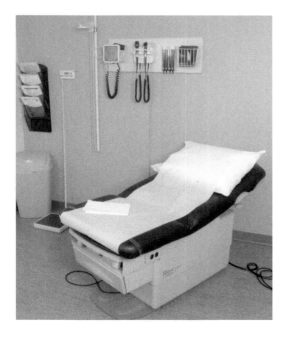

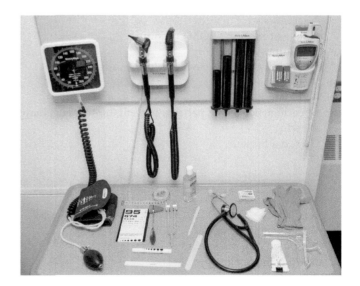

Sequence	Selected Photos

The patient walks into the room, sits; the examiner sits facing the patient; the patient remains in street clothes. Allowing the patient to remain in street clothes helps establish rapport during the interview. (NOTE: Position changes are in **bold** lines.)

The Health History

Collect the history, complete or limited as visit warrants. While obtaining the history and throughout the examination, note the person's general appearance.

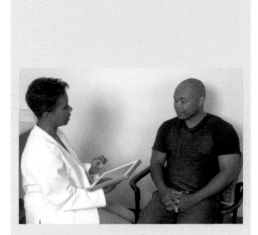

General Appearance

1. Appears stated age
2. Level of consciousness
3. Skin color
4. Nutritional status
5. Posture and position comfortably erect
6. Obvious physical deformities
7. Mobility
   Gait
   Use of assistive devices
   Range of motion (ROM) of joints
   Involuntary movement
   Able to rise from a seated position easily
8. Facial expression
9. Mood and affect
10. Speech: articulation, pattern, content appropriate, native language
11. Hearing
12. Personal hygiene

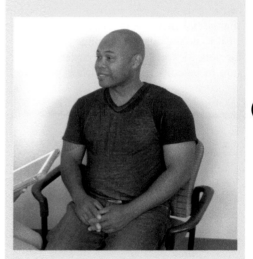

Measurement

1. Weight
2. Height
3. Waist circumference
4. Compute body mass index
5. Vision using Snellen eye chart

Ask the person to empty the bladder (save specimen, if needed), to disrobe except for underwear, and to put on a gown. Leave the room to provide privacy while the person changes. Upon your return, ask the person to **sit with legs dangling** off the side of the bed or table; you stand in front of the person.

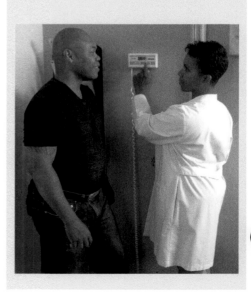

Objective Data

| **Sequence** | **Selected Photos** |

Skin

1. Examine both hands and inspect the nails.
2. For the rest of the examination, examine the skin with the corresponding regional examination.

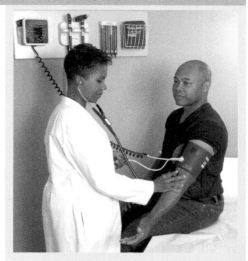

Vital Signs

1. Radial pulse
2. Respirations
3. Blood pressure (BP) in arm(s)
4. BP in lower leg; compute ankle/brachial index (if indicated)
5. Temperature (if indicated)

Head and Face

1. Inspect and palpate scalp, hair, and cranium.
2. Inspect face: expression, symmetry (cranial nerve VII).
3. Palpate the temporal artery, then the temporomandibular joint as the person opens and closes the mouth.
4. Palpate the maxillary sinuses and the frontal sinuses.

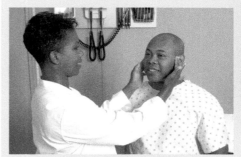

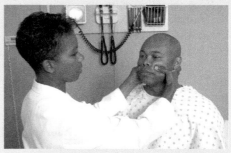

Eyes

1. Test visual fields by confrontation (cranial nerve II).
2. Test extraocular muscles: corneal light reflex, six cardinal positions of gaze (cranial nerves III, IV, VI).
3. Inspect external eye structures.
4. Inspect conjunctivae, sclerae, corneas, irides.*
5. Test pupil: size, response to light, and accommodation.

Darken room.

6. Using an ophthalmoscope, inspect ocular fundus: red reflex, disc, vessels, and retinal background.

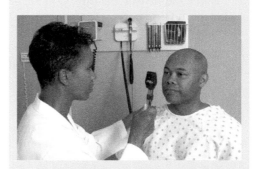

*This is the plural form of iris.

Objective Data

Sequence	Selected Photos

Ears

1. Inspect the external ear: position and alignment, skin condition, and auditory meatus.
2. Move auricle and push tragus for tenderness.
3. With an otoscope, inspect the canal, then the tympanic membrane for color, position, landmarks, and integrity.
4. Test hearing: whispered voice test.

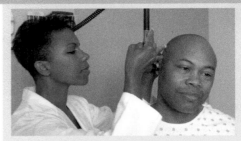

Nose

1. Inspect the external nose: symmetry, lesions.
2. Inspect facial symmetry (cranial nerve VII).
3. Test the patency of each nostril.
4. With a speculum, inspect the nares: nasal mucosa, septum, and turbinates.

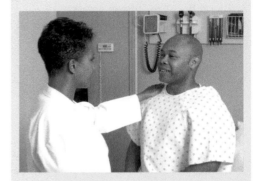

Mouth and Throat

1. Using a light, inspect the mouth: buccal mucosa, teeth and gums, tongue, floor of mouth, palate, and uvula.
2. Grade tonsils if present.
3. Note mobility of uvula as the person phonates "ahh" and test gag reflex (cranial nerves IX, X).
4. Ask the person to stick out the tongue (cranial nerve XII).
5. With a gloved hand, bimanually palpate the mouth, if indicated.

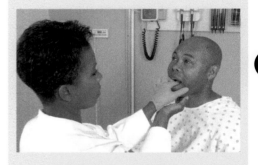

Neck

1. Inspect the neck: symmetry, lumps, and pulsations.
2. Palpate the cervical lymph nodes.
3. Inspect and palpate the carotid pulse, one side at a time. If indicated, listen for carotid bruits.
4. Palpate the trachea in midline.
5. Test ROM and muscle strength against your resistance: head forward and back, head turned to each side, and shoulder shrug (cranial nerve XI).

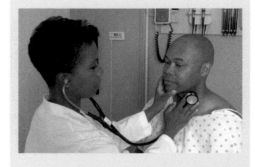

Step behind the person, taking your stethoscope with you.
6. Palpate thyroid gland, posterior approach.

Open the person's gown to expose all of the back for examination of the thorax, but leave gown on shoulders and anterior chest of female patients.

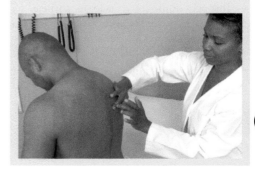

Sequence	Selected Photos

Chest, Posterior and Lateral

1. Inspect the posterior chest: configuration of the thoracic cage, skin characteristics, and symmetry of shoulders and muscles.
2. Palpate: symmetric expansion; tactile fremitus; lumps or tenderness.
3. Palpate length of spinous processes.
4. Percuss over all lung fields.
5. Percuss costovertebral angle, noting tenderness.
6. Auscultate breath sounds, comparing side to side in upper and lower lung fields; note any adventitious sounds.

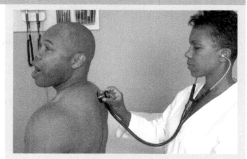

Move around to face the patient; the patient remains sitting. For a female breast examination, let the patient know you are going to the lift the gown and drape it on the shoulders, exposing the anterior chest; for a male, lower the gown to the lap.

Chest, Anterior

1. Inspect: respirations and skin characteristics.
2. Palpate: symmetric expansion, tactile fremitus, lumps, or tenderness.
3. Percuss anterior lung fields.
4. Auscultate breath sounds, comparing side to side in upper and lateral lung fields; note any adventitious sounds.

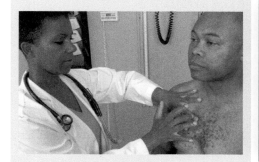

Heart

1. Ask the person to lean forward and exhale briefly; auscultate cardiac base for any murmurs.

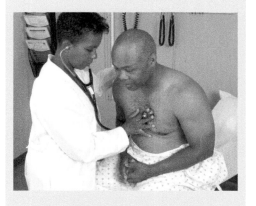

Upper Extremities

1. Test ROM and muscle strength of hands, wrists, arms, and shoulders.
2. Palpate the epitrochlear nodes.
3. Palpate temperature, capillary refill.
4. Compare radial and brachial pulses.

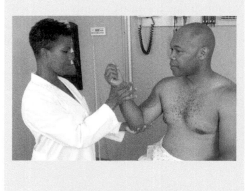

Objective Data

Sequence	Selected Photos

Objective Data *(sidebar)*

Female Breasts

1. Inspect for symmetry, mobility, and dimpling as the woman lifts arms over the head, pushes the hands on the hips, and leans forward.
2. Inspect supraclavicular and infraclavicular areas.

Help the woman to **lie supine with head at a flat** to 30-degree angle. Stand at the person's *right* side. Drape the gown up across shoulders and place an extra sheet across lower abdomen.

3. Palpate each breast, lifting the same-side arm up over head. Include the tail of Spence and areola.
4. Palpate each nipple for discharge.
5. Support the person's arm and palpate the axilla and regional lymph nodes.
6. Teach breast self-examination.

Male Breasts

1. Inspect and palpate while palpating the anterior chest wall.
2. Supporting each arm, palpate the axilla and regional nodes.

Neck Vessels

1. Inspect the neck for a jugular venous pulse, turning the person's head slightly to the left.
2. Estimate jugular venous pressure, if indicated.

Heart

1. Inspect the precordium for any pulsations or heave (lift).
2. Palpate the apical impulse and note the location.
3. Palpate the precordium for any abnormal thrill.
4. Auscultate apical rate and rhythm.
5. Auscultate with the diaphragm of the stethoscope to study heart sounds, inching from the apex up to the base, or vice versa in a rough "Z" pattern.
6. Auscultate the heart sounds with the bell of the stethoscope, again inching through all locations, noting any murmurs or abnormal sounds.
7. Turn the person over to the left side while again auscultating the apex with the bell.

The person should be **supine,** with the bed or table flat; arrange drapes to expose the abdomen from the chest to the pubis.

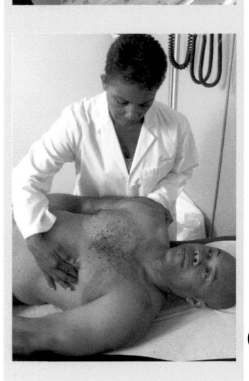

Sequence	Selected Photos

Abdomen

1. Inspect: contour, symmetry, skin characteristics, umbilicus, and pulsations.
2. Auscultate bowel sounds.
3. Auscultate for vascular sounds over the aorta, renal arteries, iliac and femoral arteries.
4. Percuss all quadrants.

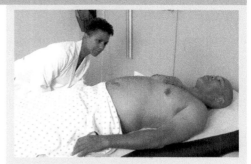

5. Palpate: light palpation in all quadrants, then deep palpation in all quadrants.
6. Palpate for liver, spleen, and kidneys.
7. Palpate aortic pulsation if indicated.

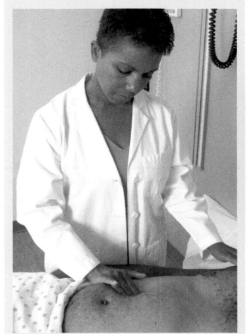

Inguinal Area

1. Palpate each groin for the femoral pulse and the inguinal nodes. Lift the drape to expose the legs.

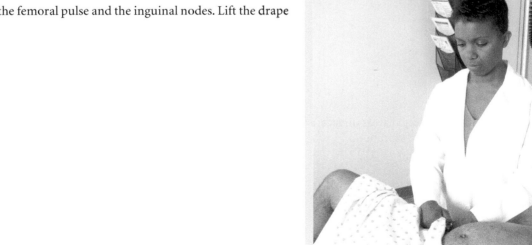

Objective Data

Sequence	Selected Photos

Lower Extremities

1. Inspect: symmetry, skin characteristics, and hair distribution.
2. Palpate pulses: popliteal, posterior tibial, dorsalis pedis.
3. Palpate for temperature and pretibial edema.
4. Separate toes and inspect.
5. Test ROM and muscle strength of hips, knees, ankles, and feet.

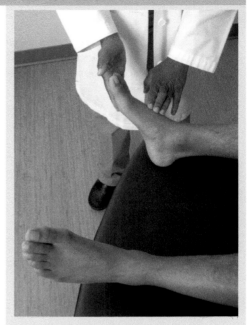

Ask the person to **sit up and to dangle** the legs off the bed or table. Keep the gown on and the drape over the lap.

Musculoskeletal

1. Note muscle strength as person sits up.

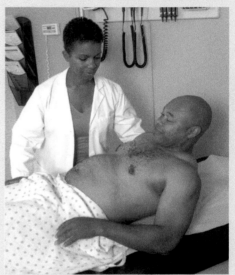

Neurologic

1. Test sensation in selected areas on face, arms, hands, legs, and feet: superficial pain, light touch, and vibration.

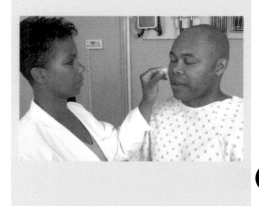

Objective Data

Sequence	Selected Photos

2. Test position sense of fingers.
3. Test stereognosis, using a familiar object.
4. Test cerebellar function of the upper extremities using finger-to-nose test or rapid–alternating movements test.

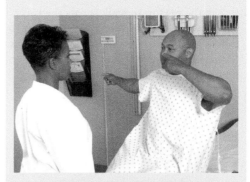

5. Elicit deep tendon reflexes: biceps, triceps, brachioradialis.

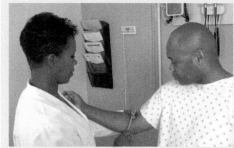

6. Test the cerebellar function of the lower extremities by asking the person to run each heel down the opposite shin.
7. Elicit deep tendon reflexes: patellar and Achilles.
8. Test the Babinski reflex.

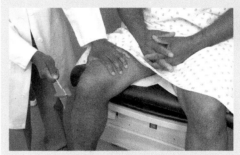

Ask the person to **stand** with the gown on. Stand close to the person.

Lower Extremities

1. Inspect legs for varicose veins.

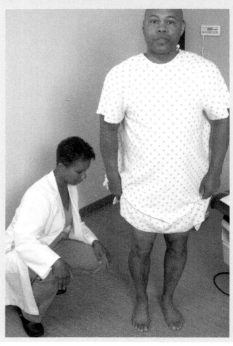

Sequence	Selected Photos

Musculoskeletal

1. Ask the person **to walk** across the room in his or her regular walk, turn, and then walk back toward you in heel-to-toe fashion.
2. Ask the person to walk on the toes for a few steps, then to walk on the heels for a few steps.
3. Stand close and check Romberg sign.

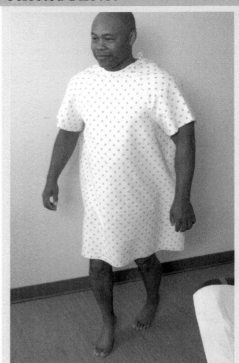

4. Ask the person to hold the edge of the bed and perform a shallow knee bend, one for each leg.
5. Stand behind and check the spine as the person touches the toes.
6. Stabilize the pelvis and test the ROM of the spine as the person hyperextends, rotates, and laterally bends.

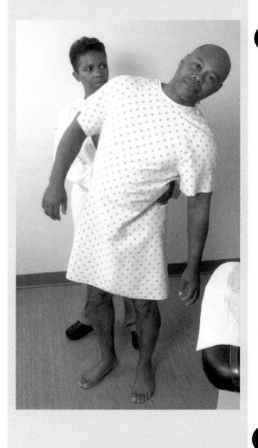

Objective Data

Sequence	Selected Photos

For the male patient, sit on a stool in front of him. The person stands.

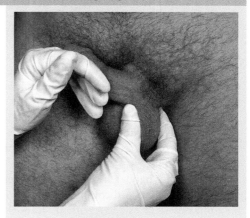

Male Genitalia

1. Inspect the penis and scrotum.
2. Palpate the scrotal contents. If a mass exists, transilluminate.
3. Check for inguinal hernia.
4. Teach testicular self-examination.

For an adult male, ask him to bend over the examination table, supporting the torso with forearms on the table. Assist the bedfast male to a left lateral position with the right leg drawn up.

Male Rectum

1. Inspect the perianal area.
2. With a gloved lubricated finger, palpate the rectal walls and prostate gland.
3. Save a stool specimen for an occult blood test.

Assist the female back to the examination table and help her assume **the lithotomy position**. Drape her appropriately. You sit on a stool at the foot of the table for the speculum examination and then stand for the bimanual examination.

Female Genitalia

1. Inspect the perineal and perianal areas.

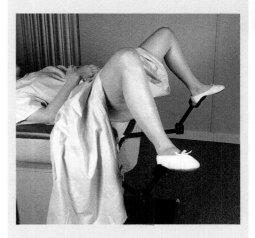

2. With a vaginal speculum inspect the cervix and vaginal walls.
3. Procure specimens.
4. Perform a bimanual examination: cervix, uterus, and adnexa.
5. Continue the bimanual examination, checking the rectum and rectovaginal walls.
6. Save a stool specimen for an occult blood test.
7. Provide tissues for the female to wipe the perineal area and help her up to a **sitting position**.

Tell the person that you are finished with the examination and that you will leave the room as he or she gets dressed. Return to discuss the examination and further plans and to answer any questions. Thank the person for his or her time.

For the hospitalized person, return the bed and any room equipment to their original position. Make sure that the call light and telephone are within easy reach.

Objective Data

DOCUMENTATION AND CRITICAL THINKING

Recording the Data

Record the data from the history and physical examination as soon after the event as possible. Memory fades as the day develops, especially when you are responsible for the care of more than one person. If you are using an electronic medical record and there is a computer at the bedside, document before leaving the room. You may also find that documenting as you move through the examination works well for you. Just make sure you do not ignore the person as you focus on the computer.

It is difficult to strike a balance between recording too much and too little data. It is important to remember that from a legal perspective, if it is not documented, it was not done. Data important for the diagnosis and treatment of the person's health should be recorded, as well as data that contribute to your decision-making process. This includes charting relevant normal or negative findings.

On the other hand, a listing of every assessment parameter described in this text yields an unwieldy, unworkable record. One way to keep your record complete yet succinct is to study your writing style. Use short, clear phrases. Avoid redundant introductory phrases such as "The patient states that…." Avoid redundant descriptions such as "No inguinal, femoral, or umbilical hernias." Just write, "No hernias."

Use simple line drawings to describe your findings. You do not need artistic talent; draw a simple sketch of a tympanic membrane, breast, abdomen, or cervix and mark your findings on it. A clear picture is worth many words.

Study the following complete history and physical examination for a sample write-up. Note the many health problems emerging through this history and examination.

Health History

BIOGRAPHIC DATA

Name: E. K.
Address: 123 Center St.
Relationship Status: Single

Birth date: 1/18/
Birthplace: Springfield

E.K. is a 23-year-old single female, currently unemployed for 6 months.

Source. E.K., seems reliable.

Reason for Seeking Care. "I'm coming in for alcohol treatment."

History of Present Illness. First alcoholic drink, age 16. First intoxication, age 17, drinking 1 or 2 times per week, a 6-pack per occasion. Attending high school classes every day, but grades slipping from A–B+ average to C– average. At age 20 drinking 2 times per week, 6 to 9 beers per occasion. At age 22 drinking 2 times per week, a 12-pack per occasion, and occasionally a 6-pack the next day to "help with the hangover." During this year experienced blackouts, failed attempts to cut down on drinking, was physically sick the morning after drinking, and was unable to stop drinking once started. Also incurred three driving-under-the-influence (DUI) legal offenses. Last DUI 1 month PTA; last alcohol use just before DUI, 18 beers that occasion. Abstinent since that time.

PAST HEALTH

Childhood Illnesses. Chickenpox at age 6. No measles, mumps, croup, pertussis. No rheumatic fever, scarlet fever, or polio. Received childhood vaccinations recommended at that time. No HPV vaccine series.

Accidents. (1) Auto accident, age 12; father driving; thrown from car, right leg crushed. Hospitalized at Memorial; surgery for leg pinning to repair multiple compound fractures. (2) Auto accident, age 21; not wearing seatbelt, head hit dashboard, no loss of consciousness, treated and released at Memorial Hospital ED. (3) Auto accident, age 23; "car hit median strip," no injuries, not seen at hospital.

Chronic Illnesses. None.

Hospitalizations. Age 12, Memorial Hospital, surgery to repair right leg as described; Dr. M.J. Carlson, surgeon.

Obstetric History. Gravida 0/Para 0/Abortion 0.

Immunizations. Childhood immunizations up-to-date. Last tetanus "probably high school." No TB skin test.

Last Examinations. Annual pelvic examinations at health department since age 15, told "normal and healthy." High school sports physical as sophomore. Last dental examination as high school junior; last vision test for driver's license age 16; never had ECG, chest x-ray.

Allergies. No known allergies.

Current Medications. Birth control pills, low-estrogen type, 1/day, for 5 years. No other prescription or over-the-counter medications.

FAMILY HISTORY

E.K. is youngest of two children; parents divorced 8 years ago; father has chronic alcoholism. See family genogram that follows.

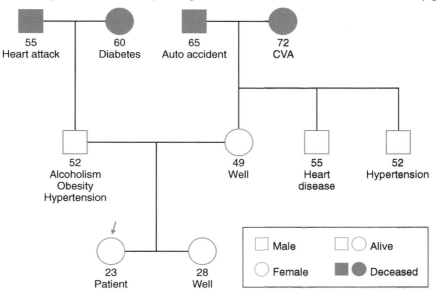

REVIEW OF SYSTEMS

General Health. Reports usual health "OK." No recent weight change; no fatigue, weakness, fever, sweats.

Skin. No change in skin color, pigmentation, or nevi. No pruritus, rash, lesions. Has bruise now over right eye; struck by boyfriend 1 week PTA. No history of skin disease. Hair: no loss, change in texture. Nails: no change.
Self-care: stays in sun "as much as I can." No use of sunscreen. Goes to tanning bed at hair salon twice/week during winter.

Head. No unusually frequent or severe headaches; no head injury, dizziness, syncope, or vertigo.

Eyes. No difficulty with vision or diplopia. No eye pain, inflammation, discharge, lesions. No history of glaucoma or cataracts. Wears no corrective lenses.

Ears. No hearing loss or difficulty. No earaches; no infections now or as child; no discharge, tinnitus, or vertigo.
Self-care: no exposure to environmental noise; cleans ears with washcloth.

Nose. No discharge; has 2 or 3 colds per year; no sinus pain, nasal obstruction, epistaxis, or allergy.

Mouth and Throat. No mouth pain, bleeding gums, toothache, sores or lesions in mouth, dysphagia, hoarseness, or sore throat. Has tonsils.
Self-care: brushes teeth twice/day, no flossing.

Neck. No pain, limitation of motion, lumps, or swollen glands.

Breasts. No pain, lumps, nipple discharge, rash, swelling, or trauma. No history of breast disease in self, mother, or sister. No surgery.
Self-care: does not do breast self-examination.

Respiratory. No history of lung disease; no chest pain with breathing; no wheezing or shortness of breath. Colds sometimes "go to my chest"; treats with over-the-counter cough medicine and aspirin. Occasional early-morning cough, nonproductive. Smokes cigarettes 2 PPD × 2 years; prior use 1 PPD × 4 years. Pack years = 8. Never tried to quit.

Cardiovascular. No chest pain, palpitation, cyanosis, fatigue, dyspnea with exertion, orthopnea, paroxysmal nocturnal dyspnea, nocturia, edema. No history of heart murmur, hypertension, coronary artery disease, or anemia. Paternal grandfather died of MI at age 55, father has history of hypertension. One paternal uncle with heart disease and one paternal uncle with hypertension.

Peripheral Vascular. No pain, numbness, tingling, or swelling in legs. No coldness, discoloration, varicose veins, infections, or ulcers. Legs are unequal in length as sequelae of accident age 12.
Self-care: previous work as cashier involved standing for 8-hour shifts; no support hose.

Documentation and Critical Thinking

Gastrointestinal. Appetite good with no recent change. No food intolerance, heartburn, indigestion, pain in abdomen, nausea, or vomiting. No history of ulcers, liver or gallbladder disease, jaundice, appendicitis, or colitis. Bowel movement 1/day, soft, brown; no rectal bleeding or pain.

Self-care: no use of vitamins, antacids, laxatives. Diet recall—see *Functional Assessment.*

Urinary. No dysuria, frequency, urgency, nocturia, hesitancy, or straining. No pain in flank, groin, suprapubic region. Urine color yellow; no history of kidney disease.

Genitalia. Menarche age 11. Last menstrual period April 18. Cycle usually q 28 days, duration 2 to 4 days, flow small amount, no dysmenorrhea. No vaginal itching, discharge, sores, or lesions.

Sexual health. In relationship for 2 years with a male partner that includes intercourse. One previous male sexual partner. Uses birth control pills to prevent pregnancy; partner uses no condoms. Concerned that partner may be having sex with other women but has not confronted him. Not aware of any STI contact. Never been tested for STIs including HIV/AIDS. History of sexual abuse by father from ages 12 to 16 years; abuse did not include vaginal or anal intercourse. E.K. is unwilling to discuss further at this time.

Musculoskeletal. No history of arthritis, gout. No joint pain, stiffness, swelling, deformity, or limitation of motion. No muscle pain or weakness. Bone trauma at age 12; has sequela of unequal leg lengths, right leg shorter, walks with limp.

Self-care: no walking or running for sport or exercise "because of leg." Able to stand during previous job as cashier. Uses lift pad in right shoe to equalize leg length.

Neurologic. No history of seizure disorder, stroke, fainting. Has had blackouts with alcohol use. No weakness, tremor, paralysis, problems with coordination, difficulty speaking or swallowing. No numbness or tingling. Not aware of memory problem, nervousness or mood change. Had counseling for sexual abuse in the past. Denies any suicidal ideation or intent during adolescent years or now.

Hematologic. No bleeding problems; no excessive bruising. Not aware of exposure to toxins, never had blood transfusion, never used needles for drug use.

Endocrine. Paternal grandmother with diabetes. No increase in hunger, thirst, or urination; no problems with hot or cold environments; no change in skin or appetite; no nervousness.

FUNCTIONAL ASSESSMENT

Self-Concept. Graduated from high school. Trained "on-the-job" as bartender; also worked as cashier in tavern. Unemployed now, on public aid, does not perceive she has enough money for daily living. Lives with older sister. Raised as Presbyterian, believes in God; does not attend church. Believes self to be "honest, dependable." Believes limitations are "smoking, weight, drinking."

Activity-Exercise. Typical day: arises 9 AM; light chores or TV; spends day looking for work, running errands, or with friends; bedtime at 11 PM. No sustained physical exercise. Believes self able to perform all ADLs; limp poses no problem in bathing, dressing, cooking, household tasks, mobility, driving a car, or previous work as cashier. No mobility aids. Hobbies are fishing, boating, snowmobiling; however, currently has no finances to engage in most of these.

Sleep-Rest. Bedtime 11 PM. Sleeps 9 to 10 hours. No sleep aids.

Nutrition. 24-hour recall: breakfast—none; lunch—bologna sandwich, chips, diet soda; dinner—hamburger, french fries, coffee; snacks—peanuts, pretzels, potato chips, "bar food." This menu is typical of most days. Eats lunch at home alone. Most dinners at fast-food restaurants or in tavern. Shares household grocery expenses and cooking chores with sister. No food intolerances.

Alcohol. See *History of Present Illness.* Denies use of illicit drugs.

Cigarettes. Smokes 2 PPD × 2 years; prior use 1 PPD × 4 years. Never tried to quit. Boyfriend smokes cigarettes.

Interpersonal Relationships. Describes family life growing up as chaotic. Father physically abusive toward mother and sexually abusive toward E.K. Parents divorced because of father's continual drinking. Few support systems currently. Estranged from mother; "Didn't believe me about my father." Father estranged from entire family. Gets along "OK" with sister. Relationship with boyfriend chaotic; has hit her twice in the past. E.K. never pressed legal charges. No close friends. Most friends are "drinking buddies" at tavern.

Coping and Stress Management. Believes housing adequate, adequate heat and utilities, and neighborhood safe. Believes home has no safety hazards. Does not use seatbelts. No travel outside 60 miles of hometown.

Identifies current stresses to be drinking, legal problems with DUIs, unemployment, financial worries. Considers her drinking to be problematic.

PERCEPTION OF HEALTH

Identifies alcohol as a health problem for herself; feels motivated for treatment. Never been interested in physical health and own body before; "Now I think it's time I learned." Expects health care providers to "Help me with my drinking. I don't know beyond that." Expects to stay at this agency for 6 weeks; "Then I don't know what."

MEASUREMENT

Height: 163 cm (5 ft, 4 in.). Weight: 68.6 kg (151 lb). Waist circumference: 32 inches. BMI: 26.

BP: 142/100 mm Hg right arm, sitting. 140/96 mm Hg right arm, lying. 138/98 mm Hg left arm, lying.

Temp: 98.6°F (37°C). Pulse 76 bpm, regular. Resp 16/min, unlabored.

General Survey. E.K. is a 23-year-old female who appears stated age, not currently under the influence of alcohol or other drugs, who articulates clearly, ambulates without difficulty, and is in no distress.

HEAD-TO-TOE EXAMINATION

Skin. Uniformly tan-pink in color, warm, dry, intact; turgor good. No lesions, birthmarks, edema. Resolving 2-cm yellow-green hematoma present over right eye; no edema; ocular structures not involved. Hair: normal distribution and texture; no pest inhabitants. Nails: no clubbing, biting, or discolorations. Nail beds: pink and firm with prompt capillary refill.

Head. Normocephalic, no lesions, lumps, scaling, parasites, or tenderness. Face: symmetric, no weakness, no involuntary movements.

Eyes. Acuity by Snellen chart: right eye 20/20; left eye 20/20–1. Visual fields full by confrontation. EOMs intact; no nystagmus. No ptosis, lid lag, discharge, or crusting. Corneal light reflex symmetric; no strabismus. Conjunctivae clear. Sclerae white; no lesion or redness. Pupils: 3 mm resting, 2 mm constricted, and = bilaterally. PERRLA.

Fundi: discs flat with sharp margins. Vessels present in all quadrants without crossing defects. Background has even color, no hemorrhage or exudates.

Ears. Pinna: no mass, lesions, scaling, discharge, or tenderness to palpation. Canals clear. Tympanic membrane: pearly gray, landmarks intact, no perforation. Whispered words heard bilaterally.

Nose. No deformities or tenderness to palpation. Nares patent. Mucosa pink; no lesions. Septum midline; no perforation. No sinus tenderness.

Mouth. Mucosa and gingivae pink; no lesions or bleeding. Right lower 1st molar missing; multiple dark spots on most teeth; gums receding on lower incisors. Tongue symmetric, protrudes midline, no tremor. Pharynx pink; no exudate. Uvula rises midline on phonation. Tonsils 1+. Gag reflex present.

Neck. Neck supple with full ROM. Symmetric; no masses, tenderness, lymphadenopathy. Trachea midline. Thyroid nonpalpable, not tender. Jugular veins flat @45 degrees. Carotid arteries 2+ and = bilaterally; no bruits.

Spine and Back. Normal spinal profile; no scoliosis. No tenderness over spine; no CVA tenderness.

Thorax and Lungs. AP < transverse diameter. Chest expansion symmetric. Tactile fremitus equal bilaterally. Lung fields resonant. Breath sounds diminished bilaterally. Expiratory wheeze and scattered rhonchi in posterior chest bilateral bases; not cleared with coughing.

Breasts. Symmetric; no retraction, discharge, or lesions. Contour and consistency firm and homogeneous. No masses or tenderness; no lymphadenopathy.

Heart. Precordium: no abnormal pulsations, no heaves. Apical impulse at 5th ICS in left MCL, no thrills. S_1–S_2 are not diminished or accentuated, no S_3 or S_4. Systolic murmur, grade 2/6, loudest at left lower sternal border; no radiation; present supine and sitting.

Abdomen. Flat, symmetric. Skin smooth with no lesions, scars, or striae. Bowel sounds present; no bruits. Tympany predominates in all quadrants. Abdomen soft; no organomegaly; no masses or tenderness; no inguinal lymphadenopathy.

Extremities. Color tan-pink; no redness, cyanosis, lesions other than surgical scar. Scar right lower leg, anterior, 28 cm × 2 cm wide, well healed. No edema, varicosities. No calf tenderness. All peripheral pulses present, 2+ and = bilaterally. Asymmetric leg length—right leg 3 cm shorter than left.

Musculoskeletal. Temporomandibular joint: no slipping or crepitation. Neck: full ROM, no pain. Vertebral column: no tenderness; no deformity or curvature; full extension, lateral bending, rotation. Arms symmetric, legs measure as described, extremities have full ROM, no pain or crepitation. Muscle strength: able to maintain flexion against resistance and without tenderness.

Neurologic. Mental status: appearance, behavior, speech appropriate. Alert and oriented to person, place, time. Thought coherent. Remote and recent memories intact. Cranial nerves II through XII intact. Sensory: pinprick, light touch, vibration intact. Stereognosis: able to identify key. Motor: no atrophy, weakness, or tremors. Gait: has limp, able to tandem walk with shoes on. Negative Romberg sign. Cerebellar: finger-to-nose smoothly intact. DTRs: see *stick gram*.

Genitalia. External genitalia: no lesion, discharge. Internal genitalia: vaginal walls pink; no lesion. Cervix: pink; nulliparous os; no lesions; small amount nonodorous clear discharge. Specimens for Pap test, GC/chlamydia, trichomoniasis, moniliasis obtained. Swabbing mucosa with acetic acid shows no acetowhitening.

Bimanual: no pain on moving cervix; uterus midline; no enlargement, masses, or tenderness. Adnexa: ovaries not enlarged, no tenderness. Anus: no hemorrhoids, fissures, or lesions. Rectal wall intact; no masses or tenderness. Stool soft, brown; Hematest negative.

ASSESSMENT

Alcohol dependence, severe, with physiologic dependence
Nicotine dependence with physiologic dependence
Hypertension
Systolic heart murmur
Decreased gas exchange
Right orbital contusion (resolving)
Overweight (approximately 10 lb)
Dental: missing tooth, probable caries
Potential for trauma
Need for health teaching: alcoholism disease process, treatment options, support systems
Need for health teaching: balanced diet
Dysfunctional family
Decreased self-esteem

CHAPTER 29

The Complete Physical Assessment: Infant, Young Child, and Adolescent

http://evolve.elsevier.com/Jarvis/

Sequence	Selected Photos

The Neonate and Infant

Review Chapter 8 for the steps on preparation and positioning and on developmental principles of the infant. The 1- and 5-minute Apgar results will give important data on the neonate's immediate response to extrauterine life but should be combined with a thorough assessment immediately after birth. The following sequence will provide important information. You may reorder this sequence as the infant's sleep and wakefulness state or physical condition warrants. A thorough assessment should be done with each well-child appointment throughout infancy.

The infant is **supine** on a warming or examination table with an overhead heating element. The infant may be nude except for a diaper.*

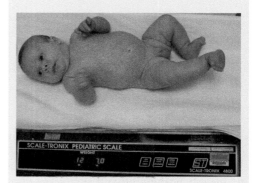

Vital Signs

Note pulse, respirations, and temperature.

Measurement

Weight, length, and head circumference are measured and plotted on growth curves for the infant's age.

General Appearance

1. Body symmetry, spontaneous position, flexion of head and extremities, and spontaneous movement.
2. Skin color and characteristics; any obvious deformities.
3. Symmetry and positioning of the facial features.
4. Alert, responsive affect.
5. Strong, lusty cry.

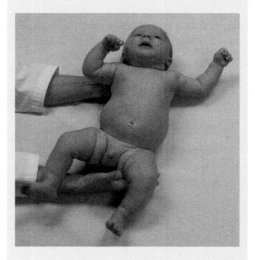

Chest and Heart

1. Inspect the skin condition over the chest and abdomen, chest configuration, and nipples and breast tissue.
2. Note movement of the abdomen with respirations, and note any chest retraction.
3. Palpate apical impulse and note its location; chest wall for thrills; tactile fremitus if the infant is crying.
4. Auscultate breath sounds, heart sounds in all locations, and bowel sounds.

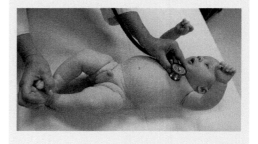

*Note: The diaper was removed to show body position and symmetry.

Sequence	Selected Photos

Abdomen

1. Inspect the shape of the abdomen and skin condition.
2. Inspect the umbilicus; count vessels (newborn); note condition of cord or stump (immediate neonatal period); note any hernia.
3. Palpate skin turgor.
4. Palpate lightly for muscle tone, liver, spleen tip, and bladder.
5. Palpate deeply for kidneys, any mass.
6. Palpate femoral pulses, inguinal lymph nodes.
7. Percuss all quadrants.

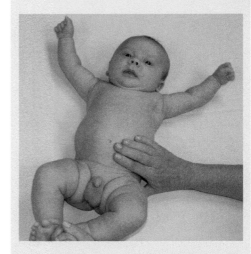

Head and Face

1. Note molding after delivery, any swelling on cranium, bulging of fontanel with crying or at rest.
2. Palpate fontanels, suture lines, and any swellings.
3. Inspect positioning and symmetry of facial features at rest and while the infant is crying.

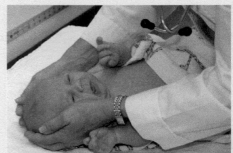

To open the neonate's eyes, support the head and shoulders and gently lower the baby backward or ask the parent to hold the baby over his or her shoulder while you stand behind the parent.

Eyes

1. Inspect the lids (edematous in the neonate), palpebral slant, conjunctivae, any nystagmus, and any discharge.
2. Using a penlight, elicit the pupillary reflex, blink reflex, and corneal light reflex; assess tracking of moving light.
3. Using an ophthalmoscope, elicit the red reflex.

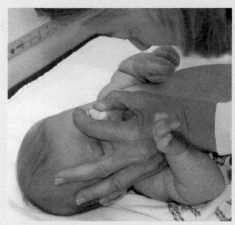

Ears

1. Inspect size, shape, alignment of auricles, patency of auditory canals, any extra skin tags or pits.
2. Note the startle reflex in response to a loud noise.
3. Palpate flexible auricles.

(Defer otoscopic examination until the end of the complete examination.)

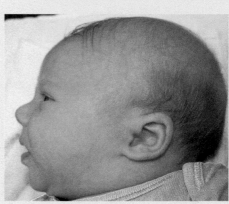

Sequence	Selected Photos

Nose

1. Determine the patency of the nares.
2. Note the nasal discharge, sneezing, and any flaring with respirations.

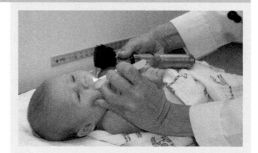

Mouth and Throat

1. Inspect the lips and gums, high-arched intact palate, buccal mucosa, tongue size, and frenulum of tongue; note absent or minimal salivation in neonate.
2. Note the rooting reflex.
3. Insert a gloved little finger, note the sucking reflex, and palpate the palate.

Neck

1. Lift the shoulders and let the head lag to inspect the neck: note midline trachea, any skinfolds, and any lumps.
2. Palpate the lymph nodes, the thyroid, and any masses.
3. While the infant is supine, elicit the tonic neck reflex; note a supple neck with movement.

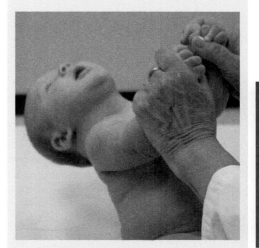

Upper Extremities

1. Inspect and manipulate, noting ROM, muscle tone, and absence of scarf sign (elbow should not reach midline).
2. Count fingers, count palmar creases, and note color of hands and nail beds.
3. Place your thumbs in the infant's palms to note the grasp reflex; then wrap your hands around infant's hands to pull up and note the head lag.

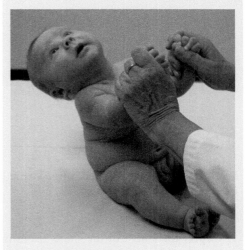

Lower Extremities

1. Inspect and manipulate the legs and feet, noting ROM, muscle tone, and skin condition.
2. Note alignment of feet and toes, look for flat soles, and count toes; note any syndactyly.
3. Test Ortolani sign for hip stability.
4. Check plantar grasp reflex (present until 8 to 10 months).
5. Check Babinski → fanning of toes until 24 months.

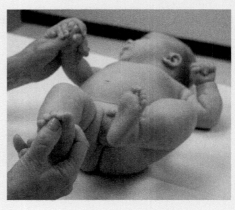

Objective Data

Sequence	Selected Photos

Genitalia

1. *Females.* Inspect labia and clitoris (edematous in the newborn), vernix caseosa between labia, and patent vagina.
2. *Males.* Inspect position of urethral meatus (do not retract foreskin), strength of urine stream if possible, and rugae on scrotum.
3. *Males.* Palpate the testes in the scrotum.

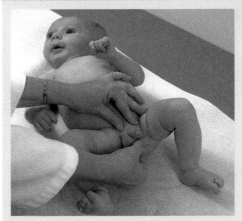

Lift the infant under the axillae and hold him or her facing you at eye level.

Neuromuscular

1. Note shoulder muscle tone and the infant's ability to stay in your hands without slipping.
2. Rotate the neonate slowly side to side; note the doll's eye reflex.
3. Turn the infant around so that his or her back is to you; elicit the stepping reflex and the placing reflex against the edge of the examination table.

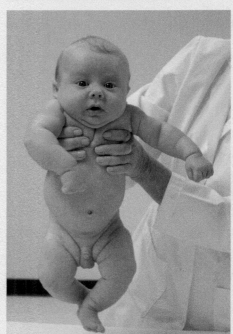

Turn the infant over and hold him or her prone in your hands, or place the infant prone on the examination table.

Spine and Rectum

1. Inspect the length of the spine, trunk incurvation reflex, and symmetry of gluteal folds.
2. Inspect intact skin; note any sinus openings, protrusions, or tufts of hair.
3. Note patent anal opening. Check for passage of meconium stool during the first 24 to 48 hours after birth.

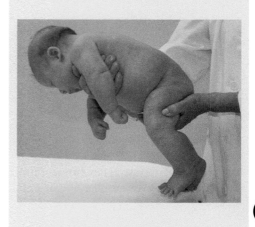

Sequence	Selected Photos

Final Procedures

1. With an otoscope, inspect the auditory canals and tympanic membranes. Ask the caregiver to hold the infant during the otoscopic exam.
2. Elicit the Moro reflex by letting the infant's head and trunk drop back a short way, jarring crib sides, or making a loud noise.

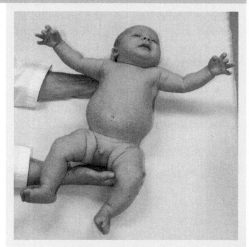

The Young Child

Review the developmental considerations in preparing for an examination of the young child in Chapter 8. The preschool child displays developing initiative and takes on tasks independently. This child is cooperative, helpful, and easy to involve. However, he or she fears body injury and may recoil from invasive procedures (e.g., tongue depressor, otoscope). The young schoolchild is developing industry. During the examination the child is cooperative and interested in learning about the body.

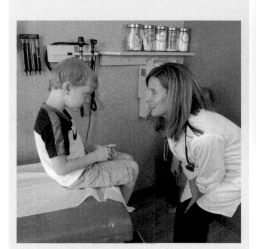

The Health History

1. Collect the history, including developmental data. Include the child in history taking as appropriate.
2. During the history note data on general appearance.

General Appearance

1. Note child's ability to amuse himself or herself while the caregiver speaks.
2. Note caregiver and child interaction.
3. Note gross- and fine-motor skills as the child plays with toys.

Gradually focus on and involve yourself with the child, at first in a "play" period.
4. Evaluate developmental milestones by using a Denver II test: gait, jumping, hopping, standing on one foot, building a tower, and throwing a ball.
5. Evaluate posture while the child is sitting and standing. Evaluate alignment of the legs and feet while the child is walking.
6. Evaluate speech acquisition.
7. Evaluate vision, hearing ability.
8. Evaluate social interaction.

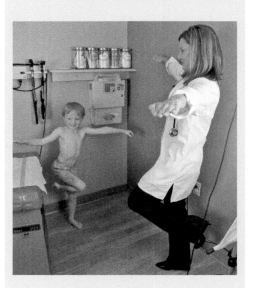

Sequence	Selected Photos

The preschooler and young schoolchild are willing to undress. Leave shorts and underpants on until the genital examination. Talk to the child and explain the steps in the examination. Use games. Have the child blow on the pinwheel as you listen to lung sounds. The pinwheel can go home as a present. The young child usually feels comfortable on the examination table. With the school-age child, talk about school, family, friends, music, sports. Demonstrate equipment to this curious child. Allow the child to sit on a caregiver's lap if he/she is uncomfortable on the exam table.

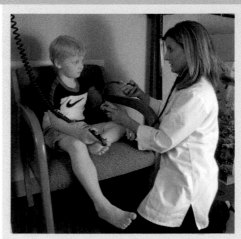

Measurement

Height, weight, temperature, blood pressure.

Upper Extremities

1. Inspect arms and hands for alignment, skin condition; inspect fingers and note palmar creases.
2. Palpate and count the radial pulse.
3. Test biceps and triceps reflexes with a reflex hammer.

Head, Face, and Neck

1. Inspect the size and shape of the head and symmetry of facies.
2. Palpate the cervical lymph nodes, trachea, and thyroid gland.

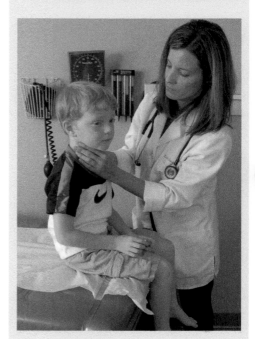

Eyes

1. Inspect the external structures. Note any palpebral slant.
2. With a penlight, test the corneal light and pupillary light reflexes.
3. Ask the child to follow your finger or a moving penlight for cardinal positions of gaze.
4. If indicated, perform the cover test, covering the eye with your thumb in a young child or using an index card.
5. Inspect conjunctivae and sclerae.
6. With an ophthalmoscope, check the red reflex. Inspect the fundus as much as possible.

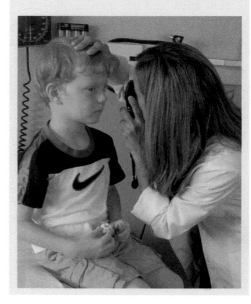

Sequence	Selected Photos

Nose

1. Inspect the external nose and skin condition.
2. With a penlight, inspect the nares for foreign body, mucosa, septum, and turbinates.

Mouth and Throat

1. With a light source, inspect the mouth, buccal mucosa, teeth and gums, tongue, palate, and uvula. Use a tongue blade as the last resort.

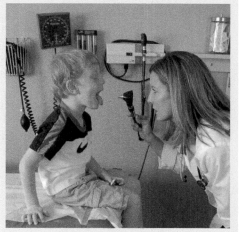

Ears

1. Inspect and palpate the auricles. Note any discharge from the auditory meatus. Check for any foreign body.
2. With an otoscope, inspect the ear canals and tympanic membranes. Gain cooperation by encouraging the child to handle the equipment or to look in the parent's ear as you hold the otoscope. Inspect the canal, then the tympanic membrane for color, position, landmarks, and integrity.

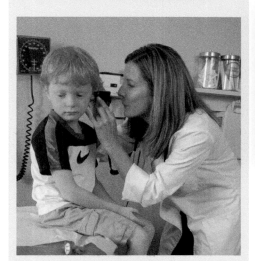

Posterior Thorax

1. Inspect the posterior chest: configuration, skin characteristics, symmetry of shoulders and muscles.
2. Palpate for lumps or tenderness, length of spinous processes.
3. Percuss over lung fields.
4. Auscultate breath sounds, comparing side to side in upper and lower lung fields; note any adventitious sounds.

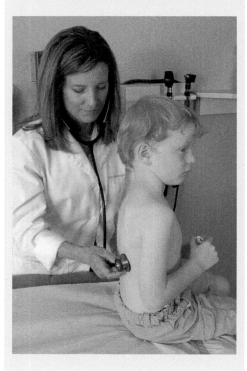

Objective Data

| **Sequence** | **Selected Photos** |

Objective Data

Anterior Thorax, Heart, and Lungs

1. Inspect size, shape, and configuration of chest cage. Assess respiratory movement.
2. Inspect pulsations on the precordium. Note nipple and breast development.
3. Palpate apical impulse and note location, chest wall for thrills, any tactile fremitus.
4. Auscultate breath sounds and heart sounds in all locations; count respiratory rate and heart rate.
5. Listen to S_1 and S_2 across the precordium; note any murmurs.

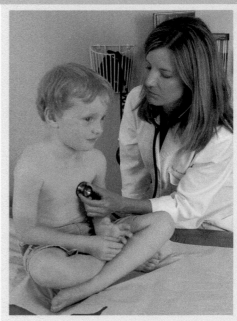

Abdomen

1. Inspect shape of abdomen, skin condition, and periumbilical area.
2. Auscultate bowel sounds.
3. Palpate skin turgor, muscle tone, liver edge, spleen, kidneys, and any masses.
4. Palpate the femoral pulses. Compare strength with radial pulses.
5. Palpate inguinal lymph nodes.

Genitalia

1. Inspect the external genitalia.
2. On males palpate the scrotum for testes. If masses are present, transilluminate.

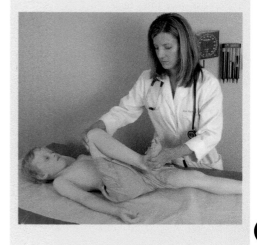

Lower Extremities

1. Note alignment of legs and skin condition.
2. Note alignment of feet. Inspect toes and longitudinal arch.
3. Check range of motion of hips, knees, ankles.
4. Palpate the dorsalis pedis pulse.
5. Gain cooperation with reflex hammer. Elicit plantar, Achilles, and patellar reflexes.

Sequence	Selected Photos

Examining Young Children

The examination is rewarding and fun. At the end you will have made a new friend.

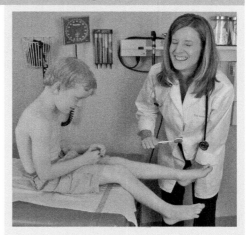

The Adolescent

The sequence for the examination is the head-to-toe format described in the adult section. Recall that the major task of adolescence is to develop a self-identity. The adolescent is increasingly self-conscious and introspective. For a well-person exam, keep the adolescent in street clothes and work around them.

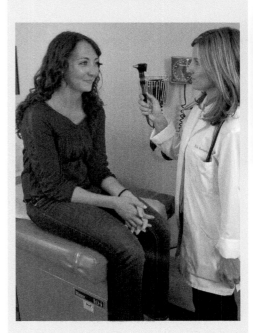

Position Sitting Up

Proceed with the head, eyes, ears, neck, and thoracic exam with the adolescent upright at the edge of the exam table.

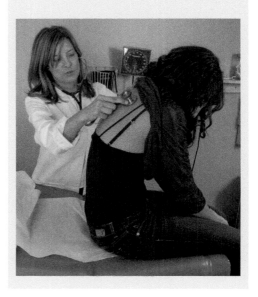

Objective Data

Sequence	Selected Photos

Position Supine

Conduct the cardiac, abdomen, and lower extremity examination next.

For the inguinal area place a drape over the lower abdomen and ask the adolescent to unzip and lower the jeans under the drape. Pant legs can be pulled up to examine the lower legs and feet.

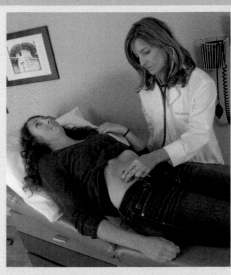

CHAPTER 30

Bedside Assessment and Electronic Documentation

http://evolve.elsevier.com/Jarvis/

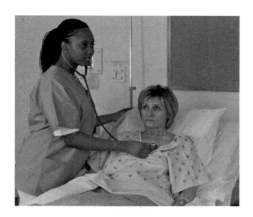

In a hospital setting the patient requires a complete head-to-toe physical examination upon admission but does not require subsequent complete head-to-toe assessments every day of his or her stay. He or she *does* require a consistent specialized examination that focuses on certain parameters. You will need to check the policy within your facility to identify frequency of these specialized assessments. In high-acuity units such as an intensive care unit, the assessment may be completed every 4 hours, whereas on a basic medical-surgical unit the frequency may be every 12 hours. Note that some measurements such as daily weights, abdominal girth, or the circumference of a limb must be taken very carefully.

The utility of such measurements depends entirely on the consistency of the procedure from nurse to nurse.

Also remember that many assessments must be done frequently throughout the course of a shift. This chapter outlines the initial assessment that will allow you to get to know your patient. As you perform this sequence, take note of anything that will need continuous monitoring, such as an abnormal blood pressure or pulse oximetry reading, or adventitious breath sounds. If there is no protocol in place for a particular assessment situation, then use your nursing judgment to determine how often you need to check on the person's status; it is very easy to be distracted by call lights and alarms as the shift progresses.

The need for multiple assessments of each patient highlights the need for efficiency in the hospital setting. Your assessments must be thorough and accurate, yet you must be able to complete them rapidly without seeming hurried.

The basic assessment applies to adults in medical, surgical, and step-down care areas. In the intensive care setting additional assessments are necessary based on patient acuity and additional lifesaving equipment that may be in use. Each assessment must be individualized to each adult, and the findings must be integrated into your complete knowledge base regarding the patient. This includes what you read in the chart, what you hear in report, and the results of any laboratory tests and diagnostic imaging that are available.

Sequence	Selected Photos

Wash your hands immediately in front of the patient upon entry to the room. If the person is not already in bed, help the person into bed. Raise the bed to a level that is comfortable for you. Remember proper body mechanics.

The Health History

On your way into the room, verify that any necessary markers or flags are in place at the doorway regarding conditions such as isolation precautions, latex allergies, or fall precautions. Once in the room, introduce yourself as the nurse, and let the patient know how long you will be the nurse.

Make direct eye contact, and do not allow yourself to be distracted by intravenous (IV) pumps or other equipment as you ask how he or she is feeling and how he or she spent the previous shift. Refer to what you have heard from the previous shift in the process of your own questioning; this alleviates the patient's frustration at answering the same questions every time he or she encounters a new staff member. Assess for pain: "Are you currently having any pain or discomfort?" Be sure to ask follow-up questions as appropriate. You

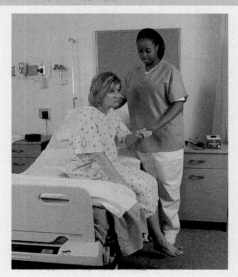

Normal Range of Findings	Abnormal Findings

should know when the last pain medication was given and what is ordered for pain management. Determine whether further dosing is needed or whether you need to contact the provider for additional orders. Confirm IV solution and rate, patient-controlled analgesia pump settings (if applicable), or epidural setting (if applicable). Assess the IV site, epidural site (if applicable), and any indwelling drains (if applicable). Assessment of the epidural site and drains can be combined with the appropriate body system.

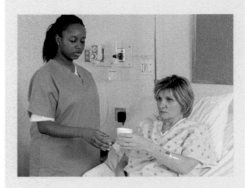

Offer water as a courtesy (if appropriate), but also note the physical data this gives you: the person's ability to hear, to follow directions, to cross the midline, and especially to swallow. Note data on the General Appearance in the following list. Complete your initial overview by verifying that the correct name band has been applied to the wrist, and ask the patient to state his or her name and date of birth.

General Appearance

1. Facial expression: Appropriate to the situation.
2. Body position: Relaxed and comfortable or tense, in pain.
3. Level of consciousness: Alert and oriented, attentive to your questions, responds appropriately.
4. Skin color: Even tone consistent with racial heritage.
5. Nutritional status: Weight appears in healthy range, fat distribution even, hydration appears healthy.
6. Speech: Articulation clear and understandable, pattern fluent and even, content appropriate.
7. Hearing: Responses and facial expression consistent with what you have said.
8. Personal hygiene: Ability to attend to basic hygiene needs such as brushing teeth and bathing.

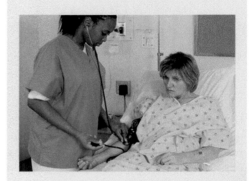

Measurement

1. Measure baseline vital signs (VS): Temperature, pulse, respirations, blood pressure (BP). Note which arm to avoid for BP because of surgery or IV access. Collect and document VS more frequently if patient is unstable or if patient condition changes. Know that VS are the ultimate responsibility of the nurse—the nursing assistant is not responsible for interpretation.
2. Pulse oximetry—Maintain ≥92% unless otherwise specified. Check pulse oximetry as ordered and as needed per nursing judgment. May need to monitor oxygen saturation continuously if patient is lethargic, receiving oxygen, or receiving narcotic medications for pain management.
3. Ask patient to rate pain level on a 0-to-10 scale at this and every subsequent visit or VS measure. Note patient's ability to tolerate pain.
4. If pain medication given, note response in 15 minutes for IV administration or 1 hour for oral dosing.

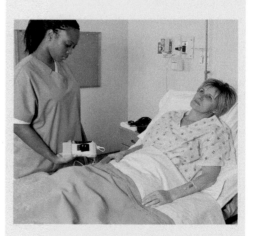

Neurologic System

1. Eyes open spontaneously to name.
2. Motor response is strong and equal bilaterally.
3. Verbal response makes sense; speech is clear and articulate.
4. Pupil size in mm and reaction, R and L.
5. Muscle strength, R and L upper, using hand grips.
6. Muscle strength, R and L lower, pushing feet against your palms.
7. Any ptosis, facial droop.
8. Sensation (omit unless indicated).
9. Communication.
10. Ability to swallow.

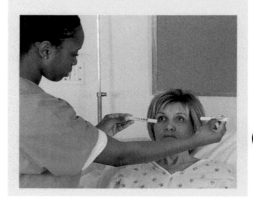

Sequence	Selected Photos

Objective Data

Respiratory System

1. Oxygen by mask, nasal cannula; check fitting and patient comfort.
2. Note FIO_2.
3. Respiratory effort.
4. Auscultate breath sounds, comparing side to side:
   Posterior lobes: Left upper, right upper, left lower, right lower.
   NOTE: If patient is unable to sit up, have patient roll or ask for help to turn patient to the side.
   Anterior lobes: Right upper, left upper, right middle and lower, left lower.
5. Cough and deep breathe. Any mucus? Check color and amount.
6. Incentive spirometer if ordered—Encourage patient to use every hour for 10 inspirations. If pulse oximetry percentage drops or adventitious sounds are heard, encourage use more frequently.

Cardiovascular System

1. Auscultate rhythm at apex: Regular, irregular? (Do NOT listen over gown.)
2. Check apical pulse against radial pulse, noting perfusion of all beats.
3. Assess heart sounds in all auscultatory areas: First with diaphragm, repeat with bell.
4. Check capillary refill for prompt return.

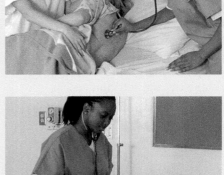

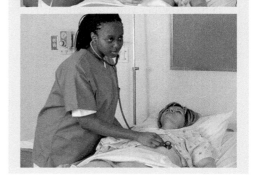

Sequence	Selected Photos

5. Check pretibial edema.
6. Palpate posterior tibial pulse, right and left.
7. Palpate dorsalis pedis pulse, right and left.
   NOTE: Be prepared to assess pulses in the lower extremities by Doppler if you cannot find them by palpation.

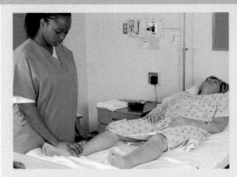

Skin

1. Note skin color, consistent with person's racial or ethnic heritage.
2. Palpate skin temperature; expect warm and dry.
3. Pinch a fold of skin under the clavicle or on the forearm to note mobility and turgor.
4. Note skin integrity, any lesions, and the condition of any dressings. Note any bleeding or infection, but do not change dressing until after physical examination.
5. Assess IV site, and note surrounding skin condition.
6. Complete any standardized scales used to quantify the risk for skin breakdown.
7. Verify that any air loss or pressure loss surfaces being used are properly applied and operating at the correct settings.

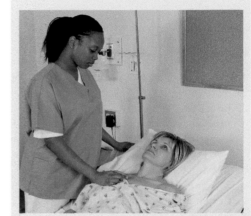

Abdomen

1. Assess contour of abdomen: Flat, rounded, protuberant.
2. Listen to bowel sounds.
3. Check any drains for color and amount of drainage and insertion site integrity.
4. Inquire whether passing flatus or stool.
5. Knowing diet orders, determine whether patient is tolerating ice chips, liquids, solids. Order correct diet as it is advanced. Note whether patient is at high risk for nutrition deficit.

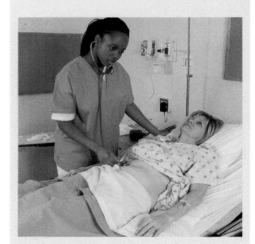

Genitourinary

1. Inquire whether voiding regularly. NOTE: Needs to void within 4 to 6 hours after surgery.
2. Check urine for color, clarity.
3. If Foley catheter in place, check color, quantity, clarity of urine with every VS check.
4. If urine output is below the expected amount, perform a bladder scan according to agency protocol. Is the problem in the production of urine or its retention?

Sequence	Selected Photos

Activity

1. Know activity orders; if on bed rest, head of bed should be elevated. Is patient at high risk for skin breakdown?
2. Are sequential compression devices (SCDs) or thromboembolic disease (TED) hose in place? SCDs must be on patient 22 out of 24 hours to be effective.
3. If ambulatory, assist patient as he or she sits up and transfers to a chair.
4. Note any assistance needed, how movement is tolerated, distance walked to chair, ability to turn and sit.
5. Assess need for any ambulatory aid or equipment.
6. Complete any standardized scales used to quantify the patient's risk for falling.
7. Initiate or continue appropriate Plan of Care. Check whether any core measures apply, such as heart failure. Implement core measures as appropriate.
8. Document assessment findings before leaving the room if possible.
9. Note examination findings requiring immediate attention[a]:
   - High or low BP (≤90 or ≥160 mm Hg systolic)
   - High or low temperature (≤97° or ≥100° F)
   - High or low heart rate (≤60 or ≥90 bpm)
   - High or low respirations (≤12 or ≥28/min)
   - O_2 saturations ≤92%
   - Low or no urine output (≤30 mL/hr or ≤240 mL/8 hr)
   - Dark amber or bloody urine (except for urology patients)
   - Postop nausea and/or vomiting
   - Pain not controlled with medication; any unusual pain such as chest pain
   - Bleeding
   - Altered level of consciousness (LOC), confusion, or difficulty arousing
   - Sudden restlessness and/or anxiety

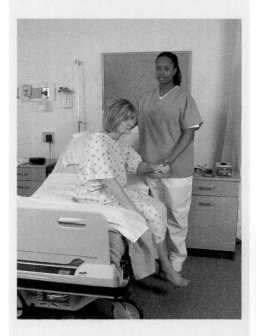

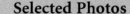

Objective Data

[a]Use nursing judgment and refer to agency policy and provider orders to determine when immediate follow up is necessary.

ELECTRONIC HEALTH RECORDING

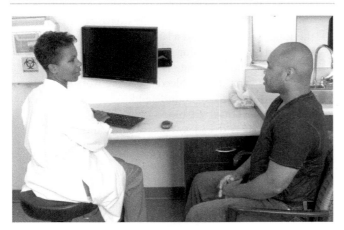

The use of technology at the bedside extends far beyond the standard equipment. Most hospitals and clinics use an electronic health record (EHR) system. EHRs replace the paper medical record, placing all relevant patient information in an easily accessible electronic system. EHRs do not include billing and scheduling systems, but focus instead on patient information. EHRs allow clinicians to access a lifetime of data to treat patients more effectively. Traditional medical records may be in a variety of locations, limiting availability; and poor penmanship can make older medical records illegible.

The federal government encourages the adoption and meaningful use of EHRs through the Health Information Technology for Economic and Clinical Health Act of 2009. The use of EHRs has increased steadily since 2008, with a ninefold increase in basic EHR adoption.[2] Basic EHR adoption includes the use of the EHR in at least one clinical unit, whereas comprehensive adoption requires each function (e.g., clinical notes, medication records, consultation requests, nursing orders, and laboratory results) to be adopted by all clinical units. EHR adoption is more prevalent among larger community and academic medical centers. Rural hospital use of EHR systems has increased significantly with at least 8 in 10 small, rural, and critical access hospitals adopting basic EHRs.[2]

Patient Safety

The meaningful use of EHRs, which include provider order entry and clinical decision support, may increase patient safety and quality care. EHRs allow all providers, regardless of geographic location, to access the health information, place orders, and receive timely patient status updates. No longer does a provider have to be on the clinical unit to retrieve test results, vital signs, or the most recent nurse's or provider's note. EHRs improve the coordination of care, facilitate safe and effective care, and assure the use of evidence-based guidelines.[4]

Many health care organizations also require providers to enter their own orders instead of allowing nurses to accept verbal or telephone orders. Computer provider order entry (CPOE) has decreased prescribing errors.[6] Well-designed EHR systems can notify providers of potential medication interactions, dosage adjustments for renal patients or advanced age, and additional required testing (e.g., laboratory tests). Nurses can benefit from EHR use in medication administration through the use of bar-code scanners, which identify both the patient and the medication. Checklists built into EHR systems can help clinicians identify health care–associated infections or patients at risk for these infections. Checklists are also used for depression and suicide screening.[5,7] Although no system is perfect, a well-designed EHR system can increase patient safety when successfully integrated into the workflow of a clinic or hospital. Unfortunately, EHRs are not always developed with the end user in mind, which can lead to issues with patient safety.[3] As EHR use becomes the standard of care, more research is needed to determine the specific factors that contribute to patient safety and increased quality of care.

USING SBAR FOR STAFF COMMUNICATION

Throughout this text we have used the SOAP acronym (**Sub**jective, **O**bjective, **A**ssessment, **P**lan) to organize assessment findings into written or charted communication. Now we turn to organizing assessment data for *verbal* communication (e.g., calls to providers, nursing shift reports, patient transfers to other units). For all these verbal reports we use the SBAR framework: **S**ituation, **B**ackground, **A**ssessment, **R**ecommendation.

SBAR was first developed by the U.S. military to standardize communication and prevent misunderstandings. In the hospital, communications errors contribute to sentinel events and are responsible, in part, for 30% of malpractice claims.[1] Standardized hand-off tools such as SBAR improve verbal communication and reduce medical errors. SBAR is a standardized framework to transmit important in-the-moment information. Using SBAR will keep your message concise and focused on the immediate problem yet give your colleague enough information to grasp the current situation and make a decision. To formulate your verbal message, use these four points:

Situation. What is happening right now? Why are you calling? State your name, your unit, patient's name, room number, patient's problem, when it happened or when it started, how severe it is.

Background. Do not recite the patient's full history since admission. Do state the data pertinent to this moment's problem: admitting diagnosis, when admitted, and appropriate immediate assessment data (e.g., vital signs,

pulse oximetry, change in mental status, allergies, current medications, IV fluids, laboratory results).

Assessment. What do YOU think is happening in regard to the current problem? If you do not know, at least state which body system you think is involved. How severe is the problem?

Recommendation. What do you want the provider to do to improve the patient's situation? Here you offer probable solutions. Order more pain medication? Come and assess the patient?

Review the following examples of SBAR communication.

Situation 1

S: This is Bill on the Oncology Unit. I'm calling about Daniel Meyers in room 8417. He has refused all oral medications since 0800.

B: Daniel is a 59-year-old male with multiple myeloma. He was admitted for an autologous stem cell transplant and received chemotherapy 10 days ago. Now he is 5 days' post auto transplant. Vital signs are stable. He is alert and oriented. IVs are dextrose 5% water running at 50 mL/hr. As of 1 hour ago, he is feeling extreme nausea, refusing all food and oral meds.

A: I think the chemo he had pre-transplant is hitting him now. Nausea is getting worse despite giving Zofran.

R: I'm concerned that he cannot stay hydrated, and he needs his meds. I need you to please change the IV rate and change all scheduled oral meds to IV. I also think we need to add an additional PRN antiemetic.

Situation 2

S: This is Andrea. I'm the nurse taking care of Max Goodson in 6443. His condition has changed, and his most recent vital signs show a significant drop in blood pressure.

B: Max is 40 years old with a history of alcoholism. He was admitted through the ED last night with abdominal pain and a suspected GI bleed. His BPs have been running in the 130s/80s. He just had a large amount of liquid maroon stool and reported feeling dizzy. I rechecked his vitals; his BP is 88/50 and heart rate is 104.

A: I'm worried that his GI bleed is getting worse.

R: Will you order a STAT complete blood count and place an order to transfuse red blood cells if his hemoglobin is below 8 g/dL? Also can you please come and assess? I think we may need to drop an NG tube and lavage him.

REFERENCES

1. Bronk, K. L. (2017). *The Joint Commission issues new sentinel event alert on inadequate hand-off communication.* https://www.jointcommission.org/the_joint_commission_issues_new_sentinel_event_alert_on_inadequate_hand-off_communication/.
2. Henry, J., Pylypchuk, Y., Searcy, T., et al. (2016). *Adoption of electronic health record systems among the U.S. non-federal acute care hospitals: 2008-2015.* ONC Data Brief, no. 35. Office of the National Coordinator for Health Information Technology: Washington, DC.

3. Kellogg, K. M., Fairbanks, R. J., & Ratwani, R. M. (2017). EHR usability: Get it right from the start. *Biomed Instrum Technol,* *51*(3), 197–199.

4. Krenn, L., & Schlossman, D. (2017). Have electronic health records improved quality of patient care? *PM R, 9,* S41–S50.

5. Loudon, H., Nentin, F., & Silverman, M. E. (2016). Using clinical decision support as a means of implementing a universal postpartum depression screening program. *Arch Womens Ment Health, 19,* 501–505.

6. Prgomet, M., Li, L., Niazkhani, Z., et al. (2016). Impact of commercial computerized provider order entry (CPOE) and clinical decision support systems (CDSSs) on medication errors, length of stay, and mortality in intensive care units: A systematic review and meta-analysis. *J Am Med Inform Assoc, 24,* 413–422.

7. Sudhanthar, S., Thakur, K., Sigal, Y., et al. (2015). Improving validated depression screen among adolescent population in primary care practice using electronic health records (EHR). *BMJ Qual Improv Rep, 21*(4).

CHAPTER 31

The Pregnant Woman

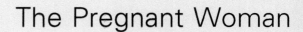
STRUCTURE AND FUNCTION

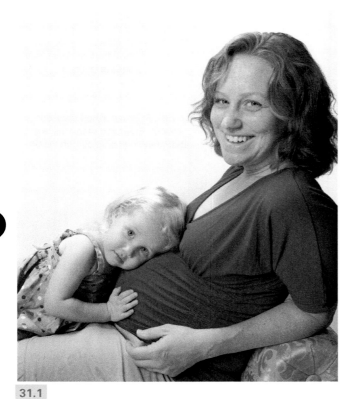

31.1

THE ENDOCRINE PLACENTA

So much happens inside the pregnant uterus before the new family can feel fetal movements (Fig. 31.1).

When the fertilized ovum enters the uterus, it is called the **blastocyst** and continues to divide, differentiate, and grow rapidly. Specialized cells in the blastocyst produce human chorionic gonadotropin (hCG), which stimulates the corpus luteum to continue to make progesterone. The blastocyst implants into the wall of the uterus, which may cause a small amount of vaginal bleeding. A specialized layer of cells becomes the **placenta,** which produces progesterone to support the pregnancy at 7 weeks and takes over this function completely from the corpus luteum at about 10 weeks.

The placenta functions as an endocrine organ and produces several hormones. These hormones help in the growth and maintenance of the fetus, and they direct changes in the woman's body to prepare for birth and lactation. The hCG stimulates the rise in progesterone during pregnancy, supports the corpus luteum, supports deep implantation of the placenta into the uterine wall, and helps maintain viability of the fetus.[14] Progesterone maintains the endometrium around the fetus, increases the alveoli in the breasts, and keeps the uterus in a quiescent state. Estrogen stimulates the duct formation in the breasts, increases the weight of the uterus, and increases certain receptors in the uterus that are important at birth.

The average length of pregnancy is 280 days from the first day of the last menstrual period (LMP), which is equal to 40 weeks, 10 lunar months, or 9 calendar months. Note that this includes the 2 weeks when the follicle was maturing but before conception actually occurred. Pregnancy is divided into three trimesters: (1) the first 12 weeks, (2) from 13 to 27 weeks, and (3) from 28 weeks to delivery.

A woman who is pregnant for the first time is called a **primigravida.** After she delivers, she is called a **primipara.** A **multigravida** is a pregnant woman who has previously been pregnant; she is a **multipara** after delivery. Any pregnant woman might be called a *gravida.* Commonly used abbreviations are G (gravida), P (para), T (term), PT (preterm deliveries), A (abortion—missed, therapeutic, voluntary), L (living children). It may be written as $G_5 \ P_4 \ T_3 \ PT_0 \ A_2 \ L_3$.

CHANGES DURING NORMAL PREGNANCY

Pregnancy is diagnosed by three types of signs and symptoms. **Presumptive signs** are those that the woman experiences, such as amenorrhea, breast tenderness, nausea, fatigue, and increased urinary frequency. **Probable signs** are those detected by the examiner such as an enlarged uterus. **Positive signs** of pregnancy are those that are direct evidence of the fetus, such as the auscultation of fetal heart tones (FHTs) or positive cardiac activity on ultrasound (US). During pregnancy, a woman's body goes through a variety of physical changes that affect nearly every system in the body (Fig. 31.2).

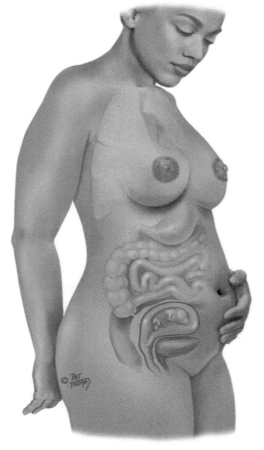

CARDIORESPIRATORY: Respiration more efficient, cardiac output increases, blood volume increases with oxygen and nutrient needs of the fetus.

HORMONAL: hCG from developing placenta detected in mother's urine. Extra fat is laid down in hips and thighs as energy source for breastfeeding.

URINARY: Increased frequency of urination as growing fetus presses on bladder.

BREASTS: Swelling, tenderness, visible veins, prominent tubercles, areolae enlarged and dark.

GASTROINTESTINAL: Nausea and vomiting, "morning sickness" common at any time of day. Constipation common.

METABOLIC: Calcium, iron, and folate are drawn from mother's stores for baby's bones and blood.

UTERUS: Amenorrhea (missed periods). Enlarging uterus rises in the abdomen beginning at 12th week.

31.2

(©Pat Thomas, 2018.)

First Trimester

After the blastocyst (developing fertilized ovum) implants in the uterus, the serum hCG becomes positive when it is first detectable in maternal serum at approximately 8 to 11 days after conception.

The following menstrual period is missed, and then hCG can be detected in the urine. Breast tingling and tenderness begin as the rising estrogen levels promote mammary growth and development of the ductal system; progesterone stimulates both the alveolar system and mammary growth. More than half of all pregnant women have nausea and vomiting. The cause is unclear but may involve the hormonal changes of pregnancy, low blood sugar, gastric overloading, slowed peristalsis, and an enlarging uterus. Fatigue is common and may be related to the initial fall in metabolic rate that occurs in early pregnancy.[9]

Estrogen and possibly progesterone cause hypertrophy of the uterine muscle cells, and uterine blood vessels and lymphatics enlarge. The uterus becomes globular in shape and compresses the bladder, which results in urinary frequency.

Early first-trimester blood pressures (BP) reflect pre-pregnancy values. In the 7th gestational week BP begins to drop until midpregnancy as a result of falling peripheral vascular resistance. Systemic vascular resistance decreases from the vasodilatory effect of progesterone and prostaglandins and possibly because of the low resistance of the placental bed.[12] The BP gradually returns to the nonpregnant baseline by term.

At the end of 9 weeks the embryonic period ends, and the fetal period begins, at which time major structures are present.[15] FHTs can be heard by Doppler US between 9 and 12 weeks. The uterus may be palpated just above the symphysis pubis at about 12 weeks.

Second Trimester

After weeks 12 to 16, the nausea, vomiting, fatigue, and urinary frequency of the first trimester improve. The woman recognizes fetal movement ("quickening") at approximately 18 to 20 weeks (the multigravida earlier). Breast enlargement continues, and **colostrum,** the precursor of milk, may be expressed from the nipples. Colostrum is yellow in color and contains more minerals and protein but less sugar and fat than mature milk. It also contains antibodies, which are protective for the newborn during its first days of life until mature milk production begins.[11]

The areolae and nipples darken because estrogen and progesterone have a melanocyte-stimulating effect, and melanocyte-stimulating hormone levels escalate from the 2nd month of pregnancy until delivery. For the same reason the midline of the abdominal skin becomes pigmented and is called the **linea nigra.** You may note **striae gravidarum** ("stretch marks") on the breast, abdomen, and other areas of weight gain.

During the second trimester systolic BP may be 2 to 8 mm Hg lower and diastolic BP 5 to 15 mm Hg lower than prepregnancy levels.[11] This drop is most pronounced at 20 weeks and may cause symptoms of dizziness and faintness, particularly after rising quickly. Stomach displacement from the enlarging uterus and altered esophageal sphincter and gastric tone as a result of progesterone predispose the woman to heartburn. Intestines are also displaced by the growing uterus, and tone and motility are decreased because of the action of progesterone, often causing constipation. The gallbladder, possibly resulting from the action of progesterone on its smooth muscle, empties sluggishly and may become distended. The stasis of bile, together with the increased cholesterol saturation of pregnancy, predisposes some women to gallstone formation.

Progesterone and, to a lesser degree, estrogen cause increased respiratory effort during pregnancy by increasing tidal volume. Hemoglobin, and therefore oxygen-carrying capacity, also increases. Increased tidal volume causes a slight drop in partial pressure of arterial carbon dioxide ($PaCO_2$), causing the woman to occasionally have dyspnea.[11]

With the rise of hCG in the first trimester, there is a transient decrease in thyroid-stimulating hormone (TSH) levels between 8 and 14 weeks' gestation. Plasma iodine levels decrease, allowing a transient increase in thyroid gland size in approximately 15% of pregnant women.

Cutaneous blood flow is augmented during pregnancy, caused by decreased vascular resistance, presumably helping to dissipate heat generated by increased metabolism. Gums may hypertrophy and bleed easily. This condition is called **gingivitis** or **epulis of pregnancy** because of growth of the capillaries of the gums.[11] For the same reason nosebleeds may occur more frequently than usual.

FHTs are audible by fetoscope (as opposed to Doppler imaging) at approximately 17 to 19 weeks. The fetal outline is palpable through the abdominal wall at approximately 20 weeks.

Third Trimester

Blood volume, which increased rapidly during the 2nd trimester, peaks in the middle of the 3rd trimester at approximately 45% greater than the prepregnancy level and plateaus thereafter. This volume is greater in multiple gestations.[12] Erythrocyte mass increases by 20% to 30% (caused by an increase in erythropoiesis and mediated by progesterone, estrogen, and placental chorionic somatomammotropin). However, plasma volume increases slightly more, causing a slight hemodilution and a small drop in hematocrit.

BP slowly rises again to approximately the prepregnancy level.[11]

Uterine enlargement causes the diaphragm to rise and the shape of the rib cage to widen at the base. Decreased space for lung expansion may cause a sense of shortness of breath. The rising diaphragm displaces the heart up and to the left. Cardiac output, stroke volume, and force of contraction are increased. The pulse rate rises 15 to 20 beats/min.[12] Because of the increase in blood volume, a functional systolic murmur, grade 2/6 or less, can be heard in more than 95% of pregnant women.[12]

Edema of the lower extremities may occur as a result of the enlarging fetus impeding venous return and from lower colloid osmotic pressure. The edema worsens with dependency, such as prolonged standing. Varicosities, which have a familial tendency, may form or enlarge from progesterone-induced vascular relaxation. Also causing varicosities is the engorgement caused by the weight of the full uterus compressing the inferior vena cava and the vessels of the pelvic area, resulting in venous congestion in the legs, vulva, and rectum. Hemorrhoids are varicosities of the rectum that are worsened by constipation, which occurs from relaxation of the large bowel by progesterone.

Progressive lordosis (an inward curvature of the lumbar spine) occurs to compensate for the shifting center of balance caused by the anteriorly enlarging uterus, predisposing the woman to backaches (Fig. 31.3). Slumping of the shoulders and anterior flexion of the neck from the increasing weight of the breasts may cause aching and numbness of the arms and hands as a result of compression of the median and ulnar nerves in the arm,[15] commonly referred to as *carpal tunnel syndrome.*

Approximately 2 weeks before going into labor, the primigravida experiences engagement (also called *lightening* or

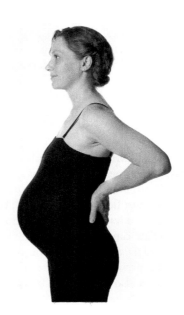

31.3

Structure and Function

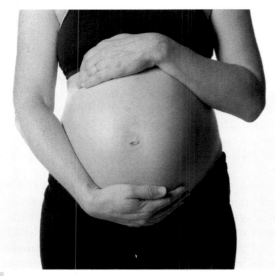

31.4

dropping), when the fetal head moves down into the pelvis (Fig. 31.4). Symptoms include a lower-appearing and smaller-measuring fundus, urinary frequency, increased vaginal secretions from increased pelvic congestion, and increased lung capacity. In the multigravida the fetus may move down at any time in late pregnancy or often not until labor. In preparation for labor the cervix begins to thin (efface) and open (dilate). A thick **mucus plug,** formed in the cervix as a mechanical barrier during pregnancy, is expelled at variable times before or during labor.

From 37 0/7 weeks to 38 6/7 weeks a pregnancy is considered *early term*, 39 0/7 weeks to 40 6/7 weeks is considered *full term*, and 41 0/7 weeks to 41 6/7 weeks is considered *late term*.[1] Elective early-term delivery should be avoided unless medically indicated due to increased risk of neonatal complications such as respiratory distress, hypoglycemia, and neonatal mortality.[3] Medical indications for early-term delivery include placental/uterine issues (e.g., placenta previa), fetal issues (e.g., growth restriction), maternal issues (e.g., hypertension, diabetes), and obstetric issues (e.g., premature preterm rupture of membranes).[2]

Determining Weeks of Gestation

The expected date of delivery, or EDD, being 280 days from the first day of the LMP, may be calculated by using **Nägele's rule.** That is, determine the first day of the last normal menstrual period (normal in timing, length, premenstrual symptoms, and amount of flow and cramping). Using the first day of the LMP, add 7 days and subtract 3 months. This date is the EDD. This date can then be used with a pregnancy wheel on which the EDD arrow is set; the present date will be pointing to the present week's gestation. The number of weeks of gestation also is estimated by physical examination, by measurement of the hCG, and most accurately by ultrasound (US) +/−2 to 3 days.

 DEVELOPMENTAL COMPETENCE

The number of teen pregnancies in the United States continues to decline; however, over 200,000 babies are born annually to teens ages 15 to 19 years. The majority (73%) of teen pregnancies occur in teens who are 18 to 19 years of age.[13] African-American and Latina teens have the highest rate of pregnancies, at nearly twice the rate of non-Hispanic white teens. Socioeconomic factors (e.g., low income and low educational level) appear to influence teen pregnancy rates, and teens in the child welfare system (e.g., foster children) are more than twice as likely to become pregnant.[10]

Teen pregnancies pose serious medical risks for both mother and fetus, such as toxemia and low-birth-weight infants; it is unclear whether these risks are the result of biologic or social factors, prolonged labor, or postpartum complications. Unfortunately, women who are under 20 years old at the time of conception are the least likely age-group to seek early prenatal care.[19]

Other risks for the pregnant adolescent are psychosocial. This young woman is at risk for the downward cycle of poverty, beginning with an incomplete education, failure to limit family size, and continuing with failure to establish a vocation and become independent. She may be unprepared emotionally to be a mother. Her social situation may be stressful. She may not have the support of her family, her partner, or his family. Medical risks for the pregnant adolescent are generally related to poverty, inadequate nutrition, substance abuse, sometimes sexually transmitted infections (STIs), poor health before pregnancy, and emotional and physical abuse from her partner, family, and peers.

On the other hand, many women are delaying childbearing, and since the advent of assisted fertility, more women older than 35 years are now becoming pregnant. Women after age 35 years are often more prepared emotionally and financially to parent; however, they are more at risk for infertility and age-related anomalies. Fertility declines with advancing maternal age because of a decrease in the number and health of eggs to be ovulated, a decrease in ovulation, endometriosis, and early-onset menopause.

The risk for Down syndrome increases from about 1 in 1340 at age 25 to 1 in 940 at age 30, 1 in 353 at age 35, 1 in 85 at age 40, and 1 in 35 at age 45.[18] Women ages 35 years and older or with a history of a genetic abnormality may be offered genetic counseling and a variety of prenatal diagnostic and screening tests. Three invasive prenatal diagnostic options are chorionic villi sampling (CVS), performed between weeks 11 and 13; amniocentesis, performed between weeks 15 and 20; and percutaneous umbilical blood sampling, performed between weeks 18 and 22. All are associated with a small risk of complications and miscarriage.

A variety of noninvasive testing options are available. The noninvasive options are considered screening tests because none can definitively diagnose anomalies in the fetus. US nuchal translucency measures the clear space in the tissues of the back of the baby's neck. It is used in combination with maternal serum levels of pregnancy-associated plasma protein-A and hCG. Free-cell DNA testing can also be done. Because a small amount of fetal DNA is found circulating in the maternal bloodstream, the test involves drawing the woman's blood and testing for a variety of fetal anomalies, including trisomy 21, trisomy 18, trisomy 13, and a variety of sex chromosome abnormalities.[7]

Prenatal screening in all women typically includes a fetal anatomy US during the second trimester and maternal blood tests. All screening and diagnostic tests should be an informed choice after pretest counseling. A positive result on any of the screening tests should be followed by appropriate counseling so that the mother can make an informed decision about next steps, including the need for further diagnostic testing.

Because the incidence of chronic diseases increases with age, women older than 35 years who are pregnant may have medical complications such as diabetes, obesity, and hypertension.[11] The increased incidence of hypertension causes an increase in placental abruption and preeclampsia. Hypertension in turn increases intrauterine growth restriction (IUGR). More women of advanced maternal age have placenta previa, placental abruption, uterine rupture, and cesarean deliveries. They have more spontaneous abortions, in part because of the increase in genetically abnormal embryos.

CULTURE AND GENETICS

Genetic disorders are diseases or defects that the baby inherits from the genes or chromosomes of one or both parents. As mentioned previously, the risk of having certain chromosomal disorders such as Down syndrome increases as a woman ages. Parents may also be carriers of genetic defects: cystic fibrosis is an inherited disorder of respiratory and gastrointestinal sequelae; Jews of Eastern European descent may have the risk of having children with Tay-Sachs, a metabolic disorder; African-American parents may pass sickle cell anemia on to a child. Also, a pregnant woman may be exposed to toxins such as alcohol or cigarette smoke that increase the risk of birth defects. It is beyond our scope here to describe all aspects of genetic counseling. There are many options for prenatal testing either before or after conception. It is important that the parents make an informed choice about whether to pursue such testing, and their choice must be respected.

The obesity epidemic in the United States affects maternal and fetal outcomes. Women who are obese (BMI ≥30 kg/m^2) have reproductive challenges. Obese women have more difficulty becoming pregnant and sustaining pregnancy, and they are more likely than their normal-weight counterparts to suffer from a variety of complications, including gestational diabetes and gestational hypertension. Obesity in pregnancy also leads to an increased risk for neonatal complications.[11] Racial disparities in obesity are well documented, with nearly 75% of non-Hispanic black women of childbearing age being classified as overweight or obese. One study found that approximately 10% of the racial disparity in birth outcomes between non-Hispanic white and non-Hispanic black women can be explained by obesity.[17] Obesity and excessive weight gain during pregnancy also increase the risk of cesarean delivery in all age-groups.[8]

Gestational diabetes mellitus (GDM) disproportionately affects certain racial and ethnic groups with Asians, African Americans, and Hispanics having the highest prevalence. While obesity is a risk factor for developing GDM, the majority of Asian Americans diagnosed with GDM are normal weight, so it appears that other factors affect their risk of developing GDM. Family history and advanced maternal age increase the risk of GDM in all ethnic groups but disproportionately affect certain groups.[23] Asian Americans with GDM are more likely to develop diabetes later in life than other ethnic groups.[24] Based on racial and ethnic differences in the prevalence of GDM, the American College of Obstetricians and Gynecologists now recommends early GDM screening for women who are African American, American Indian, Asian American, Hispanic, or Pacific Islander.[6]

OPIOID EPIDEMIC AND PREGNANCY

The use of tobacco, alcohol, or illicit drugs during pregnancy has significant consequences on the fetus because many of the drugs pass easily through the placenta. The use of tobacco, marijuana, prescription pain medications, or illegal drugs is associated with a 2 to 3 times greater risk of stillbirth, and regular use of drugs can lead to dependence in the newborn.[20]

Screening for drug and alcohol use is an essential part of the initial prenatal visit for all pregnant women. Making screening a routine part of care reduces stigmatization and can improve maternal and neonatal outcomes. Appropriate referrals are important to help the woman with an opioid use disorder during pregnancy. A nonjudgmental attitude is essential when treating a pregnant woman with an opioid use disorder. A multidisciplinary approach, without criminal sanctions, improves outcomes.[5]

The opioid epidemic in the United States is of grave concern for the health of women and infants. Infants born to pregnant woman who abuse opioid pain medications or illicit drugs (e.g., heroin) are at risk for neonatal abstinence syndrome (NAS). NAS increased fivefold between 2000 and 2012, which translates to an infant with NAS born every 25 to 30 minutes in the United States.[16,22] Clinical characteristics of NAS may include poor feeding, jitteriness, high-pitched crying, irritability, diarrhea, unstable temperature, and even seizures.[21,22] NAS can be treated with medications and supportive therapy.

Appropriate prenatal care is imperative in mothers who are addicted to substances or who report drug use during pregnancy. The use of methadone or buprenorphine in the pregnant woman addicted to heroin or opioid pain medications is preferred to medically supervised withdrawal. The use of methadone or buprenorphine provides a steady state of the drug to the fetus, reduces risk-taking behavior by the woman (e.g., reusing needles), improves compliance with prenatal care, and improves neonatal outcomes. Untreated addiction during pregnancy places the woman and fetus at risk.

Some pregnant women may rely on prescription opioid therapy for the treatment of chronic pain. In the case of medically necessary pain management, it is important to help the woman minimize opioid use by considering alternative therapies (e.g., physical therapy, behavioral approaches) and using nonopioid pain medications.[5]

SUBJECTIVE DATA

1. Menstrual history
2. Gynecologic history
3. Obstetric history
4. Current pregnancy
5. Medical history
6. Review of systems
7. Nutritional history
8. Environment/hazards

Examiner Asks	Rationale
1. Menstrual history • When was the first day of your last menstrual period (LMP) that was normal in timing, premenstrual symptoms, length, amount of flow, cramping? • Number of days in cycle? Certainty of LMP?	Using Nägele's rule, calculate the expected date of delivery (EDD) using date of LMP. With a pregnancy wheel, determine the current number of weeks of gestation. LMP may be uncertain because of hormone contraceptives or irregular menses.
2. Gynecologic history • Ever had surgery of the cervix (colposcopy, biopsy, loop electrosurgical excision [LEEP] procedure)? Uterus? Fallopian tubes?	Cervical surgery may increase the risk for cervical insufficiency, preterm cervical dilation, and preterm delivery. Uterine surgery increases the risk for uterine rupture during pregnancy and labor.
• Pap tests: Any history of abnormal? Tested for HPV?	Because more women delay childbearing, there may be an increase in gynecologic cancers during pregnancy.
• Any history of genital herpes, gonorrhea, chlamydia, syphilis, pelvic inflammatory disease (PID)?	STIs increase the risk for premature rupture of membranes, preterm labor/preterm delivery (PTL/PTD), postpartum maternal and fetal infections, or birth defects (herpes).
• Have you been tested for HIV? When? What was the result? Ever had a blood transfusion? Used a needle to take street drugs? Had a sexual partner who had any HIV risk factors?	HIV screening *must* be offered to all pregnant women to decrease the risk for transmission to the fetus. Breastfeeding is contraindicated for the HIV-positive mother because the virus is in breast milk.
• What is your sexual preference?	Woman with same-sex partner may use assisted reproduction; thus important to support this couple.
• Have you had a mammogram, breast biopsy, breast surgery?	As U.S. women delay childbearing, incidence of breast cancer may increase, posing difficult treatment options.

Examiner Asks	Rationale
3. Obstetric history[a] • Number of times pregnant? Number of term or preterm deliveries? Preterm labor? Number of spontaneous miscarriages, elective abortions, or ectopic pregnancies? • How were previous pregnancies and deliveries for you? • Ever had a cesarean section? If so, what was the indication? What type of uterine incision was made? Have you ever had a vaginal birth after a cesarean section (VBAC)?	An obstetric history helps guide prenatal care. The subjective quality of previous experiences affects current pregnancy. The vertical, or "classical," incision has increased risk for rupture and mandates that all deliveries be by cesarean birth. The "low transverse" or horizontal incision carries a low risk, and subsequent deliveries may be vaginal. Note that the direction of the skin scar does not necessarily tell how the uterus was incised.
4. Current pregnancy • Was the pregnancy planned? How do you feel about it? How does the baby's father or your partner feel about the pregnancy? Other family members? • Experienced any vaginal bleeding? When? How much? What color? Accompanied by any pain? Occurs after sex? (Affirm here that sex is safe during uncomplicated pregnancy.) • How have you been feeling? • Experienced abdominal pain? When? Where in your abdomen? Accompanied by vaginal bleeding? • Experiencing any edema? Where and under what circumstances? • How does the baby move on a daily basis?	The woman may need help in gathering her support group. Inviting significant others to future visits affirms their importance and supports involvement. Vaginal bleeding may indicate threatened abortion, cervicitis, or ectopic pregnancy in 1st trimester and must be investigated. However, a friable cervix may bleed harmlessly after sex and not hurt the fetus. Breast tenderness or fatigue is normal during pregnancy. Nausea and vomiting usually begin between weeks 4 and 5, peak between weeks 8 and 12, and resolve. Persistent severe nausea and vomiting are hyperemesis and may require medical treatment. Common causes in early pregnancy are spontaneous abortion, ectopic pregnancy, urinary tract infection (UTI), and round ligament discomfort. Late pregnancy causes are premature labor, placental abruption, and HELLP syndrome (see Table 31.1, Preeclampsia, p. 821). In the 3rd trimester differentiate the normal weight-dependent edema of pregnancy from the edema of preeclampsia. Fetal movement is an excellent indicator of fetal health. In the 3rd trimester clinicians assign women to count fetal movements.

[a]This information is recorded best in a grid format. See sample forms in the Laboratory Manual. It is separated here to include the rationale.

Examiner Asks	Rationale

• What are your plans for breastfeeding this baby?

Arrange reading, classes, and other support for the woman who is breastfeeding for the first time or the woman with an unsuccessful earlier experience.

5. Medical history

• Do you take any prescribed, over-the-counter, or herbal medications?

Screen all medications to establish safety during pregnancy.
Prevents prescribing error.

• Do you have allergies to medications or foods? If so, which type of reaction? Latex?
• Ever had German measles (rubella)?

This disease is highly teratogenic, especially in 1st trimester. Instruct the woman who has not had rubella to avoid small children who are ill.

• Ever had chickenpox?

Rarely, varicella causes congenital anomalies. The nonimmune woman should avoid exposure.

• Do you smoke cigarettes? How many? For how many years? Ever tried to quit? Drink any alcohol? How many times per week? Use any street drugs?

Explain the danger of these substances in pregnancy. Smoking increases the risk for ectopic pregnancy, spontaneous abortion, low birth weight, prematurity, preterm premature rupture of membranes, HTN in pregnancy, placental abruption, and sudden infant death syndrome. Alcohol increases the risk to the fetus for fetal alcohol syndrome (see Table 14.2, p. 268). Cocaine use is associated with congenital anomalies, a fourfold increased risk for abruptio placentae, and fetal addiction. Narcotic-addicted infants may have developmental delays or behavioral disturbances. Refer to a counseling/support program and periodic toxicology screening. Refer to a smoking-cessation program.

• Do you have a regular exercise program? Which type?

Regular exercise in pregnancy may reduce risk for gestational HTN.

• Have you ever had your vitamin D level checked?

Vitamin D is essential for maternal response to the calcium demands of the fetus for growth and bone development.

6. Review of systems
• Your weight before pregnancy? (Calculate BMI.)
• When did you last see the dentist? Need any dental work?

Baseline needed to evaluate changes.
Gums may be puffy or bleed easily in pregnancy, predisposing caries. Poor dental hygiene can lead to PTD, low-birth-weight babies, and neonatal death. Dental care is an important part of prenatal care.

• Have you had HTN or kidney disease?

Renal disease or HTN increases risk for preeclampsia.

Examiner Asks	Rationale
• Do you have diabetes? On oral hypoglycemics, insulin injection, or insulin pump? Did you have diabetes during a previous pregnancy?	Diabetes is carefully managed during pregnancy to avoid serious complications such as a macrosomic infant and cesarean delivery. Consider early screening and nutritional interventions.
• Have you had UTIs?	The hormonal milieu of pregnancy predisposes the woman to UTIs. Pregnancy may mask symptoms. A serious UTI may irritate the uterus, threatening preterm labor. Educate the woman in measures to prevent UTIs.
• Have you had depression or any other mental disorder? Have you taken any medications for mental health disorders?	Increases risk for pregnancy and postpartum depression. Some medications prescribed for mental health disorders negatively affect the fetus. Help her to prepare a support network. Counseling helps navigate the developmental challenges of becoming a mother.
• Do you feel safe in your relationship or home environment?	Intimate partner violence may escalate during pregnancy.
• Are you in a relationship with someone who physically or emotionally abuses or threatens you?	Most women will not freely offer this information. You must ask these questions at the appropriate time and in a nonthreatening manner.
• Has anyone forced you to have sexual activities against your will?	Incest or other abuse increases risk for dysfunctional labor and cesarean delivery.
7. Nutritional history	
• Do you follow a special diet? Are you vegetarian? Eat fish? What types? Teach her to avoid sea fish (swordfish, mackerel) because of mercury concentration. Also teach her to avoid raw eggs, soft cheeses, and unpasteurized dairy foods and sliced meats from delicatessens because of risk of *Listeria, Salmonella,* and toxoplasmosis.	A special diet may have nutritional risk. Help achieve adequate nutrition within the confines of her diet. Refer to dietitian.
• Any food intolerance? Or food craving? Taking prenatal vitamins, folic acid, iron?	A food intolerance, such as lactose intolerance limiting calcium intake, might affect the woman's and fetus's nutrition.
8. Environment/hazards	
• What is your occupation? What are the physical demands of the work? Are you exposed to any strong odors, chemicals, radiation, or other harmful substances? Or potentially harmful physical contact?	Hazards? Possible teratogenic exposures? The woman who is rubella nonimmune may be advised not to continue working in a daycare center. Suitability for pregnancy? The woman whose job requires long hours of standing or heavy lifting may be unable to work if signs of PTL occur.
• Do you consider your food and housing adequate?	Refer for state and federal programs to help with food, housing, or other needs.
• How do you wear your seatbelt when driving?	For maternal and fetal safety, instruct the woman to place the lap belt below the uterus and to use the shoulder strap.

OBJECTIVE DATA

PREPARATION

Many women are anxious during the pelvic exam. Verbally prepare the woman for what will happen during the examination before touching her. Save the pelvic examination for last; by that time the woman will be more comfortable with your gentle, informing manner. Communicate all findings as you go along to demonstrate your respectful affirmation of her control and responsibility in her own health and health care and that of her child.

Ask the woman to empty her bladder before the examination, reserving a clean-catch specimen for dipping for protein and glucose and for urinalysis, if required. Before the examination weigh her on the office scale and compute the BMI. Provide the woman with an escort or chaperone during examinations.

Give the woman a gown and drape. Begin the examination with the woman sitting on the exam table, wearing the gown, her lap covered by a drape.

Help her to a seated position to check her BP. Help her lie down for the breast, abdominal, and extremity examination. Use the lithotomy position for the pelvic examination (see Chapter 27). In the 2nd and 3rd trimesters keep her back elevated to a 30- or 45-degree angle. This increases comfort by avoiding the compression of the descending aorta and inferior vena cava by the pregnant uterus.

EQUIPMENT NEEDED

Stethoscope, BP cuff
Centimeter measuring tape
Doppler fetal heart rate (FHR) monitor and gel
Reflex hammer
Urine collection containers
Dipsticks for checking urine for glucose and protein
Equipment needed for pelvic examination as noted in Chapter 27.

Normal Range of Findings	Abnormal Findings

General Survey

Observe the woman's state of nourishment; a healthy BMI is 19 to 25. Note her grooming, posture, mood, and affect, which reflect her mental state. Throughout the examination observe her maturity and ability to attend and learn so you can plan your teaching of the information that she needs to successfully complete a healthy pregnancy.

Before beginning the exam, obtain vital signs and a current weight. Weight should be measured at each prenatal visit to monitor for appropriate weight gain.

Undernourished or obese. A 1st-trimester weight loss of ≥5% prepregnancy weight is worrisome and may indicate hyperemesis gravidarum.

Poor grooming, a slumped posture, and a flat affect may be signs of depression and risk for postpartum depression. Poor grooming may reflect a lack of resources and need for a social service referral.

Monitor for signs of preeclampsia throughout pregnancy.

Weight gain monitored throughout pregnancy. Provide counseling on appropriate weight gain as needed. Adequate nutrition is important throughout pregnancy.

Skin

Note any scars (particularly those of previous cesarean delivery). Many women have skin changes, such as acne or skin tags, during pregnancy that may spontaneously resolve after the pregnancy. Vascular spiders may be present on the upper body. Some women have **chloasma,** known as the *mask of pregnancy,* which is a butterfly-shaped pigmentation of the face. Note the presence of the **linea nigra,** a hyperpigmented line that begins at the sternal notch and extends down the abdomen through the umbilicus to the pubis (Fig. 31.5). Also note **striae,** or stretch marks, in areas of weight gain, particularly on the abdomen and breasts of multiparous women. These marks are bright red when they first form, but they will shrink and lighten to a silvery color (in the lightly pigmented woman) after the pregnancy.

Multiple bruises suggest physical abuse.

Note any facial edema after 20 weeks' gestation, which may signal preeclampsia.

Tracks (scars along easily accessed veins) may indicate IV drug use. Dilated breast veins may be used during pregnancy for IV drug use.

Objective Data

Normal Range of Findings	Abnormal Findings

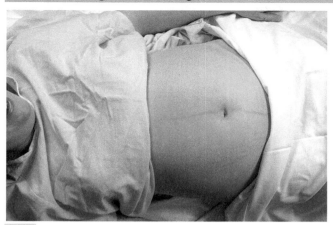

31.5

PUPPP *(p*ruritic *u*rticarial *p*apules and *p*laques of *p*regnancy) is the most common pruritic skin rash during pregnancy, more common in white and nulliparous women. It has an intensely pruritic erythematous eruption that appears late in pregnancy in the abdomen and thighs. The incidence is about 1 in 160 pregnancies. Women who are primiparas or have multiple fetuses are at higher risk.[12]

Mouth

Mucous membranes should be dark pink and moist. Gum hypertrophy (surface looks smooth, and stippling disappears) may occur normally during pregnancy (pregnancy gingivitis). Bleeding gums may be from estrogen stimulation, which causes increased vascularity and fragility.

Neck

The thyroid may be palpable and feel full but smooth during the normal pregnancy of a euthyroid woman. It is stimulated by hCG.

Breasts

The breasts are enlarged (Fig. 31.6), perhaps with resulting striae, and may be very tender. The areolae and nipples enlarge and darken in pigmentation, the nipples become more erect, and "secondary areolae" (mottling around the areolae) may develop. The blood vessels of the breasts enlarge and may shine blue through a seemingly more translucent than usual chest wall. When auscultating, blood flow through these blood vessels can be heard and may be mistaken for a cardiac murmur. This sound is called the *mammary souffle* (SOO-FL). Montgomery tubercles, located around the areolae and responsible for skin integrity of the areolae, enlarge. Colostrum, a thick yellow fluid, may be expressed from the nipples.

Complaints of nasal irritation, nasal crusting, nasal stuffiness, or recurrent nosebleeds may indicate drug inhaling. Note that some nasal congestion and nosebleeds are normal during pregnancy due to increased blood volume.

Note any suspicious nevi or lesions (see Chapter 13). It is uncommon for nevi to enlarge or darken just because of pregnancy.

Pale mucous membranes indicate anemia.

Poor dental hygiene during pregnancy may lead to PTD or low-birth-weight infants.

Solitary nodules indicate neoplasm; multiple nodules usually indicate inflammation or a multinodular goiter. Significant diffuse enlargement occurs with hyperthyroidism, thyroiditis, and hypothyroidism.

Normal Range of Findings	Abnormal Findings

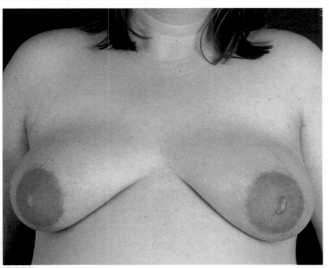

31.6 (Black, Ambros-Rudolph, Edwards, Lynch, 2008.)

Some nipples are flattened or inverted, which are common variations of normal. These can be corrected easily during pregnancy or with proper postpartum latching-on techniques. Take this opportunity in the examination to assure the pregnant woman that her breasts are "perfect breasts for breastfeeding."

The breast tissue feels nodular as the mammary alveoli hypertrophy. Take this opportunity to teach or reinforce breast self-examination (BSE). The woman should expect changes in the breast tissue during the pregnancy. Because of the lack of menses, instruct her to perform BSE periodically during her pregnancy.

Note any abnormal mass within the breast and refer for US. US of the breast(s) is used in lieu of mammograms during pregnancy and lactation.

Heart

Later in pregnancy you can palpate the apical impulse left of the midclavicular line and up to the 4th intercostal space because of the growing fetus. The pregnant woman often has a functional, soft, blowing systolic murmur that occurs as a result of increased blood volume. The murmur requires no treatment and will resolve after pregnancy.

Note any other murmur and refer. Valvular disease may need prophylactic antibiotics at delivery. Pregnancy places a large hemodynamic burden on the heart, and the woman with cardiac disease is managed closely.

Lungs

The lungs are clear bilaterally to auscultation with no crackles or wheezing. Shortness of breath is common in the 3rd trimester from pressure on the diaphragm from the enlarged uterus.

Women with asthma exacerbations during pregnancy may have an expiratory (and possibly inspiratory) wheeze.

Note any signs of respiratory infection: dyspnea, crackles, congested cough.

Peripheral Vascular

The legs may show diffuse, symmetric, bilateral pitting edema, particularly in the 3rd trimester and if the examination is occurring later in the day when the woman has been on her feet. Varicose veins in the legs are common in the 3rd trimester.

Edema, together with increased BP and proteinuria, is a sign of preeclampsia. Edema and pain in one leg occur with deep vein thrombosis (DVT) and warrant Doppler studies. Carefully evaluate any redness or red, hot, tender swelling to

Normal Range of Findings	Abnormal Findings

rule out phlebitis. Varicosities increase the risk for thrombophlebitis; she should not wear restrictive clothing or sit without moving legs for a long period. Varicosities will worsen with the weight and volume of pregnancy; support hose help minimize them.

Neurologic

Using the reflex hammer, check the biceps, patellar, and ankle deep tendon reflexes (DTRs). Normally these are 1+ or 2+ and equal bilaterally.

Brisk or greater than 2+ DTRs and clonus may be associated with elevated BP and cerebral edema in the preeclamptic woman.

Inspect and Palpate the Abdomen

Observe the shape and contours of the abdomen to discern signs of fetal position. As the woman lifts her head, you may see the **diastasis recti,** the separation of the abdominal muscles, which occurs during pregnancy, with the muscles returning together after pregnancy with abdominal exercise. When palpating, note the abdominal muscle tone, which grows more relaxed with each subsequent pregnancy. Note any tenderness; the uterus is normally nontender.

The fundus should be palpable abdominally from 12 weeks' gestation. Use the side of your hand and begin palpating centrally on the abdomen higher than you expect the uterus to be. Palpate down until you feel the fundus (the top of the uterus). Alternatively stand at the woman's right side facing her head (Fig. 31.7). Place the palm of your right hand on the curve of the uterus in the left lower quadrant and your left palm on the curve of the uterus in the right lower quadrant. Moving from hand to hand, allowing the curve of the uterus to guide you, "walk" your hands to where they meet centrally at the fundus.

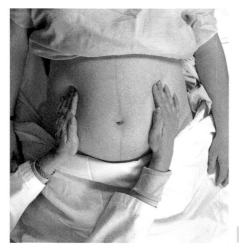

31.7

Use the centimeter measuring tape to measure the height of the fundus in centimeters from the superior border of the symphysis to the fundus (Fig. 31.8). After 20 weeks the number of centimeters should approximate the number of weeks of gestation in a woman with healthy body size and a singleton pregnancy. Beginning at 20 weeks you may feel fetal movement.

A lagging fundal height ≥2 cm may indicate intrauterine growth restriction (IUGR), transverse lie, or oblique presentation of the fetus. (See Table 31.2, Fetal Size Inconsistent With Dates, p. 822.)

Normal Range of Findings	Abnormal Findings

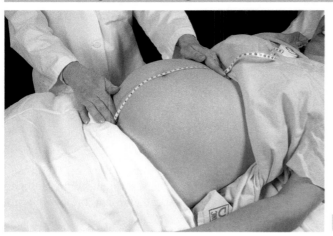

31.8

Leopold Maneuvers

In the 3rd trimester perform Leopold maneuvers to determine fetal lie, presentation, attitude, position, variety, and engagement. **Fetal lie** is the orientation of the fetal spine to the maternal spine and may be longitudinal, transverse, or oblique. **Presentation** describes the part of the fetus that is entering the pelvis first (i.e., vertex [head], breech, foot). **Attitude,** the position of fetal parts in relation to one another, may be flexed, military (straight), or extended. **Position** designates the location of a fetal part to the right or left of the maternal pelvis. **Variety** is the location of the fetal back to the anterior, lateral, or posterior part of the maternal pelvis. **Engagement** occurs when the widest diameter of the presenting part has descended into the pelvic inlet—specifically to the imagined plane at the level of the ischial spines.

Leopold's first maneuver is performed by facing the gravida's head and placing your fingertips around the top of the fundus (Fig. 31.9). Note its size, consistency, and shape. Imagine which fetal part is in the fundus. The breech feels large and firm. Because it is attached to the fetus at the waist, moving it between the thumb and fingers of the hand results in moving it slowly and with difficulty. In contrast, the fetal head feels large, round, and hard. When it is ballotted, it feels hard as you push it away and hard again as it bobs back against your fingers in an "answer." Note that the "bobbing" or "ballotting" sensation of the movement occurs because the head is attached at the neck and moves easily. If there is no part in the fundus, the fetus is in the transverse lie.

A fundal height >4 cm than expected occurs with multiple fetuses, excess amniotic fluid, or uterine myoma. Both conditions warrant US.

In patients who are obese, those with excessive amniotic fluid, or an anteriorly implanted placenta, Leopold's maneuvers are difficult to perform and interpret correctly.[11]

Malpresentations are confirmed by US (see Table 31.3, p. 823).

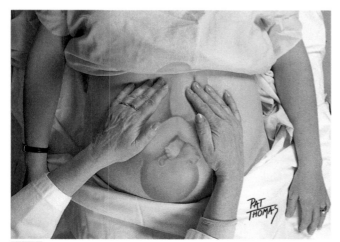

31.9 Leopold's first maneuver.

Normal Range of Findings	Abnormal Findings

For **Leopold's second maneuver,** move your hands to the sides of the uterus (Fig. 31.10). Note whether small parts or a long, firm surface is palpable on the woman's left or right side. The long, firm surface is the back. Note whether the back is anterior, lateral, or out of reach (posterior). The small parts, or limbs, indicate a posterior position when they are palpable all over the abdomen.

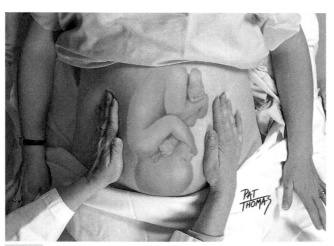

31.10   Leopold's second maneuver.

In **Leopold's third maneuver,** also called *Pawlik's maneuver,* ask the woman to bend her knees up slightly for comfort (Fig. 31.11). Grasp the lower abdomen just above the symphysis pubis between the thumb and fingers of one hand to determine which part of the fetus is there. If the presenting part is beginning to engage, it will feel "fixed." With this maneuver alone, it may be difficult to differentiate the shoulder from the vertex.

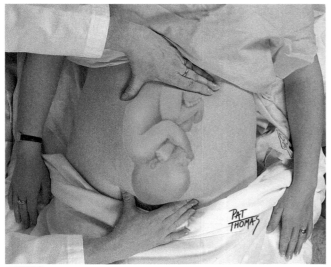

31.11   Leopold's third maneuver.

The **fourth maneuver** helps to determine engagement and, in the vertex presentation, to differentiate shoulder from vertex (Fig. 31.12). The woman's knees are still bent. Facing her feet, place your palms, with fingers pointing toward the feet, on either side of the lower abdomen. Pressing your fingers firmly, move slowly down toward the pelvic inlet. If your fingers meet, the presenting part is not engaged. If your fingers diverge at the pelvic rim, meeting a hard

Normal Range of Findings	Abnormal Findings

prominence on one side, this prominence is the occiput. This indicates that the vertex is presenting with a deflexed head (the face presenting). If your fingers meet hard prominences on both sides, the vertex is engaged in either a military or a flexed position. If your fingers come to the pelvic brim diverged but with no prominences palpable, the vertex is "dipping" into the pelvis or is engaged. In this case the firm object felt above the symphysis pubis in the third maneuver is the shoulder.

See Table 31.3, Malpresentations, p. 823.

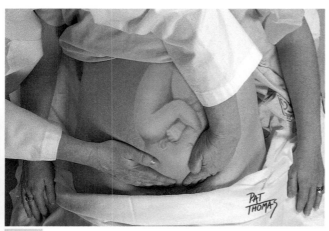

31.12 Leopold's fourth maneuver.

Auscultate the Fetal Heart Tones

FHTs are a positive sign of pregnancy. They can be heard by Doppler US at 8 to 10 weeks' gestation. They are auscultated best over the back of the fetus. After identifying the position of the fetus, use the heart tones to confirm your findings. Count the FHTs for 6 seconds and multiply by 10 to obtain the rate (Fig. 31.13). The normal rate is between 110 and 160 beats/min. Spontaneous accelerations of FHTs indicate fetal well-being.

If no FHTs are heard by Doppler by 12 weeks, verify fetal cardiac activity with US.

Further investigate any FHTs that are <110/minute or >160/minute or are irregular.

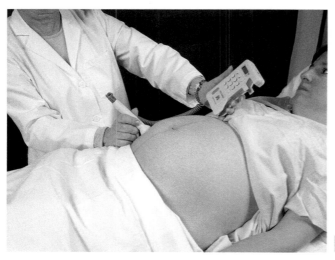

31.13

Differentiate the FHTs from the slower rate of the maternal pulse and the uterine souffle (the soft, swishing sound of the placenta receiving the pulse of maternal arterial blood) by palpating the mother's pulse while you listen.

All the abdominal findings are of interest to the woman; share them with her. Often she will want to listen to FHTs with her significant others.

Normal Range of Findings	Abnormal Findings

Pelvic Examination

Genitalia

Use the procedure for the pelvic examination described in Chapter 27. The enlargement of the labia minora is common in multiparous women. Labial varicosities may be present. The perineum may be scarred from a previous episiotomy or from lacerations. Note any hemorrhoids. Note any lesions on the symphysis pubis, labia, or perianal area.

Lesions may indicate an infection, condyloma, or genital herpes infection.

Speculum Examination

When examining the vagina, you may see **Chadwick sign,** the bluish, purplish discoloration and congested look of the vaginal wall and cervix from increased vascularity and engorgement (Fig. 31.14). Note the vaginal discharge. Vaginal discharge in pregnancy may be heavier in amount but should be similar in description to the woman's nonpregnant discharge and should not be associated with itching, burning, or an unusual odor (except that occasionally chapping of the vaginal area may be seen because of excessive moisture). Perform a wet mount or culture of the discharge when you are uncertain of its normalcy.

Many cervical infections or STIs are asymptomatic. Any cervical secretions that are purulent or mucopurulent (chlamydia or gonorrhea); yellow or green frothy (trichomoniasis); thin, white, gray, or milky, with a "fishy" odor (bacterial vaginosis); or thick, white, and clumpy (candidiasis) should be treated appropriately during the pregnancy.

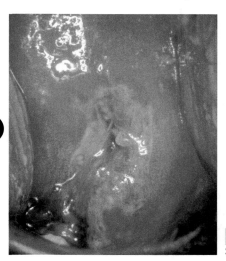

31.14 Chadwick sign. (Apgar, Brotzman, Spitzer, 2008.)

Note whether the cervix appears open. Note whether it is the smooth, round cervix with a dotlike external os of the nulliparous woman or the irregular multiparous cervix with an external os that appears more like a crooked line, the result of cervical dilation in a previous pregnancy. A friable cervix bleeds easily when touched with a cotton swab, cytobrush, or speculum because of increased vascularity. Advise the woman that small spotting may occur.

If you suspect cervicitis, obtain cultures.

Bimanual Examination

As described in Chapter 27, palpate the uterus between your internal and external hands. Note its position. The pregnant uterus may be rotated toward the right side as it rises out of the pelvis because of the presence of the descending colon on the left. This is called **dextrorotation.** Also, you may note **Hegar sign,** when the enlarged uterus bends forward on its softened isthmus between the 4th and 6th weeks of pregnancy.

Note the size and consistency of the uterus. In a singleton pregnancy the 6-week gestation uterus may seem only slightly enlarged and softened. The 8-week gestation uterus is approximately the size of an avocado, approximately 7 to 8 cm across the fundus. The 10-week gestation uterus is about the size of a grapefruit and may reach to the pelvic brim, but it is narrow and does not fill the pelvis from side to side; the 12-week gestation uterus will fill the pelvis. After

Objective Data

Normal Range of Findings	Abnormal Findings

12 weeks the uterus is sized from the abdomen. The multigravida uterus may be larger initially, and early sizing of this uterus may be less reliable for dating.

Softening of the cervix is called **Goodell sign.** When examining the cervix, note its position (anterior, midposition, or posterior), degree of effacement (or thinning, expressed in percentages assuming a ≥2-cm–long cervix initially), dilation (opening, expressed in centimeters), consistency (soft or firm), and the station of the presenting part (centimeters above or below the ischial plane) (Fig. 31.15).

Uterine fibroids (leiomyomas) may be felt during bimanual examination.

A shortened cervix is <2 cm and is associated with preterm labor or possible cervical insufficiency.

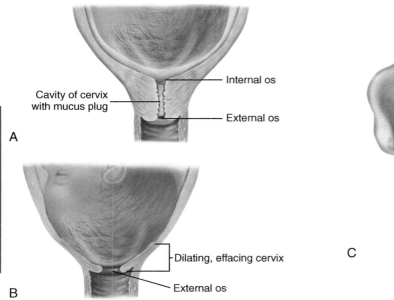

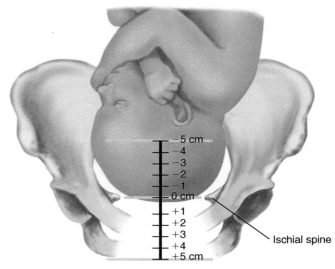

31.15 **A,** Cervix before labor. **B,** Cervix begins to efface and dilate. **C,** Station height of presenting part in relation to ischial spines.

The ovaries rise with the growing uterus. Always examine the adnexa to rule out the presence of a mass such as an ectopic pregnancy.

Adnexal enlargement and pain with palpation occur with ectopic pregnancy or ovarian mass.

To determine tone, ask the woman to squeeze your fingers as they rest in the vagina. Take this opportunity to teach the Kegel exercise, the squeezing of the vagina, which the woman can do to prepare for and recover from birth. (The woman can also identify the exercise of these muscles by stopping the flow of urine midstream, although she should do this only once and should usually let urine flow freely.) Direct the woman to squeeze slowly to a peak at the count of eight and then release slowly to the count of eight. You can prescribe this exercise to be performed 50 to 100 times a day.

Blood Pressure

After the examination take the BP when the woman is the most relaxed, in the semi-Fowler or upright position. Recheck an elevated pressure.

Gestational HTN is a persistent elevation of ≥140/90 mm Hg after the 20th week of gestation. Chronic HTN is found in women who have HTN before pregnancy or before the 20th week of gestation. These women are at higher risk for preeclampsia.[11]

Routine Laboratory and Radiologic Imaging Studies

At the first prenatal visit order a routine prenatal panel: a complete blood cell count, serology, rubella antibodies, HIV and hepatitis B screening, blood type and Rhesus factor, and antibody screening. Some providers screen for herpes

Normal Range of Findings	Abnormal Findings

simplex viruses I and II, thyroid function, and vitamin D level. Sickle-cell, cystic fibrosis, or thalassemia screening may be indicated. For some populations, a PPD/tine test may be indicated to rule out active tuberculosis or exposure to the disease. Obtain a Pap test with HPV screen at the initial visit along with cervical STI cultures.

Collect a clean-catch urinalysis at the initial prenatal visit to rule out cystitis. At each prenatal visit check the urine for protein and glucose. A clean-catch specimen is ideal for this dip because a random specimen may include vaginal secretions, which contain protein, skewing the results. For women with active substance abuse, check a urine toxicology screen.

The standard of care for US examinations is to have an US for fetal anatomic survey around 18 to 20 weeks of gestation.[4] The US is helpful in showing the age of the fetus, location of the placenta, fetal position, often the sex of the fetus, and the number of fetuses, and it may screen for certain birth defects. A cervical length measurement is recommended at 18 to 22 weeks, which can be useful to predict preterm birth. The maternal serum alpha-fetoprotein or "quad" screening is offered but is optional. Fetal nuchal translucency screening is offered as well but is optional. Women at high risk for genetic anomalies in the fetus may also be offered free cell fetal DNA testing. Regardless of the type of screening, women should be counseled on what to expect, what the results mean, and what follow-up testing may be recommended.

Antepartum fetal testing helps improve the perinatal outcome by decreasing stillbirth and long-term neurologic impairments of the fetus. This testing consists of monitoring fetal growth, amniotic fluid volume, biophysical profiling, and other potential fetal/maternal markers using ultrasonography. Fetal testing (nonstress test [NST] or contraction stress test [CST]) using electronic fetal monitors to graph and audibly hear the fetal heart rate and determine uterine activity is indicated for some conditions. The mother begins fetal movement counting at 28 weeks, which gives a good indication of fetal well-being.

DOCUMENTATION AND CRITICAL THINKING

Clinical Case Study 1

R.G. is a 27-year-old woman, gravida 2 para 1, who presents with her husband and daughter for her first prenatal visit.

SUBJECTIVE

R.G. is a full-time homemaker who completed 2 years of college. Last normal menstrual period (LNMP) was April 4 of this year (certain of date), with an expected date of delivery (EDD) of January 11 of next year, making her 10 weeks' gestation today. Her obstetric history includes a normal spontaneous vaginal delivery (NSVD) 3 years ago of a viable 7 lb, 12 oz female infant after an 8-hour labor without anesthesia, with a midline episiotomy. No complications of pregnancy, delivery, or the postpartum period. She breastfed her daughter, Ana, for 1 year. Present pregnancy was planned, and R.G. and her husband are pleased. R.G. is having breast tenderness and nausea on occasion, which resolves with crackers. No past medical or surgical conditions are present. She denies allergies. Family history is significant only for diet-controlled adult-onset diabetes in two maternal aunts.

OBJECTIVE

General: Appears well nourished and is carefully groomed. English is second language, and R.G. is fluent.
Skin: Light tan in color; surface smooth with no lesions; small tattoo noted on left forearm.
Mouth: Good dentition and oral hygiene. Oral mucosa pink; no gum hypertrophy. Thyroid gland not palpable.
Chest: Expansion equal, respirations effortless. Lung sounds clear bilaterally with no adventitious sounds. No CVA tenderness.
Heart: Rate 76 bpm, regular rhythm; S_1 and S_2 are normal, not accentuated or diminished, with soft, blowing systolic murmur Gr 2/6 at 2nd left interspace.

Breasts: Tender, without masses; with supple, everted nipples; no lesions. Breast self-exam reviewed.

Abdomen: No masses; bowel sounds present. No hepatosplenomegaly. Fundus nonpalpable. No inguinal lymphadenopathy noted.

Extremities: No varicosities, redness, or edema. Homan sign negative. DTRs 2+ and equal bilaterally. BP 110/68 mm Hg, sitting, right arm.

Pelvic: Bartholin, urethra, and Skene glands negative for discharge. Vagina: pink, with white, creamy, nonodorous discharge. Cervix: pink, closed, multiparous, 2 cm long, firm.

Uterus: 10-week size, consistent with dates, nontender, dextrorotated. FHTs heard with Doppler, rate 140s.

ASSESSMENT

Viable intrauterine pregnancy 10 weeks by reliable dates, size = dates.

R.G. and husband happy with pregnancy; she feels well.

Clinical Case Study 2

K.A. is a 30-year-old woman, gravida 9 para 7, who presents with an interpreter and her eldest daughter for her first prenatal visit.

SUBJECTIVE

K.A. is a full-time homemaker and runs a daycare facility within her home. She immigrated to the U.S. 5 years PTA with her husband and children. Her husband is employed. She lives in a one-bedroom apartment with her family. Her last menstrual period was May 28th of this year, with an EDD of March 5th of next year, making her 11 weeks' gestation today. She is a poor historian for her deliveries in Ethiopia other than one child "died in childbirth." She delivered her last child vaginally here in the U.S. without complications after 5 hours of labor. She is unsure of the baby's weight. She had a female circumcision as a child. She is having nausea with occasional vomiting, has breast tenderness, and 1 week ago experienced "pink" vaginal spotting, unrelated to intercourse. She is unsure of her family history. Both parents and all but one of her 7 siblings are deceased. This pregnancy is unexpected but okay. She is concerned about transportation to her appointments because her husband works days and she does not drive.

OBJECTIVE

General: Appears well nourished and is carefully groomed. English is 2nd language, but she understands some. Daughter who is present with her mom is well groomed and speaks English. Interpreter is present.

Skin: Dark tan in color, surface smooth, small scarring on left arm and both legs. No lesions or tattoos.

Mouth: Poor dentition. Oral mucosa pink, some gum hypertrophy. Thyroid gland palpable, but smooth, no nodules.

Chest: Expansion equal, respiration effortless. Lung sounds clear bilaterally with no adventitious sounds. No CVA tenderness.

Heart: Rate 84 bpm, regular rhythm. S_1 and S_2 are normal, not accentuated or diminished, with soft, blowing systolic murmur Gr 2/6 at 2nd left interspace.

Breasts: Tender, no masses or lesions, large everted nipples. No drainage present. Breast self-exam reviewed.

Abdomen: No masses; bowel sounds present in four quadrants. No hepatomegaly or splenomegaly. Fundus palpable 1 cm above symphysis pubis. No inguinal lymphadenopathy noted. No healed incision(s) noted.

Extremities: No lower extremity varicosities, edema, or redness noted. 1+ DTRs. BP 124/76 mm Hg, sitting, left arm.

Pelvic: Female circumcision present without infibulated scarring. Bartholin, urethra, and Skene glands negative for discharge. Vagina pink, with white, creamy, nonodorous discharge. Cervix pink, nonfriable, closed, and approximately 3 cm long and soft. Vaginal wall muscles lax. No evidence of a cystocele or rectocele.

Uterus: Approximately 13-week size and nontender. Dextrorotated. FHTs not heard with Doppler. Confirmed on ultrasound along with dating.

ASSESSMENT

Intrauterine pregnancy at 11 weeks' gestation by ultrasound today with positive fetal cardiac activity.

Aware of potential language and cultural issues. Via clinic interpreter understands advised prenatal testing, clinic routine, and warning signs and symptoms in pregnancy. Referred to social work for transportation concerns.

Physical examination normal and healthy.

ABNORMAL FINDINGS
FOR ADVANCED PRACTICE

TABLE 31.1   Preeclampsia

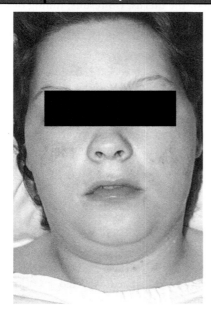

Preeclampsia is a condition specific to pregnancy that is rarely seen before 20 weeks' gestation except in the presence of a molar (gestational trophoblastic) pregnancy. It occurs in 3% to 10% of pregnancies.

Preeclampsia seems to be a culmination of maternal, placental, and fetal factors, including: (1) placenta implanted with abnormal trophoblastic invasion; (2) immunologic intolerance among maternal, placental, and fetal tissues; (3) cardiovascular or inflammatory changes; (4) genetic factors.[11]

Predisposing factors include preeclampsia in a previous pregnancy, multifetal gestation, chronic hypertension, obesity, age 35 years or older, and African-American race.[11]

The classic symptoms of preeclampsia are hypertension and proteinuria. Hypertension is a systolic BP of ≥140 mm Hg or a diastolic BP of ≥90 mm Hg that occurs after 20 weeks' gestation in a woman with previously normal blood pressure.

The BP should be compared with the woman's 1st prenatal BP (first trimester). Hypertension is necessary for the diagnosis of preeclampsia, but preeclampsia may be seen without the edema or proteinuria.

Onset and worsening symptoms may be sudden. Subjective signs may include headaches and visual changes (spots, blurring, or flashing lights) caused by cerebral edema or right upper quadrant/epigastric pain from liver enlargement. Liver enzyme levels become elevated. Hematocrit usually increases, and the platelets drop. Serum creatinine and blood urea nitrogen elevate. Hemolysis occurs at least in part as a result of vasospasm.

A serious variant of preeclampsia, the **HELLP** syndrome, involves **H**emolysis, **E**levated **L**iver enzymes, and **L**ow **P**latelets and represents an ominous clinical picture. Untreated preeclampsia may progress to eclampsia, which is manifested by generalized tonic-clonic seizures. Eclampsia may develop as late as 10 days' postpartum.

Before the syndrome becomes clinically manifested, it is affecting the placenta through vasospasm and a series of small infarctions. The capacity of the placenta to deliver oxygen and nutrients may be seriously diminished, and fetal growth may be restricted.

See Illustration Credits for source information.

TABLE 31.2	Fetal Size Inconsistent With Dates

Size Small for Dates

Fundal height measures smaller than expected for dates.

Inaccuracy of Dates

Conception may have occurred later than originally thought. Reconsider the woman's menstrual history; sexual history; contraceptive use; early pregnancy testing; early sizing of the uterus; US results; timing of pregnancy symptoms, including the date of quickening; and the fundal height measurements. If, after this review, the expected date of delivery (EDD) is correct, further investigation is required.

Preterm Labor

Contractions causing cervical change at <37 weeks' gestation. Other than delivery, preterm labor is the leading cause of hospital admission during pregnancy. Risk factors for preterm birth include vaginal bleeding in early pregnancy, cigarette smoking, low maternal weight gain, illicit drug use, young or advanced maternal age, poverty, strenuous working conditions, psychological factors (depression, anxiety, chronic stress), prior preterm delivery, and intrauterine infection.[11]

Size Large for Dates

Fundal height measures larger than expected for dates.

Inaccuracy of Dates

Review the same findings as listed previously.

Multiple Fetuses

The frequency of multiple fetuses increases with advanced maternal age and is enhanced by the increasing use of fertility drugs. The uterus enlarges where the fundal height may be beyond the calculated/expected gestational age. US examination confirms the diagnosis.

Leiomyoma (Myoma or "Fibroids")

These are preexisting benign tumors of the uterine wall, which then are stimulated to enlarge by the estrogen levels of pregnancy. Myomata may be located anywhere in the uterine wall (see Table 27.6, p. 762). When they grow in the outer uterine wall, the myometrium, they may affect the clinician's judgment of where the fundus of the uterus should be measured. A myoma may grow just underneath the endometrial surface into the uterine cavity, displacing the fetus or preventing its descent into the pelvis.

Fetal Macrosomia

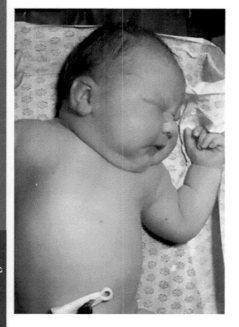

This is a condition in which the infant's weight is beyond 4000 g or 4500 g, regardless of the gestational age. Less than 8% of all live-born infants in the United States weigh more than 4000 g.[11] Risk factors associated with macrosomia include obesity, diabetes (gestational and type 2), postterm gestation, multiparity, large size of parents, advanced maternal age, previous macrosomic baby, and racial/ethnic factors.[11] Birth risks to the mother include labor abnormalities, an increased incidence for cesarean delivery, bladder trauma, and vaginal tissue trauma. Fetal risks include birth trauma such as fractured clavicle and brachial plexus nerve damage from shoulder dystocia, depressed Apgar scores, extended hospitalizations, and possible fetal mortality.

See Illustration Credits for source information.

TABLE 31.3 | **Malpresentations**

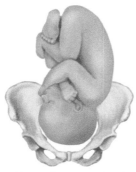

Vertex (for comparison)

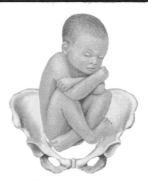

Complete breech

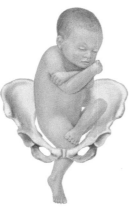

Footling breech

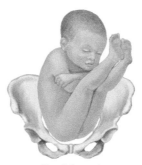

Frank breech

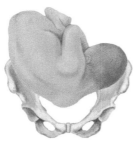

Transverse lie and
shoulder presentation

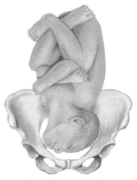

Face presentation

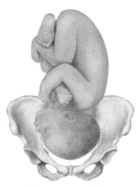

Brow presentation

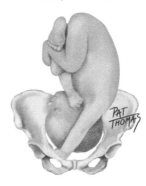

Compound presentation

Malpresentations may be detected by the hands of an experienced examiner, confirmed by the FHT location, and further confirmed by ultrasound. Before 34 weeks' gestation, any position is normal. The vertex presentation is desirable thereafter because spontaneous turning becomes less likely as the fetus grows in proportion to the amount of space and fluid in the uterus and pelvis.

Summary Checklist: The Pregnant Woman

1. Collect history.
2. Determine EDD and current number of weeks of gestation.
3. Instruct the woman to undress and empty her bladder, saving her urine to dip it for protein and glucose or culture if 1st visit.
4. Measure weight.
5. Perform a physical examination, starting with general survey.
6. Inspect skin for pigment changes, scars.
7. Check oral mucous membranes.
8. Palpate thyroid gland.
9. Inspect breast changes and palpate for masses.
10. Auscultate breath sounds, heart sounds, heart rate, and any murmurs.
11. Check lower extremities for edema, varicosities, and reflexes.
12. The abdomen: Measure fundal height, perform Leopold's maneuvers, auscultate FHTs.
13. The pelvic examination: Note signs of pregnancy, the condition of the cervix, and the size and position of the uterus.
14. Measure the BP.
15. Obtain appropriate laboratory work.

REFERENCES

1. American College of Obstetricians and Gynecologists (ACOG). (2013). Definition of term pregnancy. Committee Opinion No. 579. Reaffirmed 2017. *Obstet Gynecol, 122*, 1139–1140.
2. American College of Obstetricians and Gynecologists (ACOG). (2013). Medically indicated late-preterm and early-term deliveries. Committee Opinion No. 560. Reaffirmed 2017. *Obstet Gynecol, 121*, 908–910.
3. American College of Obstetricians and Gynecologists (ACOG). (2013). Nonmedically indicated early-term deliveries. Committee Opinion No. 561. Reaffirmed 2017. *Obstet Gynecol, 121*, 911–915.
4. American College of Obstetricians and Gynecologists (ACOG). (2016). Ultrasound in pregnancy. Practice Bulletin No. 175. *Obstet Gynecol, 128*, 1459–1460.
5. American College of Obstetricians and Gynecologists (ACOG). (2017). Opioid use and opioid use disorder during pregnancy. Committee Opinion No. 711. *Obstet Gynecol, 130*, e81–e94.
6. American College of Obstetricians and Gynecologists (ACOG). (2017). Practice Bulletin No. 180: Gestational diabetes mellitus. *Obstet Gynecol, 130*, e17–e37.
7. American College of Obstetricians and Gynecologists. (2017). *Prenatal genetic screen tests.* https://www.acog.org/Patients/FAQs/Prenatal-Genetic-Screening-Tests.
8. Beaudrot, M. E., Elchert, J. A., & DeFranco, E. A. (2016). Influence of gestational weight gain and BMI on cesarean delivery risk in adolescent pregnancies. *J Perinatol, 36*, 612–617.
9. Bossuah, K. A. (2017). Fatigue in pregnancy. *Int J Childbirth Educ, 32*(1), 10–12.
10. Centers for Disease Control and Prevention. (2017). *About teen pregnancy.* https://www.cdc.gov/teenpregnancy/about/index.htm.
11. Cunningham, F. G., Leveno, K. J., Bloom, S. L., et al. (2018). *Williams obstetrics* (25th ed.). Chicago, IL: McGraw Hill Medical Education.
12. Resnick, R., Lockwood, C., Moore, T., et al. (2018). *Creasy and Resnik's maternal-fetal medicine: Principles and practice* (8th ed.). Philadelphia: Elsevier.
13. HHS Office of Adolescent Health. (2016). *Trends in teen pregnancy and childbearing.* https://www.hhs.gov/ash/oah/adolescent-development/reproductive-health-and-teen-pregnancy/teen-pregnancy-and-childbearing/trends/index.html.
14. Kessenich, C. R., & Erigo-Backman, R. C. (2012). Using hCG testing in pregnancy and beyond. *Nurse Pract, 37*(5), 18–19.
15. King, T. L., Brucker, M. C., Jevitt, C. M., et al. (2019). *Varney's midwifery* (6th ed.). Burlington, MA: Jones & Bartlett Learning.
16. Krans, E. E., & Patrick, S. W. (2016). Opioid use disorder in pregnancy: Health policy and practice in the midst of an epidemic. *Obstet Gynecol, 128*, 4–10.
17. Lemon, L. S., Naimi, A. I., Abrams, B., et al. (2016). Prepregnancy obesity and the racial disparity in infant mortality. *Obesity (Silver Spring), 24*, 2578–2584.
18. March of Dimes. (2016). *Down syndrome.* https://www.marchofdimes.org/complications/down-syndrome.aspx.
19. Martin, J. A., Hamilton, B. E., Osterman, M. J. K., et al. (2018). Births: Final data for 2016. *Natl Vital Stat Rep, 67*(1), 1–55. https://www.cdc.gov/nchs/data/nvsr/nvsr67/nvsr67_01.pdf.
20. National Institute on Drug Abuse. (2016). *Substance use while pregnant and breastfeeding.* https://www.drugabuse.gov/publications/research-reports/substance-use-in-women/substance-use-while-pregnant-breastfeeding.
21. Patrick, S. W., Dudley, J., Martin, P. R., et al. (2015). Prescription opioid epidemic and infant outcomes. *Pediatrics, 135*, 842–850.
22. Pryor, J. R., Maalouf, F. I., Krans, E. E., et al. (2017). The opioid epidemic and neonatal abstinence syndrome in the USA: A review of the continuum of care. *Arch Dis Child Fetal Neonatal Ed, 102*, F183–F187.
23. Pu, J., Zhao, B., Wang, E. J., et al. (2015). Racial/ethnic differences in gestational diabetes prevalence and contribution of common risk factors. *Paediatr Perinat Epidemiol, 29*, 436–443.
24. Yuen, L., & Wong, V. W. (2015). Gestational diabetes mellitus: Challenges for different ethnic groups. *World J Diabetes, 6*, 1024–1032.

CHAPTER 32

Functional Assessment of the Older Adult

@http://evolve.elsevier.com/Jarvis/

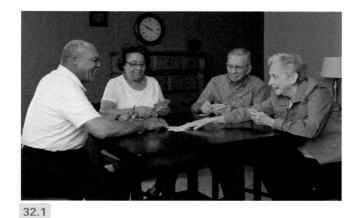

32.1

The United States has a large and expanding population of older adults. By 2040, older adults will represent over 20% of the population and the number of Americans over the age of 65 years is expected to surpass 82 million[3] (Fig. 32.1). Adults over the age of 65 are responsible for more hospital stays and clinic visits than younger adults.[3]

Many older Americans live with disabilities or have activity limitations, often because of multiple chronic conditions that may include sensory, physical, or mental impairments. Approximately 30% of older adults report difficulty in performing at least one activity of daily living (ADL), while an additional 12% report difficulty with one or more instrumental activities of daily living (IADLs).[3] Because of difficulty in performing activities of daily living, some older adults rely on caregivers. Personal caregiving can be formal (hired, paid caregivers) or informal (family, friends). Informal services accounted for approximately 37 billion hours of care and were valued at $470 billion in 2013.[2]

Aging or *older adult* is often defined as 65 years or older; however, it is important to remember that older adults are heterogeneous, and differences exist among biological, social, physical, and emotional rates of aging.[14] Older age-groups are often categorized as young-old (65 to 74 years), middle-old (75 to 84 years), and old-old (85 years and older). Although the number of chronic diseases does increase with aging, remember that a substantial number of older adults enjoy aging and report good-to-excellent health.[3]

The comprehensive assessment of an older adult requires knowledge of not only normal aging changes but also the consequences of chronic diseases, genetic makeup, and lifestyle. A comprehensive **geriatric assessment** is multidimensional and incorporates the physical examination and assessments of mental status, functional status, social and economic status,

pain, and examination of the physical environment for safety concerns. Multiple disciplines may participate in this assessment, including physicians; nurses; physical, occupational, and speech therapists; social workers; case managers; nutritionists; and pharmacists. Early recognition of disabilities and treatable conditions is instrumental in preserving function and quality of life for older adults.

The normal changes of aging presented in previous chapters do not represent pathology, but they may predispose an older adult to a disability. Older adults may present to clinics or hospitals not only with an acute illness such as pneumonia, but also with ongoing chronic geriatric syndromes such as urinary incontinence, fragile skin, confusion, problems with eating or feeding, falls, or sleep disorders. Geriatric syndromes represent a heterogeneous group of syndromes experienced by older adults; these syndromes are multifactorial and may lead to functional decline and decreased quality of life.

Normal aging changes and the development of disease may precipitate transition from home to a variety of settings where nursing-focused assessments are performed. Care may be provided in hospitals; skilled nursing, long-term care, assisted-living, and acute rehabilitation facilities; homes; and clinics (Fig. 32.2). The setting where care is provided usually determines the types of assessment and the instruments used. However, the goal of the geriatric assessment remains the same: to identify an older adult's strengths and any limitations so that appropriate interventions can be used to promote independence and prevent functional decline.

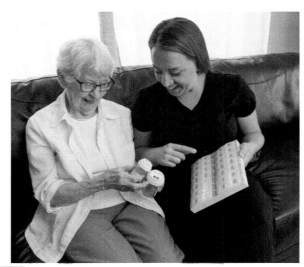

32.2

FUNCTION

Functional ability refers to one's ability to perform activities of daily living, including bathing and toileting, and independent living skills such as shopping and housework. *Functional status* is a person's ability to perform self-care, the ability to negotiate the social and physical environment, and functions needed to support independent living.[19] For example, arthritis may affect individuals' ability to dress themselves. A condition such as Alzheimer disease may affect problem solving, safety, and motivation, which in turn affects function. Lack of social support or a safe physical setting is an environmental issue that affects functional status and possibly the ability to live independently. Functional status is not static; older adults may move continuously through varying stages of independence and disability.

The assessment of function is important to provide a baseline for continuing comparison, to predict prognosis, and to provide objective measures on the efficacy of treatments. Knowing only the person's medical diagnosis is not sufficient to predict functional abilities. Older adults may not experience the usual symptoms of an acute illness, and often a decline in functional status may herald the presence of another process. For example, a urinary tract infection may present as acute confusion in the older adult.

A functional assessment is the basis for care planning, goal setting, and discharge planning. It is needed for eligibility to obtain durable medical equipment, home modifications, and inpatient or outpatient rehabilitation services. For the older adult and family, a functional assessment can identify areas for current and future planning such as the most appropriate living situation.

A functional assessment typically includes self-care (activities of daily living), self-maintenance (instrumental activities of daily living), and physical mobility.[14] Functional status is influenced by the health of the individual; it can be monitored to identify response to treatment, and it can be prognostic in identifying long-term needs.[21] Functional assessments should be completed in a systematic way. There are two approaches to use for performing a functional assessment: (1) *asking individuals* about their abilities to perform the tasks (using self-reports), or (2) actually *observing* their ability to perform the tasks. For people with memory problems, the use of surrogate reporters such as family members or caregivers may be necessary, but keep in mind that surrogates may overestimate or underestimate actual abilities.

Activities of Daily Living

ADLs are tasks necessary for self-care (Fig. 32.3). Typically, ADLs include domains of eating/feeding, bathing, grooming (the individual tasks of washing face, combing hair, shaving, cleaning teeth), dressing (lower body and upper body), toileting (bowel and bladder), walking (including propelling a wheelchair), using stairs (ascending and descending), and transferring (e.g., bed to chair). The ADL instruments are designed as either self-report, observation of tasks, or proxy/surrogate report.

The Katz Index of Independence in ADL

The Katz Index of ADL[11] is based on the concept of physical disability and measures physical function in older adults and the chronically ill. It is widely used with basic ADLs to measure performance, evaluate treatment outcomes, and predict the need for continuing supervised care.[21] Activities assessed are bathing, dressing, toileting, transferring from bed to chair, continence, and feeding. The Katz ADL uses dichotomous scoring for each category. Patients are scored as dependent or independent for each task. The Katz ADL is valuable for planning specific types of assistance that the older person may need. For example, a person may be unable to bathe independently on hospital discharge but is independent in other ADLs. In this case, plan for a home health aide to go twice a week to the home to assist the older adult with bathing.

The Katz ADL scale is a useful instrument in many settings and takes only 5 minutes to administer, but it has limitations. In an ambulatory clinic setting, the provider cannot observe the older adult perform the activity and must rely on a self-report or surrogate report. In the hospital, nursing staff may be assisting with transferring or grooming activities and may underestimate the ability for self-care. In addition, small changes in the ability to perform these activities may not be identified. A variety of other instruments are available to measure ADLs, but some require formal training and additional time to administer.

Instrumental Activities of Daily Living

IADLs refer to functional abilities necessary for independent community living. Typically IADL tasks include shopping, meal preparation, housekeeping, laundry, managing finances, taking medications, and using transportation (Fig. 32.4). Tasks such as yard work or home maintenance and leisure activities such as reading and other hobbies are included in some but not all IADL instruments. IADL instruments measure tasks historically done by women (e.g., doing laundry, cooking, housework), and many do not address activities done primarily by men such as home repairs and yard work.

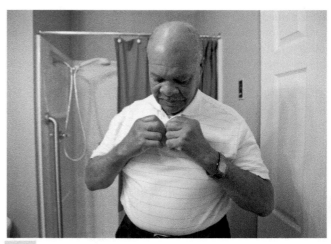

32.3

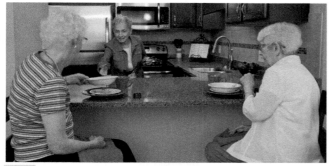

32.4

Lawton Instrumental Activities of Daily Living

The Lawton IADL scale was originally developed to determine the most suitable living situation for an older adult—that is, determining competence and maintenance of life skills such as shopping, cooking, and managing finances in a meaningful way (Fig. 32.5). IADLs are a prerequisite for independent living. The Lawton IADL scale (https://consultgeri.org/try-this/general-assessment/issue-23.pdf) contains 8 items: use of telephone, shopping, meal preparation, housekeeping, laundry, transportation, self-medication, and management of finances.

The Lawton IADL instrument is a self-report measure of performance rather than ability. Direct testing is often not feasible (e.g., demonstrating the ability to prepare food while a hospital inpatient). Attention to the final score is less important than identifying a person's strengths and areas where assistance is needed. The instrument is useful for discharge planning in acute hospital settings and for ongoing measure-

ment of function in outpatient settings. It would not be useful for those residing in institutional settings because many of the tasks are already being managed for the resident. Other IADL instruments are available, with some being direct observation versus self-report; however, some instruments take over 90 minutes to complete and are not feasible in many settings.

Advanced Activities of Daily Living

Advanced activities of daily living (AADLs) are activities that an older adult performs as a member of a family, society, and community, including occupational and recreational activities.[14] Various AADL instruments commonly include self-care, mobility, work (either paid or volunteer), recreational activities/hobbies, and socialization. Occupational therapists often perform assessment of AADLs. It is important to have the older adult set priorities for AADL activities so that interventions can be individualized.

Measuring Physical Performance

A disadvantage of many of the ADL and IADL instruments is the self-report or proxy report of functional activities. Incorporating an objective standardized measure of performance prevents overestimation or underestimation of abilities. Many physical performance measures also incorporate balance, gait, motor coordination, and endurance. Although there are clear advantages to directly observing the older adult perform the activities, there are some disadvantages. The instruments can be very time consuming, require training and special equipment, and carry the risk that the individual might fall or sustain an injury during the testing.

The **Timed Up and Go (TUG) Test**[17] is a reliable and valid test to quantify functional mobility. The test is quick, requires little training and no special equipment, and is appropriate for use in many settings, including hospitals and clinics. The practitioner observes and times the patient as he or she rises from a chair, walks 10 feet, turns, walks back to the chair, and sits down. Factors to note are sitting balance, transferring from sitting to standing (e.g., does the person need to push off the armrest to rise), pace and stability of gait, ability to turn without staggering, and sitting back down in the chair. The person should be encouraged to wear his or her usual footwear and to use any assistive device that is typically used. An elderly person who takes longer than 12 seconds to complete the test is at high risk for falling and may need further evaluation.[8]

Assessment of Risk for Functional Decline During Hospitalization

Losing the ability to perform ADLs and IADLs as a result of acute illness, and hospitalization is common in older adults and can have significant negative consequences. Functional decline is attributable to the imposition of acute illness on an aging body with diminished physiologic reserve and to limited mobility commonly experienced during a hospital admission. Ideally, all patients should be screened for functional decline while hospitalized. Multiple instruments are

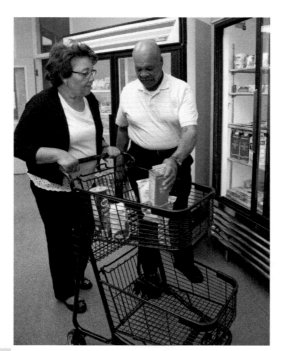

32.5

available to assess risk for functional decline, each with similar applicability to a variety of cultures and a range of older populations.[4] A person identified as being at high risk for functional decline can be referred to restorative services (e.g., physical/occupational therapy and inpatient rehabilitation services) and multidisciplinary discharge planning at the beginning of the hospital stay.

Assessment of Cognition

Cognitive impairment resulting from disease may be attributed by patients, families, and health care providers to normal changes with aging and can delay diagnostic workup. In general, a gradual and mild-to-moderate decline in short-term memory may be attributable to aging; an older adult may need more time to learn new material or a new task or may need a system for reminders. Cognition can be improved through cognitive training interventions.[12] Cognitive training interventions include brain teasers, video games, word games, and sudoku (Fig. 32.6). Domains of cognition included in most mental status assessments are attention, memory, orientation, language, visuospatial skills, and higher cognitive functions such as the ability to plan and make decisions.

Altered cognition in older adults is commonly attributed to three disorders—**dementia, delirium,** and **depression**—although other disorders such as normal pressure hydrocephalus may contribute. Depressed persons often complain of memory impairment. Delirium presents as an acute change in cognition, affecting the domain of attention. Delirium is usually attributable to an acute illness such as an infection or a medication side effect, whereas people with dementia have alterations in word finding and naming objects in addition to memory problems. Dementia, delirium, and depression may occur simultaneously with an acute illness and can complicate assessments. For example, people with dementia

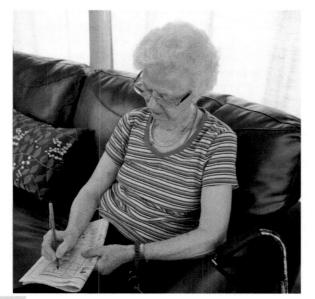

32.6

are at higher risk for delirium and, in the early stages of dementia, may also be depressed.

Cognitive assessments provide continuing comparisons with the individual's baseline to detect any acute changes such as with delirium. The assessments are not diagnostic but rather are for screening purposes and identify the need for a more comprehensive workup. Cognitive assessments are important for discharge planning (e.g., will the person remember to take the prescribed medications) and to assess for readiness for learning. As with screening for ADLs and IADLs, assessment of cognition helps with determining the best discharge plan. Many instruments are available to screen for cognitive impairment. Two commonly used instruments are the Mini-Mental State Examination (MMSE) and the Montreal Cognitive Assessment (MoCA). Both instruments can be completed in approximately 10 minutes and require only a pen and paper. While the MMSE has been used for decades, the MoCA is more sensitive in detecting mild cognitive impairment.[10] Both instruments assess multiple cognitive domains, including immediate and delayed memory and visuospatial capability, but the MoCA includes assessments of frontal executive function and spatial inattention. Patients with low educational levels tend to score poorly on the MMSE regardless of cognitive impairment.[9,20]

Depression and Function

The majority of older adults do not experience major depression. Current assessments of community dwelling older adults estimate that just 1% to 5% of them experience depression; however, approximately 13.5% of older adults who require home health care experience depression. Depression risk increases in those older adults who have at least one chronic condition.[7] Although older adults with physical impairments are at greater risk for depression, depression is not an inevitable consequence of functional impairment. Emotional experiences of sadness, grief, response to loss, and temporary "blue" moods are considered normal, but persistent depression that interferes significantly with ability to function is not. Fortunately, mood disorders, including depression, are highly treatable.

It is vital to screen and identify those older adults who have depressive symptoms. Several short screening instruments have been developed and validated for depression screening in the older adult. One example is the Geriatric Depression Scale, Short Form (Fig. 32.7).[18] Depression tends to be long-lasting and can recur; therefore, early intervention is warranted.

Social Domain

The quality of life that an older person experiences is closely linked to the success of social function. The social domain focuses on relationships within family, social groups, and the community and comprises multiple dimensions, including the sources of formal and informal assistance available. Knowledge of the day-to-day routines can give you baseline information and a reference point to detect functional decline during future encounters. A comprehensive social assessment

Geriatric Depression Scale (Short Form)		
1. Are you basically satisfied with your life?	Yes	No
2. Have you dropped many of your activities and interests?	Yes	No
3. Do you feel that your life is empty?	Yes	No
4. Do you often get bored?	Yes	No
5. Are you in good spirits most of the time?	Yes	No
6. Are you afraid that something bad is going to happen to you?	Yes	No
7. Do you feel happy most of the time?	Yes	No
8. Do you often feel helpless?	Yes	No
9. Do you prefer to stay at home rather than go out and do new things?	Yes	No
10. Do you feel you have more problems with memory than most?	Yes	No
11. Do you think it is wonderful to be alive now?	Yes	No
12. Do you feel pretty worthless the way you are now?	Yes	No
13. Do you feel full of energy?	Yes	No
14. Do you feel that your situation is hopeless?	Yes	No
15. Do you think that most people are better off than you are?	Yes	No

*Score:*____/15. One point for "no" to questions 1, 5, 7, 11, 13; one point for "yes" to other questions. Normal: 3 ± 2; mildly depressed: 7 ± 3; very depressed: 12 ± 2.

32.7

(Sheikh, Yesavage, 1986.)

is spread over several evaluation periods and assesses caregivers as well as the older adult.

Social networks consist of informal supports that are accessed by the older adult. Informal support is partly based on cultural beliefs regarding who should be providing care, prior relationships, and the location and availability of caregivers. Informal support includes family and friends and is usually provided free of charge. Nearly 40 million people provide unpaid caregiving services to an adult over 50 years old in the United States.[15] Services provided include tasks such as ADLs, shopping, and paying bills. Formal supports range from social services such as meal programs to health care services such as home health care.

The availability of assistance from family or friends frequently determines whether a functionally dependent older adult remains at home or is institutionalized. Knowing who is available to help the person if he or she becomes ill is important to document, even for healthy older adults. Knowing the social support network is an important part of the discharge plan for older adults. Several standardized assessment instruments are available to measure social support.

CAREGIVER ASSESSMENT

Most older adults with functional impairment live in the community with the help of informal support (commonly a spouse or other family member). Many spousal caregivers are as frail as the person for whom they are caring, and adult children may be older than 65 years with their own chronic illnesses. Although many caregivers experience satisfaction from providing care, caregiving is linked to physical and emotional stress, which can lead to caregiver burnout, depression, and worsening health.[15]

An older person's need for institutionalization often is better predicted from assessment of the caregiver characteristics and stress than from the severity of the patient's illness. The health and well-being of the patient and caregiver are closely linked. For these reasons part of assessing an older adult involves paying attention to the well-being of the caregiver. A health care provider may help identify programs such as support groups, respite programs, adult daycare, or hired home health aides (Fig. 32.8).

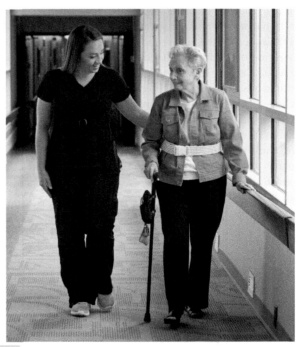

32.8

Assessment of Caregiver Burden

As a health care provider, it is imperative that you include caregivers in your assessment. Caregivers providing care for older adults may experience increased stress, anxiety, and burnout due to overwhelming demands. The level of care that the older adult requires may exceed caregiver ability. *Caregiver burden* is the perceived strain by the person who cares for an elderly, chronically ill, or disabled person. It is linked to the caregiver's ability to cope and handle stress. Signs of possible caregiver burnout include multiple somatic complaints, increased stress and anxiety, social isolation, depression, and weight loss. Several formal screening tools are available that identify caregivers of any age who need a more comprehensive assessment. Caregiver stress can lead to elder mistreatment; a thorough assessment may identify opportunities for prevention of elder abuse (see Chapter 7).

CONTEXTS OF CARE

Older adults reside in and enter the health care system along multiple levels or contexts of care, including acute-care hospitals, inpatient nursing facilities, the community, and at home. The location of the care setting affects the ability to perform a comprehensive functional assessment. During an acute illness, it may be more difficult to perform a thorough functional assessment. In addition, if a resident resides in the home environment, the parameters of assessment will be broader than if he or she is in an inpatient long-term living situation.

Acute Care Setting

While hospitalization may be necessary to treat acute illness, it puts older adults at an increased risk for functional decline, iatrogenic complications, and potential discharge to a skilled nursing facility. Hospitals appreciate the increased risk for functional decline and adverse outcomes in older adults. Many hospitals use targeted interventions to prevent functional decline related to hospitalization in older adults. One model of care is the Acute Care for Elders (ACE) unit, which is a dedicated unit within a hospital setting focused toward preventing functional decline in older adults through the design of the physical environment (e.g., bright lights, flooring to help prevent falls), collaboration among interdisciplinary teams, patient-centered care, and nursing protocols for clinical care (e.g., indwelling urinary catheter removal, reduction of restraint use, early mobilization). Acute care nurses equipped with specialized knowledge and skills have an impact on improving outcomes for the hospitalized older adult.

Community

The vast majority of older adults reside in the community, and fewer than 5% of older adults live in skilled nursing facilities. The percentage of older adults residing in skilled nursing facilities increases from 1% of those ages 65 to 74 years to about 9% of those older than 85 years.[3]

One of the goals of community-based services is to help the older adult remain at home. Assessment of functional status helps to determine the type of services that an older adult needs to maintain independent living at home. A low or negative result on a screening tool during assessment does not necessarily lead to the need for institutionalization, but instead may lead a health care provider to identify appropriate support services to help the older adult maintain independence.

Home Care

Home care refers to a range of supportive social and health services provided in the home environment. Services include nursing care, primary care, therapy (physical, occupational, and speech), social work, nutrition, case management, ADL assistance, and durable medical equipment. The home care nurse is tending not only to the illness of the older adult but also to the home safety considerations, family dynamics, and functional ability. Because of advances in health care technology, equipment is smaller and more portable. As a result, people who once were limited to hospitalization can now be treated or managed at home. In addition to cost advantages with home care versus hospitalization, older adults have been shown to recover faster when at home in familiar settings than when placed in institutions and also can avoid the risk for hospital-acquired infection.

Assisted Living

Assisted-living facilities are a popular choice for older adults and typically are considered for adults who can no longer reside at home yet do not need a skilled nursing facility. Most facilities provide apartment-style living, although some single-family dwellings are licensed to provide care. Facilities offer homelike environments where residents have the opportunity for social interaction through group dining and activities (Fig. 32.9). Some offer assistance with personal care, support with ADLs, and/or basic nursing care along with transportation and recreational activities as part of an overall package.

Continuing-Care Retirement Communities

The unique feature of continuing-care retirement communities is that all care needs for the older adult can be met in one community, supporting the concept of aging in place. These facilities feature independent living arrangements,

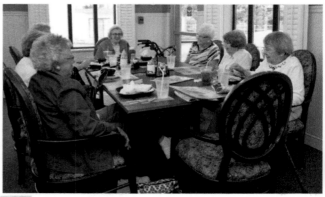

32.9

assisted-living care, and skilled nursing care, along with a variety of social and recreational activities. In these communities residents can progress through the continuum of care while residing in the same community. An older adult can enter at the independent level of living and then, as illness and/or functional limitations occur, can move to a higher level of support. Some older adults may never leave the independent living level, whereas others may progress to skilled nursing as the need for care arises.

MAINTAINING INDEPENDENCE

Exercise

Exercise and activity are essential for health promotion and maintenance in the older adult and to achieve an optimal level of functioning. A sedentary lifestyle is an important contributor to the loss in the ability to independently perform ADLs. Exercise does not prevent the process of aging, but it increases functional ability, helping to maximize the older adult's independence.

Exercise can improve cardiovascular function, postural stability, range of motion, flexibility, and muscle mass in older adults.[22] Because of these positive effects, fall risk and fractures may be decreased. In addition, participation in physical exercise has shown to reduce depressive symptoms and improve feelings of psychosocial well-being[22] (Table 32.1).

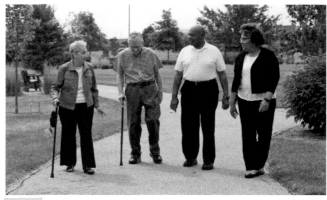

32.10

To help with compliance, physical activities should be readily available and have minimal cost associated with participation. Because pathology, both known and undiscovered, may be present in older adults (e.g., osteoporosis), the physical activity chosen should not put excessive stress on the skeletal system. Walking is a popular mode of exercise for cardiovascular endurance (Fig. 32.10). Water activities or stationary cycling may be alternative modes for individuals when walking is not feasible. Developing an activity plan, particularly for older adults with chronic health conditions, may warrant clearance and input from a health care provider or referral to a specialty program (e.g., cardiac rehabilitation).

Health Care Maintenance

Functional decline and a loss of independence are not inevitable consequences of aging. Although the prevalence of chronic disease increases with age, most older people remain functionally independent. However, evidence-based interventions for screening and detection of health conditions and disease are important given the prevalence of chronic disease in older adults. The Agency for Healthcare Research and Quality in partnership with AARP provides recommendations to promote good health, screening tests, and medications for adults over 50 years.

ENVIRONMENTAL ASSESSMENT

Common environmental hazards include inadequate lighting, loose throw rugs, curled carpet edges, obstructed hallways, cords in walkways, lack of grab bars, and low or loose toilet seats. Environmental modification can promote mobility and reduce the likelihood of a fall.

During your environmental assessment, inquire about the safety of the neighborhood and ask whether older persons have transportation and/or services available in geographic proximity to where they live. Access to basic services such as food and clothing stores, pharmacies, financial institutions, health care facilities, and social service agencies is necessary. The community environment needs to provide safety conditions such as street lamps, sidewalks, and police and fire

TABLE 32.1 **WHO Recommended Levels of Physical Activity for Adults Ages 65 and Older**
To improve cardiorespiratory function, muscular fitness, bone, and functional health and to reduce the risk of noncommunicable diseases, depression, and cognitive decline: • Older adults should do at least 150 minutes of moderate-intensity aerobic physical activity throughout the week (e.g., housework, dancing, brisk walking), at least 75 minutes of vigorous-intensity aerobic physical activity throughout the week (e.g., fast swimming, fast cycling, running), or an equivalent combination of moderate- and vigorous-intensity activity. • Aerobic activity should be performed in bouts of at least 10 minutes' duration. • For additional health benefits, older adults should increase their moderate-intensity aerobic physical activity to 300 minutes per week or engage in 150 minutes of vigorous-intensity aerobic physical activity per week or an equivalent combination of moderate- and vigorous-intensity activity. • Older adults with poor mobility should perform physical activity on 3 or more days per week to enhance balance and prevent falls. • Muscle-strengthening activities involving major muscle groups should be done on 2 or more days a week. • When older adults cannot do the recommended amounts of physical activity because of health conditions, they should be as physically active as their abilities and conditions allow.[22]

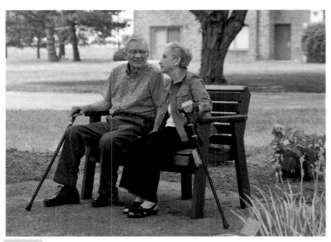

32.11

protection (Fig. 32.11). These are especially important for community dwelling older adults who need help with IADLs.

Older persons often have challenges not easily detected during an office visit. A home visit can reveal difficulties in the living situation such as household and bathing hazards, social isolation, family/caregiver stress, and nutrition issues. For example, a walk through the kitchen can assess the food preferences of the older adult. An empty refrigerator and/or kitchen cabinets may give clues to previously unrecognized functional impairment such as dementia, mobility challenges, or a decline in the ability to perform IADLs, which would warrant further assessment. Interventions such as home health assistance, transportation services, and shopping services may support the older adult to maintain community living.

Falls

Each year millions of older adults experience a fall, and approximately 20% of falls result in a serious injury, such as a head injury or broken bone.[6] A fall may also lead to serious psychological consequences. The fear of falling again may lead to a reduction in physical activity, which will cause further decline and increase the risk of a subsequent fall. Falls in older adults have multiple contributing factors such as gait and balance problems, poor vision, syncope, diabetic neuropathy, home hazards (e.g., throw rugs, uneven steps), and dementia. Most falls are caused by a combination of factors. Health care providers can reduce the risk of falls by assessing risk factors and taking corrective action as appropriate.

Older-Adult Drivers

Older-adult drivers account for 18% of all licensed drivers in the United States and 18% of all traffic fatalities.[16] Safe driving requires intact cognitive functioning, sensory perception, good physical abilities (e.g., strength to turn the steering wheel and use pedals; enough range of motion to turn head), alertness, and suitable reflexes. Early and routine attention to health care maintenance activities such as vision and hearing checks, exercise to maintain flexibility and range of motion,

and workup of any cognitive abnormalities may allow the older adult to continue to drive safely.

Driving represents independence, freedom, and control and is often a necessary part of functioning in daily life, such as getting to work or shopping for groceries. It also facilitates remaining connected socially with family and friends. Driving cessation has been linked to functional decline and depression in older adults.[1] If driving must be limited or cease altogether, it is important to establish a plan of action to enhance independence and maintain normal activity levels. This might mean accessing public transportation, carpooling, or increased involvement of family and friends for activities that require motor transportation.

Older adults often recognize that their driving abilities have changed and adjust their habits accordingly (e.g., limiting driving to daytime, good weather conditions, or only local driving). However, when this is not the case, family members, friends, or health care providers may be concerned enough about the safety of the older driver and others in the community that they need to intervene. One practical approach is a checklist of warning signs for when to stop driving (Table 32.2). In addition, the American Automobile Association provides an online driver self-assessment test, and local departments of motor vehicles and area agencies on aging can provide additional resources to help older adults and their families with ongoing assessment and planning. Health care providers also have an obligation to discuss safe driving with older adults; in many states providers are required to report certain sensory or neurodegenerative conditions.

TABLE 32.2 Warning Signs for When to Stop Driving

1. Almost crashing, with frequent close calls
2. Finding dents and scrapes on the car, fence, mailbox, etc.
3. Getting lost easily; having issues with memory
4. Having trouble seeing or following traffic signals, road signs, and pavement markings
5. Responding more slowly to unexpected situations; having trouble moving the foot from the gas to the brake pedal; confusing the two pedals
6. Misjudging gaps in traffic at intersections and on highway entrance and exit ramps
7. Driving too slow or too fast for conditions
8. Easily becoming distracted or having difficulty concentrating while driving
9. Physical limitations such as having a hard time turning around while backing up or changing lanes
10. Having trouble maintaining the correct lane or switching lanes while driving

Data from Rakow, K. We need to talk: The difficult driving conversation. https://www.aarp.org/auto/driver-safety/info-2016/when-to-stop-driving-in-older-age.html; and Staplin, L., Lococo, K.H., & Mastromatto, T. Can your older patients drive safely? *Am J Nurs, 117*(9), 34-44.

TABLE 32.3   Nonpharmacologic Interventions to Promote Sleep

CATEGORY	INTERVENTION	RATIONALE
Dietary	Limit caffeine to 2 caffeinated drinks per day, none after lunch.	Caffeine promotes wakefulness by blocking adenosine receptors in the brain.
	Restrict alcohol to 1 drink per day, none after dinner.	Alcohol may shorten the time it takes to fall asleep; but it is metabolized quickly, and withdrawal occurs in the last half of the night, producing lighter sleep and aggravating obstructive sleep apnea, restless legs syndrome, sympathetic arousal, and sweating.
	Restrict fluid intake in the evening.	This reduces nighttime awakening resulting from a full bladder.
	Avoid heavy, spicy meals near bedtime.	This reduces nighttime awakening caused by heartburn.
	Have a light bedtime snack of milk or cheese and crackers.	This promotes sleep by reducing hypoglycemia.
Schedule	Adhere to a regular schedule for meals and sleep, using an alarm, if necessary, to ensure rising at a regular time. Limit naps to one 30-minute, early-afternoon nap.	Maintaining temporal patterns of rest and activity enhances synchrony with circadian rhythms. Excessive daytime napping weakens the homeostatic drive to sleep.
Environment	Maintain daytime light and nighttime dark. Open drapes and blinds; increase the wattage in lamps. Increase sunlight exposure to at least $\frac{1}{2}$ hour per day. Keep the sleep environment dark.	Circadian rhythms are established primarily by patterns of light and dark.
	Use the bed only for sleep or sex, not for work or watching television. Limit time spent in bed to the average time spent asleep. If not asleep after 30 minutes, get up and engage in a relaxing activity until the need to sleep is felt.	The bed becomes an environmental cue for sleep.
	Promote uninterrupted sleep.	Limiting noise minimizes sleep disruption.
Activities	Maintain an active physical and social daytime schedule. Avoid passive activities such as watching television.	Vigorous activity promotes daytime arousal, prevents napping, and lessens depression, which can disrupt sleep.
	Keep to a relaxing bedtime ritual.	Relaxing activities augment one's readiness for sleep. A warm bath enhances a drop in core temperature.
Delirium	Frequently reorient the patient by keeping a clock and calendar in the room and maintaining a regular schedule and associated light and dark patterns.	These measures decrease anxiety.

From Cole, C., & Richards, K. (2007). Sleep disruption in older adults. *Am J Nurs, 107*(5), 40-49.

Sleep

Sleep architecture changes with aging (e.g., more difficulty falling and staying asleep); however, significantly altered sleep patterns are not a normal part of aging. Most adults of all ages need about 8 hours of sleep per night to feel alert and rested. The primary causes of altered sleep in older adults are physiologic (e.g., cardiovascular disease, pulmonary disease) and psychiatric illnesses (e.g., depression), as well as side effects of the medications to treat these disorders (beta-blockers, corticosteroids, diuretics). Detrimental consequences of poor sleep in older adults include poor health outcomes, falls, and impaired cognition.[13]

Because medications used to treat insomnia such as sedatives and hypnotics have many side effects for older adults, a nonpharmacologic approach to managing sleep is recommended (Table 32.3). In the home, the use of relaxing music, exposure to sunlight during the day, consistent bedtime routines, the limiting of food and drink after early evening, whole-body relaxation, and reduced light, noise, and room temperature may improve sleep.

SPIRITUAL ASSESSMENT

Spirituality provides personal answers about the meaning and purpose of one's own life and how to interpret life events. Spiritual health may improve with age, even as physical and mental health deteriorate. The aging process is a part of one's journey, with capability for growth. Views on spirituality vary greatly from one adult to another and among people of the same faith or belief system. It is important to acknowledge spirituality as a powerful coping mechanism during stressful life events and during illness to the end of life.

Spiritual assessment is highly individual and should be addressed with each person. Open-ended questions provide a foundation for future dialogue. A sample question posed during the initial assessment might be "Do you consider yourself to be a spiritual person?" If the person says "yes," a follow-up question could be "How does that spirituality relate to your health or health care decisions?" Involving chaplains or clergy members when possible and appropriate can provide the older adult with support and serve as a resource to the clinician.

SPECIAL CONSIDERATIONS

Assessment of the functional status of an older adult can be more time consuming than for younger adults. For hospitalized or institutionalized older adults, consider assessing function during normal activities such as grooming, at mealtimes, or during toileting.

Understand that a person with multiple medical problems may tire early and easily and that many medications have side effects that contribute to fatigue or affect attention span. Provide directions in written format if necessary. Have the older adult use sensory assistive devices such as glasses if necessary, and have hearing amplifiers and page magnifiers available. Face the person as much as possible, speak slowly in a lower-pitched voice, and enunciate words clearly.

Including the older adult in decision making about how the interview or testing is to be done establishes rapport and promotes self-esteem. Be aware of body language and behaviors, and be prepared to modify your approach. Touch can also help in establishing rapport and can reduce anxiety. Remember to slow down your approach and provide breaks as necessary.

A functional assessment can be intimidating for older adults. Frustration or embarrassment may arise if some physical maneuvers cannot be performed or questions cannot be answered during cognitive testing. Older adults may also be fearful about the consequences of functional testing such as losing independent living or having a caregiver move into the home. Try to provide reassurance that not everyone can complete all of the tasks or answer all of the questions and that, to the extent possible, confidentiality will be honored.

Ensure adequate space if doing tests of mobility. An aging adult may need room to maneuver an assistive device. When testing mobility, stand close to him or her to prevent a fall. The environment should be well lighted; avoid high-gloss, shiny, slippery surfaces. Minimize extraneous noise such as those from intercoms, televisions, or high-traffic areas. Warm rooms, access to fluids, proximity to a bathroom, and privacy are important.

Assessing Those in Pain

If the older adult is feeling pain or discomfort, the depth of knowledge gathered through the assessments will suffer. Alleviating pain should be a priority. It may be necessary to administer premedication before parts of the assessment, especially if the assessment requires movement. Another strategy is to use positioning to decrease pain. Ask which position is most comfortable. Providing comfort can help maximize the information gathered. It is paramount to remember that older adults with cognitive impairment do not experience less pain. Older adults with cognitive impairment suffer from conditions typically associated with pain (e.g., arthritis, osteoporosis, shingles) just as frequently as cognitively intact persons.

Assessing Older Adults With Altered Cognition

Cognitive impairment poses unique challenges. The older adult may not be able to actively participate in the evaluation and/or provide consistent answers. Gathering information from the older adult firsthand is always the best method but is not always feasible. To ensure the collection of reliable information, one strategy is to interview the caregiver and/or family to obtain subjective assessment data. Another is to arrange opportunities to assess the person when he or she identifies being most alert.

Adults with cognitive impairment may need questions or directions broken down into single commands, with ongoing verbal or physical cueing. Never assume that he or she cannot respond to questions even when there is known cognitive impairment. Using *yes* or *no* questions may prevent frustration. Be relaxed and patient because a person with dementia may mirror your emotions. If a family member or caregiver needs to provide collateral information, avoid doing this in front of the older adult.

REFERENCES

1. AAA Foundation. (2015). https://www.aaafoundation.org/sites/default/files/2015DrivingCessationFS.pdf.
2. AARP Public Policy Institute. (2015). *Valuing the invaluable: 2015 update.* http://www.aarp.org/content/dam/aarp/ppi/2015/valuing-the-invaluable-2015-update-new.pdf.
3. Administration on Aging. (2016). *A profile of older Americans.* https://www.acl.gov/sites/default/files/Aging%20and%20Disability%20in%20America/2016-Profile.pdf.
4. Beaton, K., & Grimmer, K. (2013). Tools that assess functional decline: Systematic literature review update. *Clin Interv Aging, 8*, 485–494.
5. Reference deleted in proofs.
6. CDC. (2017). *Home and recreational safety.* https://www.cdc.gov/homeandrecreationalsafety/falls/adultfalls.html.
7. CDC. (2017). *Healthy aging.* https://www.cdc.gov/aging/mentalhealth/depression.htm.
8. CDC. (2017). *STEADI Materials for healthcare providers.* https://www.cdc.gov/steadi/materials.html.
9. Devenney, E., & Hodges, J. R. (2017). The Mini-Mental State Examination: Pitfalls and limitations. *Pract Neurol, 17*, 79–80.
10. Finney, G. R., Minagar, A., & Heilman, K. M. (2016). Assessment of mental status. *Neurol Clin, 34*, 1–16.
11. Katz, S., Ford, A. B., Moskowitz, R. W., et al. (1963). Studies of illness in the aged: the index of ADL, a standardized measure of biological and psychosocial functioning. *JAMA, 185*, 94–101.

12. Kelly, M. E., et al. (2014). The impact of cognitive training and mental stimulation on cognitive and everyday functioning of healthy older adults: A systematic review and meta-analysis. *Ageing Res Rev, 15,* 28–43.

13. Lo, J. C., et al. (2016). Self-reported sleep duration and cognitive performance in older adults: A systematic review. *Sleep Med, 17,* 87–98.

14. Mauk, K. L. (2014). *Gerontological nursing: Competencies for care.* Boston: Jones & Bartlett.

15. National Alliance for Caregiving; AARP. (2015). *Caregiving in the U.S.: Executive summary.* Bethesda, MD: National Alliance for Caregiving. http://www.aarp.org/content/dam/aarp/ppi/2015/caregiving-in-the-united-states-2015-report-revised.pdf.

16. National Highway Traffic Safety Administration's National Center for Statistics and Analysis. (2017). *2015 data—traffic safety facts: Older population (DOT HS 812 372).* Washington, DC: National Highway Traffic Safety Administration.

17. Podsiadlo, D., & Richardson, S. (1991). The timed "Up & Go": A test of basic functional mobility for frail elderly persons. *J Am Geriatr Soc, 39*(2), 142–148.

18. Sheikh, J. I., & Yesavage, J. A. (1986). Geriatric depression scale: Recent evidence and development of a shorter version. *Clin Gerontol, 5,* 165–172.

19. Touhy, T. A., & Jett, K. F. (2016). *Ebersole & Hess' Toward healthy aging: Human needs and nursing response* (9th ed.). Philadelphia: Elsevier.

20. Votruba, K. L., Persad, C., & Giordani, B. (2016). Cognitive deficits in healthy elderly population with "normal" scores on the Mini-Mental State Examination. *J Geriatr Psychiatry, 29*(3), 126–132.

21. Ward, K. T., & Reuben, D. B. (2017). *Comprehensive geriatric assessment.* UpToDate. https://www.uptodate.com/contents/comprehensive-geriatric-assessment#H10.

22. World Health Organization. (2011). *Global recommendations on physical activity for health: 65 years and above.* http://www.who.int/dietphysicalactivity/factsheet_olderadults/en/.

Figure 1.2 Alfaro-LeFevre, R. (2009). *Critical thinking and clinical judgment: A practical approach.* (4th ed.). Philadelphia: Saunders.

Figure 1.5 Yoder-Wise, P. S. (2015). *Leading and managing in nursing.* (6th ed.). St. Louis: Mosby.

Figure 2.2 Courtesy Holly Birch Photography.

Figure 2.3 U.S. Department of Health and Human Services, Healthy People 2020. *Social determinants of health.* https://www.healthypeople.gov/2020/topics-objectives/topic/social-determinants-of-health.

Figure 2.6 *C* and *D* Courtesy Rachel E. Spector, 2009.

Figure 2.7 Aztec healer. U.S. Department of Defense. (2015). Latino Heritage Festival photo essay. https://www.defense.gov/Photos/Essay-View/CollectionID/14493/.

Figure 4.4 American Society of Human Genetics. (2004). www.ashg.org.

Figure 4.16 Klein, D. A., Goldenring, J. M., & Adelman, W. P. (2014). HEEADSSS 3.0: The psychosocial interview for adolescents updated for a new century fueled by media. *Contemp Pediatrics.* 1-16. contemporarypediatrics.modernmedicine.com.

Figure 5.2 Kroenke, K., Spitzer, R. L., Williams, J. B., et al. (2007). Anxiety disorders in primary care: Prevalence, impairment, comorbidity, and detection. *Ann Intern Med.* 146(5), 317-325.

Figure 5.3 Spitzer, Robert L., Williams, Janet B. W., & Kroenke, Kurt, et al. (1999). Developed with an educational grant from Pfizer Inc. No permission required to reproduce, translate, display, or distribute.

Figure 6.2 Substance Abuse and Mental Health Services Administration (SAMHSA). (2016.) 2015 National Survey on Drug Use and Health (NSDUH). https://www.samhsa.gov/data/sites/default/files/NSDUH-DetTabs-2015/NSDUH-DetTabs-2015/NSDUH-DetTabs-2015.htm.

Figure 7.1 © nicolesy/iStock/Thinkstock.

Figure 7.3 Yaffe, M. J., Lithwick, M., & Wolfson, C. (2006).

Figure 7.4 Zitelli, B. J., McIntire, S. C., & Nowalk, A. J. (2012). *Atlas of pediatric physical diagnosis.* (6th ed.). Philadelphia: Saunders.

Figure 7.5 Jacquelyn C. Campbell, PhD, RN, 1985, 1988, 2001.

Table 7.2 (Immersion injury patterns), (Pattern burn injury) Jenny, C. (2011). *Child abuse and neglect: Diagnosis, treatment, and evidence.* Philadelphia: Saunders; **(Cigarette burns)** Paller, A. S., & Mancini, A. J. (2016). *Hurwitz clinical pediatric dermatology.* (5th ed.). Philadelphia: Saunders.

Table 7.3 (Thigh bruises) (Courtesy Dr. D. C. Homeier.) From Walls, R. M., Hockberger, R. S., & Gausche-Hill, M. (2018). *Rosen's emergency medicine: Concepts and clinical practice.* (9th ed.). Philadelphia: Elsevier; **(Bruising and petechiae)** Bolognia, J., Schaeffer, J., Duncan, Karyanne,

et al. (2014). *Dermatology essentials.* Philadelphia: Saunders; **(Nasal fracture)** Courtesy Dr. John D. McDowell. From Neville, B. W., Damm, D. D., Allen, C. M., et al. (2016). *Oral and maxillofacial pathology.* (4th ed.). St. Louis: Elsevier; **(Belt-loop)** Kim, P. T., & Falcone, R. A., Jr. (2017). Nonaccidental trauma in pediatric surgery. *Surg Clin North Am.* 97(1), 21-33; **(Fingers)** Lambert, S., & Lyons, C. J. (2017). *Taylor and Hoyt's pediatric ophthalmology and strabismus.* (5th ed.). St. Louis: Elsevier; **(Self-defense bruises)** Payne-James, J., & Byard, R. W. (eds.) (2016). *Encyclopedia of forensic and legal medicine.* (2nd ed.). Edinburgh: Elsevier, Ltd.

Table 7.4 (Signs of neglect) Courtesy of L. Gibbs, MD. From Gibbs, L. M. (2014). Understanding the medical markers of elder abuse and neglect: Physical examination findings. *Clin Geriatr Med.* 30(4), 687-712.

Figure 8.10 Zakus, S. M. (2001). *Mosby's clinical skills for medical assistants.* (4th ed.). St. Louis: Mosby.

Figure 9.10 Rossman, I. (1986). *Clinical geriatrics.* (3rd ed.). Philadelphia: Lippincott.

Table 9.2 (Marfan syndrome) Anderson, R. C., Baker, E. J., Redington, A., et al. (2010). *Paediatric cardiology.* (3rd ed.). Philadelphia: Churchill Livingstone; **(Acromegaly [hyperpituitarism])** Clinical Slide Collection on the Rheumatic Diseases.1991, 1995, 1997. Used by permission of the American College of Rheumatology; **(Anorexia nervosa)** Comerci, George D., MD; **(Hypopituitary dwarfism; Gigantism)** Hall, R., & Evered, D. C. (1990). *Color atlas of endocrinology.* (2nd ed.). London: Mosby; **(Achondroplastic dwarfism)** Jones, A., & Owen, R. (1995). *Color atlas of clinical orthopedics.* (2nd ed.). London: Mosby; **(Endogenous obesity—Cushing syndrome)** Wenig, B. M., Hefess, C. S., & Adair, C. F. (1997). *Atlas of endocrine pathology.* Philadelphia: Saunders.

Figure 10.11 Thomas, Pat, 2014.

Figure 11.4 Thomas, Pat, 2018.

Figure 11.5 McCaffery, M., & Pasero, C. (1999). *Pain: Clinical manual.* (2nd ed.). St. Louis: Mosby.

Figure 11.6 Acute Pain Management Guideline Panel, 1992.

Figure 11.7 Faces Pain Scale-Revised (FPS-R). Hicks, C. L., von Baeyer, C. L., Spafford, P. A., et al. (2001). Faces Pain Scale—Revised: Toward a common metric in pediatric pain measurement. *Pain.* 93(2), 173-183. © 2001 International Association for the Study of Pain (IASP).

Figure 11.8 Brady, Rick; Riva, MD.

Figure 11.9 Krechel, S. W., & Bildner, J. (1995). CRIES—a new neonatal postoperative pain measurement score: Initial testing of validity and reliability. *Paediatr Anaesth.* 5(1), 53-61.

Figure 11.10 Voepel-Lewis, T., Zanotti, J., Dammeyer, J. A., et al. (2010). Reliability and validity of the face, legs, activity, cry, consolability behavioral tool in assessing acute pain in critically ill patients. *Am J Crit Care, 19*(1), 55-61.

Figure 11.11 Warden, V., Hurley, A. C., & Voticer, L. (2003). Development and psychometric evaluation of the Pain Assessment in Advanced Dementia (PAINAD) Scale. *J Am Med Dir Assoc. 4*(1), 9-15.

Table 11.5 (Reflexive sympathetic dystrophy) Thomas, Pat, 2010.

Figure 12.1 Cavan Images.

Figure 12.2 Agricultural Research Service (ARS). (2012). Image Gallery. Beltsville, MD: U.S. Department of Agriculture.

Figure 12.3 Busch, Niels.

Table 12.3 (Marasmus) Hall, R., & Evered, D. C. (1990). *Color atlas of endocrinology.* (2nd ed.). London: Mosby; **(Kwashiorkor)** Kramer, C. V., & Allen, S. (2015). Malnutrition in developing countries. *Paediatr Child Healt. 25*(9), 422-427.

Table 12.4 (Pellagra; Rickets) Latham, M. C., et al. (1980). *Scope manual on nutrition.* Kalamazoo: The Upjohn Company, Thomas Spies, MD; **(Magenta tongue)** McLaren, D. S. (1981). *Color atlas of nutritional disorders.* London: Wolfe Medical, C. E. Butterworth, Jr.; **(Follicular hyperkeratosis, Scorbutic gums, Bitot's spots)** Taylor, K. B., & Anthony, L. E. (1983). *Clinical nutrition.* New York: McGraw-Hill.

Figure 13.4 Hurwitz, S. (1993). *Clinical pediatric dermatology: A textbook of skin disorders of childhood and adolescence.* (2nd ed.). Philadelphia: Saunders.

Figure 13.5 Patton, K. T., Thibodeau, G. A., Douglas, M. M. (2012). Essentials of anatomy & physiology. (1st ed.). St. Louis: Mosby.

Figure 13.8 Lemmi and Lemmi, 2011.

Figure 13.14 Lemmi and Lemmi, 2011.

Figure 13.15 Lemmi and Lemmi, 2011.

Figure 13.17 Lemmi and Lemmi, 2011.

Figure 13.18 Bowden, V. R., Dickey, S. B., & Greenburg, C. S. (1998). *Children and their families: The continuum of care.* Philadelphia: Saunders.

Figure 13.19 Hurwitz, S. (1993). *Clinical pediatric dermatology: A textbook of skin disorders of childhood and adolescence.* (2nd ed.). Philadelphia: Saunders.

Figure 13.20 Hurwitz, S. (1993). *Clinical pediatric dermatology: A textbook of skin disorders of childhood and adolescence.* (2nd ed.). Philadelphia: Saunders.

Figure 13.21 Cohen, B. (2013). *Pediatric dermatology.* (4th ed.). Edinburgh: Elsevier, Ltd.

Figure 13.22 Eichenfield, L. F., Frieden, I. J., Mathes, E. F., et al. (2015). *Neonatal and infant dermatology.* (3rd ed.). Philadelphia: Elsevier.

Figure 13.23 Murray, S. S., & McKinney, E. S. (2010). *Foundations of maternal-newborn and women's health nursing.* (5th ed.). St. Louis: Saunders.

Figure 13.24 Habif, T. P., Campbell, J. L., Jr., Chapman, M. S., et al. (2005). *Skin disease: Diagnosis and treatment.* (2nd ed.). St. Louis: Mosby.

Figure 13.25 Marks, J. G., & Miller, J. J. (2019). *Lookingbill and Marks' principles of dermatology.* (6th ed.). Philadelphia: Elsevier.

Figure 13.26 Lemmi and Lemmi, 2011.

Figure 13.27 Habif, T. P., Campbell, J. L., Jr., Quitadamo, M. J., et al. (2001). *Skin disease: Diagnosis and treatment.* St. Louis: Mosby.

Figure 13.28 Marks, J. G., & Miller, J. J. (2019). *Lookingbill and Marks' principles of dermatology.* (6th ed.). Philadelphia: Elsevier.

Figure 13.29 Callen, J. P., Greer, K. E., Hood, A. F., et al. (1993). *Color atlas of dermatology.* Philadelphia: Saunders.

Figure 13.31 Williams, P. A. (2020). *Basic geriatric nursing.* (7th ed.). St. Louis: Elsevier.

Table 13.4 (Wheal and urticaria [hives]) Fireman, P. (1996). *Atlas of allergies.* (2nd ed.). London: Mosby; **(Macule and patch; Papule and plaque; Nodule and tumor; Vesicle and bulla; Cyst; Pustule)** Lemmi and Lemmi, 2011; **(Primary skin lesions [line drawings])** Thomas, Pat, 2010.

Table 13.5 (Crust; Scale; Fissure; Erosion; Ulcer; Excoriation; Scar; Atrophic scar; Lichenification; Keloid) Lemmi and Lemmi, 2011; **(Secondary skin lesions [line drawings])** Thomas, Pat, 2010.

Table 13.6 (Decubitus ulcer: Stages 1-4) Potter, P. A., Perry, A. G., Stockert, P., Hall, A. (2015). *Essentials for Nursing Practice.* (8th ed.). St. Louis: Mosby.

Table 13.7 (Petechiae) Dockery, G. L. (1997). *Cutaneous disorders of the lower extremity.* Philadelphia: Saunders; **(Strawberry mark [immature hemangioma]), Cavernous hemangioma [mature]; Venous lake)** Habif, T. P., Campbell, J. L., Jr., Chapman, M. S., et al. (2005). *Skin disease: Diagnosis and treatment.* (2nd ed.). St. Louis: Mosby; **(Telangiectasia; Spider or star angioma; Ecchymosis)** Lemmi and Lemmi, 2011; **(Strawberry mark [immature hemangioma])** Lookingbill, D. P., & Marks, J. G. (1993). *Principles of dermatology.* (2nd ed.). Philadelphia: Saunders; **(Port-wine stain [Nevus flammeus]; Purpura),** Paller, A. S., & Mancini, A. J. (2011). *Hurwitz clinical pediatric dermatology: A textbook of skin disorders of childhood and adolescence.* (4th ed.). Philadelphia: Saunders.

Table 13.8 (Chickenpox [varicella]) Callen, J. P., Greer, K. E., Hood, A. F., et al. (1993). *Color atlas of dermatology.* Philadelphia: Saunders; **(Measles [rubeola] in dark skin)** Feigin, R. D., & Cherry, J. D. (1998). *Textbook of pediatric infectious diseases.* (4th ed.). Philadelphia: Saunders; **(Intertrigo [candidiasis]; Impetigo; Measles [rubeola] in light skin)** Lemmi and Lemmi, 2011; **(Diaper dermatitis; Atopic dermatitis [eczema]; German measles [rubella])** Paller, A. S., & Mancini, A. J. (2011). *Hurwitz clinical pediatric dermatology: A textbook of skin disorders of childhood and adolescence.* (4th ed.). Philadelphia: Saunders.

Table 13.9 (Primary contact dermatitis; Allergic drug reaction; Psoriasis) Lookingbill, D. P., & Marks, J. G. (1993). *Principles of dermatology.* (2nd ed.). Philadelphia: Saunders; **(Tinea pedis [ringworm of the foot]; Labial herpes**

simplex [cold sores]; Tinea versicolor; Herpes zoster [shingles]) Lemmi and Lemmi, 2011; (**Tinea corporis [ringworm of the body]**) Paller, A. S., & Mancini, A. J. (2011). *Hurwitz clinical pediatric dermatology: A textbook of skin disorders of childhood and adolescence.* (4th ed.). Philadelphia: Saunders; (**Erythema migrans of Lyme disease**) Swartz, M. H. (2005). *Textbook of physical diagnosis: History and examination.* (5th ed.). Philadelphia: Saunders.

Table 13.10 (**Metastatic malignant melanoma**) Habif, T. P, Dinulos, J. G. H., Chapman, M. S., et al. (2018). *Skin disease: Diagnosis and treatment.* (4th ed.). Philadelphia: Elsevier; (**Squamous cell carcinoma**) Habif, T. P., Campbell, J. L., Jr., Quitadamo, M. J., et al. (2001). *Skin disease: Diagnosis and treatment.* St. Louis: Mosby; (**Basal cell carcinoma; Malignant melanoma**) Lookingbill, D. P., & Marks, J. G. (1993). *Principles of dermatology.* (2nd ed.). Philadelphia: Saunders.

Table 13.11 (**Pediculosis capitis [head lice]**) Callen, J. P., Greer, K. E., Hood, A. F., et al. (1993). *Color atlas of dermatology.* Philadelphia: Saunders; (**Alopecia.**) Fitzpatrick, J. E., High, W. A., Kyle, W. L. (2018). *Urgent care dermatology: Symptom-based diagnosis.* (1st ed.). Philadelphia: Elsevier; (**AIDS-related Kaposi sarcoma: Patch stage**) Friedman-Kien, A. E. (1989). *Color atlas of AIDS.* Philadelphia: Saunders; (**Toxic alopecia; Seborrheic dermatitis [cradle cap]**) Hurwitz, S. (1993). *Clinical pediatric dermatology: A textbook of skin disorders of childhood and adolescence.* (2nd ed.). Philadelphia: Saunders; (**Folliculitis**) Paller, A. S., & Mancini, A. J. (2016). *Hurwitz clinical pediatric dermatology: A textbook of skin disorders of childhood and adolescence.* (5th ed.). Philadelphia: Saunders; (**Hirsutism**) James, W., Berger, T., Elston, D. (2012). *Andrews' diseases of the skin.* (11th ed.). Philadelphia: Saunders; (**Tinea capitis [scalp ringworm]; Furuncle and abscess),** Lookingbill, D. P., & Marks, J. G. (1993). *Principles of dermatology.* (2nd ed.). Philadelphia: Saunders.

Table 13.12 (**Beau's line; Splinter hemorrhages),** Callen, J. P., Greer, K. E., Hood, A. F., et al. (1993). *Color atlas of dermatology.* Philadelphia: Saunders; (**Late clubbing**) Clinical Slide Collection on the Rheumatic Diseases.1991, 1995, 1997. Used by permission of the American College of Rheumatology; (**Scabies; Paronychia; Onycholysis; Pitting; Habit-tic dystrophy**) Lemmi and Lemmi, 2011.

Figure 14.1 Thomas, Pat, 2018.

Figure 14.2 Thomas, Pat, 2018.

Figure 14.8 Thomas, Pat, 2006.

Figure 14.12 *B* Dean, S., Garrett, N., & Tyrrell, J. (2008). Management of enlarged cervical lymph nodes. *Paediatr Child Healt.* 118(3), 118-122.

Figure 14.14 *B* Lemmi and Lemmi, 2011.

Figure 14.16 Murray, S. S., & McKinney, E. S. (2014). *Foundations of maternal-newborn and women's health nursing.* (6th ed.). St. Louis: Saunders.

Figure 14.17 Murray, S. S., & McKinney, E. S. (2014). *Foundations of maternal-newborn and women's health nursing.* (6th ed.). St. Louis: Saunders.

Table 14.1 (**Primary headaches**) Thomas, Pat, 2014.

Table 14.2 (**Hydrocephalus**) Bowden, V. R., Dickey, S. B., & Greenburg, C. S. (1998). *Children and their families: The continuum of care.* Philadelphia: Saunders; (**Down syndrome**) Hockenberry, M. J., & Wilson, D. (2012). *Wong's essentials of pediatric nursing.* (9th ed.). St. Louis: Mosby; (**Plagiocephaly**) Pomatto, J. K., Calcaterra, J., Kelly, K. M., et al. (2006). A study of family head shape: Environment alters cranial shape. *Clin Pediatr.* 45(1), 55-64; (**Craniosynostosis**) Quiñones-Hinojosa, A. (2012). *Schmidek and Sweet operative neurosurgical techniques: Indications, methods, and results.* (6th ed.). Philadelphia: Saunders; (**Fetal alcohol syndrome**) Streissguth, A. P., Landesman-Dwyer, S., Martin, J. C., et al. (1980). Teratogenic effects of alcohol in humans and laboratory animals. *Science.* 209(4454), 353-361; (**Fetal alcohol syndrome [line drawing]**) Thomas, Pat, 2006; (**Atopic [allergic] facies; Allergic salute and crease**) Zitelli, B. J., & Davis, H. W. (2007). *Atlas of pediatric physical diagnosis.* (5th ed.). St. Louis: Mosby.

Table 14.3 (**Pilar cyst [wen]** Callen, J. P., Greer, K. E., Hood, A. F., et al. (1993). *Color atlas of dermatology.* Philadelphia: Saunders; (**Goiter**) Lemmi and Lemmi, 2011; (**Parotid gland enlargement**) Meningaud, J. P., Pitak-Arnnop, P., Fouret, P., et al. (2007). Kimura's disease of the parotid region. *J Oral Maxillofac Surg. (65)*1, 134-140; (**Thyroid—multinodular goiter**) Swartz, M. H. (2005). *Textbook of physical diagnosis: History and examination.* (5th ed.). Philadelphia: Saunders; (**Congenital torticollis**) Zitelli, B. J., & Davis, H. W. (2007). *Atlas of pediatric physical diagnosis.* (5th ed.). St. Louis: Mosby.

Table 14.4 (**Myxedema [hypothyroidism]**) Hall, R., & Evered, D. C. (1990). *Color atlas of endocrinology.* (2nd ed.). London: Mosby; (**Hyperthyroidism**) Swartz, M. H. (2005). *Textbook of physical diagnosis: History and examination.* (5th ed.). Philadelphia: Saunders; (**Hypothalamic-pituitary-thyroid axis**) Thomas, Pat, 2014.

Table 14.5 (**Parkinson syndrome**) Glynn, M., & Drake, W. M. (2012). *Hutchison's clinical methods: An integrated approach to clinical practice.* (23rd ed.). Philadelphia: Saunders/Elsevier, Ltd.; (**Cachectic appearance**) Lemmi and Lemmi, 2011; (**Acromegaly**) Liu, G. T., Volpe, N. J., & Galetta, S. L. (2010). *Neuro-ophthalmology: Diagnosis and management.* (2nd ed.). Philadelphia: Saunders; (**Stroke or "brain attack"**) Nolte, J., & Sundsten, J. (2009). *The human brain: An introduction to its functional anatomy.* (6th ed.). Philadelphia: Mosby/Elsevier; (**Bell palsy**) Studdiford, J. S., Altschuler, M., Salzman B., et al. (2009). *Images from the wards: Diagnosis and treatment.* (1st ed.). Philadelphia: Saunders; (**Cushing syndrome**) Yeh, M. W., & Duh, Q. Y. (2012). *Sabiston textbook of surgery: The biological basis of modern surgical practice.* (19th ed.). Philadelphia: Saunders.

Figure 15.1 Thomas, Pat, 2006.

Figure 15.2 Thomas, Pat, 2006.

Figure 15.3 Thomas, Pat, 2006.

Figure 15.17 Thomas, Pat, 2006.

Figure 15.21 Boyd-Monk, Heather, and Wills Eye Hospital, Philadelphia.

Figure 15.22 Lemmi and Lemmi, 2011.

Figure 15.23 Lemmi and Lemmi, 2011.

Figure 15.29 Zitelli, B. J., & Davis, H. W. (2007). *Atlas of pediatric physical diagnosis.* (5th ed.). St. Louis: Mosby.

Figure 15.30 Albert, D. M., & Jakobiec, F. A. (1994). *Principles and practice of ophthalmology.* Philadelphia: Saunders.

Figure 15.31 Lemmi and Lemmi, 2011.

Figure 15.32 Swartz, M. H. (2015). *Textbook of physical diagnosis: History and examination.* (7th ed.). Philadelphia: Saunders.

Figure 15.33 Mannis, M. J., & Holland, E. J. (2017). *Cornea.* (4th ed.). Philadelphia: Elsevier.

Figure 15.34 Freidman, N., Pineda, R. (1998). *The Massachusetts Eye and Ear Infirmary illustrated manual of ophthalmology.* Philadelphia: Saunders.

Table 15.1 (Left esotropia; Exotropia) Zitelli, B. J., & Davis, H. W. (2007). *Atlas of pediatric physical diagnosis.* (5th ed.). St. Louis: Mosby.

Table 15.2 (Ectropion; Entropion) Friedman, N. J., Kaiser, P. K., & Pineda, R. (2014). *The Massachusetts Eye and Ear Infirmary illustrated manual of ophthalmology.* (4th ed.). Philadelphia: Saunders Elsevier; **(Upward palpebral slant)** Hockenberry, M. J., & Wilson, D. (2013). *Wong's essentials of pediatric nursing.* (9th ed.). St. Louis: Mosby; **(Periorbital edema)** Ibsen, O. A. C., & Phelan, J. A. (1992). *Oral pathology for the dental hygienist.* (2nd ed.). Philadelphia: Saunders; **(Exophthalmos [protruding eyes]; Ptosis [drooping upper lid])** Lemmi and Lemmi, 2011.

Table 15.3 (Chalazion) Boyd-Monk, Heather, and Wills Eye Hospital, Philadelphia; **(Blepharitis [inflammation of the eyelids]; Dacryocystitis [inflammation of the lacrimal sac])** Freidman, N., & Pineda, R. (1998). *The Massachusetts Eye and Ear Infirmary illustrated manual of ophthalmology.* Philadelphia: Saunders; **(Basal cell carcinoma)** Friedman, N. J., Kaiser, P. K., & Pineda, R. (2014). The Massachusetts Eye and Ear Infirmary illustrated manual of ophthalmology. (4th ed.). Philadelphia: Saunders Elsevier; **(Hordeolum [stye])** Lemmi and Lemmi, 2011.

Table 15.6 (Primary angle-closure glaucoma) Atkinson, P., Kendall, R., & Rensburg, L. V. (2011). *Emergency medicine: An illustrated color text.* (1st ed.). Philadelphia: Churchill Livingstone; **(Herpes simplex)** Friedman, N. J., Kaiser, P. K., & Pineda R. (2014). *The Massachusetts Eye and Ear Infirmary illustrated manual of ophthalmology.* (4th ed.). Philadelphia: Saunders Elsevier; **(Allergic conjunctivitis)** Holgate, S. T., Church, M. K., Broide, D. H., et al. (2012). *Allergy.* (4th ed.). Philadelphia: Saunders; **(Conjunctivitis; Subconjunctival hemorrhage)** Lemmi and Lemmi, 2011; **(Iritis [circumcorneal redness])** Scheie, H. G., & Albert, D. M. (1977). *Textbook of ophthalmology.* (9th ed.). Philadelphia: Saunders.

Table 15.7 (Corneal abrasion) Boyd-Monk, Heather, and Wills Eye Hospital, Philadelphia; **(Hypopyon)** Friedman, N. J., Kaiser, P. K., & Pineda, R. (2014). *The Massachusetts*

Eye and Ear Infirmary illustrated manual of ophthalmology. (4th ed.). Philadelphia: Saunders Elsevier; **(Pterygium; Hyphema),** Lemmi and Lemmi, 2011.

Table 15.8 (Central gray opacity—nuclear cataract; Star-shaped opacity—cortical cataract) Freidman, N., & Pineda, R. (1998). *The Massachusetts Eye and Ear Infirmary illustrated manual of ophthalmology.* Philadelphia: Saunders.

Table 15.9 (Excessive cup-disc ratio) Freidman, N., & Pineda, R. (1998). *The Massachusetts Eye and Ear Infirmary illustrated manual of ophthalmology.* Philadelphia: Saunders; **(Optic atrophy [disc pallor]; Papilledema [choked disc])** Friedman, N., Kaiser, P. K., & Pineda, R. (2009). *The Massachusetts Eye and Ear Infirmary illustrated manual of ophthalmology.* (3rd ed.). Philadelphia: Saunders.

Table 15.10 (Arteriovenous crossing [nicking]) Freidman, N., & Pineda, R. (1998). *The Massachusetts Eye and Ear Infirmary illustrated manual of ophthalmology.* Philadelphia: Saunders; **(Moderate nonproliferative diabetic retinopathy; Severe nonproliferative diabetic retinopathy)** Friedman, N. J., Kaiser, P. K., & Pineda, R. (2014). *The Massachusetts Eye and Ear Infirmary illustrated manual of ophthalmology.* (4th ed.). Philadelphia: Saunders Elsevier; **(Narrowed [attenuated] arteries: age 14 years and age 61 years)** Lemmi and Lemmi, 2011.

Figure 16.1 Thomas, Pat, 2010.

Figure 16.3 Lemmi and Lemmi, 2011.

Figure 16.4 Thomas, Pat, 2006.

Figure 16.9 Lemmi and Lemmi, 2011.

Figure 16.10 Thomas, Pat, 2006.

Table 16.1 (Hearing loss) Thomas, Pat, 2014.

Table 16.2 (Frostbite) Auerbach, P. (2007). *Wilderness medicine.* (5th ed.). St. Louis: Mosby; **(Branchial remnant and ear deformity)** Liebert, P. S. (1996). *Color atlas of pediatric surgery.* (2nd ed.). Philadelphia: Saunders; **(Otitis externa [swimmer's ear]; Cellulitis)** Lemmi and Lemmi, 2011.

Table 16.3 (Carcinoma) Ameerally, P. J., & Colver, G. B. (2007). Cutaneous cryotherapy in maxillofacial surgery. *J Oral Maxillofac Surg. 65*(9), 1785-1792; **(Chondrodermatitis nodularis helicus)** Habif, T. P., Campbell, J. L., Jr., Chapman, M. S., et al. (2005). *Skin disease: Diagnosis and treatment.* (2nd ed.). St. Louis: Mosby; **(Keloid)** Lemmi and Lemmi, 2011; **(Sebaceous cyst)** Liebert, P. S. (1996). *Color atlas of pediatric surgery.* (2nd ed.). Philadelphia: Saunders; **(Battle sign)** Zitelli, B. J., McIntire, S. C., & Nowalk, A. J. (2012). *Atlas of pediatric physical diagnosis.* (6th ed.). Philadelphia: Saunders; **(Tophi)** Clinical Slide Collection on the Rheumatic Diseases.1991, 1995, 1997. Used by permission of the American College of Rheumatology.

Table 16.4 (Ear canal abnormalities) Thomas, Pat, 2010.

Table 16.6 (Fungal infection [otomycosis]), Thomas, Pat, 2010; **(Retracted drum; Acute [purulent] otitis media [early stage]; Acute [purulent] otitis media [later stage])** Adams, G. L., Boies, L. R., Jr., & Hilger, P. A. (1989). *Boies fundamentals of otolaryngology: A textbook of ear, nose and throat diseases.* (6th ed.). Philadelphia: Saunders; **(Perforation; Blue drum [hemotympanum])** Dhillon, R. S., &

East, C. A. (2013). *Ear, nose and throat and head and neck surgery.* (4th ed.). Philadelphia: Churchill Livingstone; (**Insertion of tympanostomy tubes**) Fireman, P. (1996). *Atlas of allergies.* (2nd ed.). London: Mosby; (**Scarred drum**) Lim, E., Loke, Y. K., & Thompson, A. (2007). *Medicine & surgery: An integrated textbook.* Philadelphia: Churchill Livingstone; (**Otitis media with effusion; Cholesteatoma; Bullous myringitis**) Swartz, M. H. (2005). *Textbook of physical diagnosis: History and examination.* (5th ed.). Philadelphia: Saunders.

Figure 17.1 Thomas, Pat, 2006.

Figure 17.2 Thomas, Pat, 2006.

Figure 17.3 Thomas, Pat, 2006.

Figure 17.4 Thomas, Pat, 2010.

Figure 17.5 Thomas, Pat, 2010.

Figure 17.6 Thomas, Pat, 2006.

Figure 17.9 Fireman, P. (1996). *Atlas of allergies.* (2nd ed.). London: Mosby.

Figure 17.16 Ibsen, O. A. C., & Phelan, J. A. (1996). *Oral pathology for the dental hygienist.* (2nd ed.). Philadelphia: Saunders.

Figure 17.17 Flint, P. W, Haughey, B. H., Lund, V., et al. (2015). *Cummings otolaryngology.* (6th ed.). Philadelphia: Saunders.

Figure 17.18 Thomas, Pat, 2006.

Figure 17.22 Zitelli, B. J., McIntire, S. C., & Nowalk, A. J. (2012). *Atlas of pediatric physical diagnosis.* (6th ed.). Philadelphia: Saunders.

Figure 17.23 Lemmi and Lemmi, 2011.

Figure 17.24 Lemmi and Lemmi, 2011.

Figure 17.25 Van Schayck, O. C. P., Williams, S., Barchilon, V., et al. (2017). Treating tobacco dependence: Guidance for primary care on life-saving interventions. *NPJ Prim Care Respir Med. 27*(1), 38.

Table 17.1 (Foreign body; Allergic rhinitis; Nasal polyps) Fireman, P. (1996). *Atlas of allergies.* (2nd ed.). London: Mosby; (**Perforated septum**) Hawke, M. (1998). *Diagnostic handbook of otorhinolaryngology.* London: Martin Dunitz, reproduced by permission of Taylor & Francis Books UK.

Table 17.2 (Cleft lip) Ibsen, O. A. C., & Phelan, J. A. (1996). *Oral pathology for the dental hygienist.* (2nd ed.). Philadelphia: Saunders; (**Herpes simplex 1; Angular cheilitis**) Callen, J. P., Greer, K. E., Hood, A. F., et al. (1993). *Color atlas of dermatology.* Philadelphia: Saunders; (**Carcinoma; Retention "cyst" [mucocele]**), Hawke, M. (1998). *Diagnostic handbook of otorhinolaryngology.* London: Martin Dunitz, reproduced by permission of Taylor & Francis Books UK.

Table 17.3 (Gingivitis) Callen, J. P., Greer, K. E., Hood, A. F., et al. (1993). *Color atlas of dermatology.* Philadelphia: Saunders; (**Baby bottle tooth decay**) Ferguson, F. Department of Children's Dentistry, School of Dental Medicine, SUNY at Stony Brook, Stony Brook, NY; (**Epulis; Gingival hyperplasia**) Ibsen, O. A. C., & Phelan, J. A. (1996). *Oral pathology for the dental hygienist.* (2nd ed.). Philadelphia: Saunders; (**Dental caries**) McWhorter, A., Pediatric

Dentistry, Baylor College of Dentistry, The Texas A & M University System, Dallas, TX; (**Meth mouth**) Neville, B. W., Damm, D. D., Allen, C. M., et al. (2009). *Oral and maxillofacial pathology.* (3rd ed.). St. Louis: Saunders; (**Tooth avulsion**) Torabinejad, M., Walton, R.E., Fouad, A.F. (2015). *Endodontics: Principles and practice* (5th ed.). Philadelphia: Saunders.

Table 17.4 (Candidiasis or monilial infection) Callen, J. P., Greer, K. E., Hood, A. F., et al. (1993). *Color atlas of dermatology.* Philadelphia: Saunders; (**Koplik spots**) Feigin, R. D., & Cherry, J. D. (1998). *Textbook of pediatric infectious diseases.* (4th ed.). Philadelphia: Saunders; (**Aphthous ulcers; Herpes simplex 1**) Lemmi and Lemmi, 2011; (**Candidiasis in adult**) Peters, W., & Pasvol, G. (2007). *Atlas of tropical medicine and parasitology.* (6th ed.). Philadelphia: Churchill Livingstone; (**Leukoplakia**) Sleisinger, M. H., & Fordtran, J. S. (1993). *Gastrointestinal diseases: Pathophysiology, diagnosis, and management.* Vol. 1. (5th ed.). Philadelphia: Saunders.

Table 17.5 (Smooth, glossy tongue [atrophic glossitis]) Adams, G. L., Boies, L. R., Jr., & Hilger, P. A. (1989). *Boies fundamentals of otolaryngology: A textbook of ear, nose and throat diseases.* (6th ed.). Philadelphia: Saunders; (**Black hairy tongue**) Callen, J. P., Greer, K. E., Hood, A. F., et al. (1993). *Color atlas of dermatology.* Philadelphia: Saunders; (**Ankyloglossia**) Ibsen, O. A. C., & Phelan, J. A. (1996). *Oral pathology for the dental hygienist.* (2nd ed.). Philadelphia: Saunders; (**Geographic tongue [migratory glossitis]; Fissured or scrotal tongue**) Lemmi and Lemmi, 2011; (**Carcinoma**) Wenig, B. M., Hefess, C. S., & Adair, C. F. (1997). *Atlas of endocrine pathology.* Philadelphia: Saunders; (**Enlarged tongue [macroglossia]**) Zitelli, B. J., & Davis, H. W. (2007). *Atlas of pediatric physical diagnosis.* (5th ed.). St. Louis: Mosby.

Table 17.6 (Acute tonsillitis and pharyngitis) Douglas, G., Nicol, F., & Robertson, C. (2013). *Macleod's clinical examination.* (13th ed.). Philadelphia: Churchill Livingstone; (**Oral Kaposi sarcoma**) Flint, P. W., Haughey, B. H., Lund, V. J., et al. (2010). *Cummings otolaryngology: Head & neck surgery.* (5th ed.). Philadelphia: Saunders; (**Bifid uvula**) Hawke, M. (1998). *Diagnostic handbook of otorhinolaryngology.* London: Martin Dunitz, reproduced by permission of Taylor & Francis Books UK; (**Peritonsillar abscess**) Pfenninger, J. L., & Fowler, G. C. (2011). *Pfenninger and Fowler's procedures for primary care.* (3rd ed.). St. Louis: Mosby; (**Cleft palate**) Zitelli, B. J., & Davis, H. W. (2002). *Atlas of pediatric physical diagnosis.* (4th ed.). St. Louis: Mosby.

Figure 18.7 Callen, J.P., et al. (1993). *Color atlas of dermatology.* Philadelphia: Saunders.

Figure 18.18 Thomas, Pat, 2014.

Figure 18.20 (Adolescent gynecomastia) Hammond, D. C. (2009). *Atlas of aesthetic breast surgery.* (1st ed.). Philadelphia: Saunders.

Table 18.3 (Fixation; Deviation in nipple pointing) Mansel, R. (1995). *Color atlas of breast diseases.* London: Mosby; (**Dimpling; Peau d'orange**) Quick, C. R. G., Reed, J. B.,

Harper, S. J. F., Saeb-Parsy, K., Deakin, P. J. (2014). *Essential surgery: Problems, diagnosis and management.* (5th ed.). Edinburgh: Elsevier, Ltd.

Table 18.6 (Carcinoma) Evans, A. J., et al. (1998). *Atlas of breast disease management: 50 illustrative cases.* Philadelphia: Saunders; **(Mammary duct ectasia; Intraductal papilloma; Paget's disease [intraductal carcinoma])** Mansel, R. (1995). *Color atlas of breast diseases.* London: Mosby.

Table 18.7 (Mastitis; Breast abscess) Mansel, R. (1995). *Color atlas of breast diseases.* London: Mosby.

Table 18.8 (Male breast cancer) Elshafieya, M. E., Zeeneldinb, A. A., Elsebaia, H. I., et al. (2011). Epidemiology and management of breast carcinoma in Egyptian males: Experience of a single Cancer Institute. *J Egypt Natl Canc Inst. 23*(3), 115-122; **(Male breast abnormalities)** Lorenzo, G. D., Autorino, R., Perdonà, S., et al. (2005). Management of gynaecomastia in patients with prostate cancer: A systematic review. *Lancet Oncol. 6*(12), 972-979.

Figure 19.1 Thomas, Pat, 2010.

Figure 19.2 Thomas, Pat, 2010.

Figure 19.10 Thomas, Pat, 2010.

Figure 19.11 Thomas, Pat, 2010.

Figure 19.12 Thomas, Pat, 2006.

Figure 19.13 Nichols, F. H., & Zwelling, E. (1997). *Maternal-newborn nursing: Theory and practice.* Philadelphia: Saunders.

Unn Figure 19.1 Lung Function Questionnaire from GlaxoSmithKline, 2013.

Figure 20.3 Thomas, Pat, 2006.

Figure 20.4 Thomas, Pat, 2006.

Figure 20.6 Thomas, Pat, 2006.

Figure 20.8 Thomas, Pat, 2006.

Figure 20.9 Thomas, Pat, 2006.

Figure 20.12 Thomas, Pat, 2014.

Figure 20.15 Lakatta, E. G. (1985). Cardiovascular function in later life. *Cardiovasc Med. 10,* 37-40.

Figure 20.28 B Thomas, Pat, 2014

Table 20.9 (Abnormal pulsations on the precordium) Thomas, Pat, 2006.

Table 20.10 (Congenital heart defects) Thomas, Pat, 2006.

Table 20.11 (Murmurs due to valvular defects) Thomas, Pat, 2006.

Figure 21.1 Thomas, Pat, 2010.

Figure 21.3 Thomas, Pat, 2010.

Figure 21.4 Thomas, Pat, 2014.

Figure 21.6 Thomas, Pat, 2010.

Figure 21.20 B Bloom, A., Watkins, P. H., & Ireland, J. (1992). *Color atlas of diabetes.* (2nd ed.). St. Louis: Mosby.

Figure 21.22 B Lemmi and Lemmi, 2011.

Table 21.2 (Raynaud's phenomenon—pallor; Raynaud's phenomenon—cyanosis) Lemmi and Lemmi, 2011; **(Lymphedema)** Walsh, T. D., Fainsinger, R., Foley, K., et al. (2009). *Palliative medicine.* Philadelphia: Saunders.

Table 21.4 (Arterial-ischemic ulcer) Dockery, G. L. (1997). *Cutaneous disorders of the lower extremity.* Philadelphia: Saunders; **(Neuropathic ulcer)** Lemmi and Lemmi, 2011;

(Venous [stasis] ulcer) Lookingbill, D. P., & Marks, J. G. (1993). *Principles of dermatology.* (2nd ed.). Philadelphia: Saunders.

Table 21.5 (Deep vein thrombophlebitis [DVT]) Dockery, G. L. (1997). *Cutaneous disorders of the lower extremity.* Philadelphia: Saunders; **(Superficial varicose veins)** Lemmi and Lemmi, 2011.

Figure 22.1 Thomas, Pat, 2006.

Figure 22.2 Thomas, Pat, 2006.

Figure 22.3 Thomas, Pat, 2006.

Figure 22.4 Thomas, Pat, 2006.

Table 22.2 (Clinical portrait of intestinal obstruction) Thomas, Pat, 2014.

Table 22.3 (Common sites of referred abdominal pain) Thomas, Pat, 2006.

Table 22.4 (Diastasis recti) Clark, D. A. (2000). *Atlas of neonatology.* (7th ed.). Philadelphia: Saunders; **(Epigastric hernia)** Conroy, K., & Malata, C. M. (2012). Epigastric hernia following DIEP flap breast reconstruction: Complication or coincidence? *J Plast Reconstr Aesthet Surg. 65*(3), 387-391; **(Incisional hernia)** Lemmi and Lemmi, 2011; **(Umbilical hernia)** Zitelli, B. J., & Davis, H. W. (2007). *Atlas of pediatric physical diagnosis.* (5th ed.). St. Louis: Mosby.

Figure 23.2 Thomas, Pat, 2006.

Figure 23.8 Thomas, Pat, 2018.

Figure 23.32 C Dieppe, P. A., Cooper, C., & McGill, N. (1991). *Arthritis and rheumatism in practice.* London: Gower Medical Publishing.

Figure 23.33 B Dieppe, P. A., Cooper, C., & McGill, N. (1991). *Arthritis and rheumatism in practice.* London: Gower Medical Publishing.

Figure 23.37 Courtesy Lemmi & Lemmi, 2011.

Figure 23.44 Thomas, Pat, 2018.

Figure 23.50 Zitelli, B. J., & Davis, H. W. (2007). *Atlas of pediatric physical diagnosis.* (5th ed.). St. Louis: Mosby.

Table 23.1 (Ankylosing spondylitis) Thomas, Pat, 2018.

Table 23.2 (Joint effusion) Bunker, T., & Schranz, P. J. (1998). *Clinical challenges in orthopaedics: The shoulder.* London: Martin Dunitz, reproduced by permission of Taylor & Francis Books UK; **(Atrophy)** Chung, K. C, Yang, L. J.-S., & McGillicuddy, J. E. (2012). *Practical management of pediatric and adult brachial plexus palsies.* (1st ed.). Philadelphia: Saunders; **(Frozen shoulder—adhesive capsulitis)** Peñas C. F., Cleland, J. A., & Huijbregts, P. A. (2011). *Neck and arm pain syndromes: Evidence-informed screening, diagnosis and management.* Philadelphia: Churchill Livingstone; **(Dislocated shoulder)** Roberts, J. R., Custalow, C. B., Thomsen, T. W. (2019). *Roberts and Hedges' clinical procedures in emergency medicine and acute care.* (7th ed.). Philadelphia: Elsevier; **(Tear of rotator cuff)** Waldman, S. D. (2010). *Physical diagnosis of pain: An atlas of signs and symptoms.* (2nd ed.). Philadelphia: Saunders.

Table 23.3 (Rheumatoid nodules) Walker, B. R., Colledge, N. R., Ralston, S. H., et al. (2014). *Davidson's principles and practice of medicine.* (22nd ed.). London: Churchill

Livingstone; (**Olecranon bursitis**) Dieppe, P. A., Cooper, C., & McGill, N. (1991). *Arthritis and rheumatism in practice.* London: Gower Medical Publishing; (**Arthritis**) Polley, H. F., & Hunder, G. G. (1978). *Physical examination of the joints.* (2nd ed.). Philadelphia: Saunders; (**Epicondylitis—tennis elbow**) Skirven, T. M., Osterman, A. L., Fedorczyk, J. M., et al. (2011). *Rehabilitation of the hand and upper extremity.* (6th ed.). St. Louis: Mosby.

Table 23.4 (**Dupuytren contracture**) Asar, F. M., Beaty, J. H., & Canale, S. T. (2017). *Campbell's operative orthopaedics.* (13th ed.). St. Louis: Mosby; (**Ganglion cyst**) Waldman, S. D. (2019). *Atlas of common pain syndromes.* (4th ed.). Philadelphia: Elsevier; (**Carpal tunnel syndrome with atrophy of thenar eminence**) Clinical Slide Collection on the Rheumatic Diseases.1991, 1995, 1997. Used by permission of the American College of Rheumatology; (**Swanneck and boutonnière deformity**) Clinical Slide Collection on the Rheumatic Diseases.1991, 1995, 1997. Used by permission of the American College of Rheumatology; (**Polydactyly; Syndactyly**) Liebert, P. S. (1996). *Color atlas of pediatric surgery.* (2nd ed.). Philadelphia: Saunders; (**Ankylosis**) Slutsky, D. J. (2010). *Principles and practice of wrist surgery.* Philadelphia: Saunders; (**Ulnar deviation or drift; Degenerative joint disease, or osteoarthritis**) Walker, J. M., & Helewa, A. (1996). *Physical therapy in arthritis.* Philadelphia: Saunders.

Table 23.5 (**Mild synovitis; Prepatellar bursitis**) Dieppe, P. A., Cooper, C., & McGill, N. (1991). *Arthritis and rheumatism in practice.* London: Gower Medical Publishing; (**Osgood-Schlatter disease**) Hochberg, M. C., Silman, A. J., Smolen, J. S., et al. (2003). *Rheumatology* (3rd ed.). St. Louis: Mosby; (**Swelling of menisci**) Jones, A., & Owen, R. (1995). *Color atlas of clinical orthopedics.* (2nd ed.). London: Mosby; (**Post-polio muscle atrophy**) Lemmi and Lemmi, 2011.

Table 23.6 (**Achilles tenosynovitis; Acute gout**) Dieppe, P. A., Cooper, C., & McGill, N. (1991). *Arthritis and rheumatism in practice.* London: Gower Medical Publishing; (**Tophi with chronic gout**) Dockery, G. L. (1997). *Cutaneous disorders of the lower extremity.* Philadelphia: Saunders; (**Callus; Ingrown toenail; Plantar wart**) Lemmi and Lemmi, 2011; (**Plantar fasciitis**) Thomas, Pat, 2018; (**Hallux valgus with bunion and hammertoes**) Walker, J. M., & Helewa, A. (1996). *Physical therapy in arthritis.* Philadelphia: Saunders.

Table 23.7 (**Scoliosis**) Miller, M. D., Hart, J. A., & MacKnight, J. M. (2010). *Essential orthopaedics.* (1st ed.). Philadelphia: Saunders; (**Herniated nucleus pulposus**) Polley, H. F., & Hunder, G. G. (1978). *Physical examination of the joints.* (2nd ed.). Philadelphia: Saunders.

Table 23.8 (**Congenital dislocated hip**) Asar, F. M., Beaty, J. H., & Canale, S. T. (2017). *Campbell's operative orthopaedics.* (13th ed.). St. Louis: Mosby; (**Talipes equinovarus**) Chudley, A. E., MD; (**Spina bifida**) Thompson, D. N. P. (2010). Spinal dysraphic anomalies; classification, presentation and management. *Paediatr Child Healt.* 20(9), 397-403.

Figure 24.1 Thomas, Pat, 2006.
Figure 24.2 Thomas, Pat, 2006.
Figure 24.3 Thomas, Pat, 2006.
Figure 24.4 Thomas, Pat, 2006.
Figure 24.5 Thomas, Pat, 2010.
Figure 24.7 Thomas, Pat, 2006.
Figure 24.45 Glasgow Coma Scale from Teasdale, G., & Jennett, B. (1974). Assessment of coma and impaired consciousness. A practical scale. *Lancet.* 304(7872), pp. 81-84. Images Thomas, Pat, 2014.
Figure 24.60 *B* Braddom, R. L. (2011). *Physical medicine and rehabilitation.* (4th ed.). Philadelphia: Saunders.
Table 24.1 (**10 warning signs of Alzheimer's disease**) Leifer, B. P. (2009). Alzheimer's disease: Seeing the signs early. *J Acad Nurse Pract.* 21(11), 588-595.**Table 24-5** (**Ischemic and hemorrhagic stroke**) Thomas, Pat, 2014.
Table 24.8 (**Patterns of motor system dysfunction**) Thomas, Pat, 2010.
Table 24.10 (**Abnormal postures**) Thomas, Pat, 2006.
Table 24.12 (**Frontal release signs**) Thomas, Pat, 2006.
Figure 25.1 Thomas, Pat, 2010.
Figure 25.2 Thomas, Pat, 2010.
Figure 25.3 Thomas, Pat, 2010.
Figure 25.4 Cooper, Connie.
Figure 25.9 *B* Lemmi and Lemmi, 2011.
Table 25.1 (**Sexual maturity rating in boys**) Tanner, J. M. (1962). *Growth at adolescence.* Oxford, England: Blackwell Scientific.
Table 25.2 (**Urine color and discolorations**) Cooper, Connie.
Table 25.3 (**Urethritis [urethral discharge and dysuria]**) Edmond, R., Rowl, H. A. K., & Welsby, P. (1995). *Colour atlas of infectious diseases.* (3rd ed., p. 161). London: Mosby; (**Renal calculi**) Gould, B. E., & Dyer, R. (2011). *Pathophysiology for the health professions.* (4th ed.). Philadelphia: Saunders; (**Acute urinary retention and urinary tract infection; Urethral stricture**) Thomas, Pat, 2018.
Table 25.4 (**Carcinoma**) Callen, J. P., Greer, K. E., Hood, A. F., et al. (1993). *Color atlas of dermatology.* Philadelphia: Saunders; (**Syphilitic chancre**) Edmond, R., Rowl, H. A. K., & Welsby, P. (1995). *Colour atlas of infectious diseases.* (3rd ed., p. 161). London: Mosby. (**Genital warts**) Habif, T. P., Campbell, J. L., Jr., Chapman, M. S., et al. (2005). *Skin disease: Diagnosis and treatment.* (2nd ed.). St. Louis: Mosby; (**Tinea cruris**) Lemmi and Lemmi, 2011; (**Genital herpes—HSV-2 infection**) Pfizer Laboratories Division, Pfizer Inc., New York. A close look at VD: A slide presentation produced as a public service.
Table 25.5 (**Epispadias**) Frimberger, D. (2011). Diagnosis and management of epispadias. *Semin Pediatr Surg.* 20(2), 85-90; (**Paraphimosis**) Keys, C., & Lam, J. P. H. (2013). Foreskin and penile problems in childhood. *Surgery* (Oxford). 31(3), 130-134; (**Phimosis**) Liebert, P. S. (1996). *Color atlas of pediatric surgery.* (2nd ed.). Philadelphia: Saunders; (**Hypospadias**) Wein, A. J., Kavoussi, L. R., Partin, A. W., et al. (2016). *Campbell-Walsh urology.* (11th ed.). Philadelphia: Elsevier; (**Peyronie disease**) Wein, A. J.,

Kavoussi, L. R., Partin, A. W., Peters, C. A. (2016). *Campbell-Walsh urology.* (11th ed.). Philadelphia: Elsevier.

Table 25.6 (Abnormalities in the scrotum) Thomas, Pat, 2006.

Table 25.7 (Inguinal and femoral hernias) Thomas, Pat, 2006.

Figure 27.2 Thomas, Pat, 2018.

Figure 27.12 *A* Courtesy Lemmi & Lemmi, 2011.

Table 27.1 (Sexual maturity rating in girls) Tanner, J. M. (1962). *Growth at adolescence.* Oxford, England: Blackwell Scientific.

Table 27.2 (Pediculosis pubis) James, W. D., Elston, D. M., & McMahon, P. J. (2018). *Andrews' diseases of the skin clinical atlas.* (1st ed.). Philadelphia: Elsevier; **(Syphilitic chancre; Abscess of Bartholin's gland)** Edmond, R., Rowl, H. A. K., & Welsby, P. (1995). *Colour atlas of infectious diseases.* (3rd ed., p. 161). London: Mosby; **(Human papillomavirus genital warts)** Habif, T. P. (2016). *Clinical dermatology.* (6th ed.). Philadelphia: Elsevier; **(Herpes simplex virus—type 2)** Jenny, C. (2011). *Child abuse and neglect: Diagnosis, treatment, and evidence.* Philadelphia: Saunders; **(Red rash—contact dermatitis)** Pfizer Laboratories Division, Pfizer Inc., New York. A close look at VD: A slide presentation produced as a public service; **(Urethral caruncle)** Rimsza, M. E. (1989). An illustrated guide to adolescent gynecology. *Pediatr Clin N Am. 36*(3), 641.

Table 27.3 (Uterine prolapse) Kostas-Polston, E. A., & Johnson-Mallard, V. (2015). Protruding mass. *J Nurse Pract. 11*(2), 373-376; **(Cystocele/rectocele)** Lemmi and Lemmi, 2011.

Table 27.4 (Polyp) Lemmi and Lemmi, 2011; **(Human papillomavirus [HPV, condylomata]; Cervical cancer)**

Symonds, E. M., MacPherson, M. B. A. (1997). *Color atlas of obstetrics and gynecology.* London: Mosby-Wolfe.

Table 27.5 (Candidiasis [moniliasis]) Lemmi and Lemmi, 2011; **(Gonorrhea)** Morse, S. A., Ballard, R. C., Holmes, K. K., et al. (2010). *Atlas of sexually transmitted diseases and AIDS.* (4th ed.). Philadelphia: Saunders.

Table 27.7 (Polycystic ovary syndrome) Courtesy Andrew T. Trout, MD.

Table 27.8 (Ambiguous genitalia) Moore, K. L., & Persaud, T. V. N. (1998). *Before we are born: Essentials of embryology and birth defects.* (5th ed.). Philadelphia: Saunders; **(Vulvovaginitis in child)** Muram, D., & Simmons, K. J. (2008). Pattern recognition in pediatric and adolescent gynecology—a case for formal education. *J Pediatr Adolesc Gynecol. 21*(2), 103-108.

Figure 31.2 Thomas, Pat, 2018.

Figure 31.6 Black, M., Ambros-Rudolph, C. M., Edwards, L., et al. (2008). *Obstetric and gynecologic dermatology.* (3rd ed.). St. Louis: Mosby.

Figure 31.14 Apgar, B.S., Brotzman, G.L., Spitzer, M. (2008). *Colposcopy: Principles and practice* (2nd ed.). Philadelphia: Saunders.

Table 31.1 (Preeclampsia) Symonds, E. M., & MacPherson, M. B. A. (1997). *Color atlas of obstetrics and gynecology.* London: Mosby-Wolfe.

Table 31.2 (Fetal macrosomia) Meur, S., & Mann, N. P. (2007). Infant outcomes following diabetic pregnancies. *Paediatr Child Healt. 17*(6), 217-222.

Figure 32.7 Sheikh, J. I., & Yesavage, J. A. Geriatric Depression Scale (GDS): Recent evidence and development of a shorter version. In: Brink, T. L. (1986). *Clinical gerontology: A guide to assessment and intervention.* Binghamton, NY: Haworth Press, pp. 165-173.

b indicates boxed material, *f* indicates illustrations, and *t* indicates tables.

845

Assessment Terms: English and Spanish

ENGLISH	SPANISH	ENGLISH	SPANISH
History Taking			
How do you feel?	¿Cómo se siente?	Nausea	Náusea
Good	Bien	Does eating make you vomit?	¿El comer le hace vomitar?
Bad	Mal	How are your stools?	¿Cómo son sus heces?
Let me see ...	Déjeme ver ...	Are they regular?	¿Son regulares?
Let me feel your pulse.	Déjeme tomarle el pulso.	Have you noticed their color?	¿Se ha fijado en el color?
Is your memory good?	¿Es buena su memoria?	Are you constipated?	¿Está estreñido?
Do you have any pain in your head?	¿Le duele la cabeza?	Do you have diarrhea?	¿Tiene diarrea?
Did you fall? How did you fall?	¿Se cayó? ¿Cómo se cayó?	Have you any difficulty urinating?	¿Tiene dificultad en orinar?
Did you faint?	¿Se desmayó?	Do you urinate involuntarily?	¿Orina sin querer?
Have you ever had fainting spells?	¿Ha tenido desmayos alguna vez?	Are any of your limbs swollen?	¿Están hinchados algunos de sus miembros?
Have you slept well?	¿Ha dormido bien?	How long have they been swollen like this?	¿Desde cuándo están hinchados así?
Have you any difficulty in breathing?	¿Tiene dificultad al respirar?	Have you ever had:	¿Alguna vez usted ha padecido:
How long have you been coughing for?	¿Desde cuándo tose Usted?	cancer	del cáncer
Do you cough a little?	¿Tose poco?	diabetes	de la diabetes
Do you expectorate much?	Escupe mucho?	heart disease	de una enfermedad cardíaca
What is the color of your expectorations?	De qué color es el esputo?	respiratory disease	de una enfermedad respiratoria
Is your hearing affected?	¿Está afectado el oído?	cirrhosis	de la cirrosis
Do you have ringing in the ears?	¿Le zumban los oídos?	depression	de la depresión
When did your eyesight begin to fail you?	¿Desde cuándo ha disminuido su visión?	Do you smoke?	¿Fuma usted?
Do you sometimes see double?	¿Ve las cosas doble algunas veces?	How much do you smoke each day?	¿Cuánto fuma a diario?
Tell me what number this is.	Dígame qué número es éste.	When did you stop smoking?	¿Cuándo dejó de fumar?
Tell me what letter this is.	Dígame qué letra es ésta.	Do you drink?	¿Toma bebidas alcohólicas?
Do things look cloudy to you?	¿Ve las cosas nubladas?	How often do you drink?	¿Cuántos tragos habitualmente?
Can you see clearly?	¿Puede ver claramente?		
Better at a distance?	¿Mejor a cierta distancia?		

Assessment Terms: English and Spanish

ENGLISH	SPANISH	ENGLISH	SPANISH
Physical Assessment			
Look up.	Mire para arriba.	The gums	Las encías
Look down.	Mire para abajo.	The hand	La mano
Look toward your nose.	Mírese la nariz.	The head	La cabeza
Look at me.	Míreme.	The heart	El corazón
Take a deep breath.	Respire profundo.	The leg	La pierna
Cough.	Tosa.	The liver	El hígado
Cough again.	Tosa otra vez.	The lungs	Los pulmones
Open your mouth.	Abra la boca.	The mouth	La boca
Squeeze my hand.	Apriete mi mano.	The muscles	Los músculos
Can you do better than that?	¿No puede hacerlo más fuerte?	The neck	El cuello
Does your arm feel paralyzed?	¿Está el brazo paralizado?	The nerves	Los nervios
Raise your arm.	Levante el brazo.	The nose	La nariz
Raise it more.	Más alto.	The ribs	Las costillas
Now the other.	Ahora el otro.	The shoulder blades	Las paletillas
Show me where.	Muéstreme dónde.	The side	El costado
In the abdomen?	¿En el vientre?	The skin	La piel
Stick out your tongue.	Saque la lengua.	The tongue	La lengua
Bend over.	Inclínese hacia delante.	The throat	La garganta
Touch your toes.	Toque los dedos de pie.	The teeth	Los dientes
The ankle	El tobillo	The fingers	Los dedos
The arm	El brazo	The toes	Los dedos de pie
The back	La espalda	The scalp	El cuero cabelludo
The bones	Los huesos	The face	La cara
The chest	El pecho	The breast	El pecho
The ears	Los oídos	The anus	El ano
The elbow	El codo	The genitals	Los genitales
The eye	El ojo	The armpit	La axila
The foot	El pie	The groin	La ingle
Pain Assessment			
Do you have any pain?	¿Tiene dolor?	Do you still have a lot of pain?	¿Le duele mucho todavía?
Where does it hurt?	¿Dónde le duele?	Does it hurt when you breathe?	¿Le duele al respirar?
Do you have pain here?	¿Le duele aquí?	Shooting pains?	¿Dolores agudos?
Do you have a pain in your side?	¿Le duele el costado?	Like pins and needles?	¿Como si estuvieran pinchándole con alfileres?
Is it worse now?	¿Está peor ahora?	Did you feel much pain at the time?	¿Sintió mucho dolor entonces?
Do you still have pain?	¿Le duele todavía?		

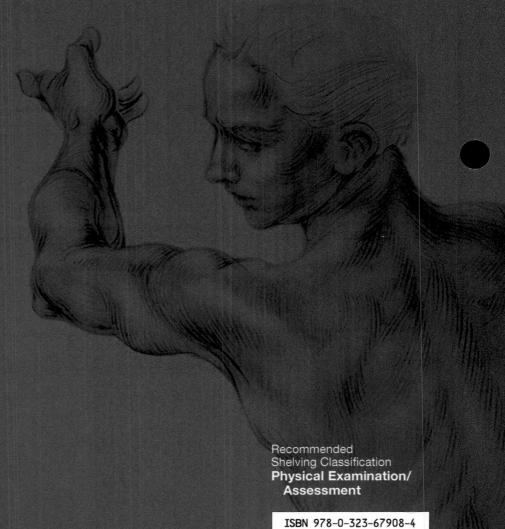

ISBN 978-0-323-67908-4

9 780323 679084

ELSEVIER elsevier.com